## Recommended Dietary Allowances (RDA) and Adequate Intakes (AI) for Vitamins

| Age (yr) | Thiamin RDA (mg/day) | Riboflavin RDA (mg/day) | Niacin RDA (mg/day)[a] | Biotin AI (µg/day) | Pantothenic acid AI (mg/day) | Vitamin $B_6$ RDA (mg/day) | Folate RDA (µg/day)[b] | Vitamin $B_{12}$ RDA (µg/day) | Choline AI (mg/day) | Vitamin C RDA (mg/day) | Vitamin A RDA (µg/day)[c] | Vitamin D RDA (IU/day)[d] | Vitamin E RDA (mg/ day)[e] | Vitamin K AI (µg/day) |
|---|---|---|---|---|---|---|---|---|---|---|---|---|---|---|
| *Infants* | | | | | | | | | | | | | | |
| 0–0.5 | 0.2 | 0.3 | 2 | 5 | 1.7 | 0.1 | 65 | 0.4 | 125 | 40 | 400 | 400 (10 µg) | 4 | 2.0 |
| 0.5–1 | 0.3 | 0.4 | 4 | 6 | 1.8 | 0.3 | 80 | 0.5 | 150 | 50 | 500 | 400 (10 µg) | 5 | 2.5 |
| *Children* | | | | | | | | | | | | | | |
| 1–3 | 0.5 | 0.5 | 6 | 8 | 2 | 0.5 | 150 | 0.9 | 200 | 15 | 300 | 600 (15 µg) | 6 | 30 |
| 4–8 | 0.6 | 0.6 | 8 | 12 | 3 | 0.6 | 200 | 1.2 | 250 | 25 | 400 | 600 (15 µg) | 7 | 55 |
| *Males* | | | | | | | | | | | | | | |
| 9–13 | 0.9 | 0.9 | 12 | 20 | 4 | 1.0 | 300 | 1.8 | 375 | 45 | 600 | 600 (15 µg) | 11 | 60 |
| 14–18 | 1.2 | 1.3 | 16 | 25 | 5 | 1.3 | 400 | 2.4 | 550 | 75 | 900 | 600 (15 µg) | 15 | 75 |
| 19–30 | 1.2 | 1.3 | 16 | 30 | 5 | 1.3 | 400 | 2.4 | 550 | 90 | 900 | 600 (15 µg) | 15 | 120 |
| 31–50 | 1.2 | 1.3 | 16 | 30 | 5 | 1.3 | 400 | 2.4 | 550 | 90 | 900 | 600 (15 µg) | 15 | 120 |
| 51–70 | 1.2 | 1.3 | 16 | 30 | 5 | 1.7 | 400 | 2.4 | 550 | 90 | 900 | 600 (15 µg) | 15 | 120 |
| >70 | 1.2 | 1.3 | 16 | 30 | 5 | 1.7 | 400 | 2.4 | 550 | 90 | 900 | 800 (20 µg) | 15 | 120 |
| *Females* | | | | | | | | | | | | | | |
| 9–13 | 0.9 | 0.9 | 12 | 20 | 4 | 1.0 | 300 | 1.8 | 375 | 45 | 600 | 600 (15 µg) | 11 | 60 |
| 14–18 | 1.0 | 1.0 | 14 | 25 | 5 | 1.2 | 400 | 2.4 | 400 | 65 | 700 | 600 (15 µg) | 15 | 75 |
| 19–30 | 1.1 | 1.1 | 14 | 30 | 5 | 1.3 | 400 | 2.4 | 425 | 75 | 700 | 600 (15 µg) | 15 | 90 |
| 31–50 | 1.1 | 1.1 | 14 | 30 | 5 | 1.3 | 400 | 2.4 | 425 | 75 | 700 | 600 (15 µg) | 15 | 90 |
| 51–70 | 1.1 | 1.1 | 14 | 30 | 5 | 1.5 | 400 | 2.4 | 425 | 75 | 700 | 600 (15 µg) | 15 | 90 |
| >70 | 1.1 | 1.1 | 14 | 30 | 5 | 1.5 | 400 | 2.4 | 425 | 75 | 700 | 800 (20 µg) | 15 | 90 |
| *Pregnancy* | | | | | | | | | | | | | | |
| ≤18 | 1.4 | 1.4 | 18 | 30 | 6 | 1.9 | 600 | 2.6 | 450 | 80 | 750 | 600 (15 µg) | 15 | 75 |
| 19–30 | 1.4 | 1.4 | 18 | 30 | 6 | 1.9 | 600 | 2.6 | 450 | 85 | 770 | 600 (15 µg) | 15 | 90 |
| 31–50 | 1.4 | 1.4 | 18 | 30 | 6 | 1.9 | 600 | 2.6 | 450 | 85 | 770 | 600 (15 µg) | 15 | 90 |
| *Lactation* | | | | | | | | | | | | | | |
| ≤18 | 1.4 | 1.6 | 17 | 35 | 7 | 2.0 | 500 | 2.8 | 550 | 115 | 1200 | 600 (15 µg) | 19 | 75 |
| 19–30 | 1.4 | 1.6 | 17 | 35 | 7 | 2.0 | 500 | 2.8 | 550 | 120 | 1300 | 600 (15 µg) | 19 | 90 |
| 31–50 | 1.4 | 1.6 | 17 | 35 | 7 | 2.0 | 500 | 2.8 | 550 | 120 | 1300 | 600 (15 µg) | 19 | 90 |

NOTE: For all nutrients, values for infants are AI. The glossary on the inside back cover defines units of nutrient measure.

[a]Niacin recommendations are expressed as niacin equivalents (NE), except for recommendations for infants younger than 6 months, which are expressed as preformed niacin.

[b]Folate recommendations are expressed as dietary folate equivalents (DFE).

[c]Vitamin A recommendations are expressed as retinol activity equivalents (RAE).

[d]Vitamin D recommendations are expressed as cholecalciferol and assume an absence of adequate exposure to sunlight.

[e]Vitamin E recommendations are expressed as α-tocopherol.

## Recommended Dietary Allowances (RDA) and Adequate Intakes (AI) for Minerals

| Age (yr) | Sodium AI (mg/day) | Chloride AI (mg/day) | Potassium AI (mg/day) | Calcium RDA (mg/day) | Phosphorus RDA (mg/day) | Magnesium RDA (mg/day) | Iron RDA (mg/day) | Zinc RDA (mg/day) | Iodine RDA (µg/day) | Selenium RDA (µg/day) | Copper RDA (µg/day) | Manganese AI (mg/day) | Fluoride AI (mg/day) | Chromium AI (µg/day) | Molybdenum RDA (µg/day) |
|---|---|---|---|---|---|---|---|---|---|---|---|---|---|---|---|
| *Infants* | | | | | | | | | | | | | | | |
| 0–0.5 | 120 | 180 | 400 | 200 | 100 | 30 | 0.27 | 2 | 110 | 15 | 200 | 0.003 | 0.01 | 0.2 | 2 |
| 0.5–1 | 370 | 570 | 700 | 260 | 275 | 75 | 11 | 3 | 130 | 20 | 220 | 0.6 | 0.5 | 5.5 | 3 |
| *Children* | | | | | | | | | | | | | | | |
| 1–3 | 1000 | 1500 | 3000 | 700 | 460 | 80 | 7 | 3 | 90 | 20 | 340 | 1.2 | 0.7 | 11 | 17 |
| 4–8 | 1200 | 1900 | 3800 | 1000 | 500 | 130 | 10 | 5 | 90 | 30 | 440 | 1.5 | 1.0 | 15 | 22 |
| *Males* | | | | | | | | | | | | | | | |
| 9–13 | 1500 | 2300 | 4500 | 1300 | 1250 | 240 | 8 | 8 | 120 | 40 | 700 | 1.9 | 2 | 25 | 34 |
| 14–18 | 1500 | 2300 | 4700 | 1300 | 1250 | 410 | 11 | 11 | 150 | 55 | 890 | 2.2 | 3 | 35 | 43 |
| 19–30 | 1500 | 2300 | 4700 | 1000 | 700 | 400 | 8 | 11 | 150 | 55 | 900 | 2.3 | 4 | 35 | 45 |
| 31–50 | 1500 | 2300 | 4700 | 1000 | 700 | 420 | 8 | 11 | 150 | 55 | 900 | 2.3 | 4 | 35 | 45 |
| 51–70 | 1300 | 2000 | 4700 | 1000 | 700 | 420 | 8 | 11 | 150 | 55 | 900 | 2.3 | 4 | 30 | 45 |
| >70 | 1200 | 1800 | 4700 | 1200 | 700 | 420 | 8 | 11 | 150 | 55 | 900 | 2.3 | 4 | 30 | 45 |
| *Females* | | | | | | | | | | | | | | | |
| 9–13 | 1500 | 2300 | 4500 | 1300 | 1250 | 240 | 8 | 8 | 120 | 40 | 700 | 1.6 | 2 | 21 | 34 |
| 14–18 | 1500 | 2300 | 4700 | 1300 | 1250 | 360 | 15 | 9 | 150 | 55 | 890 | 1.6 | 3 | 24 | 43 |
| 19–30 | 1500 | 2300 | 4700 | 1000 | 700 | 310 | 18 | 8 | 150 | 55 | 900 | 1.8 | 3 | 25 | 45 |
| 31–50 | 1500 | 2300 | 4700 | 1000 | 700 | 320 | 18 | 8 | 150 | 55 | 900 | 1.8 | 3 | 25 | 45 |
| 51–70 | 1300 | 2000 | 4700 | 1200 | 700 | 320 | 8 | 8 | 150 | 55 | 900 | 1.8 | 3 | 20 | 45 |
| >70 | 1200 | 1800 | 4700 | 1200 | 700 | 320 | 8 | 8 | 150 | 55 | 900 | 1.8 | 3 | 20 | 45 |
| *Pregnancy* | | | | | | | | | | | | | | | |
| ≤18 | 1500 | 2300 | 4700 | 1300 | 1250 | 400 | 27 | 12 | 220 | 60 | 1000 | 2.0 | 3 | 29 | 50 |
| 19–30 | 1500 | 2300 | 4700 | 1000 | 700 | 350 | 27 | 11 | 220 | 60 | 1000 | 2.0 | 3 | 30 | 50 |
| 31–50 | 1500 | 2300 | 4700 | 1000 | 700 | 360 | 27 | 11 | 220 | 60 | 1000 | 2.0 | 3 | 30 | 50 |
| *Lactation* | | | | | | | | | | | | | | | |
| ≤18 | 1500 | 2300 | 5100 | 1300 | 1250 | 360 | 10 | 13 | 290 | 70 | 1300 | 2.6 | 3 | 44 | 50 |
| 19–30 | 1500 | 2300 | 5100 | 1000 | 700 | 310 | 9 | 12 | 290 | 70 | 1300 | 2.6 | 3 | 45 | 50 |
| 31–50 | 1500 | 2300 | 5100 | 1000 | 700 | 320 | 9 | 12 | 290 | 70 | 1300 | 2.6 | 3 | 45 | 50 |

NOTE: For all nutrients, values for infants are AI.

# NUTRITION

*Through the Life Cycle*

**Sixth Edition**


Judith E. Brown
Ph.D., M.P.H., R.D.
University of Minnesota

*with*

**Ellen Lechtenberg,** M.P.H., R.D., I.B.C.L.C.
Primary Children's Hospital

**Maureen A. Murtaugh,** Ph.D., R.D.
University of Utah School of Medicine

**Patricia L. Splett,** Ph.D., M.P.H., R.D.
Nutrition Consultant

**Jamie Stang,** Ph.D., M.P.H., R.D.
University of Minnesota

**Robyn Wong,** M.P.H., R.D., C.S.P., L.D.
Kaiser Permanente Medical Center - Hawaii

**Ellen K. Bowser,** M.S., R.D., LDN, FAND, R.N, B.S.N.
University of Florida Pediatric Pulmonary Division

**Beth L. Leonberg,** M.S., M.A., R.D., C.S.P., F.A.N.D., L.D.N.
Drexel University

**Nadine R. Sahyoun,** Ph.D., R.D.
University of Maryland



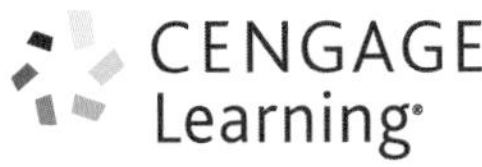


Australia • Brazil • Mexico • Singapore • United Kingdom • United States

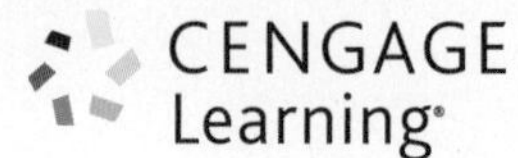

***Nutrition Through the Life Cycle*, 6e**
**Judith E. Brown**

Product Manager: Krista Mastroianni
Content Developer: Lauren Oliveira
Product Assistant: Victor Luu
Marketing Manager: Tom Ziolkowski
Content Project Manager: Carol Samet
Art Director: Michael Cook
Manufacturing Planner: Karen Hunt
Production Service: Lynn Lustberg, MPS Limited
Photo Researcher: Lumina Datamatics
Text Researcher: Lumina Datamatics
Text Designer: Ellen Pettengell Design
Cover Designer: Michael Cook
Cover Image: Gts/Shutterstock.com
Compositor: MPS Limited



Library of Congress Control Number: 2015945351
ISBN: 978-1-305-62800-7

Loose-leaf Edition:
ISBN: 978-1-305-88088-7

**Cengage Learning**
20 Channel Center Street
Boston, MA 02210
USA

Cengage Learning is a leading provider of customized learning solutions with employees residing in nearly 40 different countries and sales in more than 125 countries around the world. Find your local representative at **www.cengage.com.**

Cengage Learning products are represented in Canada by Nelson Education, Ltd.

To learn more about Cengage Learning Solutions, visit **www.cengage.com.** Purchase any of our products at your local college store or at our preferred online store **www.cengagebrain.com.**

Printed in the United States of America
Print Number: 01 Print Year: 2016

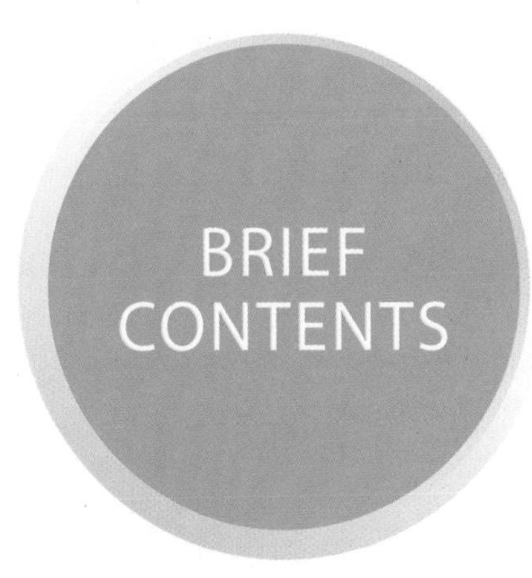
BRIEF
CONTENTS

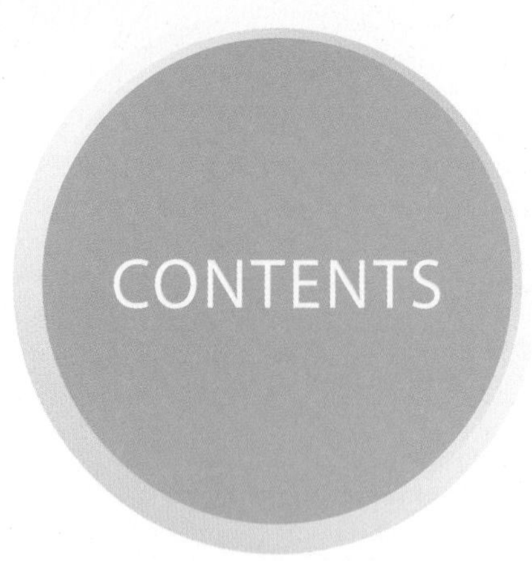

# CONTENTS

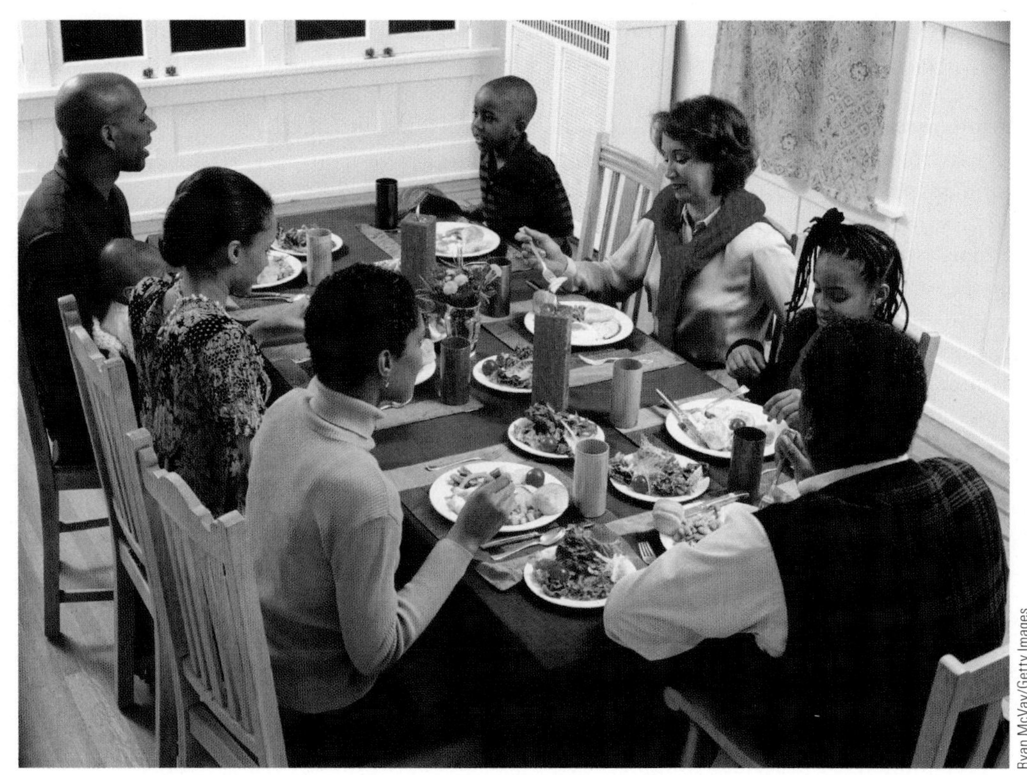

Ryan McVay/Getty Images

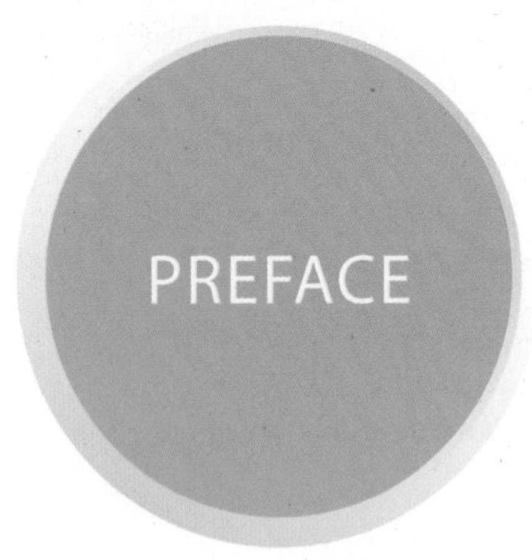

# PREFACE

It is our privilege to offer you the 6th edition of *Nutrition Through the Life Cycle*. This text was initially developed, and has been revised, to address the needs of instructors teaching, and students taking, a two- to four-credit course in life-cycle nutrition. It is written at a level that assumes students have had an introductory nutrition course. Overall, the text is intended to give instructors a tool they can productively use to enhance their teaching efforts, and to give students an engaging and rewarding educational experience they will carry with them throughout their lives and careers.

The authors of *Nutrition Through the Life Cycle* represent a group of experts with experience in clinical practice, teaching, and research related to nutrition during specific phases of the life cycle. All of us remain totally dedicated to the goals established for the text at its conception: to make the text comprehensive, logically organized, evidence-based, realistic, and relevant to the needs of instructors and students.

Chapter 1 summarizes key elements of introductory nutrition and gives students who need it a chance to update or renew their knowledge. Students can "test" their knowledge of many aspects of introductory nutrition by answering the review questions listed at the end of the chapter. Coverage of the life-cycle phases begins with preconception nutrition and continues with each major phase of the life cycle through adulthood and the special needs of the elderly. Each of these 19 chapters was developed based on a common organizational framework that includes learning objectives, prevalence statistics, physiological principles, nutritional needs and recommendations, model programs, case studies, and recommended practices. Chapters end with a list of key points and review questions.

To meet the knowledge needs of students with the variety of career goals represented in many life-cycle nutrition courses, we include two chapters for each life-cycle phase. The first chapter for each phase covers normal nutrition topics, and the second covers nutrition-related conditions and interventions. Every chapter focuses on scientifically based information and employs up-to-date resources and references. Answers to the case studies and review questions, and Internet resources that lead to reliable information on topics presented in the chapters, are now located on the web and can be accessed through www.cengagebrain.com.

## New to the Sixth Edition

Advances in knowledge about nutrition and health through the life cycle are expanding at a remarkably high rate. New research is taking our understanding of the roles played by healthy dietary patterns, nutrients, gene variants and nutrient–gene interactions, body fat, physical activity, and dietary supplements to new levels. You will see in this edition these emerging areas of direct relevance to nutrition addressed as well as updated information on dietary patterns and health generated by the 2015 Dietary Guidelines for Americans.

## Chapter-by-Chapter Changes

### Chapter 1: Nutrition Basics

- Incorporated content from the 2015 Dietary Guidelines for Americans
- Updated information on USDA's ChooseMyPlate interactive diet planning and evaluation tools
- Updated content on effects of cholesterol, added sugar, and sodium on health
- Added content on nutrition labeling requirements
- Deleted content on functional foods
- Updated content on dietary assessment
- Modified illustrations and tables

### Chapter 2: Preconception Nutrition

- Expanded content on female and male reproductive physiology
- Updated and revised content on nutrient status and fertility
- Condensed and updated content on periconcptional folate status
- Expanded dietary intake recommendations section to include preconception and early pregnancy dietary intake
- Modified illustrations and tables

### Chapter 3: Preconception Nutrition: Conditions and Interventions

- New chapter opening with content on weight status and fertility
- Added content on PKU, including a menu plan for a person with PKU
- Modified content on celiac disease
- Modified illustrations and tables

### Chapter 4: Nutrition During Pregnancy

- Revised some of the learning objectives
- Updated natality statistics
- Updated content on "Developmental Origins of Health and Disease"
- Modified illustrations and tables
- Expanded content on reproductive physiology
- Added content on metabolic effects of specific gene variants
- Extensively modified content on calcium and iron and pregnancy, and on dietary supplements
- Revised dietary recommendations to be consistent with the 2015 Dietary Guidelines

### Chapter 5: Nutrition During Pregnancy: Conditions and Interventions

- Updated content on obesity, diabetes, and hypertension in pregnancy to incorporate recent recommendations and research results
- Added content on gene variants and their effect on nutrient metabolism and disease and disorder risk during pregnancy
- Modified illustrations and tables

### Chapter 6: Nutrition During Lactation

- Added table of human milk contrasted with cow's milk–based human milk substitutes
- Updated breastfeeding prevalence in the United States
- Updated breastfeeding promotion (U.S. Surgeon General)
- Modified illustrations and tables
- Many minor updates to include current literature

### Chapter 7: Nutrition During Lactation: Conditions and Interventions

- Updated information on sore nipples
- Updated information on effectiveness of cabbage leaves
- Additional information on use of Reglan, including FDA black box warning
- Updated information on alcohol and breastfeeding
- Updated information on marijuana, caffeine, and drugs of abuse
- New section on e-cigarettes
- New section on milk sharing
- Modified illustrations and tables

### Chapter 8: Infant Nutrition

- Incorporated Nutrition Care process language
- Expanded content on infant hunger and satiety cues
- Condensed information on infant formula types and indications for use
- Updated content on sequence of infant development and feeding skills
- Expanded content on early childhood caries
- Modified illustrations and tables

### Chapter 9: Infant Nutrition: Conditions and Interventions

- Updated table on potential nutrition problems in infants with special health care needs
- Expanded section on growth in preterm infants
- Expanded content on brain development in early life and vital role of protein and iron
- Updated table comparing term, post-discharge, and premature formulas
- Modified illustrations and tables

### Chapter 10: Toddler and Preschooler Nutrition

- Updated poverty rates for children and deleted sentence on health insurance rates for children
- Updated information on dental caries rate in children and included ethnic information
- Updated information on CDC lead exposure in children
- Added AAP recommendation on consumption of pasteurized milk and milk products for pregnant women and children
- Updated data on overweight and obesity rates in toddlers and preschoolers and included ethnic breakdowns of such
- Updated data on the use of supplements by children ages 1–3 and 4–8
- Included FDA information on which fish young children should avoid due to mercury content
- Updated WIC and SNAP enrollment characteristics

- Discussed WIC changes to meet the Dietary Guidelines for Americans
- Revised case study to include more cultural implications
- Modified illustrations and tables

### Chapter 11: Toddler and Preschooler Nutrition: Conditions and Interventions

- Updated data on children with special health care needs
- Updated information on autism and use of gluten and/or casein free diets, and the "Combating Autism Act of 2006."
- Revised information on asthma and nutrition
- Expanded information on bronchopulmonary dysplasia
- Expanded information on food allergies including resources for families
- Modified illustrations and tables

### Chapter 12: Child and Preadolescent Nutrition

- Incorporated results of meta-analysis on the importance of family mealtime to nutritional status
- Included evidence analysis of the influence of media and screen time on children's food choices
- Updated information on trends in childhood overweight and obesity prevalence
- Included recent recommendations for expanding physical education in schools
- Provided most recent recommendations for hydration for children in organized sports
- Updated and expanded information on recommended changes to the school food environment
- Modified tables and illustrations

### Chapter 13: Child and Preadolescent Nutrition: Conditions and Interventions

- Updated information on prevalence of Autism Spectrum Disorders
- Provided most recent data on increasing prevalence of types 1 and 2 diabetes mellitus
- Expanded content on nutrition and growth in children with attention deficit hyperactivity disorder
- Expanded information on resources for families of children with chronic health conditions
- Modified tables and illustrations

### Chapter 14: Adolescent Nutrition

- Updated information related to frequency of snacking, meal skipping, and consuming family meals
- Updated information regarding current intake of nutrients compared to DRI/EAL values
- Updated information regarding current intake of food groups
- Updated information on school meals program regulations and requirements
- Included description of a new model program for community-engaged nutrition education for teens
- Modified illustrations and tables

### Chapter 15: Adolescent Nutrition: Conditions and Interventions

- Updated information on prevalence and treatment of overweight and obesity among teens
- Updated information about the use of tobacco, alcohol, and illicit substances among teens
- Expanded content related to screening and intervention for chronic health conditions
- Updated information on eating disorders to be consistent with DSM V criteria
- Modified illustrations and tables

### Chapter 16: Adult Nutrition

- Updated statistics in tables with most current data from national surveys
- Revised definition of determinants of health as used by Healthy People 2020
- Added description of accumulation of adipose tissue
- Added section on the gut microbiome
- Updated section on risk nutrients and added choline and iron
- Revised recommendations for beverage selections
- Included new illustration to represent the complexity of factors influencing nutrition and health
- Added table of Nutrient and Fluid Considerations for Intensive Physical Activity

### Chapter 17: Adult Nutrition: Conditions and Interventions

- Reorganized sections for greater continuity throughout chapter
- Updated statistics on disease prevalence and Healthy People 2020 objectives

- Expanded information about the metabolic and hedonistic origins of obesity and included new race-specific waist circumferences criteria for obesity
- Included links to risk calculators for cardiovascular disease and diabetes
- Incorporated new guidelines for cardiovascular diseasing screening and prevention
- Incorporated the latest standard for diabetes management, including criteria for diagnosis of prediabetes and diabetes, and the more flexible approach to dietary management
- Added self-management education and support, replaced exchange lists with carbohydrate counting as the preferred approach for dietary self-management, and updated antihyperglycemic drug information
- Incorporated updated research on cancer and nutrition
- Revised the HIV section to address the impact of newer medications on nutrition needs and intervention throughout the phases of HIV and AIDS
- Included new and updated references
- Modified illustrations and tables

### Chapter 18: Nutrition and Older Adults

- Revised the introductory section
- Updated life expectancy information
- Revised the section on calorie restriction
- Updated all statistics—prevalence, incidence
- Deleted Table 18–7, medication use among older adults
- Revised section on folate, nutrient supplement
- Revised section on federal nutrition programs for older adults

### Chapter 19: Nutrition and Older Adults: Conditions and Interventions

- New illustration added—Decline in mortality by leading causes of deaths
- Updated statistics on all disease prevalence
- Revised sections to reflect new guidelines issued in 2013–2015 on heart disease, stroke, diabetes, hypertension, and lifestyle modifications
- Revised sections to include new information on periodontal disease, vitamin $B_{12}$, obesity, and unintentional weight loss

## Instructor Resources

Updated for the 6th edition is the Instructor Companion site that contains Microsoft PowerPoint™ lecture presentations with artwork, chapter outlines, and discussion questions. The Instructor's Manual, images from the text, videos, and animations, and more can also be found on this site. The Test Bank is offered through Cengage Learning Testing Powered by Cognero and contains multiple-choice, true/false, matching, and discussion exercises. Cengage Learning Testing is a flexible, online system that allows you to author, edit, and manage test bank content, create multiple test versions, and deliver tests from your LMS, your classroom or wherever you want.

## Acknowledgments

This edition introduces four new chapter authors: Robyn Wong, MPH, RD, CSP, Nutrition Specialist—NICU and Pediatrics, Kaiser Permanente Medical Center in Honolulu (Chapters 8, 9); Ellen Bowser, MS, RDN, LDN, RN, an associate in pediatrics who is a faculty nutritionist with the University of Florida Pediatric Pulmonary Division (Chapters 10, 11); Beth L. Leonberg, MS, RDN, CSP, FAND, LDN, an assistant clinical professor and director, Didactic Program in Dietetics at Drexel University (Chapters 12, 13); and Nadine Sahyoun, PhD, RD, a professor and director of the graduate program in Nutrition and Food Science Department of Nutrition and Food Science at the University of Maryland, College Park (Chapters 18, 19). We are very fortunate to have such high-caliber authors continue work on the comprehensive and instructive chapters begun by Janet Isaacs, Nancy Wooldridge, and Bea Krinke five editions ago. Thank you Janet, Nancy, and Bea for bringing your intelligence, experience, and dedicated efforts to these chapters.

It takes the combined talents and efforts of authors, editors, assistants, and the publisher to develop a new edition of a textbook and its instructional resources. We have had the pleasure of working with an ambitious and thorough group of professionals at Cengage, including Yolanda Cossion and Krista Mastroianni, product managers; and Lauren Oliveira, content developer of Life Sciences. Their careful and complete work on the development and implementation of this new edition is appreciated greatly. Lynn Lustberg, project manager from MPS Limited, once again served as the textbook producer. She kept us on time and on target in an effective and thoughtful way.

## Reviewers

Many thanks to the following reviewers, whose careful reading and thoughtful comments helped enormously in shaping revisions to the 6th edition.

Theresa Loomis
SUNY Oneonta

Beverly Moellering
University of Saint Francis

Cydne Perry
Shepherd University

Dean Chiarelli
Arizona State University

Laura Horn
Cincinnati State Technical and Community College

Bruce Rengers
Metropolitan State University of Denver

Allison Childress
Texas Tech University

Christen Harris
Bastyr University

Wendy Buchan
California State University Sacramento

Karen Kubena
Texas A&M University

Betty Alford
Texas Woman's University

Leta Aljadir
University of Delaware

Clint Allred
Texas A&M University

Dea Hanson Baxter
Georgia State University

Janet Colson
Middle Tennessee State University

Kathleen Davis
Texas Women's University

Shelley R. Hancock
The University of Alabama

Laura Horn
Cincinnati State Community College

Dr. Mary Jacob
California State University, Long Beach

Pera Jambazian
California State University, Los Angeles

Tay Seacord Kennedy
Oklahoma State University

Younghee Kim
Bowling Green State University

Barbara Kirks
California State University, Chico

Kaye Stanek Krogstrand
University of Nebraska

Karen Kubena
Texas A&M University

Sally Ann Lederman
Columbia University

Richard Lewis
University of Georgia

Marcia Magnus
Florida International University

J. Harriett McCoy
University of Arkansas

Sharon McWhinney
Prairie View A&M University

Janis Mena
University of Florida

Robert Reynolds
University of Illinois at Chicago

Sharon Nickols-Richardson
Virginia Polytechnic Institute and State University

Lisa Roth
University of Florida

Claire Schmelzer
Eastern Kentucky University

Adria Sherman
Rutgers University

Carmen R. Roman-Shriver
Texas Tech University

Joanne Slavin
University of Minnesota

Joanne Spaide
Professor Emeritus, University of Northern Iowa

Diana-Marie Spillman
Miami University, Oxford, Ohio

Wendy Stuhldreher Slippery Rock
University of Pennsylvania

Anne VanBeber
Texas Christian University

Phyllis Moser-Veillon
University of Maryland

Janelle Walter
Baylor University

Doris Wang
University of Minnesota Crookston

Suzy Weems, Ph.D.
Stephen F. Austin State University

Kay Wilder
Point Loma Nazarene College

Angela Stiegemeyer
Southeast Missouri State University

Janelle M. Walter
Baylor University

Virginia A. Bennett
Central Washington University

Mark S. Meskin
California State Polytechnical University–Pomona

May you enjoy using this text as much as the authors relish the opportunity of making it available to you.

Judith Brown *with*

Ellen Lechenberg

Maureen Murtaugh

Patricia Splett

Jamie Stang

Robyn Wong

Ellen Bowser

Beth L. Leonberg

Nadine Sahyoun

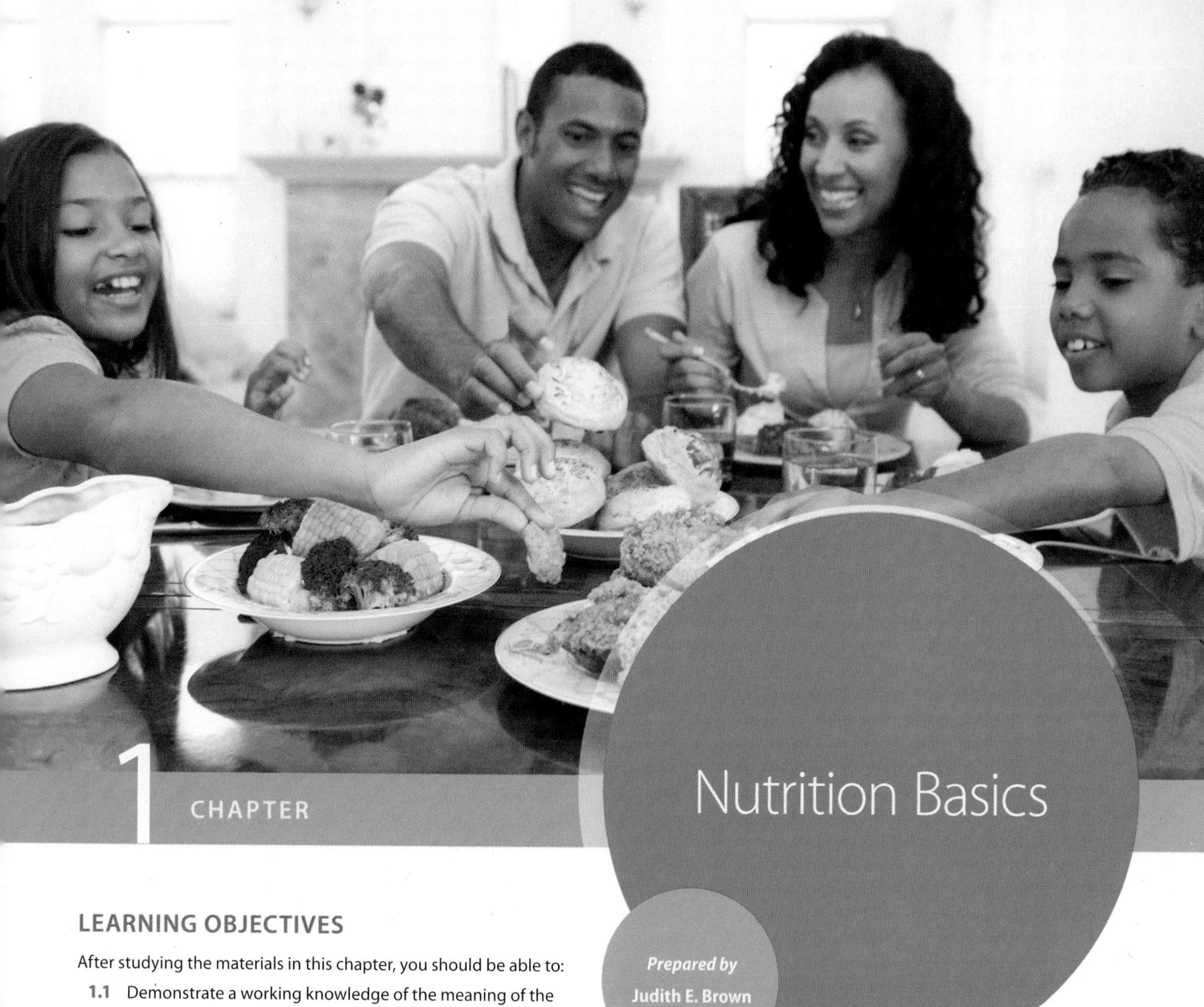

1 CHAPTER

# Nutrition Basics

*Prepared by*
**Judith E. Brown**

## LEARNING OBJECTIVES

After studying the materials in this chapter, you should be able to:

**1.1** Demonstrate a working knowledge of the meaning of the 10 nutrition concepts presented.

**1.2** Apply knowledge about the elements of nutrition labeling to decisions about the nutritional value of foods.

**1.3** Cite two examples of how nutrient needs change during the life cycle and how nutritional status at one stage during the life cycle can influence health status during another.

**1.4** Describe the components of individual-level nutrition assessment.

**1.5** Identify the basic elements of four public food and nutrition programs.

**1.6** Apply the characteristics of healthy dietary patterns to the design of one.

iStockphoto.com/Catherine Yeulet

# Introduction

Need to freshen up your knowledge of nutrition? Or, do you need to get up to speed on basic nutrition for the course? This chapter presents information about nutrition that paves the way to understanding specific needs and benefits related to nutrition by life-cycle stage.

Nutrition is an interdisciplinary science focused on the study of how foods, ***nutrients***, and other food constituents affect health. The body of knowledge about nutrition is large and is growing rapidly, changing views on what constitutes the best nutrition advice. You are encouraged to stay up-to-date on the best nutrition advice for diet and health-related issues.

This chapter centers on (1) the principles of the science of nutrition, (2) nutrients and other constituents of food, (3) healthy dietary patterns, (4) public food and nutrition programs, (5) nutritional assessment, and (6) nationwide priorities for improvements in the *public's nutritional health*.

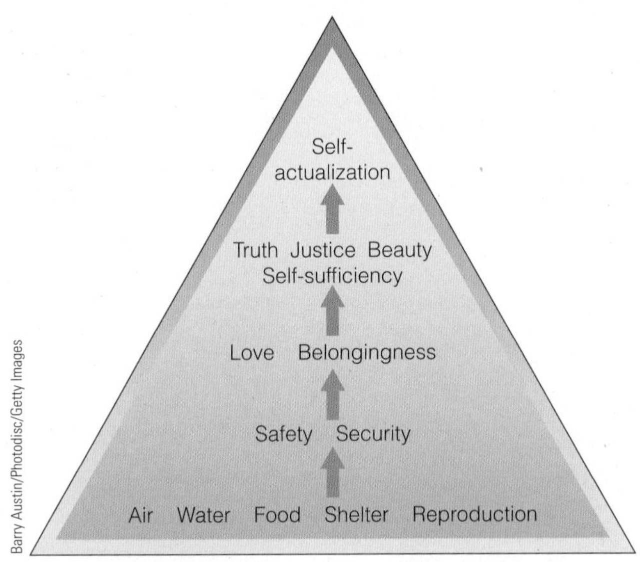


ILLUSTRATION 1.1 ▸ The need for food is part of Maslow's hierarchy of needs.

# Principles of the Science of Nutrition

LO 1.1 Demonstrate a working knowledge of the meaning of the 10 nutrition concepts presented.

Every field of science is governed by a set of principles that provides the foundation for growth in knowledge. These principles change little with time. Knowledge of the principles of nutrition listed in Table 1.1 will serve as a springboard to greater understanding of the nutrition and health relationships explored in the chapters to come.

TABLE 1.1 ▸ Principles of human nutrition

| | |
|---|---|
| **PRINCIPLE #1** | Food is a basic need of humans. |
| **PRINCIPLE #2** | Foods provide energy (calories), nutrients, and other substances needed for growth and health. |
| **PRINCIPLE #3** | Health problems related to nutrition originate within cells. |
| **PRINCIPLE #4** | Poor nutrition can result from both inadequate and excessive levels of nutrient intake. |
| **PRINCIPLE #5** | Humans have adaptive mechanisms for managing fluctuations in food intake. |
| **PRINCIPLE #6** | Malnutrition can result from poor diets and from disease states, genetic factors, or combinations of these causes. |
| **PRINCIPLE #7** | Some groups of people are at higher risk of becoming inadequately nourished than others. |
| **PRINCIPLE #8** | Poor nutrition can influence the development of certain chronic diseases. |
| **PRINCIPLE #9** | Adequacy, variety, and balance are key characteristics of healthy dietary patterns. |
| **PRINCIPLE #10** | There are no "good" or "bad" foods. |



**Principle #1** Food is a basic need of humans.

Humans need enough food to live and the right assortment of foods for optimal health (Illustration 1.1). People who have enough food to meet their needs at all times experience ***food security***. They are able to acquire food in socially acceptable ways—without having to scavenge or steal food. ***Food insecurity*** exists when the availability of safe, nutritious foods, or the ability to acquire them in socially acceptable ways, is limited or uncertain.[1] It exists in 14.3 percent of United States and 7.7 percent of Canadian households.[2,3]

**Principle #2** Foods provide energy (calories), nutrients, and other substances needed for growth and health.

People eat foods for many different reasons. The most compelling reason is the requirement for ***calories*** (energy), nutrients, and other substances supplied by foods for growth and health.

A calorie is a measure of the amount of energy transferred from food to the body. Because calories are a unit of measure and not a substance actually present in food, they are not considered to be nutrients.

Nutrients are chemical substances in food that the body uses for a variety of

**nutrients** Chemical substances in foods that are used by the body for growth and health.

**food security** Access at all times to a sufficient supply of safe, nutritious foods.

**food insecurity** Limited or uncertain availability of safe, nutritious foods, or the ability to acquire them in socially acceptable ways.

**calorie** A unit of measure of the amount of energy supplied by food. Also known as the "kilocalorie" (kcal), or the "large Calorie."

TABLE 1.2 ▸ The six categories of nutrients

1. **Carbohydrates** Chemical substances in foods that consist of a single sugar molecule or multiples of sugar molecules in various forms. Sugar and fruit, starchy vegetables, and whole grain products are good dietary sources.
2. **Proteins** Chemical substances in foods that are made up of chains of amino acids. Animal products and dried beans are examples of protein sources.
3. **Fats (Lipids)** Components of food that are soluble in fat but not in water. They are more properly referred to as "lipids." Most fats are composed of glycerol attached to three fatty acids. Oil, butter, sausage, and avocado are examples of rich sources of dietary fats.
4. **Vitamins** Fourteen specific chemical substances that perform specific functions in the body. Vitamins are present in many foods and are essential components of the diet. Vegetables, fruits, and grains are good sources of vitamins.
5. **Minerals** In the context of nutrition, minerals consist of 15 elements found in foods that perform particular functions in the body. Milk, dark, leafy vegetables, and meat are good sources of minerals.
6. **Water** An essential component of the diet provided by food and fluid.

functions that support growth, tissue maintenance and repair, and ongoing health. Essentially, every part of our body was once a nutrient consumed in food. There are six categories of nutrients (Table 1.2). Each category except water consists of a number of different substances.

## Essential and Nonessential Nutrients

Of the many nutrients required for growth and health, some must be provided by the diet while others can be made by the body.

**Essential Nutrients** Nutrients the body cannot manufacture, or generally produce in sufficient amounts, are referred to as ***essential nutrients***. Here *essential* means "required in the diet." All of the following nutrients are considered essential:

- Carbohydrates
- Certain amino acids (the ***essential amino acids***: histidine, isoleucine, leucine, lysine, methionine, phenylalanine, threonine, tryptophan, and valine)
- Linoleic acid and alpha-linolenic acid (essential fatty acids)
- Vitamins
- Minerals
- Water

**Nonessential Nutrients** Cholesterol, creatine, and glucose are examples of nonessential nutrients. ***Nonessential nutrients*** are present in food and used by the body, but they do not have to be part of our diets. Many of the beneficial chemical substances in plants are not considered essential, for example, yet they play important roles in maintaining health.

**Requirements for Essential Nutrients** All humans require the same set of essential nutrients, but the amount of nutrients needed varies based on:

- Age
- Body size
- Gender
- Genetic traits
- Growth
- Illness
- Physical activity
- Medication use
- Pregnancy and lactation

Amounts of essential nutrients required each day vary a great deal, from cups (for water) to micrograms (e.g., for folate and vitamin $B_{12}$).

## Dietary Intake Standards

Dietary intake standards developed for the public cannot take into account all of the factors that influence nutrient needs, but they do account for the major ones of age, gender, growth, and pregnancy and lactation. Intake standards are called Dietary Reference Intakes (DRIs).

- *Dietary Reference Intakes (DRIs)*. This is the general term used for the nutrient intake standards for healthy people.
- *Recommended Dietary Allowances (RDAs)*. These are levels of essential nutrient intake judged to be adequate to meet the known nutrient needs of practically all (98 percent) of healthy people while decreasing the risk of certain chronic diseases.
- *Adequate Intakes (AIs)*. These are "tentative" RDAs. AIs are based on less conclusive scientific information than are the RDAs.
- *Estimated Average Requirements (EARs)*. These are nutrient intake values that are estimated to meet the requirements of half the healthy individuals in a group. The EARs are used to assess adequacy of intakes of population groups.
- *Tolerable Upper Intake Levels (ULs)*. These are upper limits of

**essential nutrients** Substances required for growth and health that cannot be produced, or produced in sufficient amounts, by the body. They must be obtained from the diet.

**essential amino acids** Amino acids that cannot be synthesized in adequate amounts by humans and therefore must be obtained from the diet. Also called *indispensible amino acids*.

**nonessential nutrients** Nutrients required for growth and health that can be produced by the body from other components of the diet.

nutrient intake compatible with health. The ULs do not reflect desired levels of intake. Rather, they represent total, daily levels of nutrient intake from food, fortified foods, and supplements that should not be exceeded.

DRIs have been developed for most of the essential nutrients and will be updated periodically. (These are listed on the inside front covers of this text.) Current DRIs were developed through a joint U.S.–Canadian effort, and the standards apply to both countries. The DRIs are levels of nutrient intake intended for use as reference values for planning and assessing diets for healthy people. They consist of the RDAs and the other categories of intake standards described in Illustration 1.2. It is recommended that individuals aim for nutrient intakes that approximate the RDAs or AI levels. Additional tests are required to confirm inadequate nutrient intakes and status.[4]

## Standards of Nutrient Intake for Nutrition Labels

The Nutrition Facts panel on packaged foods uses standard levels of nutrient intakes based on an earlier edition of recommended dietary intake levels. The levels are known as ***Daily Values*** (***DVs***) and are used to identify the amount of a nutrient provided in a serving of food compared to the standard level.

The "% DV" listed on nutrition labels represents the percentages of the standards obtained from one serving of the food product. Table 1.3 lists DV standard amounts for nutrients that are mandatory or voluntary components of nutrition labels. Additional information on nutrition labeling is presented later in this chapter.

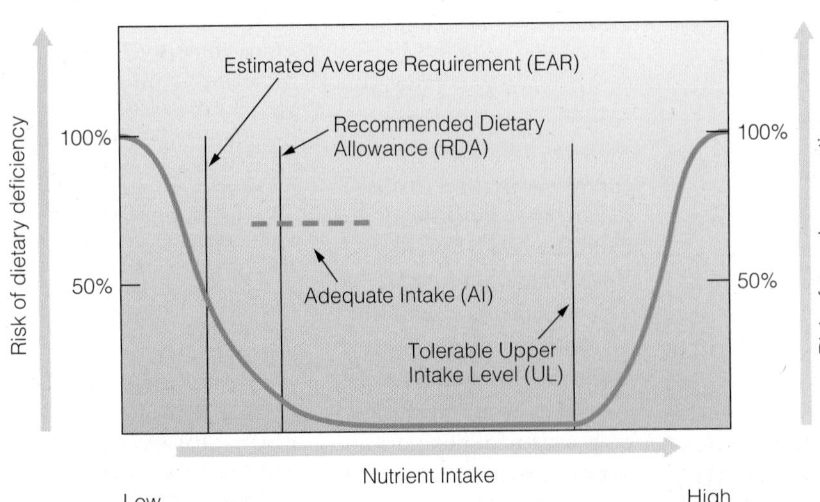


ILLUSTRATION 1.2 ▸ Theoretical framework, terms, and abbreviations used in the Dietary Reference Intakes.

TABLE 1.3 ▸ Daily Values (DVs) for nutrition labeling based on intakes of 2000 calories per day in adults and children aged 4 years and above

| MANDATORY COMPONENTS OF THE NUTRITION LABEL | |
|---|---|
| FOOD COMPONENT | DAILY VALUE (DV) |
| Total fat | 65 g[a] |
| Saturated fat | 20 g |
| Cholesterol | 300 mg[a] |
| Sodium | 2400 mg |
| Total carbohydrate | 300 g |
| Dietary fiber | 25 g |
| Vitamin A | 5000 IU[a] |
| Vitamin C | 60 mg |
| Calcium | 1000 mg |
| Iron | 18 mg |

[a]g = grams; mg = milligrams; IU = International Units

## Carbohydrates

Carbohydrates are used by the body mainly as a source of readily available energy. They consist of the simple sugars (monosaccharides and disaccharides), complex carbohydrates (the polysaccharides), most dietary sources of fiber, and alcohol sugars. Alcohol (ethanol) is closely related chemically to carbohydrates and is usually considered to be part of this nutrient category. Illustration 1.3 shows the similarity in the chemical structure of basic carbohydrate units. The most basic forms of carbohydrates are single molecules called monosaccharides.

Glucose (also called "blood sugar" and "dextrose"), fructose ("fruit sugar"), and galactose are the most common monosaccharides. Molecules containing two monosaccharides are called disaccharides. The most common disaccharides are:

- Sucrose (glucose + fructose, or common table sugar)
- Maltose (glucose + glucose, or malt sugar)
- Lactose (glucose + galactose, or milk sugar)

Complex carbohydrates (also called polysaccharides) are considered "complex" because they have more elaborate chemical structures than the simple sugars. They include:

**daily values (DVs)** Scientifically agreed-upon standards for daily intakes of nutrients from the diet developed for use on nutrition labels.

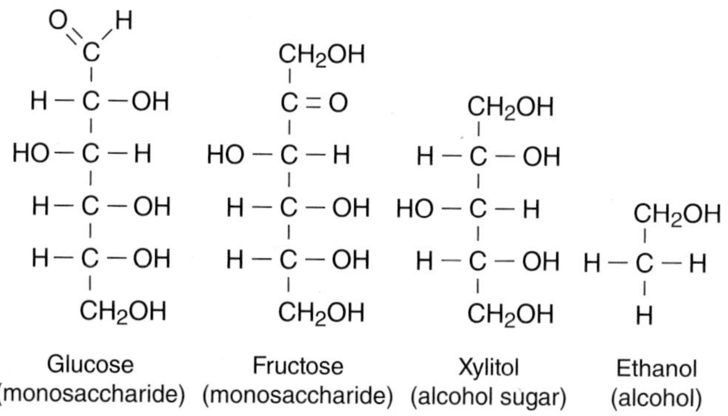

| Glucose | Fructose | Xylitol | Ethanol |
|---|---|---|---|
| O=C–H | $CH_2OH$ | | |
| H–C–OH | C=O | $CH_2OH$ | |
| HO–C–H | HO–C–H | H–C–OH | |
| H–C–OH | H–C–OH | HO–C–H | $CH_2OH$ |
| H–C–OH | H–C–OH | H–C–OH | H–C–H |
| $CH_2OH$ | $CH_2OH$ | $CH_2OH$ | H |
| (monosaccharide) | (monosaccharide) | (alcohol sugar) | (alcohol) |

ILLUSTRATION 1.3 ▸ Chemical structures of some simple carbohydrates.

- Starches (the plant form of stored carbohydrate)
- Glycogen (the animal form of stored carbohydrate)
- Most types of fiber

Each type of simple and complex carbohydrate, except fiber, provides four calories per gram. Dietary fiber supplies two calories per gram on average, even though fiber cannot be broken down by human digestive enzymes. Bacteria in the large intestine can digest some types of dietary fiber, however. These bacteria excrete fatty acids as a waste product of fiber digestion. The fatty acids are absorbed and used as a source of energy. The total contribution of fiber to our energy intake is modest (around 50 calories), and supplying energy is not a major function of fiber.[5] The main function of fiber is to provide "bulk" for normal elimination. It has other beneficial properties, however. High-fiber diets reduce the rate of glucose absorption (a benefit for people with diabetes) and may help prevent cardiovascular disease and obesity.[10]

Alcohol sugars (nonalcoholic in the beverage sense) are like simple sugars, except they include a chemical component of alcohol. Xylitol, mannitol, and sorbitol are common forms of alcohol sugars. Some are very sweet, and only small amounts are needed to sweeten commercial beverages, gums, yogurt, and other products. Unlike the simple sugars, alcohol sugars do not promote tooth decay.

Alcohol (consumed as ethanol) is considered to be part of the carbohydrate family because its chemical structure is similar to that of glucose. It is a product of the fermentation of sugar with yeast. With seven calories per gram, alcohol has more calories per gram than do other carbohydrates.

**Glycemic Index of Carbohydrates and Carbohydrates in Foods** In the not-too-distant past, it was assumed that "a carbohydrate is a carbohydrate is a carbohydrate." If all types of carbohydrates had the same effect on blood glucose levels and health, then it didn't matter what type was consumed. As is the case with many untested assumptions, this one fell by the wayside. It is now known that some types of simple and complex carbohydrates in foods elevate blood glucose levels more than do others. Such differences are particularly important to people with disorders such as ***insulin resistance*** and ***type 2 diabetes***.[6]

Carbohydrates and carbohydrate-containing foods are now being classified by the extent to which they increase blood glucose levels. This classification system is called the ***glycemic index***. Carbohydrates that are digested and absorbed quickly have a high glycemic index and raise blood glucose levels to a higher extent than do those with lower glycemic index values (Table 1.4).

**Recommended Intake Level** Recommended intake of carbohydrates is based on their contribution to total energy intake. It is recommended that 45–65 percent of calories come from carbohydrates. Added sugar should constitute no more than 25 percent of total caloric intake. It is recommended that adult females consume between 21 and 25 grams, and males 30–38 grams of total dietary fiber daily.[7]

**Food Sources of Carbohydrates** Carbohydrates are widely distributed in plant foods, while milk is the only important animal source of carbohydrates (lactose). Table 1.5 lists selected food sources by type of carbohydrate.

## Protein

Protein in foods provides the body with ***amino acids*** used to build and maintain protein-based components of the body such as muscle, bone, enzymes, and red blood cells. The body can also use protein as a source of energy—it provides four calories per gram. However, this is not a primary function of protein. Of the common types of amino acids, nine must be provided by the diet and are classified as essential amino acids. Amino acids that the body needs but can manufacture from other amino acids and components of the diet are classified as ***nonessential amino acids***.

**insulin resistance** A condition in which cell membranes have a reduced sensitivity to insulin so that more insulin than normal is required to transport a given amount of glucose into cells.

**type 2 diabetes** A disease characterized by high blood glucose levels due to the body's inability to use insulin normally, to produce enough insulin, or both.

**glycemic index** A measure of the extent to which blood glucose levels are raised by consumption of an amount of food that contains 50 grams of carbohydrate compared to 50 grams of glucose. A portion of white bread containing 50 grams of carbohydrate is sometimes used for comparison.

**amino acids** The "building blocks" of protein. Unlike carbohydrates and fats, amino acids contain nitrogen.

**nonessential amino acids** Amino acids that can be readily produced by humans from components of the diet. Also referred to as *dispensable amino acids*.

TABLE 1.4 ▸ Glycemic Index (GI) of selected foods[71,72]

| HIGH GI | (70 AND HIGHER) | MEDIUM GI | (56–69) | LOW GI | (55 OR LOWER) |
|---|---|---|---|---|---|
| Glucose | 100 | Breadfruit | 69 | Honey | 55 |
| French bread | 95 | Fruit Loops | 69 | Oatmeal | 54 |
| Scone | 92 | Orange soda | 68 | Corn | 53 |
| Sticky rice | 87 | Pita bread | 68 | Cracked wheat bread | 53 |
| Broken rice | 86 | Sucrose | 68 | Orange juice | 52 |
| Potato, baked | 85 | Taco shells | 68 | Banana | 52 |
| Potato, instant mashed | 85 | Croissant | 67 | Mango | 51 |
| Special K, rice | 84 | Angel food cake | 67 | Potato, boiled | 50 |
| Corn Chex | 83 | Fruit punch | 67 | Corn tortilla | 49 |
| Pretzel | 83 | Cherries | 66 | Green peas | 48 |
| Rice Krispies | 82 | Cream of Wheat | 66 | Pasta | 48 |
| Cornflakes | 81 | Brown rice | 66 | Carrots, raw | 47 |
| Corn Pops | 80 | Couscous | 65 | Lactose | 46 |
| Gatorade | 78 | Quaker Quick Oats | 65 | Milk chocolate | 43 |
| Jelly beans | 78 | Raisins | 64 | All-Bran | 42 |
| Cocoa pops | 77 | Chapati | 62 | Orange | 42 |
| Doughnut, cake | 76 | French bread with butter and jam | 62 | Peach | 42 |
| Waffle, frozen | 76 | Raisin Bran | 61 | Apple juice | 40 |
| Doughnuts | 75 | Sweet potato | 61 | Apple | 38 |
| French fries | 75 | Bran muffin | 60 | Pear | 38 |
| Grape Nuts | 75 | Just Right cereal | 60 | Tomato juice | 38 |
| Shredded Wheat | 75 | Blueberry muffin | 59 | Yam | 37 |
| White rice | 75 | Mini Wheats | 59 | Yogurt | 31 |
| Cheerios | 74 | Coca-Cola | 58 | Flour tortilla | 30 |
| Popcorn | 72 | Power Bar | 56 | Dried beans | 25 |
| Watermelon | 72 | Special K | 56 | Grapefruit | 25 |
| Carrots, diced, cooked | 70 | | | Milk | 25 |
| Wheat bread | 70 | | | Fructose | 19 |
| White bread | 70 | | | Pinto beans | 14 |
| | | | | Hummus | 6 |

Food sources of protein (Table 1.6) differ in quality based on the types and amounts of amino acids they contain. Foods of high protein quality include a balanced assortment of all of the essential amino acids. Protein from milk, cheese, meat, eggs, and other animal products is considered high quality. Plant sources of protein, with the exception of soybeans for adults, do not provide all nine essential amino acids in amounts needed to support growth in children and tissue maintenance. Combinations of plant foods, such as grains or seeds with dried beans, however, yield high-quality protein. The variety of amino acids found in these foods complement each other, thus providing a source of high-quality protein.

**Recommended Protein Intake** DRIs for protein are shown on the inside front cover of this text. In general, proteins should contribute 10–35 percent of total energy intake.[7] Protein deficiency, although rare in economically developed countries, leads to loss of muscle tissue, growth failure, weakness, reduced resistance to disease, and kidney and heart problems. It contributes to the development of a severe form of protein-energy malnutrition in young children known as ***kwashiorkor***.

**Kwashiorkor** A severe form of protein-energy malnutrition in young children. It is characterized by swelling, fatty liver, susceptibility to infection, profound apathy, and poor appetite. The cause of kwashiorkor is unclear.

TABLE 1.5 ▸ Food sources of carbohydrates

| A. SIMPLE SUGARS (MONO- AND DISACCHARIDES) THE SIMPLE SUGAR CONTENT OF SOME COMMON FOODS | | | | | |
|---|---|---|---|---|---|
| | PORTION SIZE | GRAMS OF CARBOHYDRATES | | PORTION SIZE | GRAMS OF CARBOHYDRATES[a] |
| **Sweeteners** | | | **Beverages** | | |
| Corn syrup | 1 tsp | 5 | Fruit drinks | 1 cup | 29 |
| Honey | 1 tsp | 6 | Soft drinks | 12 oz | 38 |
| Maple syrup | 1 tsp | 4 | Skim milk | 1 cup | 12 |
| Table sugar | 1 tsp | 4 | Whole milk | 1 cup | 11 |
| **Fruits** | | | **Candy** | | |
| Apple | 1 medium | 16 | Gumdrops | 1 oz | 25 |
| Peach | 1 medium | 8 | Hard candy | 1 oz | 28 |
| Watermelon | 1 wedge (4″ × 8″) | 25 | Caramels | 1 oz | 21 |
| Orange | 1 medium | 14 | Fudge | 1 oz | 21 |
| Banana | 1 medium | 21 | Milk chocolate | 1 oz | 16 |
| **Vegetables** | | | **Breakfast cereals** | | |
| Broccoli | ½ cup | 2 | Apple Jacks | 1 oz | 13 |
| Corn | ½ cup | 3 | Raisin Jacks | 1 oz | 19 |
| Potato | 1 cup | 1 | Cheerios | 1 oz | 14 |

| B. COMPLEX CARBOHYDRATES (STARCHES) COMPLEX | | | | | |
|---|---|---|---|---|---|
| | PORTION SIZE | GRAMS OF CARBOHYDRATES | | PORTION SIZE | GRAMS OF CARBOHYDRATES |
| **Grain and grain products** | | | **Dried beans (cooked)** | | |
| Rice (white), cooked | ½ cup | 21 | Lima beans | ½ cup | 11 |
| Pasta, cooked | ½ cup | 15 | White beans | ½ cup | 13 |
| Cornflakes | 1 cup | 11 | Kidney beans | ½ cup | 12 |
| Oatmeal, cooked | ½ cup | 12 | **Vegetables** | | |
| Cheerios | 1 cup | 11 | Potato | 1 medium | 30 |
| Whole wheat bread | 1 slice | 7 | Corn | ½ cup | 10 |
| | | | Broccoli | ½ cup | 2 |

| C. DIETARY FIBER | | | | | |
|---|---|---|---|---|---|
| | PORTION SIZE | GRAMS OF FIBER | | PORTION SIZE | GRAMS OF FIBER |
| **Grain and grain products** | | | **Fruits** | | |
| Bran Buds | ½ cup | 12.0 | Raspberries | 1 cup | 8.0 |
| All Bran | ½ cup | 11.0 | Avocado | ½ medium | 7.0 |
| Raisin Bran | 1 cup | 7.0 | Mango | 1 medium | 4.0 |
| Granola (homemade) | ½ cup | 6.0 | Pear (with skin) | 1 medium | 4.0 |
| Bran Flakes | ¾ cup | 5.0 | Apple (with skin) | 1 medium | 3.3 |
| Oatmeal | 1 cup | 4.0 | Banana | 6″ long | 3.1 |
| Spaghetti noodles | 1 cup | 4.0 | Orange (no peel) | 1 medium | 3.0 |
| Shredded Wheat | 1 biscuit | 2.7 | Peach (with skin) | 1 medium | 2.3 |
| Whole wheat bread | 1 slice | 2.0 | Strawberries | 10 medium | 2.1 |
| Bran (dry; wheat, oat) | 2 Tbsp | 2.0 | | | |

*(Continued)*

TABLE 1.5 ▸ Food sources of carbohydrates (*Continued*)

| | PORTION SIZE | GRAMS OF FIBER |
|---|---|---|
| **Vegetables** | | |
| Lima beans | ½ cup | 6.6 |
| Green peas | ½ cup | 4.4 |
| Potato (with skin) | 1 medium | 3.5 |
| Brussels sprouts | ½ cup | 3.0 |
| Broccoli | ½ cup | 2.8 |
| Carrots | ½ cup | 2.8 |
| Green beans | ½ cup | 2.7 |
| Collard greens | ½ cup | 2.7 |
| Cauliflower | ½ cup | 2.5 |
| Corn | ½ cup | 2.0 |
| **Nuts** | | |
| Almonds | ¼ cup | 4.5 |
| Peanuts | ¼ cup | 3.3 |
| Peanut butter | 2 Tbsp | 2.3 |
| **Dried beans (cooked)** | | |
| Pinto beans | ½ cup | 10.0 |
| Peas, split | ½ cup | 8.2 |
| Black beans (turtle beans) | ½ cup | 8.0 |
| Lentils | ½ cup | 7.8 |
| Kidney or navy beans | ½ cup | 6.9 |
| Black-eyed peas | ½ cup | 5.3 |
| **Fast foods** | | |
| Big Mac | 1 | 3 |
| French fries | 1 regular serving | 3 |
| Whopper | 1 | 3 |
| Cheeseburger | 1 | 2 |
| Taco | 1 | 2 |
| Chicken sandwich | 2 | 1 |
| Egg McMuffin | 1 | 1 |
| Fried chicken, drumstick | 1 | 1 |

[a]4 grams sucrose = 1 teaspoon.

TABLE 1.6 ▸ Food sources of protein

| | PORTION SIZE | GRAMS OF PROTEIN |
|---|---|---|
| **Meats** | | |
| Beef, lean | 3 oz | 26 |
| Tuna, in water | 3 oz | 24 |
| Hamburger, lean | 3 oz | 24 |
| Chicken, no skin | 3 oz | 24 |
| Lamb | 3 oz | 22 |
| Pork chop, lean | 3 oz | 20 |
| Haddock, broiled | 3 oz | 19 |
| Egg | 1 med | 6 |
| **Dairy Products** | | |
| Cottage cheese, low fat | ½ c | 14 |
| Yogurt, low fat | 1 c | 13 |
| Milk, skim | 1 c | 9 |
| Milk, whole | 1 c | 8 |
| Swiss cheese | 1 oz | 8 |
| Cheddar cheese | 1 oz | 7 |
| **Grain Products** | | |
| Oatmeal, cooked | ½ cup | 4 |
| Pasta, cooked | ½ cup | 4 |
| Bread | 1 slice | 2 |
| Rice, white or brown | ½ cup | 2 |

## Fats (Lipids)

Fats in food share the property of being soluble in fats but not in water. They are actually a subcategory of *lipids,* but this category of macronutrient is referred to as fat in the DRIs.[7] Lipids include fats, oils, and related compounds such as cholesterol. Fats are generally solid at room temperature, whereas oils are usually liquid. Fats and oils are made up of various types of triglycerides (triacylglycerols), which consist of three ***fatty acids*** attached to ***glycerol*** (Illustration 1.4). The number of carbons contained in the fatty acid component of triglycerides varies from 8 to 22.

Fats and oils are a concentrated source of energy, providing nine calories per gram. Fats perform a number of important functions in the body. They are needed for cholesterol and sex-hormone synthesis, components of cell membranes, vehicles for carrying certain vitamins that are soluble in fats only, and suppliers of the ***essential fatty acids*** required for growth and health.

**fatty acids** The fat-soluble components of fats in foods.

**glycerol** A component of fats that is soluble in water. It is converted to glucose in the body.

**essential fatty acids** Components of fat that are a required part of the diet (i.e., linoleic and alpha-linolenic acids). Both contain unsaturated fatty acids.

**Essential Fatty Acids** There are two essential fatty acids: linoleic acid and alpha-linolenic acid. Because

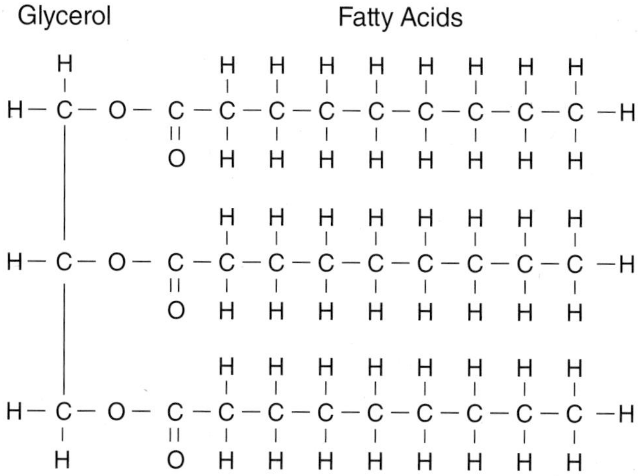

```
Glycerol                  Fatty Acids

   H           H   H   H   H   H   H   H   H
   |           |   |   |   |   |   |   |   |
H— C— O— C —C —C —C —C —C —C —C —C —H
   |       ||  |   |   |   |   |   |   |   |
   |       O   H   H   H   H   H   H   H   H
   |
   |           H   H   H   H   H   H   H   H
   |           |   |   |   |   |   |   |   |
H— C— O— C —C —C —C —C —C —C —C —C —H
   |       ||  |   |   |   |   |   |   |   |
   |       O   H   H   H   H   H   H   H   H
   |
   |           H   H   H   H   H   H   H   H
   |           |   |   |   |   |   |   |   |
H— C— O— C —C —C —C —C —C —C —C —C —H
   |       ||  |   |   |   |   |   |   |   |
   H       O   H   H   H   H   H   H   H   H
```

ILLUSTRATION 1.4 ▸ Basic structure of a triglyceride.

these fatty acids are essential, they must be supplied in the diet. The central nervous system is particularly rich in derivatives of these two fatty acids. They are found in phospholipids, which—along with cholesterol—are the primary lipids in the brain and other nervous system tissue. Biologically active derivatives of essential fatty acids include ***prostaglandins***, ***thromboxanes***, and ***prostacyclins***:

***Linoleic Acid*** Linoleic acid is the parent of the omega-6 (or n-6) fatty acid family. One of the major derivatives of linoleic acid is arachidonic acid. Arachidonic acid serves as a primary structural component of the central nervous system. Most vegetable oils and meats, as well as human milk, are good sources of linoleic acid. American diets tend to provide sufficient to excessive levels of linoleic acid, and considerable amounts are stored in body fat.

***Alpha-Linolenic Acid*** Alpha-linolenic acid is the parent of the omega-3 (n-3) fatty acid family. It is present in many types of dark green vegetables, vegetable oils, and flaxseed. Derivatives of this essential fatty acid include eicosapentaenoic acid (EPA) and docosahexaenoic acid (DHA). Relatively small amounts of EPA and DHA are produced in the body from alpha-linolenic acid because the conversion is low.[7] EPA and DHA also enter the body through intake of fatty, cold-water fish, shellfish, and human milk. Regular consumption of fish (two or more servings per week) reduces chronic inflammation and the risk of heart disease and sudden cardiac death.[11] DHA is found in large amounts in the central nervous system, the retina of the eye, and the testes. The body stores only small amounts of alpha-linolenic acid, EPA, and DHA.[12] On average, adults in the United States and Canada consume around 100 mg of EPA plus DHA daily, far short of the estimated need of 300–500 mg daily.[13]

**Saturated and Unsaturated Fats** Fats (lipids) come in two basic types: ***saturated*** and ***unsaturated***. Whether a fat is saturated or not depends on whether it has one or more double bonds between carbon atoms in one or more of its fatty acid components. If one double bond is present in one or more of the fatty acids, the fat is considered ***monounsaturated***; if two or more are present, the fat is ***polyunsaturated***.

Some unsaturated fatty acids are highly unsaturated. Alpha-linolenic acid, for example, contains three double bonds, arachidonic acid four, EPA five, and DHA six. These fatty acids are less stable than fatty acids with fewer double bonds, because double bonds between atoms are weaker than single bonds.

Saturated fats contain no double bonds between carbons and tend to be solid at room temperature. Animal products such as butter, cheese, and meats and two plant oils (coconut and palm) are rich sources of saturated fats. Fat we consume in our diets, whether it contains primarily saturated or unsaturated fatty acids, is generally in the triglyceride (or triacylglyceride) form.

Although most foods contain both saturated and unsaturated fats, animal foods tend to contain more saturated and less unsaturated fat than plant foods. Saturated fatty acids tend to increase blood levels of LDL cholesterol (the lipoprotein that is associated with heart-disease risk when present in high levels), whereas unsaturated fatty acids tend to decrease LDL cholesterol levels.[11,14]

▸ ***Hydrogenation and Trans Fats*** Oils can be made solid by adding hydrogen to the double bonds of their unsaturated fatty acids. This process, called hydrogenation, makes some of the fatty acids in oils saturated and enhances storage life and baking qualities. Hydrogenation may alter the molecular structure of the fatty acids; however,

**prostaglandins** A group of physiologically active substances derived from the essential fatty acids. They are present in many tissues and perform such functions as the constriction or dilation of blood vessels and stimulation of smooth muscles and the uterus.

**thromboxanes** Biologically active substances produced in platelets that increase platelet aggregation (and therefore promote blood clotting), constrict blood vessels, and increase blood pressure.

**prostacyclins** Biologically active substances produced by blood vessel walls that inhibit platelet aggregation (and therefore blood clotting), dilate blood vessels, and reduce blood pressure.

**saturated fats** Fats in which adjacent carbons in the fatty acid component are linked by single bonds only (e.g., –C–C–C–C–).

**unsaturated fats** Fats in which adjacent carbons in one or more fatty acids are linked by one or more double bonds (e.g., –C–C=C–C=C–).

**monounsaturated fats** Fats in which only one pair of adjacent carbons in one or more of its fatty acids is linked by a double bond (e.g., –C–C=C–C–).

**polyunsaturated fats** Fats in which more than one pair of adjacent carbons in one or more of its fatty acids are linked by two or more double bonds (e.g., –C–C=C–C=C–).

changing the naturally occurring *cis* structure to the *trans* form. Trans fatty acids raise blood LDL-cholesterol levels to a greater extent than do saturated fatty acids. They are naturally present in dairy products and meats, but the primary dietary sources are products made from hydrogenated fats. Due to nutrition labeling requirements and public uproar, the ***trans fat*** content of bakery products, chips, fast foods, and other products made with hydrogenated fats has decreased substantially.

**Cholesterol** Dietary ***cholesterol*** is a fatlike, clear liquid substance primarily found in lean and fat components of animal products. Cholesterol is a component of all animal cell membranes, the brain, and the nerves. It is the precursor of estrogen, testosterone, and vitamin D, which is manufactured in the skin upon exposure to sunlight. The body generally produces only one-third of the cholesterol our bodies use because more than sufficient amounts of cholesterol are provided in most people's diet. The extent to which dietary cholesterol intake modifies blood cholesterol level appears to vary a good deal based on genetic tendencies.[14,15] Leading sources of dietary cholesterol are egg yolks, meat, milk and milk products, and fats such as butter.

**Recommended Intake of Fats** Scientific evidence and opinions related to the effects of fat on health have changed substantially in recent years—and so have recommendations for fat intake. In the past, it was recommended that Americans aim for diets providing less than 30 percent of total calories from fat. Concerns that high-fat diets encourage the development of obesity have been eased by studies demonstrating that excessive caloric intakes—and not diets high in fat—are related to weight gain. Current advice indicates that dietary fat intake should be within the range of 20 to 35 percent of total calories. Average intake of fat among adults in the United States is 33 percent of total calories.[11]

There is no recommended level of cholesterol intake, because there is no evidence that cholesterol is required in the diet. The body is able to produce enough cholesterol, and people do not develop a cholesterol deficiency disease if it is not consumed.

Overall, it is recommended that ***dietary patterns*** emphasize food sources of polyunsaturated fats, that intake of *trans* fats should be as low as possible, and that consumption of EPA and DHA should be increased by eating fish at least twice a week. Reduced intake of foods high in saturated fat intake is also recommended.[11]

**Food Sources of Fat** The fat content of many foods can be identified by reading the nutrition information labels on food packages. The amount of total fat, saturated fat, *trans* fat, and cholesterol in a serving of food is listed on the label. Table 1.7 lists the total fat, saturated fat, unsaturated fat, cholesterol, and omega-3 fatty acid contents (EPA and DHA) of selected foods.

## Vitamins

Vitamins are chemical substances in foods that perform specific functions in the body. Fourteen have been discovered so far. They are classified as either fat soluble or water soluble (Table 1.8).

The B-complex vitamins and vitamin C are soluble in water and found dissolved in water in foods. The fat-soluble vitamins consist of vitamins A, D, E, and K and are present in the fat portions of foods. (To remember the fat-soluble vitamins, think of "DEKA" for vitamins D, E, K, and A.) Only these chemical substances are truly vitamins. Substances such as coenzyme $Q_{10}$, inositol, provitamin $B_5$ complex, and pangamic acid (vitamin $B_{15}$) may be called vitamins, but they are not. Except for vitamin $B_{12}$, water-soluble vitamin stores in the body are limited and run out within a few weeks to a few months after intake becomes inadequate. Fat-soluble vitamins are stored in the body's fat tissues and the liver. These stores can be sizable and last from months to years when intake is low.

Excessive consumption of the fat-soluble vitamins from supplements, especially of vitamins A and D, produces various symptoms of toxicity. High intake of the water-soluble vitamins from supplements can also produce adverse health effects. Toxicity symptoms from water-soluble vitamins, however, tend to last a shorter time and are more quickly remedied. Vitamin overdoses are very rarely related to food intake.

Vitamins do not provide energy or, with the exception of choline, serve as structural components of the body. Some play critical roles as ***coenzymes*** in chemical changes that take place in the body, known as ***metabolism***. Vitamin A is needed to replace the cells that line the mouth and esophagus, thiamin is needed for maintenance of normal appetite, and riboflavin and folate are needed for the synthesis of body proteins. Other vitamins (vitamins C and E, and beta-carotene—a precursor of vitamin A) act as

***trans* fat** A type of unsaturated fat present in hydrogenated oils, margarine, shortenings, pastries, and some cooking oils that increase the risk of heart disease. Fats containing fatty acids in the *trans* versus the more common *cis* form are generally referred to as *trans* fat.

**cholesterol** A fat-soluble, colorless liquid primarily found in animals products.

**dietary pattern** The quantities, proportions, variety, or combination of different foods, drinks, and nutrients in diets, and the frequency with which they are habitually consumed.

**coenzymes** Chemical substances that activate enzymes.

**metabolism** The chemical changes that take place in the body. The conversion of glucose to energy or body fat is an example of a metabolic process.

TABLE 1.7 ▸ Food sources of fats

**A. TOTAL FAT**

| | PORTION SIZE | GRAMS OF TOTAL FAT | | PORTION SIZE | GRAMS OF TOTAL FAT |
|---|---|---|---|---|---|
| **Fats and Oils** | | | Milk, 2% | 1 cup | 5.0 |
| Mayonnaise | 1 Tbsp | 11.0 | Hamburger, 21% fat | 3 oz | 15.0 |
| Ranch dressing | 1 Tbsp | 6.0 | Hamburger, 16% fat | 3 oz | 13.5 |
| Vegetable oils | 1 tsp | 4.7 | Steak, rib-eye | 3 oz | 9.9 |
| Butter | 1 tsp | 4.0 | Bacon | 3 strips | 9.0 |
| Margarine | 1 tsp | 4.0 | Steak, round | 3 oz | 5.2 |
| **Meats, Fish** | | | Chicken, baked, no skin | 3 oz | 4.0 |
| Sausage | 4 links | 18.0 | Flounder, baked | 3 oz | 1.0 |
| Hot dog | 2 oz | 17.0 | Shrimp, boiled | 3 oz | 1.0 |
| **Fast Foods** | | | Milk, 1% | 1 cup | 2.9 |
| Whopper | 8.9 oz | 32.0 | Milk, skim | 1 cup | 0.4 |
| Big Mac | 6.6 oz | 31.4 | Yogurt, frozen | 1 cup | 0.3 |
| Quarter Pounder with Cheese | 6.8 oz | 28.6 | **Other Foods** | | |
| Veggie pita | 1 | 17.0 | Avocado | ½ | 15.0 |
| Subway meatball sandwich | 1 | 16.0 | Almonds | 1 oz | 15.0 |
| Subway turkey sandwich | 1 | 4.0 | Cashews | 1 oz | 13.2 |
| **Milk and Milk Products** | | | French fries | 14 | 10.0 |
| Cheddar cheese | 1 oz | 9.5 | Taco chips | 1 oz (10 chips) | 10.0 |
| Milk, whole | 1 cup | 8.5 | Potato chips | 1 oz (14 chips) | 7.0 |
| American cheese | 1 oz | 6.0 | Peanut butter | 1 Tbsp | 6.1 |
| Cottage cheese, regular | ½ cup | 5.1 | Egg | 1 | 6.0 |

**B. SATURATED FATS**

| | PORTION SIZE | GRAMS OF SATURATED FAT | | PORTION SIZE | GRAMS OF SATURATED FAT |
|---|---|---|---|---|---|
| **Fats and Oils** | | | Hot dog | 1 | 4.9 |
| Margarine | 1 tsp | 2.9 | Chicken, fried, with skin | 3 oz | 3.8 |
| Butter | 1 tsp | 2.4 | Salami | 3 oz | 3.6 |
| Salad dressing, ranch | 1 Tbsp | 1.2 | Haddock, breaded, fried | 3 oz | 3.0 |
| Peanut oil | 1 tsp | 0.9 | Rabbit | 3 oz | 3.0 |
| Olive oil | 1 tsp | 0.7 | Pork chop, lean | 3 oz | 2.7 |
| Salad dressing, thousand island | 1 Tbsp | 0.5 | Steak, round, lean | 3 oz | 2.0 |
| Canola oil | 1 tsp | 0.3 | Turkey, roasted | 3 oz | 2.0 |
| **Milk and Milk Products** | | | Chicken, baked, no skin | 3 oz | 1.7 |
| Cheddar cheese | 1 oz | 5.9 | Prime rib, lean | 3 oz | 1.3 |
| American cheese | 1 oz | 5.5 | Venison | 3 oz | 1.1 |
| Milk, whole | 1 cup | 5.1 | Tuna, in water | 3 oz | 0.4 |
| Cottage cheese, regular | ½ cup | 3.0 | **Fast Foods** | | |
| Milk, 2% | 1 cup | 2.9 | Croissant w/egg, bacon, & cheese | 1 | 16.0 |
| Milk, 1% | 1 cup | 1.5 | Sausage croissant | 1 | 16.0 |
| Milk, skim | 1 cup | 0.3 | Whopper | 1 | 11.0 |
| **Meats, Fish** | | | Cheeseburger | 1 | 9.0 |
| Hamburger, 21% fat | 3 oz | 6.7 | Bac'n Cheddar Deluxe | 1 | 8.7 |
| Sausage, links | 4 | 5.6 | | | |

(Continued)

TABLE 1.7 ▸ Food sources of fats (*Continued*)

| | PORTION SIZE | GRAMS OF SATURATED FAT | | PORTION SIZE | GRAMS OF SATURATED FAT |
|---|---|---|---|---|---|
| Taco, regular | 1 | 4.0 | Peanuts, dry-roasted | 1 oz | 1.9 |
| Chicken breast sandwich | 1 | 3.0 | Sunflower seeds | 1 oz | 1.6 |
| **Nuts and Seeds** | | | | | |
| Macadamia nuts | 1 oz | 3.2 | | | |

**C. UNSATURATED FATS**

| | PORTION SIZE | GRAMS OF UNSATURATED FAT | | PORTION SIZE | GRAMS OF UNSATURATED FAT |
|---|---|---|---|---|---|
| **Fats and Oils** | | | Haddock, breaded, fried | 3 oz | 6.5 |
| Canola oil | 1 tsp | 4.1 | Chicken, baked, no skin | 3 oz | 6.0 |
| Vegetable oils | 1 tsp | 3.6 | Pork chop, lean | 3 oz | 5.3 |
| Margarine | 1 tsp | 2.9 | Turkey, roasted | 3 oz | 4.5 |
| Butter | 1 tsp | 1.3 | Tuna, in water | 3 oz | 0.7 |
| **Milk and Milk Products** | | | Egg | 1 | 5.0 |
| Cottage cheese, regular | ½ cup | 3.0 | **Nuts and Seeds** | | |
| Cheddar cheese | 1 oz | 2.9 | Sunflower seeds | 1 oz | 16.6 |
| American cheese | 1 oz | 2.8 | Almonds | 1 oz | 12.6 |
| Milk, whole | 1 cup | 2.8 | Peanuts | 1 oz | 11.3 |
| **Meats, Fish** | | | Cashews | 1 oz | 10.2 |
| Hamburger, 21% fat | 3 oz | 10.9 | | | |

**D. CHOLESTEROL**

| | PORTION SIZE | MILLIGRAMS CHOLESTEROL | | PORTION SIZE | MILLIGRAMS CHOLESTEROL |
|---|---|---|---|---|---|
| **Fats and Oils** | | | Ostrich, ground | 3 oz | 63 |
| Butter | 1 tsp | 10.3 | Pork chop, lean | 3 oz | 60 |
| Vegetable oils, margarine | 1 tsp | 0 | Hamburger, 10% fat | 3 oz | 60 |
| **Meats, Fish** | | | Venison | 3 oz | 48 |
| Brain | 3 oz | 1476 | Wild pig | 3 oz | 33 |
| Liver | 3 oz | 470 | Goat, roasted | 3 oz | 32 |
| Egg | 1 | 186 | Tuna, in water | 3 oz | 25 |
| Veal | 3 oz | 128 | **Milk and Milk Products** | | |
| Shrimp | 3 oz | 107 | Ice cream, regular | 1 cup | 56 |
| Prime rib | 3 oz | 80 | Milk, whole | 1 cup | 34 |
| Chicken, baked, no skin | 3 oz | 75 | Milk, 2% | 1 cup | 22 |
| Salmon, broiled | 3 oz | 74 | Yogurt, low fat | 1 cup | 17 |
| Turkey, baked, no skin | 3 oz | 65 | Milk, 1% | 1 cup | 14 |
| Hamburger, 20% fat | 3 oz | 64 | Milk, skim | 1 cup | 7 |

**E. OMEGA-3 (N-3) FATTY ACIDS**

| | PORTION SIZE | MILLIGRAMS EPA + DHA | | PORTION SIZE | MILLIGRAMS EPA + DHA |
|---|---|---|---|---|---|
| **Fish and Seafood** | | | Anchovies | 3 oz | 1747 |
| Fish oil | 1 tsp | 2796 | Herring | 3 oz | 1712 |
| Shad | 3 oz | 2046 | Salmon, wild | 3 oz | 1564 |
| Salmon, farmed | 3 oz | 1825 | Whitefish | 3 oz | 1370 |

| | PORTION SIZE | MILLIGRAMS EPA + DHA | | PORTION SIZE | MILLIGRAMS EPA + DHA |
|---|---|---|---|---|---|
| Mackerel | 3 oz | 1023 | Catfish, wild | 3 oz | 201 |
| Sardines | 3 oz | 840 | Crawfish | 3 oz | 187 |
| Whiting | 3 oz | 440 | Sheepshead | 3 oz | 162 |
| Flounder | 3 oz | 426 | Tuna, light, and in oil | 3 oz | 109 |
| Trout, freshwater | 3 oz | 420 | Lobster | 3 oz | 71 |
| Oysters | 3 oz | 375 | Egg yolk | 1 | 40 |
| Snapper | 3 oz | 273 | DHA-fortified egg | 1 | 150 |
| Shrimp | 3 oz | 268 | Human milk | 4 oz | 126 |
| Clams | 3 oz | 241 | DHA-fortified beverages | 4 oz | 32 |
| Haddock | 3 oz | 202 | | | |

*Mercury content <0.2 ppm as given in *Mercury levels in commercial fish and shellfish*, 2006 update, U.S. Environmental Protection Agency, www.epa.gov.

***antioxidants*** and perform other functions. By preventing or repairing damage to cells due to oxidation, these vitamins help maintain body tissues and prevent disease. Primary functions, consequences of deficiency and overdose, primary food sources, and comments about each vitamin are listed in Table 1.9

**Recommended Intake of Vitamins** Recommendations for levels of intake of vitamins are presented in the tables on the inside front covers of this text. Note that Tolerable Upper Levels of Intake (ULs) for many vitamins are also given; they represent levels of intake that should not be exceeded. Table 1.10 lists food sources of each vitamin.

## Phytochemicals

There are many substances in foods in addition to nutrients that affect health. Some foods contain naturally occurring toxins, such as poison in puffer fish and solanine in green sections near the skin of some potatoes. Consuming the poison in puffer fish can be lethal; large doses of solanine can interfere with nerve impulses. Some plant pigments, hormones, and other naturally occurring substances that protect plants from insects, oxidization, and other damaging exposures also appear to benefit human health. These substances in plants are referred to as ***phytochemicals***, and knowledge about their effects on human health is advancing rapidly. Many of the phytochemicals that benefit health are pigments that act as antioxidants in the human body. Table 1.11 shows a list of the good food sources of antioxidants. Notice that most of the foods listed are colorful.

Consumption of foods rich in specific pigments and other phytochemicals, rather than consumption of isolated phytochemicals, may help prevent certain types of cancer, cataracts, type 2 diabetes, hypertension, infections, and heart disease. High intakes of certain phytochemicals from vegetables, fruits, nuts, seeds, and whole-grain products may partially account for lower rates of heart disease and cancer observed in people with high intakes of these foods.[16,17]

TABLE 1.8 ▸ Vitamin solubility

| WATER-SOLUBLE VITAMINS | FAT-SOLUBLE VITAMINS |
|---|---|
| B-complex vitamins | Vitamin A (retinol, beta-carotene) |
| Thiamin ($B_1$) | Vitamin D (1,25 dihydroxy-cholecalciferol) |
| Riboflavin ($B_2$) | Vitamin E (alpha-tocopherol) |
| Niacin ($B_3$) | Vitamin K |
| Vitamin $B_6$ | |
| Folate | |
| Vitamin $B_{12}$ | |
| Biotin | |
| Pantothenic acid | |
| Choline | |
| Vitamin C (ascorbic acid) | |

## Minerals

Humans require the 15 minerals listed in Table 1.12. Minerals are unlike other nutrients in that they consist of single atoms and carry a charge in solution. The charge (resulting from having an unequal number of electrons and protons) carried by minerals allows them to combine with other minerals to form stable complexes in bone, teeth, cartilage, and other tissues. In body fluids, charged minerals serve as a source of electrical power that stimulates muscles to contract (e.g., the heart to beat) and nerves to react. Minerals also help the body maintain an adequate

**antioxidants** Chemical substances that prevent or repair damage to cells caused by exposure to oxidizing agents such as oxygen, ozone, and smoke and to other oxidizing agents normally produced in the body. Many different antioxidants are found in foods; some are made by the body.

**phytochemicals** (phyto = plants) Chemical substances in plants, some of which affect body processes in humans that may benefit health. Also called phytonutrients.

TABLE 1.9 ▸ Summary of the vitamins

| THE WATER-SOLUBLE VITAMINS | | |
|---|---|---|
| | PRIMARY FUNCTIONS | CONSEQUENCES OF DEFICIENCY |
| **Thiamin (vitamin $B_1$)**<br>AI[a] women: 1.1 mg<br>men: 1.2 mg | • Coenzyme in the metabolism of carbohydrates, alcohol, and some amino acids<br>• Required for the growth and maintenance of nerve and muscle tissues<br>• Required for normal appetite | • Fatigue, weakness<br>• Nerve disorders, mental confusion, apathy<br>• Impaired growth<br>• Swelling<br>• Heart irregularity and failure |
| **Riboflavin (vitamin $B_2$)**<br>AI women: 1.1 mg<br>men: 1.3 mg | • Coenzyme involved in energy metabolism of carbohydrates, proteins, and fats<br>• Coenzyme function in cell division<br>• Promotes growth and tissue repair<br>• Promotes normal vision | • Reddened lips, cracks at both corners of the mouth<br>• Fatigue |
| **Niacin (vitamin $B_3$)**<br>RDA women: 14 mg<br>men: 16 mg<br>UL: 35 mg (from supplements and fortified foods) | • Coenzyme involved in energy metabolism<br>• Coenzyme required for the synthesis of body fats<br>• Helps maintain normal nervous system functions | • Skin disorders<br>• Nervous and mental disorders<br>• Diarrhea, indigestion<br>• Fatigue |
| **Vitamin $B_6$ (pyridoxine)**<br>AI women: 1.3 mg<br>men: 1.3 mg<br>UL: 100 mg | • Coenzyme involved in amino acid, glucose, and fatty acid metabolism and neurotransmitter synthesis<br>• Coenzyme in the conversion of tryptophan to niacin<br>• Required for normal red blood cell formation<br>• Required for the synthesis of lipids in the nervous and immune systems | • Irritability, depression<br>• Convulsions, twitching<br>• Muscular weakness<br>• Dermatitis near the eyes<br>• Anemia<br>• Kidney stones |
| **Folate (folacin, folic acid)**<br>RDA women: 400 mcg<br>men: 400 mcg<br>UL: 1000 mcg (from supplements and fortified foods) | • Required for the conversion of homocysteine to methionine<br>• Methyl ($CH_3$) group donor and coenzyme in DNA synthesis, gene expression and regulation<br>• Required for the normal formation of red blood and other cells | • Megaloblastic cells and anemia<br>• Diarrhea, weakness, irritability, paranoid behavior<br>• Red, sore tongue<br>• Increased blood homocysteine levels<br>• Increased risk of neural tube defects and other malformations, low birthweight and preterm delivery (in pregnancy) |
| **Vitamin $B_{12}$ (cyanocobalamin)**<br>AI women: 2.4 mcg<br>Men: 2.4 mcg | • Coenzyme involved in the synthesis of DNA, RNA, and myelin<br>• Required for the conversion of homocysteine to methionine<br>• Needed for normal red blood cell development | • Neurological disorders (nervousness, tingling and numbness in fingers, brain degeneration)<br>• Pernicious anemia characterized by large, oval-shaped red blood cells<br>• Sore, beefy red, smooth tongue<br>• Fatigue |

| THE WATER-SOLUBLE VITAMINS *(Continued)* | | |
|---|---|---|
| CONSEQUENCES OF OVERDOSE | PRIMARY FOOD SOURCES | HIGHLIGHTS AND COMMENTS |
| • High intakes of thiamin are rapidly excreted by the kidneys. Oral doses of 500 mg/day or less considered safe. | • Grains and grain products (cereals, pasta, bread)<br>• Pork | • Need increases with carbohydrate intake.<br>• There is no "e" on the end of *thiamin.*<br>• Deficiency rare in the U.S.; may occur in people with alcoholism.<br>• Enriched grains and cereals prevent thiamin deficiency. |
| • None known; high doses are rapidly excreted by the kidneys. | • Milk, yogurt, cheese<br>• Grains and grain products (cereals, rice, pasta, bread)<br>• Liver, fish, beef<br>• Eggs | • Destroyed by exposure to light. |
| • Flushing, headache, cramps, rapid heartbeat, nausea, diarrhea, decreased liver function with doses above 0.5 g per day | • Meats, fish<br>• Grains and grain products (cereals, rice, pasta, bread) | • Niacin has a precursor—tryptophan. Tryptophan, an amino acid, is converted to niacin by the body. Much of our niacin intake comes from tryptophan.<br>• High doses raise HDL cholesterol levels, decrease LDL cholesterol, and lower triglyceride levels. |
| • Bone pain, loss of feeling in fingers and toes, muscular weakness, numbness, loss of balance (mimicking multiple sclerosis) | • Breakfast cereals<br>• Brussels sprouts, sweet peppers, potatoes<br>• Meats (all types) | • Vitamins go from $B_3$ to $B_6$ because $B_4$ and $B_5$ were found to be duplicates of vitamins already identified. |
| • May mask signs of vitamin $B_{12}$ deficiency (pernicious anemia), especially in older adults | • Ready-to-eat cereals, fortified grain products<br>• Dark green, leafy vegetables<br>• Dried beans | • Folate means "foliage." It was first discovered in leafy green vegetables.<br>• This vitamin is easily destroyed by heat.<br>• Synthetic form (folic acid) added to fortified grain products is better absorbed than naturally occurring folates.<br>• Some individuals are genetically susceptible to folate deficiency.<br>• Folate status has improved since folic acid fortification of refined grain products. |
| • None known. Excess vitamin $B_{12}$ is rapidly excreted by the kidneys or is not absorbed into the bloodstream.<br>• Vitamin $B_{12}$ injections may cause a temporary feeling of heightened energy. | • Fish, seafood, meats<br>• Milk, cheese<br>• Ready-to-eat cereals | • Older people, people who malabsorb $B_{12}$, and vegans are at risk for vitamin $B_{12}$ deficiency.<br>• Vitamin $B_{12}$ is found in animal products and microorganisms only. |

*(Continued)*

TABLE 1.9 ▸ Summary of the vitamins (*Continued*)

| THE WATER-SOLUBLE VITAMINS | | |
|---|---|---|
| | PRIMARY FUNCTIONS | CONSEQUENCES OF DEFICIENCY |
| **Biotin**<br>AI women: 30 mcg<br>men: 30 mcg | • Required by enzymes involved in fat, protein, and glycogen metabolism | • Seizures, vision problems<br>• Hearing loss<br>• Weakness |
| **Pantothenic acid (pantothenate)**<br>AI women: 5 mg<br>men: 5 mg | • Coenzyme involved in energy metabolism of carbohydrates and fats<br>• Coenzyme in protein metabolism | • Fatigue, sleep disturbances, numbness, impaired coordination<br>• Vomiting, nausea |
| **Vitamin C (ascorbic acid)**<br>RDA women: 75 mg<br>men: 90 mg<br>UL: 2000 mg | • Required for collagen synthesis<br>• Acts as an antioxidant; protects LDL cholesterol, eye tissues, sperm proteins, DNA, and lipids against oxidation<br>• Required for the conversion of Fe$^{11}$ to Fe1$^{11}$<br>• Required for neurotransmitters and steroid hormone synthesis | • Bleeding and bruising easily due to weakened blood vessels, cartilage, and other tissues containing collagen<br>• Slow recovery from infections and poor wound healing<br>• Fatigue, depression |
| **Choline**<br>AI women: 425 mg<br>AI men: 550 mg<br>UL: 3.5 g | • Serves as a structural and signaling component of cell membranes<br>• Required for the normal development of memory and attention processes during early life<br>• Required for the transport and metabolism of fat and cholesterol | • Fatty liver<br>• Infertility<br>• Hypertension |
| **THE FAT-SOLUBLE VITAMINS** | | |
| **Vitamin A**<br>RDA women: 700 mcg<br>men: 900 mcg<br>UL: 3000 mcg | • Needed for the formation and maintenance of mucous membranes, skin, bone<br>• Needed for vision in dim light | • Increased incidence and severity of infection (including measles)<br>• Impaired vision, xerophthalmia, blindness<br>• Inability to see in dim light |
| **Vitamin E (alpha-tocopherol)**<br>RDA women: 15 mg<br>men: 15 mg<br>UL: 1000 mg | • Acts as an antioxidant, prevents damage to cell membranes in blood cells, lungs, and other tissues by repairing damage caused by free radicals<br>• Participates in the regulation of gene expression | • Muscle loss, nerve damage<br>• Anemia<br>• Weakness |

| THE WATER-SOLUBLE VITAMINS (*Continued*) | | |
|---|---|---|
| CONSEQUENCES OF OVERDOSE | PRIMARY FOOD SOURCES | HIGHLIGHTS AND COMMENTS |
| • None known. Excesses are rapidly excreted. | • Grain and cereal products<br>• Meats, dried beans, cooked eggs<br>• Vegetables | • Deficiency is extremely rare. May be induced by the overconsumption of raw eggs. |
| • None known. Excesses are rapidly excreted. | • Many foods, including meats, grains, vegetables, fruits, and milk | • Deficiency is very rare. |
| • Regular intake of 1 g or more per day of supplemental vitamin C can cause nausea, cramps, diarrhea; and increase the risk of kidney stones. | • Fruits: oranges, lemons, limes, strawberries, cantaloupe, honeydew melon, grapefruit, kiwi fruit, mango, papaya<br>• Vegetables: broccoli, green and red peppers, collards, cabbage, tomatoes, asparagus, potatoes<br>• Ready-to-eat cereals | • Need increases among smokers (to 110–125 mg per day).<br>• Is fragile; easily destroyed by heat and exposure to air.<br>• Supplements may decrease severity of symptoms of colds.<br>• Deficiency may develop within 3 weeks of very low intake. |
| • Low blood pressure<br>• Sweating, diarrhea<br>• Fishy body odor<br>• Liver damage | • Beef<br>• Eggs<br>• Pork<br>• Dried beans<br>• Fish<br>• Milk | • Most of the choline we consume from foods comes from its location in cell membranes.<br>• Lecithin, an additive commonly found in processed foods, is a rich source of choline.<br>• Choline is primarily found in animal products.<br>• It is considered a B-complex vitamin. |
| THE FAT-SOLUBLE VITAMINS (*Continued*) | | |
| • Vitamin A toxicity (hypervitamosis A) with acute doses of 500,000 IU, or long-term intake of 50,000 IU per day.<br>• Nausea, irritability, blurred vision, weakness<br>• Increased pressure in the skull, headache<br>• Liver damage<br>• Hair loss, dry skin<br>• Birth defects | • Vitamin A is found in animal products only<br>• Liver, clams<br>• Low-fat milk, American cheese<br>• Ready-to-eat cereals | • Beta-carotene is a vitamin A precursor or "provitamin"; it functions as an antioxidant.<br>• Symptoms of vitamin A toxicity may mimic those of brain tumors and liver disease.<br>• 1 mcg vitamin A = 3.33 IU vitamin A. |
| • Intakes of up to 800 IU per day are unrelated to toxic side effects; over 800 IU per day may increase bleeding (blood-clotting time).<br>• Avoid supplement use if aspirin, anticoagulants, or fish oil supplements are taken regularly. | • Vegetable oil<br>• Salad dressings, mayonnaise<br>• Whole grains, wheat germ<br>• Leafy, green vegetables, asparagus<br>• Nuts and seeds | • Vitamin E is destroyed by exposure to oxygen and heat.<br>• Oils naturally contain vitamin E; it's there to protect the fat from breakdown due to free radicals.<br>• Eight forms of vitamin E exist, and each has different antioxidant strengths.<br>• 1 mg vitamin E = 1.49 IU. |

(*Continued*)

TABLE 1.9 ▸ Summary of the vitamins (*Continued*)

| THE WATER-SOLUBLE VITAMINS (*Continued*) | | |
|---|---|---|
| | PRIMARY FUNCTIONS | CONSEQUENCES OF DEFICIENCY |
| **Vitamin D (Vitamin $D_2$ = ergocalciferol, Vitamin $D_3$ = cholicalciferol)**<br>RDA women: 15 mcg (600 IU)<br>men: 15 mcg (600 IU)<br>UL: 100 mcg (4000 IU) | • Required for calcium and phosphorus absorption and for metabolism in the intestines and bone, and for their utilization in bone and teeth formation, nerve and muscle activity<br>• Inhibits inflammation<br>• Participates in insulin secretion and blood glucose level maintenance | • Weak, deformed bones (children)<br>• Loss of calcium from bones (adults), osteoporosis<br>• Increased risk of inflammation-related diseases and death from all causes |
| **Vitamin K (phylloquinone, menaquinone)**<br>AI women: 90 mcg<br>men: 120 mcg | • Regulation of synthesis of blood-clotting proteins<br>• Aids in the incorporation of calcium into bones | • Bleeding, bruises<br>• Decreased calcium in bones<br>• Deficiency is rare; may be induced by the long-term use (months or more) of antibiotics |

[a]AI (Adequate Intakes) and RDAs (Recommended Dietary Allowances) are for 19–30-year-olds; UL (Upper Limits) are for 19–70-year-olds.

TABLE 1.10 ▸ Food sources of vitamins

| THIAMIN | | | | | |
|---|---|---|---|---|---|
| FOOD | SERVING SIZE | THIAMIN (MG) | FOOD | SERVING SIZE | THIAMIN (MG) |
| **Meats:** | | | Macaroni | ½ cup | 0.2 |
| Ham | 3 oz | 0.6 | Rice | ½ cup | 0.2 |
| Pork | 3 oz | 0.5 | Bread | 1 slice | 0.1 |
| Beef | 3 oz | 0.4 | **Vegetables:** | | |
| Liver | 3 oz | 0.2 | Peas | ½ cup | 0.2 |
| **Nuts and seeds:** | | | Lima beans | ½ cup | 0.2 |
| Pistachios | ¼ cup | 0.3 | Corn | ½ cup | 0.2 |
| Macadamia nuts | ¼ cup | 0.2 | **Fruits:** | | |
| Peanuts, dry roasted | ¼ cup | 0.2 | Orange juice | 1 cup | 0.2 |
| **Grains:** | | | Orange | 1 | 0.1 |
| Breakfast cereals | 1 cup | 0.3–1.4 | Avocado | ½ | 0.1 |
| Flour tortilla | 1 | 0.2 | | | |

| RIBOFLAVIN | | | | | |
|---|---|---|---|---|---|
| FOOD | SERVING SIZE | RIBOFLAVIN (MG) | FOOD | SERVING SIZE | RIBOFLAVIN (MG) |
| **Milk and milk products:** | | | **Vegetables:** | | |
| Milk | 1 cup | 0.5 | Collard greens | ½ cup | 0.3 |
| 2% milk | 1 cup | 0.5 | Spinach, cooked | ½ cup | 0.2 |
| Yogurt, low-fat | 1 cup | 0.5 | Broccoli | ½ cup | 0.1 |
| Skim milk | 1 cup | 0.4 | Yogurt | 1 cup | 0.4 |
| Tuna | 3 oz | 0.1 | American cheese | 1 oz | 0.1 |
| | | | Cheddar cheese | 1 oz | 0.1 |

| THE FAT-SOLUBLE VITAMINS (*Continued*) | | |
|---|---|---|
| **CONSEQUENCES OF OVERDOSE** | **PRIMARY FOOD SOURCES** | **HIGHLIGHTS AND COMMENTS** |
| • Mental retardation in young children, severe illness and dementia in adults<br>• Abnormal bone growth and formation<br>• Nausea, diarrhea, irritability, weight loss<br>• Deposition of calcium in organs such as the kidneys, liver, and heart | • Vitamin D–fortified milk, breakfast cereals, and other foods<br>• Fish and shellfish | • Vitamin $D_3$ is the most active form of this vitamin.<br>• Vitamin D is synthesized from a form of cholesterol in skin cells upon exposure of the skin to UV rays from the sun.<br>• Inadequate vitamin D status is common, individuals with dark skin are at higher risk.<br>• Breastfed infants with little sun exposure can benefit from vitamin D supplements.<br>• 1 mcg vitamin D = 40 IU. |
| • Toxicity is a problem only when synthetic forms of vitamin K are taken in excessive amounts; that may cause liver disease. | • Leafy, green vegetables<br>• Grain products | • Vitamin K is produced to some extent by gut bacteria.<br>• Newborns are given a vitamin K because they have "sterile" guts and consequently no vitamin K–producing bacteria. |

| RIBOFLAVIN | | | | | |
|---|---|---|---|---|---|
| **FOOD** | **SERVING SIZE** | **RIBOFLAVIN (MG)** | **FOOD** | **SERVING SIZE** | **RIBOFLAVIN (MG)** |
| **Meats:** | | | **Grains:** | | |
| Liver | 3 oz | 3.6 | Breakfast cereals | 1 cup | 0.1–1.7 |
| Pork chop | 3 oz | 0.3 | Macaroni | ½ cup | 0.1 |
| Beef | 3 oz | 0.2 | Bread | 1 slice | 0.1 |
| **Eggs:** | | | | | |
| Egg | 1 | 0.2 | | | |

| NIACIN | | | | | |
|---|---|---|---|---|---|
| **FOOD** | **SERVING SIZE** | **NIACIN (MG)** | **FOOD** | **SERVING SIZE** | **NIACIN (MG)** |
| **Meats:** | | | Almonds | ¼ cup | 1.3 |
| Liver | 3 oz | 14.0 | **Vegetables:** | | |
| Tuna | 3 oz | 7.0 | Asparagus | ½ cup | 1.2 |
| Turkey | 3 oz | 4.0 | Corn | ½ cup | 1.2 |
| Chicken | 3 oz | 11.0 | Green beans | ½ cup | 1.2 |
| Salmon | 3 oz | 6.9 | **Grains:** | | |
| Veal | 3 oz | 6.4 | Breakfast cereals | 1 cup | 5.0–20.0 |
| Beef (round steak) | 3 oz | 4.0 | Brown rice | ½ cup | 1.5 |
| Pork | 3 oz | 4.0 | Noodles, enriched | ½ cup | 1.0 |
| Haddock | 3 oz | 3.9 | Rice, white, enriched | ½ cup | 1.2 |
| Shrimp | 3 oz | 2.2 | Bread, enriched | 1 slice | 1.1 |
| **Nuts and seeds:** | | | | | |
| Peanuts, dry roasted | ¼ cup | 4.9 | | | |

(*Continued*)

TABLE 1.10 ▸ Food sources of vitamins (*Continued*)

| VITAMIN $B_6$ | | | | | |
|---|---|---|---|---|---|
| FOOD | SERVING SIZE | VITAMIN $B_6$ (MG) | FOOD | SERVING SIZE | VITAMIN $B_6$ (MG) |
| **Meats:** | | | **Fruits:** | | |
| Liver | 3 oz | 0.8 | Banana | 1 | 0.4 |
| Fish | 3 oz | 0.3–0.6 | Avocado | ½ cup | 0.3 |
| Chicken | 3 oz | 0.4 | Watermelon | 1 cup | 0.3 |
| Ham | 3 oz | 0.4 | **Vegetables:** | | |
| Hamburger | 3 oz | 0.4 | Brussels sprouts | ½ cup | 0.2 |
| Veal | 3 oz | 0.4 | Potato | ½ cup | 0.4 |
| Pork | 3 oz | 0.3 | Sweet potato | ½ cup | 0.3 |
| Beef | 3 oz | 0.2 | Carrots | ½ cup | 0.2 |
| **Grains:** | | | Sweet peppers | ½ cup | 0.2 |
| Breakfast cereals | 1 cup | 0.5–7.0 | | | |

| FOLATE | | | | | |
|---|---|---|---|---|---|
| FOOD | SERVING SIZE | FOLATE (MCG) | FOOD | SERVING SIZE | FOLATE (MCG) |
| **Vegetables:** | | | Romaine lettuce | 1 cup | 65 |
| Garbanzo beans | ½ cup | 141 | Peas | ½ cup | 47 |
| Spinach, cooked | ½ cup | 131 | **Grains:**[a] | | |
| Navy beans | ½ cup | 128 | Ready-to-eat cereals | 1 cup/1 oz | 100–400 |
| Asparagus | ½ cup | 120 | Rice | ½ cup | 77 |
| Lima beans | ½ cup | 76 | Noodles | ½ cup | 45 |
| Collard greens, cooked | ½ cup | 65 | Wheat germ | 2 Tbsp | 40 |

| VITAMIN $B_{12}$ | | | | | |
|---|---|---|---|---|---|
| FOOD | SERVING SIZE | VITAMIN $B_{12}$ (MCG) | FOOD | SERVING SIZE | VITAMIN $B_{12}$ (MCG) |
| **Fish and seafood:** | | | **Milk and milk products:** | | |
| Oysters | 3 oz | 13.8 | Skim milk | 1 cup | 1.0 |
| Scallops | 3 oz | 3.0 | Milk | 1 cup | 0.9 |
| Salmon | 3 oz | 2.3 | Yogurt | 1 cup | 0.8 |
| Clams | 3 oz | 2.0 | Cottage cheese | ½ cup | 0.7 |
| Crab | 3 oz | 1.8 | American cheese | 1 oz | 0.2 |
| Tuna | 3 oz | 1.8 | Cheddar cheese | 1 oz | 0.2 |
| **Meats:** | | | **Grains:** | | |
| Liver | 3 oz | 6.8 | Breakfast cereals | 1 cup | 0.6–12.0 |
| Beef | 3 oz | 2.2 | **Eggs:** | | |
| Veal | 3 oz | 1.7 | Egg | 1 | 0.6 |

| VITAMIN C | | | | | |
|---|---|---|---|---|---|
| FOOD | SERVING SIZE | VITAMIN C (MG) | FOOD | SERVING SIZE | VITAMIN C (MG) |
| **Fruits:** | | | Cranberry juice cocktail | 1 cup | 90 |
| Guava | ½ cup | 180 | Orange | 1 | 85 |
| Orange juice, vitamin C-fortified | 1 cup | 108 | Strawberries, fresh | 1 cup | 84 |
| | | | Cantaloupe | ¼ whole | 63 |
| Kiwi fruit | 1 | 108 | Grapefruit | 1 medium | 51 |
| Grapefruit juice, fresh | 1 cup | 94 | | | |

| VITAMIN C | | | | | |
|---|---|---|---|---|---|
| FOOD | SERVING SIZE | VITAMIN C (MG) | FOOD | SERVING SIZE | VITAMIN C (MG) |
| Raspberries, fresh | 1 cup | 31 | Green peppers | ½ cup | 60 |
| Watermelon | 1 cup | 15 | Collard greens | ½ cup | 48 |
| **Vegetables:** | | | Vegetable (V-8) juice | ¾ cup | 45 |
| Sweet red peppers | ½ cup | 142 | Tomato juice | ¾ cup | 33 |
| Cauliflower, raw | ½ cup | 75 | Cauliflower, cooked | ½ cup | 30 |
| Broccoli | ½ cup | 70 | Potato | 1 medium | 29 |
| Brussels sprouts | ½ cup | 65 | Tomato | 1 medium | 23 |

| CHOLINE | | | | | |
|---|---|---|---|---|---|
| FOOD | SERVING SIZE | CHOLINE (MG) | FOOD | SERVING SIZE | CHOLINE (MG) |
| **Meats:** | | | Collards, cooked | ½ cup | 39 |
| Beef | 3 oz | 111 | Black-eyed-peas (Cowpeas) | ½ cup | 39 |
| Pork chop | 3 oz | 94 | | | |
| Lamb | 3 oz | 89 | Chickpeas (garbanzo beans) | ½ cup | 35 |
| Ham | 3 oz | 87 | | | |
| Beef | 3 oz | 85 | Brussels sprouts | ½ cup | 32 |
| Turkey | 3 oz | 70 | Broccoli | ½ cup | 32 |
| Salmon | 3 oz | 56 | Collard greens | ½ cup | 30 |
| **Eggs:** | | | Refried beans | ½ cup | 29 |
| Egg | 1 large | 126 | **Milk and milk products:** | | |
| **Vegetables:** | | | Milk, 2% | 1 cup | 40 |
| Baked beans | ½ cup | 50 | Cottage cheese, low-fat | ½ cup | 37 |
| Navy beans, boiled | ½ cup | 41 | Yogurt, low-fat | 1 cup | 35 |

| VITAMIN A | | | | | |
|---|---|---|---|---|---|
| FOOD | SERVING SIZE | VITAMIN A RETINOL (MCG) | FOOD | SERVING SIZE | VITAMIN A RETINOL (MCG) |
| **Meats:** | | | **Milk and milk products:** | | |
| Liver | 3 oz | 9,124 | American cheese | 1 oz | 114 |
| Clams | 3 oz | 145 | Fat-free/low-fat milk | 1 cup | 100 |
| **Fortified breakfast cereals** | 1 cup | 150 | Whole milk | 1 cup | 58 |
| | | | Egg | 1 | 84 |

| BETA-CAROTENE | | | | | |
|---|---|---|---|---|---|
| FOOD | SERVING SIZE | BETA-CAROTENE MCG RETINOL EQUIVALENTS, RE | FOOD | SERVING SIZE | BETA-CAROTENE MCG RETINOL EQUIVALENTS, RE |
| **Vegetables:** | | | Beet greens, cooked | ½ cup | 276 |
| Sweet potatoes | ½ cup | 961 | Swiss chard, cooked | ½ cup | 268 |
| Pumpkin, canned | ½ cup | 953 | Winter squash, cooked | ½ cup | 268 |
| Carrots, raw | ½ cup | 665 | | | |
| Spinach, cooked | ½ cup | 524 | Vegetable juice | 1 cup | 200 |
| Collard greens, cooked | ½ cup | 489 | Romaine lettuce | 1 cup | 162 |
| | | | **Fruit:** | | |
| Kale, cooked | ½ cup | 478 | Cantaloupe | ½ cup | 135 |
| Turnip greens, cooked | ½ cup | 441 | Apricots, fresh | 4 | 134 |

*(Continued)*

TABLE 1.10 ▸ Food sources of vitamins (*Continued*)

**VITAMIN E**

| FOOD | SERVING SIZE | VITAMIN E (MG) | FOOD | SERVING SIZE | VITAMIN E (MG) |
|---|---|---|---|---|---|
| **Nuts and seeds:** | | | Salad dressing | 2 Tbsp | 1.5 |
| Sunflower seeds | 1 oz | 7.4 | **Fish and seafood:** | | |
| Almonds | 1 oz | 7.3 | Crab | 3 oz | 4.5 |
| Hazelnuts (filberts) | 1 oz | 4.3 | Shrimp | 3 oz | 3.7 |
| Mixed nuts | 1 oz | 3.1 | Fish | 3 oz | 2.4 |
| Pine nuts | 1 oz | 2.6 | **Grains:** | | |
| Peanut butter | 2 Tbsp | 2.5 | Wheat germ | 2 Tbsp | 4.2 |
| Peanuts | 1 oz | 2.2 | Whole wheat bread | 1 slice | 2.5 |
| **Vegetable oil:** | | | **Vegetables:** | | |
| Sunflower oil | 1 Tbsp | 5.6 | Spinach, cooked | ½ cup | 3.4 |
| Safflower oil | 1 Tbsp | 5.6 | Yellow bell pepper | 1 | 2.8 |
| Canola oil | 1 Tbsp | 2.4 | Turnip greens, cooked | ½ cup | 2.2 |
| Peanut oil | 1 Tbsp | 2.1 | | | |
| Corn oil | 1 Tbsp | 1.9 | Swiss chard, cooked | ½ cup | 1.7 |
| Olive oil | 1 Tbsp | 1.9 | Asparagus | ½ cup | 1.5 |
| | | | Sweet potato | ½ cup | 1.5 |

**VITAMIN D**

| FOOD | SERVING SIZE | VITAMIN D (MCG) | VITAMIN D IU | FOOD | SERVING SIZE | VITAMIN D (MCG) | VITAMIN D IU |
|---|---|---|---|---|---|---|---|
| **Fish and seafoods:** | | | | Crispix, Kellogg's | 1 cup | 1.2 | 48 |
| Swordfish | 3 oz | 14 | 566 | **Other vitamin D-fortified foods:** | | | |
| Trout | 3 oz | 13 | 502 | | | | |
| Salmon | 3 oz | 11 | 447 | Orange juice | 1 cup | 2.5 | 100 |
| Tuna, light, canned in oil | 3 oz | 5.7 | 228 | Rice milk | 1 cup | 2.5 | 100 |
| | | | | Soy milk | 1 cup | 2.5 | 100 |
| Halibut | 3 oz | 4.9 | 196 | Yogurt | 1 cup | 2.0 | 80 |
| Tuna, light, canned in water | 3 oz | 3.8 | 152 | Margarine | 2 tsp | 1.2 | 48 |
| | | | | **Milk:** | | | |
| Tuna, white, canned in water | 3 oz | 1.7 | 68 | Milk, whole | 1 cup | 3.2 | 128 |
| | | | | Milk, 2% | 1 cup | 2.9 | 116 |
| **Vitamin D-fortified breakfast cereals:** | | | | Milk, 1% | 1 cup | 2.9 | 116 |
| Whole grain Total | 1 cup | 3.3 | 132 | Milk, skim (nonfat) | 1 cup | 2.9 | 116 |
| Total Raisin Bran | 1 cup | 2.6 | 104 | | | | |
| Corn Pops, Kellogg's | 1 cup | 1.2 | 48 | | | | |

**VITAMIN K**

| FOOD | SERVING SIZE | VITAMIN K (MCG) | FOOD | SERVING SIZE | VITAMIN K (MCG) |
|---|---|---|---|---|---|
| **Vegetables and fruits** | | | Spinach, raw | ½ cup | 73 |
| Kale, cooked | ½ cup | 531 | Lettuce, leafy green | 1 cup | 71 |
| Spinach, cooked | ½ cup | 444 | Asparagus, cooked | 4 spears | 48 |
| Turnip greens, cooked | ½ cup | 426 | Kiwifruit | ½ cup | 37 |
| | | | Berries, blue or black | 1 cup | 29 |
| Broccoli, cooked | ½ cup | 110 | | | |
| Brussels sprouts, cooked | ½ cup | 109 | Okra, cooked | ½ cup | 23 |
| | | | Peas, cooked | ½ cup | 21 |
| Mustard greens, cooked | ½ cup | 105 | Leeks | 1 | 16 |
| Cabbage, cooked | ½ cup | 82 | | | |

[a]Fortified, refined grain products such as bread, rice, pasta, and crackers provide approximately 60 micrograms of folic acid per standard serving.

TABLE 1.11 ▸ Good sources of antioxidant-rich foods[73,74]

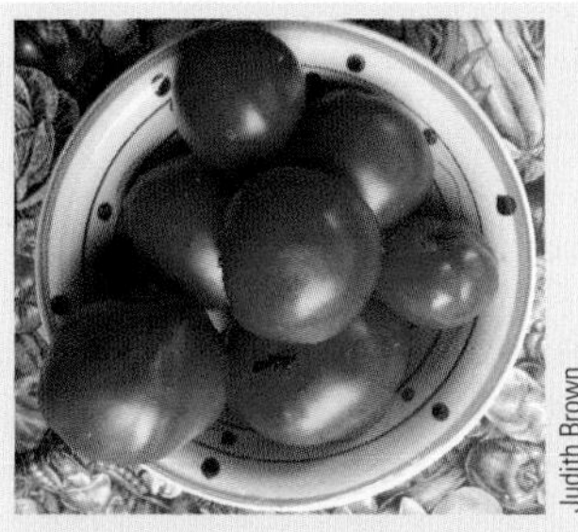


| | |
|---|---|
| | Artichokes |
| | Cranberries |
| | Blueberries, domestic |
| | Coffee, brewed |
| | Red cabbage |
| | Pecans |
| | Cloves, ground |
| | Grape juice |
| Pomegranate | Chocolate, dark |
| Blackberries | Cranberry juice |
| Tomatoes | Wine, red |
| Blueberries, wild | Pineapple juice |
| Strawberries | Guava nectar |
| Raspberries | Mango nectar |

amount of water in tissues and control how acidic or basic body fluids remain.

The tendency of minerals to form complexes has implications for the absorption of minerals from food. Calcium and zinc, for example, may combine with other minerals in supplements or with dietary fiber and form complexes that cannot be absorbed. Therefore, in general, the proportion of total mineral intake that is absorbed is less than for vitamins.

Functions, consequences of deficiency and overdose, primary food sources, and comments about the 15 minerals needed by humans are summarized in Table 1.13.

**Recommended Intake of Minerals** Recommendations for intake of minerals are presented in the tables on the inside front covers of this text. Note that Tolerable Upper Levels of Intake for many minerals are also given in a separate table. Table 1.14 lists food sources of each essential mineral.

## Water

Water is the last, but not the least, nutrient category. Adults are about 60–70 percent water by weight. Water provides the medium in which most chemical reactions take place in the body. It plays a role in energy transformation, the excretion of wastes, and temperature regulation.

TABLE 1.12 ▸ Minerals required by humans

| | | |
|---|---|---|
| Calcium | Fluoride | Chromium |
| Phosphorus | Iodine | Molybdenum |
| Magnesium | Selenium | Sodium |
| Iron | Copper | Potassium |
| Zinc | Manganese | Chloride |

People need enough water to replace daily losses from perspiration, urination, and exhalation. In normal weather conditions with normal physical activity levels, the total water requirement of adult males is 15–16 cups from foods and fluids per day. The corresponding figure for females is 11 cups. Total water intake includes drinking water, water in beverages, and water that is a part of food. People generally consume about 75 percent of their water intake from water and other fluids and 25 percent from foods. The need for water is generally met by consuming sufficient fluids to satisfy thirst, and the need for water is greater in hot and humid climates or when physical activity levels are high. Adequate consumption of water is indicated by the excretion of urine that is pale yellow and normal in volume.[20]

**homeostasis** Constancy of the internal environment. The balance of fluids, nutrients, gases, temperature, and other conditions needed to ensure ongoing, proper functioning of cells and, therefore, all parts of the body.

**Dietary Sources of Water** The best sources of water are tap and bottled water; nonalcoholic beverages such as fruit juice, milk, and vegetable juice; and brothy soups. Alcohol tends to increase water loss though urine, so beverages such as beer and wine are not as "hydrating" as water is. Caffeinated beverages are hydrating in people who are accustomed to consuming them.[21]

**Principle #3** Health problems related to nutrition originate within cells.

## Nutrient Functions at the Cellular Level

The functions of each cell are maintained by the nutrients it receives. Problems arise when a cell's need for nutrients differs from the amounts that are available. Cells (Illustration 1.5) are the building blocks of tissues (such as bones and muscles), organs (the heart, kidney, and liver, for example), and systems (such as the circulatory and respiratory systems). Normal cell health and functions are maintained when a nutritional and environmental utopia exists within and around cells. This state of optimal cellular nutrient conditions supports ***homeostasis*** in the body.

Disruptions in the availability of nutrients, or the presence of harmful substances in the cell's environment, initiate diseases and disorders that eventually affect tissues, organs, and systems. For example, folate, a B vitamin, is required for protein synthesis within cells. When too little folate is available, cells produce proteins with abnormal shapes and functions. Abnormalities in the shape of red blood cell proteins lead to functional changes that produce loss of appetite, weakness, and irritability.

**Principle #4** Poor nutrition can result from both inadequate and excessive levels of nutrient intake.

TABLE 1.13 ▸ Summary of minerals

| | PRIMARY FUNCTIONS | CONSEQUENCES OF DEFICIENCY |
|---|---|---|
| **Calcium**<br>AI* women: 1000 mg<br>men: 1000 mg<br>UL: 2500 mg | • Component of bones and teeth<br>• Required for muscle and nerve activity, blood clotting | • Poorly mineralized, weak bones (osteoporosis)<br>• Rickets in children<br>• Osteomalacia (rickets in adults)<br>• Stunted growth in children<br>• Convulsions, muscle spasms |
| **Phosphorus**<br>RDA women: 700 mg<br>men: 700 mg<br>UL: 4000 mg | • Component of bones and teeth<br>• Component of certain enzymes and other substances involved in energy formation<br>• Required for maintenance of acid-base balance of body fluids | • Loss of appetite<br>• Nausea, vomiting<br>• Weakness<br>• Confusion<br>• Loss of calcium from bones |
| **Magnesium**<br>RDA women: 310 mg<br>men: 400 mg<br>UL: 350 mg<br>(from supplements only) | • Component of bones and teeth<br>• Needed for nerve activity<br>• Activates hundreds of enzymes involved in metabolism | • Stunted growth in children<br>• Weakness<br>• Muscle spasms<br>• Personality changes |
| **Iron**<br>RDA women: 18 mg<br>men: 8 mg<br>UL: 45 mg | • Transports oxygen as a component of hemoglobin in red blood cells<br>• Component of myoglobin (a muscle protein)<br>• Required for certain reactions involving energy formation | • Iron deficiency<br>• Iron-deficiency anemia<br>• Weakness, fatigue<br>• Hair loss<br>• Pale appearance<br>• Reduced attention span and resistance to infection<br>• Mental retardation, developmental delay in children<br>• Ice craving<br>• Decreased resistance to infection |
| **Zinc**<br>RDA women: 8 mg<br>men: 11 mg<br>UL: 40 mg | • Required for the activation of many enzymes involved in the reproduction of proteins<br>• Component of insulin, many enzymes | • Growth failure<br>• Delayed sexual maturation<br>• Slow wound healing<br>• Loss of taste and appetite<br>• In pregnancy, low-birth-weight infants and preterm delivery |
| **Fluoride**<br>AI women: 3 mg<br>men: 4 mg<br>UL: 10 mg | • Component of bones and teeth (enamel) | • Tooth decay and other dental diseases |
| **Iodine**<br>RDA women: 150 mcg<br>men: 150 mcg<br>UL: 1100 mcg | • Required for the synthesis of thyroid hormones that help regulate energy production and growth<br>• Required for normal brain development | • Goiter<br>• Cretinism (mental retardation, hearing loss, growth failure) |

| CONSEQUENCES OF OVERDOSE | PRIMARY FOOD SOURCES | HIGHLIGHTS AND COMMENTS |
|---|---|---|
| • Drowsiness<br>• Calcium deposits in kidneys, liver, and other tissues<br>• Suppression of bone remodeling<br>• Decreased zinc absorption | • Milk and milk products (cheese, yogurt)<br>• Calcium-fortified foods | • The average intake of calcium among U.S. women is approximately 60% of the DRI.<br>• One in four women and one in eight men in the U.S. develop osteoporosis.<br>• Adequate calcium and vitamin D status must be maintained to prevent bone loss. |
| • Muscle spasms | • Milk and milk products (cheese, yogurt)<br>• Meats<br>• Seeds, nuts | • Deficiency is generally related to disease processes. |
| • Diarrhea<br>• Dehydration<br>• Impaired nerve activity due to disrupted utilization of calcium | • Plant foods (dried nuts, peanuts, potatoes, green vegetables)<br>• Ready-to-eat cereals | • Magnesium is primarily found in plant foods.<br>• Average intake among U.S. adults is below the RDA. |
| • Hemochromatosis ("iron poisoning")<br>• Vomiting, abdominal pain, diarrhea<br>• Blue coloration of skin<br>• Iron deposition in liver and heart<br>• Decreased zinc absorption<br>• Oxidation-related damage to tissues and organs | • Liver, beef, pork<br>• Dried beans<br>• Iron-fortified cereals<br>• Prunes, apricots, raisins<br>• Spinach<br>• Bread | • Cooking foods in iron and stainless steel pans increases the iron content of the foods.<br>• Vitamin C, meat, and alcohol increase iron absorption.<br>• Iron deficiency is the most common nutritional deficiency in the world.<br>• Average iron intake of young children and women in the U.S. is low. |
| • Over 25 mg/day is associated with nausea, vomiting, weakness, fatigue, susceptibility to infection, copper deficiency, and metallic taste in mouth.<br>• Increased blood lipids | • Meats (all kinds)<br>• Grains<br>• Nuts<br>• Dried beans<br>• Ready-to-eat cereals | • Like iron, zinc is better absorbed from meats than from plants<br>• Marginal zinc deficiency may be common, especially in children.<br>• Zinc supplements may decrease duration and severity of the common cold. |
| • Fluorosis<br>• Brittle bones<br>• Mottled teeth<br>• Nerve abnormalities | • Fluoridated water and foods and beverages made with it<br>• White grape juice | • Toothpastes, mouth rinses, and other dental care products may provide fluoride.<br>• Fluoride overdose has been caused by ingestion of fluoridated toothpaste. |
| • Over 1 mg/day may produce pimples, goiter, and decreased thyroid function. | • Iodized salt<br>• Milk and milk products<br>• Seaweed, seafoods<br>• Bread from commercial bakeries | • Iodine deficiency remains a major health problem in some developing countries.<br>• Amount of iodine in plants depends on iodine content of soil.<br>• The need for iodine increases 50% during pregnancy. |

*(Continued)*

TABLE 1.13 ▸ Summary of minerals (*Continued*)

| | PRIMARY FUNCTIONS | CONSEQUENCES OF DEFICIENCY |
|---|---|---|
| **Selenium**<br>RDA women: 55 mcg<br>men: 55 mcg<br>UL: 400 mcg | • Acts as an antioxidant in conjunction with vitamin E (protects cells from damage due to exposure to oxygen)<br>• Needed for thyroid hormone production | • Anemia<br>• Muscle pain and tenderness<br>• Keshan disease (heart failure), Kashin-Beck disease (joint disease) |
| **Copper**<br>RDA women: 900 mcg<br>men: 900 mcg<br>UL: 10,000 mcg | • Component of enzymes involved in the body's utilization of iron and oxygen<br>• Functions in growth, immunity, cholesterol and glucose utilization, brain development | • Anemia<br>• Seizures<br>• Nerve and bone abnormalities in children<br>• Growth retardation |
| **Manganese**<br>AI women: 2.3 mg<br>men: 1.8 mg | • Required for the formation of body fat and bone | • Weight loss<br>• Rash<br>• Nausea and vomiting |
| **Chromium**<br>AI women: 35 mcg<br>men: 25 mcg | • Required for the normal utilization of glucose and fat | • Elevated blood glucose and triglyceride levels<br>• Weight loss |
| **Molybdenum**<br>RDA women: 45 mcg<br>men: 45 mcg<br>UL: 2000 mcg | • Component of enzymes involved in the transfer of oxygen from one molecule to another | • Rapid heartbeat and breathing<br>• Nausea, vomiting<br>• Coma |
| **Sodium**<br>AI adults: 1500 mg<br>UL adults: 2300 mg | • Regulation of acid-base balance in body fluids<br>• Maintenance of water balance in body tissues<br>• Activation of muscles and nerves | • Weakness<br>• Apathy<br>• Poor appetite<br>• Muscle cramps<br>• Headache<br>• Swelling |
| **Potassium**<br>AI adults: 4700 mg | • Same as for sodium | • Weakness<br>• Irritability, mental confusion<br>• Irregular heartbeat<br>• Paralysis |
| **Chloride**<br>AI adults: 2300 mg<br>UL: 3,600 mg | • Component of hydrochloric acid secreted by the stomach (used in digestion)<br>• Maintenance of acid-base balance of body fluids<br>• Maintenance of water balance in the body | • Muscle cramps<br>• Apathy<br>• Poor appetite<br>• Long-term mental retardation in infants |

*AIs and RDAs are for women and men 19–30 years of age; ULs are males and females 19–70 years of age.

| CONSEQUENCES OF OVERDOSE | PRIMARY FOOD SOURCES | HIGHLIGHTS AND COMMENTS |
|---|---|---|
| • "Selenosis"; symptoms of selenosis are hair and fingernail loss, weakness, liver damage, irritability, and "garlic" or "metallic" breath. | • Meats and seafoods<br>• Eggs | • Content of foods depends on amount of selenium in soil, water, and animal feeds.<br>• Selenium supplements have not been found to prevent cancer. |
| • Wilson's disease (excessive accumulation of copper in the liver and kidneys).<br>• Vomiting, diarrhea<br>• Tremors<br>• Liver disease | • Potatoes<br>• Grains<br>• Dried beans<br>• Nuts and seeds<br>• Seafood | • Toxicity can result from copper pipes and cooking pans.<br>• Average intake in the U.S. is below the RDA. |
| • Infertility in men<br>• Disruptions in the nervous system, learning impairment<br>• Muscle spasms | • Whole grains<br>• Coffee, tea<br>• Dried beans<br>• Nuts | • Toxicity is related to overexposure to manganese dust in miners or contaminated ground water. |
| • Kidney and skin damage | • Whole grains<br>• Wheat germ<br>• Liver, meat<br>• Beer, wine<br>• Oysters | • Toxicity usually results from exposure in chrome-making industries or overuse of supplements.<br>• Supplements do not build muscle mass, increase endurance, or reduce blood glucose levels. |
| • Loss of copper from the body<br>• Joint pain<br>• Growth failure<br>• Anemia<br>• Gout | • Dried beans<br>• Grains<br>• Dark green vegetables<br>• Liver<br>• Milk and milk products | • Deficiency is extraordinarily rare. |
| • High blood pressure in susceptible people<br>• Kidney disease<br>• Heart problems | • Foods processed with salt<br>• Cured foods (corned beef, ham, bacon, pickles, sauerkraut)<br>• Table and sea salt<br>• Milk, cheese<br>• Salad dressing | • Very few foods naturally contain much sodium; processed foods are the leading source.<br>• High-sodium diets are associated with hypertension, particularly in "salt-sensitive" people.<br>• Kidney disease, excessive water consumption are related to sodium depletion. |
| • Irregular heartbeat, heart attack | • Plant foods (potatoes, squash, lima beans, tomatoes, plantains, bananas, oranges, orange juice, avocados)<br>• Meats<br>• Milk and milk products<br>• Coffee | • Content of vegetables is often reduced in processed foods.<br>• Diuretics (water pills), vomiting, diarrhea may deplete potassium.<br>• Salt substitutes often contain potassium.<br>• Potassium intake tracks with vegetables and fruit intake. |
| • Vomiting | • Same as for sodium (most of the chloride in our diets comes from salt) | • Excessive vomiting and diarrhea may cause chloride deficiency.<br>• Legislation regulating the composition of infant formulas was enacted in response to formula-related chloride deficiency and subsequent mental retardation in infants. |

TABLE 1.14 Food sources of minerals

| MAGNESIUM | | | | | |
|---|---|---|---|---|---|
| FOOD | AMOUNT | MAGNESIUM (MG) | FOOD | AMOUNT | MAGNESIUM (MG) |
| **Legumes:** | | | **Vegetables:** | | |
| Lentils, cooked | ½ cup | 134 | Bean sprouts | ½ cup | 98 |
| Split peas, cooked | ½ cup | 134 | Black-eyed peas | ½ cup | 58 |
| Tofu | ½ cup | 130 | Spinach, cooked | ½ cup | 48 |
| **Nuts:** | | | Lima beans | ½ cup | 32 |
| Peanuts | ¼ cup | 247 | **Milk and milk products:** | | |
| Cashews | ¼ cup | 93 | Milk | 1 cup | 30 |
| Almonds | ¼ cup | 80 | Cheddar cheese | 1 oz | 8 |
| **Grains:** | | | American cheese | 1 oz | 6 |
| Bran buds | 1 cup | 240 | **Meats:** | | |
| Wild rice, cooked | ½ cup | 119 | Chicken | 3 oz | 25 |
| Breakfast cereal, fortified | 1 cup | 85 | Beef | 3 oz | 20 |
| Wheat germ | 2 Tbsp | 45 | Pork | 3 oz | 20 |

| CALCIUM[a] | | | | | |
|---|---|---|---|---|---|
| FOOD | AMOUNT | CALCIUM (MG) | FOOD | AMOUNT | CALCIUM (MG) |
| **Milk and milk products:** | | | Ice milk | 1 cup | 180 |
| Yogurt, low-fat | 1 cup | 413 | American cheese | 1 oz | 175 |
| Milk shake (low-fat frozen yogurt) | 1¼ cup | 352 | Custard | ½ cup | 150 |
| Yogurt with fruit, low-fat | 1 cup | 315 | Cottage cheese | ½ cup | 70 |
| Skim milk | 1 cup | 301 | Cottage cheese, low-fat | ½ cup | 69 |
| 1% milk | 1 cup | 300 | **Vegetables:** | | |
| 2% milk | 1 cup | 298 | Spinach, cooked | ½ cup | 122 |
| 3.25% milk (whole) | 1 cup | 288 | Kale | ½ cup | 47 |
| Swiss cheese | 1 oz | 270 | Broccoli | ½ cup | 36 |
| Milk shake (whole milk) | 1¼ cup | 250 | **Legumes:** | | |
| Frozen yogurt, low-fat | 1 cup | 248 | Tofu | ½ cup | 260 |
| Frappuccino | 1 cup | 220 | Dried beans, cooked | ½ cup | 60 |
| Cheddar cheese | 1 oz | 204 | **Foods fortified with calcium:** | | |
| Frozen yogurt | 1 cup | 200 | Orange juice | 1 cup | 350 |
| Cream soup | 1 cup | 186 | Frozen waffles | 2 | 300 |
| Pudding | ½ cup | 185 | Soy milk | 1 cup | 200–400 |
| Ice cream | 1 cup | 180 | Breakfast cereals | 1 cup | 150–1000 |

| SELENIUM | | | | | |
|---|---|---|---|---|---|
| FOOD | AMOUNT | SELENIUM (MCG) | FOOD | AMOUNT | SELENIUM (MCG) |
| **Seafood:** | | | Egg | 1 medium | 37 |
| Lobster | 3 oz | 66 | Ham | 3 oz | 29 |
| Tuna | 3 oz | 60 | Beef | 3 oz | 22 |
| Shrimp | 3 oz | 54 | Bacon | 3 oz | 21 |
| Oysters | 3 oz | 48 | Chicken | 3 oz | 18 |
| Fish | 3 oz | 40 | Lamb | 3 oz | 14 |
| **Meats/Eggs:** | | | Veal | 3 oz | 10 |
| Liver | 3 oz | 56 | | | |

| ZINC | | | | | |
|---|---|---|---|---|---|
| FOOD | AMOUNT | ZINC (MG) | FOOD | AMOUNT | ZINC (MG) |
| **Meats:** | | | Oatmeal, cooked | 1 cup | 1.2 |
| Liver | 3 oz | 4.6 | Bran flakes | 1 cup | 1.0 |
| Beef | 3 oz | 4.0 | Brown rice, cooked | ½ cup | 0.6 |
| Crab | ½ cup | 3.5 | White rice | ½ cup | 0.4 |
| Lamb | 3 oz | 3.5 | **Nuts and seeds:** | | |
| Turkey ham | 3 oz | 2.5 | Pecans | ¼ cup | 2.0 |
| Pork | 3 oz | 2.4 | Cashews | ¼ cup | 1.8 |
| Chicken | 3 oz | 2.0 | Sunflower seeds | ¼ cup | 1.7 |
| **Legumes:** | | | Peanut butter | 2 Tbsp | 0.9 |
| Dried beans, cooked | ½ cup | 1.0 | **Milk and milk products:** | | |
| Split peas, cooked | ½ cup | 0.9 | Cheddar cheese | 1 oz | 1.1 |
| **Grains:** | | | Whole milk | 1 cup | 0.9 |
| Breakfast cereal, fortified | 1 cup | 1.5–4.0 | American cheese | 1 oz | 0.8 |
| Wheat germ | 2 Tbsp | 2.4 | | | |

| SODIUM | | | | | |
|---|---|---|---|---|---|
| FOOD | AMOUNT | SODIUM (MG) | FOOD | AMOUNT | SODIUM (MG) |
| **Miscellaneous:** | | | Meat loaf | 3 oz | 555 |
| Salt | 1 tsp | 2,132 | Sausage | 3 oz | 483 |
| Dill pickle | 1 (4½ oz) | 1,930 | Hot dog | 1 | 477 |
| Sea salt | 1 tsp | 1,716 | Fish, smoked | 3 oz | 444 |
| Ravioli, canned | 1 cup | 1,065 | Bologna | 1 oz | 370 |
| Spaghetti with sauce, canned | 1 cup | 955 | **Milk and milk products:** | | |
| Baking soda | 1 tsp | 821 | Cream soup | 1 cup | 1070 |
| Beef broth | 1 cup | 810 | Cottage cheese | ½ cup | 455 |
| Chicken broth | 1 cup | 770 | American cheese | 1 oz | 405 |
| Gravy | ¼ cup | 720 | Cheese spread | 1 oz | 274 |
| Italian dressing | 2 Tbsp | 720 | Parmesan cheese | 1 oz | 247 |
| Pretzels | 5 (1 oz) | 500 | Gouda cheese | 1 oz | 232 |
| Green olives | 5 | 465 | Cheddar cheese | 1 oz | 175 |
| Pizza with cheese | 1 wedge | 455 | Skim milk | 1 cup | 125 |
| Soy sauce | 1 tsp | 444 | Whole milk | 1 cup | 120 |
| Cheese twists | 1 cup | 329 | **Grains:** | | |
| Bacon | 3 slices | 303 | Bran flakes | 1 cup | 363 |
| French dressing | 2 Tbsp | 220 | Cornflakes | 1 cup | 325 |
| Potato chips | 1 oz (10 pieces) | 200 | Croissant | 1 medium | 270 |
| Catsup | 1 Tbsp | 155 | Bagel | 1 | 260 |
| **Meats:** | | | English muffin | 1 | 203 |
| Corned beef | 3 oz | 808 | White bread | 1 slice | 130 |
| Ham | 3 oz | 800 | Whole wheat bread | 1 slice | 130 |
| Fish, canned | 3 oz | 735 | Saltine crackers | 4 squares | 125 |

*(Continued)*

TABLE 1.14 Food sources of minerals (*Continued*)

| IRON | | | | | |
|---|---|---|---|---|---|
| FOOD | AMOUNT | IRON (MG) | FOOD | AMOUNT | IRON (MG) |
| **Meat and meat alternatives:** | | | Rye bread | 1 slice | 1.0 |
| Liver | 3 oz | 7.5 | Whole wheat bread | 1 slice | 0.8 |
| Round steak | 3 oz | 3.0 | White bread | 1 slice | 0.6 |
| Hamburger, lean | 3 oz | 3.0 | **Fruits:** | | |
| Baked beans | ½ cup | 3.0 | Prune juice | 1 cup | 9.0 |
| Pork | 3 oz | 2.7 | Apricots, dried | ½ cup | 2.5 |
| White beans | ½ cup | 2.7 | Prunes | 5 medium | 2.0 |
| Soybeans | ½ cup | 2.5 | Raisins | ¼ cup | 1.3 |
| Pork and beans | ½ cup | 2.3 | Plums | 3 medium | 1.1 |
| Fish | 3 oz | 1.0 | **Vegetables:** | | |
| Chicken | 3 oz | 1.0 | Spinach, cooked | ½ cup | 2.3 |
| **Grains:** | | | Lima beans | ½ cup | 2.2 |
| Breakfast cereal, iron-fortified | 1 cup | 8.0 (4–18) | Black-eyed peas | ½ cup | 1.7 |
| | | | Peas | ½ cup | 1.6 |
| Oatmeal, fortified, cooked | 1 cup | 8.0 | Asparagus | ½ cup | 1.5 |
| Bagel | 1 | 1.7 | | | |
| English muffin | 1 | 1.6 | | | |

| PHOSPHOROUS | | | | | |
|---|---|---|---|---|---|
| FOOD | AMOUNT | PHOSPHOROUS (MG) | FOOD | AMOUNT | PHOSPHOROUS (MG) |
| **Milk and milk products:** | | | **Grains:** | | |
| Yogurt | 1 cup | 327 | Bran flakes | 1 cup | 180 |
| Skim milk | 1 cup | 250 | Shredded wheat | 2 large biscuits | 81 |
| Whole milk | 1 cup | 250 | Whole wheat bread | 1 slice | 52 |
| Cottage cheese | ½ cup | 150 | Noodles, cooked | ½ cup | 47 |
| American cheese | 1 oz | 130 | Rice, cooked | ½ cup | 29 |
| **Meats:** | | | White bread | 1 slice | 24 |
| Pork | 3 oz | 275 | **Vegetables:** | | |
| Hamburger | 3 oz | 165 | Potato | 1 medium | 101 |
| Tuna | 3 oz | 162 | Corn | ½ cup | 73 |
| Lobster | 3 oz | 125 | Peas | ½ cup | 70 |
| Chicken | 3 oz | 120 | French fries | ½ cup | 61 |
| **Nuts and seeds:** | | | Broccoli | ½ cup | 54 |
| Sunflower seeds | ¼ cup | 319 | **Other:** | | |
| Peanuts | ¼ cup | 141 | Milk chocolate | 1 oz | 66 |
| Pine nuts | ¼ cup | 106 | Cola | 12 oz | 51 |
| Peanut butter | 1 Tbsp | 61 | Diet cola | 12 oz | 45 |

| POTASSIUM | | | | | |
|---|---|---|---|---|---|
| FOOD | AMOUNT | POTASSIUM (MG) | FOOD | AMOUNT | POTASSIUM (MG) |
| **Vegetables:** | | | Broccoli | 1/2 cup | 205 |
| Potato | 1 medium | 780 | **Fruits:** | | |
| Winter squash | ½ cup | 327 | Avocado | ½ medium | 680 |
| Tomato | 1 medium | 300 | Orange juice | 1 cup | 469 |
| Celery | 1 stalk | 270 | Banana | 1 medium | 440 |
| Carrots | 1 medium | 245 | Raisins | ¼ cup | 370 |

| POTASSIUM | | | | | |
|---|---|---|---|---|---|
| FOOD | AMOUNT | POTASSIUM (MG) | FOOD | AMOUNT | POTASSIUM (MG) |
| Prunes | 4 large | 300 | Bran flakes | 1 cup | 248 |
| Watermelon | 1 cup | 158 | Raisin bran | 1 cup | 242 |
| **Meats:** | | | Wheat flakes | 1 cup | 96 |
| Fish | 3 oz | 500 | **Milk and milk products:** | | |
| Hamburger | 3 oz | 480 | Yogurt | 1 cup | 531 |
| Lamb | 3 oz | 382 | Skim milk | 1 cup | 400 |
| Pork | 3 oz | 335 | Whole milk | 1 cup | 370 |
| Chicken | 3 oz | 208 | **Other:** | | |
| **Grains:** | | | Salt substitutes | 1 tsp | 1,300–2,378 |
| Bran buds | 1 cup | 1080 | | | |

| FLUORIDE | | | | | |
|---|---|---|---|---|---|
| FOOD | AMOUNT | FLUORIDE (MG) | FOOD | AMOUNT | FLUORIDE (MG) |
| Grape juice, white | 6 oz | 350 | French fries, McDonald's | 1 medium | 130 |
| Instant tea | 1 cup | 335 | Dannon's Fluoride to Go | 8 oz | 178 |
| Raisins | 3½ oz | 234 | Municipal water, U.S. | 8 oz | 186 |
| Wine, white | 3½ oz | 202 | Bottled water, store brand | 8 oz | 37 |
| Wine, red | 3½ oz | 105 | Iodized salt | 1 tsp | 400 |

| IODINE | | | | | |
|---|---|---|---|---|---|
| FOOD | AMOUNT | IODINE (MCG) | FOOD | AMOUNT | IODINE (MCG) |
| Haddock | 3 oz | 125 | Cottage cheese | ½ cup | 50 |
| Cod | 3 oz | 87 | Egg | 1 | 22 |
| Shrimp | 3 oz | 30 | Cheddar cheese | 1 oz | 17 |
| Bread | 1 oz (1 slice) | 35–142 | | | |

[a]Actually, the richest source of calcium is alligator meat; 3½ ounces contain about 1,231 milligrams of calcium, but just try to find it on your grocer's shelf!

Each nutrient has a range of intake levels that corresponds to optimum functioning of that nutrient (Illustration 1.6). Intake levels below and above this range are associated with impaired functions.

Inadequate intake of an essential nutrient, if prolonged, results in obvious deficiency diseases. Marginally deficient diets produce subtle changes in behavior or physical condition. If the optimal intake range is exceeded (usually by overdoses of supplements), mild to severe changes in mental and physical functions occur, depending on the amount of the excess and the nutrient involved. Overt vitamin C deficiency, for example, produces irritability, bleeding gums, pain upon being touched, and failure of bone growth. Marginal deficiency may cause delayed wound healing. The length of time a deficiency or toxicity takes to develop depends on the type and amount of the nutrient consumed and the extent of body nutrient reserves. Intakes of 32 mg/day of vitamin C, or about one-third of the RDA for adults (75 mg and 90 mg per day for women and men, respectively), lower blood vitamin C levels to the deficient state within three weeks. On the excessive side, too much supplemental vitamin C causes diarrhea and increases the risk of kidney stone formation.[22,23] For nutrients, enough is as good as a feast.

**Steps in the Development of Nutrient Deficiencies and Toxicities** Poor nutrition due to inadequate diet generally develops in the stages outlined in Illustration 1.7.

After a period of deficient intake of an essential nutrient, tissue reserves become depleted, and subsequently, blood levels of the nutrient decline. When the blood level can no longer supply cells with optimal amounts of nutrients, cell processes change. These changes have a negative effect on the cell's ability to form proteins appropriately, regulate energy formation and use, protect itself from oxidation, or carry out other normal functions. If the deficiency continues, groups of cells malfunction, which leads to problems related to tissue and organ functions. Physical signs of the deficiency may then develop, such as growth failure with protein deficiency or an inability to walk as a result of beriberi (thiamin deficiency). Eventually, some problems produced by the deficiency can no longer be

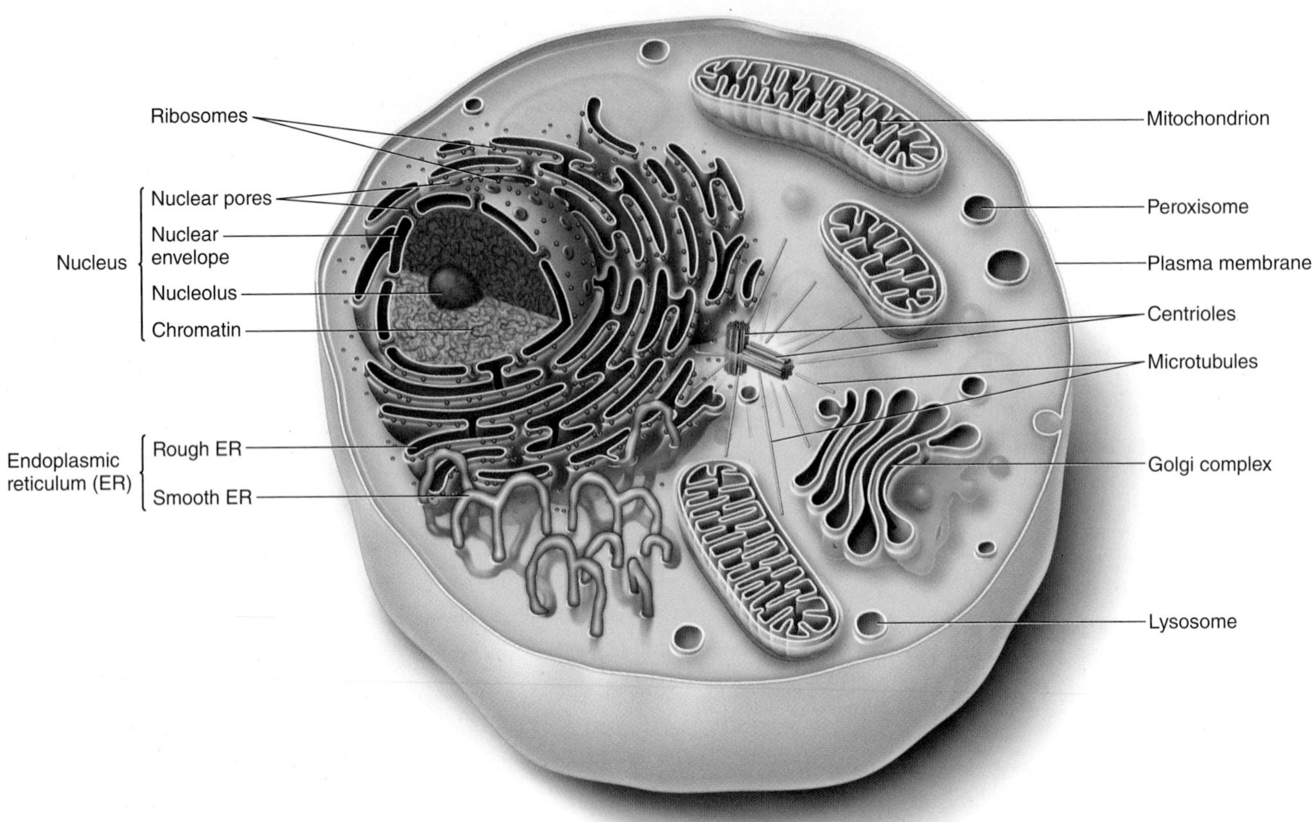


ILLUSTRATION 1.5 ▸ Schematic representation of the structure and major components of a human cell.

reversed by increased nutrient intake. Blindness that results from serious vitamin A deficiency, for example, is irreversible.

Excessively high intakes of many essential nutrients produce toxicity diseases. Excessive vitamin A, for example, produces hypervitaminosis A, and selenium overdose leads to selenosis. Signs of toxicity stem from an increased level of the nutrient in the blood and the subsequent oversupply of the nutrient to cells. The high nutrient load upsets the balance needed for optimal cell function. These changes in

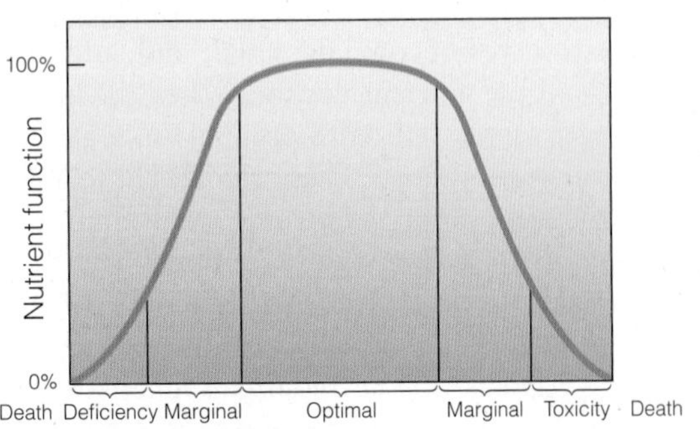


ILLUSTRATION 1.6 ▸ Nutrient function and consequences by level of intake.

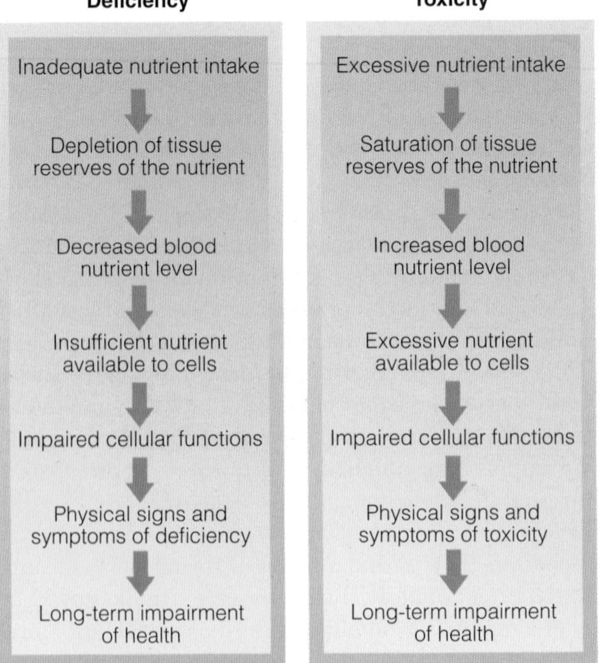


ILLUSTRATION 1.7 ▸ Usual steps in the development of nutrient deficiencies and toxicities.

cell function lead to the signs and symptoms of a toxicity disease.

For both deficiency and toxicity diseases, the best way to correct the problem is at the level of intake. Identifying and fixing intake problems prevents related health problems from developing.

**Nutrient Deficiencies Are Usually Multiple** Most foods contain many nutrients, so poor diets are generally inadequate in a number of nutrients. Calcium and vitamin D, for example, are present in milk. Deficiencies of both of these nutrients may develop from a low milk intake and an otherwise poor diet.

***The "Ripple Effect"*** Dietary changes affect the level of intake of many nutrients. Switching from a high-fat to a low-fat diet, for instance, may result in a lower intake of calories and higher intake of dietary fiber and vitamins. Consequently, dietary changes introduced for the purpose of improving intake of a particular nutrient produce a "ripple effect" on the intake of other nutrients.

**Principle #5** Humans have adaptive mechanisms for managing fluctuations in food intake.

Healthy humans have adaptive mechanisms that partially protect the body from poor health due to fluctuations in nutrient intake. These mechanisms act to conserve nutrients when dietary supply is low and to eliminate them when excessively high amounts are present. Dietary surpluses of nutrients such as iron, calcium, vitamin A, and vitamin $B_{12}$ are stored within tissues for later use. In the case of iron and calcium, absorption is also regulated so that the amount absorbed changes in response to the body's need for these nutrients. The body has a low storage capacity for other nutrients, such as vitamin C and water, and excesses are eliminated through urine or stools. Fluctuations in energy intake are primarily regulated by changes in appetite. If too few calories are consumed, however, the body will obtain energy from its glycogen and fat stores. If caloric intakes remain low and a significant amount of body weight is lost, the body down-regulates its need for energy by lowering body temperature and the capacity for physical work. When energy intake exceeds need, the extra is converted to fat—and to a lesser extent, to glycogen—and stored for later use.

**Principle #6** Malnutrition can result from poor diets and from disease states, genetic factors, or combinations of these causes.

***Malnutrition*** ***Malnutrition*** means "poor nutrition" and results from either inadequate or excessive availability of energy or nutrients within cells. Niacin toxicity, obesity, and iron deficiency are examples of malnutrition.

Malnutrition can result from poor diets as well as from diseases that interfere with the body's ability to use the nutrients consumed. ***Primary malnutrition*** results when a poor nutritional state is dietary in origin. ***Secondary malnutrition***, on the other hand, is precipitated by a disease state, surgical procedure, or medication. Diarrhea, alcoholism, AIDS, and gastrointestinal tract bleeding are examples of conditions that may cause secondary malnutrition.

IN FOCUS

### Nutrigenomics

**Definition:** The study of nutrient–gene interactions and the effects of these interactions on health. Also called nutritional genomics.

Nutrigenomics covers the study of the effects of genes on how the body uses nutrients and the ways in which dietary components affect gene expression, function, and health status.

As our understanding of the specific influences of food components on genes, gene functions, and health through the life cycle progresses, nutritional advice will become individualized based on knowledge of a person's genetic makeup.

**Nutrient–Gene Interactions** Advances in knowledge about nutrient–gene interactions in health and disease are revolutionizing the science and practice of nutrition. This new field of nutrition science is called ***nutrigenomics*** and is highlighted in the "In Focus" box. Genes provide the codes for enzyme and other protein synthesis, and they consequently affect body functions in a huge number of ways. Although individuals are 99.9 percent genetically identical, the 0.1 percent difference in genetic codes makes everyone unique. Variations in gene types (or genotypes) contribute to disease resistance and development, and to the way individuals respond to various drugs.[24,25]

Thousands of rare diseases related to a defect in a single gene have been identified,

**malnutrition** The cellular imbalance between the supply of nutrients and energy and the body's demand for them to ensure growth, maintenance, and specific functions.

**primary malnutrition** Malnutrition that results directly from inadequate or excessive dietary intake of energy or nutrients.

**secondary malnutrition** Malnutrition that results from a condition (e.g., disease, surgical procedure, medication use) rather than primarily from dietary intake.

**nutrigenomics** The study of diet- and nutrient-related functions and interactions of genes and their effects on health and disease.

and many of these affect nutrient needs. Such defects can alter the absorption or utilization of nutrients such as amino acids, iron, zinc, and the vitamins $B_{12}$, $B_6$, or folate. Phenylketonuria (PKU), galaçostemia, and hemochromatosis are three examples of single-gene defects that substantially affect nutrient needs or utilization (Table 1.15).[26–28]

Most diseases related to genetic traits are not as well defined as are single-gene defects. They are more likely to represent an interwoven mesh of multiple gene variants and environmental factors.

Food and nutrient intake is a prominent environmental factor that interacts with genotype and gene function. Lack of adequate nutrition during pregnancy, for example, can program gene functions for life in ways that increase or decrease the risk of chronic disease development.[29] Throughout life, components of foods consumed affect gene function by turning specific genes "on" or "off," thereby affecting what metabolic reactions occur within the body. Newly identified relationships between dietary components and genes are being announced regularly. Here are a few examples of effects of nutrient–gene interactions on health status:

- Consumption of high glycemic index carbohydrates appears to increase the risk of type 2 diabetes in individuals with a certain form of a gene involved in insulin production and secretion.[30]
- High alcohol intake during pregnancy in some women sharply increases the risk of fetal alcohol syndrome in her fetus, but the fetuses of other women with different genetic traits are not affected by high alcohol intake.[31]
- Regular consumption of green tea reduces the risk of prostate cancer in certain individuals with particular genetic traits.[32]

Genetic factors alone cannot explain the rapid rise in obesity and type 2 diabetes in the United States, but they do provide clues about needed preventive and therapeutic measures.

**Principle #7** Some groups of people are at higher risk of becoming inadequately nourished than others.

Women who are pregnant or breastfeeding, infants, children, people who are ill, and frail elderly persons have a greater need for nutrients than healthy adults and elderly people do. As a result, they are at higher risk of becoming inadequately nourished than others. Within these groups, those at highest risk of nutritional insults are the poor. In cases of widespread food shortages, such as those induced by war or natural disaster, the health of these nutritionally vulnerable groups is compromised the soonest and the most.

**Principle #8** Poor nutrition can influence the development of certain chronic diseases.

**Shared Dietary Risk Factors** Today, the major causes of death among Americans are slow-developing, lifestyle-related ***chronic diseases*** (Illustration 1.8). Based on government survey data, 44 percent of Americans have a chronic condition such as diabetes, heart disease, cancer, ***hypertension***, or high cholesterol levels, and 13 percent have three or more of these conditions.[33]

**chronic disease** Slow-developing, long-lasting diseases that are not contagious (e.g., heart disease, cancer, diabetes). They can be treated but not always cured.

**hypertension** High blood pressure. It is defined in adults as blood pressure exerted inside blood vessel walls that typically exceeds 140/90 mmHg (millimeters of mercury).

**hypertension** High blood pressure. It is defined in adults as blood pressure exerted inside blood vessel walls that typically exceeds 140/90 mmHg (millimeters of mercury).

TABLE 1.15 ▸ Examples of single-gene disorders that affect nutrient need[75-77]

| | |
|---|---|
| **PKU (phenylketonuria)** | A rare disorder caused by the lack of the enzyme phenylalanine hydroxylase. Lack of this enzyme causes phenylalanine, an essential amino acid, to build up in the blood. High blood levels of phenylalanine during growth lead to mental retardation, poor growth, and other problems. PKU is treated by low-phenylalanine diets. |
| **Galactosemia** | Galactosemia is a single-gene-defect disorder that interferes with the body's utilization of the sugar galactose found in lactose ("milk sugar"). The signs and symptoms of galactosemia result from an inability to use galactose to produce energy. If infants with classic galactosemia are not treated promptly with a low-galactose diet, life-threatening complications appear within a few days after birth. People with this condition must avoid all milk, milk-containing products (including dry milk), and other foods that contain galactose for life. It occurs in approximately 1 in 30,000 to 60,000 newborns. |
| **Hemochromatosis** | A single-gene defect disorder affecting 1 in 300 and occurring most commonly in Caucasians. It is caused by a defect in a gene that produces a protein that controls how much iron is absorbed from food. Individuals with hemochromatosis absorb more iron than normal and have excessive levels of body iron. High levels of body iron have toxic effects on tissues such as the liver and heart. Hemochromatosis is treated with medications and a low-iron and vitamin C diet. A high intake of vitamin C can make hemochromatosis worse because vitamin C increases the absorption of iron. |

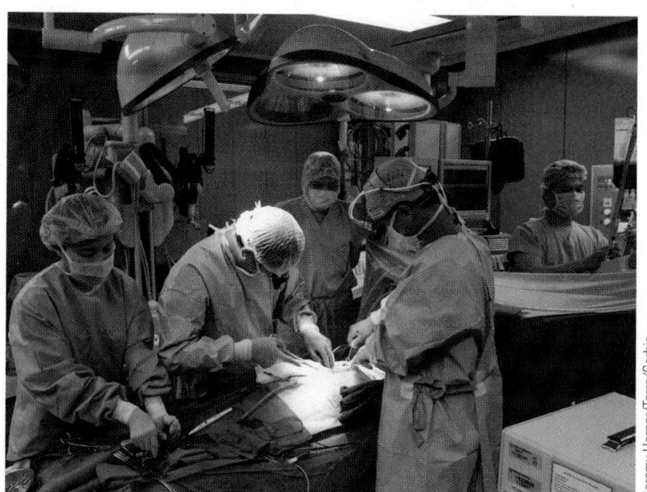
Jeremy Horner/Terra/Corbis

ILLUSTRATION 1.8 ▸ Poor nutrition increases the risk of many chronic diseases.

The leading causes of death among Americans are heart disease and cancer. Together they account for 47 percent of all deaths.[34] Western-type dietary patterns high in food sources of saturated fats, *trans* fats, sugars, and sodium; and low in vegetables, fruits, legumes, and whole grain products are linked to the development of heart disease, obesity, and type 2 diabetes.[11] Six types of cancer, including colon, pancreatic, and breast cancer, are related to obesity, habitually low intakes of vegetables and fruits, and high levels of intake of processed meats.[35]

Diet is related to three other leading causes of death: diabetes, ***stroke***, and ***Alzheimer's disease***. Example of relationships between diseases and disorders and diet are overviewed in Table 1.16. A number of these diseases and disorders share the common dietary risk factors of low intakes of vegetables, fruits, and whole grains; and excess calorie and sugar intake. These risk factors are associated with the development of ***chronic inflammation*** and ***oxidative stress***, conditions that are strongly related to the development of chronic diseases.[11,42]

**stroke** An event that occurs when a blood vessel in the brain ruptures or becomes blocked. Stroke is often associated with "hardening of the arteries" in the brain. Also called cerebral vascular accident.

**Alzheimer's disease** A brain disease that represents the most common form of dementia. It is characterized by memory loss for recent events that expands to more distant memories over the course of 5 to 10 years. It eventually produces profound intellectual decline characterized by dementia and personal helplessness.

Inadequate and excessive nutrient intakes may contribute to the development of more than one disease and produce disease by more than one mechanism. The effects of habitually poor diets on chronic disease development often take years to become apparent.

**Principle #9** Adequacy, variety, and balance are key characteristics of healthy dietary patterns.

**Healthy Dietary Patterns** Healthy diets correspond to a dietary pattern associated with normal growth and development, a healthy body weight, health maintenance, and disease prevention. One such pattern is represented by the USDA's ChooseMyPlate food group intake guide.

TABLE 1.16 ▸ Examples of diseases and disorders linked to diet[78-81]

| DISEASE OR DISORDER | DIETARY CONNECTIONS |
|---|---|
| **Heart disease** | Excessive body fat, high intakes of *trans* fat, added sugar, and salt; low vegetable, fruit, fish, nuts, and whole grain intakes |
| **Cancer** | Low vegetable and fruit intakes; excessive body fat and alcohol intake; regular consumption of processed meats |
| **Stroke** | Low vegetable and fruit intake; excessive alcohol intake; high animal-fat diets |
| **Diabetes** (type 2) | Excessive body fat; low vegetable, whole grain, and fruit intake; high added sugar intake |
| **Cirrhosis of the liver** | Excessive alcohol consumption; poor overall diet |
| **Hypertension** | Excessive sodium (salt) and low potassium intake, excess alcohol intake; low vegetable and fruit intake; excessive levels of body fat |
| **Iron-deficiency anemia** | Low iron intake |
| **Tooth decay and gum disease** | Excessive and frequent sugar consumption; inadequate fluoride intake |
| **Osteoporosis** | Inadequate calcium and vitamin D, low intakes of vegetables and fruits |
| **Obesity** | Excessive calorie intake, overconsumption of energy-dense, nutrient-poor foods |
| **Chronic inflammation and oxidative stress** | Excessive calorie intake; excessive body fat; high animal-fat diets; low intake of whole grains, vegetables, fruit, and fish |
| **Alzheimer's disease** | Regular intake of high-fat animal products; low intake of olive oil, vegetables, fruits, fish, wine, and whole grains |

Several other types of dietary patterns, including the Healthy Mediterranean-Style Dietary Pattern and the Healthy U.S.-Style Dietary Pattern, have also been found to promote health and foster disease prevention.[11] Healthy dietary patterns are characterized by the regular consumption of moderate portions of a variety of foods from each of the basic food groups. No specific foods or food preparation techniques are excluded in a healthy dietary pattern.

Healthy dietary patterns are plant-food based and include the regular consumption of vegetables, fruits, dried beans, fish and seafood, low-fat dairy products, poultry and lean meats, nuts and seeds, and whole grains. Dietary patterns that include large or frequent servings of foods containing high amounts of *trans* fat, added sugars, salt, or alcohol miss the healthy dietary pattern mark. Healthy dietary patterns supply needed nutrients and beneficial phytochemicals through food rather than through supplements or special dietary products.[43]

**Energy and Nutrient Density** Most Americans consume more calories than needed, become overweight as a result, *and* consume inadequate diets. This situation is partly due to overconsumption of ***energy-dense foods*** such as processed and high-fat meats, chips, candy, many desserts, and full-fat dairy products. Energy-dense foods have relatively high-calorie values per unit weight of the food. Intake of energy-dense diets is related to the consumption of excess calories and to the development of overweight and diabetes.[11]

Many energy-dense foods are nutrient poor, or contain low levels of nutrients given their caloric value. These foods are sometimes referred to as ***empty-calorie foods*** and include products such as soft drinks, sherbet, hard candy, alcohol, and cheese twists. Excess intake of energy-dense and empty-calorie foods increases the likelihood that calorie needs will be met or exceeded before nutrients needs are met. Diets most likely to meet nutrient requirements without exceeding calorie need contain primarily ***nutrient-dense foods***, or foods with high levels of nutrients and relatively low calorie value. Nutrient-dense foods such as nonfat milk and yogurt, lean meat, dried beans, vegetables, and fruits provide relatively high amounts of nutrients compared to their calorie value.[11]

**Principle #10** There are no "good" or "bad" foods.

People tend to classify foods as being "good" or "bad," but such opinions about individual foods oversimplify the potential contribution of these foods to a diet.[43] Although opinions about which foods are good or bad vary, hot dogs, ice cream, candy, bacon, and french fries are often judged to be bad, whereas vegetables, fruits, and whole-grain products are given the "good" stamp. Unless we're talking about spoiled stew, poisonous mushrooms, or something similar, however, no food can be firmly labeled as good or bad. Ice cream can be a "good" food for physically active, normal-weight individuals with high calorie needs who have otherwise met their nutrient requirements by consuming nutrient-dense foods. Some people who only eat what they consider to be "good" foods, like vegetables, fruits, whole grains, and tofu, may still miss the healthful diet mark due to inadequate consumption of essential fatty acids and certain vitamins and minerals. All foods can fit into a healthful diet as long as nutrients needs are met at calorie-intake levels that maintain a healthy body weight.[43]

# Nutritional Labeling

**LO 1.2** Apply knowledge about the elements of nutrition labeling to decisions about the nutritional value of foods.

In 1990, the U.S. Congress passed legislation establishing requirements for nutrition information, nutrient content claims, and health claims presented on food and dietary supplement labels. This legislation, called the Nutrition Labeling and Education Act, requires that almost all multiple-ingredient foods and ***dietary supplements*** be labeled with a Nutrition Facts panel (Illustration 1.9). The act also requires that nutrient content and health claims appearing on package labels, such as "*trans* fat–free" and "helps prevent cancer," qualify based on criteria established by the Food and Drug Administration (FDA).

In 2014, the FDA proposed modifying the requirements for nutrition labelling to include added sugars on the Nutrition Facts Panel, and to state serving sizes as those generally consumed.[44]

**chronic inflammation** Low-grade inflammation that lasts weeks, months, or years. Inflammation is the first response of the body's immune system to infectious agents, toxins, or irritants. It triggers the release of biologically active substances that promote oxidation and other reactions to counteract the infection, toxin, or irritant. A side effect of chronic inflammation is that it also damages lipids, cells, and tissues.

**oxidative stress** A condition that occurs when cells are exposed to more oxidizing molecules (such as free radicals) than to antioxidant molecules that neutralize them. Over time, oxidative stress causes damage to lipids, DNA, cells, and tissues. It increases the risk of heart disease, type 2 diabetes, cancer, and other diseases.

**energy-dense foods** Food that have relatively high-calorie values per unit weight of the food.

**empty-calorie foods** Foods that provide an excess of calories relative to their nutrient content.

**nutrient-dense foods** Foods that contain relatively high amounts of nutrients compared to their caloric value.

**dietary supplements** Any product intended to supplement the diet, including vitamin and mineral supplements, proteins, enzymes, amino acids, fish oils, fatty acids, hormones and hormone precursors, and herbs and other plant extracts. In the United States, such products must be labeled "Dietary Supplement."

**Nutrition Facts**
Serving Size 1 Entree
Serving Per Container 1

| **Amount Per Serving** | | | |
|---|---|---|---|
| **Calories** 380 Calories from Fat 170 | | | |
| | | | %Daily Value |
| **Total Fat** 19g | | | **29%** |
| Saturated Fat 10g | | | **50%** |
| Trans Fat 2g | | | |
| **Cholesterol** 85mg | | | **28%** |
| **Sodium** 810mg | | | **34%** |
| **Total Carbohydrate** 33g | | | **11%** |
| Dietary Fiber 3g | | | **12%** |
| Sugars 5g | | | |
| **Protein** 20g | | | |
| Vitamin A 10% | | Vitamin C 0% | |
| Calcium 10% | | Iron 15% | |

Percent Daily Values are based on a 2000 calorie diet. Your daily values may be higher or lower depending on your calorie needs:

| | Calories | 2000 | 2500 |
|---|---|---|---|
| Total Fat | Less Than | 65g | 80g |
| Sat Fat | Less Than | 20g | 25g |
| Cholesterol | Less Than | 300mg | 300mg |
| Sodium | Less Than | 2400mg | 2400mg |
| Total Carbohydrate | | 300g | 375g |
| Dietary Fiber | | 25g | 30g |

**Alternate Format**

**Nutrition Facts**
**8 servings per container**
Serving size 2/3 cup (55g)

Amount per 2/3 cup
**Calories 230**

% Daily Value*

| **QUICK FACTS:** | |
|---|---|
| 12% | **Total Fat** 8g |
| 12% | **Total Carbs** 37g |
| | **Sugars 1g** |
| | **Protein 3g** |
| **AVOID TOO MUCH:** | |
| 5% | **Saturated Fat 1g** |
| | ***Trans*** **Fat** 0g |
| 0% | **Cholesterol 0mg** |
| 7% | **Sodium 160mg** |
| | **Added Sugars 0g** |
| **GET ENOUGH:** | |
| 14% | **Fiber 4g** |
| 10% | **Vitamin D** 2mcg |
| 20% | **Calcium** 260mg |
| 45% | **Iron** 8mg |
| 5% | **Potassium** 235mg |

* Footnote on Daily Values (DV) and calorie reference to be inserted here.

It is available at www.fda.gov/downloads/Food/GuidanceRegulation/GuidanceDocumentsRegulatoryInformation/LabelingNutrition/UCM387451.pdf, and can be found as Ill. 4.14 on p. 4-12 in NN8e.

ILLUSTRATION 1.9 ▸ Example of a Nutrition Facts panel. The existing (left) and the proposed Nutrition Facts panels (right).

www.fda.gov/Food/GuidanceRegulation/GuidanceDocumentsRegulatoryInformation/LabelingNutrition/ucm385663.htm#images

Consequently, the nutrition information labels you see on food packing will likely be a bit different by the end of 2016 than the one shown in Illustration 1.9.

Concern about rising rates of overweight and type 2 diabetes among children and youth prompted senators in the United States to propose national menu labeling standards for fast food and other restaurants in 2009. Legislation passed in 2011 requires restaurant chains with 20 or more outlets to post calories on menus or menu boards and make additional information about the fat, saturated fat, carbohydrate, sodium, protein, and fiber content available in writing upon request.

## Nutrition Facts Panel

For foods, the Nutrition Facts panel must list the content of fat, saturated fat, *trans* fat, cholesterol, sodium, total carbohydrates, fiber, sugars, protein, vitamins A and C, calcium, and iron in a standard serving. Additional nutrients may be listed on a voluntary basis. If a health claim about a particular nutrient is made for the product, the product's content of the nutrient addressed in the claim must be shown. Nutrition Facts panels contain a column that lists the percentage Daily Value (% DV) for each relevant nutrient. This information helps consumers decide, for example, whether the carbohydrate content of a serving of a specific food product is a lot or a little.

Nutrient content claims made on food package labels must meet specific criteria. Products labeled "no *trans* fat" or "*trans* fat–free," for example, must contain less than 0.5 grams of *trans* fat and of saturated fat. Products labeled "low sodium" must contain less than 140 mg of sodium per serving.

## Ingredient Label

Food products must list ingredients in an "ingredient label." The list must begin with the ingredient that contributes the greatest amount of weight to the product and continue with the other ingredients on a weight basis.

The FDA now requires that ingredient labels note the presence of common food allergens in products. Potential food allergens that must be listed are milk, eggs, fish, shellfish, tree nuts, wheat, peanuts, and soybeans. These eight foods account for 90 percent of food allergies.

## Dietary Supplement Labeling

Dietary supplements such as herbs, amino acid pills and powders, and vitamin and mineral supplements must show a "Supplement Facts" panel that lists serving size, ingredients, and % DV of essential nutrients contained. Because they do not have to be shown to be safe and effective before they are sold, labels on dietary supplements cannot claim to treat, cure, or prevent disease. They can be labeled with standardized nutrition content claims such as "high in calcium" or "a good source of fiber." They can also be labeled with health claims such as "may reduce the risk of heart disease" if the product qualifies based on nutrition labeling requirements. Dietary supplements can make other claims on product labels not approved by the FDA, such as "supports the immune system" or "helps maintain mental health," as long as the label doesn't state or imply that the product will prevent, cure, or treat disease. If a health claim is made on a dietary supplement label, the label also must present the FDA disclaimer:

*This product has not been evaluated by the FDA. This product is not intended to diagnose, treat, cure, or prevent any disease.*

**Enrichment and Fortification** Some foods are labeled as "enriched" or "fortified." These two terms have specific definitions. ***Enrichment*** pertains only to refined grain products and covers some of the vitamins and one of the minerals lost when grains are refined. By law, producers of bread, cornmeal, crackers, flour tortillas, white rice, and other products made with refined grains must use flours enriched with thiamin, riboflavin, niacin, and iron.

Any food can be fortified with added vitamins

**enrichment** The replacement of thiamin, riboflavin, niacin, and iron lost when grains are refined.

and minerals, and its manufacturers most often do so on a voluntary basis to enhance product sales. However, some foods must be fortified. Refined grain flours must be fortified with folic acid, milk with vitamin D, and low-fat and skim milk with vitamin D and vitamin A. Although fortification is not required for salt, it is often fortified with iodine. ***Fortification*** of these foods has contributed substantially to reductions in the incidence of diseases related to inadequate intakes.[45]

## Herbal Remedies

The FDA considers herbal products to be dietary supplements; they are taken by many people during various stages of the life cycle. Thousands of types of herbal products are available (Illustration 1.10). Some herbal remedies act like drugs and have side effects, but they are not considered to be drugs and are loosely regulated. They do not have to be shown to be safe or effective before they are marketed. Herbs vary substantially in safety and effectiveness—they can have positive, negative, or neutral effects on health. Knowledge of the effects of herbal remedies is far from complete, making it difficult to determine appropriateness of their use in many cases. The extent to which herbs pose a risk to health depends on the amount taken, the duration of use, and the user's age, lifecycle stage, and health status.

**Prebiotics and Probiotics** The terms *prebiotics* and *probiotics* were derived from *antibiotics* due to their probable effects on increasing resistance to various diseases. Prebiotics and probiotics are in a class of functional foods by themselves. ***Prebiotics*** are fiberlike, indigestible carbohydrates that are broken down by bacteria in the colon. The breakdown products foster the growth of beneficial bacteria. The digestive tract generally contains over 500 species of microorganisms and 100 trillion bacteria. Some species of bacteria such as *E. coli* 0157:H7 may cause disease; others, such as strains of lactobacillus and bifidobacteria, may help prevent certain diseases.[46] Because they foster the growth of beneficial bacteria, prebiotics are considered "intestinal fertilizer." ***Probiotic*** is the term for live, beneficial ("friendly") bacteria that enter food products during fermentation and aging processes. Those that survive digestive enzymes and acids may start colonies of beneficial bacteria in the digestive tract. Table 1.17 lists foods and other sources of pre- and probiotics.

**fortification** The addition of one or more vitamins or minerals to a food product.

**prebiotics** Certain fiberlike forms of indigestible carbohydrates that support the growth of beneficial bacteria in the lower intestine. Nicknamed "intestinal fertilizer."

**probiotics** Strains of lactobacillus and bifidobacteria that have beneficial effects on the body. Also called "friendly bacteria."

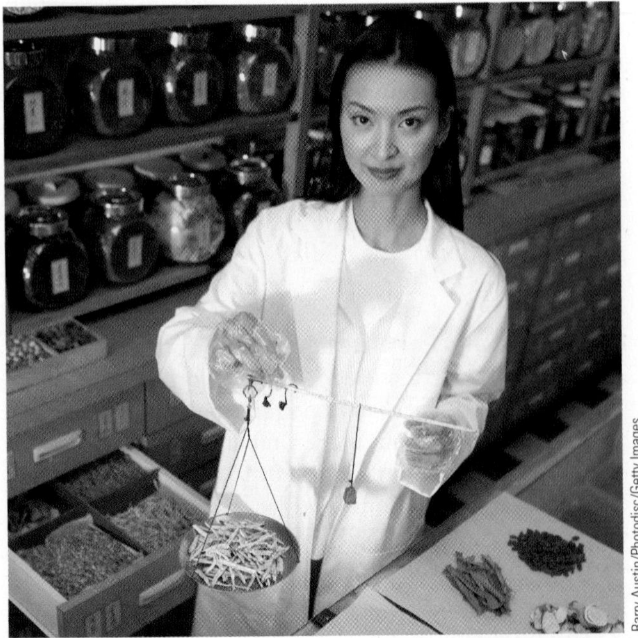

Barry Austin/Photodisc/Getty Images

ILLUSTRATION 1.10 ▸ Herbal products are widely available on the market.

TABLE 1.17 ▸ Food and other sources of prebiotics and probiotics

| PROBIOTICS |
|---|
| **Fermented or aged milk and milk products** |
| • Yogurt with live culture |
| • Buttermilk |
| • Kefir |
| • Cottage cheese |
| • Dairy spreads with added inulin |
| **Other fermented products** |
| • Soy sauce |
| • Tempeh |
| • Fresh sauerkraut |
| • Miso |
| **Breast milk** |
| Probiotic tablets, powders, and nutritional beverages |
| **PREBIOTICS** |
| Chicory |
| Jerusalem artichokes |
| Wheat |
| Barley |
| Rye |
| Onions |
| Garlic |
| Leeks |
| Prebiotic tablets, powders, and nutritional beverages |

Prebiotics and probiotics have been credited with important benefits, such as the prevention and treatment of diarrhea and other infections in the gastrointestinal tract; prevention of colon cancer; decreased blood levels of triglycerides, cholesterol, and glucose; and decreased dental caries.[46] Prebiotics appear to be safe in general; however, probiotics may be harmful to specific individuals who may develop blood infections.[47] The primary side effects associated with prebiotic and probiotic use are flatulence, bloating, and constipation.[46]

Availability of foods containing prebiotics and probiotics is much more common in Japan and European countries than in Canada or the United States. However, availability of such products is increasing in these countries as research results shed light on their safety and effectiveness.[48]

# The Life-Course Approach to Nutrition and Health

**LO 1.3** Cite two examples of how nutrient needs change during the life cycle and how nutritional status at one stage during the life cycle can influence health status during another.

Nutritional needs should be met at every stage of the life cycle because nutritional status at one stage influences health status in the next ones. Lack of adequate nutrition during pregnancy, for example, can program gene functions for life in ways that set the stage for lifelong metabolic changes that increase the risk of chronic-disease development. Iron deficiency experienced by young children can decrease intellectual capacity later in life, and adequate vitamin D status during adolescence and early adulthood decreases the risk of breast cancer in older women.[49] Disease prevention and health promotion, rather than repair of health problems, requires a focus on meeting nutritional and other health needs of individuals during every stage of the life cycle.

## Meeting Nutritional Needs Across the Life Cycle

Healthy individuals require the same nutrients throughout life, but amounts of nutrients needed vary based on age, growth, and development. Nutrient needs during each stage of the life cycle can be met through a variety of foods and food practices. There is no one best diet for everyone. Traditional diets defined by diverse cultures and religions provide the foundation for meeting individuals' nutritional needs and the framework for dietary modification when needed.[11,50] Although it is inaccurate to say that all or most members of a particular cultural group or religion follow the same dietary practices, groups of individuals may share common beliefs about food and food-intake practices.

## Dietary Considerations Based on Ethnicity

People immigrating to the United States and other countries both preserve dietary traditions of their cultural group and integrate cross-cultural adaptations into their dietary practices. The extent to which culturally based food habits change depends to some extent on income, food cost, and ethnic food availability. Immigrant families from El Salvador who live in urban areas of the United States, for example, maintain many cultural food practices from their homeland:

- Breakfast generally consists of fried beans, corn tortillas, occasionally eggs, and sweetened coffee with boiled milk.
- Lunch consists of soup, fried meat, rice or rice with vegetables, corn tortillas, and fruit juice.
- Dinner will offer fried beef or chicken, corn tortillas, rice, dried beans, fruit juice, and black coffee.

Cross-cultural adaptations made by a portion of Salvadorans immigrating to the United States include the addition of french fries, hamburgers, American cheeses, salad dressing, tacos, flour tortillas, and peanut butter to their diets.[51]

Sometimes diets of native populations change when their numbers become overwhelmed by other population groups. A primary example of this phenomenon is represented by changes in traditional dietary practices of American Indians. In general, traditional diets of American Indians in the United States consisted of foods such as buffalo, deer, wild berries and other fruits, corn, turnips, squash, wild potato, and wild rice. Loss of land and buffalo, discrimination, poverty, and food programs that offered refined flour, sugar, salt pork, and other high-fat meats drastically changed what American Indians ate, how they lived, and their health status. Activities aimed at bringing back traditional foods and dietary practices are under way among many American Indians groups.[52]

Food preferences of African Americans vary widely but may stem from their cultural food heritage. Historically important foods include corn bread, pork, buttermilk, rice, sweet potatoes, greens, cabbage, salt pork, and fried fish. These "soul foods" make up less of the African American diet now than in the past but remain foods of choice for special occasions.[53]

## Dietary Considerations Based on Religion

Many religions have special dietary laws and practices. For example:

- Some Hindus may not consume foods such as garlic and onions, which are believed to hinder spiritual development.
- Buddhists in certain countries tend to be vegetarian or to eat fish as their only choice of meat. In countries

such as Tibet and Japan, vegetarianism is rare among Buddhists.

- Alcohol is prohibited as part of Sikhism, and meat prepared by kosher or halal methods is avoided.
- The Church of Latter Day Saints, or the Mormon Church, prohibits alcohol and discourages consumption of caffeine. Mormons may eat meat and prize wheat.
- Seventh-Day Adventists tend to follow a strict lacto-ovo vegetarian diet and exclude alcohol and caffeine. Whole grains, vegetables, and fruits are considered to be the base of diets, and dried beans, low-fat dairy products, and eggs may be consumed infrequently.
- Jewish dietary laws require that foods consumed must be kosher, or fit to eat according to Judaic law. Organizations are certified as supplying foods that are kosher. The Jewish calendar includes six fasting days that call for total abstinence from food or drink.
- The Muslim religion has dietary laws that require foods to be halal, or permitted for consumption by Muslims. Pork consumption is not allowed, nor is the consumption of animals slaughtered in the name of any god other than Allah. Slaughterhouses must be under the supervision of a halal certifier in order for meat to be considered fit to eat, although some Muslims will eat other meats. Consuming alcohol is prohibited.[54]

Additional information about cultural and religious food practices and beliefs can be obtained directly by getting to know people from a variety of cultures and their dietary preferences. This information can be of great benefit in nutrition education and counseling situations.

# Nutrition Assessment

**LO 1.4** Describe the components of individual-level nutrition assessment.

Nutrition assessment of groups and individuals is a prerequisite to planning for the prevention or solution of nutrition-related health problems. It represents a broad area within the field of nutrition and is highlighted here.

Nutritional status may be assessed for a population group or for an individual. Community-level assessment identifies a population's status using broad nutrition and health indicators, whereas individual assessment provides the baseline for anticipatory guidance and nutrition intervention.

## Community-Level Assessment

A target community's "state of nutritional health" can generally be estimated using existing vital statistics data, seeking the opinions of target group members and local health experts, and making observations. Knowledge of average household incomes; the proportion of families participating in SNAP (formerly called the Food Stamp Program), soup kitchens, school breakfast programs, or food banks; and the age distribution of the group can help identify key nutrition concerns and issues. In large communities, rates of infant mortality, heart disease, and cancer can reveal whether the incidence of these problems is unusually high.

Information gathered from community-level nutrition assessment can be used to develop community-wide programs addressing specific problem areas, such as childhood obesity or iron-deficiency anemia. Nutrition programs should be integrated into community-based health programs.

## Individual-Level Nutrition Assessment

Nutrition assessment of individuals has four major components:

1. Clinical/physical assessment
2. Dietary assessment
3. Anthropometric assessment
4. Biochemical assessment

Data from all of these areas are needed to describe a person's nutritional status. Data on height and weight provide information on weight status, for example, and knowledge of blood iron levels tells you something about iron status. It cannot be concluded that people who are normal weight or have good iron status are "well nourished." Single measures do not describe a person's nutritional status.

## Clinical/Physical Assessment

A clinical/physical assessment involves visual inspection of a person by a trained ***registered dietitian nutritionist (RDN)*** or other qualified professional to note features that may be related to malnutrition. Excessive or inadequate body fat, paleness, bruises, and brittle hair are examples of features that may suggest nutrition-related problems. Physical characteristics are nonspecific indicators, but they can support other findings related to nutritional status. They cannot be used as the sole criterion upon which to base a decision about the presence or absence of a particular nutrition problem.

## Dietary Assessment

Many methods are used for assessing dietary intake. For clinical purposes, computerized 24-hour dietary recalls and food records are most common. Single 24-hour recalls and food

**registered dietitian nutritionist (RDN)**
An individual who has acquired food and nutrition knowledge and skills necessary to pass a national registration examination and who participates in continuing professional education.

frequency questionnaires are most useful for estimating dietary intakes for groups, whereas multiple recalls and dietary histories are generally used for assessments of individual diets.

**24-Hour Dietary Recalls and Records** Becoming proficient at administering 24-hour recalls takes training and practice. Food records, on the other hand, are completed by clients themselves. These are more accurate if the client has also received some training. Generally, the purpose of assessing an individual's diet is to estimate the person's overall diet quality so that strengths and weaknesses can be identified, or to assess intake of specific nutrients that may be involved in disease states. Information on multiple days of dietary intake is needed to obtain a reliable estimate of intake by food group, calories, and nutrients.[83]

**Dietary History** Dietary histories have been used for decades and represent a quantitative method of dietary assessment. They require an interview by a trained professional that is about 1½ hours long and includes a 24-hour dietary recall modified to represent usual intake, careful deliberations over food types and portions, and a cross-check food frequency questionnaire that confirms 24-hour usual dietary intake information. Results must be coded, checked, and processed. Although expensive, diet histories provide more complete and accurate data than most other dietary assessment methods.[55]

**Food Frequency Questionnaires** Food frequency questionnaires are often used in epidemiological studies to estimate food and nutrient intake of groups of people. These tools are considered semiquantitative because they force people into describing food intake based on a limited number of food choices and portion sizes (Illustration 1.11). Validated food frequencies are relatively inexpensive to administer and tabulate, and they provide good enough estimates of dietary intake to rank people by their food and nutrient intake levels. They tend to underestimate food intake and provide data that are more likely to fail to identify nutrient and health relationships than are quantitative assessment techniques such as the dietary history.[55,56]

**Internet Dietary Assessment Resources** Several high-quality Internet resources are available for dietary assessment. Food Tracker, available from the MyPlate.gov site and developed by the U.S. Department of Agriculture (USDA), is an example of a high-quality Internet resource. This interactive program provides an analysis of nutrient and food group intake.

**USDA's Automated Multiple-Pass Method** An interactive method for collecting 24-hour dietary recalls either in person, online, or by telephone has been validated by several studies.[57] It's the Automated Multiple-Pass Dietary Recall and is being used in government-sponsored nutrition studies such as the large "What We Eat in America" surveys. It utilizes a five-step, multiple-pass 24-hour recall. The term *multiple pass* refers to the repeated use of questions that hone the accuracy of information provided by interviewees about the food they ate the previous day.

The five-step interview process used by the automated multiple-pass method consists of the following:

1. **The Quick List** Quickly collect a list of foods and beverages consumed the previous day.

| | Frequency of Consumption | | | | | | | | |
|---|---|---|---|---|---|---|---|---|---|
| **Food** | **Never or less than once per month** | **1–3 per month** | **1 per week** | **2–4 per week** | **5–6 per week** | **1 per day** | **2–3 per day** | **4–5 per day** | **6+ per day** |
| **1. a.** Broth-type soups, 1 cup | | | | | | | | | |
| **b.** Tap water, 1 cup | | | | | | | | | |
| **c.** Sparkling or mineral water, 1-cup serving | | | | | | | | | |
| **d.** Decaffeinated black tea, iced or hot, 1 cup | | | | | | | | | |
| **e.** Herbal tea, (no caffine) iced or hot, 1 cup | | | | | | | | | |
| **2.** Custard or pudding, 1/2 cup | | | | | | | | | |
| **3.** Onions, 1/4 cup, alone or in combination | | | | | | | | | |

ILLUSTRATION 1.11 ▸ Example component of a food frequency questionnaire.

SOURCE: J. Brown, University of Minnesota; Diana Project form, adapted from W. Willett's Food Frequency Questionnaire.

2. **The Forgotten Foods List** Probe for foods forgotten during development of the Quick List.
3. **Time and Occasion List** Collect information on the time and eating occasion for each food.
4. **The Detail Cycle** Collect detailed information on the description and amount of food consumed using the USDA's interactive Food Model Booklet and measuring guides.
5. **Final Probe Review** Review 24-hour recall and ask about anything else consumed.

An automated, self-administered 24-hour recall known the ASA24 is a freely available Web-based tool that enables automated self-administered 24-hour recalls and analysis.[58]

**The Healthy Eating Index** The HEI (Healthy Eating Index) assesses a person's reported dietary intake based on 10 dietary components that cover intake of the USDA's basic food groups informed by the Dietary Guidelines for Americans recommendations. The components are assigned scores based on the extent to which diets meet recommended standards of intake. The HEI is primarily used for population monitoring of dietary quality, evaluation of interventions, and research. It has been shown to be a valid tool for assessing dietary quality.[59]

## Anthropometric Assessment

Individual measures of body size (e.g., height, weight, percent body fat, bone density, and head and waist circumferences) are useful in the assessment of nutritional status—if done correctly. Each measure requires use of standard techniques and calibrated instruments by trained personnel. Unfortunately, ***anthropometric*** measurements are frequently performed and recorded incorrectly in clinical practice. Training on anthropometric measures is often available through public health agencies and programs such as WIC (Special Supplemental Nutrition Program for Women, Infants, and Children), and courses and training sessions at colleges and universities.

## Biochemical Assessment

Nutrient and enzyme levels, gene characteristics, and other biological markers are components of the biochemical assessment of nutritional status. Which nutrition biomarkers are measured depends on what problems are suspected, based on other evidence. For example, a young child who tires easily, has a short attention span, and does not appear to be consuming sufficient iron based on dietary assessment results may have blood taken for analyses of hemoglobin and serum ferritin (markers of iron status). Suspected inborn errors of metabolism that may underlie nutrient malabsorption may be identified through genetic or other tests. Such results provide specific information on a component of a person's nutritional status and are very helpful in the diagnosis and treatment of particular condition.

A number of references on normal levels of nutrition biomarkers in women and men are available.[60-63] Nutrient biomarker levels are reported in conventional units (such as ng/mL), or SI units, (such as ng/mL). The second page of Appendix A shows you how to convert conventional units of measure to SI units, and visa versa. Nutritional biomarker values and reference ranges are affected by many variables, including sample and method of analysis used and population characteristics. They may change as more information becomes known about nutrient biomarker concentrations and health relationships. In the future, biochemical assessments will include a nutrigenomics profile to identify health risks due to interactions among an individual's genetic makeup, gene functions, and components of food.

After the fact-finding phase of nutrition assessment, the dietitian nutritionist or other qualified professionals must apply their brains to their clients' problems. There is no one-size-fits-all approach to solving nutrition problems—each has to be figured out individually.

## Monitoring the Nation's Nutritional Health

Food availability, dietary intake, weight status, and nutrition-related disease incidence are investigated regularly in the United States by the National Nutrition Monitoring System. This wide-ranging system is primarily responsible for the conduct of ***nutrition surveillance*** and ***nutrition monitoring*** studies.

The first U.S. nutrition survey began in 1936 when hunger, poor growth in children, and vitamin and mineral deficiencies were common. Today's surveys monitor rates of obesity, diabetes, and other nutrition-related disorders; the safety of the food supply (e.g., the mercury content of fish and pesticide residues in vegetables and fruits); and food and nutrient intake.

The major, ongoing U.S. studies related to diet, the food supply, and nutritional health are overviewed in Table 1.18. Together with findings from studies conducted by university researchers and others, the results give direction to food and nutrition policies and programs aimed at safeguarding the food supply, improving the population's nutritional health, and maintaining a successful agricultural economy.[64]

**Anthropometry** The science of measuring the human body and its parts.

**nutrition surveillance** Continuous assessment of nutritional status for the purpose of detecting changes in trend or distribution in order to initiate corrective measures.

**nutrition monitoring** Assessment of dietary or nutrition status at intermittent times with the aim of detecting changes in the dietary or nutritional status of a population.

TABLE 1.18 ▸ U.S. National nutrition monitoring systems

| SURVEY | PURPOSE |
|---|---|
| 1. National Health and Nutrition Examination Survey (NHANES) | Assesses dietary intake, health, and nutritional status in a sample of adults and children in the United States on a continual basis |
| 2. Nationwide Food Consumption Survey (NFCS) | Performs regular surveys of food and nutrient intake and understanding of diet and health relationships among national sample of individuals in the United States |
| 3. Total Diet Study (sometimes called Market Basket Study) | Ongoing studies that determine the levels of various pesticide residues, contaminants, and nutrients in foods and diets |

TABLE 1.19 ▸ Income eligibility standards for the WIC program (≤185% of poverty income, July 1, 2015, through June 30, 2016)[66]

| HOUSEHOLD SIZE | HOUSEHOLD INCOME PER YEAR |
|---|---|
| 1 | $21,775 |
| 2 | $29,471 |
| 3 | $37,167 |
| 4 | $44,863 |
| 5 | $52,559 |
| 6 | $60,255 |
| 7 | $67,951 |
| 8 | $75,647 |
| Each additional member | $7,696 |

# Public Food and Nutrition Programs

**LO 1.5** Identify the basic elements of four public food and nutrition programs.

A variety of federal, state, and local programs are available to provide food and nutrition services to families and individuals. Many communities have nutrition coalitions or partnership groups that collaborate on meeting the food and nutritional needs of community members. Programs representing church-based feeding sites, food shelves, Second Harvest Programs, the Salvation Army, missions, and others are usually a part of local coalitions. These central resources can be identified by contacting the local public health or cooperative extension agency. State-level programs are generally part of large national programs.

About one in five Americans participates in at least one of the USDA's 15 food assistance programs at some point during the year. The Supplemental Nutrition Assistance Program (SNAP) is the nation's largest food assistance program. The program also serves as a source of demand for the products of American farmers and food companies.[65] Some programs, such as the School Breakfast and Lunch Program, benefit many children. Other programs are targeted to families and individuals in need. *Need* is generally defined as including individual and household incomes below the poverty line. Some programs, such as WIC, have eligibility standards of up to 185 percent of the poverty line (Table 1.19). Income guidelines change periodically and are higher for people in Alaska and Hawaii.[66]

## WIC

The Special Supplemental Nutrition Program for Women, Infants, and Children (WIC) was established in 1972 and is administered by the USDA. The program provides nutrition education and counseling as well as food vouchers for low-income pregnant, postpartum, and breastfeeding women and for low-income children under the age of five years. Food vouchers apply to nutritious foods such as fortified breakfast cereals, iron-fortified infant cereals and formula, milk, cheese, eggs, peanut butter, dried beans whole grain products, fruits, vegetables, and 100 percent fruit and vegetable juices. Some WIC programs offer vouchers for the purchase of produce at farmers' markets. WIC staff also provides breastfeeding support and referrals to health-care and social-service providers.

Eligibility for WIC is based on low-income status and the presence of a nutritional risk, such as iron deficiency or being underweight. WIC services are provided through approximately 10,000 clinic sites throughout the United States and in American Samoa, Guam, Puerto Rico, and the Virgin Islands. The program serves more than 7 million women and children each year. Nearly half of all infants and a quarter of all young children in the United States participate in the WIC program.[84]

The WIC program has been shown to have a number of positive effects on the health of participants. Infants born to women participating in WIC while pregnant are less likely to be small at birth or to be born before term than the infants of nonparticipating low-income women. Children served by WIC tend to consume more nutritious diets and experience lower rates of iron deficiency than children who are low-income but not enrolled in WIC. WIC is cost effective: every dollar invested in WIC prenatal nutrition services saves $3.13 on Medicaid costs for infants during the first two years of life.[67]

Table 1.20 presents information on existing federal food and nutrition programs. You can get more information on these programs online at www.fns.usda.gov.

TABLE 1.20 ▶ Examples of federal food and nutrition programs

| PROGRAM | ACTIVITY |
|---|---|
| **Child and Adult Care Food Program (CACFP)** | Reimburses child and adult care organizations in low-income areas for provision of nutritious foods. |
| **Summer Food Service Program** | Provides foods to children in low-income areas during the summer. |
| **School Breakfast and Lunch Programs** | Provide free breakfasts and reduced-cost or no-cost lunches to children from families who cannot afford to buy them. |
| **SNAP (Food Stamp Program)** | Subsidizes food purchases of low-income families and individuals. |
| **WIC** | Serves low-income, pregnant, and breastfeeding women and children up to 5 years of age. Participants must have a nutritional risk factor to qualify. Provides supplemental nutritious foods and nutrition education as an adjunct to health care. |
| **Head Start Program** | Includes nutrition education for children and parents and supplies meals for children in the program. |

### Nationwide Priorities for Improvements in Nutritional Health

Public health initiatives involving population-based improvements in food safety, food availability, and nutritional status have led to major gains in the health status of the country's population. Among the important components of this success story are programs that have expanded the availability of: housing; safe food and water; foods fortified with iodine, iron, vitamin D, or folate; fluoridated public water; food assistance; and nutrition education. Today's priorities for improvements in the public's health and longevity center on reducing obesity, type 2 diabetes, and physical inactivity. Goals for dietary changes are a central part of the nation's overall plan for health improvements.[68]

Objectives related to the goals for improving the nutritional health of the nation are summarized in the document "Healthy People 2020" (Table 1.21). Because the seeds of many chronic diseases are planted during pregnancy and childhood, major emphasis is placed on diet and nutritional status early in life.

TABLE 1.21 ▶ Examples of the *Healthy People 2020* nutrition objectives for the nation

| HEALTHIER FOOD ACCESS |
|---|
| • Increase the proportion of schools that offer nutritious foods and beverages outside of school meals. |
| • Increase the proportion of Americans who have access to a food retail outlet that sells a variety of foods that are encouraged by the dietary guidelines. |
| **WEIGHT STATUS** |
| • Increase the proportion of adults who are at a healthy weight. |
| • Reduce the proportion of adults who are obese. |
| • Reduce the proportion of children and adolescents who are considered obese. |
| • Prevent inappropriate weight gain in youths and adults. |
| **FOOD INSECURITY** |
| • Eliminate very low food security among children. |
| • Reduce household food insecurity and in doing so reduce hunger. |
| **FOOD AND NUTRIENT CONSUMPTION** |
| • Increase the variety and contribution of vegetables to diets. |
| • Increase the contribution of whole grains to diets. |
| • Reduce the consumption of calories from solid fats and added sugars. |
| • Reduce the consumption of saturated fat. |
| • Reduce the consumption of sodium. |
| • Increase the consumption of calcium. |
| • Reduce the consumption of sodium. |
| **IRON DEFICIENCY** |
| • Reduce iron deficiency among young children and females of childbearing age. |
| • Reduce iron deficiency among pregnant females. |
| **HEALTH CARE AND WORKSITE SETTINGS** |
| • Increase the proportion of physician office visits that include counseling or education related to nutrition and weight. |

## Nutrition and Health Guidelines for Americans

LO 1.6 Apply the characteristics of healthful diets to the design of one.

In the United States and Canada, the national guidelines for diet and health are called the "Dietary Guidelines for Americans," and the major educational tools for consumers based on the guidelines can be found at MyPlate.gov (Illustration 1.12).

### Dietary Guidelines for Americans

The Dietary Guidelines for Americans provide science-based recommendations to promote health and to reduce the risk for major chronic diseases through diet and physical activity. Due to its credibility and focus on health promotion and disease prevention for the public, the Dietary Guidelines form the basis of federal food and nutrition education programs and policies. Under legislative mandate, the Dietary Guidelines for Americans must be updated every five years.[11]

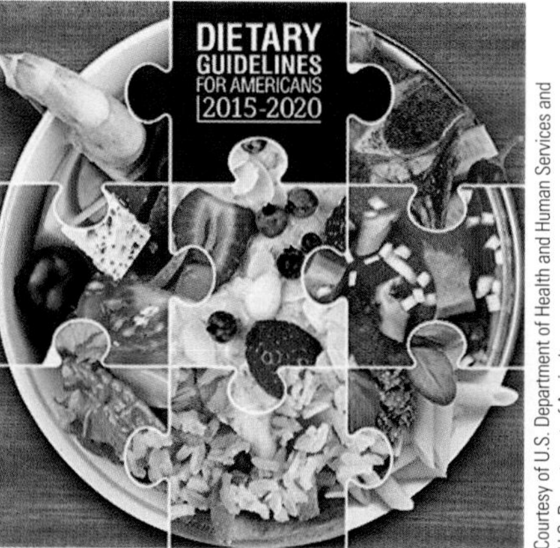


Courtesy of U.S. Department of Health and Human Services and U.S. Department of Agriculture

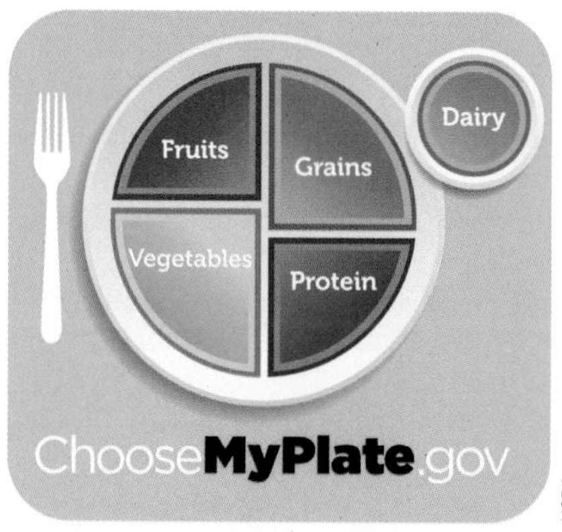


USDA

ILLUSTRATION 1.12 ▸ The major diet and health guides for Americans.

The 2015 Dietary Guidelines highlight dietary patterns associated with decreased risk of obesity, heart disease, and diabetes; nutrient inadequacies; and physical activity.[85] The 2015 Dietary Guidelines Advisory Committee, which consisted of scientific experts on nutrition and health, concluded that the health of the U.S. population could be improved, and common chronic diseases and disorders prevented, if Americans consume a healthy dietary pattern (shown in Table 1.22) and exercise regularly. Key elements of the 2015 Dietary Guidelines related to food and nutrient intake, dietary pattern, and food safety and sustainability are listed in Table 1.23.

Types and combinations of foods included in the Healthy Mediterranean-Style Dietary Pattern, the Healthy U.S.-Style Dietary Pattern, and the Healthy Vegetarian-Style Dietary Pattern are recommended by the guidelines.[85] Healthy dietary patterns are characterized by regular consumption of moderate portions of a variety of foods from each of the basic food groups.

## MyPlate.gov

MyPlate supports the healthy eating messages in the Dietary Guidelines through offering the following key pieces of advice:

- Make at least half your plate fruits and vegetables.
- Make half your grains whole grains.
- Eat fewer foods that are high in saturated fat, *trans* fats, added sugar, and sodium.
- Avoid oversized portions.
- Switch to fat-free or low-fat (1 percent) milk.
- Drink water instead of sugary drinks.
- Compare sodium in foods like soup, bread, and frozen meals—and choose the foods with lower numbers.

The importance of consuming enough calories for growth and health while not consuming extra calories and gaining weight is also stressed. Regular physical activity (60 minutes per day for children and adolescents and 2½ hours or more per week of moderate activity for adults weekly) is stressed because it contributes to health maintenance and weight control.

## USDA's Food Groups

The USDA's long tradition of offering consumers a list of basic food groups is upheld in the current recommendations. Grains, vegetables, fruits, dairy, and protein foods are the designated groups. Interactive, educational material provided by MyPlate.gov includes details about the types of foods that belong to each group. Unlike previous food

TABLE 1.22 ▸ Characteristics of Healthy Dietary Patterns[11,69,82]

Healthy dietary patterns include the regular consumptions of:

- Fruits and vegetables
- Whole grains and whole grain products, and other high-fiber foods
- Nuts, all types
- Oils (such as olive oil, seed, and vegetable oils)
- Legumes (such as navy and pinto beans)
- Low-fat dairy products
- Poultry, lean meats
- Fish and seafood
- Alcohol in moderation (by adults who chose to drink).

Healthy dietary patterns are *not* characterized by the regular consumptions of:

- Foods and beverages high in added sugar such as sugar-sweetened soft drinks, fruit drinks, and sweetened teas
- Foods high in sodium such as some fast- and processed foods
- Refined grain products such as white bread, rice cakes, pasta
- Processed meats such as salami and bologna
- Foods high in saturated fats, such as animal fat and tropical oils

**TABLE 1.23** ▸ Key elements of the 2015 Dietary Guidelines for Americans[85]

1. Nutrient intake of the U.S. population over the age of 2 years:
    - Intake of vitamin D, calcium, potassium, and fiber should be increased.
    - Intake of iron is low in females.
    - Intake of sodium, added sugar, saturated fat, and calories are too high.
    - Saturated fats should be replaced with unsaturated fats, especially polyunsaturated fats, and not with carbohydrates.
    - Limit added sugar intake to ≤10% of total calorie intake.
    - Current levels of caffeine intakes do not exceed safe levels for any age group.
    - Cholesterol intake is not considered a nutrient of concern for overconsumption.
    - Total fat intake does not need to be reduced. The type of fat is more important than the amount.
    - Moderate alcohol intake (1-2 drinks per day) by adults who chose to drink is included in a healthy dietary pattern.
2. Healthy dietary pattern
    - Obesity and common disease and disorder risks are reduced if people follow a healthy dietary pattern (see Table 6.1).
3. Food Safety and Sustainability (recommendation is from the 2015 Dietary Guidelines Advisory Committee report[11])
    - Moderate coffee/caffeine consumption (3 to 5 cups or up to 400 mg caffeine per day by adults, 200 mg or 2 cups of coffee by pregnant women) is not associated with disease risk and may decrease the risk of certain health problems.
    - High caffeine intakes are inappropriate for children, and caffeine should not be combined with alcohol.
    - Low-calorie sweeteners (artificial sweeteners) appear to be safe but should not be used as a primary replacement for sugar in foods and beverages.
    - Water is the preferred beverage of choice.
    - A dietary pattern high in plant-based foods is associated with a lower environmental impact that is the current U.S. dietary pattern.
4. Physical Activity
    - Regular physical activity benefits the health of nearly all people, including individuals with physical disabilities, pregnant women, and children.
    - Americans should engage in at least 150 minutes per week of moderate intensity physical activity unless medically unable to do so.
5. Promising strategies for facilitating individual behavioral changes that promote improved diets and physical activity levels include:
    - Decrease screen time.
    - Expand access to a healthy food environment.
    - Increase family meals, decrease fast-food meals.
    - Label food in a way that helps target healthy food choices.
    - Self-monitor diet and physical activity.
    - Increase opportunities for physical activity.

group guides, the current version does not recommend serving sizes or numbers of servings individuals in general should consume from the food groups. This information is provided if requested using a personalized interactive tool on menu planning such as the "Daily Food Plan." The personalized information generated shows amounts of each food group to consume and food portion sizes that correspond to that amount.

Information on amounts of basic foods contained in a cup or an ounce is provided separately in the ChooseMyPlate materials. Table 1.24 highlights examples of this information. You can get additional examples of serving size equivalents by highlighting a food group shown on the daily food plan output and clicking on "What counts as an ounce?" or "What counts as a cup?"

**Example Menus** What does an eating pattern based on the USDA's food group guidelines look like? Seven days of menus based on a 2,000-calorie diet that meet the USDA's food group recommendations and nutrient needs are available from the "Tips & Resources" link on the ChooseMyPlate.gov homepage. Three days of the menus and the food group and nutrient analysis for the menu are shown in Illustration 1.13. The menus are intended to give consumers specific and

**TABLE 1.24** ▸ How much food counts as a cup or an ounce?

| | |
|---|---|
| **Vegetables:** | 1 cup = 1 cup raw or cooked vegetables or vegetable juice or 2 cups leafy salad greens |
| **Fruits:** | 1 cup = 1 cup raw or cooked fruit or 100% fruit juice, or ½ cup dried fruit |
| **Dairy:** | 1 cup = 1 cup milk, yogurt, or fortified soy milk; or 1½ ounces natural or 2 ounces processed cheese |
| **Grains:** | 1 oz = 1 slice of bread, ½ cup cooked rice, cereal, or pasta; or 1 oz ready-to-eat cereal |
| **Protein:** | 1 oz = 1 oz lean meat, poultry, or fish; 1 egg, 1 Tbsp peanut butter, ½ oz nuts or seeds; ¼ cup cooked dried beans or peas |

## Sample menus for a 2000 Calorie Food Pattern

### DAY 1

**BREAKFAST**
Creamy oatmeal (cooked in milk):
*½ cup uncooked oatmeal*
*1 cup fat-free milk*
*2 Tbsp raisins*
*2 tsp brown sugar*
Beverage: 1 cup orange juice

**LUNCH**
Taco salad:
*2 ounces tortilla chips*
*2 ounces cooked ground turkey*
*2 tsp corn/canola oil (to cook turkey)*
*¼ cup kidney beans**
*½ ounce low-fat cheddar cheese*
*½ cup chopped lettuce*
*½ cup avocado*
*1 tsp lime juice (on avocado)*
*2 Tbsp salsa*
Beverage:
1 cup water, coffee, or tea**

**DINNER**
Spinach lasagna roll-ups:
*1 cup lasagna noodles(2 oz dry)*
*½ cup cooked spinach*
*½ cup ricotta cheese*
*1 ounce part-skim mozzarella cheese*
*½ cup tomato sauce**
1 ounce whole wheat roll
*1 tsp tub margarine*
Beverage:1 cup fat-free milk

**SNACKS**
2 Tbsp raisins
1 ounce unsalted almonds

### DAY 2

**BREAKFAST**
Breakfast burrito:
*1 flour tortilla (8" diameter)*
*1 scrambled egg*
*⅓ cup black beans**
*2 Tbsp salsa*
½ large grapefruit
Beverage:
1 cup water, coffee, or tea**

**LUNCH**
Roast beef sandwich:
*1 small whole grain hoagie bun*
*2 ounces lean roast beef*
*1 slice part-skim mozzarella cheese*
*2 slices tomato*
*¼ cup mushrooms*
*1 tsp corn/canola oil (to cook mushrooms)*
*1 tsp mustard*
Baked potato wedges:
*1 cup potato wedges*
*1 tsp corn/canola oil (to cook potato)*
*1 Tbsp ketchup*
Beverage:1 cup fat-free milk

**DINNER**
Baked salmon on beet greens:
*4 ounce salmon filet*
*1 tsp olive oil*
*2 tsp lemon juice*
*⅓ cup cooked beet greens (sauteed in 2 tsp corn/canola oil)*
Quinoa with almonds:
*½ cup quinoa*
*½ ounce slivered almonds*
Beverage:1 cup fat-free milk

**SNACKS**
1 cup cantaloupe balls

### DAY 3

**BREAKFAST**
Cold cereal:
*1 cup ready-to-eat oat cereal*
*1 medium banana*
*½ cup fat-free milk*
1 slice whole wheat toast
*1 tsp tub margarine*
Beverage: 1 cup prune juice

**LUNCH**
Tuna salad sandwich:
*2 slices rye bread*
*2 ounces tuna*
*1 Tbsp mayonnaise*
*1 Tbsp chopped celery*
*½ cup shredded lettuce*
1 medium peach
Beverage: 1 cup fat-free milk

**DINNER**
Roasted chicken:
*3 ounces cooked chicken breast*
1 large sweet potato, roasted
½ cup succotash (limas & corn)
*1 tsp tub margarine*
1 ounce whole wheat roll
*1 tsp tub margarine*
Beverage:
1 cup water, coffee, or tea**

**SNACKS**
¼ cup dried apricots
1 cup flavored yogurt (chocolate)

## Sample Menus for a 2000 Calorie Food Pattern

**Average amounts for weekly menu:**

| Food group | Daily average over 1 week |
|---|---|
| **GRAINS** | **6.2 oz eq** |
| Whole grains | 3.8 |
| Refined grains | 2.4 |
| **VEGETABLES** | **2.6 cups** |
| Vegetable subgroups (amount per week) | |
| Dark green | 1.6 cups per week |
| Red/Orange | 5.6 |
| Starchy | 5.1 |
| Beans and Peas | 1.6 |
| Other Vegetables | 4.1 |
| **FRUITS** | **2.1 cups** |
| **DAIRY** | **3.1 cups** |
| **PROTEIN FOODS** | **5.7 oz eq** |
| Seafood | 8.8 oz per week |
| **OILS** | **29 grams** |
| **CALORIES FROM ADDED FATS AND SUGARS** | 245 calories |

| Nutrient | Daily average over 1 week |
|---|---|
| Calories | 1975 |
| Protein | 96 g |
| Protein | 19% kcal |
| Carbohydrate | 275 g |
| Carbohydrate | 56% kcal |
| Total fat | 59 g |
| Total fat | 27% kcal |
| Saturated fat | 13.2 g |
| Saturated fat | 6.0% kcal |
| Monounsaturated fat | 25 g |
| Polyunsaturated fat | 16 g |
| Linoleic Acid | 13 g |
| Alpha-linolenic Acid | 1.8 g |
| Cholesterol | 201 mg |
| Total dietary fiber | 30 g |
| Potassium | 4701 mg |
| Sodium | 1810 mg |
| Calcium | 1436 mg |
| Magnesium | 468 mg |
| Copper | 2.0 mg |
| Iron | 18 mg |
| Phosphorus | 1885 mg |
| Zinc | 14 mg |
| Thiamin | 1.6 mg |
| Riboflavin | 2.5 mg |
| Niacin Equivalents | 24 mg |
| Vitamin B6 | 2.4 mg |
| Vitamin B12 | 12.3 mcg |
| Vitamin C | 146 mg |
| Vitamin E | 11.8 mg (AT) |
| Vitamin D | 9.1 mcg |
| Vitamin A | 1090 mcg (RAE) |
| Dietary Folate Equivalents | 530 mcg |
| Choline | 386 mg |

ILLUSTRATION 1.13 ▸ ChooseMyPlate.gov sample menus and food group and nutrient analysis report for a 2,000-calorie food pattern.

SOURCE: www.choosemyplate.gov/food-groups /downloads /Sample_Menus-2000Cals-DG2010.pdf general ideas about the types of foods to include in meals on a daily basis.

**USDA's Interactive Diet Planning Tools** Want to lose weight? Learn about healthful foods for your preschooler or when you are pregnant? Look up information on the calorie value of different foods or keep track of your food intake? You can access this information and more on the website ChooseMyPlate.gov. To help lose weight, for example, access the "Daily Food Plan" interactive tool. This feature can be used to identify the amount of each food group you should consume daily to gradually move toward a healthier weight (Illustration 1.13). An allowance for teaspoons of oil, and an "empty calorie" allowance for extra fats and sugars are included in the Daily Food Plan results.

Access "Super Tracker" and an analysis of your calorie and nutrient intake will be generated based on your age, weight, height, and physical activity level. You can save and update this information to track your progress toward meeting healthier goals.

**The DASH Diet** This is a well-established healthy dietary pattern that has been described in detail. The pattern served as the basis for the development of the Healthy U.S.-Style Dietary Pattern. Originally published as a diet that helps control mild and moderate high blood pressure in experimental studies, the DASH Diet also reduces the risk of some types of cancer, osteoporosis, and heart disease. Improvements in blood pressure are generally seen within two weeks of starting this dietary pattern.[70]

The DASH dietary pattern emphasizes fruits, vegetables, low-fat dairy foods, whole-grain products, poultry, fish, and nuts. Only low amounts of animal fat, red meats, sweets, and sugar-containing beverages are included. This dietary pattern provides ample amounts of potassium, magnesium, calcium, fiber, and protein and limited amounts of saturated and *trans* fats. Recommendations for types and amounts of food included in this eating plan for a 2,000-calorie diet are shown in Table 1.25.

TABLE 1.25 ▸ A DASH eating plan for a 2,000-calorie diet

| FOOD GROUP | DAILY SERVINGS (EXCEPT AS NOTED) | SERVING SIZES |
|---|---|---|
| Grains & grain products | 7–8 | 1 slice bread<br>1 cup ready-to-eat cereal*<br>cup cooked rice, pasta, or cereal |
| Vegetables | 4–5 | 1 cup raw leafy vegetable<br>cup cooked vegetable<br>6 ounces vegetable juice |
| Fruits | 4–5 | 1 medium fruit<br>cup dried fruit<br>cup fresh, frozen, or canned fruit<br>6 oz fruit juice |
| Low-fat or fat free dairy foods | 2–3 | 8 oz milk<br>1 cup yogurt<br>1 ounce cheese |
| Lean meats, poultry, and fish | 2 or less | 3 oz cooked lean meats, skinless poultry, or fish |
| Nuts, seeds, and dry beans | 4–5 per week | ⅓ cup or 1 oz nuts<br>1 Tbsp or 1 oz seeds<br>½ cup cooked dry beans |
| Fats & oils** | 2–3 | 1 tsp soft margarine<br>1 Tbsp low-fat mayonnaise<br>2 Tbsp light salad dressing<br>1 tsp vegetable oil |
| Sweets | 5 per week | 1 Tbsp sugar<br>1 Tbsp jelly or jam<br>ounce jelly beans<br>8 oz lemonade |

*Serving sizes vary. Check the product's nutrition label.

**Fat content changes serving counts for fats and oils: For example, 1 Tbsp of regular salad dressing equals 1 serving; 1 Tbsp of a low-fat dressing equals 1 serving; 1 Tbsp of a fat free dressing equals 0 servings.

SOURCE: Dietary Guidelines for Americans, Appendix A-1: The DASH Eating Plan at 1,600-, 2,000-, 2,600-, and 3,100- Caloric Levels (www.health.gov/dietaryguidelines/dga2005/document/pdf/Appendix_A.pdf).

## REVIEW QUESTIONS

1. Nutrition is defined as "the study of foods, their nutrients and other chemical constituents, and the effects that food constituents have on health."
   _____True _____False
2. The word *nonessential,* as in *nonessential nutrient,* means that the nutrient is *not* required for growth and health.
   _____True _____False
3. Nutrients are classified into five basic groups: carbohydrates, protein, fats, vitamins, and water.
   _____True _____False
4. Tissue stores of nutrients decline after blood levels of the nutrients decline.
   _____True _____False
5. An individual's genetic traits play a role in how nutrient intake affects disease risk.
   _____True _____False
6. Groups of people at higher risk than others of becoming inadequately nourished include _______ and ______.
7. Almost all multiple-ingredient foods must be labeled with nutrition information.
   _____True _____False
8. In general, % DV of 10 percent or more listed for nutrients in Nutrition Facts panels are considered "low," and those listed as 50 percent or more are considered "high."
   _____True _____False
9. An overriding principle of nutrition labeling regulations is that nutrient content and health claims made about a food on the packaging must be truthful.
   _____True _____False
10. The term *enriched* on a food label means that extra vitamins and minerals have been added to the food to bolster its nutritional value.
    _____True _____False
11. _____ You see a yogurt product at the grocery store labeled "fat free." This nutrient content claim means that a standard serving of the yogurt contains:
    a. No fat, or negligible amounts of fat
    b. No, or negligible amounts of, fat, *trans* fat, and sodium
    c. Fewer than 10 grams of fat and 4.5 grams of saturated fat
    d. Three grams of fat or less
12. Healthy individuals require the same nutrients throughout life, but the amounts of nutrients needed vary based on age, growth, and development.
    _____True _____False
13. Iron deficiency during childhood may decrease a child's ability to learn early in life but does not have a lasting affect on intellectual capacity.
    _____True _____False
14. The primary components of individual-level nutrition assessment consist of visual physical assessment, food frequency questionnaire administration, body weight measurement, and a blood draw.
    _____True _____False
15. Semiquantitative measures of dietary assessment provide good enough estimates of dietary intake to rank individuals by their food and nutrient intakes. Quantitative dietary assessment methods are needed to evaluate an individual's dietary intake.
    _____True _____False
16. The Supplemental Nutrition Assistance Program (SNAP), formerly called the "Food Stamp Program," subsidizes food purchases of low-income families.
    _____True _____False
17. Individuals participating in the WIC program have one or more nutritional risk factors.
    _____True _____False

Questions 18–20 refer to the following case scenario:

Assume you are attending a family picnic and are staring at a table full of food. Your choices from the table are: fried chicken, cold-cut platter (bologna, salami), whole grain rolls, shrimp, jello, spinach salad, fruit salad, baked beans, potato chips, zucchini squash, cake, and low-fat milk.

18. _____ From the food options available, which three foods would you put on your plate if you wanted to consume the basic foods?
    a. fried chicken, fruit salad, and baked beans
    b. zucchini squash, jello, and baked beans
    c. spinach salad, cold cuts, and shrimp
    d. spinach salad, zucchini squash, and shrimp
19. _____ Which of the following sets of foods would *not* be considered basic foods?
    a. potato chips and cold cuts
    b. cake and spinach salad
    c. jello and fruit salad
    d. fried chicken and zucchini squash
20. _____ You decide to have a glass of milk along with shrimp, fruit salad, baked beans, and spinach salad. Which basic food group is missing from your plate?
    a. vegetables c. grains
    b. fruits d. protein foods

**Visit www.cengagebrain.com to access MindTap, a complete digital course that includes additional resources.**

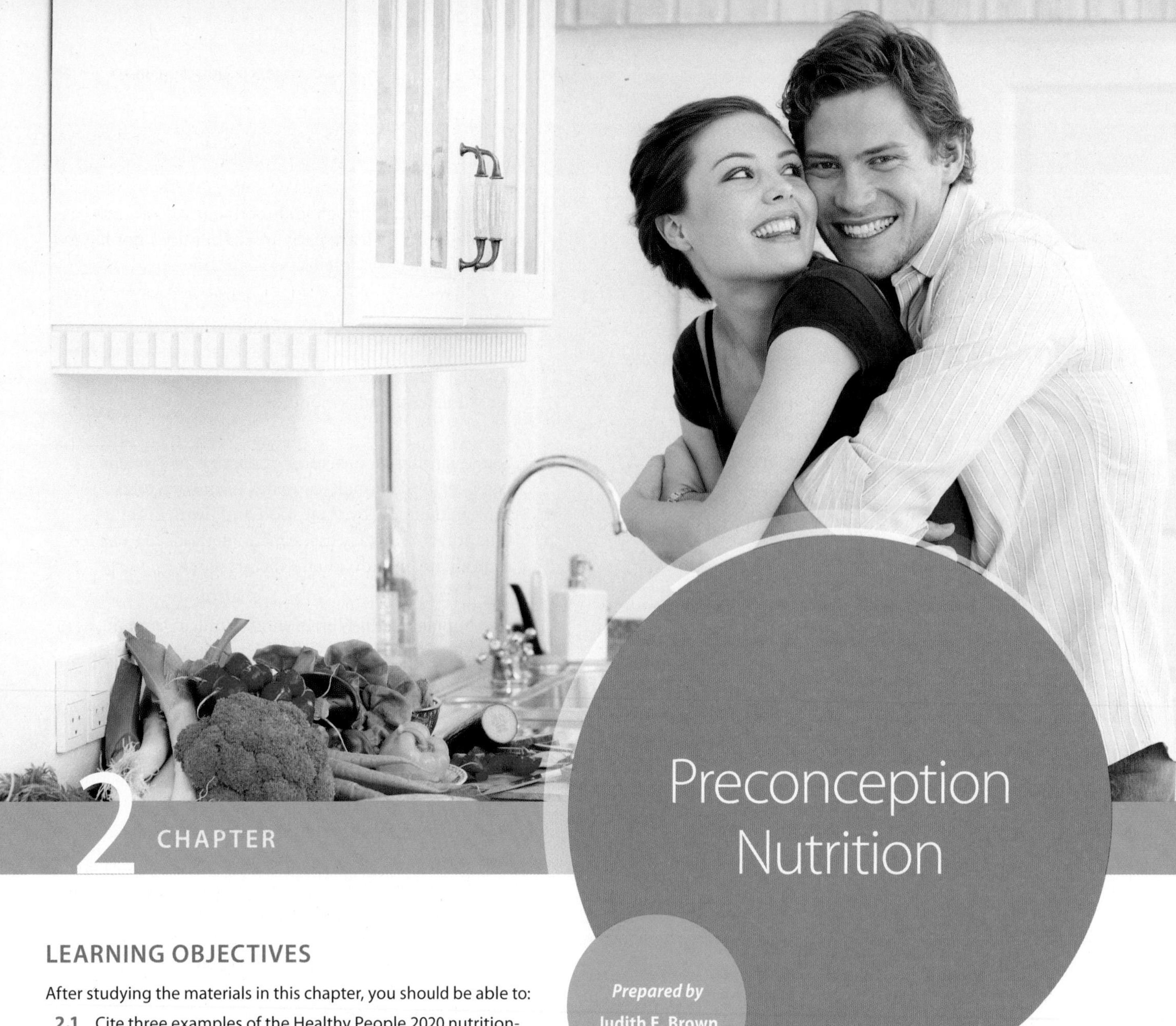

# 2 CHAPTER Preconception Nutrition

*Prepared by*
**Judith E. Brown**

## LEARNING OBJECTIVES

After studying the materials in this chapter, you should be able to:

**2.1** Cite three examples of the Healthy People 2020 nutrition-related objectives for the preconception period.

**2.2** Identify six major hormones involved in the regulation of male and female fertility processes, and identify their source and effects on the regulation of fertility processes.

**2.3** Describe the potential effects of nutrition-related factors such as body fat content, iron status, and alcohol intake on fertility in females and males.

**2.4** Cite four examples of relationships between nutrient intake and nutritional status during the periconceptional period and the outcome of pregnancy.

**2.5** Develop a one-day menu for a preconceptional woman and a man based on the ChooseMyPlate.gov food guidance materials.

**2.6** Identify three nutrition-related consequences that may be related to the use of combination hormonal contraceptives, and a consequence that is related to the use of estrogen or progestin contraceptives only.

**2.7** Cite three important nutrition-related components of preconceptional health care.

**2.8** Describe the four steps of the Nutrition Care Process.

# Introduction

Human reproduction is the result of a superb orchestration of complex and interrelated genetic, biological, environmental, and behavioral processes.[1] In healthy individuals these processes occur smoothly for females and males, and set the stage for successful reproduction. However, in less than healthy individuals, brought about by conditions such as acute undernutrition or high levels of alcohol intake, for example, can disrupt these finely tuned processes and diminish reproductive capacity. Sometimes conception occurs in the presence of poor nutritional or health status. Such events increase the likelihood that fetal growth and development, the health of the mother during pregnancy, and the future health of the offspring, will be compromised.[2,3]

This chapter first highlights vital statistics related to the preconception period and presents background information on reproductive physiology. Then the focus turns to the effects of nutrition on fertility, the importance of nutritional factors during the periconceptional period, preconceptional nutritional status and the course and outcome of pregnancy, dietary recommendations for preconception, nutritional effects of contraceptives, and model programs that promote preconceptional nutritional health. The chapter ends with an overview and case study related to the "Nutrition Care Process," an emerging system for the delivery of nutrition services to individuals before pregnancy and to others. The following chapter addresses the role of nutrition in specific conditions—such as premenstrual syndrome, diabetes, eating disorders, obesity, celiac disease, and polycystic ovary syndrome—that affect preconceptional health and fertility.

# Preconception Overview

LO 2.1 Cite three examples of the Healthy People 2020 nutrition-related objectives for the preconception period.

About 15 percent of all couples fail to conceive within 12 months of attempting pregnancy.[4] They are generally considered to be ***infertile***, or more correctly ***infecund. Fertility*** refers to the actual production of children, whereas ***fecundity*** addresses the biological capacity to bear children. The actual production of children within population groups is assessed as the fertility rate, or the number of births per 1000 women of childbearing age (15–44 years in most statistical reports). For example, in 2013 the fertility rate in the United States was 62.5 births per 1000 women aged 15 to 44 years.[5] Even scientists and clinicians rarely use these terms correctly, however, so to avoid confusion, the familiar meanings of *fertility* and *infertility* are used in this chapter.

Infertility is generally defined as the lack of conception after 1 year of unprotected intercourse. This definition leads to a "yes/no" answer about fertility that is misleading. Approximately 44 percent of couples qualifying as infertile will eventually conceive a child without the help of fertility treatments.[6] Chances of conception decrease the longer infertility lasts as women and men age beyond 35 years.[7]

Healthy couples having regular, unprotected intercourse have a 20–25 percent chance of a diagnosed pregnancy within a given menstrual cycle.[8] However, many more conceptions probably occur. Studies show that 30–50 percent of conceptions are lost by resorption into the uterine wall within the first 6 weeks after conception. Another 9 percent are lost by ***miscarriage*** in the first 20 weeks of pregnancy.[9] The most common known cause of miscarriage is the presence of a severe defect in the ***fetus***. Miscarriages can also be caused by maternal infection, structural abnormalities of the uterus, ***endocrine*** or ***immunological*** disturbances, and unknown, random events.[10]

Women who experience multiple miscarriages (variously defined as two or three), men who have sperm abnormalities (such as low sperm count or density, malformed sperm, or immobile sperm), and women who ovulate infrequently are considered ***subfertile***. It is estimated that 18 percent of married couples in the United States are subfertile due to delayed time to conception (over 12 months) or repeated pregnancy losses.[11] A silver lining to subfertility is that the reproductive capacity of one individual can compensate for diminished potential in the other. In addition, subfertility can be diminished by improvements in diet, weight status, and lifestyle.[6]

## 2020 Nutrition Objectives for the Nation Related to Preconception

National priorities for improvement in health status during the preconception period include those related to nutrition (Table 2.1). The objectives

**infertility** Involuntary absence of production of children.

**infecundity** Biological inability to bear children after one year of unprotected intercourse.

**fertility** Actual production of children. The word best applies to specific vital statistic rates, but it is commonly taken to mean the ability to bear children.

**fecundity** Biological ability to bear children.

**miscarriage** Generally defined as the loss of a conceptus in the first 20 weeks of pregnancy. Also called spontaneous abortion.

**fetus** The developing organism from 8 weeks after conception to the moment of birth.

**endocrine** A system of ductless glands, such as the thyroid, adrenal glands, ovaries, and testes, that produces secretions that affect body functions.

**immunological** Having to do with the immune system and its functions in protecting the body from bacterial, viral, fungal, or other infections and from foreign proteins (i.e., those proteins that differ from proteins normally found in the body).

**subfertility** Reduced level of fertility characterized by unusually long time to conception (over 12 months) or repeated pregnancy losses.

TABLE 2.1 ▸ Healthy People 2020 nutrition-related objectives for the nation for preconception[116]

- Increase the proportion of women who are at a healthy weight prior to pregnancy by 10%.
- Reduce the proportion of women aged 18 to 44 years who have impaired fecundity by 10%.
- Reduce the proportion of men aged 18 to 44 years who have impaired fecundity by 10%.
- Increase the proportion of women who did not drink alcohol prior to pregnancy by 10%.
- Reduce iron deficiency among females of childbearing age by 10%.
- Increase the proportion of women of childbearing potential with intake of at least 400 mcg of folic acid from fortified foods or dietary supplements by 10%.
- Reduce the proportion of women of childbearing potential who have low red cell folate concentrations by 10%.
- Increase the proportion of women delivering a live birth who received preconception care services and practiced key recommended preconception health behaviors by 10%.



represent priority problem areas that focus policy development and program and service initiatives at the local, state, and national levels. Progress in meeting the health objectives for the nation is monitored on a regular basis.

# Reproductive Physiology

LO 2.2 Identify six major hormones involved in the regulation of male and female fertility processes, and identify their source and effects on the regulation of fertility processes.

The reproductive systems of females and males (Illustration 2.1) begin developing in the first months after conception and continue to grow in size and complexity of function through ***puberty.*** Females are born with a complement of immature ***ova*** and males with sperm-producing capabilities. The capacity for reproduction is established during puberty when hormonal changes cause the maturation of the reproductive system over the course of 3–5 years.

Approximately 7 million immature ova, or *primordial follicles,* are formed during early fetal development, but only about one-half million per ovary remain by the onset of puberty. During a woman's fertile years, some 400–500 ova will mature and be released for possible fertilization. Due to losses in viable ova over time, very few remain by ***menopause.*** For men, sperm numbers and viability decrease somewhat after approximately 35 years of age, but sperm are produced from puberty until death. For both men and women, the quality of eggs and sperm decrease somewhat with age as damage to these cells' DNA accumulates.[10]

## Female Reproductive System

During puberty females develop monthly ***menstrual cycles,*** the purpose of which is to prepare an ovum for fertilization by sperm and the uterus for implantation of a fertilized egg. Menstrual cycles result from complex interactions among hormones secreted by the ***hypothalamus*** the ***pituitary gland,*** and the ovary. This section focuses on the nutritional effects on hormonal changes in the menstrual cycle and on fertility.

Menstrual cycles tend to 26–29 days long, but it is not uncommon for cycles to be several days shorter or longer. About 12% of cycles are the commonly self-reported 28 days long. Length of cycles vary from cycle-to-cycle and with increasing age.[11] The first day of the cycle is when menses, or blood flow, begins. The first half of the cycle is called the *follicular phase;* the last 14 days is the *luteal phase.* (Illustration 2.2.)

**Hormonal Effects During the Menstrual Cycle** At the beginning of the follicular phase, estrogen stimulates the hypothalamus to secrete *gonadotropin-releasing hormone* (GnRH), which causes the pituitary gland to release the *follicle-stimulating hormone* (FSH) and *luteinizing hormone* (LH). (See Table 2.2.) FSH prompts the growth and maturation of 6 to 20 follicles, or capsules in the surface of the ovary in which ova mature. The presence of FSH stimulates the production of *estrogen* by cells within the follicles. Estrogen and FSH further stimulate the growth and maturation of follicles while rising LH levels cause cells within the follicles to secrete *progesterone.* Estrogen and progesterone also prompt the uterine wall (or endometrium) to store glycogen and other nutrients and to expand the growth of blood vessels and connective tissue. These changes prepare the uterus for nourishing a conceptus

**puberty** The period in life during which humans become biologically capable of reproduction.

**ova** Eggs of the female produced and stored within the ovaries (singular is *ovum*).

**menopause** Cessation of the menstrual cycle and reproductive capacity in females.

**menstrual cycle** An approximately 4-week interval in which hormones direct a build up of blood and nutrient stores within the wall of the uterus and ovum maturation and release. If the ovum is fertilized by a sperm, the stored blood and nutrients are used to support the growth of the fertilized ovum. If fertilization does not occur, they are released from the uterine wall over a period of 3 to 7 days. The period of blood flow is called the *menses,* or the menstrual period.

**hypothalamus** A section of the brain responsible for the production of many hormones and other chemical substances that affect body functions such as temperature regulation, thirst, hunger, sleep, mood, reproduction, and the release of other hormones within the body.

**pituitary gland** A pea-sized gland located at the base of the brain. It is connected to the hypothalamus and produces and secretes growth hormone, prolactin, oxytocin, follicle-stimulating hormone, luteinizing hormone, and other hormones in response to signals from the hypothalamus.

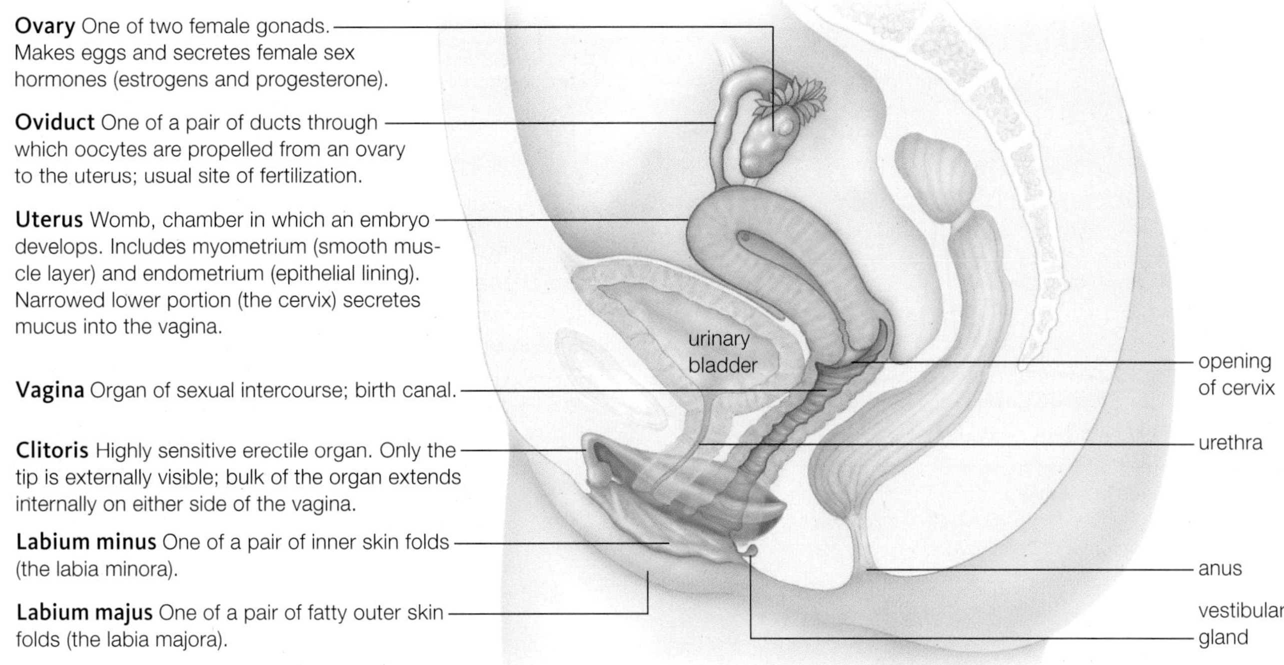


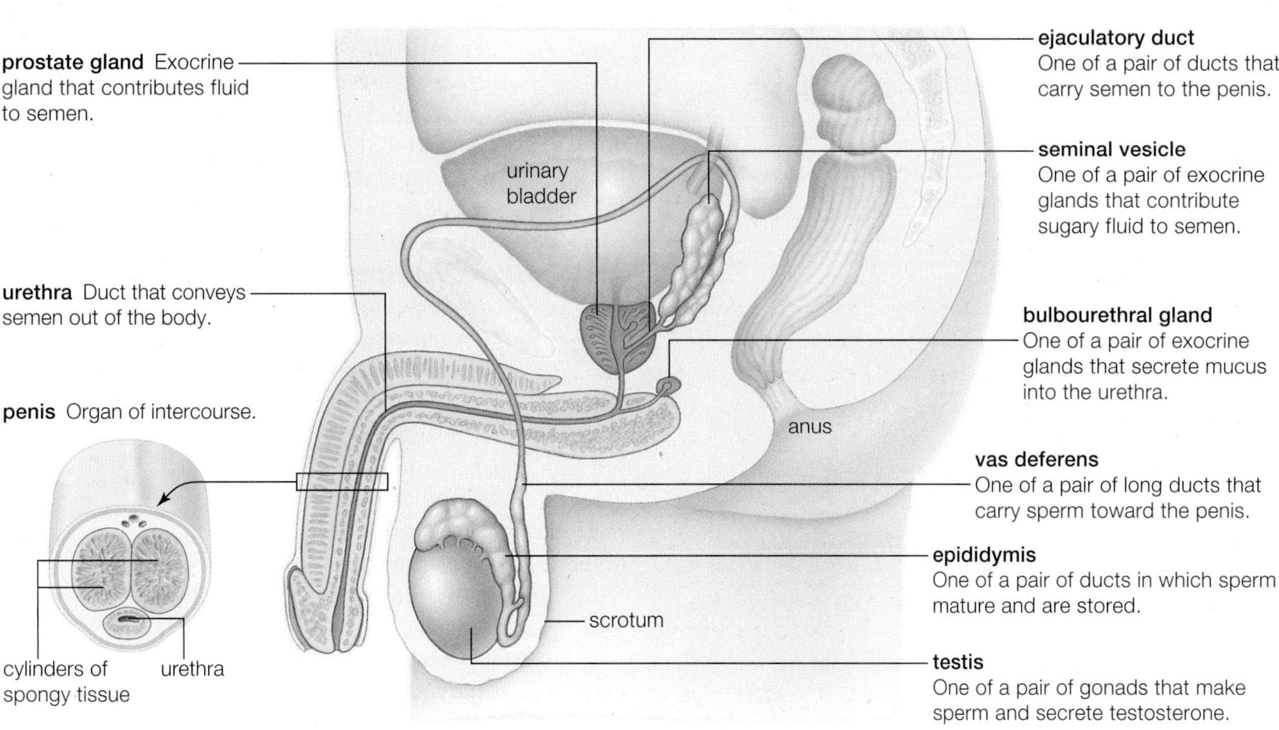


ILLUSTRATION 2.1 ▸ Mature (a) female and (b) male reproductive systems.

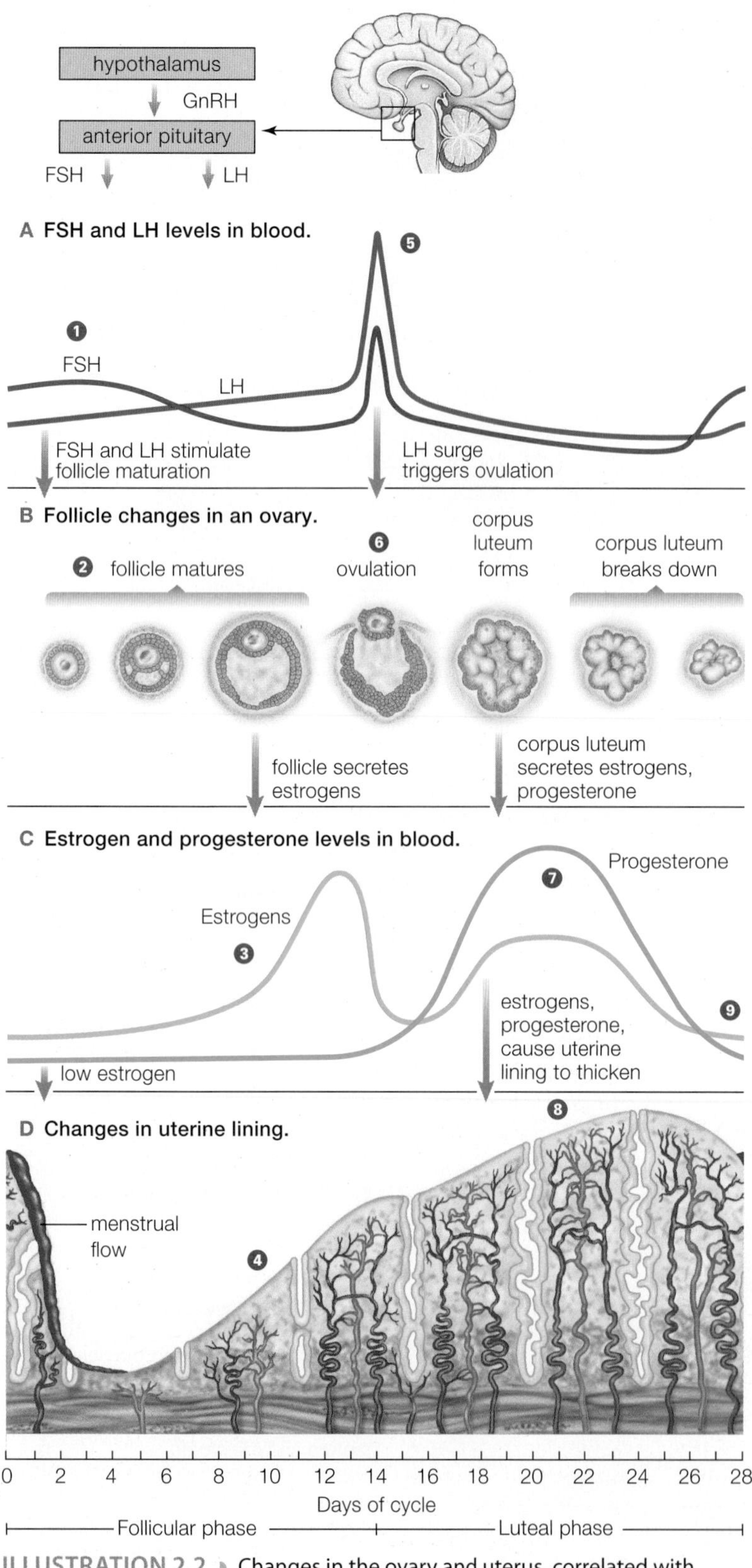


ILLUSTRATION 2.2 ▸ Changes in the ovary and uterus, correlated with changing hormone levels during the follicular and luteal phases of the menstrual cycle.

after implantation. Just prior to ovulation, which usually occurs on day 14 of a 28-day menstrual cycle, blood levels of FSH and LH peak. The surge in LH level results in the release of an ovum from a follicle, and voilà! Ovulation occurs.

The luteal phase of the menstrual cycle begins after ovulation. Much of the hormonal activity that regulates biological processes during this half of the cycle is initiated by the cells in the follicle left behind when the egg was released. These cells grow in number and size and form the ***corpus luteum*** from the original follicle. The corpus luteum secretes large amounts of progesterone and some estrogen. These hormones now inhibit the production of GnRH, and thus the secretion of FSH and LH. Without sufficient FSH and LH, ova within follicles do not mature and are not released. (This is also how estrogen and progesterone in some birth control pills inhibit ova maturation and release.) Estrogen and progesterone secreted by the corpus luteum further stimulate the development of the endometrium. If the ovum is not fertilized, the production of hormones by the corpus luteum declines, and blood levels of progesterone and estrogen fall. This decline removes the inhibitory effect of these hormones on GnRH release, and GnRH is again able to stimulate release of FSH for the next cycle of follicle development, and of LH for the stimulation of progesterone and estrogen production. Decreased levels of progesterone and estrogen also cause blood vessels in the uterine wall to constrict, allowing the uterine wall to release its outer layer in the *menstrual flow*. Cramps and other side effects of menstruation can be traced to the production of ***prostaglandins*** by the uterus. These substances cause the uterus to contract and release the blood and nutrients stored in the uterine wall.

**corpus luteum** (*corpus* = body, *luteum* = yellow) A tissue about 12 mm in diameter formed from the follicle that contained the ovum prior to its release. It produces estrogen and progesterone. The "yellow body" derivation comes from the accumulation of lipid precursors of these hormones in the corpus luteum.

**prostaglandins** A group of physiologically active substances derived from the essential fatty acids. They are present in many tissues and perform such functions as the constriction or dilation of blood vessels and stimulation of smooth muscles and the uterus.

TABLE 2.2 ▸ Hormones that regulate fertility processes

| HORMONE | ABBREVIATION | SOURCE | ACTION |
|---|---|---|---|
| Gonadotropin-releasing hormone | GnRH | Hypothalamus | Stimulates release of FSH and LH |
| Follicle-stimulating hormone | FSH | Pituitary | Stimulates ovarian follicle growth and maturation, estrogen secretion, and endometrial changes characteristic of the first portion of the menstrual cycle in females. It stimulates sperm production in males. |
| Luteinizing hormone | LH | Pituitary | Stimulates ovulation, the development of the corpus luteum (which secretes progesterone), and the production of testosterone in males. |
| Estrogen (most abundant form is estradiol) | | Ovaries, testes, fat cells, corpus luteum, and placenta (during pregnancy) | Stimulates release of GnRH in follicular phase and inhibits in luteal phase; stimulates thickening of uterine wall during menstrual cycle |
| Progesterone (progestin, progestogen, and gestagon are similar) | | Ovaries and placenta | "Progestational," it prepares uterus for fertilized ovum and to maintain a pregnancy; stimulates uterine lining buildup during menstrual cycle; helps stimulate cell division of fertilized ova; inhibits action of testosterone |
| Testosterone | | Mostly by the testes, ovaries | Stimulates maturation of male sex organs and sperm, formation of muscle tissue, and other functions |

If the ovum is fertilized, it will generally implant in the lining of the uterus within 8 to 10 days. Hormones secreted by the dividing, fertilized egg signal the corpus luteum to increase in size and to continue to produce enough estrogen and progesterone to maintain the nutrient and blood vessel supply in the endometrium. The corpus luteum ceases to function within the first few months of pregnancy, when it is no longer needed for hormone production.

## Male Reproductive System

Reproductive capacity in males is established by complex interactions among the hypothalamus, pituitary gland, and ***testes.*** The process in males is ongoing rather than cyclic. Fluctuating levels of GnRH signal the release of FSH and LH, which trigger the production of testosterone (Table 2.2) by the testes. Testosterone and other ***androgens*** stimulate the maturation of sperm, which takes 70–80 days. When mature, sperm are transported to the ***epididymis*** for storage. Upon ejaculation, sperm mix with secretions from the testes, seminal vesicle, prostate, and bulbourethral gland to form ***semen.*** Just as some aspects of female reproductive processes remain unclear, scientists have yet to fully elucidate hormonal and other processes involved in male reproduction.

**Sources of Disruptions in Fertility** The intricate mechanisms that regulate fertility can be disrupted by many factors, including adverse nutritional exposures, severe stress, infection, tubal damage and other structural problems, and chromosomal abnormalities (Table 2.3).[2,4,12-15] Conditions that modify fertility appear to affect hormones that regulate ovulation, the presence or length of the luteal phase, sperm production, or the tubular passageways that ova and sperm must travel for conception to occur. Sexually transmitted infections, for example, can result in ***pelvic inflammatory disease (PID),*** which may lead to scarring and blockage of the fallopian tubes.[16] ***Endometriosis*** is also a common cause of reduced fertility. It develops when portions of the endometrial wall that build up during menstrual cycles leave the uterus and become embedded within other body tissues.[17] Endocrine abnormalities that modify hormonal regulation of fertility are the leading diagnoses related to infertility. "Unknown cause" is the next most common diagnosis, applied to about 10% of all cases of male and female infertility.[12,18]

**testes** Male reproductive glands located in the scrotum. Also called testicles.

**androgens** Types of steroid hormones produced in the testes, ovaries, and adrenal cortex from cholesterol. Some androgens (testosterone, dihydrotestosterone) stimulate development and functioning of male sex organs.

**epididymis** Tissues on top of the testes that store sperm.

**semen** The penile ejaculate containing a mixture of sperm and secretions from the testes, prostate, and other glands. It is rich in zinc, fructose, and other nutrients. Also called seminal fluid.

**pelvic inflammatory disease (PID)** A general term applied to infections of the cervix, uterus, fallopian tubes, or ovaries. Occurs predominantly in young women and is generally caused by infection with a sexually transmitted disease, such as gonorrhea or Chlamydia.

**endometriosis** A disease characterized by the presence of endometrial tissue in abnormal locations, such as deep within the uterine wall, in the ovary, or in other sites within the body. The condition is quite painful and is associated with abnormal menstrual cycles and infertility in 30–40 percent of affected women.

TABLE 2.3 ▸ Factors related to altered fertility in women and men[2,4,12,13–15]

| FEMALES AND MALES | FEMALES | MALES |
|---|---|---|
| • Weight loss >10 to 15% of normal weight<br>• Inadequate antioxidant status (selenium, vitamins C and E)<br>• Inadequate body fat<br>• Excessive body fat, especially central fat<br>• Extreme levels of exercise<br>• High alcohol intake<br>• Endocrine disorders (e.g., hypothyroidism, Cushing's disease)<br>• Structural abnormalities of the reproductive tract<br>• Chromosomal abnormalities in sperm and eggs<br>• Celiac disease<br>• Oxidative stress and chronic inflammation<br>• Severe psychological stress<br>• Infection (sexually transmitted diseases)<br>• Diabetes, cancer, other disorders<br>• Some medications | • Recent oral contraceptive use (within 2 months)<br>• Anorexia nervosa, bulimia nervosa<br>• Vegan diets<br>• Age >35 years<br>• Metabolic syndrome<br>• Pelvic inflammatory disease (PID)<br>• Endometriosis<br>• Polycystic ovary syndrome<br>• Poor iron stores<br>• High-fiber diet | • Inadequate zinc status<br>• Heavy metal exposure (lead, mercury, cadmium, manganese)<br>• Halogen (in some pesticides) and glycol (in antifreeze, de-icers) exposure<br>• Estrogen exposure (in DDT, PCBs)<br>• Sperm defects (quality, motility)<br>• Excessive heat to testes<br>• Steroid abuse<br>• High intake of soy foods |

# Nutrition and Fertility

LO 2.3 Describe the potential effects of nutrition-related factors such as body fat content, iron status, and alcohol intake on fertility in females and males.

In the past few decades there has been an explosion in research reports related to the effects of nutrition and other lifestyle factors on fertility. Nutrition and lifestyles are now viewed as core components of the prevention and treatment of many cases of infertility.

Nutrient intake from food and dietary supplements, calorie intake, and body fat affect fertility primarily by (1) altering the environment in which eggs and sperm develop, and (2) modifying levels of hormones involved in reproductive processes.[12,19] Nutrient intake and body fat before conception also influence the mother's health during pregnancy and the growth and development of the fetus. Nutritional factors generally exert a temporary influence on fertility; normal fertility returns once the problem is corrected.

## Undernutrition and Fertility

Undernutrition among previously well-nourished women is associated with a dramatic decline in fertility that recovers when food intake does.[18,20] Food shortages in Europe in the seventeenth and eighteenth centuries were accompanied by dramatic declines in birth rates. Famine in Holland during World War II that led to calorie intakes of about 1,000 per day among women was associated with a 50 percent decline in fertility and a 53 percent decrease in birth rate. Fertility status improved within 4 months after the end of the famine, but for many women it took as long as a year for their menstrual cycles to return to normal. Similarly, the 1974–1975 famine in Bangladesh resulted in a 40 percent decline in births.[21] More recent evidence indicates that relatively short periods of inadequate calorie intake or weight loss may temporarily decrease fertility in some women.[2,22]

## Body Fat and Fertility

Excessive and inadequate levels of body fat are related to declines in fertility in women and men. Fat cells produce estrogen, testosterone, and *leptin,* and their availability changes with body fat content. Changes in the availability of these hormones interfere with reproductive processes such as follicular development, ovulation, and sperm maturation and production.[13]

**Excessive Body Fat and Fertility** Obesity, or the existence of excessive body fat, is generally indicated by ***body mass index*** values over 30 kg/m$^2$. Most obese women and men are not infertile, but they are more likely to be subfertile than normal-weight individuals.[23,24] Obese women tend to have higher levels of estrogen, androgens, and leptin than nonobese

**leptin** A protein secreted by fat cells that, by binding to specific receptor sites in the hypothalamus, decreases appetite, increases energy expenditure, and stimulates gonadotropin secretion. Leptin levels are elevated by high, and reduced by low, levels of body fat.

**body mass index (BMI)** Weight in kg/height in m$^2$. BMIs < 18.5 are considered underweight, 18.5–24.9 normal weight, 25–29.9 overweight, and BMIs of 30 and higher obesity.

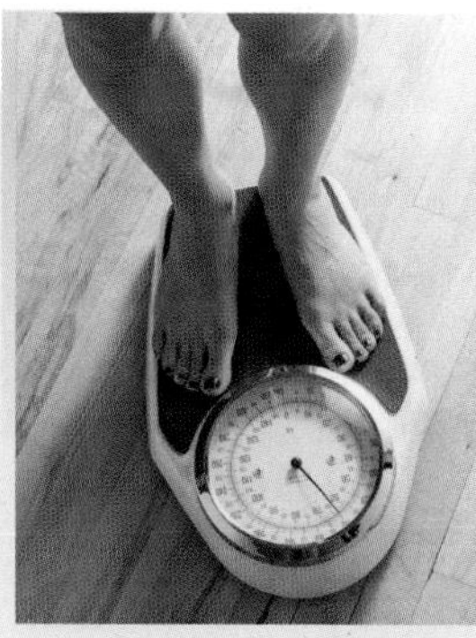
Duncan Smith/Photodisc/Getty Images

# CASE STUDY 2.1

## Cyclic Infertility with Weight Loss and Gain

After four years of experiencing amenorrhea, Tonya seeks medical care to help her become pregnant. She is convinced that her lack of menstrual periods is the cause of her infertility. Tonya's height is 5 feet 5 inches; her weight is 107 pounds, which she has maintained for 4 years (she previously weighed 121 pounds). Her FSH and LH levels are both abnormally low, and she is not ovulating. When the importance and methods of weight gain are explained to her, Tonya agrees to gain some weight. After she regains 7 pounds, her LH level is normal, but her FSH level is still low, and the luteal phase of her cycles is abnormally short. When her weight reaches 119 pounds, Tonya's LH and FSH levels, ovulation, and menstrual cycles are normal.

### Questions

1. Was Tonya underweight or normal weight based on her body mass index (BMI, kg/m$^2$) when she weighed 107 pounds?
2. Can you determine Tonya's body fat content based on her BMI?
3. Why isn't Tonya ovulating?
4. What likely happened to Tonya's average estrogen level when her weight decreased from 121 to 107 pounds?
5. What are two likely reasons Tonya was advised to gain weight to improve her chances of conception rather than being given Clomid or another ovulation-inducing drug?

women.[23,25] These hormonal changes favor the development of menstrual-cycle irregularity (it occurs in 30 to 47 percent of overweight and obese women), ovulatory failure and ***anovulatory cycles,*** and ***amenorrhea.***[12,24] Obesity in men is associated with lower levels of testosterone and increased estrogen and leptin levels.[26] These changes in hormonal status are related to reduced sperm production in 16 percent of obese men and higher-than-average rates of erectile dysfunction.[20] Loss of body fat is related to improvements in hormone levels, oxidative stress and chronic inflammation, and conception rates in both men and women.[23]

Approximately one in three men and women in the United States is obese, making subfertility related to excess body fat a common problem and an important health and quality-of-life concern.[27] The multiple and complex effects of obesity on fertility and early pregnancy are addressed in more detail in Chapter 3.

**Inadequate Body Fat and Fertility** It appears that a critical level of body fat (usually indicated by a body mass index over 20 kg/m$^2$) is needed to trigger and sustain normal reproductive functions in women.[12,28,29] Low levels of body fat during adolescence is related to delays in the age of onset of menstruation and to reduced fertility later in life. Impaired fertility in underweight women often takes the form of delayed time to conception and amenorrhea. Lowered libido and reduced sperm production have been identified in underweight men with low levels of body fat.[28,30]

**Weight Loss and Fertility in Normal-Weight Women and Men** In normal-weight women, weight loss that exceeds approximately 10–15 percent of usual weight decreases estrogen, LH, and FSH concentrations.[20,22,31] Consequences of these hormonal changes include amenorrhea, anovulatory cycles, and short or absent luteal phases. It is estimated that about 30 percent of cases of impaired fertility are related to simple weight loss. In the past, this form of amenorrhea was called *weight-related amenorrhea*. It is now called *hypothalamic amenorrhea*.[22] Hormone levels tend to return to normal when weight is restored to within 95 percent of previous weight.[20] Case Study 2.1 provides an example of the effect of weight loss on fertility.

Weight gain is the recommended first-line treatment for amenorrhea related to low body weight.[22] In many cases, however, the advice is more easily given than applied. About 10 percent of underweight women will not consider weight gain and may change health care providers in search of a different solution to infertility.[15]

Treatment of underweight women with Clomid (clomiphene citrate, a drug that induces ovulation) generally does not improve fertility until weight is gained.[22] Fertility may be improved through the use of GnRH, FSH, and other hormones. However, twice as many infants born to underweight women receiving such therapy are small for gestational age compared to infants born

**anovulatory cycles** Menstrual cycles in which ovulation does not occur.

**amenorrhea** Absence of menstrual cycle.

to underweight women who gain weight and experience unassisted conception.[20]

Weight loss decreases fertility in men just as it does in women. In the classic starvation experiments by Keys during World War II, men experiencing a 50 percent reduction in caloric intake reported substantially reduced sexual drive. Sperm viability and motility decreased as weight reached 10 to 15 percent below normal, and sperm production ceased entirely when weight loss exceeded 25 percent of normal weight. Sperm production and libido returned to normal after weight was regained.[30]

## Nutrient Status and Fertility

A growing body of evidence indicates that intake of ***antioxidants*** such as vitamin E, vitamin C, beta-carotene, selenium, and antioxidant-rich pigments in vegetables and fruits play important roles in fertility in women and men (Illustration 2.3).[32] Antioxidant nutrients are needed to protect cells of the reproductive system, including eggs and sperm, from damage due to oxidative stress. Oxidative stress occurs when the production of potentially destructive reactive oxygen molecules ***free radicals***) exceeds the body's own antioxidant defenses. Reactive oxygen molecules attack polyunsaturated fatty acids in sperm membranes, and that decreases sperm motility and reduces the ability of sperm to fuse with an egg. Once the membrane surrounding sperm is damaged, reactive oxygen molecules can enter the sperm cell and damage DNA. This can result in the passage of defective DNA on to the conceptus.[32,36,37] Oxidative stress is observed in approximately half of all infertile men.[34] In women, oxidative stress can harm egg and follicular development and can interfere with corpus luteum function and implantation of the egg in the uterine wall.[32,35]

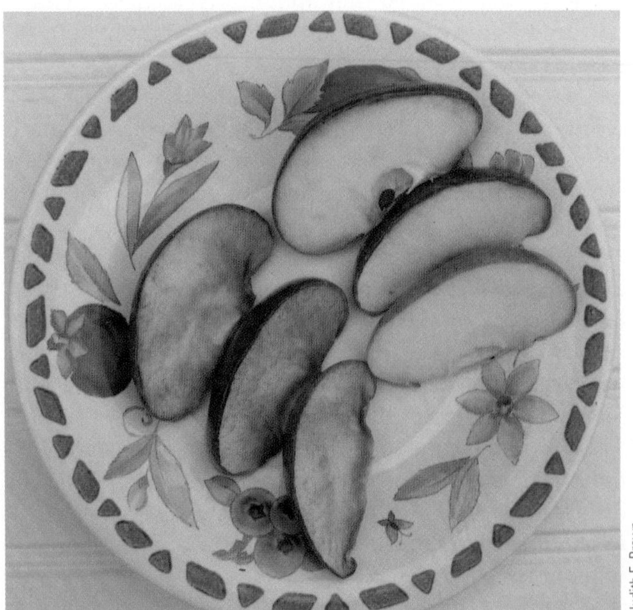


ILLUSTRATION 2.3 ▸ Apple slices exposed to air will turn brown due to oxidation reactions. The oxidation reactions are prevented if the slices are coated with a vitamin C–rich solution such as lemon juice.

**Antioxidant Status and Fertility** A number of studies have shown lower intakes of antioxidant nutrients in infertile than fertile women and men. Other studies have noted that higher average intakes of antioxidants are associated with improvements in levels of oxidative stress in infertile women and improved sperm maturation, motility, concentration, and reduced DNA and chromosome damage in men.[35–37] A number of studies addressing the effects of antioxidant supplements on fertility have been undertaken but due to weaknesses in study designs no reliable conclusions about the effects can be stated.[14,18] It appears that dietary sources of antioxidants and correction of specific deficiencies with nutrient supplements may be beneficial.[39–42]

**Zinc Status and Fertility in Men** Zinc plays important roles in the reduction of oxidative stress, sperm maturation, and testosterone synthesis. It has been investigated for its potential role in infertility. Zinc deficiency in men has been found to be related to poorer sperm quality and sperm concentrations, and to abnormal sperm shapes.[43–45] Although it is clear that zinc deficiency can impair normal reproductive functions, it is not clear that supplemental zinc improves fertility in the absence of zinc deficiency.[38,41]

**Soy Isoflavones and Fertility** Soy isoflavones are chemically similar to estrogen and are known to induce infertility in sheep consuming high amounts of soy.[46] In humans, regular intake of soy foods such as tofu, soymilk, tempeh, and textured soy protein is related to reduced sperm count in men[47] and decreased fertility in women.[48] Effects of high soy-food diets on fertility may be related to the influence of isoflavones on levels or the activity of estradiol, or possibly on other hormones such as progesterone and luteinizing hormone.[46,49]

**Iron Status and Fertility** Poor iron status prior to pregnancy is a fairly common problem in women of childbearing age and is related to reduced fertility. Between 9 and 16 percent of women of childbearing age in the United States have iron deficiency and 14 percent have low iron stores.[50,51] Results of a

**antioxidants** Chemical substances that prevent or repair damage to molecules and cells caused by oxidizing agents. Vitamins C (see Illustration 2.3) and E, selenium, and certain components of plants function as antioxidants.

**free radicals** Chemical substances (often oxygen-based) that are missing electrons. The absence of electrons makes the chemical substance reactive and prone to oxidizing nearby molecules by stealing electrons from them. Free radicals can damage lipids, cell membranes, DNA, and tissues by altering their chemical structure and functions. They also form as a normal part of metabolism. Over time, oxidative stress causes damage to lipids, cell membranes, DNA, cells, and tissues.

large prospective study of nurses indicate that infertility due to a lack of ovulation is related to iron intake. In this study, women who regularly used iron supplements and consumed plant sources of iron were 60 percent less likely to develop ovulatory infertility than women who did not. Mechanisms underlying the link between iron status and ovulation are not yet established.[52]

**Caffeine and Fertility** Should women concerned about infertility consume coffee and other beverages with caffeine? The evidence-based answer to the question is uncertain because study results are mixed.[55,56]

In a study of European women, researchers found that the chance of conception within a 10-month interval of unprotected intercourse was half as likely among women who consumed over 4 cups of coffee per day (500 mg caffeine) versus the conception rate of women who consumed a cup of coffee or less.[56] Another study reported that intake of over 300 mg of caffeine daily from coffee, sodas, and tea decreased the chance of conceiving by 27 percent per cycle compared to negligible caffeine intake.[57] In both studies, the effect of caffeine on time to conception was stronger in women who smoked. Other studies have failed to find effects of caffeine intake prior to pregnancy on the amount of time it takes to become pregnant, or indicators of ovarian function.[53,54]

Results of research on the effects of caffeine or coffee intake on fertility in women are conflicting, and overall effects are likely weak. Effects of coffee or caffeine consumption on fertility may be due to one or more of the hundreds of other biologically active substances in coffee, or to characteristics of women who consume lots of coffee and other sources of caffeine. Nonetheless, neither coffee nor caffeine are essential components of diets, and individuals who are concerned should likely not be dissuaded from cutting back on coffee or caffeine if they choose to do so (Table 2.4).

TABLE 2.4 ▸ Caffeine content of foods and beverages

| SOURCE | CAFFEINE (MG) |
|---|---|
| **Coffee, one cup** | |
| Drip | 115–175 |
| Decaffeinated (ground or instant) | 0.5–4.0 |
| Instant | 61–70 |
| Percolated | 97–140 |
| Espresso (2 oz) | 100 |
| **Tea, one cup** | |
| Black, brewed 5 minutes, U.S. brands | 32–144 |
| Black, brewed 5 minutes, imported brands | 40–176 |
| Green, brewed 5 minutes | 25 |
| Instant | 40–80 |
| **Soft drinks** | |
| Coca-Cola (12 oz) | 47 |
| Cherry Coke (12 oz) | 47 |
| Diet Coca-Cola (12 oz) | 47 |
| Dr. Pepper (12 oz) | 40 |
| Ginger ale (12 oz) | 0 |
| Mountain Dew (12 oz) | 54 |
| Pepsi-Cola (12 oz) | 38 |
| Diet Pepsi-Cola (12 oz) | 37 |
| 7-Up (12 oz) | 0 |
| **Energy drinks** | |
| Rockstar Energy Shot (2.5 oz) | 229 |
| Five-Hour Energy (2 oz) | 215 |
| Full Throttle (8 oz) | 210 |
| Ripped Force (8 oz) | 120 |
| Monster Energy (8 oz) | 92 |
| Red Bull (8 oz) | 80 |
| Full Throttle (8 oz) | 72 |
| Jolt (12 oz) | 72 |
| Surge (8 oz) | 35 |
| **Chocolate** | |
| Cocoa, chocolate milk, one cup | 10–17 |
| Milk chocolate candy, 1 oz | 1–15 |
| Chocolate syrup, one ounce (2 Tbsp) | 4 |



**Alcohol and Fertility** Alcohol intake has been found to affect fertility in men and women. In men, intakes of 5–25 drinks per week appear to increase testosterone levels and reduce sperm concentration, total sperm count, and the percent of sperm with normal shape.[4] In a study of 430 Danish couples attempting pregnancy for 6 months, consumption of from 1 to 5 alcohol-containing drinks per week by women was related to a 39 percent lower chance of conception. Consumption of over 10 alcoholic beverages per week was related to a 66 percent reduction in the probability of conception during the 6-month period.[58] Consumption of 7 or more drinks a week has been associated with a doubling of risk for infertility in women over the age of 30 only.[59] Individual genetic characteristics may be involved in the relationship between alcohol intake and fertility. Alcohol intake has been found to reduce fertility only in women with a specific ***gene variant*** that reduces the rate of alcohol breakdown in the body.[53]

**Heavy-Metal Exposure and Fertility** Exposure to high levels of lead is related to decreased sperm production and abnormal sperm motility and shape.[60] Inhaled or ingested lead is transported to the pituitary gland, where it appears to disrupt hormonal communications with the testes. The result is lowered testosterone levels and decreased sperm production and motility. The men most likely to be exposed to excess lead tend to be workers in smelting and battery factories.[61,62]

Exposure to excess levels of cadmium, molybdenum, manganese, boron, cobalt, copper, nickel, silver, or tin may also affect male fertility.[63,64] These metals may build up in male reproductive systems through the inhalation of fumes or dust

**Gene variant** An alteration in the normal sequence of a gene. The different forms of the same genes are considered "alleles."

TABLE 2.5 ▸ Estimates of the incidence of irregular or absent menstrual cycles in female athletes and sedentary women[31,66]

| | INCIDENCE OF IRREGULAR OR ABSENT MENSTRUAL CYCLES |
|---|---|
| Joggers (5 to 30 miles per week) | 23% |
| Runners (over 30 miles per week) | 34% |
| Long-distance runners (over 70 miles per week) | 43% |
| Competitive bodybuilders | 86% |
| Noncompetitive bodybuilders | 30% |
| Volleyball players | 48% |
| Ballet dancers | 44% |
| Sedentary women | 13% |

containing particles or through long-term use of dietary supplements, industrial pollution, or consumption of contaminated water.[64,65]

**Physical Activity and Fertility** The adverse effects of intense levels of physical activity on fertility were observed over 40 years ago in female competitive athletes. Since then, a number of studies have shown that young female athletes may experience delayed age of puberty and lack menstrual cycles. Average age of menarche for competitive female athletes and ballet dancers is often delayed by 2 to 4 years.[12] The delay in menarche increases if females begin training for events that require thinness (such as gymnastics) before menarche normally would begin. Very high levels of exercise can also interrupt previously established, normal menstrual cycles. The presence of abnormal cycles reportedly ranges from about 23 percent in joggers to 86 percent in female bodybuilders (Table 2.5).[31,66]

Delays and interruptions in normal menstrual cycles appear to result from hormonal and metabolic changes primarily related to caloric deficits rather than intense exercise.[12,67] Metabolic and hormonal status generally reverts to normal after high levels of training and caloric deficits end. Some of the hormones involved in fertility impairments perform other important functions in the body, which may also be disrupted. Reduced levels of estrogen that accompany low levels of body fat and amenorrhea, for example, may decrease bone density and increase the risk of shortness, bone fractures, and osteoporosis.[66,67]

# Nutrition During the Periconceptional Period

LO 2.4 Cite four examples of relationships between nutrient intake and nutritional status during the periconceptional period and the outcome of pregnancy.

The time around conception is considered the ***periconceptional period.*** It represents a critical period of time when nutritional and other exposures can impact conception, pregnancy maintenance, and the growth, development, and future health of the offspring.[2] It has been variously defined as one month before conception through three months after conception in a study of the effects of alcohol intake on outcomes, to three months prior to pregnancy to one month post-conception in an investigation of the effects of folic acid on outcomes.[68,69]

Most of the periconceptional period occurs before pregnancy is recognized or prenatal care has begun.[1] However, an extensive level of growth and development occurs within the early part of pregnancy. Approximately 8 to 10 days after an ovum is fertilized, it implants into the uterine wall. Within the first month after conception, the developing ***embryo*** will have grown from a single cell to millions of cells, basic structures of organs will have formed, and the blueprint for future growth and development will have been established.

Gene function in the embryo and fetus can be modified during early pregnancy by ***DNA methylation.*** Modifications in DNA functional status can affect growth, development, and disease risk later in life by a mechanism known as "metabolic programming."[70] Low-energy intakes during the periconceptional period due to food restriction, weight loss, eating disorders; or exposure to high amount of vitamin A in the form of retinol or retinoic acid from supplements or drugs used to treat acne for example, can modify gene functions in a developing embryo in ways that produce metabolic changes that influence the future health of the offspring (Table 2.6).[2,71,72] This chapter addressed the importance of adequate folate and iron intake during the periconceptional period, and Chapter 4 expands on the discussion of nutrition and fetal development.

## Periconceptional Folate Status

Folate status prior to conception is an important concern because inadequate folate very early in pregnancy is related to the development of approximately 50 percent of cases of ***neural tube defects (NTDs)***, such

**periconceptional period** The time period around conception, variously measured in weeks or months depending on the pregnancy outcomes of interest.

**embryo** The developing organism from conception through 8 weeks.

**DNA methylation** The modification of a replicated strand of DNA by addition of a methyl group ($CH_3$) to specific regions of the strand. Methylation can suppress the activity of certain genes in ways that affect metabolic processes and disease risk. It is a normal part of development and is needed for cellular differentiation and organ development but can also be influenced by nutritional and other environmental exposures.

**neural tube defects (NTDs)** A group of birth defects that are caused by incomplete development of the brain, spinal cord, or their protective coverings. Spina bifida is one of the most common types of neural tube defects.

TABLE 2.6 ▸ Periconceptional nutritional exposures that may disrupt fetal growth and development[2,71,93]

**Weight Status**

- Being underweight increases the risk of maternal complications during pregnancy and the delivery of small and early newborns.
- Obesity increases the risk of clinical complications during pregnancy and delivery of newborns with neural tube defects or excessive body fat.

**Nutrient Status**

- Excessive vitamin A intake (retinol, retinoic acid) increases the risk the fetus will develop facial and heart abnormalities.
- High maternal blood levels of lead increase the risk of intellectual disability in the offspring.
- Iodine deficiency early in pregnancy increases the risk that children will experience impaired mental and physical development.
- Iron deficiency increases the risk of early delivery and development of iron deficiency in the child within the first few years of life.

**Alcohol**

- Regular intake of alcohol increases the risk of *fetal alcohol syndrome* and *fetal alcohol effects*, both of which include impaired mental and physical development.

**Diabetes**

- Poorly controlled blood glucose levels early in pregnancy increase the risk of fetal malformations, excessive infant size at birth, and the development of diabetes in the offspring later in life.

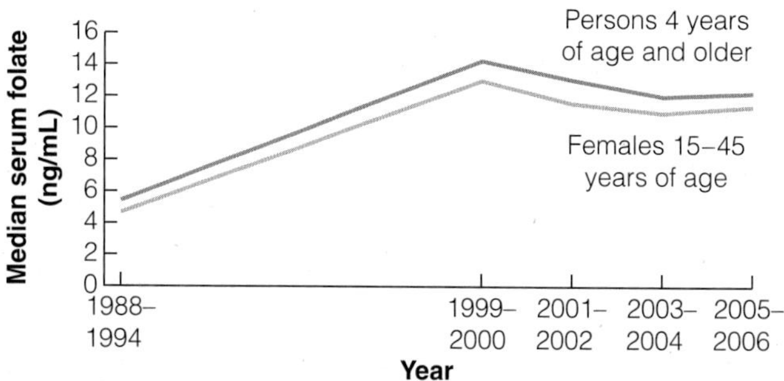


ILLUSTRATION 2.4 ▸ Mean serum folate levels of women of childbearing age (15–45 years) between 1999 and 2006.

NOTE: Statistically significant differences between 1988–1994 and 1999–2000 and between 1999–2000 and 2001–2002 for both groups. Statistically significant difference between 2001–2002 and 2003–2004 for persons 4 years of age and older.

SOURCE: www.cdc.gov/nchs/data/databriefs/db06.htm

as spina bifida. NTDs develop between the third and fourth week after conception—or before many women even know they are pregnant, and well before prenatal care generally begins.[72] Folate is an essential nutrient required for DNA replication and as a component of enzymatic reactions involved in amino acid synthesis and vitamin metabolism.[73] Knowledge of the folate–neural tube defect relationship, and awareness that folate intake was inadequate in many women of childbearing age, prompted public health efforts to increase folate intake. In particular, efforts are focused on encouraging women to consume folic acid, a highly absorbable, synthetic form of this B vitamin. In 1998, that task was made easier when the Food and Drug Administration mandated that refined grain products such as white bread, grits, crackers, rice, and pasta be fortified with folic acid. Many countries now fortify refined grain products with folic acid, and rates of NTDs have decreased significantly in these countries.[76] Rates of NTDs in countries that have not instituted folic acid fortification programs have not improved.[74,75]

There's another benefit related to improvements in folate status before conception: It lowers the risk of delivery of a baby that is ***small for gestational age***. Risk reduction does not appear to occur when inadequate folate status is improved after conception.[78,79]

Intake of folic acid and folate status have increased substantially in most US population groups since fortification. Average folate intake of women between the ages of 20 and 39 years in the United States is 527 DFE ***dietary folate equivalents***) per day, which is above the RDA of 400 DFE per day for folate for women in 20- to 39-years-old.[77] Serum folate (a short-term indicator of folate status; see Illustration 2.4) and red-blood-cell folate concentrations (a marker of longer-term folate status) increased significantly after the institution of folic acid fortification and have remained fairly stable since 2006.[76]

The recommended intake of 400 mcg folic acid daily for preconceptional women can be obtained by consuming a serving of a breakfast cereal fortified with 400 mcg folic acid and other folic acid fortified refined grain products (Table 2.7). Foods containing refined grains formulated to be gluten-free may not be fortified with folic acid.

***Gene Variants and Folate Status*** Some individuals have an increased need for folate due to specific gene variants involved in folate metabolism. These gene variants can impair the conversion of folate to its active form and increase folate requirement.[80] One of the best-studied and most common gene variants affects 5, 10-methylenetetrahydrofolate reductase (MTHFR) activity. This enzyme is responsible for production of the major circulating form of folate used by the body. The C677T ***allele*** of the gene that encodes for MTHFR produces an enzyme that has reduced activity. Women with this gene variant are at increased risk of having an NTD-affected newborn.[81] Some population groups have higher incidence of the MTHFR gene variants associated with increased folate need and risk of NTD.[74]

**small for gestational age** Newborn weight is less than 10th percentile for gestational age.

**dietary folate equivalents (DFE)** A measure of folate availability used by the Reference Dietary Intakes. 1 DFE = 1 mcg food folate, which is equivalent to 0.6 mcg. folic acid.

**allele** A different version of the same gene. Alleles have a different arrangement of bases than the usual version of the gene.

TABLE 2.7 ▸ Examples of breakfast cereals that contain 400 mcg folic acid per serving and other food sources of folic acid[a,117,118]

| FULLY FORTIFIED BREAKFAST CEREALS (400 MG FOLIC ACID PRESERVING) |
|---|
| All-Bran® |
| All-Bran Bran Buds |
| Bran Buds® |
| Cap'n Crunch Original ® |
| Cap'n Crunch's Crunch Berries® |
| Cap'n Crunch's Peanut Butter Crunch® |
| Cinnamon Life |
| Crispy Rice |
| Fiber One |
| Honey Toasted Oats |
| Life |
| Life Oatmeal Squares |
| Low-Fat Granola with Raisins |
| Malt-O-Meal® |
| Mueslix Smart Start® |
| Multi-Bran Chex® |
| Oat Flakes & Blueberry Clusters |
| Original Low-Fat Granola without Raisins |
| Product 19® |
| Special K® Original |
| Total Raisin Bran |
| Wheat Chex® |
| Wheat Flakes |
| Whole Grain Total |

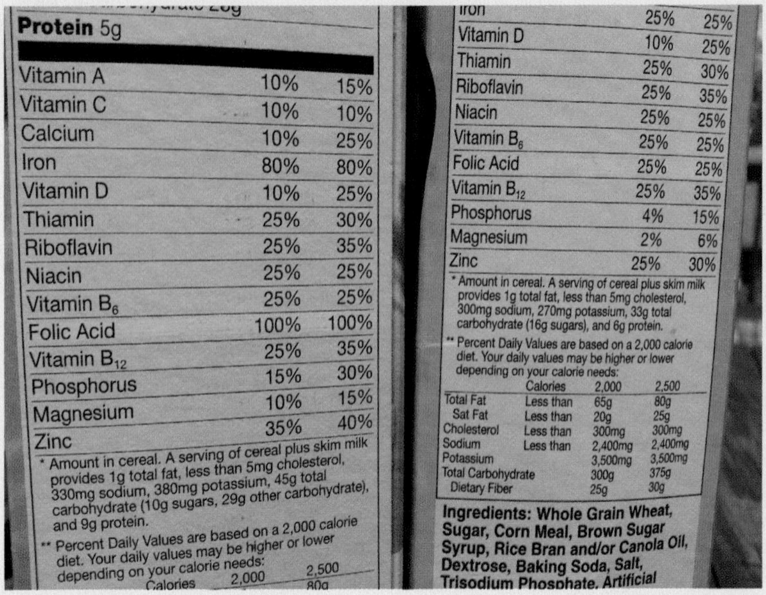

Judith E. Brown

| FOLIC ACID CONTENT OF OTHER FORTIFIED FOODS | mcg folic acid |
|---|---|
| Rice, white, cooked; 1 cup | 104 |
| Other breakfast cereals, 1 cup/1 oz | 100 |
| Pasta, cooked, 1 cup | 92 |
| Tortilla, flour. 1 large/2 oz | 49 |
| Bread, white, 1 slice/1 oz | 46 |
| Grits, cooked, 1 cup | 36 |

[a]Product formulations may change. Confirm folic acid amount by checking the Nutrition Facts panel.

***Remaining Risk Group for Neural Tube Defects*** Although the incidence of neural tube defects in the United States declined by 36 percent post-folic acid fortification, some women are still at risk. Risk groups for folate inadequacy and neural tube defects include Hispanic Americans, particularly women from Mexico and Central America, women who take the anti-seizure drug valproate without appropriate folic acid supplementation, and women who have previously delivered an infant with a neural tube defect.[76,82,83] The increased risk of neural tube defects in Hispanic Americans appears to be related to low intake of folic acid. Additionally, Hispanic Americans as a group have a higher prevalence of a MTHFR gene variant that interferes with folate metabolism and increases folate need.[84] Low folic acid intakes have been related to the regular consumption of corn tortillas (Illustration 2.5) and other foods made from corn masa flour (corn dough flour) that is not fortified with folic acid. The FDA is currently reviewing a proposal to allow folic acid fortification of corn masa flour.[85]

In 1992, the Public Health Service issued a recommendation that women who have had a prior NTD-affected pregnancy take a 4.0 mg folic acid supplement before and early in pregnancy to help prevent recurrence. This recommendation was implemented prior to folic acid fortification and may be reconsidered. Current research indicates that 4.0 mg of folic acid per day is a suprathreshhold dose related to high levels of folic acid excretion in urine. The high folic acid dose does not appear to improve folic acid functions beyond that achieved by intakes of 400 mcg per day before conception and during the first trimester of pregnancy.[72,86,87]

## Periconceptional Iron Status

Iron deficiency is the most common nutritional deficiency worldwide.[88] Iron deficiency prior to pregnancy increases the

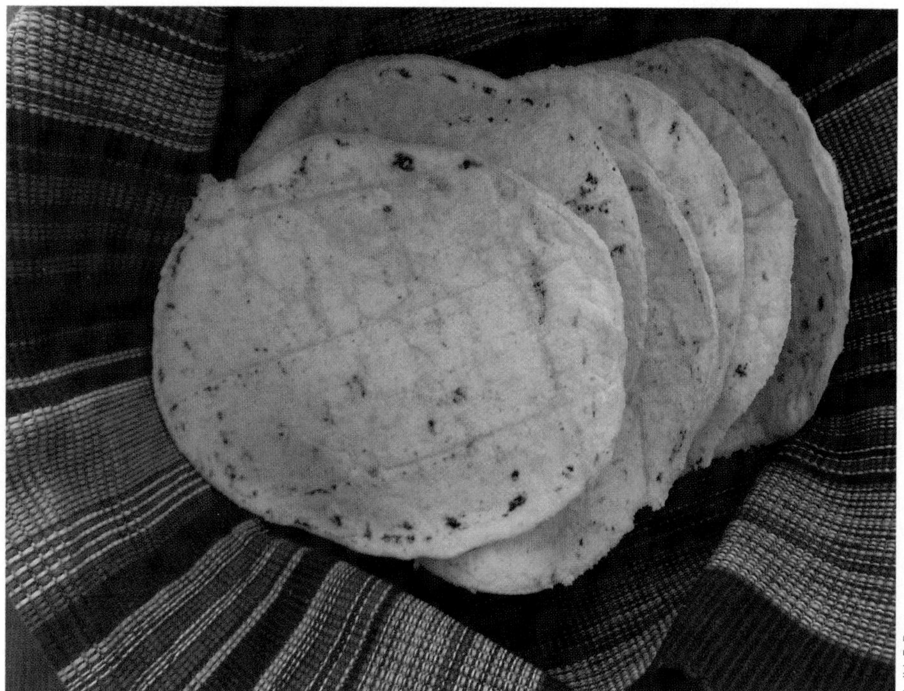

Judith E. Brown

ILLUSTRATION 2.5 ▸ Corn tortillas, a staple food in Mexico and Central America, is made from corn masa flour, which is not fortified with folic acid.

risk that iron-deficiency anemia will occur during pregnancy and that infants will be born with low stores of iron. Iron deficiency before pregnancy is also related to increased rates of preterm delivery.[89] It is easier and more efficient to build up iron stores before pregnancy than during pregnancy. Iron status has been found to improve by 15 weeks of pregnancy when women start increasing iron intake 2–3 months prior to conception. Women who start to increase iron intake a month after conception do not experience the same benefit.[90]

Iron status can generally be improved by the regular consumption of vitamin C–rich fruits and vegetables along with plant sources of iron, iron-fortified cereals, and lean meats, and by the use of modest doses of iron supplements (18 mg a day) if needed. Ideally, women would enter pregnancy with a sufficient level of stored iron to last throughout pregnancy.[91]

# Recommended Dietary Intake and Healthy Dietary Patterns for Preconceptional Women

LO 2.5 Develop a one-day menu for a preconceptional woman and a man based on the ChooseMyPlate.gov food guidance materials.

It is recommended that women who may become pregnant (1) consume 400 mcg of folic acid from fortified foods or supplements in addition to dietary folate from a variety of foods, (2) take no more than 10,000 IU of vitamin A (retinol or retinoic acid) from supplements daily; and (3) limit or omit alcohol-containing beverages. Recommendations for nutrient intake given in the Dietary Reference Intakes (DRIs) should be applied in making food and dietary supplement decisions while paying specific attention to the Tolerable Upper Intake Levels for nutrients.[92,93] For both women and men, energy and nutrients requirements should be met by foods rather than supplements if possible.[94]

Healthy dietary patterns are described by the 2015 Dietary Guidelines Advisory Committee as those that focus on basic, nutrient-dense foods including fish, poultry, lean meats, vegetables, fruits, legumes, whole grains and whole grain products, oils, and nuts.[94] These types of dietary patterns, combined with healthy lifestyles, are associated with a reduced risk of poor pregnancy outcomes, improved infant and child health and development, and decrease the risk of chronic health problems later in life.[70] Dietary patterns prior to pregnancy generally continue during pregnancy, so it is helpful to enter pregnancy while consuming a healthy one.[95]

Food selection prior to pregnancy can be based on USDA's ChooseMyPlate.gov healthy dietary pattern guidance information (see Table 2.8). The types and number of servings recommended from each food group are determined primarily by a person's calorie and nutrient needs based on age, sex, height, weight, and physical activity level. A balanced

TABLE 2.8 ▸ ChooseMyPlate.gov 2,200 calorie plan for a 28-year-old woman and a 2,800 calorie plan for a 28-year-old male[a]

| | FOOD GROUP | | | | | | |
|---|---|---|---|---|---|---|---|
| | CALORIES | GRAINS | VEGETABLES | FRUITS | DAIRY | PROTEIN | OILS |
| For a 28-year-old woman weighing 130 pounds, 5′6″ tall, and physically active 30–60 minutes per day: | 2,200 | 7 oz | 3 c | 2 c | 3 c | 6 oz | 6 tsp |
| For a 28-year-old man weighing 164 pounds, 5′10″ tall, and physically active 30–60 minutes per day: | 2,800 | 10 oz | 3.5 cup | 2.5 cup | 3 cup | 7 oz | 8 tsp |

**Advice:**

- Make half your grains whole grains
- Vary your vegetables; include dark green, red, and orange vegetables
- Drink fat-free or 1% milk
- Go lean with protein
- How much food counts as a cup or an ounce?

| | |
|---|---|
| Vegetables: | 1 cup = 1 cup raw or cooked vegetables or vegetable juice, or 2 cups leafy salad greens |
| Fruits: | 1 cup = 1 cup raw or cooked fruit or 100% fruit juice, or ½ cup dried fruit |
| Dairy: | 1 cup = 1 cup milk, yogurt, or fortified soy milk; or 1½ ounces natural or 2 oz processed cheese |
| Grains: | 1 ounce = 1 slice of bread, ½ cup cooked rice, cereal, or pasta; or 1 oz ready-to-eat cereal |
| Protein: | 1 oz = 1 oz lean meat, poultry, or fish; 1 egg, 1 Tbsp peanut butter, ½ oz nuts or seeds; ¼ cup cooked dried beans or peas |

[a]Visit SuperTracker at MyPlate.gov to identify food group recommendations based on various levels of calorie need.

diet high in nutrient-dense foods promotes general health and normal weight status, and helps prepare women for the nutrient needs of pregnancy (Table 2.9).[96]

TABLE 2.9 ▸ Example 2,000 calorie, 1-day menu from ChooseMyPlate.gov

**Breakfast**
1 whole wheat English muffin
1 Tbsp all-fruit preserves
1 hard-cooked egg
Beverage: 1 cup water, coffee, or tea

**Lunch**
White bean-vegetable soup:
1¼ cup chunky vegetable soup with pasta, ½ cup white beans
6 saltine crackers
½ cup celery sticks
Beverage: 1 cup fat-free milk

**Dinner**
Rigatoni with meat sauce:
1 cup rigatoni pasta (2 oz dry)
2 ounces cooked ground beef (95% lean)
2 tsp corn/canola oil (to cook beef)
½ cup tomato sauce
3 Tbsp grated parmesan cheese
Spinach salad:
1 cup raw spinach leaves, ½ cup tangerine sections, ½ oz chopped walnuts, 4 tsp oil and vinegar dressing
Beverage: 1 cup water, coffee, or tea

**Snack**
1 cup nonfat fruit yogurt

# Influence of Contraceptives on Preconceptional Nutrition Status

LO 2.6 Identify three nutrition-related consequences that may be related to the use of combination hormonal contraceptives, and a consequence that is related to the use of estrogen or progestin contraceptives only.

Many types of contraceptives are available by prescription. These contraceptives contain forms of estrogen, mainly estradiol, and/or progestin (the term used for progesterone, the natural hormone), and progestogen (the synthetic form). Estradiol is always combined with progestin, but some contraceptives employ progestin only for women who, for health reasons, cannot take estrogen. When used together, estradiol and progestin suppress the action of LH and FSH and thereby ovulation. Progestin blocks LH and ovulation, and, by causing the cervical mucus to become thick and sticky, it induces a barrier to sperm. Hormonal contraceptives are available as pills, patches, implants, and injections. All are effective at preventing pregnancy if used correctly.[97]

## Nutritional Side Effects of Hormonal Contraception

The estradiol and progestin content of contraceptives in the current third generation of contraceptives is lower than earlier generations of contraceptive[98] and the forms of the hormones used have become more targeted.[99] Their use is associated with far fewer side effects than the earlier versions, and complications related to their use are rare.[100] Combination hormonal contraceptives, such as most oral contraceptives, do not appear to be associated with weight gain.[101,102] Progestin-only hormonal contraceptives such as Depo-Provera are associated with weight gain. Women using progestin for contraception gain, on average, around 10 pounds within the first 5 years of use. The gain has been found to be related to increased fat storage rather than to fluid or lean tissues. Progestin-only contraceptives have been found to decrease bone mineral accretion in adolescents.[102,103]

Estradiol and progestin contraceptive use appears to be associated with altered blood lipid levels and glucose metabolism, as well as other changes in health status.[104] Combination contraceptives tend to decrease HDL cholesterol, increase LDL cholesterol and triglyceride concentrations, increase blood glucose and insulin levels, and increase inflammation somewhat.[99] Metabolic changes associated with estradiol appear to increase the risk of stroke due to blood clots and heart attack in some users.[105] Whether combined contraceptives increase the risk of type 2 diabetes is not yet clear.[106]

Hormonal contraceptives may not be recommended for women at risk of cardiovascular disease or blood clots, and women with high blood pressure. Women who use these contraceptives are advised not to smoke.[104,105] Fertility usually resumes within 3–6 months after contraceptive use stops, but some women regain it sooner.[97]

Effective and safe hormonal forms of contraception for males have been developed but are not yet approved for use. Male hormonal contraception is currently based on the use of testosterone alone or in combination with progestin. Testosterone administration to males suppresses the secretion of LH and FSH, depriving the testes of the signals required for spermatogenesis and thereby markedly reducing sperm production. Studies have shown that sperm counts return to normal in most men within 6 months of discontinuing the hormonal contraceptives.[107]

# Model Preconceptional Health and Nutrition Programs

LO2.7 Cite three important nutrition-related components of preconceptional health care.

This section highlights two model programs that benefit preconceptional women. One is the Special Supplemental Nutrition Program for Women, Infants, and Children—better known as the WIC program—and the other an iron supplement program in Indonesia.

The WIC program serves to safeguard the health of low-income pregnant, postpartum, and breastfeeding women, infants, and children up to age 5 who are at nutritional risk by providing nutritious foods to supplement diets, information on healthy eating including breastfeeding promotion and support, and referrals to health care. It serves nearly 9 million pregnant and breastfeeding women, infants, and young children in the United States.[108] Through services provided to postpartum women and nutrition education delivered during infancy and early childhood, WIC is in a position to benefit preconceptional women in the next pregnancy even through they are not a specific target audience for the program.[109]

## Preconceptional Benefits of WIC

Potential benefits of WIC services to pregnant women during pregnancy, as well as between consecutive pregnancies, were assessed in a study in California. One group of women received WIC benefits during one pregnancy through the first two months of the next pregnancy. The control group received WIC services during pregnancy only. Women who received WIC services through to a subsequent pregnancy had better iron status and delivered newborns with higher birthweights and greater lengths than did women who received WIC benefits during pregnancy only.[110] The study indicates that low-income women at nutritional risk benefit from WIC services from one pregnancy to the next.

In 2012, the USDA launched a grants program in collaboration with the University of California at Los Angeles that is evaluating the impact of the existing WIC program on periconceptional nutrition. The intention of the research is to measure the cost and benefits of WIC services on outcomes such as ovulatory infertility, birth defects, complications during pregnancy, preterm birth, and low birthweight.[109] Depending on the results of these studies, preconceptional women may become eligible for WIC services.

## Decreasing Iron Deficiency in Preconceptional Women in Indonesia

Approximately one in every two women in Indonesia experiences iron-deficiency anemia during pregnancy. In a unique effort to prevent this problem, the Ministry of Health initiated regulations that require a couple applying for a marriage license to receive advice on iron status from those dispensing the license. All women are now advised to take 30–60 mg of iron along with folic acid in a supplement. Of 344 women studied after the program was initiated, 98 percent reported that they had purchased and taken iron folate tablets; 56 percent had taken at least 30 tablets. The incidence of iron deficiency in this group of women dropped by almost half.[111]

## Preconception Care: Preparing for Pregnancy

Increasingly, routine preconceptional health care visits and educational sessions are being recommended and introduced into health care services. Services focus on risk assessment of behaviors such as weight status, dietary and alcohol intake, folate and iron status, and vitamin, mineral, and herbal supplement use, as well as on the presence of diseases such as diabetes, hypertension, infections, and genetic traits that may be transmitted to offspring.[112,113] Psychosocial needs should also be addressed as part of preconceptional care, and referrals made to appropriate services for issues such as eating disorders, abuse, violence, or lack of food or shelter.[114] The desire of couples planning for pregnancy to have a healthy newborn makes the preconceptional period a prime time for positive behavioral changes. It presents opportunities to make lasting improvements in the health and well-being of individuals and families.

**CDC's Preconception Health Initiative** Efforts to boost the availability and utilization of preconception health care services now have the backing of the Centers for Disease Control and Prevention (CDC). In 2006, the CDC released a report highlighting recommendations for improving preconception health and health care services.[114] The report was developed in response to the slow progress the United States had made in improving rates of poor pregnancy outcomes, and in achieving the 2010 Health Objectives set in 2000 for the Nation related to preconception health. Additionally, the recommendations address the persistent problem of higher rates of poor pregnancy outcomes in African Americans, Hispanic Americans, and other groups compared to Caucasians.

The report concludes that preconception health care should be delivered at regularly scheduled primary care visits and include education about preconception health and pregnancy outcome; screening for vaccination, weight, and iron and folate status; assessment of alcohol use; and management of disorders such as diabetes and celiac disease. The CDC recommends that preconception services include counseling to modify individual health behaviors that, if left unchanged, would negatively impact fertility and pregnancy outcomes. Initiatives such as this one are increasing public awareness of the importance of preconception health and of planning pregnancy.[114]

Starting pregnancy in the best health status possible can make an important difference to reproductive outcomes. Even in ideal conditions, continued infertility, early pregnancy loss, fetal malformations, and maternal complications will sometimes occur.

# The Nutrition Care Process

LO 2.8 Describe the four steps of the Nutrition Care Process.

The National Academy of Nutrition and Dietetics (formerly known as the American Dietetic Association) has developed nutrition care standards intended to serve as guidelines for the delivery of nutrition services.[115] The standards are called the Nutrition Care Process (NCP), and they are part of new technology-based systems being developed to facilitate health-services delivery and cost evaluation, electronic charting, coding, and outcome measurement. The process is being evaluated and will be revised and updated as needed on an ongoing basis.

The Nutrition Care Process focuses on the delivery of effective nutrition care through the use of:

- A common approach to, and standardized methods for, nutrition assessment.
- Specific terms to describe nutrition diagnoses identified by the nutrition assessment. Nutrition diagnoses are treated independently by a nutrition practitioner.
- Effective intervention plans and goals related to treating the specific nutrition diagnoses.
- Nutrition monitoring and evaluation techniques that identify client/patient outcomes relevant to the nutrition diagnoses and the intervention plans and goals.

The Nutrition Care Process in practice consists of four steps:

1. Nutrition assessment
2. Nutrition diagnosis
3. Nutrition intervention
4. Nutrition monitoring and evaluation

Table 2.10 summarizes components of these four steps.

## The Nutrition Care Process Related to the Preconception Period

Components of the Nutrition Care Process vary to some extent based on the life-cycle stage of the individuals being served. Preconception services are tailored to the nutritional needs of women before pregnancy, and to the nutrition and reproductive health needs of men. Topics such as weight status; folic acid, iron, and antioxidant intake; dietary supplement use; reproductive history; contraceptive use; and effects of existing disorders on early fetal development would be addressed as part of the nutrition care process. Case Study 2.2 addresses a preconception health problem related to nutrition and asks students to use the Nutrition Care Process to formulate responses to questions asked about the case.

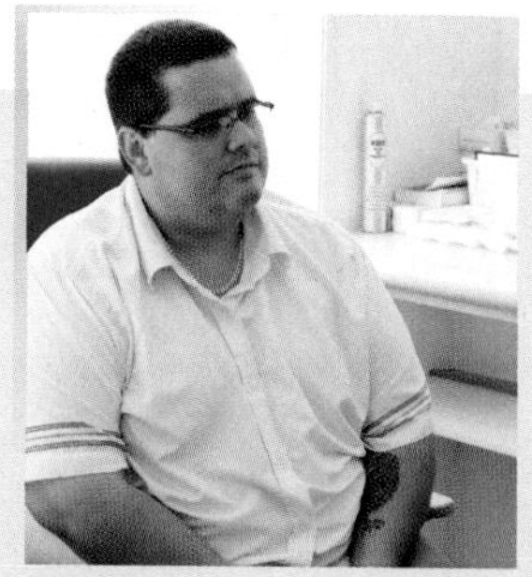
Life in View/Science Source

# NUTRITION CARE PROCESS (NCP) CASE STUDY 2.2

## Male Infertility

This case study requires use of the American Dietetic Association's Nutrition Care Process.

Mr. Trigger, a 29-year old male, and his healthy 32-year-old wife have been unable to conceive after two years of unprotected intercourse. Results of medical tests led Mr. Trigger to be diagnosed with male-factor infertility due to low sperm production. No other health problems were identified. His weight was assessed to be 260 lbs. (118 kg) and his height measured 5 ft. 10 in. (1.78 m). Mr. Trigger was referred to a registered dietitian for nutritional assessment, diagnoses, intervention, and follow-up.

Results of the nutritional assessment revealed that Mr. Trigger was physically inactive and consumed an average of 145 calories more per day than recommended based on his weight, height, and physical activity level. Results of assessments of Mr. Trigger's dietary and supplement intake; nutrition-focused physical findings; nutrition knowledge, behaviors, and beliefs; and food availability revealed no additional problem areas.

### Questions

1. What is Mr. Trigger's BMI?
2. Name an appropriate priority nutrition diagnosis for this case.
3. Name one potential nutrition intervention that addresses the nutrition diagnosis.
4. Cite one nutrition-related indicator that could be used to monitor and evaluate the intervention.

(Answers are located in the Instructor's Manual for the 6th edition of *Nutrition Through the Life Cycle.*)

TABLE 2.10 ▸ Summary of the components of the four steps of the Nutrition Care Process[115]

**Step 1: Nutrition Assessment**

- Food/Nutrition-Related History
  - Food and nutrient intake (e.g., diet history, fat intake)
  - Medicinal/dietary supplement intake (e.g., medications, supplement use)
  - Knowledge/beliefs/attitudes (e.g., level of nutrition knowledge, unscientific beliefs, attitudes)
  - Nutrition-related behaviors (e.g., binge-eating behavior, willingness to try new foods)
  - Food and supplies availability (e.g., eligibility for and utilization of government/community food and nutrition programs)
  - Physical activity (e.g., physical activity history, intensity)
- Biochemical Data, Medical Tests, and Procedures
  - Tests (e.g., resting metabolic rate, bone density)
- Anthropometric Measurements
  - Body size, growth (BMI, growth pattern)
- Client History
  - Medical history, treatments, use of alternative/complementary medicine, social history

**Step 2: Nutrition Diagnosis**

- Identification of nutrition-specific problem(s) based on results of the nutrition assessment. Diagnoses are classified as being related to:
  - Food and nutrient intake (e.g., food and nutrient amounts consumed relative to need, such as "excessive energy intake," "underweight," "excess fat intake")
  - Clinical (e.g., nutrition problems related to medical and physical conditions such as "swallowing difficulties due to [name the factor, e.g., lack of saliva]," "breastfeeding difficulty due to [name the factor, e.g., failure to obtain a let-down reflex]," "altered lab value, low vitamin D due to [name the factor, e.g., sun sensitivity]")
  - Behavioral-environmental (e.g., problem related to behavior, knowledge, beliefs, and access to food such as "food-and nutrition-related knowledge deficit," "limited access to food")

*(Continued)*

TABLE 2.10 ▸ Summary of the components of the four steps of the Nutrition Care Process[115] *(Continued)*

| Step 3: Nutrition Intervention |
|---|
| • Identify and implement effective, individually tailored nutrition interventions that will resolve or improve the nutrition problems identified. Nutrition intervention strategies are organized into four categories:<br>1. Food and/or nutrient delivery<br>2. Nutrition education<br>3. Nutrition counseling<br>4. Coordination of nutrition care |
| **Step 4: Nutrition Monitoring and Evaluation** |
| – Measure and monitor changes in the client's nutrition-related health status and evaluate the effectiveness of the intervention based on client nutrition and health outcomes. |

## KEY POINTS

1. Preconceptional nutritional status influences maternal health and the course and outcome of pregnancy.
2. The Healthy People 2020 nutrition objectives for preconception focus on improving weight status prior to pregnancy, decreasing alcohol consumption around the time of conception, deceasing inadequate iron and folate status, and expanding the utilization of preconceptional care services.
3. Dietary intake, supplement use, weight status, and body fat content affect the development and maintenance of a person's biological capacity to reproduce.
4. The major hormones involved in the regulation of fertility processes in females and males are gonadtropin-releasing hormone (GnRH), follicle-stimulating hormone (FSH), leutinizing hormone (LH), estrogen, progesterone, and testosterone. These hormones can be affected by nutritional status.
5. Inadequate and excessive levels of body fat, weight loss in normal-weight individuals, oxidative stress and chronic inflammation, low antioxidant intake from vegetables and fruits, high alcohol intake, eating disorders, certain chronic health problems, high soy-food diets, inadequate zinc status, and heavy-metal exposure are related to fertility.
6. The effects of hormonal contraceptives on body weight and on blood lipid, insulin, and glucose concentrations depend on the estradiol and progestin content of the contraceptive.
7. Adequate folate status prior to pregnancy substantially reduces the risk of neural-tube and other defects in newborns. Some cases of inadequate folate status are related to gene variants that increase the need for folate.
8. Low iron stores prior to pregnancy increase the risk of iron deficiency during pregnancy, preterm delivery, and low iron stores in the infant. Iron stores can be more effectively accumulated prior to rather than during pregnancy.
9. A healthy, preconceptional dietary pattern for women and men is described by the ChooseMyPlate.gov food guidance material.
10. The periconceptional period represents a critical period of time when nutritional and other exposures can impact conception, pregnancy maintenance, and the growth, development, and future health of the offspring.
11. Preconception health services should be a part of primary health care and would likely improve fertility and pregnancy outcomes.
12. The process by which nutrition care service should be provided to preconceptional women and men (and others) has been defined by the American Academy of Nutrition and Dietetics.

## REVIEW QUESTIONS

1. ____ Which of the following is a nutrition objective for preconception included in the Healthy People 2020 document?
   a. Decrease the proportion of men who consume soy products before conception by 10 percent.
   b. Increase the proportion of women of childbearing potential by 10 percent with intake of at least 400 mcg of folic acid from fortified foods or dietary supplements.
   c. Increase the proportion of women and men who consume less than 30 percent of total calories as fat prior to pregnancy.
   d. Increase the proportion of men and women who regularly take a multivitamin and mineral supplement prior to pregnancy by 10 percent.
2. Nutrient intake from food, calorie intake, and body fat affect fertility primarily by altering the environment in which eggs and sperm develop, and modifying levels of hormones involved in reproductive processes.
   ____ True ____ False
3. Estrogen is produced by fat cells, the pituitary gland, and the testes.
   ____ True ____ False
4. The maturation of sperm takes 70–80 days.
   ____ True ____ False

Match the term listed in Column A with its definition from Column B

| Column A | Column B |
|---|---|
| 5. ____ Puberty | a. A tissue about 12 mm in diameter formed from the follicle that contained the ovum prior to its release. It produces estrogen and progesterone. |
| 6. ____ Corpus luteum | b. Biological ability to bear children. |
| 7. ____ Subfertility | c. Generally defined as the loss of a conceptus in the first 20 weeks of pregnancy. |
| 8. ____ Fecundity | d. The period in life during which humans become biologically capable of reproduction. |
| 9. ____ Miscarriage | e. Menstrual cycles in which ovulation does not occur. |
| 10. ____ Luteinizing hormone | f. A hormone that prepares the uterus for a fertilized ovum and helps to maintain a pregnancy; stimulates uterine lining buildup during menstrual cycle. |
| 11. ____ Progesterone | g. Absence of menstrual cycle. |
| 12. ____ Anovulatory cycles | h. A hormone that stimulates secretion of estrogen, progesterone, and testosterone and growth of the corpus luteum. |
| 13. ____ Amenorrhea | i. Reduced level of fertility characterized by unusually long time to conception (over 12 months) or repeated early pregnancy losses. |

14. Weight loss of 10–15 percent of body weight in normal-weight men, but not in normal-weight women, decreases fertility.
    ____ True ____ False
15. Both inadequate and excessive levels of body fat affect fertility.
    ____ True ____ False
16. Studies have consistently shown that high intakes of caffeine or coffee reduce fertility.
    ____ True ____ False
17. ____ Although the incidence of neural tube defects in the United States declined post-folic acid fortification, some women are still at risk. Which of the following options represents a risk group for inadequate folate status and a neural tube defect affected pregnancy?
    a. Non-Hispanic Black women
    b. Non-Hispanic White women
    c. Asian Americans
    d. Hispanic Americans
18. It is recommended that preconceptional women consume 400 mcg of folic acid from fortified foods or supplements, in addition to dietary folate from a variety of foods.
    ____ True ____ False

19. Low energy intakes during the periconceptional period due to food restriction, weight loss, or eating disorders may modify gene functions in the embryo in ways that influence the future health of the offspring.

    _____ True _____ False

20. Some individuals have an increased need for folate due to the gene variant 5, 10-methylenetetrahydrofolate reductase that blocks the absorption of folate from food.

    _____ True _____ False

21. Women should enter pregnancy with a good level of stored iron because it is easier to build up iron stores before than during pregnancy.

    _____ True _____ False

22. The basic food groups presented in ChooseMyPlate are milk, meat and beans, vegetables, fruits, and breads and cereals.

    _____ True _____ False

23. Menus generated by ChooseMyPlate include basic foods that are nutrient dense. The amounts of basic foods included in menus are primarily based on a person's age, sex, height, weight, and physical activity level.

    _____ True _____ False

24. The current generation of oral contraceptives increases the risk of iron deficiency.

    _____ True _____ False

25. Combination hormonal contraceptive use is associated with weight gain.

    _____ True _____ False

26. Progestin-only contraceptives are related to increased blood glucose and LDL cholesterol levels.

    _____ True _____ False

27. Women who received WIC services from one pregnancy through to a subsequent pregnancy appear to gain more weight during the subsequent pregnancy than do women who receive WIC benefits during pregnancy only.

    _____ True _____ False

28. The CDC recommends that preconceptional health programs include education about weight, iron, and folate status; assessment of alcohol use; and services related to the management of disorders such as diabetes and celiac disease.

    _____ True _____ False

29. _____ Which of the following is *not* a step in the Nutrition Care Process?

    a. nutrition assessment
    b. nutrition diagnosis
    c. nutrition supplementation
    d. nutrition intervention

**Visit www.cengagebrain.com to access MindTap, a complete digital course that includes additional resources.**

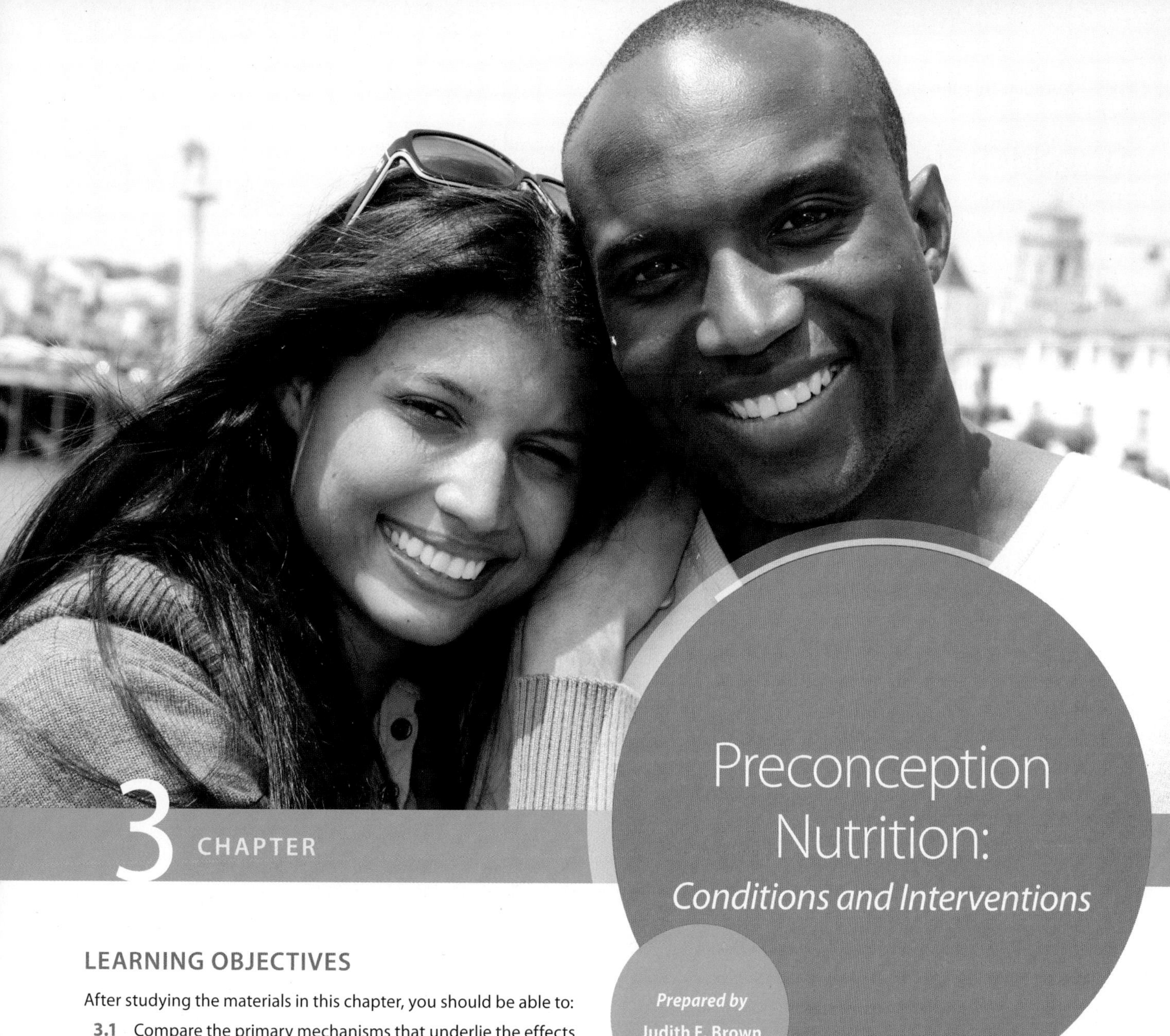

3 CHAPTER

# Preconception Nutrition: *Conditions and Interventions*

*Prepared by*
Judith E. Brown

## LEARNING OBJECTIVES

After studying the materials in this chapter, you should be able to:

**3.1** Compare the primary mechanisms that underlie the effects of obesity and underweight on fertility in women and men.

**3.2** Identify two mechanisms by which a negative energy balance can influence fertility.

**3.3** Illustrate two ways in which good blood glucose control during the periconceptional period can benefit fetal growth and development.

**3.4** Cite three key components of the nutritional management of PCOS.

**3.5** Summarize the major reasons why dietary control of PKU is particularly important prior to pregnancy.

**3.6** Describe three nutritional consequences of untreated celiac disease.

**3.7** Identify four common symptoms of premenstrual syndrome and the proposed effects of dietary supplements on the symptoms of premenopausal dysphoric disorder (PMDD).

Goodluz/Shutterstock.com

# Introduction

This chapter addresses specific preconceptional and *periconceptional* nutrition-related conditions that may influence fertility or the course and outcome of pregnancy. Evidence related to the role of diet, dietary supplements, and nutrition interventions on the development and management of the conditions is presented. We begin with a discussion of obesity and then progress to underweight, negative energy balance, eating disorders, the female athlete triad, diabetes, polycystic ovary syndrome, phenylketonuria, celiac disease, and premenstrual syndrome.

# Weight Status and Fertility

LO 3.1 Compare the primary mechanisms that underlie the effects of obesity and underweight on fertility in women and men.

Rates of reproductive health problems related to high levels of body fat are increasing in the United States and other countries along with rising rates of obesity. Currently, 35.1 percent of adults in the United States are obese and 33.9 percent are overweight.[1] Only 1.7 percent of adults are underweight.[2]

Metabolic and hormonal changes induced by very high or low levels of body fat appear to be largely responsible for disruptions in fertility associated with obesity and underweight. These metabolic and hormonal changes influence fertility primarily by interfering with ovulation or sperm development.[3] Some of the metabolic and hormonal changes occurring with obesity and underweight prior to conception also influence pregnancy outcomes.

## Obesity, Body Fat Distribution, and Fertility

Obesity is now classified as a disease because its tends to shorten life span and is related to metabolic conditions that encourage development of health problems such as heart disease, type 2 diabetes, and impaired fertility. Overweight appears to impact fertility and pregnancy in women with metabolic abnormalities such as insulin resistance and ***chronic inflammation***. Associations between overweight and poor health outcomes are much weaker than those for obesity in the absence of high levels of ***intra-abdominal fat*** (also called visceral fat).[4-6]

Obesity marked by excess intra-abdominal fat is related to ***insulin resistance***, elevated levels of insulin, chronic inflammation, oxidative stress, and ***metabolic syndrome***. Metabolic syndrome is referred to again in this and other chapters and is overviewed in the In Focus: Metabolic Syndrome box. These conditions can interfere with reproductive processes in women and men.[3,5] In women, elevated blood insulin levels reduce ***sex hormone binding globulin*** (SHBG) and that prompts the ovaries to increase production of testosterone. Excess testosterone disrupts egg development.[3] Ovulatory disorders produced by testosterone and other androgen excesses are related to irregular menstrual cycles, ***anovulation***, and delayed time to conception. High levels of intra-abdominal fat in women contribute to anovulation, ***amenorrhea***, delayed conception, and a reduced response to fertility treatments.[3]

Men with high levels of body fat can experience fertility problems because of hormonal changes related to the metabolism of testosterone in fat tissue. Fat tissue contains an enzyme (aromatase) that converts testosterone to estradiol, and this conversion may be abnormally high in people with high body fat. Consequently, obese men tend to have low testosterone and elevated estradiol levels. Increased blood levels of estradiol inhibit secretion of ***luteinizing hormone*** (LH) and ***follicle stimulating hormone*** (FSH) by the pituitary. Alterations in LH and FSH can lower testosterone synthesis. Low levels of testosterone decrease sperm production and promote infertility and subfertility.[10]

High levels of intra-abdominal fat in men are directly related to oxidative stress, a condition that can damage unsaturated fats and DNA. Specifically, oxidative stress can lead to the breakdown of polyunsaturated fatty acids in sperm membranes and damage sperm DNA. Damage to sperm can reduce fertility by impairing sperm functions and motility.[11] Insulin resistance and oxidative stress in men is also associated with impaired sexual functions.[3,9] Results from a large study recently found that paternal obesity is associated with an increased risk of autism spectrum disorder in offspring.[7]

**periconceptional period** The time period around conception, variously measured in weeks or months, depending on the pregnancy outcomes of interest.

**chronic inflammation** Low-grade inflammation that lasts weeks, months, or years. Inflammation is the first response of the body's immune system to infectious agents, toxins, or irritants. It triggers the release of biologically active substances that promote oxidation and other reactions to counteract the infection, toxin, or irritant. A side effect of chronic inflammation is that it also damages lipids, cells, and tissues.

**intra-abdominal fat** Fat located within the abdominal cavity around organs such as the liver, pancreas, and intestines. Intra-abdominal fat is referred to as visceral fat and is much more metabolically active than fat stored in other parts of the body.

**insulin resistance** A condition in which cell membranes have reduced sensitivity to insulin so that more insulin than normal is required to transport a given amount of glucose into cells.

**metabolic syndrome** A constellation of metabolic abnormalities that increase the risk of heart disease, hypertension, type 2 diabetes, and other disorders. Metabolic syndrome is characterized by insulin resistance, abdominal obesity, high blood pressure and triglycerides levels, low levels of HDL cholesterol, and impaired glucose tolerance. It is also called *insulin resistance syndrome*.

**sex hormone binding globulin (SHBG)** A protein that binds with the sex hormones testosterone and estrogen. These hormones are inactive when bound to SHBG, but are available for use when needed. Low levels of SHBG are related to increased availability of testosterone and estrogen in the body.

**anovulation** The absence of ovulation.

**amenorrhea** Absence of menstrual cycles.

IN FOCUS

## Metabolic Syndrome

**Definition: Metabolic syndrome** is not a specific disease but, rather, a cluster of abnormal metabolic and other health indicators. It is diagnosed when three of the following five conditions exist:

1. Waist circumference > 40″ in men, > 35″ in women (These are an indicator of the presence of insulin resistance. Other population-based definitions of elevated waist circumference may also be used.)
2. Blood triglycerides ≥ 150 mg/dL
3. HDL cholesterol < 40 mg/dL in men and < 50 mg/dL in women
4. Blood pressure of ≥ 130/85 mm Hg
5. Fasting blood glucose ≥ 100 mg/d[103]

**Prevalence:** It is estimated that 32 percent of U.S. adults and 20 percent of Canadian adults have metabolic syndrome.[104]

**Major physiological aspects and consequences:** The cluster of metabolic risk factors found in people with metabolic syndrome greatly increases the risk of development of cardiovascular disease and type 2 diabetes. Metabolic syndrome is also characterized by chronic inflammation and oxidative stress. Over time, chronic inflammation and oxidative stress cause damage to cells and body functions, and can impair reproductive functions in both women and men.[105]

The first-line therapy for metabolic syndrome is lifestyle changes that emphasize dietary modifications, weight reduction, and exercise. Diets high in antioxidant-rich fruits, vegetables, whole-grain products, fiber, and low-fat dairy products are recommended. Such diets decrease inflammation, plasma triglyceride levels, body weight, plasma glucose levels, and blood pressure and increase HDL cholesterol levels.[12,106]

**Risk factors:** People with metabolic syndrome are often obese, have high levels of central body fat, and are insulin resistant. Specific gene variants appear to play important roles in the development of MS due to their influence on glucose utilization, insulin activity, chronic inflammation, and the formation of intra-abdominal fat stores.[107,108]

SOURCE: Alberti, K. G. et al. Harmonizing the metabolic syndrome. A joint statement of the International Diabetes Federation Task Force on Epidemiology and Prevention; National Heart, Lung, and Blood Institute; American Heart Association; World Heart Federation; International Atherosclerosis Society; and the International Association for the Study of Obesity. Circulation 2009; 120:1640–5.

Oxidative stress can be decreased by the regular consumption of colorful vegetables, fruits, whole grains and whole grain products, and limited intake of sugar-sweetened beverages and foods.[12] Weight loss and moderate-intensity exercise, such as brisk walking, for 150 minutes a week also help reduce oxidative stress.[13]

**Metabolically Healthy Individuals** Not all individuals with high or low levels of body fat are at risk of fertility problems. Whether obese (or non-obese) individuals are at risk for health problems primarily depends on their metabolic profile. Metabolically healthy individuals, or those with no evidence of elevated blood pressure, glucose intolerance, abnormal blood lipid levels, or increased markers of inflammation and oxidative stress, are at lower risk of disease development than are metabolically unhealthy individuals. About one-in-four obese individual are metabolically healthy, and some normal weight individuals with excess abdominal fat can have metabolic disorders.[17,18] Increasing physical fitness, even in the absence of weight loss, decreases the negative, metabolic effects of obesity.[19]

**Weight Loss Benefits** Fertility problems in obese women and men can often be reduced or eliminated by weight loss. It is the treatment of first choice.[21] Read more about one woman's experience with weight loss and fertility in Case Study 3.1. Weight reduction methods focused on behavioural goals and skills such as meal planning, food preparation, snack choices, and portion sizes; and regular participation in enjoyable physical activities are recommended.[22] Aerobic exercise, such as walking and jogging, appears to be particularly helpful for improving insulin resistance. Approaches to weight loss that stigmatize or shame obese individuals may be counterproductive. Strategies that work tend to be supportive and individualized.[23]

Medications are available that may restore fertility in the absence of weight loss in obese individuals, and weight loss surgery may be indicated to recover fertility status if weight-loss efforts fail. Women who lose weight prior to pregnancy due to bariatric surgery are at lower risk of developing diabetes and hypertension during pregnancy than are obese women who do not lose weight.[24] They are, however, at increased risk of developing deficiencies of thiamin, vitamin $B_6$ and vitamin $B_{12}$, and D; and calcium, iron, copper, and zinc.[25,26] Assessment of micronutrient status and vitamin and mineral supplementation should be included as routine components of care post-bariatric surgery.[27] Conception is not recommended during the first year after bariatric surgery when weight loss is most rapid.[29]

Conception may follow the return of fertility in women who reduce dietary intake and lose weight. It is important to monitor

**luteinizing hormone (LH)** A hormone produced by the pituitary gland that stimulates ovulation, the development of the corpus luteum (which secretes progesterone), and the production of testosterone in males.

**follicle stimulating hormone (FSH)** A hormone produced by the pituitary gland that stimulates ovarian follicle growth and maturation, estrogen secretion, and endometrial changes characteristic of the first portion of the menstrual cycle in females. It stimulates sperm production in males.

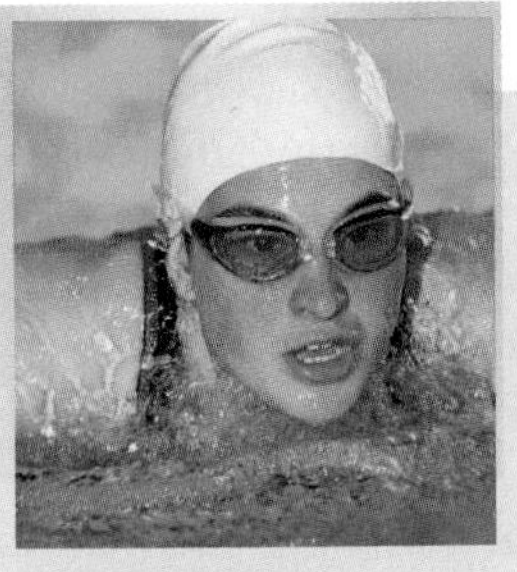
Westend 61 GmbH/Alamy

## CASE STUDY 3.1

### Anna Marie's Tale

Exercise can be bad for you—or at least it is for Anna Marie. She and her husband Mark already have two delightful children, full-time jobs, and hectic schedules. Mark wants more children, but Anna Marie is dead set against it. Mark refuses to use contraception and has made Anna Marie promise not to use any, either. Anna Marie makes the promise because she thinks she can avoid pregnancy by staying at her weight of 210 pounds. At this weight, Anna Marie seldom has a menstrual period and figures the odds of conception are slim. For 2 years, Anna Marie's plan for avoiding conception has worked.

Now that the children are older, Anna Marie finds she has a bit of free time, which she uses to indulge her love of swimming. Within months of beginning her program of swimming regularly, however, Anna Marie abandons it. Her menstrual periods have become regular, and her contraception method is lost.

Anna Marie's weight at 210 pounds has remained stable during the months she has been swimming. It appears that her improved level of physical fitness and body fat has improved her fertility status.

#### Questions

1. What was likely the reason for Anna Marie's infertility when she was inactive?
2. Give an example of a hormonal change that may have occurred after Anna Marie began exercising regularly.
3. Name a possible health consequence related to Anna Marie's high weight and lack of menstrual cycles.

nutritional status during weight loss. Poor status of iron, vitamin D, folate, and other nutrients during the periconceptional period may impair maternal health and fetal development.[28]

### Underweight and Fertility

Ovulatory processes are sensitive to energy balance and can be disrupted by weight loss and low levels of body fat.[14] Women with low BMIs (<20 kg/m$^2$) may develop anovulation and amenorrhea due to reduced hypothalamic production of ***gonadotropin releasing hormone*** (GnRH). GnRH stimulates the release of follicle-stimulating hormone (FSH) and luteinizing hormone (LH) from the anterior pituitary. Both are needed for egg maturation and release.[15] Serum FSH tends to be higher, and sperm concentration and sperm count lower, in men with a BMI of less than 20 kg/m$^2$.[16]

## Negative Energy Balance and Fertility

LO 3.2 Identify two mechanisms by which a negative energy balance can influence fertility.

Caloric restriction that produces a negative energy balance in underweight, and normal weight, menstruating females is related to the development of ***hypothalamic amenorrhea***. This condition produces a loss of menstrual cycles due to the absence of ovulation and is most likely to occur in women with restricting-type eating disorders and females athletes who maintain a low body weight.[30,31] It is suggested that these mechanisms come into effect to prevent pregnancy in women who are malnourished and poorly prepared for the calorie and nutrient costs of fetal growth and development.[31]

Energy deficits that characterize hypothalamic amenorrhea appear to suppress the activity of gonadotropin releasing hormone (GnRH). Other mechanisms in addition to suppression of GnRH may play a role in the development of anovulation in women with anorexia nervosa and the ***female athlete triad***.[30]

### Anorexia Nervosa, Bulimia Nervosa, and Fertility

***Anorexia nervosa*** and ***bulimia nervosa*** are both related to the development of hypothalamic amenorrhea in some, but not all, women with these disorders.[32] Women with these conditions who became pregnant, however, are more likely to miscarry, experience preterm

**gonadotropin releasing hormone (GnRH)** A hormone produced in the hypothalamus that is responsible for the release of follicle stimulating hormone and luteinizing hormone by the pituitary gland.

**hypothalamic amenorrhea** A condition characterized by cessation of menstruation due to changes in hypothalamic signals that maintain ovulation. Changes in hypothalamic function appear to be triggered by an energy deficit. Also called *functional hypothalamic amenorrhea* and *weight-related amenorrhea*.

**female athlete triad** A condition marked by the simultaneous presence of an eating disorder, menstrual dysfunction, and osteoporosis in otherwise healthy female athletes. It is characterized by the interrelated factors of energy deficit, menstrual dysfunction, and loss of bone mineral density.

**anorexia nervosa** An eating disorder characterized by extreme weight loss, poor body image, and irrational fears of weight gain and obesity.

delivery, and deliver newborns that are low birthweight (or less than 5.5 pounds or 2500 grams).[33] Very low levels of body fat are related to reduced estrogen production in fat cells. In addition, suppressed activity of GnRH leads to a decrease in estrogen production by the ovaries. Inadequate estrogen leads to the loss of bone mineral accretion and density, and increases the risk for osteoporosis and fractures.[31,34]

Ovulation and menstruation resume in most women with eating disorders with a return to normal eating behaviors and weight gain.[34] It is often difficult for women with eating disorders to achieve and maintain weight gain. Appropriate care entails the use of evidence-based practices utilizing an interdisciplinary group of experienced health professionals that includes a dietitian, nurse, social worker, and psychiatrist.[32] Additional information about eating disorders can be found in Chapter 15.

### Women, Exercise, and Fertility

Improved opportunities for female participation in sports in recent decades have been followed by an upsurge in the number of females who are competitive athletes.[34] Although this is a healthy trend, some who are involved in sports that emphasize a lean body type are compromising their health (Illustration 3.1).[34] Chronic energy deficits combined with very high levels of physical activity can place women at risk of developing the *female athlete triad.* It is called a triad because it consists of three conditions: amenorrhea, an eating disorder, and osteoporosis.

Amenorrhea associated with the female athlete triad appears to be triggered when energy intake is about 30 percent less than energy requirement.[35] This level of energy deficit leads to a loss of normal secretion of LH and FSH, a lack of estrogen production, and other hormonal changes seen in hypothalamic amenorrhea. Metabolic changes triggered by hormonal shifts result in decreased bone density and an increased susceptibility to stress fractures in affected athletes.[35]

Treatment of the female athlete triad focuses on correction of the negative energy balance and on restoration of ovulation and bone mass accretion.[36] Peak bone mass is established before age 30, so it is particularly important that interruptions in bone development be prevented or short in duration.[31] Vitamin D, calcium, and other supplements may be needed in addition to a balanced and adequate diet to facilitate bone development.[127] Restoration of energy balance can reverse disruptions in reproductive hormones and bone formation.[34]

The effect of high levels of physical activity on reproductive hormones in overweight females appears to be different from that experienced by lean athletes. Overweight females who engage in long-distance running, fast cycling, and other aerobic physical activities tend to experience improvements in reproductive hormone levels and increased fertility compared to overweight women who are sedentary.[6]

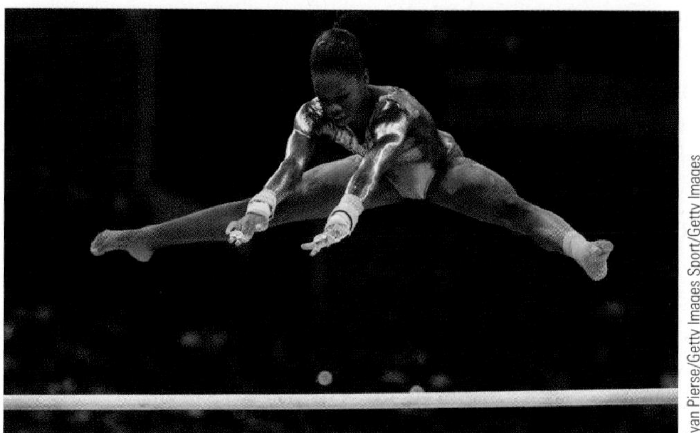

Ryan Pierse/Getty Images Sport/Getty Images

ILLUSTRATION 3.1 ▸ Female athletes most likely to develop the female athlete triad participate in sports like gymnastics that emphasize a lean body.

## Diabetes Prior to Pregnancy

**LO 3.3** Illustrate two ways in which good blood glucose control during the periconceptional period can benefit fetal growth and development.

Poorly controlled blood glucose levels during the periconceptional period increase the risk of maternal and fetal complications during pregnancy. High blood glucose levels during the first two months of pregnancy are ***teratogenic***; they are associated with a two- to threefold increase in the incidence of ***congenital abnormalities*** in newborns, including malformations of the pelvis, central nervous system, and heart. Exposure to high blood glucose during the first two months increases the risk of miscarriage.[37,38]

Management approaches to blood glucose control in diabetes depends, in part, on whether women have ***type 1 diabetes*** or ***type 2 diabetes***. Once thought of as a disease of older

**bulimia nervosa** An eating disorder characterized by recurrent episodes of rapid, uncontrolled eating of large amounts of food in a short period of time. Episodes of binge eating are followed by compensatory behaviors such as such as self-induced vomiting, dieting, excessive exercise, or misuse of laxatives, to prevent weight gain.

**teratogenic** Exposures that produce malformations in embryos or fetuses.

**congenital abnormality** A structural, functional, or metabolic abnormality present at birth. Also called congenital anomalies. These may be caused by environmental or genetic factors, or by a combination of the two. Structural abnormalities are generally referred to as congenital malformations, and metabolic abnormalities as inborn errors of metabolism.

**type 1 diabetes** A disease characterized by high blood glucose levels resulting from destruction of the insulin-producing cells of the pancreas. This type of diabetes was called juvenile-onset diabetes and insulin-dependent diabetes in the past, and its official name is type 1 diabetes mellitus.

**type 2 diabetes** A disease characterized by high blood glucose levels due to the body's inability to use insulin normally, or to produce enough insulin. This type of diabetes was called adult-onset diabetes and non-insulin-dependent diabetes in the past. Its official name is type 2 diabetes mellitus.

IN FOCUS

## Diabetes

**Definition:** There are three major types of diabetes mellitus: type 1, type 2, and gestational. All types of diabetes are characterized by abnormally high blood glucose levels, or fasting levels of 126 mg/dL (7 mmol/L) or higher.[109] People with diabetes are considered to be "carbohydrate intolerant" because carbohydrate consumption tends to raise blood glucose levels.

Type 1 diabetes is carbohydrate intolerance resulting from destruction of insulin-producing cells of the pancreas. Individuals with type 1 diabetes require an external supply of insulin. It is considered an ***autoimmune disease***. About 10 percent of cases of diabetes are of this type.

Type 2 diabetes is carbohydrate intolerance due to the body's inability to produce enough insulin. About 90 percent of cases of diabetes are of this type.

Gestational diabetes is carbohydrate intolerance that begins or is first recognized during pregnancy. It is closely related to type 2 diabetes. (Additional information about gestational diabetes is presented in Chapter 5.)

**Prevalence:** Approximately 12 percent of U.S. adults have type 2 diabetes and less than 1 percent of youth and adults have type 1. Gestational diabetes is diagnosed in 4–9 percent of pregnancies. Rates of gestational and type 2 diabetes are increasing worldwide due to escalating rates of obesity.[110,111]

**Major physiological aspects and consequences:** Major signs and symptoms of diabetes are frequent urination, increased thirst and fluid intake, increased appetite, and elevated blood glucose levels.

People with gestational diabetes or type 2 are generally obese and have insulin resistance. Insulin resistance that develops with obesity partly originates from metabolic changes initiated in fat cells. High amounts of body fat are related to an increased release of fatty acids from fat cells into blood. High circulating levels of fatty acids stimulate the production of free radicals and other proinflammatory molecules and the development of oxidative stress and chronic inflammation. These and other changes are related to the development of insulin resistance in liver and muscle cells, excessive fat storage in the liver, and increased insulin output by beta cells of the pancreas. Over time, insulin resistance can lead to the exhaustion of beta cells and decreased insulin production, elevated blood glucose levels, and the onset of type 2 diabetes.[112]

Elevated blood glucose levels in people with diabetes have many adverse consequences in the short- and long-term. Such consequences can be limited or postponed by tightly managed blood glucose levels. Diabetes increases the risk of coronary heart disease, kidney disease, vision problems and blindness, nerve problems, and loss of limbs.

Types 1 and 2 diabetes are chronic diseases that require lifelong management. Patient education, nutritional support, and blood-glucose monitoring are important for long-term blood glucose control. Some people with type 2 diabetes can control the disease through dietary and physical activity changes and weight loss.[41]

**Risk factors:** Exposure to certain infectious diseases, drugs, and other environmental agents can trigger the onset of type 1 diabetes in genetically susceptible individuals. Obesity, especially central obesity, is a primary risk factor for gestational and type 2 diabetes.[113]

adults, type 2 diabetes is becoming increasingly common in young adults and children due to the obesity epidemic. Approximately four of five U.S. adults with type 2 diabetes are overweight or obese.[39] Background information on diabetes is presented in the In Focus: Diabetes box.

## Nutritional Management of Diabetes Prior to Pregnancy

The main goals of the management of diabetes are blood glucose control, resolution of coexisting health problems, and health maintenance. The healthy dietary pattern recommended for people with diabetes is basically the same as for others. People with diabetes, however, are counseled to reduce intake of beverages with artificial sweeteners.[40] It is not recommended that individual with diabetes exclude all sources of sugar from their diets.[41] Foods low in ***glycemic index*** and high in fiber are encouraged, as are brightly colored fruits and vegetables, whole grains and whole grain products, low-fat dairy products, poultry, fish, dried beans, nuts and seeds.[12,42] (Table 1.4 lists the GI of a variety of foods.) Foods with high GI tend to raise blood glucose and insulin levels more than do foods with low GI, and high-GI foods lead to more episodes of hyperglycemia (high blood glucose level) than do diets providing mainly low-GI

**autoimmune disease** Diseases that result from a failure of an organism to recognize its own constituent parts as "self." The organism attempts to defend itself from the perceived foreign substance through actions of its immune system. These actions can damage molecules, cells, tissues, and organs. Type 1 diabetes, lupus, and rheumatoid arthritis are examples of autoimmune disease.

carbohydrate foods.[43] Ample intake of dietary fiber (14 grams per 1,000 calories) appear to be particularly helpful for glucose control.[41,44] Reduced-calorie diet and behavioral change plans should be included as part of the care for individuals with diabetes who would benefit from weight loss.

Physical activity is generally part of a diabetes care plan because it improves blood glucose levels, physical fitness, and insulin utilization. Both strength and aerobic exercise are recommended.[45] Individualized dietary and physical activity plans and follow-up care for individuals with diabetes should be provided by an experienced health care team that includes a registered dietitian-nutritionist.[46] The blood glucose response to diet composition varies somewhat among individuals, so dietary advice must be tailored for every person.[47]

There is no clear evidence of benefit from vitamin or mineral supplementation in people with diabetes who do not have underlying deficiencies. Routine supplementation with antioxidants, such as vitamin E, vitamin C, and beta-carotene, or with chromium is not recommended because of a lack of evidence of any benefit.[41]

**Prevention of Gestational and Type 2 Diabetes** Gestational diabetes is considered a form of type 2 diabetes. Its occurrence during pregnancy substantially increases the risk that type 2 diabetes will occur later in life.[48] In the best of all worlds, the risk of developing diabetes would be reduced prior to pregnancy. Several effective approaches to risk reduction have been identified for gestational diabetes and for type 2 diabetes.

Weight loss if overweight, increased dietary fiber intake, consumption of a healthy dietary pattern, and regular exercise prior to pregnancy are related to a reduced risk of gestational diabetes.[12,49] Weight loss should be achieved before pregnancy because it is not recommended during pregnancy.[50] Regardless of prepregnancy weight status, women adhering to a healthy dietary pattern are 24 to 46 percent less likely to develop gestational diabetes than women who consume a typical western-type diet containing high-glycemic-index carbohydrate foods, refined grains, and meats high in saturated fat.[51]

The risk of type 2 diabetes can be decreased by weight loss, low-glycemic-index sources of carbohydrates, exercise, and consumption of a healthy dietary pattern.[12,49,55] A large study that took place over a three-year period found that losses in body weight of about 7 percent of original weight combined with 150 minutes per week of exercise reduced the risk of type 2 diabetes development by 50 percent.[52] Dietary patterns containing primarily low-glycemic-index sources of carbohydrates such as whole grains and whole grain products, vegetable, and fruits are associated with lower fasting blood glucose levels. Exercise improves physical fitness levels, general health, and insulin sensitivity.[53,54] Factors associated with reduced risk of developing gestational diabetes, type 2 diabetes, or both are summarized in Table 3.1.

**TABLE 3.1** Factors associated with reduced risk of developing gestational diabetes, type 2 diabetes, or both[12]

- Weight loss (if needed)
- Regular exercise
- Healthy dietary pattern
- High fiber intake
- Intake of low GI carbohydrate sources
- Regular vegetable and fruit consumption

# Polycystic Ovary Syndrome and Fertility

**LO 3.4** Cite three key components of the nutritional management of PCOS.

**Case scenario:** Lupe is a 28-year-old woman who is 5 feet 3 inches tall and weighs 208 pounds. She and her husband want to start a family, but her highly irregular periods and a failure to become pregnant as soon as desired have brought her to see her doctor. At the clinic it is determined that Lupe's waist circumference is 38 inches and her body mass index (BMI) is 37 kg/m$^2$. Laboratory tests show that her blood levels of insulin and triglycerides are high and that she is not ovulating. Lupe is diagnosed as having ***polycystic ovary syndrome,*** or ***PCOS.***

Many women with undiagnosed PCOS seek care due to concerns about missing menstrual cycles or an inability to become pregnant. Between 5 and 10 percent of women of reproductive age have PCOS, and it is a leading cause of female infertility.[56] PCOS is not a disease but, rather, a syndrome that consists of a variety of clinical signs. Infertility in women with PCOS is primarily related to the absence of ovulation. Characteristically, the outer layer of the ovaries of women with PCOS is thick and hard, and it may look yellowish.[57]

About half of women with PCOS are overweight or obese, but even in women with PCOS who are normal weight, levels of intra-abdominal fat are usually high.[58] Some women with PCOS have excess body hair (also known as hirsutism, Illustration 3.2), acne, high blood levels of insulin, triglycerides, and ***androgens***; and low levels of HDL cholesterol

**glycemic index (GI)** A measure of the extent to which blood glucose levels are raised by consumption of an amount of food that contains 50 grams of carbohydrate compared to 50 grams of glucose. A portion of white bread containing 50 grams of carbohydrate is sometimes used for comparison instead of 50 grams of glucose.

**Polycystic ovary syndrome (PCOS)** (polycysts = many cysts; i.e., abnormal sacs with membranous linings). A condition in females generally characterized by insulin resistance, high blood insulin levels, obesity, polycystic ovaries, menstrual dysfunction, amenorrhea, infertility, hirsutism (excess body hair), and acne.

**androgens** Types of steroid hormones produced in the testes, ovaries, and adrenal cortex from cholesterol. Some androgens (testosterone, dihydrotestosterone) stimulate development and functioning of male sex organs.

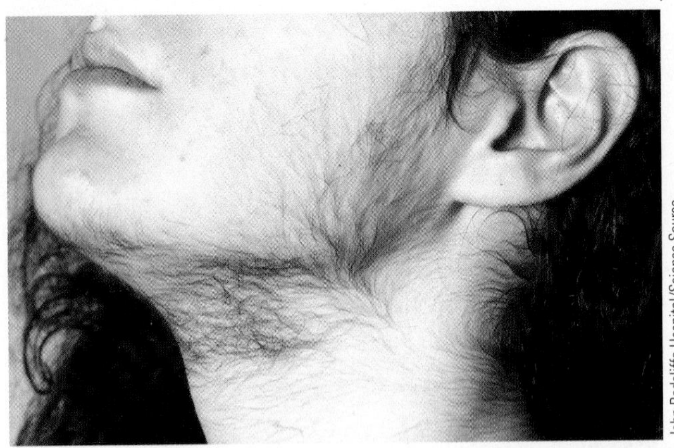


ILLUSTRATION 3.2 ▸ The appearance of hirsutism (abnormal facial or body hair) in a woman with PCOS.

(Table 3.2). PCOS appears to have a genetic component, and its development is influenced by environment-gene interactions.[59] It tends to run in families where females have a history of infertility, menstrual problems, type 2 diabetes, central obesity, and hirsutism. In utero exposures that affect fetal gene programming may be a factor in its development. It appears that the onset of PCOS is related to specific gene variants that lead to overproduction of androgens such as testosterone.[20] PCOS is sometimes difficult to diagnose (and may therefore not be treated) because signs and symptoms of the disorder vary among individual women.[60]

The cause of PCOS is still debated, but insulin resistance is a leading candidate because it plays a pivotal role in most cases of PCOS regardless of body weight.[58] Less commonly, PCOS is caused by androgen-secreting tumors in the ovaries or adrenal gland, other disorders, and certain medications.[61] High blood levels of insulin stimulate the ovaries to produce androgens (such as testosterone), and excess androgens disrupt development of follicles.[62] High blood levels of androgens can lead to excess hair growth on the face and other parts of the body, while high insulin levels increase intra-abdominal fat stores and raise triglyceride and lower HDL cholesterol levels.[63]

TABLE 3.2 ▸ Variation in clinical signs associated with PCOS[120]

| CLINICAL SIGN | PERCENT OF WOMEN WITH PCOS AFFECTED |
|---|---|
| Menstrual irregularities | 90% |
| Polycystic ovaries | 67–86% |
| Excess abdominal fat | 80% |
| Insulin resistance | 80% |
| Overweight, obesity | 80% |
| Abnormal facial and body hair | 70% |
| High testosterone levels | 70% |
| Infertility | 70% |
| Low HDL cholesterol levels | 64% |
| High triglycerides | 47% |

Although obesity does not cause PCOS, it exacerbates reproductive and metabolic problems associated with it. Rates of PCOS in teens and women increase with of the rise of overweight and obesity.[63] Women with PCOS are at increased risk of spontaneous abortions, gestational and type 2 diabetes, hypertension, and cardiovascular disease.[57]

### Nutritional Management of PCOS

The primary goal in the treatment of PCOS is to increase insulin sensitivity. A number of insulin-sensitizing drugs, including metformin, can be used to lower blood insulin levels and reduce the excess production of androgens by the ovaries.[57] Other drugs may be used to stimulate ovulation. The preferred first-line treatment for women with PCOS, however, is dietary modification, weight loss if needed, and exercise.[64] Weight loss and exercise improve insulin sensitivity, benefit blood lipids and insulin levels, and lower fasting glucose and testosterone levels in women with PCOS. Care must be taken to individualize eating and exercise plans if weight loss is to succeed. PCOS is a long-term health problem that requires a sustainable approach to weight loss and exercise. In addition, women may benefit from knowing more about PCOS, long-term health risks, and why weight loss and exercise may be needed.[65]

Dietary recommendations for females with PCOS emphasize lean sources of protein, whole grains, fruits and vegetables high in antioxidants, ample fiber intake, regular meals, nonfat dairy products, vitamin D adequacy, and low-GI carbohydrates.[66,67] Basic foods such as whole grains and high-fiber, low-GI carbohydrates are encouraged to limit blood glucose surges and insulin production. Weight loss is recommended (if needed), as is aerobic and strength-building exercise (30 minutes or more per day).[68] If drugs are used to treat the symptoms of PCOS, they should be used in conjunction with diet and exercise.[69]

Symptoms of PCOS tend to improve substantially in overweight and obese women with weight loss of 5–10 percent of initial body weight.[68] Symptoms generally worsen if diet, weight loss, and exercise recommendations are not followed.[60] Most women with PCOS are able to modify eating and exercise behaviors, and to have children.[59]

## Phenylketonuria (PKU)

LO 3.5 Summarize the major reasons why dietary control of PKU is particularly important during pregnancy.

**phenylketonuria (PKU)** An inherited error in phenylalanine metabolism most commonly caused by a deficiency of phenylalanine hydroxylase, which converts the essential amino acid phenylalanine to the nonessential amino acid tyrosine. Also called hyperphenylalaninemia.

***Phenylketonuria*** (also called hyperphenylalaninemia) is the most frequently inherited disorder of amino-acid metabolism and is an important, preventable cause of intellectual disability. It occurs in roughly 1 in 10,000 individuals.[74]

Phenylketonuria (PKU) derives its name from the characteristic presence of phenylalanine in the urine of people with this condition. PKU is an inherited problem that causes elevation in blood phenylalanine levels due to very low levels or lack of the enzyme phenylalanine hydroxylase. Lack of this enzyme diminishes the conversion of the essential amino acid phenylalanine to tyrosine, a nonessential amino acid, and causes phenylalanine to accumulate in blood. High levels of phenylalanine impair nerve functions and interfere with amino acid transport.[70]

If present during early pregnancy, high levels of phenylalanine accumulate in the embryo and fetus and impair normal central nervous system development. Elevated phenylalanine levels in the first 8 weeks of pregnancy increase the risk of heart defects. The risk increases if high blood levels of phenylalanine are combined with low-protein diets early in pregnancy.[71] Untreated women with PKU have a 92 percent chance of delivering a newborn with mental retardation and a 73 percent chance that the infant will be born with an abnormally small head (microcephaly).[72,73] Infants born to women with high blood levels of phenylalanine during pregnancy are at elevated risk of seizures, hyperactivity, and abnormal behavioral patterns later in life.[74]

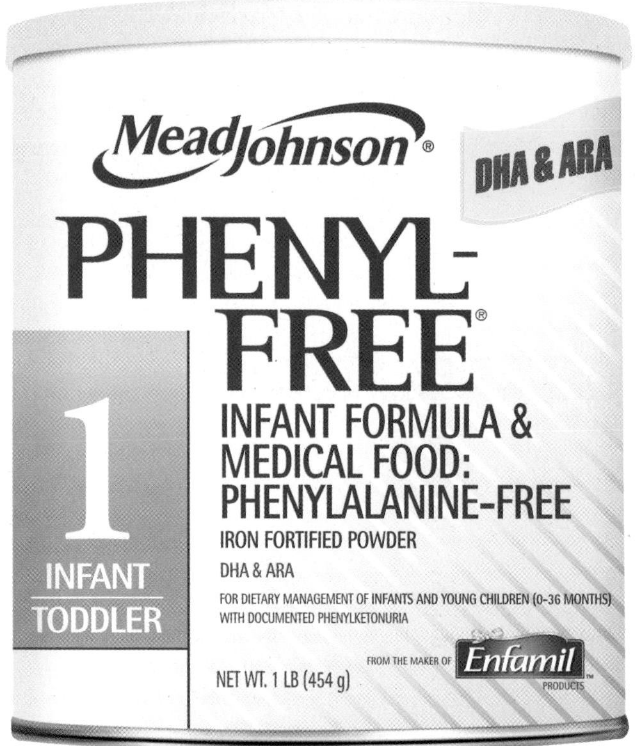


Courtesy of Mead Johnson & Company, LLC

ILLUSTRATION 3.3 ▸ An example of a phenylalanine-free formula.

TABLE 3.3 ▸ One Person's PKU Experience

Margaret was a healthy newborn but during her first year of life she started to experience seizures and difficulty in standing and walking. When she was 13 months old, she was diagnosed with PKU and started on a low-phenylalanine diet. Her development improved until the age of 8 years, when she was taken off the diet. It was reasoned that she no longer needed the low-phenylalanine diet because "her brain had grown." Around the age of 19, Margaret became violent, destructive, hysterical, and self-abusive. Her family put her back on the PKU diet, and although she continued to have seizures and remained profoundly retarded, her behaviors and quality of life improved.[121]

Not all infants born to a parent with PKU inherit the disorder, and some infants inherit it from parents who do not have PKU. It is important that infants born with PKU be identified and started on low-phenylalanine formula (Illustration 3.3) as soon after birth as possible. Because phenylalanine is an essential amino acid, some phenylalanine must be included in the diet. To meet this need, the phenylalanine-free formula will be mixed with an amount of breast milk or formula that supplies enough phenylalanine to meet needs while controlling blood phenylalanine levels. Table 3.3 presents a condensed story about the journey of a woman born with PKU that was identified late and inadequately controlled. Individuals born with PKU who adhere to an adequate, low-phenylalanine diet during childhood and later in life tend to develop normally or at levels that are somewhat below normal (Illustration 3.4).[75]

People with undiagnosed PKU may self-select low-protein foods because meat and other rich sources of protein make them light-headed and easily confused. They may find it difficult to comprehend all the information they receive after the inborn error is diagnosed.[76,77]

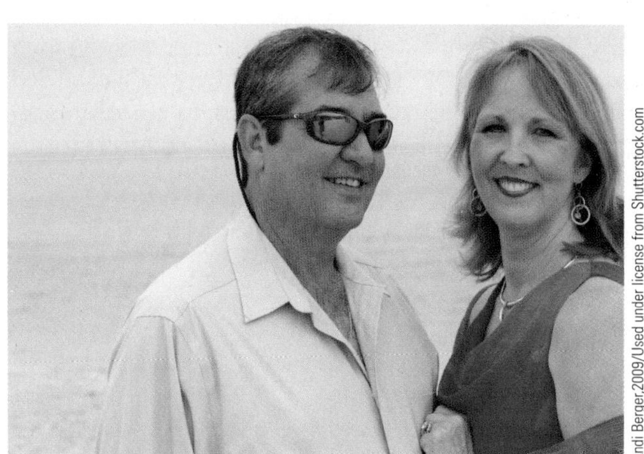

Andi Berger,2009/Used under license from Shutterstock.com

ILLUSTRATION 3.4 ▸ You can't pick a person with well-controlled PKU out of a crowd.

### Maternal PKU

In the past, it was thought that children with PKU could safely go off the PKU diet after the brain developed. Later, it was made abundantly clear that PKU diets should be maintained through adolescents and continue into adulthood in individuals who have intellectual disabilities.[77] Women with PKU who are not on a PKU diet before pregnancy are at risk for a condition called maternal PKU. Uncontrolled PKU in women represents risks for the fetus during pregnancy, even if the fetus did not inherit the disorder. The extent of the harm caused to the fetus increases with high maternal phenylalanine levels. Adverse effects on the fetus can be minimized if maternal phenylalanine levels are well controlled before and throughout pregnancy, and energy and nutrient needs of the mother are met.[74,78]

In the 1960s, the United States adopted newborn screening programs that test infants for a variety of genetic disorders including PKU.[78] States track individuals testing positive for PKU to ensure they are provided with medical and nutrition services, a prescription low-phenylalanine formula, and are made aware of the potential adverse effects of uncontrolled PKU throughout pregnancy. Not all women are able to follow the diet, however, because it is expensive and unpalatable to them, while others may get confused and have trouble staying on the diet.[78] Many speciality foods products for PKU diets, such as specially processed pastas, breads, imitation cheese, and baking mixes are available, and some are fortified with tyrosine, other amino acids, and vitamins minerals, and fat for calories. Alternatives to diet therapy for PKU management are being developed and tested. In the future, it is likely that PKU will be managed largely by techniques such as cell transplantation, gene therapy, or injectable forms of the missing enzyme.[77]

### Nutritional Management of PKU

PKU can be successfully managed by a low-phenylalanine diet, instituted and monitored with the help of an experienced registered dietitian-nutritionist, nurses, and physicians. Table 3.4 shows an example of a one-day menu for a person following a PKU diet. PKU diets are individualized based on blood phenylalanine response to protein foods. Successful PKU diets maintain blood concentrations of phenylalanine in the range of 120–360 μmol/L (2–6 mg/dL).[78] High phenylalanine protein foods such as meat, fish, eggs, and wheat are excluded from the diet. Supplemental DHA (200 mg per day) should be consumed because PKU diets lack dietary sources of this important omega-3 fatty acid.[79]

For many individuals, the PKU diet is beneficial throughout life, but it is critical that it be adhered to prior to conception and maintained throughout pregnancy. It usually takes about 4 to 6 months to learn and implement the PKU diet and to lower blood phenylalanine levels.[80]

**TABLE 3.4** ▸ A one-day menu for a person following a PKU diet[77,128]

Breakfast: Puffed rice with nondairy coffee creamer, a peach, and phenylalanine-free formula
Lunch: Vegetarian vegetable soup, low-protein crackers, apple
Snack: phenylalanine-free formula
Dinner: Broccoli, baked potato, margarine, cranberry juice, phenylalanine-free formula, fruit ice

# Celiac Disease

**LO 3.6** Describe three nutritional consequences of untreated celiac disease.

Celiac disease, highlighted in the In Focus: Celiac Disease box, is related to somewhat higher rates of infertility and to substantially higher rates of subfertility.[81] In males, untreated celiac disease is related to alterations in the actions of androgens, delayed sexual maturation, and hypogonadism. Hypogonadism is marked by a deficiency of sex hormones, and poor development and functioning of the reproductive system. In females, untreated celiac disease is associated with amenorrhea, increased rates of miscarriage, fetal growth restriction, low birth-weight deliveries, and a short duration of lactation. It is hypothesized that the effects of celiac disease on reproductive functions in males and females is related to malabsorption-induced deficiencies of nutrients such as zinc, folate, and iron; and direct effects of inflammation on intestinal and other tissues.[82,83] Table 3.5 lists vitamin and mineral deficiencies and other potential health consequences of untreated celiac disease. Normal reproductive functions generally

**TABLE 3.5** ▸ Vitamin and mineral deficiencies and other health consequences that may occur in people with untreated celiac disease[122,123]

| VITAMIN DEFICIENCIES | OTHER POTENTIAL HEALTH PROBLEMS |
|---|---|
| Folate | Lactose maldigestion, intolerance |
| Vitamin $B_{12}$ | Weight loss |
| Vitamin A | Anemia |
| Vitamin D | Osteoporosis |
| Vitamin E | Subfertility |
| Vitamin K | Growth failure (in children and adolescents) |
| | Irritable bowel disease |
| **MINERAL DEFICIENCIES** | |
| Calcium | |
| Iron | |

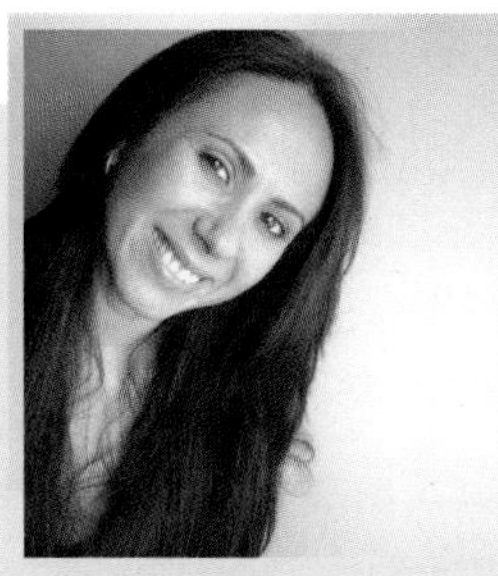
Joeysworld.com/Alamy

# CASE STUDY 3.2

## Celiac Disease

Chloe, age 30, has not had a period for over 2 years. Her gynecological exam turns up no abnormalities, but the hormones she is given to stimulate her menstrual periods do not work. Since the age of 10, Chloe has had painful stomach cramps, frequent diarrhea or constipation, and periodic iron-deficiency anemia. Multiple visits to doctors have failed to find the cause of Chloe's health problems. At around the age of 20, Chloe had begun to wonder if she was a medical anomaly or a hypochondriac.

Still bothered by her health problems and about to be married, Chloe seeks care again. This time she is seen by a nurse practitioner who has just read an article on celiac disease. The nurse sends Chloe to a registered dietitian, who advises Chloe on a gluten-free diet. After faithfully following the diet for a week, Chloe feels better. The cramps, diarrhea, and constipation are much improved, and later on, her menstrual cycles return. She returns to her doctor for a checkup and requests a test for celiac disease. By that time, however, her intestinal biopsy comes back normal because she has been on the diet for months.

### Questions

1. What should have been the first clue that Chloe might have celiac disease?
2. What facts provide other clues to the possibility of celiac disease?
3. How long will Chloe have to stay on a gluten-free diet?

return after celiac disease has been stabilized with a nutritionally adequate gluten-free diet.[83,84]

Not all individuals with celiac disease have overt symptoms, so it may be missed as an underlying cause of infertility.[85] It should be considered in unexplained cases of infertility, early pregnancy loss, and poor pregnancy outcomes.[86,87] Case Study 3.2 describes the experience of a woman ultimately diagnosed with celiac disease.

TABLE 3.6 ▸ Examples of foods that do or do not contain gluten

| GLUTEN-CONTAINING FOODS | GLUTEN-FREE FOODS[a] |
|---|---|
| Beer, ale | Fruit |
| Barley | Vegetables |
| Broth, bouillon powder/cubes | Dried beans |
| Brown rice syrup | Amaranth |
| Bulgur | Cassava, millet |
| Commercial soups, salad dressings | Grits, corn, cornmeal |
| Breads, cereals, pastas | Quinoa |
| Imitation seafood | Oatmeal (gluten-free) |
| Cakes, pies, cookies | Fats |
| Processed meats | Fresh meats, fish |
| Soy sauce | Soy flour, cereals, tofu |
| Wheat starch | Rice, wild rice |
| Pizza | Eggs |
| Macaroni and cheese | Nuts, seeds |
| Seasonings | Cheese (not processed) |
| Marinades, gravies | Popcorn |
| Rye-containing products | Milks |
| Vegetarian meat substitutes | Chips (100% corn, potato) |
| Flavored-rice packaged products | |

[a]Assumes foods have not been contaminated with gluten during processing and are free of gluten-containing ingredients

### Nutritional Management of Celiac Disease

Treatment of celiac disease focuses on the goals of elimination of gluten from the diet, correction of vitamin and mineral deficiencies, and the long-term maintenance of health. The cornerstone of treatment—elimination of gluten—can be challenging. Gluten is found in a variety of nongrain foods, including hot dogs, deli meats, some vitamin and mineral supplements, flavored potato chips, bouillon, and salad dressing. Table 3.6 lists foods that contain gluten and others that do not. An example of a gluten-free one-day diet for an adult with celiac disease is shown in Table 3.7.

People with celiac disease are generally avid food-label readers and eventually become skilled at selecting gluten-free foods. In 2008, the Food and Drug Administration started allowing gluten-free foods to be labeled "gluten-free" if they qualify according to a standard definition.[108] Many different food-product labels announce "gluten-free," "without gluten," and "no gluten," but there are no federal inspections in place to guarantee that food so labeled actually qualifies as gluten free. The Gluten-Free Certification Organization tests food products for gluten content and certifies them with a GF mark (Illustration 3.5) if found to contain less than 10 ppm, or 3 mg, gluten per serving.

IN FOCUS

## Celiac Disease

**Definition:** An autoimmune disease characterized by chronic inflammation of the small intestine due to an inherited sensitivity to the gliadin portion of gluten in wheat, rye, and barley. It is associated with the malabsorption of nutrients, nutrient deficiencies, and an increased risk of other immune disorders. Also called gluten-sensitive enteropathy, celiac sprue, and nontropical sprue.[114]

**Diagnosis:** Blood tests for celiac antibodies and genetic markers of celiac disease are used to help identify the presence of celiac disease. The gold-standard diagnostic test for celiac disease, however, is small bowel biopsy and examination of cells for signs of damage due to the disease.[115] The test has to be undertaken while individuals are consuming their normal diet and not a gluten-free one. Removal of gluten from the diet corrects intestinal cell damage and may lead to an incorrect diagnosis.

**Prevalence:** Celiac disease occurs in approximately 1 percent of the population of the United States. It is three times more common in women than men,[116] and most likely to occur in non-Hispanic White Americans.[117] The incidence of celiac disease appears to be increasing. Although awareness of, and screening for, celiac disease is increasing, far more individuals have the disease than have been diagnosed with it. It is estimated that only 17 percent of individuals with celiac disease in the United States have been diagnosed.[85]

**Major physiological aspects and consequences:** The presence of gliadin in the small intestine triggers an autoimmune response that causes an inflammatory reaction to occur in the inside lining of the small intestine. Over time, the inflammation causes the lining of the small intestine to become flattened and to absorb nutrients poorly (Illustration 3.6). The damage produced by chronic inflammation in the small intestine may lead to a variety of vitamin and mineral deficiencies and other health consequences.

Symptoms of celiac disease range from none or very mild to severe and vary by age and sex. Diarrhea, abdominal pain, nutrient malabsorption, bloating, weight loss, iron-deficiency anemia, infertility, fatigue, and growth failure in children often characterize the disease. Many cases of celiac disease are clinically silent—presenting no clear, related symptoms.[85] Long-standing, untreated celiac disease predisposes individuals to other autoimmune diseases. The only effective treatment is a lifelong gluten-free diet.[118]

**Risk factors:** The primary risk factor for celiac disease is a genetic predisposition toward reacting to gliadin as a foreign protein.[114] Repeated exposure to certain types of infectious agents, such as ***rotavirus***, may also trigger the onset of the disease in genetically susceptible people.[119]

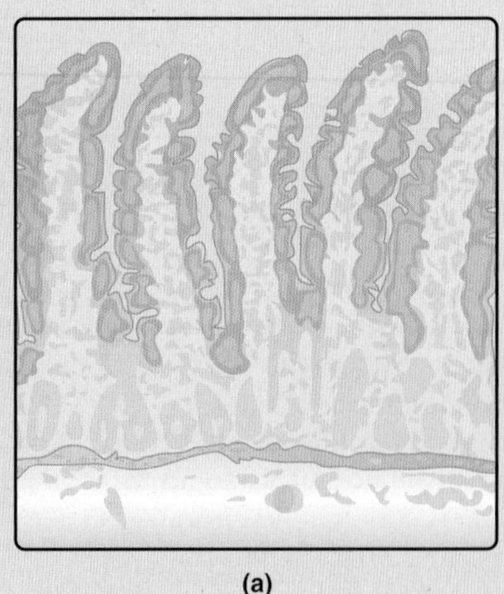

(a)

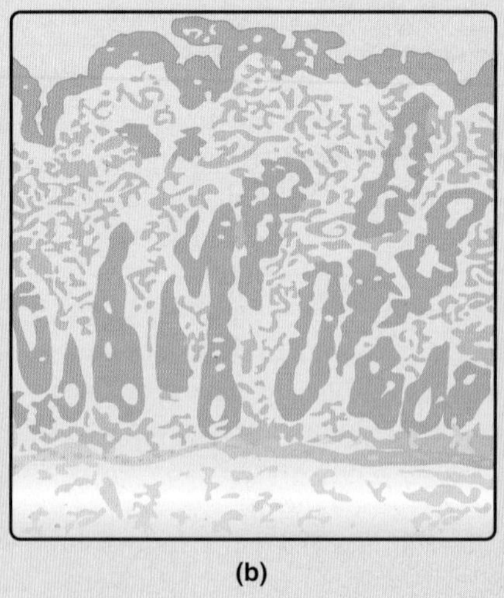

(b)



ILLUSTRATION 3.6 ▸ Sections of the small intestine showing normal villi structures of a person without celiac disease (a) and the flattened villi that develops in people with untreated celiac disease (b).

TABLE 3.7 ▸ Example of one day's diet and snack options for an adult with celiac disease

| BREAKFAST | DINNER |
|---|---|
| Gluten-free bagel with nut butter<br>Sliced bananas in yogurt<br>Tea | Lamb stew (thickened with potato starch) with carrots and lentils<br>Rice<br>Gluten-free cake<br>Low-fat milk |
| **LUNCH** | **SNACK OPTIONS** |
| Gluten-free pasta salad with chicken, broccoli, and tomatoes<br>Oil and vinegar dressing<br>Gluten-free roll with margarine<br>Fresh fruit<br>Low-fat milk | Popcorn<br>Spring rolls with rice paper<br>Ice cream<br>Fruit<br>Dark chocolate<br>Gluten-free cookies<br>String cheese<br>Rice cakes |

TABLE 3.8 ▸ Key features of the Nutrition Care Process for individuals with celiac disease[124]

**A. Nutrition Assessment**

1. Assessment of food/nutrition-related history
   - Food and nutrient intake with focus on vitamins and minerals listed in Table 3.5
   - Knowledge, skills, attitudes about celiac and dietary change
   - Access to food
2. Assessment of biochemical data and medical results
   - Severity of intestinal lining damage
   - Presence of anemia, osteoporosis, other diseases

**B. Nutrition Intervention**

1. Provide education and guidance on nutritionally adequate, gluten-free diet
2. Advise on the use of gluten-free multivitamin and mineral supplement as required
3. Provide resources and education on label reading, food cross-contamination, and support groups

**C. Nutrition Monitoring and Evaluation**

1. Monitor dietary intake, gluten intake from all sources, celiac antibody levels
2. Monitor persistent gastrointestinal symptoms not eliminated by a gluten-free diet, coordinate care
3. Monitor nutrition risks for poor pregnancy outcomes

**Evidence-Based Nutrition Practice Guidelines for Celiac Disease** Evidence-based nutrition practice guidelines and the Nutrition Care Process for celiac disease have been developed by the American Dietetic Association.[88] Major components of nutrition care services and the Nutrition Care Process are highlighted in Table 3.8. Monitoring individuals for abnormalities in nutritional status that may impact reproductive outcomes is an important part of the Nutrition Care Process for celiac disease.

Certified GF ® Gluten-Free

Courtesy of the Gluten-Free Certification Program

ILLUSTRATION 3.5 ▸ The Gluten-Free Certification Organization tests and certifies products as gluten-free and awards qualifying products this mark.

**Wheat Allergy and Non-Celiac Gluten Sensitivity** Wheat allergy and non-celiac gluten sensitivity, in addition to celiac disease, are related to gluten ingestion. Table 3.9 summarizes characteristics of each of these conditions. Diagnostic criteria for, and mechanisms involved in non-celiac gluten sensitivity require additional study because gaps in knowledge about this condition exist and there are no diagnostic standards. People reporting the condition often test negatively for celiac disease but often report that a gluten-free diet helps them feel better.[89]

Gluten-free diets are becoming increasingly popular in the United States and are most often followed by individuals who have not been diagnosed with celiac disease.[90] Whether adherence to a gluten-free diet by individuals who do not have celiac disease or wheat allergy benefits health is not clear. It is recommended that underlying causes of

**rotavirus** A virus that is the most common cause of severe diarrhea among children. Diarrhea caused by rotavirus generally lasts 2 days, and recovery is full in otherwise healthy children. The rotavirus is generally spread from an infected person's stools to food.

TABLE 3.9 Characteristics of disorders related to sensitivity to gluten[89,125,126]

| **Celiac disease** |
|---|
| • Onset of symptoms gradual (months or years after gluten introduction).<br>• Risk of nutrient deficiencies and other autoimmune disorders.<br>• Celiac disease–related antibodies present in serum; celiac-related genes also present.<br>• Tissue damage is to lining of small intestine present, abdominal pain, diarrhea.<br>• Symptom relief and small intestine damage recovery comes with gluten-free diet. |
| **Wheat allergy** |
| • Allergic reaction onset within minutes to hours after wheat ingestion.<br>• Symptoms (which can be severe) include rash, gastrointestinal upsets, and respiratory problems.<br>• Damage to the small intestine is not present.<br>• Wheat-specific antibodies are identified in serum.<br>• Wheat versus a placebo blind food challenge produces symptoms. |
| **Non-celiac gluten sensitivity**[a] |
| • Adverse reactions are similar to those of celiac disease occur when gluten consumed.<br>• Symptoms include behavioral changes, bone and joint pain, muscle cramps, leg numbness, weight loss, chronic fatigue, diarrhea, and "foggy mind."<br>• Is not related to damage to the small intestine, higher risk of nutrient deficiencies, or other immune disorders.<br>• Absence of antibodies related to gluten intolerance or allergy in blood serum.<br>• Gluten versus placebo food challenge may produce symptoms in response to gluten.<br>• May not need to restrict rye or barley from the diet; only wheat. |

[a] Additional studies are needed to confirm the characteristics and mechanisms that may underlie gluten sensitivity.

symptoms be identified prior to self-treatment with a gluten-free diet.[91]

# Premenstrual Syndrome

LO 3.7 Identify four common symptoms of premenstrual syndrome and the proposed effects of dietary supplements on the symptoms of premenopausal dysphoric disorder (PMDD).

It wasn't until 1987 that PMS, or ***premenstrual syndrome***, moved from the psychogenic disorder section of medical textbooks to chapters on physiologically based problems. PMS is characterized by life-disrupting physiological and psychological changes that begin in the ***luteal phase*** of the menstrual cycle and end with menses (menstrual bleeding). Symptoms of PMS disappear within two days after the onset of menses and return with the next luteal phase. It is a fairly common condition among menstruating women.[92,93]

A standardized, self-administered questionnaire about symptoms completed for three menstrual cycles is the primary tool used for the diagnosis of PMS. Individuals reporting the presence of one or more of the behavioral and of the physical symptoms shown in Table 3.10 during the 5 days before menses over three consecutive menstrual cycles meet the criteria for the diagnosis PMS.[94]

Premenstrual dysphoric disorder (PMDD) is a severe form of PMS that occurs in about 5 percent of menstruating women.[95] It is characterized by marked mood swings, anxiety, anger, irritability, depression, disruptions of personal relationships, and physical symptoms (breast tenderness, headache, joint or muscle pain). Some women with PMDD develop a marked increase in appetite, overeat, and crave certain foods. PMDD is diagnosed when five or more of the common symptoms of PMDD occur during most menstrual cycles.[92]

The cause of PMS and PMDD are not yet clear. However, the symptoms appear to be related to enhanced responsiveness to normal changes in ovarian hormone levels that produce ovulation, and to alterations in the availability of the neurotransmitter ***serotonin***.[96,97]

## Treatment of PMS

Prevention of ovulation, either through the use of estrogen patches or implants, gonadotropin-releasing hormone blockers, certain types of oral contraceptive pills, or removal of the ovaries can greatly diminish or abolish PMS symptoms. Serotonin reuptake inhibitors, which

**premenstrual syndrome** (*premenstrual* = the period of time preceding menstrual bleeding; *syndrome* = a constellation of symptoms). A condition occurring among women of reproductive age that includes a group of physical and psychological symptoms with onset in the luteal phase and subsiding with menstrual bleeding. Premenstrual dysphoric disorder (PMDD) is a severe form of PMS.

**luteal phase** The second half of the menstrual cycle (usually days 14 to 28) that occurs after ovulation.

**serotonin** A neurotransmitter derived from the amino acid tryptophan that affects nerve cell activities that excite or inhibit various behaviors and body functions. It plays a role in mood, appetite regulation, food intake, respiration, pain transmission, blood vessel constriction, sleep, and other body functions.

TABLE 3.10 Common symptoms of PMS[92]

| PHYSICAL | PSYCHOLOGICAL |
|---|---|
| • Tender breasts<br>• Abdominal bloating<br>• Swelling<br>• Headache | • Angry outbursts<br>• Depression<br>• Irritability<br>• Confusion<br>• Anxiety<br>• Social withdrawal |

are the active ingredient in some types of antidepressants, and anti-inflammation medications effectively reduce PMS symptoms in many women.[95,98] However, about a fourth of women with PMDD do not benefit sufficiently from established medical therapies. A few types of dietary supplements, including vitamin $B_6$ (50–100 mg/day), calcium (1,000 mg/day), and chasteberry extract (20 mg/day), may be useful as adjuncts in the treatment of PMDD. Doses of vitamin $B_6$ and calcium should not exceed the tolerable upper intake level (UL) for these nutrients. The UL for vitamin $B_6$ is 100 mg/day and for calcium it's 2,500 mg/day. Chasteberry extract may not be safe for women who may become pregnant or who use hormonal contraceptives.[99–101] Many other dietary supplements claiming to treat PMS and PMDD are available on the market but appropriate studies demonstrating their effectiveness and safety are not available.[102]

## KEY POINTS

1. Nutrition and other lifestyle changes are a core component of the treatment of a variety of common health problems of women and men prior to conception.
2. Nutrition and health status during the periconceptional period influences embryonic development and the risk of complications during pregnancy.
3. Obesity is related to a number of hormonal and metabolic changes that may compromise fertility and health status in men and women.
4. Modest levels of weight loss in obese women and men, and weight gain in underweight individuals, improve fertility.
5. Rates of diseases and disorders associated with obesity such as metabolic syndrome, polycystic ovary syndrome, gestational diabetes, and type 2 diabetes are increasing in the United States and other countries. Obesity-related health problems affecting fertility and the course and outcome of pregnancy are being seen increasingly in clinical practice.
6. Oxidative stress and chronic inflammation are related to impaired fertility and are important components of disorders such as diabetes, infertility, metabolic syndrome, polycystic ovary syndrome, and celiac disease. Antioxidant nutrients, healthful dietary patterns, weight loss, and regular exercise play key roles in reducing adverse effects of oxidative stress and chronic inflammation.
7. Insulin resistance is a key feature of obesity, gestational and type 2 diabetes, metabolic syndrome, and polycystic ovary syndrome.
8. Some obese and underweight individuals are metabolically healthy.
9. Energy deficits in individuals with hypothalamic amenorrhea, eating disorders, and the female athlete triad are related to reduced fertility.
10. Estrogen deficits in women with the female athlete triad can lead to reduced bone formation in young women.
11. PKU is a genetic disorder that causes blood phenylalanine levels to rise to toxic concentrations in untreated individuals. Untreated PKU can produce malformations, neurological disorders, and severe mental retardation in children and adults. It is treated with a low-phenylalanine diet for life.
12. Untreated celiac disease is related to multiple vitamin and mineral deficiencies, impaired fertility, fetal growth disruptions, and other adverse pregnancy outcomes. Standard treatment for celiac disease is a gluten-free diet.

## REVIEW QUESTIONS

1. Most of the treatments for PMS are based on the prevention of ovulation.

   _____True _____False

2. A wide variety of dietary supplements, ranging from evening primrose oil to St. John's Wort, have been found to effectively and safely treat the symptoms of PMS.

   _____True _____False

3. The presence of excess intra-abdominal fat is related to insulin resistance, elevated levels of insulin, chronic inflammation, oxidative stress, and the metabolic syndrome.

   _____True _____False

4. Obesity is related to impaired fertility and chronic inflammation in men only.

   _____True _____False

5. Weight loss surgery is the recommended, first-line treatment for obesity in adults.

   _____True _____False

6. Men with high amounts of body fat tend to have low levels of testosterone and elevated estradiol levels. These hormonal changes do not appear to effect sperm production, however.

   _____True _____False

7. Caloric restriction that produces a negative energy balance in underweight and normal weight, menstruating females is related to the development of hypothalamic amenorrhea.

   _____True _____False

8. Energy deficits that characterize hypothalamic amenorrhea appear to suppress the activity of gonadotropin releasing hormone (GnRH).

   _____True _____False

9. A lack of body fat and low levels of estrogen can lead to the loss of bone mineral accretion and density, and increases the risk for osteoporosis and fractures.

   _____True _____False

10. Health problems related to anorexia nervosa resolve after the eating disorder is successfully treated.

    _____True _____False

Questions 11–14 refer to this scenario and appropriate components of the nutritional management of type 2 diabetes.

Scenario: Lois was diagnosed with type 2 diabetes two months before she planned to become pregnant. To get her blood glucose under control before pregnancy, Lois worked with a dietitian-nutritionist who specializes in diabetes, and together they developed a plan to reduce Lois's blood glucose levels.

11. As part of the plan, Lois would have to exclude from her diet sugar and foods containing sugar.

    _____True _____False

12. Assume Lois will attempt to consume 2,000 calories a day. Based on that level of calorie intake, her fiber intake should total approximately 28 grams daily.

    _____True _____False

13. Lois plans to perform aerobic exercise 25 minutes daily because it will help improve insulin resistance, lower blood glucose levels, and improve her blood lipid levels.

    _____True _____False

14. Lois should take a chromium supplement to help lower her blood glucose levels.

    _____True _____False

15. Poorly controlled blood glucose levels before pregnancy is a risk factor for congenital malformation in newborns.

    _____True _____False

16. Weight loss, healthy dietary patterns, and exercise prior to pregnancy are related to a reduced risk of gestational diabetes.

    _____True _____False

17. Weight loss of 7 percent of body weight and exercise reduce the risk of type 2 diabetes.

    _____True _____False

18. Excess visceral fat and insulin resistance are shared characteristics among women with PCOS.

    _____True _____False

19. Weight loss and exercise improve insulin sensitivity, benefit blood lipids and insulin levels, and lower fasting glucose and testosterone levels in women with PCOS.

    _____True _____False

20. Infants born to women with high blood levels of phenylalanine during pregnancy are at elevated risk of seizures, intellectual disability, and abnormal behavioral patterns beginning in the teen years.

    _____True _____False

21. Individuals with PKU can safely consume high-protein foods such as beef, chicken, or eggs once a day.

    _____True _____False

22. Individuals born with PKU who adhere to an adequate, low-phenylalanine diet during childhood and later in life tend to develop normally or at levels that are somewhat below normal.

    _____True _____False

23. Individuals with celiac disease have overt symptoms that are easily identified. Consequently, the existence of celiac disease tends to be strongly suspected in cases of infertility.

    _____True _____False

24. Individuals with active celiac disease share the problems of abdominal pain, headache, nutrient malabsorption, and iron deficiency.

    _____True _____False

**Visit www.cengagebrain.com to access MindTap, a complete digital course that includes additional resources.**

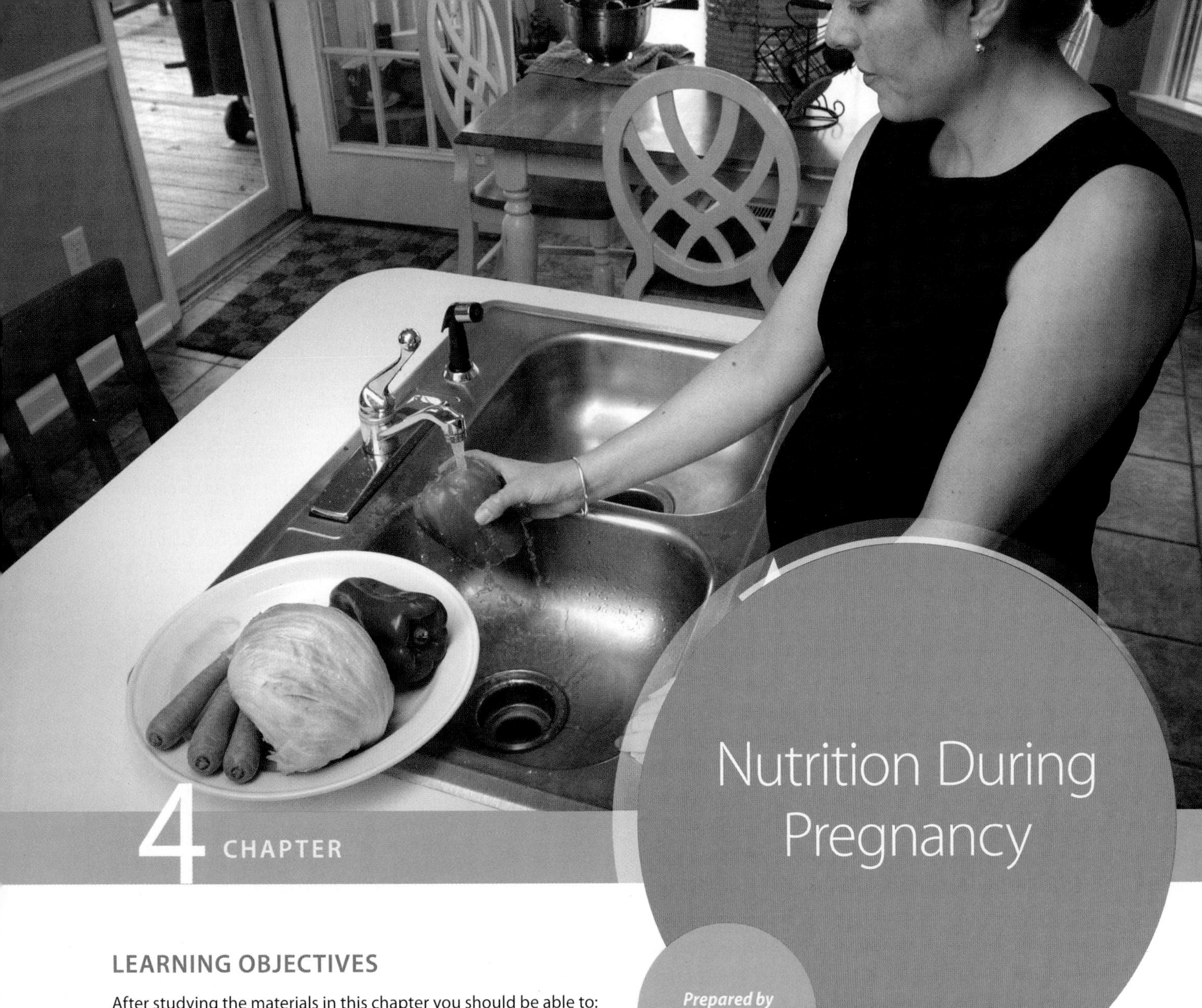

4 CHAPTER

# Nutrition During Pregnancy

*Prepared by*
Judith E. Brown

## LEARNING OBJECTIVES

After studying the materials in this chapter you should be able to:

**4.1** Identify three problem areas related to pregnancy outcomes in the United States.

**4.2** Describe five physiological changes that normally occur during pregnancy that would be considered abnormal if they did not occur during pregnancy.

**4.3** Correlate critical periods of growth and development and the potential consequences of inadequate energy and nutrient availability during these periods on future health status.

**4.4** Identify recommended weight gain ranges for women who enter pregnancy underweight, normal weight, overweight, and obese.

**4.5** Correlate three examples of relationships between nutritional status during pregnancy and long-term health outcomes in offspring.

**4.6** Provide five examples of how the need for energy and specific nutrients change due to pregnancy.

**4.7** Identify three factors that influence dietary intake during pregnancy that are not related to food availability.

**4.8** Develop a one-day diet for pregnancy based on ChooseMyPlate.gov food intake recommendations for pregnancy.

**4.9** Describe two reasons why pregnant women and their fetuses are particularly vulnerable to certain foodborne illnesses.

**4.10** Identify the basic components of a nutritional assessment of pregnant women.

**4.11** Identify three health benefits to women of regular exercise during pregnancy.

**4.12** Assess three common health problems during pregnancy and the evidence on the effectiveness of dietary interventions for their treatment or amelioration.

**4.13** Describe the nutrition service components of a model nutrition program during pregnancy.

CDC/PHIL

# Introduction

The nine months of pregnancy represent the most intense period of growth and development humans ever experience. How well these processes go depends on many factors, most of which are modifiable. Of the factors affecting fetal growth and development that are within our control to change, nutritional status stands out. At no other time in life are the benefits of optimal nutritional status more obvious than during pregnancy.

This chapter addresses the status of pregnancy outcomes in the United States and other countries. It covers physiological changes that take place to accommodate pregnancy, and the impact of these changes on maternal nutritional needs. The chapter presents the roles of nutrition in fostering fetal growth, development, and long-term health; it also covers dietary supplement use and weight-gain recommendations. The discussion goes on to consider common problems during pregnancy that can be addressed with nutritional remedies. Chapter 5 addresses clinical conditions and nutrition interventions during pregnancy. We begin this chapter by highlighting vital statistics reports that clearly show a need for improving pregnancy outcomes in the United States.

# The Status of Pregnancy Outcomes

LO 4.1 Identify three problem areas related to pregnancy outcomes in the United States.

The status of reproductive outcomes in the United States and other economically developed countries is routinely assessed through examination of a particular set of vital statistics; data called *natality* statistics (*natality* means "related to birth"). Natality statistics summarize important information about the occurrence of pregnancy complications and harmful behaviors, in addition to infant mortality (death) and morbidity (illness) rates within a specific population. Illustration 4.1 presents a time line of key intervals and events before, during, and after pregnancy. Table 4.1 provides natality statistics for the periods and outcomes shown in Illustration 4.1. These data are used to identify problems in need of resolution and to identify progress in meeting national goals for improvement in the course and outcome of pregnancy. (Note: A table of measurement abbreviations and equivalents is located in Appendix A.)

## Infant Mortality

Infant mortality reflects the general health and socioeconomic status of a population. The reason for this is because so many of the socioeconomic and environmental factors that influence the health of pregnant women and newborns also affect the health of the rest of the population (Illustration 4.2).[1] This historical view of infant mortality rates indicates that population-wide improvements in social circumstances, infectious disease control, and availability of safe and nutritious foods have corresponded to greater reductions in infant mortality than have technological advances in medical care.[2,3] Small improvements in infant mortality in the past few decades in the United States are largely due to technological advances in, and access to health care. Even though the United States spends more money on health care than any other nation, the infant mortality rate ranks 56th among countries of the world (Illustration 4.3).[2,4]

A standard definition of a ***liveborn infant*** is implemented internationally

**liveborn infant** A liveborn infant is the outcome of delivery when a completely expelled or extracted fetus breathes, or shows any sign of life such as beating of the heart, pulsation of the umbilical cord, or definite movement of voluntary muscles, whether or not the cord has been cut or the placenta is still attached.

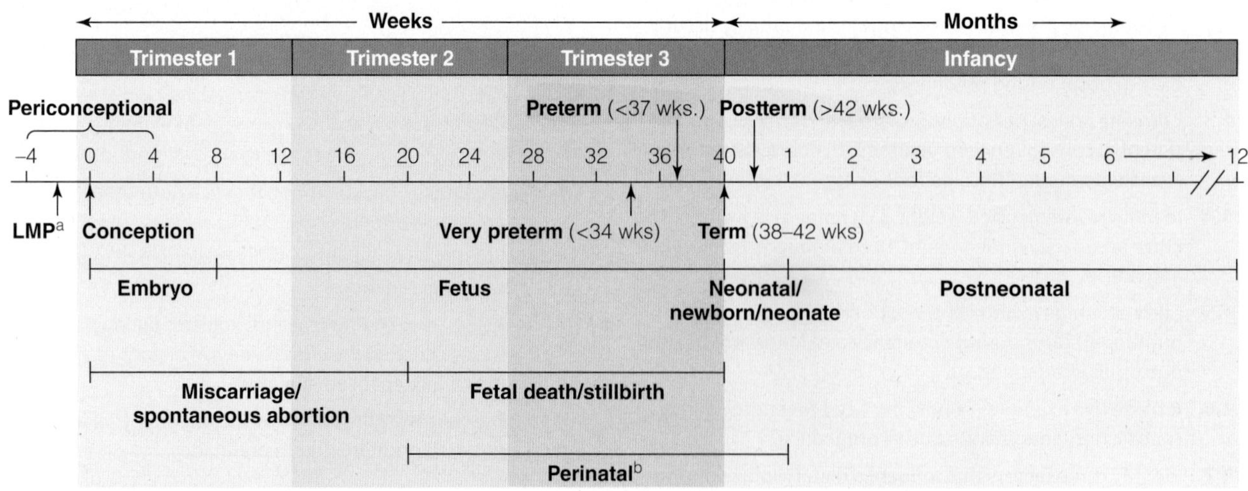


ILLUSTRATION 4.1 Time-related terms before, during, and after pregnancy.

TABLE 4.1 ▸ Natality statistics: rates, definitions, and trends in the United States[3,288-290]

| | RATES | | |
|---|---|---|---|
| | 1995 | 2013 | DEFINITION |
| Maternal mortality | 7.1 | 18.5 | Deaths/100,000 live births |
| Fetal deaths (stillbirths) | 7.0 | 6.1 | Deaths/1000 pregnancies over 20 weeks gestation |
| Perinatal mortality | 7.6 | 6.3 | Deaths/1000 deliveries over 20 weeks gestation to 7 days after birth |
| Neonatal mortality | 4.9 | 4.0 | Deaths from delivery to 28 days/1000 live births |
| Postneonatal mortality | 2.7 | 2.2 | Deaths from 28 days after birth to 1 year/1000 live births |
| Infant mortality | 7.6 | 6.1 | Deaths from birth to age 1 year/1000 live births |
| Preterm | 11.0 | 11.4 | Births <37 weeks gestation/100 live births |
| Very preterm | 1.9 | 3.5 | Births <34 weeks gestation/100 live births |
| Low birthweight | 7.3 | 8.0 | Newborn weights <2500 g (5 lb 8 oz)/100 live births |
| Very low birthweight | 1.4 | 1.5 | Newborn weights <1500 g (3 lb 4 oz)/100 live births |
| Multifetal pregnancies | | | |
| Twins | 1 in 40 | 1 in 30 | Number of twin births/total live births |
| Triplets + | 1 in 784 | 1 in 652 | Number of triplets plus higher-order multiple births/total live births |
| Adolescent pregnancies | 56.8 | 26.5 | Births/1000 females aged 15 to 19 years |

to identify infant live births. It is unlikely that differences in the definition or reporting of infant mortality among countries account for the relatively high ranking of the United States.[5] Two-thirds of deaths of liveborn infants occur within the first month after birth, the neonatal period.[3]

## Low Birthweight, Preterm Delivery, and Infant Mortality

Infants born at low birthweight or preterm are at substantially higher risk of dying in the first year of life than are larger and older newborns. Low-birthweight infants make up 8 percent of all births, yet comprise 66 percent of all infant deaths. The 11.4 percent of newborns delivered prior to 37 weeks of pregnancy similarly account for a disproportionately large number of infant deaths.[6] Low-birthweight and preterm infant outcomes are intertwined in that the shorter the pregnancy, the less newborns tend to weigh (Table 4.2).

Rates of preterm delivery and low birthweight in the United States have trended slowly downward in the last decade but remain higher in non-Hispanic Black infants than in other infants (Table 4.3). The relatively high rates of preterm

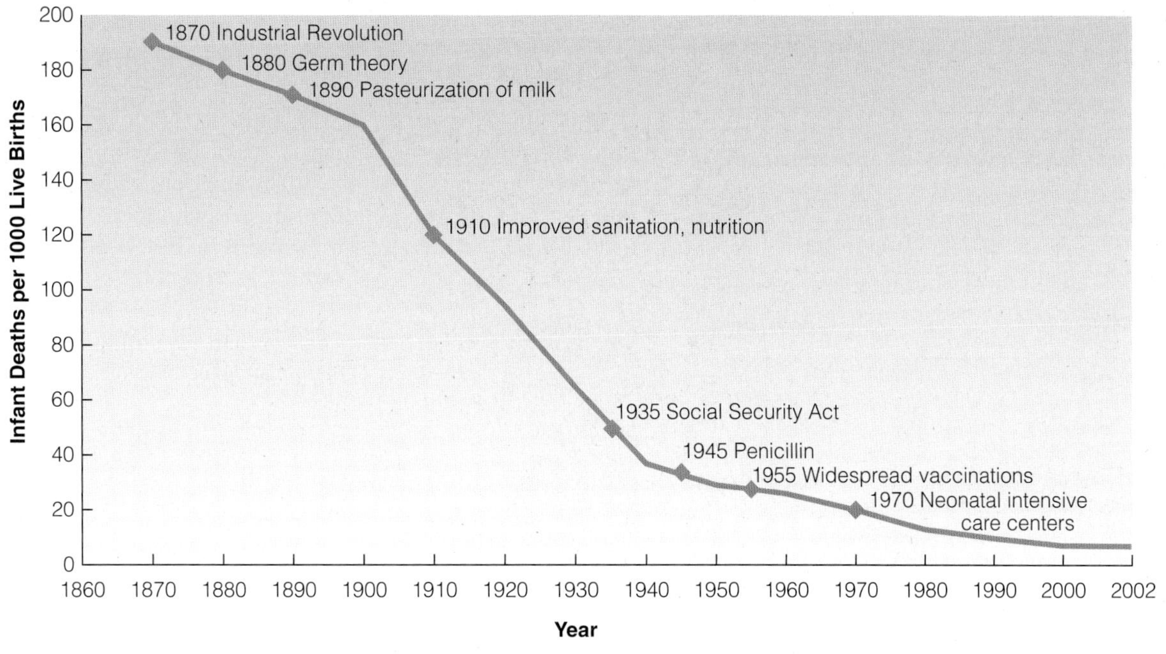


ILLUSTRATION 4.2 ▸ Chronology of events related to declines in infant mortality in the United States.

SOURCE: Judith E. Brown, 2003

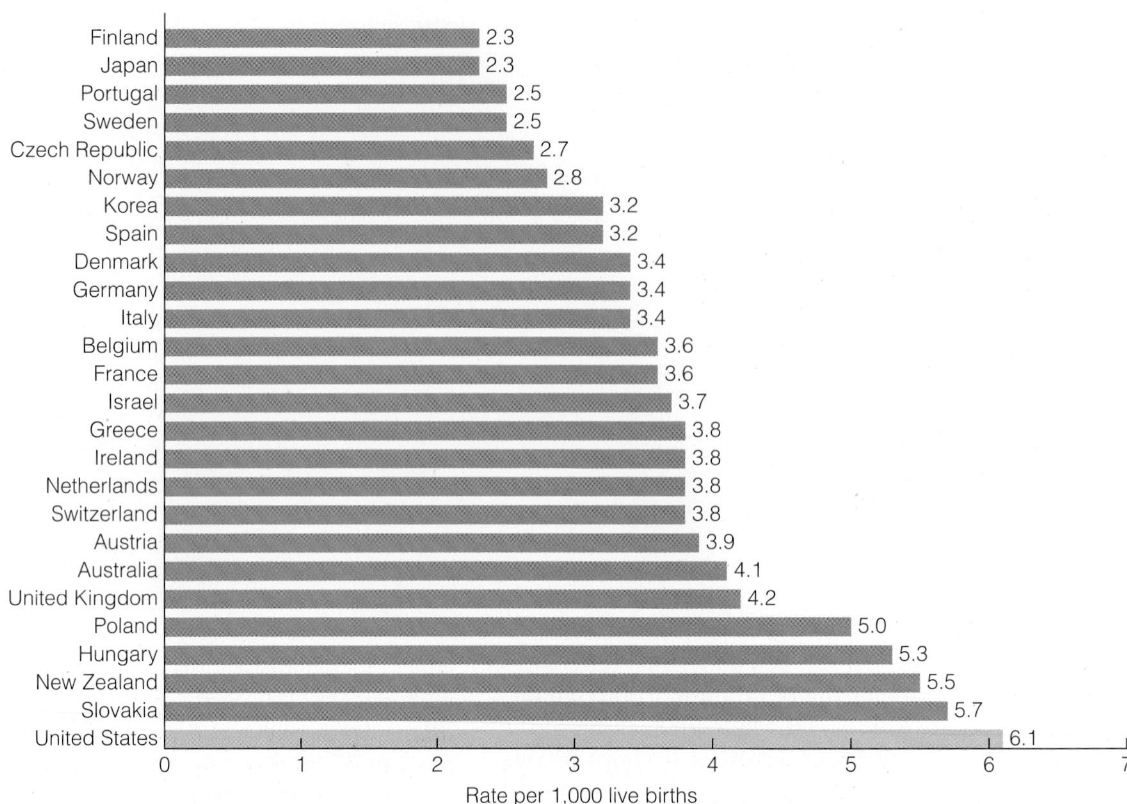


ILLUSTRATION 4.3 ▸ Infant mortality rates in United States and Europe, 2010.
Illustration shows a graph of infant mortality rate by country. Figure 1. Infant mortality from the National Vital Statistics Reports, 63(5), September 24, 2014.

SOURCE: MacDorman, M. F., et al. (2010). International Comparisons of Infant Mortality and Related Factors: United States and Europe. Available at: www.cdc.gov/nchs/data/nvsr/nvsr63/nvsr63_05.pdf

and low birthweight in non-Hispanic Black infants clearly represents a health disparity in need of resolution. Racial discrimination, poor access to nutritious foods, lack of access to health care, and poverty appear to account for a portion of the differences in infant mortality among non-Hispanic Blacks in the United States.[5,7]

TABLE 4.2 ▸ U.S. range of birthweights by gestational age[291,292]

| BIRTHWEIGHT | | WEEKS GESTATION | INFANT MORTALITY RATE |
|---|---|---|---|
| POUNDS (LB) AND OUNCES (OZ) | GRAMS | | |
| <1 lb 2 oz | <500 | <22 | 846 |
| 1 lb 2 oz–2 lb 3 oz | 500–999 | 22–27 | 316 |
| 2 lb 3 oz–3 lb 5 oz | 1000–1499 | 27–29 | 62 |
| 3 lb 5 oz–4 lb 6 oz | 1500–1999 | 29–31 | 28 |
| 4 lb 6 oz–5 lb 8 oz | 2000–2499 | 31–33 | 12 |
| 5 lb 8 oz–6 lb 10 oz | 2500–2999 | 33–36 | 4.6 |
| 6 lb 10 oz–7 lb 11 oz | 3000–3499 | 36–40 | 2.4 |
| 7 lb 11 oz–8 lb 13 oz | 3500–3999 | 40+ | 1.7 |
| 8 lb 13 oz–9 lb 14 oz | 4000–4499 | 40+ | 1.5 |
| 9 lb 14 oz–11 lb | 4500–4999 | 40+ | 2.5 |
| >11 lb | 5000+ | 40+ | — |

## Reducing Infant Mortality and Morbidity

Deaths and illnesses associated with low-birthweight and preterm infants can be reduced to an important extent through improvements in the birthweight of newborns. Infants weighing 3500 to 4500 grams at birth (or 7 lb 12 oz to 10 lb) are least likely to die within the first year of life,

TABLE 4.3 ▸ Rates of preterm delivery and low birthweight for the U.S. population and by ethnic/racial background, 2013[293]

| | PRETERM | LOW BIRTHWEIGHT |
|---|---|---|
| All | 11.4 | 8.0 |
| Non-Hispanic Blacks | 16.3 | 13.1 |
| Non-Hispanic Whites | 10.8 | 7.0 |
| American Indian/ Alaskan Native | 13.6 | 7.6 |
| Asian/Pacific Islander | 10.7 | 8.5 |
| Hispanic | 11.3 | 7.1 |

TABLE 4.4 ▸ 2020 health objectives for the nation related to pregnant women and infants

- Reduce the rates of fetal and infant deaths.
- Reduce the rate of maternal mortality.
- Reduce low birthweight and very low birthweight.
- Reduce preterm births.
- Reduce the rate of fetal and infant deaths.
- Increase the proportion of pregnant women who receive early and adequate prenatal care.
- Increase abstinence from alcohol during pregnancy.
- Increase the proportion of women who gain weight appropriately during pregnancy.

as well as in the perinatal, neonatal, and postneonatal periods.[8] Newborns weighing 3500 to 4500 grams are also at an advantage as a group in relation to overall health status and subsequent mental development.[9] They are less likely to develop heart disease, diabetes, lung disease, hypertension, and other disorders later in life.[10] Reducing the proportion of infants born small, early, or both would clearly decrease infant mortality.

**2020 Health Objectives for the Nation** National health objectives for pregnant women and newborns focus on the reduction of low birthweight, preterm delivery, and infant mortality. A number of the objectives are related to improvements in nutritional status (Table 4.4). U.S. public health efforts are also being targeted at improving prenatal weight gain, access to care, and behaviors that adversely affect the course and outcome of pregnancy in all population groups.

# Physiology of Pregnancy

LO 4.2 Describe five physiological changes that normally occur during pregnancy that would be considered abnormal if they did not occur during pregnancy.

Conception triggers thousands of complex and sequenced biological changes that transform two united cells into a member of the next generation of human beings. The rapidity with which structures and functions develop in mother and fetus and the time-critical nature of energy and nutrient needs make maternal nutritional status a key element of successful reproduction.[11]

Pregnancy begins at conception; that occurs approximately 14 days before a woman's next menstrual period is scheduled to begin and ovulation occurs. Assessed from conception, pregnancy averages 38 weeks, or 266 days, in length. Most commonly, however, pregnancy duration is given as 40 weeks (280 days) because it is measured from the date of the first day of the last menstrual period (LMP). Consequently, the common way of measuring pregnancy duration includes two nonpregnant weeks at the beginning. The anticipated date of delivery is denoted by the ancient terminology of *estimated date of confinement*, or EDC. Assessment of duration of pregnancy as weeks from conception is correctly termed *gestational age*, whereas time in pregnancy estimated from LMP reflects *menstrual age*. It is particularly important to get these terms straight during early fetal development, when a 2-week error in duration of pregnancy may mean miscalculating the timing of nutrient-related events in pregnancy.

## Maternal Physiology

Changes in maternal physiology during pregnancy are so profound that they were previously considered abnormal and in need of correction. Doctors routinely advised pregnant women to follow low-sodium diets to reduce fluid retention, restricted their patients' weight gain and dietary intake to prevent complications at delivery, and prescribed excessive levels of iron and other supplements to bring blood nutrient levels back up to "normal." We now know that what is considered normal physiological status of nonpregnant women cannot be considered normal for women who are pregnant. Fortunately, it is now understood that attempts to bring maternal physiological changes back to nonpregnant levels may cause more harm than good to the pregnancy.

Changes in maternal body composition and functions occur in a specific sequence during pregnancy. The order of the sequence is absolute because the successful completion of each change depends on the one before it. Because maternal physiological changes set the stage for fetal growth and development, they begin in earnest within a week after conception.[12]

The sequence of physiological changes taking place during pregnancy is listed in Table 4.5. To provide the fetus with sufficient energy, nutrients, and oxygen for growth, the mother must first expand the volume of plasma that can be circulated. Maternal nutrient stores are accumulated next. These stores are established in advance of the time they will be needed to support large gains in fetal

TABLE 4.5 ▸ Sequence of tissue development and approximate gestational week of maximal rates of change in maternal systems, the placenta, and fetus during pregnancy[14]

| TISSUE | SEQUENCE OF DEVELOPMENT | GESTATIONAL WEEK OF MAXIMAL RATE OF GROWTH |
|---|---|---|
| Maternal plasma volume | 1 | 20 |
| Maternal nutrient stores | 2 | 20 |
| Placental weight | 3 | 31 |
| Uterine blood flow | 4 | 37 |
| Fetal weight | 5 | 37 |

TABLE 4.6 ▸ Summary of maternal anabolic and catabolic phases of pregnancy[11,16]

| MATERNAL ANABOLIC PHASE 0–20 WEEKS | MATERNAL CATABOLIC PHASE 20+ WEEKS |
|---|---|
| Blood volume expansion, increased cardiac output | Mobilization of fat and nutrient stores |
| Buildup of fat, nutrient, and liver glycogen stores | Increased production and blood levels of glucose, triglycerides, and fatty acids; decreased liver glycogen stores |
| Growth of some maternal organs | Accelerated fasting metabolism |
| Increased appetite, food intake (positive caloric balance) | Increased appetite and food intake decline somewhat near term |
| Decreased exercise tolerance | Increased levels of catabolic hormones |
| Increased levels of anabolic hormones | |

weight. Similarly, the maximal rate of placental growth is timed to precede that of fetal weight gain. This sequence of events ensures that the ***placenta*** is fully prepared for the high level of functioning that will be needed as fetal weight increases most rapidly. Fetuses depend on the functioning of multiple systems, established well in advance of their maximal rates of growth and development. Abnormalities in the development of any of these physiological systems can modify subsequent fetal growth and development.

## Normal Physiological Changes During Pregnancy

Physiological changes in pregnancy can be divided into two basic groups: those occurring in the first half of pregnancy and those in the second half. In general, physiological changes in the first half are considered *maternal anabolic* changes because they build the capacity of the mother's body to deliver relatively large quantities of blood, oxygen, and nutrients to the fetus in the second half of pregnancy. The second half is a time of "maternal catabolic" changes in which energy and nutrient stores, and the heightened capacity to deliver stored energy and nutrients to the fetus, predominate (Table 4.6). Approximately 10 percent of fetal growth is accomplished in the first half of pregnancy, and the remaining 90 percent occurs in the second half.[11]

The list of physiological changes that normally occur during pregnancy is extensive (Table 4.7), and such changes affect

**placenta** A disk-shaped organ of nutrient and gas interchange between mother and fetus. At term, the placenta weighs about 15 percent of the weight of the fetus.

TABLE 4.7 ▸ Normal changes in maternal physiology during pregnancy[12,294]

**Blood Volume Expansion**
- Blood volume increases 20%
- Plasma volume increases 50%
- Edema (occurs in 60–75% of women)

**Hemodilution**
- Concentrations of many vitamins and minerals in blood decrease

**Blood Lipid Levels**
- Increased concentrations of cholesterol, LDL cholesterol, triglycerides, HDL cholesterol

**Blood Glucose Levels**
- Increased insulin resistance (increased plasma levels of glucose and insulin)

**Maternal Organ and Tissue Enlargement**
- Heart, thyroid, liver, kidneys, uterus, breasts, adipose tissue

**Circulatory System**
- Increased cardiac output through increased heart rate and stroke volume (30–50%)
- Increased heart rate (16% or 6 beats/min)
- Decreased blood pressure in the first half of pregnancy (29%), followed by a return to nonpregnancy levels in the second half

**Respiratory System**
- Increased tidal volume, or the amount of air inhaled and exhaled (30–40%)
- Increased oxygen consumption (10%)

**Food Intake**
- Increased appetite and food intake; weight gain
- Taste and odor changes, modification in preference for some foods
- Increased thirst

**Gastrointestinal Changes**
- Relaxed gastrointestinal tract muscle tone
- Increased gastric and intestinal transit time
- Nausea (70%), vomiting (40%)
- Heartburn
- Constipation

**Kidney Changes**
- Increased glomerular filtration rate (50–60%)
- Increased sodium conservation
- Increased nutrient spillage into urine; protein is conserved
- Increased risk of urinary tract infection

**Immune System**
- Suppressed immunity
- Increased risk of urinary, reproductive tract, and other infections

**Basal Metabolism**
- Increased basal metabolic rate in second half of pregnancy
- Increased body temperature

**Hormones**
- Placental secretions of large amounts of hormones needed to support physiological changes of pregnancy

every maternal organ and system. Changes that are most directly related to maternal energy and nutrient needs are discussed here.

**Body Water Changes** A woman's body gains a good deal of water during pregnancy, primarily due to increased volumes of plasma and extracellular fluid, as well as amniotic fluid. The primary purpose of increased body water composition is to expand blood flow and nutrient transfer to the placenta and fetus.[13] Total body water increases in pregnancy range from 7 to 10 liters (approximately 7 to 10 quarts, or about 2 to 2½ gallons). About two-thirds of the expansion is intracellular (blood and body tissues) and one-third is extracellular (fluid in spaces between cells).[14] Plasma volume begins to increase within a few weeks after conception and reaches a maximum at approximately 34 weeks. Early pregnancy surges in plasma volume appear to be the primary reason that pregnant women feel tired and become exhausted easily when undertaking exercise performed routinely prior to pregnancy. Fatigue associated with plasma-volume increases in the second and third months of pregnancy declines as other compensatory physiological adjustments are made.

Gains in body water vary a good deal among women during normal pregnancy. High gains are associated with increasing degrees of ***edema*** and weight gain. If not accompanied by hypertension, edema generally reflects a healthy expansion of plasma volume. Birthweight is strongly related to plasma volume: generally, the greater the expansion, the greater the newborn size. The increased volume of water in the blood is responsible for the "dilution effect" of pregnancy on blood concentrations of some vitamins and minerals. Blood levels of fat-soluble vitamins tend to increase in pregnancy, whereas levels of the water-soluble vitamins tend to decrease. Vitamin supplement use can modify these relationships.[14,33]

**Hormonal Changes** Many of the normal physiological changes that occur during pregnancy are modulated by hormones produced by the placenta (Illustration 4.4). The placenta serves many roles (they are presented later in this chapter), but a key one is the production of ***steroid hormones***, such as progesterone and estrogen. The placenta is also the main supplier of many other hormones needed to support the physiological changes of pregnancy (Table 4.8).

**Maternal Nutrient Metabolism** Adjustments in maternal nutrient metabolism are apparent within the first few weeks after conception and progress throughout pregnancy.[12] Many of the adjustments are directed toward ensuring that nutrients will be available to the fetus during periods of high nutrient need. The amount and types of nutrients required depend on what is needed for specific metabolic pathways to function and for fetal structures to develop. Because normal fetal tissue growth and development are genetically timed, nutrients must be available at the same time that genes controlling fetal growth and development are expressed.[10]

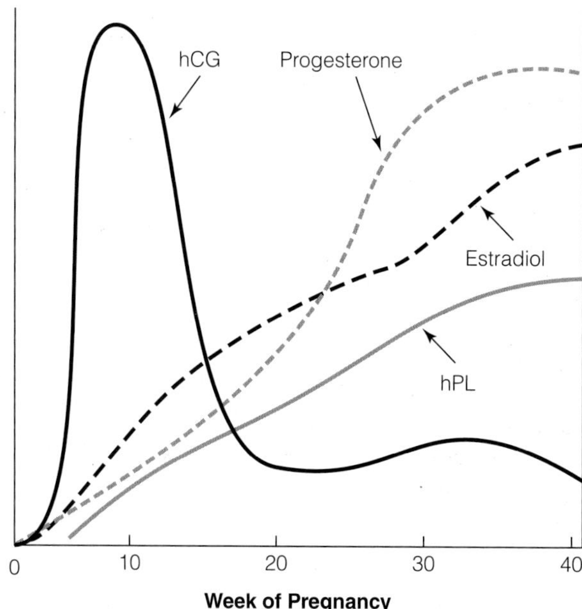


ILLUSTRATION 4.4 ▸ Patterns of changes in maternal plasma levels of hormones during pregnancy.

SOURCE: Graph sketched by J. E. Brown.

***Carbohydrate Metabolism*** Many adjustments in carbohydrate metabolism are made during pregnancy that promote the availability of glucose to the fetus. Glucose is

TABLE 4.8 ▸ Key placental hormones and examples of their roles in pregnancy[33,295]

|  |
|---|
| **Human chorionic gonadotropin (hCG)** |
| Maintains early pregnancy by stimulating the corpus luteum to produce estrogen and progesterone. It stimulates growth of the endometrium. The placenta produces estrogen and progesterone after the first 2 months of pregnancy. |
| **Progesterone** |
| Maintains the implant; stimulates growth of the endometrium and its secretion of nutrients; relaxes smooth muscles of the uterine blood vessels and gastrointestinal tract; stimulates breast development; promotes lipid deposition. |
| **Estrogen** |
| Increases lipid formation and storage, protein synthesis, and uterine blood flow; prompts uterine and breast duct development; promotes ligament flexibility. |
| **Human chorionic somatotropin (hCS)** |
| Increases maternal insulin resistance to maintain glucose availability for fetal use; promotes protein synthesis and the breakdown of fat for energy for maternal use. |
| **Human placental lactogen** |
| Supports fetal growth and development by triggering metabolic changes that increase the availability of glucose and amino acids. |
| **Leptin** |
| May participate in the regulation of appetite and lipid metabolism, weight gain, and utilization of fat stores. |

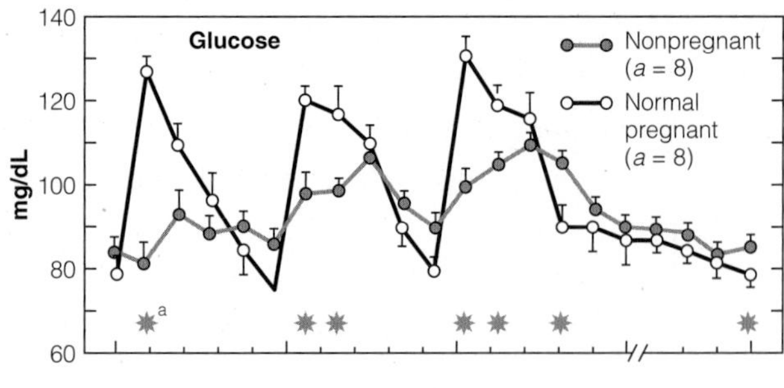


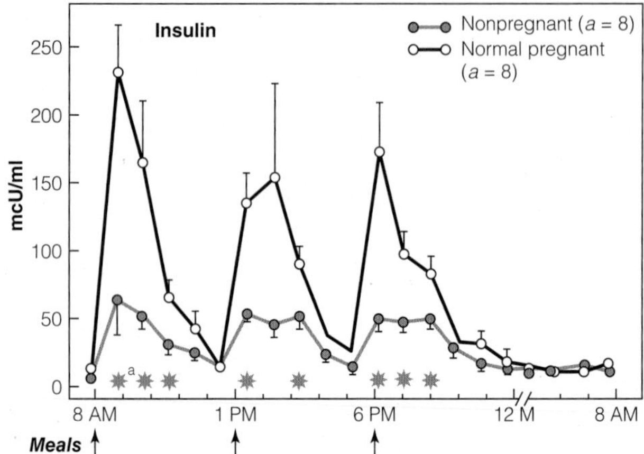


ILLUSTRATION 4.5 ▸ Plasma glucose and insulin levels in nonpregnant women and in women near term.

SOURCE: Reprinted from *American Journal of Obstetrics and Gynecology* 140(6): 730–736. R. L. Phelps et al., © 1981, with permission from Elsevier; a * indicates statistical significance.

the fetus's preferred fuel, even though fats can be utilized for energy. Continued availability of a fetal supply of glucose is accomplished primarily through metabolic changes that promote maternal insulin resistance. These changes, sometimes referred to as the *diabetogenic effect of pregnancy*, make normal pregnant women slightly carbohydrate intolerant in the third trimester of pregnancy (Illustration 4.5).[16]

Carbohydrate metabolism in the first half of pregnancy is characterized by estrogen- and progesterone-stimulated increases in insulin production and conversion of glucose to glycogen and fat. In the second half, rising levels of hCS and prolactin from the mother's pituitary gland inhibit the conversion of glucose to glycogen and fat. At the same time, insulin resistance builds in the mother, increasing her reliance on fats for energy. Decreased conversion of glucose to glycogen and fat, lowered maternal utilization of glucose, and increased liver production of glucose help to ensure that a constant supply of glucose for fetal growth and development is available in the second half of pregnancy.[16]

Fasting maternal blood glucose levels decline in the third trimester due to increased utilization of glucose by the rapidly growing fetus. However, post-meal blood glucose concentrations are elevated and remain higher longer than before pregnancy.[16]

***Accelerated Fasting Metabolism*** Maternal metabolism is rapidly converted toward ***glucogenic amino acid*** utilization, fat oxidation, and increased production of ***ketones*** with fasts that last longer than 12 hours. Decreased levels of plasma glucose and insulin and increased levels of triglycerides, free fatty acids, and ketones are seen hours before they occur in nonpregnant fasting women. The rapid conversion to fasting metabolism allows pregnant women to use primarily stored fat for energy while sparing glucose and amino acids for fetal use.[17]

Although these metabolic adaptations help ensure a constant fetal supply of glucose, fasting eventually increases the dependence of the fetus on ketone bodies for energy. Prolonged fetal utilization of ketones, such as occurs in women with poorly controlled diabetes or in those who lose weight during part or all of pregnancy, is associated with abnormal growth and impaired intellectual development of the offspring.[12,17]

***Protein Metabolism*** Nitrogen and protein are needed in increased amounts during pregnancy for synthesis of new maternal and fetal tissues. It is estimated that 925 grams (2 lb) of protein are accumulated during pregnancy.[18] To some extent, the increased need for protein is met through reduced levels of nitrogen excretion and the conservation of amino acids for protein tissue synthesis. There is no evidence, however, that the mother's body stores protein early in pregnancy in order to meet fetal needs for protein later in pregnancy. Maternal and fetal needs for protein are primarily fulfilled by the mother's intake of protein during pregnancy.[11]

***Fat Metabolism*** Multiple changes occur in the body's utilization of fats during pregnancy. Overall, changes in lipid metabolism promote the accumulation of maternal fat stores in the first half of pregnancy and enhance fat mobilization in the second half.[19] Increased fat mobilization causes blood lipid levels to increase dramatically (Table 4.9). Plasma triglyceride levels increase first, more than doubling nonpregnant levels by term.[20] Cholesterol-containing lipoproteins, phospholipids, and fatty acids also increase, but to a lesser extent than do triglycerides. The increased cholesterol supply is used by the placenta for steroid hormone synthesis, and by the fetus for nerve and cell membrane formation.[17]

High concentrations of cholesterol and triglycerides observed during

**edema** Swelling (usually of the legs and feet, but can also extend throughout the body) due to an accumulation of extracellular fluid.

**steroid hormones** Hormones such as progesterone, estrogen, and testosterone produced primarily from cholesterol.

**glucogenic amino acids** Amino acids such as alanine and glutamate that can be converted to glucose.

**ketones** Metabolic byproducts of the breakdown of fatty acids in energy formation. b-hydroxybutyric acid, acetoacetic acid, and acetone are the major ketones, or *ketone bodies*.

TABLE 4.9 ▸ Approximate changes in cholesterol and triglyceride levels during normal pregnancy[23, 20, 296]

| TRIMESTER | CHOLESTEROL MMOL/L | (MG/DL) | TRIGLYCERIDES MMOL/L | (MG/DL) |
|---|---|---|---|---|
| 1 | 4.53 | (175) | 1.19 | (105) |
| 2 | 5.18 | (200) | 1.32 | (117) |
| 3 | 6.22 | (240) | 2.58 | (228) |
| Nonpregnant | 4.27 | (165) | 1.05 | (93) |

normal pregnancy have not been found to promote the development of atherosclerosis (hardening of the arteries).[21] However, evidence suggests that abnormally high levels of cholesterol and triglycerides may indicate the prepregnancy existence of insulin resistance or another disorder. Insulin resistance before conception increases the risk that diabetes and hypertension will develop during pregnancy.[16,29]

By the third trimester of pregnancy, most women have a lipid profile that would be considered atherogenic if not for pregnancy. Although a cholesterol-lowering diet during pregnancy has been found to lower maternal cholesterol levels somewhat, it does not appear to alter cord and neonatal cholesterol levels.[22] Increases in HDL cholesterol in pregnancy, as well as other changes in serum lipids appear to revert to prepregnancy levels postpartum.[23]

***Mineral Metabolism*** Impressive changes in maternal mineral metabolism occur during pregnancy in order to support plasma volume expansion and the transfer of minerals to the growing fetus. To provide the fetus with calcium needed for bone formation, maternal absorption of calcium and the rate of calcium mobilization from bone increase.[24]

Elevated levels of body water and tissue synthesis during pregnancy are accompanied by increased requirements for sodium and other minerals. Sodium metabolism is delicately balanced during pregnancy to promote an accumulation of sodium by the mother, placenta, and fetus.[25] This is accomplished by changes in the kidneys that increase aldosterone secretion and the retention of sodium. Low-salt or low-sodium diets are not recommended during pregnancy because they may be harmful and have not been shown to reduce the risk of hypertension.[26] Sodium restriction may overstress mechanisms that act to conserve sodium and lead to functional and growth impairments due to sodium depletion.[27]

## The Placenta

The word *placenta* is derived from the Latin word for cake. The placenta, with its round, disk-like shape (Illustration 4.6), looks somewhat like a cake—with some imagination. The placenta develops from embryonic tissue and is larger than the fetus for most of pregnancy. Development of the placenta precedes fetal development.

Functions of the placenta include the following:

- Hormone and enzyme production
- Nutrient and gas exchange between the mother and fetus
- Removal of waste products from the fetus[28]

Its structure, including three to four layers of cells separating maternal and fetal blood, acts as a barrier to many harmful compounds, and it governs the rate of passage of nutrients and other substances into and out of the fetal circulation (Illustration 4.7). The barrier role of the placenta is better described as a fence than as a filter that guards the fetus against all things harmful. Many potentially harmful substances (alcohol, excessive levels of some vitamins, drugs, and certain bacteria such as listeria, for example) do pass through the placenta to the fetus.[29] The placenta is a barrier to the passage of many types of bacteria and viruses, maternal red blood cells, and large proteins. The placenta prevents the mixing of fetal and maternal blood until delivery, when ruptures in blood vessels may occur.[30]

**Nutrient Transfer** The placenta uses 30–40 percent of the glucose delivered by the maternal circulation. If nutrient supply is low, the placenta fulfills its own needs before nutrients are made available to the fetus. If nutrient

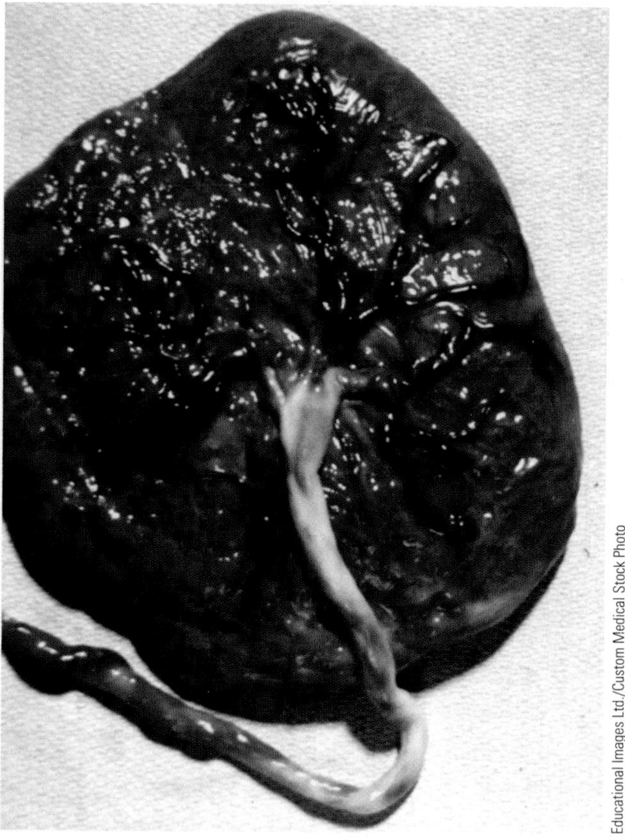

Educational Images Ltd./Custom Medical Stock Photo

ILLUSTRATION 4.6 ▸ A placenta.

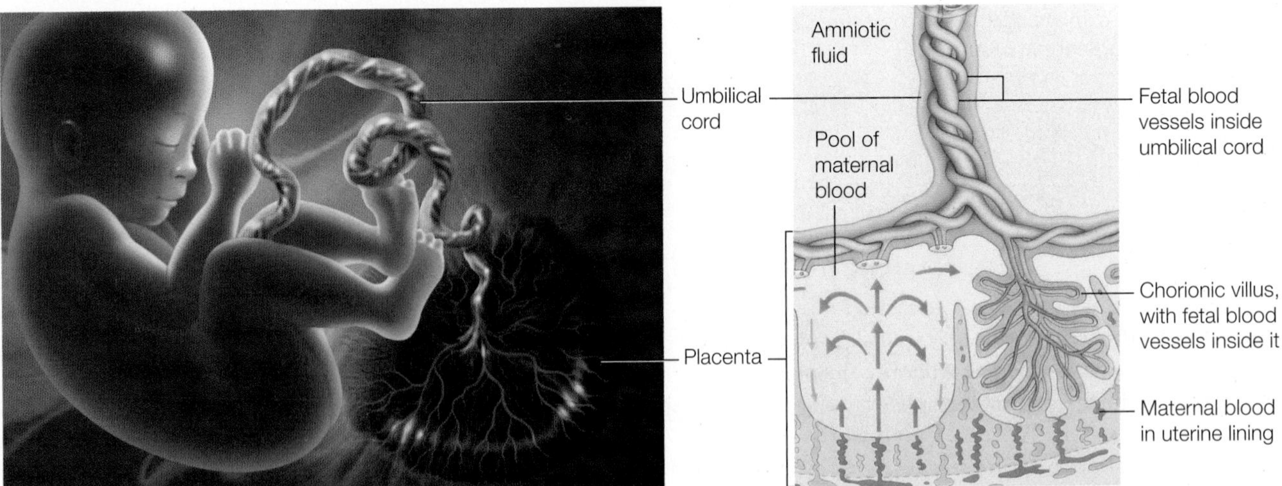


Artist's depiction of the view inside the uterus, showing a fetus connected by an umbilical cord to the pancake-shaped placenta.

The placenta consists of maternal and fetal tissue. Fetal blood flowing in vessels of chorionic villi exchanges substances by diffusion with maternal blood around the villi. The bloodstreams do not mix.

**ILLUSTRATION 4.7** ▶ **Structure of the placenta. Maternal arteries and veins are part of the maternal circulation, whereas umbilical arteries and veins are part of the fetal circulation. Blood enters the fetus through umbilical veins and exits through umbilical arteries.**

Starr, C., Evers, C., and Starr, L. (2016). Biology: The Unity and Diversity of Life, 14th ed., Cengage Learning, Boston Mass.

supplies fall short of meeting placental needs, functioning of the placenta is compromised to sustain the nutrient supply and health of the mother.[31]

Nutrient transfer across the placenta depends on a number of factors, including:

- The size and the charge of molecules available for transport
- Lipid solubility of the particles being transported
- The concentration of nutrients in maternal and fetal blood

Small molecules with little or no charge (water, for example) and lipids (cholesterol and ketones, for instance) pass through the placenta most easily, while large molecules (e.g., insulin and enzymes) aren't transferred at all. Nutrient exchange between the mother and fetus is unregulated for some nutrients, oxygen, and carbon dioxide; it is highly regulated for other nutrients. Nutrient transfer based on concentration gradients determined by the levels of the nutrient in the maternal and the fetal blood is unregulated. In these cases, nutrients cross placenta membranes by simple diffusion from blood with high concentration of the nutrient to blood with lower concentration. Three primary mechanisms regulate nutrient transfer: facilitated diffusion, active transport, and endocytosis (or pinocytosis) (Table 4.10).

The fetus receives small amounts of water and other nutrients from ingestion of ***amniotic fluid***. By the second half of pregnancy, the fetus is able to swallow

**amniotic fluid** The fluid contained in the amniotic sac that surrounds the fetus in the uterus.

**TABLE 4.10** ▶ **Mechanisms of nutrient transport across the placenta**[33,28,297]

| MECHANISM | EXAMPLES OF NUTRIENTS |
|---|---|
| **Passive diffusion** (also called *simple diffusion*) Nutrients transferred from blood with higher concentration levels to blood with lower concentration levels | Water, some amino acids and glucose, free fatty acids, ketones, vitamins E and K,[a] some minerals (sodium, chloride), gases |
| **Facilitated diffusion** Receptors ("carriers") on cell membranes increase the rate of nutrient transfer | Some glucose, iron, vitamins A and D |
| **Active transport** Energy (from ATP) and cell membrane receptors | Water-soluble vitamins, some minerals (calcium, zinc, iron, potassium) and amino acids |
| **Endocytosis** (also called *pinocytosis*) Nutrients and other molecules are engulfed by placenta membrane and released into fetal blood supply | Immunoglobulins, albumin |

[a]Vitamin K crosses the placenta slowly and to a limited degree.

and absorb water, minerals, nitrogenous waste products, and other substances in amniotic fluid.[32]

**The Fetus Is Not a Parasite** Contrary to popular wisdom, the fetus cannot take whatever nutrients it needs from the mother's body at the mother's expense. When maternal nutrient intakes fall below optimum levels or adjustment thresholds, fetal growth and development are compromised more than maternal health.[11] In general, nutrients will first be used to support maternal nutrient needs for her health and physiological changes, and next for placental development, before they become available at optimal levels to the fetus. For example:

- Underweight women gaining the same amount of weight as normal-weight women tend to deliver smaller infants and to retain more of the weight gained during pregnancy at the expense of fetal growth.[33]
- Fetal growth tends to be reduced in pregnant teenagers who gain height during pregnancy compared to fetal growth in teens who do not grow during pregnancy.[34]
- Vitamin and mineral deficiencies and toxicities in newborns have been observed in women who showed no signs of deficiency or toxicity diseases during pregnancy.[38]

If the fetus did act as a parasite, it would harm the mother for its own benefit. Rather, the fetus is generally harmed more by poor maternal nutritional status than the mother.[33]

# Embryonic and Fetal Growth and Development

**LO 4.3** Correlate critical periods of growth and development and the potential consequences of inadequate energy and nutrient availability during these periods on future health status.

The rate of human ***growth*** and ***development*** is higher during gestation than at any time thereafter (Table 4.11). If the rate of weight gain achieved in the 9 months of gestation continued after delivery, infants would weigh about 160 pounds at their first birthdays and be 20 feet tall by age 20!

## Critical Periods of Growth and Development

Fetal growth and development proceed along genetically determined pathways in which cells are programmed to multiply, ***differentiate***, and establish long-term functional levels during set time intervals. Such time intervals,

**growth** Increase in an organism's size through cell multiplication (hyperplasia) and enlargement of cell size (hypertrophy).

**development** Progression of the physical and mental capabilities of an organism through growth and differentiation of organs and tissues, and integration of functions.

**differentiation** Cellular acquisition of one or more characteristics or functions different from that of the original cells.

TABLE 4.11 Notes on normal embryonic and fetal growth and development[11,14,33]

| | | | |
|---|---|---|---|
| **Day 1** | Conception; one cell called the zygote exists. | **Week 9** | Embryo now considered a fetus. |
| **Day 2–3** | Eight cells have formed (called the morula) and enter the uterine cavity. | **Month 3** | Weighs 1 oz; primitive egg and sperm cells developed, hard palate fuses, breathes in amniotic fluid. |
| **Day 6–8** | The morula becomes fluid-filled and is renamed the blastocyst. The blastocyst is comprised of 250 cells, and cell differentiation begins. | **Month 4** | Weighs about 6 oz; placenta diameter is 3 in. |
| **Day 10** | Embryo implants into the uterine wall, where glycogen is accumulating. | **Month 5** | Weighs about 1 lb, 11 in. long; skeleton begins to calcify, hair grows. |
| **Day 12** | Embryo is composed of thousands of cells; differentiation well under way. Utero placental circulation being formed. | **Month 6** | 14 in. long; fat accumulation begins, permanent teeth buds form; lungs, gastrointestinal tract, and kidneys formed but are not fully functional. |
| **Week 4 (21–28 days)** | ¼ inch long; rudimentary head, trunk, arms; heart "practices" beating; spinal cord and two major brain lobes present. | **Month 7** | Gains ½–1 oz per day. |
| **Week 5 (28–35 days)** | Rudimentary kidney, liver, circulatory system, eyes, ears, mouth, hands, arms, and gastrointestinal tract; heart beats 65 times per minute, circulating its own newly formed blood. | **Months 8 and 9** | Gains about 1 oz per day; stores fat, glycogen, iron, folate, $B_6$ and $B_{12}$, riboflavin, calcium, magnesium, vitamins A, E, D; functions of organs continue to develop. Growth rate declines near term. Placenta weighs 500–650 g (1–1½ lb) at term. |
| **Week 7 (49–56 days)** | ½ inch long, weighs 2–3 g (less than a teaspoon of sugar); brain sends impulses, gastrointestinal tract produces enzymes, kidney eliminates some waste products, liver produces red blood cells, muscles work. | | |

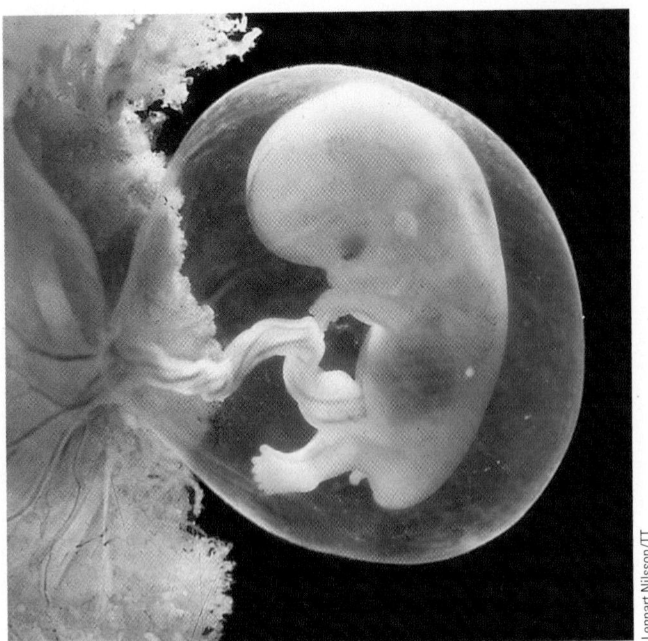


ILLUSTRATION 4.8 ▸ An embryo at 8 weeks after conception within the amniotic sac and attached by the umbilical cord to the placenta. At only 1″ long and weighing 3-4 grams, all major organs have begun to form, as well as arms, legs, and toes.

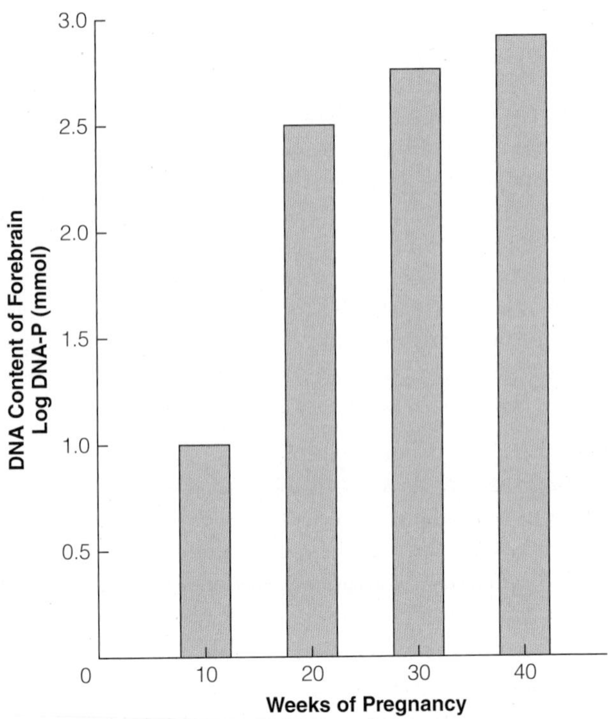


ILLUSTRATION 4.9 ▸ The critical period of cell multiplication of the forebrain. Growth in cell numbers is indicated by increases in DNA content of a given amount of tissue.

SOURCE: Bar graph developed by author from data in Dobbing, J., Sands, J. (1973). Quantitative growth and development of the human brain. *Arch Dis Child, 48*, 757–767.

known as ***critical periods,*** are most intense during the first 2 months after conception, when a majority of organs and tissues begin to form (Illustration 4.8). On the whole, critical periods represent a "one-way street," because it is not possible to reverse directions and correct errors in growth or development that occurred during a previous critical period. Consequently, adverse effects of nutritional and other insults occurring during critical periods of growth and development persist throughout life.[35]

**Hyperplasia** Critical periods of growth and development are characterized by hyperplasia, or an increase in cell multiplication. Because every human cell has a specific amount of DNA, periods of hyperplasia can be determined by noting times during gestation when the DNA content of specific organs and tissues increases sharply. The critical period of rapid cell multiplication of the forebrain, for example, is between 10 and 20 weeks of gestation (Illustration 4.9).

The brain is the first organ that develops in humans, and along with the rest of the central nervous system, it is given priority access to energy, nutrient, and oxygen supplies. Thus, in conditions of low energy, nutrient, and oxygen availability, the needs of the central nervous system will be met before those of other fetal tissues such as the liver or muscles. The heart and adrenal glands come next after the central nervous system in the hierarchy of targets for preferential nutrient delivery.[31]

Deficits or excesses in nutrients supplied to the embryo and fetus during critical periods of cell multiplication can produce lifelong defects in organ and tissue structure and function. The organ or tissue undergoing critical periods of growth at the time of the adverse exposure will be affected most.[35] For example, the neural tube develops into the brain and spinal cord during weeks 3 and 4 after conception. If folate supplies are inadequate during this critical period of growth, permanent defects in brain or spinal cord formation occur, regardless of folate availability at other times. Other tissues—such as the pancreas, which does not undergo rapid cell multiplication until the third trimester of pregnancy—do not appear to be affected by the early shortage of folate.

Some degree of hyperplasia takes place in a number of organs and tissues in the first year or two after birth and during the adolescent growth spurt. Cells of the central nervous system, for instance, continue to multiply for about 2 years after birth, but at a much slower pace than early in pregnancy. Skeletal and muscle cells increase in number during the adolescent growth spurt.[36]

*In utero* and early life changes in DNA content of the brain have been investigated in fetuses, infants, and young children dying from non-nutritional causes and from undernutrition. Deficits in DNA

**critical periods**
Pre-programmed time periods during embryonic and fetal development when specific cells, organs, and tissues are formed and integrated, or functional levels established. Also called *sensitive periods.*

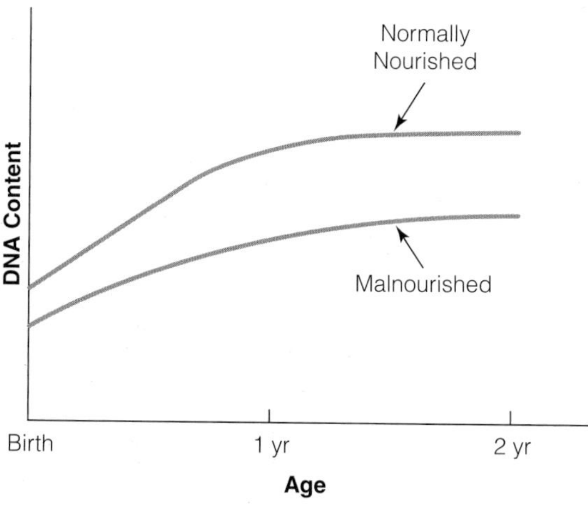


ILLUSTRATION 4.10 ▸ Patterns of change in the DNA content of the cerebellum of the brains of young children dying from non-nutritional causes and from undernutrition.

SOURCE: Patterns drawn by Judith Brown from data in Winick, M. (1969). Malnutrition and brain development. *Journal of Pediatrics* 74(6): 667–679.

content (or cell number) in the brains of children dying of protein-energy malnutrition is different than those dying from accidents (Illustration 4.10). Deficits in DNA were apparent a few months after birth, indicating that severe malnutrition early in pregnancy reduced brain cell number *in utero*.[37]

**Hyperplasia and Hypertrophy** Cell multiplication continues at a lower rate after critical periods of cell multiplication and is accompanied by increases in the size of cells. This phase of growth can be seen in Illustration 4.11, where it begins around 20 weeks in the forebrain when the rate of increase in DNA content slows. Cell size increases mainly due to an accumulation of protein and lipids inside of cells. Consequently, increases in cell size can be determined by measuring the protein or lipid content of cells. Specialized functions of cells, such as production of digestive enzymes by cells within the small intestine or neurotransmitters by nerve cells, occur along with increases in cell number and size.[33]

**Hypertrophy** Periods of hyperplasia-hypertrophy are followed by hypertrophy only. During this phase, cells continue to accumulate protein and lipids, and functional levels continue to grow in sophistication, but cells no longer multiply. Reductions in cell size caused by unfavorable nutrient environments or other conditions are associated with deficits in organ and tissue functions, such as reduced mental capabilities or declines in muscular coordination. Such functional changes can often be reduced or reversed later if deficits are corrected.[35]

**Maturation** The last phase of growth and development is maturation—the stabilization of cell number and size.

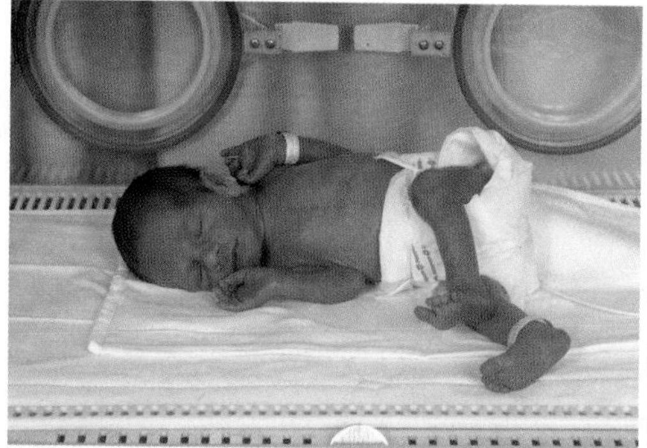

Publiphoto/Science Source

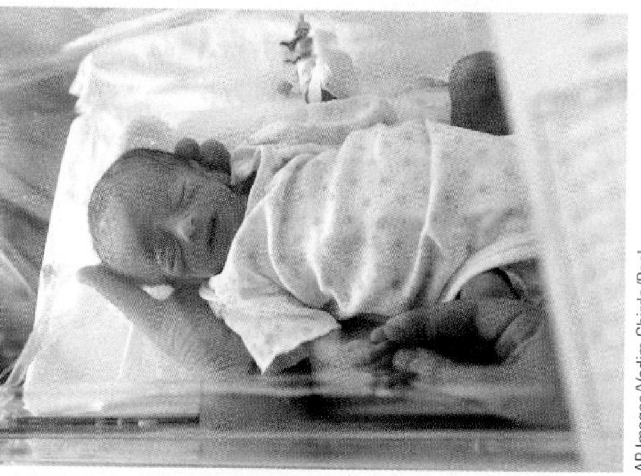

AP Images/Vadim Ghirda/Pool

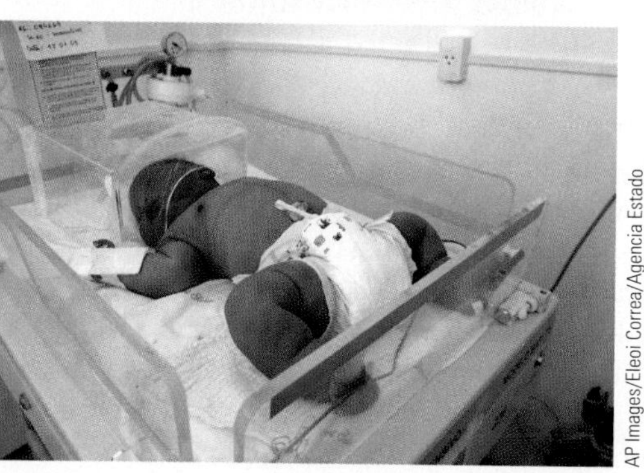

AP Images/Eleoi Correa/Agencia Estado

ILLUSTRATION 4.11 ▸ The newborn on the top is disproportionately small for gestational age, the middle newborn is proportionately small for gestational age, and the newborn on the bottom is large for gestational age.

This phase occurs after tissues and organs are fully developed later in life.

## Fetal Body Composition

The fetus undergoes marked changes in body composition during pregnancy (Table 4.12). The general trend is toward progressive increases in fat, protein, and mineral content. Some of the most drastic changes take place in the last 5 weeks of pregnancy, when body fat, glycogen stores, and mineral content increase substantially.

**Variation in Fetal Growth** Given a healthy mother and fetal access to needed amounts of energy, nutrients, and oxygen; and freedom from toxins, fetal genetic

TABLE 4.12 ▸ Estimated changes in body composition of the fetus by time in pregnancy[48,299]

| COMPONENT | 10 WEEKS | 20 WEEKS | 30 WEEKS | 40 WEEKS |
|---|---|---|---|---|
| Body weight, g | 10 | 300 | 1667 | 3450 |
| Water, g | < 9 | 263 | 1364 | 700 |
| Protein, g | < 1 | 22 | 134 | 446 |
| Fat, g | < 1 | 26 | 66 | 525 |
| Sodium, meq | < 1 | 32 | 136 | 243 |
| Potassium, meq | < 1 | 12 | 75 | 170 |
| Calcium, g | < 1 | 1 | 10 | 28 |
| Magnesium, mg | < 1 | 5 | 31 | 76 |
| Iron, mg | < 1 | 17 | 104 | 278 |
| Zinc, mg | < 1 | 6 | 26 | 53 |

growth potential is achieved.[38] However, as evidenced by the relatively high rate of low birthweight in the United States, optimal conditions required for achievement of genetic growth potential often do not exist during pregnancy. Variations in fetal growth and development are not generally due to genetic causes but, rather, to environmental factors such as energy, nutrient, and oxygen availability, and to conditions that interfere with genetically programmed growth and development. Insulin-like growth factor-1 (IGF-1) is the primary growth stimulator of the fetus. It promotes uptake of nutrients by the fetus and inhibits fetal tissue breakdown. Levels of IGF-1 are sensitive to maternal nutrition; its levels are decreased by undernutrition. Low levels of IGF-1 decrease muscle and skeletal mass and produce asymmetrical growth.[31] Factors such as prepregnancy underweight and shortness, low weight gain during pregnancy, poor dietary intakes, smoking, drug abuse, and certain clinical complications of pregnancy are associated with reduced fetal growth.[39]

Risk of illness and death varies substantially with size at birth and is particularly high for newborns experiencing intrauterine growth retardation (IUGR).[39] For a portion of newborns, smallness at birth is normal and may reflect familial genetic traits. Because IUGR is complicated to determine, it is usually approximated by assessment of size for gestational age using a reference standard (Table 4.13). Infants are generally considered likely to have experienced intrauterine growth retardation if their weight for gestational age or length is low. Newborns whose weight is less than the 10th percentile for gestational age are considered ***small for gestational age***, or **SGA**. This determination is further categorized into ***disproportionately small for gestational age (dSGA)*** and ***proportionately small for gestational age (pSGA)***. Newborns who weigh less than the 10th percentile of weight for gestational age but have normal length and head circumference for age are considered dSGA. If weight, length, and head circumference are less than the 10th percentile for gestational age, then the newborn is considered pSGA (Illustration 4.11). Approximately two-thirds of SGA newborns in the United States are disproportionately small, and one-third are proportionately small.[38]

**small for gestational age (SGA)** Newborn weight is less than 10th percentile for gestational age. Also called *small for date* (SFD).

**disproportionately small for gestational age (dSGA)** Newborn weight is less than 10th percentile of weight for gestational age; length and head circumference are normal. Also called *asymmetrical* SGA.

**proportionately small for gestational age (pSGA)** Newborn weight, length, and head circumference are less than 10th percentile for gestational age. Also called *symmetrical* SGA.

**dSGA** Infants who are disproportionately small for gestational age look skinny, wasted, and wrinkly. They tend to have small abdominal circumferences, reflecting a lack of glycogen stores in the liver, and little body fat. It appears

TABLE 4.13 ▸ Percentiles of weight in grams for newborn gestational age

| GESTATIONAL AGE (WK) | 5TH PCTL | 10TH PCTL | 50TH PCTL | 90TH PCTL | 95TH PCTL |
|---|---|---|---|---|---|
| 20 | 249 | 275 | 412 | 772 | 912 |
| 21 | 280 | 314 | 433 | 790 | 957 |
| 22 | 330 | 376 | 496 | 826 | 1023 |
| 23 | 385 | 440 | 582 | 882 | 1107 |
| 24 | 435 | 498 | 674 | 977 | 1223 |
| 25 | 480 | 558 | 779 | 1138 | 1397 |
| 26 | 529 | 625 | 899 | 1362 | 1640 |
| 27 | 591 | 702 | 1035 | 1635 | 1927 |
| 28 | 670 | 798 | 1196 | 1977 | 2237 |
| 29 | 772 | 925 | 1394 | 2361 | 2553 |
| 30 | 910 | 1085 | 1637 | 2710 | 2847 |
| 31 | 1088 | 1278 | 1918 | 2986 | 3108 |
| 32 | 1294 | 1495 | 2203 | 3200 | 3338 |
| 33 | 1513 | 1725 | 2458 | 3370 | 3536 |
| 34 | 1735 | 1950 | 2667 | 3502 | 3697 |
| 35 | 1950 | 2159 | 2831 | 3596 | 3812 |
| 36 | 2156 | 2354 | 2974 | 3668 | 3888 |
| 37 | 2357 | 2541 | 3117 | 3755 | 3956 |
| 38 | 2543 | 2714 | 3263 | 3867 | 4027 |
| 39 | 2685 | 2852 | 3400 | 3980 | 4107 |
| 40 | 2761 | 2929 | 3495 | 4060 | 4185 |
| 41 | 2777 | 2948 | 3527 | 4094 | 4217 |
| 42 | 2764 | 2935 | 3522 | 4098 | 4213 |
| 43 | 2741 | 2907 | 3505 | 4096 | 4178 |
| 44 | 2724 | 2885 | 3491 | 4096 | 4122 |

NOTE: Pctl = percentile

SOURCE: Alexander G, et al. (1996). A United States National Reference for Fetal Growth. *Obstet Gynecol*, 87, 163–168, table 2. Reprinted with permission from Wolters Kluwer Health.

that these infants have experienced *in utero* malnutrition in the third trimester of pregnancy and that it compromised liver glycogen and fat storage. Short-term episodes of malnutrition, such as maternal weight loss or low weight gain late in pregnancy that compromise energy, nutrient, or oxygen availability appear to be related to dSGA.[38] These infants generally have smaller organ sizes but the normal number of cells in organs and tissues.

Infants who are dSGA are at risk of developing the "hypos" after birth (hypoglycemia, hypocalcemia, hypomagnesiumenia, and hypothermia). If the period of maternal undernutrition was short, dSGA infants tend to experience good catch-up growth with nutritional rehabilitation.[31] Unfortunately, disproportionately small infants tend to perform less well academically and are at greater risk than other infants for heart disease, hypertension, and type 2 diabetes in the adult years.[19,40]

**pSGA** Proportionately SGA newborns look small but well proportioned. It is believed that these infants have experienced long-term malnutrition *in utero*, due to factors such as prepregnancy underweight, consistently low rates of maternal weight gain in pregnancy and the corresponding inadequate dietary intake, maternal disease, or chronic exposure to alcohol.[33]

Because nutritional insults existed during critical periods of growth early in pregnancy, pSGA infants generally have a reduced number of cells in organs and tissues. These babies tend to exhibit fewer health problems at birth than do dSGA infants, but catch-up growth is poorer, even with nutritional rehabilitation. On average, pSGA infants remain shorter and lighter and have smaller head circumferences throughout life than do infants born ***appropriate for gestational age (AGA)*** or ***large for gestational age (LGA)***.[41]

The goal of nutritional rehabilitation for pSGA infants should be catch-up in weight and length, and not just weight. This goal appears to be easier to reach if pSGA infants are breastfed. Excessive weight gain by pSGA infants appears to increase the risk of obesity, hypertension, heart disease, and type 2 diabetes later in life.[42]

**LGA** Newborns with weights greater than the 90th percentile for gestational age are considered to be large for gestational age. Although it is difficult to predict LGA, it appears to be related to prepregnancy obesity, poorly controlled diabetes in pregnancy, excessive weight gain in pregnancy, and possibly other factors.[43,44]

Except for infants born to women with poorly controlled diabetes during pregnancy or other health problems, LGA newborns experience far lower illness and death rates than do SGA infants, and they tend to be taller later in life.[45] Delivery and postpartum complications in mothers, however, tend to be higher with LGA newborns, and these include increased rates of operative delivery, ***shoulder dystocia***, and postpartum hemorrhage.

## Nutrition, Miscarriage, and Preterm Delivery

Several other pregnancy outcomes are related in part to maternal nutrition. Highlighted here are the roles played by nutrition in miscarriage and preterm delivery.

**Miscarriages** Over 30 percent of implanted embryos are lost by reabsorption into the uterus or expulsion before 20 weeks of pregnancy. Roughly a third of these losses are recognized as a miscarriage and the remaining occur before the pregnancy is realized by the mother.[46] Such early losses of embryos and fetuses are thought to be primarily caused by noninherited chromosomes abnormalities, immunological disorders, thyroid disorders, hormonal imbalances, reproductive tract infections, and drug or alcohol abuse.[47]

The presence of nausea and vomiting early in pregnancy is related to a low risk of miscarriage. Nausea and vomiting may occur as a side effect of healthy changes in hormone levels.[48] Women who enter pregnancy underweight are at higher risk of miscarriage than are normal and overweight women.[49] High levels of oxidative stress in women in the first half of pregnancy, and in men prior to conception, have been linked to a substantial increase in the risk of miscarriage.[50,51] Vitamin D and vitamin E deficiency in the first trimester of pregnancy have been found to increase the risk of miscarriage.[52]

Miscarriage often generates feelings of guilt and women may blame themselves for the loss, even though chances are very high that it was not due to anything they did. Miscarriages are common and reflect the fact that human reproduction is far from perfectly efficient.[53,54]

**Preterm Delivery** Infants born preterm are at greater risk than other infants of death, neurological problems reflected later in low IQ scores, attention deficit-hyperactivity disorders, enrollment in special education, congenital malformations, and chronic health problems such as ***cerebral palsy***. The risk for these outcomes increases as gestational age at birth decreases.[55] Infants born very preterm (less than 34 weeks) commonly have problems related to growth, digestion, respiration, and other conditions due to immaturity.[56] Low stores of fat, essential fatty acids, glycogen, calcium, iron, zinc, and other nutrients in very preterm infants may also interfere with

**appropriate for gestational age (AGA)** Weight, length, and head circumference are between the 10th and 90th percentiles for gestational age.

**large for gestational age (LGA)** Weight for gestational age exceeds the 90th percentile for gestational age. Also defined as birthweight greater than 4500 g (10 lb) and referred to as *excessively sized for gestational age*, or *macrosomic*.

**shoulder dystocia** Blockage or difficulty of delivery due to obstruction of the birth canal by the infant's shoulders.

**cerebral palsy** A group of disorders characterized by impaired muscle activity and coordination present at birth or developed during early childhood.

growth and health after delivery.[57] Additionally, breast-milk content of riboflavin and vitamins A, C, and $B_{12}$ may be low in women who have inadequate intake of these vitamins during the third trimester of pregnancy.[58-60]

Use of multivitamin or folic acid supplements and adequate folate intake before and during early pregnancy appear to be associated with a decreased risk of preterm delivery.[61,62] Caffeine intake of up to 300 mg per day (the equivalent of 2–3 cups of coffee) does not appear to be related to the risk of preterm delivery,[238] while intake of one to three fish meals a week appears to be protective.[63,64] Healthy dietary patterns, characterized by the regular consumption of foods such as fish, chicken, whole grains, vegetables, fruits, and legumes, are associated with a lower risk of preterm versus a high-fat, high added sugar, and refined grain products dietary pattern.[65–67]

Underweight women who gain less than the recommended amount of weight during pregnancy are at particularly high risk for preterm delivery. Women entering pregnancy obese are also at increased risk, but to a lesser extent than is the case for underweight women.[68] Additionally, it appears that women who exercise during pregnancy are at lower risk of preterm delivery than are women who do not exercise.[69]

Within the past few years, a number of studies have identified increased levels of cholesterol, triglycerides, or free fatty acids and elevated levels of markers of inflammation and oxidative stress in the first half of pregnancy in women delivering preterm.[51,70,71] Higher than average cholesterol levels have been observed as early as 8 weeks of pregnancy in women delivering preterm.[51] Elevated levels of these lipids appear to be present early in pregnancy, before major increases in blood lipid levels generally occur. This result is raising the question of whether women with high levels of lipids coming into pregnancy are at increased risk of preterm delivery. Indications of increased inflammatory markers and oxidative stress early in pregnancy suggest that chronic inflammation and oxidative stress may be involved in the development of physiological conditions that favor preterm delivery.[51] Whether diets rich in antioxidant nutrients and measures that reduce lipid levels and oxidative stress decrease the risk for preterm delivery is not currently known.

Although preterm delivery is a major health problem in the United States, its etiology remains unclear, and the search for effective prevention programs continues. A portion of preterm deliveries appears to be related to genital tract infections, insufficient uterine-placental blood flow, placental abruption (bleeding into the uterus), prepregnancy underweight, low weight gain in pregnancy, short interpregnancy interval (less than 6 months), and high levels of psychological or social stress. It is also fairly common in women who have previously delivered preterm.[57]

## Developmental Origins of Health and Disease

Rather amazing discoveries about nutrition and embryonic and fetal growth and development are being made currently. Not that long ago it was assumed that the fetus would take whatever nutrients and other substances it needed for normal growth and development from the mother. It was widely assumed that only extremely poor diets were hazardous to the fetus, and that the mother's health would be compromised by poor diets rather than fetal health.[72] Advances in knowledge have changed old assumptions. They point to the critical importance of maternal nutrition during every phase of pregnancy on fetal growth, development, and noncommunicable, chronic disease risk.[73,74] It is now widely concluded that chronic disease does not begin to develop during childhood or the adult years, but rather *in utero*.

**TABLE 4.14** Examples of noncommunicable diseases related to smallness or thinness at birth[19,77]

| | |
|---|---|
| Allergies | Mood disorders |
| Autoimmune diseases | Obesity |
| Bronchitis | Osteoporosis |
| Cardiovascular disease | Ovarian cancer |
| Decreased bone mineral content | Polycystic ovary syndrome |
| | Schizophrenia |
| Gestational diabetes | Short stature |
| Hypertension | Stroke |
| Irritable bowel syndrome | Subfertility in males |
| Kidney disease | Suicide |
| Metabolic syndrome | Type 2 diabetes |

Relationships between maternal and fetal exposures during pregnancy and later disease risk in offspring are now generally referred to as *developmental origins of health and disease*. In the past, it was referred to as the *fetal origins hypothesis, developmental programming*, and the *Barker hypothesis*. (The terms used to describe this area of knowledge are evolving almost as rapidly as the research.)

Much of the evidence that relates *in utero* exposures to later disease in humans comes from studies showing increased risk for high levels of visceral fat, obesity, heart disease, hypertension, type 2 diabetes, gestational diabetes, and chronic bronchitis in small, short, and thin newborns (Table 4.14). Each of these conditions reflect less than optimal fetal growth and development.[42,75] Maternal nutrition appears to play key roles in mechanisms that lead to later disease risk because it is a major factor affecting fetal growth and development.[10] Although smallness and thinness at birth are recognized as risk factors for later disease development, specific aspects of maternal nutrition unrelated to size at birth have also been related to disease development later in life.[76]

Relatively small reductions in weight or disproportions in newborn size have been related to increased later disease risk. Risk of cardiovascular disease (heart disease and stroke), for instance, is associated with birthweights below 7.5 lb (3360 g)—weights that are often considered "normal" (Table 4.15) .[77]

TABLE 4.15 ▸ Association of birthweight with the risk of cardiovascular disease in the U.S. Nurses Study[75]

| BIRTHWEIGHT | RELATIVE RISK OF: | |
|---|---|---|
| | HEART DISEASE | STROKE |
| < 5 lb (2240 g) | 1.5 | 2.3 |
| 5–5½ lb (2240–2500 g) | 1.3 | 1.4 |
| 5½–7 lb (2500–3136 g) | 1.1 | 1.3 |
| 7–8½ lb (3136–3808 g) | 1.0 | 1.0 |
| 8½–10 lb (3808–4480 g) | 1.0 | 1.0 |
| > 10 lb (> 4480 g) | 0.7 | 0.7 |

### Mechanisms Underlying Developmental Programming

The process of human growth and development *in utero* and during the first year of life is not inflexible or solely determined by genes. It is also influenced by environmental exposures. This characteristic of early growth and development has been termed ***developmental plasticity***. The term reflects the ability of the fetus to modify gene functions when exposed to adverse conditions that threaten its immediate chances of survival. These modifications can foster fetal survival *in utero* and later in life, given the same set of environmental circumstances. They can increase the risk of certain diseases, however, if environmental conditions change.[10]

Environmental exposures modify development through ***epigenetic*** mechanisms that program gene function while not changing DNA structure. Epigenetic mechanisms influence growth and development by silencing certain genes (or turning them off) and activating (turning on) others. Epigenetic changes may last throughout all cell divisions for the remainder of the cell's life and for multiple generations.[10]

#### *Examples of Developmental Programming Effects*

Results of studies during human pregnancy, and laboratory studies involving animals, point to ways in which *in utero* energy and nutrient exposures may prompt fetal adaptations that affect gene function programming and later disease risk. Energy availability has been a major focus of many of these studies because of its importance to fetal growth and development. In human studies, energy available for fetal growth and development is often assessed by pregnancy weight change and newborn birth size.

An inadequate availability of glucose during fetal growth and development would hinder central nervous system (CNS) development and threaten fetal survival. Mechanisms are set in place, however, that triage available glucose to the central nervous system. This change represents an adaptation by the body to how glucose utilization is programmed to operate.

What adaptations are made to ensure the CNS gets priority access to glucose? Studies indicate that the expression of genes that produce insulin receptors on muscle cell membranes may be suppressed in response to a low availability of glucose. This increases insulin resistance and decreases uptake of glucose by muscle cells, and reduces their growth. It also increases the availability of glucose for CNS development.

Adaptations that decrease muscle utilization of glucose and reduce muscle size may serve the offspring well later in life if food availability and intake are limited. If food is abundant and food intake is high, however, such adaptations may lead to elevated blood levels of glucose and insulin. These changes may increase the risk of obesity, type 2 diabetes, gestational diabetes, and other disorders associated with insulin resistance.[10]

Increased susceptibility to insulin resistance and weight gain in infants experiencing nutritional insults *in utero* has been attributed to a *thrifty phenotype*, or gene functions programmed *in utero* to conserve energy.[78]

The function of genes involved in cholesterol metabolism appear to be modified in males with birthweights less than 7 lb. (3.2 kg). In these individuals, production of "good" cholesterol (HDL) tends to decrease in response to high-fat, high-saturated-fat diets. HDL cholesterol production generally increases in males with higher birthweights in response to this type of diet. High blood levels of HDL cholesterol are protective against heart disease.[79]

Some studies have shown a link between maternal nutritional exposures during pregnancy and later disease risk in infants with a wide range of birthweights. Low weight gain around mid-pregnancy, for example, has been associated with higher blood pressure in children, and low levels of maternal body fat during pregnancy with increased risk of heart disease in offspring.[80]

Maternal nutrition is thought to underlie many of the relationships between *in utero* exposures and later disease risk, but other important factors are also involved. Exposures around the time of conception and during pregnancy such as infection, preexisting conditions such as obesity, hypertension, and diabetes, drugs, and environmental toxins also affect later disease risk. Adverse exposures during infancy when organs and tissues are still developing also can affect gene programming and later disease risk.[10,81]

***Limitations in Knowledge about the Developmental Origins of and Health and Disease*** Many questions about the influence of maternal and fetal nutritional exposures on later disease risk remain. Which specific nutritional exposures are responsible for changes in gene function and increased disease risk? How do the genetic characteristics of sperm influence fetal vulnerability to developmental programming? What levels of energy and nutrient availability are

**developmental plasticity** The concept that development can be modified by particular environmental conditions experienced by a fetus or infant.

**epigenetic** (*epi* = over, above) Heritable changes in gene function that do not entail a change in DNA sequence. Epigenetic modifications play a crucial role in the silencing and expression of noncoding portions of genes.

related to the optimal functioning of genes? How can we "rescue" or repair detrimental epigenetic changes so that they correspond to a person's actual rather than *in utero* or early-life exposures? Progress is being made toward finding out answers to each of these questions. The implications of the associations between maternal, paternal, and fetal nutrition and adult disease risk are immense.[82]

Current knowledge of relationships between maternal nutrition exposures and later disease risk can be applied in practice. For example, we know that entering pregnancy in good health, a healthy dietary pattern before and during pregnancy, gaining the appropriate amount of weight, and reducing fetal exposure to potentially harmful can benefit later health in infants.[75,83]

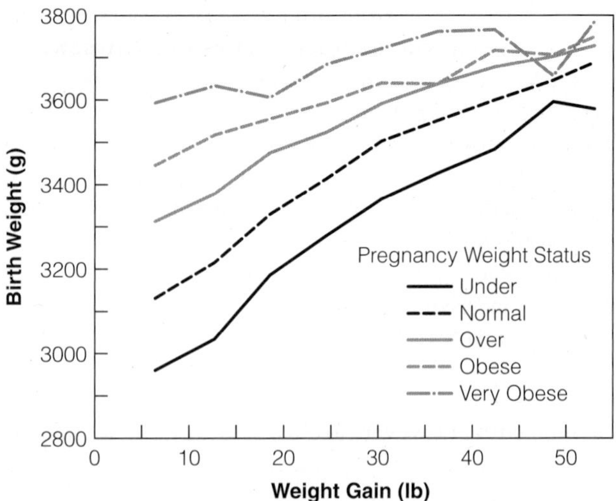


ILLUSTRATION 4.12 ▸ Pregnancy weight gain by prepregnancy weight status and birthweight.

SOURCE: Brown, J. E. (1988). *Clinical Nutrition*, 7, Fig. 1, p. 186. Reprinted by permission from Elsevier.

# Pregnancy Weight Gain

LO 4.4 Identify recommended weight gain ranges for women who enter pregnancy underweight, normal weight, overweight, and obese.

Weight gain during pregnancy is an important consideration because newborn weight and health status tend to increase with adequate weight gain. Birthweights of infants born to women with weight gains of 15 lbs. (7 kg.) for example, average 3100 grams (6 lb 14 oz). This weight is about 500 grams less than the average birthweight of 3600 grams (8 lb) in women gaining 30 pounds (13.6 kg). Rates of low birthweight are higher in women gaining too little weight during pregnancy.[84] Weight gain during pregnancy is an indicator of plasma volume expansion and positive calorie balance, and provides a rough index of dietary adequacy.[85]

Multiple studies show broad agreement on amounts of weight gain that are related to the birth of infants with weights that place them within the lowest category of risk for death or health problems.[48] Yet how much weight should be gained during pregnancy remains a socially hotly debated topic. Earlier in the last century, when gains were routinely restricted to 15 or 20 pounds, weight gain in pregnancy was seen as the cause of pregnancy hypertension, difficult deliveries, and obesity in women. Pregnant women would be placed on low-calorie diets, were prescribed diuretics and amphetamines, and urged to use saccharin to limit weight gain.[86] None of these notions have been shown to be valid. Social biases related to body weight and shape in women are an important reason to apply recommendations for weight gain in pregnancy based on scientific evidence.

## Pregnancy Weight Gain Recommendations

Current recommendations for weight gain in pregnancy are based primarily on gains associated with the birth of healthy-sized newborns.[87] Prepregnancy weight status influences the relationship between weight gain and birthweight (Illustration 4.12). The higher the weight before pregnancy, the lower the weight gain needed to produce healthy-sized infants.

Because underweight women tend to retain some of the weight gained in pregnancy for their own needs, they need to gain more weight in pregnancy than do other women. Overweight and obese women, on the other hand, are able to use a portion of their energy stores to support fetal growth, so they need to gain less (Table 4.16).[88]

Duration of gestation, smoking, maternal health status, ***gravida***, and ***parity*** also influence birthweight. Consequently, gaining a certain amount of weight during pregnancy does not guarantee that newborns will be a healthy size. It does improve the chances that this will happen, however.

Approximately 31 percent of U.S. women gain within the recommended weight ranges during pregnancy.[89] For all except the obese, women who gain within the recommended ranges are approximately half

**gravida** Number of pregnancies a woman has experienced.

**parity** The number of previous deliveries experienced by a woman; *nulliparous* = no previous deliveries, *primiparous* = one previous delivery, *multiparous* = two or more previous deliveries. Women who have delivered infants are considered to be *parous*.

TABLE 4.16 ▸ Pregnancy weight gain recommendations[91]

| PREPREGNANCY WEIGHT STATUS BODY MASS INDEX | RECOMMENDED WEIGHT GAIN |
|---|---|
| Underweight, < 18.5 kg/m² | 28–40 lb (12.7–18.2 kg) |
| Normal weight, 18.5–24.9 kg/m² | 25–35 lb (11.4–15.9 kg) |
| Overweight, 25–29.9 kg/m² | 15–25 lb (6.8–11.4 kg) |
| Obese, 30 kg/m² or higher | 11–20 lb (5.0–9.1 kg) |
| Twin pregnancy | 25–54 lb (11.4–24.5 kg) |

as likely to deliver low-birthweight or SGA newborns as are women who gain less. Rates of LGA newborns, Caesarean-section deliveries, and postpartum weight retention tend to be higher when pregnancy weight gain by women with high BMIs exceeds that recommended.[90,91] It appears that insulin resistance is related to excessive weight gain during pregnancy and some of the adverse neonatal outcomes.[92]

Concern has been expressed about the relationship between excessive weight gain during pregnancy and the risk of obesity in children. There appears to be a relationship between excessive weight gain during pregnancy and higher body fat levels in newborns.[93] The effects of weight gain, however, are dwarfed by the influence of parental obesity and environmental factors on child weight status.[94,95]

Restriction of pregnancy weight gain to levels below the recommended ranges is not recommended. It does not decrease the risk of pregnancy-related hypertension and is associated with increased infant death and low birthweight, and poorer offspring growth and development.[96] In addition, low weight gain in pregnancy may increase the risk that infants will develop heart disease, type 2 diabetes, hypertension, and other types of chronic disease later in life.[39,97]

**Rate of Pregnancy Weight Gain** Rates at which weight is gained during pregnancy appear to be as important to newborn outcomes as is total weight gain. Low rates of gain in the first trimester of pregnancy may slow fetal growth and result in reduced birthweight and thinness.[98] For underweight and normal-weight women, rates of gain of less than 0.5 pound (0.25 kg) per week in the second half of pregnancy, and of less than 0.75 pound (0.37 kg) per week in the third trimester of pregnancy, double the risk of preterm delivery and SGA newborns. For overweight and obese women, rates of gain of less than 0.5 pound (0.25 kg) per week in the third trimester also double the risk of preterm birth.[99] Third-trimester weight gains exceeding approximately 1.5 pounds a week (0.7 kg), however, add little to birthweight in normal-weight and heavier women, and may increase postpartum weight retention.[100]

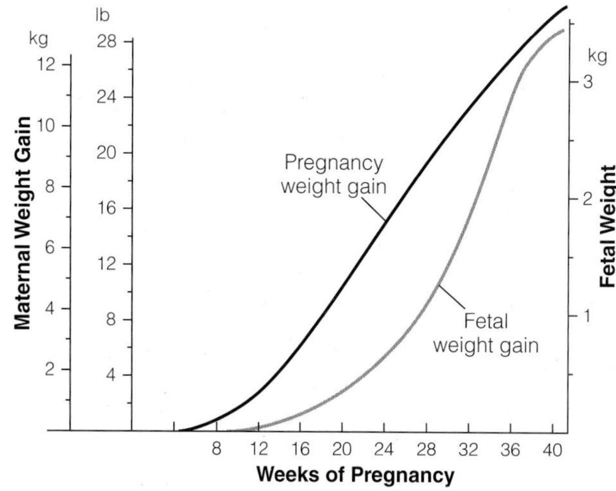


ILLUSTRATION 4.13 ▸ Rates of maternal and fetal weight gain during pregnancy.

SOURCE: Curves drawn by Judith E. Brown from research data.[98]

Rate of weight gain is generally highest around mid-pregnancy—which is prior to the time the fetus gains most of its weight (Illustration 4.13). In general, the pattern of gain should be within a few pounds of that represented by the weight-gain curves for pregnancy, an example of which is shown in Illustration 4.14.[87] Some weight (3–5 lb) should be gained in the first trimester, followed by gradual and consistent gains thereafter. The rate of weight gain often slows a bit a few weeks prior to delivery, but as is the case for the rest of pregnancy, weight should not be lost until after delivery.[98]

**Composition of Weight Gain in Pregnancy** A question often asked by pregnant women is, "Where does the weight gain go?" The fetus actually comprises only about a third of the total weight gained during pregnancy in women who enter pregnancy at normal weight or underweight. Most of the rest of the weight is accounted for by the increased weight of maternal tissues (Table 4.17).

TABLE 4.17 ▸ Components of weight gain during pregnancy for healthy, normal-weight women delivering a 3500-g (about 8-lb) infant at term[11,14,33,297]

| | WEIGHT GAIN, GRAMS | | | |
|---|---|---|---|---|
| COMPONENT | 10 WEEKS | 20 WEEKS | 30 WEEKS | 40 WEEKS |
| Fetus | 5 | 300 | 1500 | 3550 |
| Placenta | 20 | 170 | 430 | 670 |
| Uterus | 140 | 320 | 600 | 1120 |
| Amniotic fluid | 30 | 350 | 750 | 896 |
| Breasts | 45 | 180 | 360 | 448 |
| Blood supply | 100 | 600 | 1300 | 1344 |
| Extracellular fluid | 0 | 265 | 803 | 3200 |
| Maternal fat stores | 315 | 2135 | 3640 | 3500 |
| Total weight gain at term = 14.7 kg or 32 lb | | | | |

State of California — Health and Human Services Agency

California Department of Public Health

Name:

**Weight Categories for Women According to Height and Pre-pregnancy Weight (ibs)[1]:**

| Height | Under Weight (BMI <18.5) | Normal Weight (BMI 18.5–24.9) | Over Weight (BMI 25–29.9) | Obese (BMI ≥ 30) |
|---|---|---|---|---|
| 4′7″ | <80 | 80–107 | 108–128 | >128 |
| 4′8″ | <83 | 83–111 | 112–133 | >133 |
| 4′9″ | <86 | 86–115 | 116–138 | >138 |
| 4′10″ | <89 | 89–119 | 120–143 | >143 |
| 4′11″ | <92 | 92–123 | 124–148 | >148 |
| 5′ | <95 | 95–127 | 128–153 | >153 |
| 5′1″ | <98 | 98–132 | 133–158 | >158 |
| 5′2″ | <101 | 101–136 | 137–163 | >163 |
| 5′3″ | <105 | 105–140 | 141–169 | >169 |
| 5′4″ | <108 | 108–145 | 146–174 | >174 |
| 5′5″ | <111 | 111–149 | 150–179 | >179 |
| 5′6″ | <115 | 115–154 | 155–185 | >185 |
| 5′7″ | <118 | 118–159 | 160–191 | >191 |
| 5′8″ | <122 | 122–164 | 165–196 | >196 |
| 5′9″ | <125 | 125–168 | 169–202 | >202 |
| 5′10″ | <129 | 129–173 | 174–208 | >208 |
| 5′11″ | <133 | 133–178 | 179–214 | >214 |
| 6′ | <137 | 137–183 | 184–220 | >220 |
| 6′1″ | <140 | 140–189 | 190–227 | >227 |
| 6′2″ | <143 | 143–194 | 195–233 | >233 |
| 6′3″ | <148 | 149–199 | 200–239 | >239 |

BMI = Weight (lbs.)/Height (in.)² X 703

**Recommended Weight Gain[1]:**

| **Mark One:** | **Single** | **Twins** |
|---|---|---|
| ☐ Underweight | **28–40 lbs.** | N/A |
| ☐ Normal | **25–35 lbs.** | 37–54 lbs. |
| ☐ Overweight | **15–25 lbs.** | 31–50 lbs. |
| ☐ Obese | **11–20 lbs.** | 25–42 lbs. |

Pre-pregnancy Weight: ___________

Height: ___________

1
IOM,2009. *Weight Gain During Pregnancy: Reexamining the Guidelines.* Washington,DC: National Academies Press.
2
Per Personal Communication with the Committee to Reexamine IOM Pregnancy Weight Guidelines

| Date | Wt | Wk Gest. | Initials |
|---|---|---|---|
| | | | |
| | | | |
| | | | |
| | | | |
| | | | |
| | | | |
| | | | |
| | | | |
| | | | |
| | | | |
| | | | |
| | | | |
| | | | |



CDPH 4472B2 (03/10)

ILLUSTRATION 4.14 ▸ An example of a pregnancy weight gain graph based on the IOM charts for normal weight pregnant women from the California Department of Maternal and Child Health.[a]

[a]A weight gain graph for pregnant women in each of the four prepregnancy weight status groups can be located from: www.cdph.ca.gov/pubsforms/forms/Pages/MaternalandChildHealth.aspx

SOURCE: State of California—Health and Human Services Agency, California Department of Public Health www.cdph.ca.gov/pubsforms/forms/CtrldForms/cdph4472b2.pdf

**Body Fat Changes** Pregnant women store a significant amount of body fat in normal pregnancy in order to meet their own and the fetus's energy needs, and to prepare for the energy demands of lactation. Body fat stores increase the most between 10 and 20 weeks of pregnancy, or before fetal energy requirements are highest. Levels of stored fat tend to decrease before the end of pregnancy. Only 0.5 kg of the approximately 3.5 kg of fat stored during pregnancy is deposited in the fetus.[11,101]

**Postpartum Weight Retention** About 30 years ago, the average amount of weight retained by women 1 year after delivery was about 2 pounds.[101] Currently, that average is higher and reflects the fact that women are gaining more weight during pregnancy and losing less after delivery. About half of all women gain above the recommended Institute of Medicine (IOM) weight ranges during pregnancy. Underweight women are least likely to gain above the IOM range, but they tend to retain several pounds more of the weight gained postpartum.[89] Weight gains within the IOM ranges are associated with a 6.6-pound (3 kg) lower weight retention 3 years postpartum than are gains above the IOM ranges.[102]

Women of all prepregnancy weight statuses tend to lose about 14 pounds (6.4 kg) within the first 6 weeks after delivery.[103] After that, the amount of weight retained postpartum varies, mainly based on the amount of weight gained during pregnancy and prepregnancy weight status.[104] Women who gain over 44 pounds (20 kg) during pregnancy, for example, weigh on average 9–10 pounds (around 4.3 kg) more than their prepregnancy weight at 1 year postpartum.[88] The rate of weight loss beyond 6 weeks after delivery decreases, on average, among women who entered pregnancy obese compared to underweight, normal, and overweight women. Overweight and obese women are most likely to gain weight between pregnancies.[94]

***Prevention of Excessive Body Weight*** A number of pregnancy weight gain management programs have been developed to help limit excessive weight gain during pregnancy. Effective programs tend to include weight gain, diet, and exercise counseling and monitoring. On average, women participating in these programs gain 2.6–3.1 pounds (1.2–1.4 kg) less than women in control groups.[105,106]

Weight losses of 1–2 pounds per month postpartum with diet and exercise are appropriate.[102] Exclusive breastfeeding may facilitate weight loss to a small extent in postpartum women who gained within the IOM ranges. It appears to have little or no effect on weight loss in women who gain above the ranges. It is concluded that breastfeeding should not be promoted as an effective weight loss method but, rather, based on its own merits.[107]

# Nutrition and the Course and Outcome of Pregnancy

LO 4.5 Correlate three examples of relationships between nutritional status during pregnancy and long-term health outcomes in offspring.

The history of beliefs about the effects of maternal diet on the course and outcome of pregnancy is rife with superstition, ill-founded and hazardous conclusions, and unhelpful suggestions. For example, women in ancient Rome were advised to eat mice often if they wanted to have a child with dark eyes.[108] Societies have shared a belief in the importance of "eating right" during pregnancy for the child's sake, but actual knowledge about maternal nutrition and the course and outcome of pregnancy has been acquired only relatively recently.

## Famine and Pregnancy Outcome

Much of the scientific interest in the effects of maternal nutrition on the course and outcome of pregnancy comes from studies done in the first half of the twentieth century. Ecological studies on effects of famines in Europe and Japan during World War II on the course and outcome of pregnancy demonstrated potential negative, as well as positive, effects of food intake on fertility and newborn outcomes.

**The Dutch Hunger Winter, 1943–1944** As mentioned briefly in Chapter 2, people in many parts of Holland experienced severe food shortages for an 8-month period during World War II due to enemy occupation of major cities. Although people in Holland were generally well nourished and had a reasonable standard of living before the disaster, conditions rapidly deteriorated during the famine. In addition to intakes that averaged only about 1100 kcal and 34 grams of protein per day, fuel was in low supply and the winter harsh.

Carefully kept records by health officials showed a sharp decline in pregnancy rates of over 50 percent during the famine, an effect attributed to absent and irregular menstrual periods. Average birthweight declined by 372 grams (13 oz), delivery of low-birthweight infants increased by 50 percent, and rates of infant deaths increased. Birthweight did not fully "catch up" in infants born to women exposed to famine early in pregnancy, even if they received enough food later in pregnancy. This result supports the notion that the fetal growth trajectory may be established early in pregnancy and that early nutritional deprivations limit fetal growth regardless of food intake later in pregnancy.[109]

Although the Dutch famine was associated with major declines in fertility and newborn health and survival,

TABLE 4.18 ▸ Exposure to the Dutch World War II famine by time in pregnancy and adult offspring health risks[300,301]

| PERIOD OF FAMINE | | |
|---|---|---|
| FIRST TRIMESTER | FIRST AND/OR SECOND TRIMESTER | SECOND HALF OF PREGNANCY |
| Schizophrenia | Antisocial personality disorder | Decreased glucose tolerance |
| High LDL and low HDL cholesterol | | |
| High body weight and central body fat | | |
| Infertility | | |
| Neural-tube defects | | |

the rather good nutritional status of women prior to the famine likely protected pregnant women and their infants' health. Normal fertility status and newborn outcomes returned within a year after the famine ended.[110] Studies undertaken in the last 30 years on adults who were born to women during the hunger winter (the Dutch famine cohort) show relationships between the timing of famine during pregnancy and adult offspring health outcomes (Table 4.18).

**The Siege of Leningrad, 1942** Unlike people in Holland, the population in Leningrad (now called St. Petersburg) had experienced moderate deprivations in nutritional status and quality of life prior to the famine. As was the case for pregnant women in Holland, the famine in Leningrad resulted in average intakes of approximately 1100 kcal per day. Infertility and low-birthweight rates increased over 50 percent, infant death rates rose, and birthweights dropped by an average of 535 grams (1.2 lb) during the famine.[111] Rates of pSGA newborns also increased, suggesting that the poor nutritional status of women coming into pregnancy and persistent undernutrition during pregnancy interfered with critical periods of fetal growth.

**Food Shortages in Japan** Effects of World War II–associated food shortages on reproductive outcomes in Japan were similar to those observed in Holland. Japanese women tended to be well nourished prior to the shortages. Lack of food before and during pregnancy was reflected in decreased fertility status among women and in reductions in birthweight that averaged 200 grams (0.44 lb).

Social and economic improvements occurring in Japan after the war led to increased availability of many foods, including animal products. This higher plane of nutrition achieved during the postwar years in Japan was accompanied by major increases in newborn size and the "growing up" of Japanese children. In a trend that continues today, subsequent generations of Japanese adults averaged 2 inches taller than the previous generation.[112] Infant mortality in Japan, which ranked among the highest for industrialized nations prior to World War II, declined incredibly after the war and remains well below rates in the United States and in a number of other developed countries.[113]

**The Famine in China, 1959–1961** The Chinese famine of 1959–1961 was the largest in human history and mainly affected individuals living in rural areas. Little information about the diet and lifestyles of people in China during that time is available. Given available data, it is concluded that famine exposure during pregnancy was associated with a large reduction in births, an increased risk of type 2 diabetes, a three-fold increase in the odds of developing hypertension, and a two-fold increase in risk of schizophrenia in adults versus adults not born during the famine.[114] The risk of type 2 diabetes was higher in famine exposed offspring exposed to a food-rich urban environment after birth.[75]

**Food Shortages in Other Areas** Food shortages continue to occur in various parts of the world and to adversely affect fertility and the course and outcome of pregnancy. Effects have become predictable, such that declines in fertility and newborn size and vitality are viewed as part of the consequences of such disasters. For example, the siege of Sarajevo, which decreased food availability during 1993–1994, led to reduced caloric and nutrient intakes during pregnancy, reduced maternal weight gain and newborn weights, and increased rates of perinatal mortality and congenital anomalies.[115] Birthweight did not fully catch up in infants born to women exposed to famine early in pregnancy, even if they received enough food later in pregnancy. This result supports the notion that the fetal growth trajectory may be established early in pregnancy and that early nutritional deprivations limit fetal growth regardless of food intake later in pregnancy.[109] It is suspected that epigenetic mechanisms likely play important roles in relationships between prenatal famine and adverse outcomes later in life.[116]

# Energy and Nutrient Needs During Pregnancy

LO 4.6 Provide five examples of how the need for energy and specific nutrients change due to pregnancy.

Nutrient requirements during pregnancy are not static. They vary during the course of pregnancy depending on prepregnancy nutrient stores, body size and composition, physical activity levels, stage of pregnancy, and health status. For the most part, nutrient needs can be and are optimally met by consuming well balanced, adequate, and healthful diets consisting of basic foods. Healthful diets established during pregnancy can last well beyond pregnancy and benefit health for life.

Carefully conducted studies of diet and pregnancy outcome in the first half of the twentieth century began the era of scientifically based recommendations on nutrition and pregnancy. The now-classic studies conducted by Bertha Burke at Harvard in the 1940s were particularly influential.[117] These studies showed that diet quality during pregnancy, assessed using diet histories, was strongly related to newborn health status. Newborns assessed as having optimal physical condition by pediatricians were found to be much more common among women consuming high-quality diets, whereas those with the poorest physical condition were born to women with the poorest-quality diets. Average birthweight of newborns assessed as being in optimal physical condition was 7 pounds, 15 ounces in females, and 8 pounds, 8 ounces in males.[118] Although Burke's studies did not show that high-quality pregnancy diets by themselves were responsible for robust newborn health, they provided some of the first evidence that prenatal diet quality may strongly influence pregnancy outcome.

Research results recently published support the concept that healthy dietary patterns during pregnancy improve infant outcomes.[119] Decreased rates of congenital malformations and fetal growth restriction have been found to be associated with the intake of high quality diets during pregnancy. High-quality diets during pregnancy were characterized by regular intake of vegetables, fruits, legumes, nuts, fish, poultry, vegetables oils, whole grains, and adequate fiber and nutrient intakes. Lower quality diets were characterized by regular intake of high fat or processed red meats, added sugars, high-fat dairy products, sweets, and a low consumption of vegetables and fruits.[120,121] These results indicate that the quality of the overall diet during pregnancy is an important factor affecting pregnancy outcome.

Thousands of other studies on the effects of nutrition on the course and outcome of pregnancy are now available. The following sections highlight research results and recommendations related to calories, key nutrients, and other substances in food that influence the course and outcome of pregnancy.

## The Need for Energy

Energy requirements during pregnancy increase mainly due to protein and fat tissue synthesis, and the energy cost of maintaining an expanding amount of metabolically active tissues. Protein synthesis primarily occurs in fetal, placental, uterine, and breast tissues. Most of the fat synthesized during pregnancy is used to buildup maternal fat stores. Expanded metabolic activity related to the increased work of the mother's cardiovascular, respiratory, and renal systems is responsible for much of the increase in energy needed for basal metabolism. The fetus accounts for about a third of the increased energy needs of pregnancy.[14]

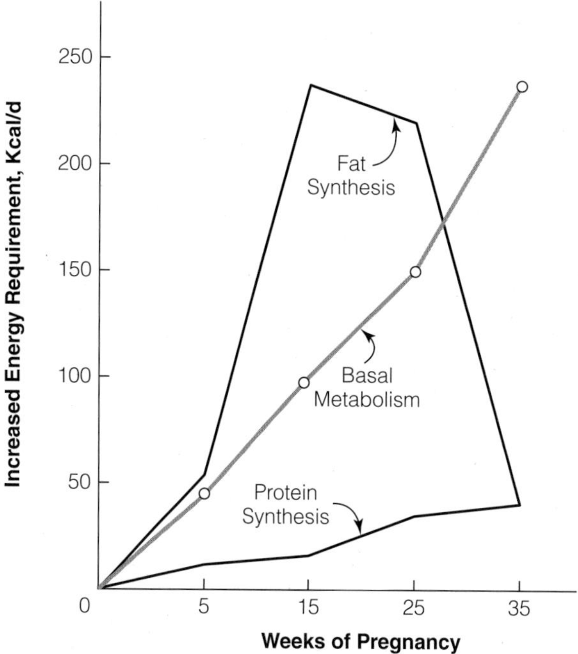


ILLUSTRATION 4.15 ▸ Components of increased oxygen consumption in normal pregnancy.

SOURCE: Graph developed by author from data presented in Durnin, JVGA. (1986). Energy requirements of pregnancy. Nestle Foundation Annual Report, Nestle Foundation, Lausanne, Switzerland, pp. 33–38; Hytten, F. E. (1980). Nutrition. Clinical physiology in Obstetrics, Oxford: Blackwell Scientific Publications, pp. 163–192; and Institute of Medicine (1990). Nutrition During Pregnancy. I. Weight gain. II. Nutrient supplements. Washington, DC: National Academy Press, pp. 137–138.

Energy requirements change during pregnancy depending on the timing of maternal and fetal tissue formation. Illustration 4.15 shows the average, estimated calorie requirements for maternal fat and protein tissue synthesis, and for basal metabolism, by time in pregnancy. The increased need for energy in pregnancy averages 300 kcal a day, or a total for pregnancy of 80,000 kcal.[14] The DRIs for energy intake for pregnancy are 1340 kcal per day for the second trimester and 1452 kcal per day for the third trimester of pregnancy. Caloric intake recommendations represent a rough estimate that by no means applies to every woman.[122]

Additional energy requirements of women have been found by different studies to range from 210–570 kcal a day.[11] The need for additional calories during pregnancy may be a good deal lower in women who perform little exercise, and higher in women who are very active. Low levels of energy expenditure from physical activity are common in the first trimester of pregnancy, and the energy savings may produce a positive caloric balance even though a woman's caloric intake hasn't changed much. Contrary to a previous belief, energy needs of pregnant women do not appear to be affected by "metabolic efficiencies" of pregnancy that decrease caloric need.[123]

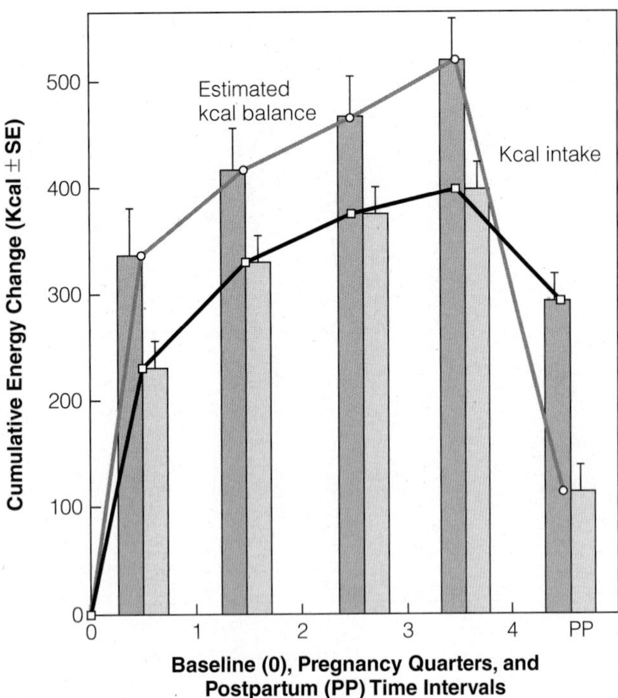


ILLUSTRATION 4.16 ▸ Estimated caloric balance in pregnancy through 6–8 weeks postpartum.

SOURCE: Based on research performed by J. E. Brown et al. (1997) and published in *Clinical Perinatology*, 24(2): 433–449.

Instead, the estimated caloric balance is higher than caloric intake throughout pregnancy and becomes negative postpartum (Illustration 4.16). The positive caloric balance observed during pregnancy is due to the fact that women consumed more calories than they expended in physical activity and basal metabolism. Adequacy of calorie intake is most easily assessed in practice by pregnancy weight gain. Rates of gain in women who do not have noticeable edema are a good indicator of caloric balance.

**The Need for Carbohydrates** As for adults, approximately 45–65 percent of total caloric intake during pregnancy should come from carbohydrates. Women should consume a minimum of 175 grams carbohydrates to meet the fetal brain's need for glucose. On average, women in the United States consume 53 percent of calories (269 g) from carbohydrates during pregnancy.[124] Basic foods such as vegetables, fruits, and whole-grain products containing fiber and a variety of other nutrients are good choices for high-carbohydrate foods. These foods provide beneficial phytochemicals, such as plant antioxidants, and protection against constipation. In addition, sources of carbohydrates that do not contain added sugars and fat tend to be less energy dense than foods that do and may help women manage pregnancy weight gain.[125]

***Artificial Sweeteners*** Evidence related to the potential affects of non-nutritive, artificial sweeteners on the course and outcome of pregnancy are sparse. Diet soft drinks and other artificially sweetened beverages and foods are often poor sources of nutrients and may displace other more nutrient-dense foods in the diet. Recent evidence indicates that artificial sweeteners may adversely affect blood glucose levels.[126]

**Alcohol and Pregnancy Outcome** Far fewer pregnant women consume alcohol than do nonpregnant women. Approximately 12 percent of pregnant non-Hispanic White and non-Hispanic Black women, and 7 percent of Hispanic women in the United States consume any alcohol during pregnancy, whereas about 54 percent of women who are not pregnant drink alcohol-containing beverages sometimes.[127,128]

Alcohol ingested by a pregnant woman readily passes through the placenta to the fetus where it can act as a toxin and interrupt normal growth and development. Adverse effects of high amounts of alcohol intake (such as several drinks per day or more and frequent binge drinking of five or more drinks at a time) include an increased risk of abnormal mental development and growth in the offspring.[129] Adverse effects of alcohol intake during pregnancy are mild or undetectable when intakes are low (such as one or two drinks per week) or when alcohol intake exists but is infrequent.[130]

There is no clearly defined safe level of alcohol intake during pregnancy for all women; therefore, it is advised that women who are or may become pregnant do not drink.[130] *In utero* alcohol exposure during the second half of the first trimester of pregnancy is the most critical time for the avoidance of alcohol during pregnancy.[131] Frequent consumption of high amounts of alcohol from early pregnancy onward is related to the development of fetal alcohol spectrum disorders. This topic is addressed in the next chapter.

## The Need for Protein

The recommended intake of protein during pregnancy is 71 grams daily. On average, pregnant women in the United States consume 73 grams of protein daily.[124] Physiological adaptations in protein metabolism during pregnancy shift in the direction of meeting maternal and fetal needs for protein. Consequently, less protein is used for energy and more is used for protein synthesis.[133]

Protein requirements increase during pregnancy primarily due to protein tissue accretion. Of the approximately 925 grams of protein (2 pounds) accumulated in protein tissues during pregnancy, 440 grams are taken up by the fetus, 216 grams are used for increases in maternal blood and extracellular fluid volume, 166 grams are consumed by the uterus, and 100 grams are accumulated by the placenta. Additional protein is also required to maintain the protein tissue developed.[134] Protein supplements do not benefit the course or outcome of pregnancy in well-nourished women.[135]

TABLE 4.19 ▸ Tool for estimating protein intake

| FOOD | PROTEIN, GRAMS | HOW MUCH PROTEIN IS THERE IN THIS USUAL DAY'S DIET? | |
|---|---|---|---|
| Milk, 1 c | 8 | 2 slices toast | 6 |
| Cheese, 1 oz | 7 | 1 cup milk | 8 |
| Egg, 1 | 7 | 3 oz tuna | 21 |
| Meat, 1 oz | 7 | 2 slices bread | 6 |
| Dried beans, 1 c | 13 | 2 oz chicken | 14 |
| Bread, 1 slice or oz | 3 | 1 oz cheese | 7 |
| | | 2 tortillas | 6 |
| | | ½ cup refried beans | 7 |
| | | Total g protein | =75 |

Protein content of nonvegetarian diets can be simply estimated by evaluating women's usual daily intake of major sources of protein (Table 4.19).

## The Need for Fat

It is estimated that pregnant women consume 33 percent of total calories on average from fat.[124] Fat consumed in foods is used as an energy source for fetal growth and development and serves as a source of fat-soluble vitamins. Fat also provides essential fatty acids that are specifically required for components of fetal growth and development. It is recommended that pregnant women consume 13 grams of linoleic acid (an essential fatty acid) daily, and 1.4 grams of the other essential fatty acid, alpha-linolenic acid. Diets in the United States tend to provide sufficient amounts of linoleic acid but too little alpha-linolenic acid and other fatty acids related to it.[124] Rich food sources of linoleic acid include safflower, corn, sunflower, and soy oil. Alpha-linolenic acid is found in good quantities in flaxseed, walnut, soybean, and canola oils, and leafy green vegetables.

Linoleic acid is the primary fatty acid of the n-6, or the omega-6, fatty acid family, and alpha-linolenic acid is the major n-3, or omega-3, fatty acid. The term "omega-6" or "omega-3" is assigned to these fatty acids based on the location of the first double bond from the end of the carbon chain of the fatty acid (Illustration 4.17). Linoleic acid and alpha-linolenic acid are considered to be long-chained, polyunsaturated fatty acids (LCPUFA) and are sometimes referred to as such.

Linoleic and alpha-linolenic acids serve as structural components of cell membranes. The brain, retina, and other neural tissues of the fetus are particularly rich in these fatty acids. Derivatives of linoleic acid and alpha-linolenic acid serve as precursors for ***eicosanoids*** that regulate numerous cell and organ functions.[136] Two members of the alpha-linolenic acid family of fatty acids, eicosapentaenoic acid (EPA) and docosahexaenoic acid (DHA), play particularly important roles in pregnancy. EPA and DHA are highly unsaturated molecules: EPA contains five double bonds between carbons, and DHA has six. The double bonds tend to break down upon exposure to light, heat, or oxygen in the air. They are the components of fish that become oxidized with time and release a "fishy" odor.[137]

### Omega-3 Fatty Acids, EPA, and DHA During Pregnancy

EPA and DHA can be derived from food sources of alpha-linolenic acid, but only in limited quantities. In pregnant women, 9 percent of alpha-linolenic acid is converted to EPA and DHA.[138] Even relatively high intakes of alpha-linolenic acid during pregnancy fail to increase maternal blood content of EPA and DHA.[139,] Consequently, adequate intake of these two omega-3 fatty acids depends on the consumption of food sources of EPA and DHA, or the use of supplements. Fish and seafood are by far the richest food sources of EPA and DHA (Table 1.7 in Chapter 1). Intakes of 500 mg to 3 grams per day of EPA + DHA do not appear to be related to excessive bleeding. Intakes of 500 mg per day are considered safe for consumption by healthy women in pregnancy.[140]

EPA and DHA are selectively transported through the placenta to the fetus and, given adequate maternal intake of these fatty acids, concentrations of EPA and DHA become higher in fetal blood than in maternal blood in the third trimester of pregnancy. Maternal stores of EPA and DHA may become depleted during pregnancy due to their increased use by the developing fetus. Preterm infants may be born with low stores of EPA and DHA.[141]

Eicosanoid derivatives of EPA reduce inflammation, dilate blood vessels, and reduce blood clotting. DHA is a major structural component of phospholipids in cell membranes in the central nervous system, including retinal photoreceptors.

**eicosanoids** Molecules synthesized from essential fatty acids. They exert complex control over many bodily systems, mainly in inflammation and immunity, and act as messengers in the central nervous system.

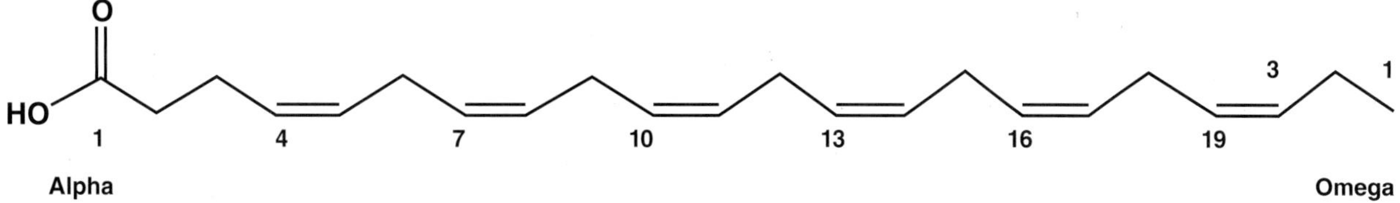


ILLUSTRATION 4.17 ▸ The structure of the omega-3 fatty acid DHA, showing the "alpha" end on the left and the "omega" end on the right.

It is accumulated into the brain of the fetus most rapidly during the last trimester of pregnancy and during the first year of life.[138] Optimal functioning of the central nervous system appears to depend on the availability of sufficient amounts of DHA during critical phases of growth and development when central nervous system tissues are being formed.[142]

Women who consume adequate amounts of EPA and DHA during pregnancy and lactation tend to deliver infants with somewhat higher levels of intelligence, better vision, and otherwise more mature central nervous system functioning than do women who consume low amounts of these fatty acids.[143,144] Sufficient intake of EPA and DHA during pregnancy has been found to prolong gestation by a few days, and to decrease the risk of preterm delivery.[145]

***Dietary Intake Recommendations for EPA and DHA*** An adequate intake of EPA and DHA during pregnancy is estimated to be 300 mg per day.[146] Most women in the United States consume about a third of this amount,[147] and vegan women are at particularly high risk of poor EPA and DHA status.[148] The Food and Drug Administration recommends that intake of EPA and DHA does not exceed 3 grams per day.

EPA and DHA are found together in fish, fish oils, and seafood (it turns out that fish really is "brain food"). Cod liver oil contains relatively high amounts of vitamins A and D (Table 4.20). DHA is available from egg yolk and DHA-fortified eggs, orange juice, snack bars and cookies, and other products, and in certain types of algae that produce it.

Due to the benefits to fetal and infant growth and development of adequate DHA and EPA, it is recommended that pregnant women consume at least two, four-ounce servings of cooked fish or seafood each week.[149] Women are encouraged to select different types of fish and seafood low in mercury such as shrimp, canned light tuna, salmon, pollock, and catfish. Fish known to generally contain high levels of mercury (swordfish, king mackerel, tilefish, and shark) should not be consumed. The Environmental Protection Agency provides information on the safety of locally caught fish on its "EPA Fish Advisory" website.

Many pregnant women avoid eating fish during pregnancy due to a concern that its content of mercury and other pollutants may harm the baby. Intake of low-mercury fish, however, has not been related to adverse outcomes.[150]

TABLE 4.20 ▸ EPA + DHA, vitamin A, and vitamin D content of cod liver oil and other fish oils[302,303]

| | EPA + DHA | VITAMIN A | VITAMIN D |
|---|---|---|---|
| Cod liver oil, 1 tsp | 810 mg | 4500 IU | 450 IU |
| Fish oil, salmon, 1 tsp | 1410 mg | 0 | 15 IU |
| Fish oil, sardines, 1 tsp | 940 mg | 0 | 0 |
| Fish oil, herring, 1 tsp | 470 mg | 0 | 0 |

For women who do not like fish, fish oil supplementation appears safe and beneficial.[144]

## The Need for Vitamins and Minerals During Pregnancy

Requirements for most vitamins and minerals increase during pregnancy due to metabolic demands associated with placental and fetal growth, expansion of maternal tissues and plasma volume, and increased nutrient needs for tissue maintenance. Maternal physiological adaptations involve changes in vitamin and mineral absorption and utilization that respond to the changing needs for these nutrients by time in pregnancy.[11]

**Folate** Inadequate folate during pregnancy has long been associated with anemia in pregnancy and reduced fetal growth.[151] Only during the last few decades, however, has the broad spectrum of effects of folate been recognized. Discoveries of the multiple effects of inadequate folate intake on the development of congenital abnormalities and clinical complications of pregnancy represent some of the most important advances in our knowledge about nutrition and pregnancy.

***Folate Background*** The term *folate* encompasses all compounds that have the properties of folic acid and includes monoglutamate and polyglutamate forms of the vitamin. The monoglutamate form of folate is represented primarily by folic acid, a synthetic form of folate used in fortified foods and supplements. A similar monoglutamate form of folate naturally occurs in a few foods. Food sources of folate contain primarily the polyglutamate form of folate. The two major types of folates are often distinguished by referring to the monoglutamates as folic acid and the polyglutamates as dietary folate.

Bioavailability of folic acid and dietary folate differs substantially. Folic acid is nearly 100 percent bioavailable if taken in a supplement on an empty stomach, and 85 percent bioavailable if consumed with food or in fortified foods. Naturally occurring folates are 50 percent bioavailable on average.[152] Folate requirements increase dramatically during pregnancy due to the extensive organ and tissue growth that takes place.

***Functions of Folate*** Folate is a methyl group ($CH_3$) donor and enzyme cofactor in metabolic reactions involved in the replication of DNA, gene expression, and amino acid metabolism. Deficiency of folate impairs these processes, leading to abnormal cell division and tissue formation.[153] Folate serves as a methyl donor in the conversion of homocysteine to the amino acid methionine. The conversion of homocysteine to methionine depends primarily on three enzymes and folate, vitamin $B_{12}$, and vitamin $B_6$ cofactors. Lack of folate in particular, and less commonly of vitamin $B_{12}$, as well as differences in functional levels of genes that affect folate metabolism can lead to an accumulation of homocysteine. This may result in methionine shortage at a crucial stage of fetal development.

A common ***gene variant*** that codes the formation of the enzyme 5,10-methylene tetrahydrofolate reductase (MTHFR) has been identified. This gene variant (MTHFR C677T) is associated with a reduction in blood folate concentration and is found in 1.2 percent of non-Hispanic Blacks, 11.6 percent of non-Hispanic Whites, and 19.4 percent of Mexican-Americans.[154] Up to 60 percent of the United States population may experience decreased folate status due to gene variants that affect the activity of MTHFR to some degree.[155] The prevalence of gene variants affecting folate metabolism varies within countries and among population groups.

***Folate and Congenital Abnormalities*** Researchers have known since the 1950s that low and high intakes of certain vitamins and minerals cause congenital abnormalities in laboratory animals. They have also known that neural-tube defects, brain and heart defects, and cleft palate can be caused by feeding pregnant rats folate-deficient diets.[156] Firmly held beliefs that only severe malnutrition affects fetal growth and that genetic errors are the sole cause of congenital abnormalities delayed recognition of the importance of folate to human pregnancy.[157]

Neural-tube defects (NTDs) are malformations of the spinal cord and brain. There are three major types of NTDs:

1. Spina bifida is marked by the spinal cord failing to close, leaving a gap where spinal fluid collects during pregnancy (see Illustration 4.18). Paralysis below the gap in the spinal cord occurs in severe cases.
2. Anencephaly is the absence of the brain or spinal cord.
3. Encephalocele is characterized by the protrusion of the brain through the skull.

It is now well accepted that inadequate availability of folate between 21 and 27 days after conception (when the embryo is only 2–3 mm in length) can interrupt normal cell differentiation and cause NTDs.[158] Neural-tube defects are among the most common types of congenital abnormalities identified in infants, with approximately 4,000 pregnancies affected each year in the United States.[159] NTDs are among the most preventable types of congenital abnormalities that exist.[160]

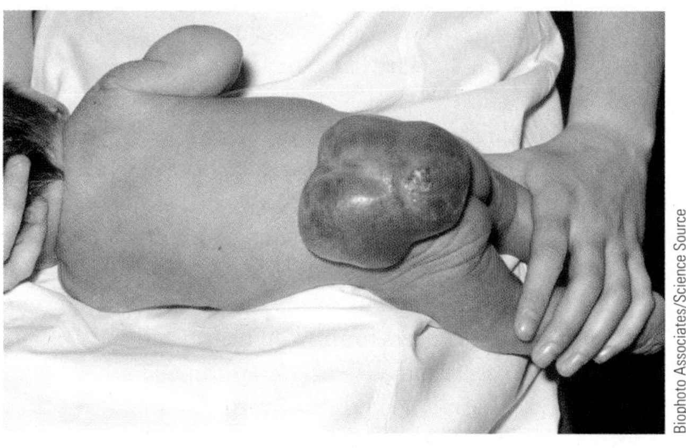


ILLUSTRATION 4.18 ▸ A newborn child with spina bifida.

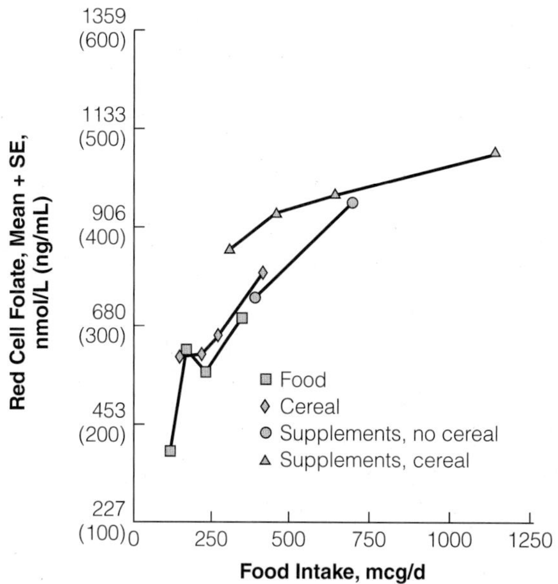


ILLUSTRATION 4.19 ▸ Mean red cell folate level in preconceptional women by level of intake of various sources of folate.
SOURCE: Brown JE et al., *JAMA*, Vol. 277, No. 6, p. 551 (Feb 19, 1997).

Preliminary evidence indicates that presence of the MTHFR variant in pregnant women may increase the risk of autism.[161] Other risk factors for neural-tube defects exist. Obesity and diabetes during pregnancy are also associated with their development.[162]

***Folate Status of Women in the United States*** Folate status is assessed by serum and red cell folate levels. Of the two measures, red cell folate levels are the preferred indicator because they represent long-term folate intake, whereas serum folate levels reflect only recent intake. Levels of red cell folate of over 300 ng/mL (or 680 nmol/L) are associated with very low risk of NTDs.[163] These levels of red cell folate can generally be achieved by folic acid intakes that average 400 mcg daily. Red cell folate levels are higher among women who consume folic-acid-fortified cereals or supplements compared to women consuming folate from food only (Illustration 4.19).

Folate status in women of childbearing age in the United States has improved since the advent of folic-acid fortification of refined grain products in 1998. Average levels of red cell folate in U.S. women have increased 150 percent since

**gene variant** An alteration in the normal coding sequence of a gene. The different forms of the same genes are considered *alleles*.

TABLE 4.21 ▸ Examples of food sources of highly available folate

| | AMOUNT | FOLIC ACID (MCG) |
|---|---|---|
| **A. Foods** | | |
| Orange | 1 | 40 |
| Orange juice | 6 oz | 82 |
| Pineapple juice | 6 oz | 44 |
| Papaya juice | 6 oz | 40 |
| Dried beans | ½ cup | 50 |
| **B. Fortified Foods** | | |
| Highly fortified breakfast cereal[a] | 1 cup or 1 oz | 400 |
| Breakfast cereal | 1 cup or 1 oz | 100 |
| Bread, roll | 1 slice or 1 oz | 40 |
| Pasta | ½ cup | 30 |
| Rice | ½ cup | 30 |

[a]Includes Product 19, Smart Start, Special K, and Total.

fortification began.[165] Countries fortifying foods with folic acid have experienced a 20 to 80 percent decline in rates of neural-tube defects.[166] Low levels of intake of folic-acid-fortified grain products and breakfast cereals still leave some women with too little folate, however.

***Dietary Sources of Folate*** Many vegetables and fruits are good sources of folate (see Table 1.9 in Chapter 1), but only a few foods contain the highly bioavailable form of folate (Table 4.21). Adequacy of folic acid intake before and during pregnancy can be estimated by adding up the amount of folic acid in foods typically consumed in the daily diet using the data in the table. Whole-grain products including breads and pastas, corn flour, corn tortillas, brown rice, oatmeal, shredded wheat, and organic grain products may or may not be fortified with folic acid. You have to check food labels to find that out.

***Recommended Intake of Folate*** Due to variation in folate bioavailability, the DRI for folate takes into consideration a measure called *dietary folate equivalents*, or DFE. One DFE equals any of the following:

- 1 mcg food folate
- 0.6 mcg folic acid consumed in fortified foods or a supplement taken with food
- 0.5 mcg of folic acid taken as a supplement on an empty stomach

Folic acid taken in a supplement without food provides twice the dietary folate equivalents as does an equivalent amount of folate from food.

It is recommended that women consume 600 mcg DFE of folate per day during pregnancy and include 400 mcg folic acid from fortified foods or supplements. The remaining 200 mcg DFE should be obtained from vegetables and fruits. These nutrient-dense foods provide an average of 40 mcg of folate per serving.[159] Because NTDs develop before women may realize they are pregnant, adequate folate should be consumed several months prior to, as well as throughout, pregnancy.

Women who have previously delivered an infant affected by an NTD have been urged to take sufficient folic acid in a supplement to reduce the risk of recurrence.[167] Currently, 4000 mcg of folic acid is recommended, but that dose is likely high because of research results showing that doses of 400 mcg are likely effective and not above the tolerable upper intake level.[167] The upper limit for intake of folic acid from fortified foods and supplements is set at 1000 mcg per day. There is no upper limit for folate consumed in its naturally occurring form in foods. The 1000 mcg level represents an amount of folic acid that may mask the neurological signs of vitamin $B_{12}$ deficiency. If left untreated, vitamin $B_{12}$ deficiency leads to irreversible neurological damage.[168]

**Choline** Choline is a B-complex vitamin that humans can produce, but not in high enough amounts to meet needs when dietary intake of choline is very limited. The need for choline increases during pregnancy due to its roles as a component of phospholipids in cell membranes and a precursor of intracellular messengers. Choline can be converted to betaine, which, like folate, serves as a source of methyl groups used to regulate gene function, neural-tube and brain development, and the conversion of homocysteine to methionine.[169] Large amounts of choline are transported via the mother's blood to the embryo and fetus during pregnancy.[170]

The RDA for choline in pregnancy is 450 mg daily. Average intake of choline by women between the ages of 20 and 39 years in the United States, however, is 280 mg per day.[124] Some experts are concerned that pregnant women may not be getting enough choline for optimal fetal brain growth and intellectual development.[171] Choline is often not included in prenatal vitamin supplements.[172] Although this is a much discussed and exciting area of research, it is not yet clear whether low dietary choline availability in women during pregnancy represents a risk factor for fetal brain and intellectual development.[173] Choline status tends to be adequate in women who regularly consume eggs and meat, the two major sources of this vitamin.[170] The top food sources of choline are listed in Table 4.22.

**Vitamin A** Vitamin A is a key nutrient in pregnancy because it plays important roles in reactions involved in cell differentiation. Deficiency of this vitamin is rare in pregnant women in industrialized countries, but it is a major problem in many developing nations. Vitamin A deficiency that occurs early in pregnancy can produce malformations of the fetal lungs, urinary tract, and heart.[174]

Of more concern than vitamin A deficiency in the United States are problems associated with excessive intakes of vitamin A in the form of retinol or retinoic acid (but not beta-carotene).[175] Intakes of these forms of vitamin A

TABLE 4.22 ▸ The ten top food sources of choline[a]

| | MG CHOLINE |
|---|---|
| 1. Egg, large | 126 |
| 2. Beef, meat only, 3 oz | 111 |
| 3. Pork chop, 3 oz | 94 |
| 4. Lamb, roasted, 3 oz | 89 |
| 5. Ham, 3 oz | 87 |
| 6. Turkey, 3 oz | 70 |
| 7. Salmon, 3 oz | 56 |
| 8. Baked beans, ½ cup | 50 |
| 9. Navy beans, boiled, ½ cup | 41 |
| 10. Milk, 2%, 1 cup | 40 |

[a]SOURCE: www.ars.usda.gov/nutrientdata

of over 10,000 IU per day, and the use of medications such as Accutane and Retin-A for acne and wrinkle treatment, increase the risk of fetal abnormalities. Effects are particularly striking in infants born to women using Accutane or Retin-A early in pregnancy (see Illustration 4.20). Fetal exposure to the high doses of retinoic acid in these drugs tends to result in "retinoic acid syndrome." Features of this syndrome include small ears or no ears, abnormal or missing ear canals, brain malformation, and heart defects.[176]

Due to the potential toxicity of retinol, it is recommended that women take no more than 5,000 IU of vitamin A as retinol from supplements during pregnancy.[27] Most supplements made today contain beta-carotene rather than retinol. High intakes of beta-carotene have not been related to birth defects.[177] Although women were issued strong warnings not to take Retin-A or Accutane if pregnancy was possible, ill-timed use continued to occur, as it did with retinoic acid.[175] Accutane is no longer on the market, but other retinoic acid–based medications for acne remain available.[178]

**Vitamin D** Vitamin D supports fetal growth, the addition of calcium to bone, and tooth and enamel formation. Lack of a sufficient supply of vitamin D during pregnancy compromises fetal as well as childhood bone development.[179] Lack of maternal vitamin D readily compromises fetal vitamin D status.[180]

Infants born to women with vitamin D deficiency tend to be smaller than average, more likely to have low blood calcium levels (hypocalcaemia) at birth, and more likely to have poorly calcified bones and abnormal enamel. They are also more likely to develop dental caries in childhood.[180-183] Miscarriage, preeclampsia, preterm birth, maternal infection, and the development of type 1 diabetes and asthma in children are under

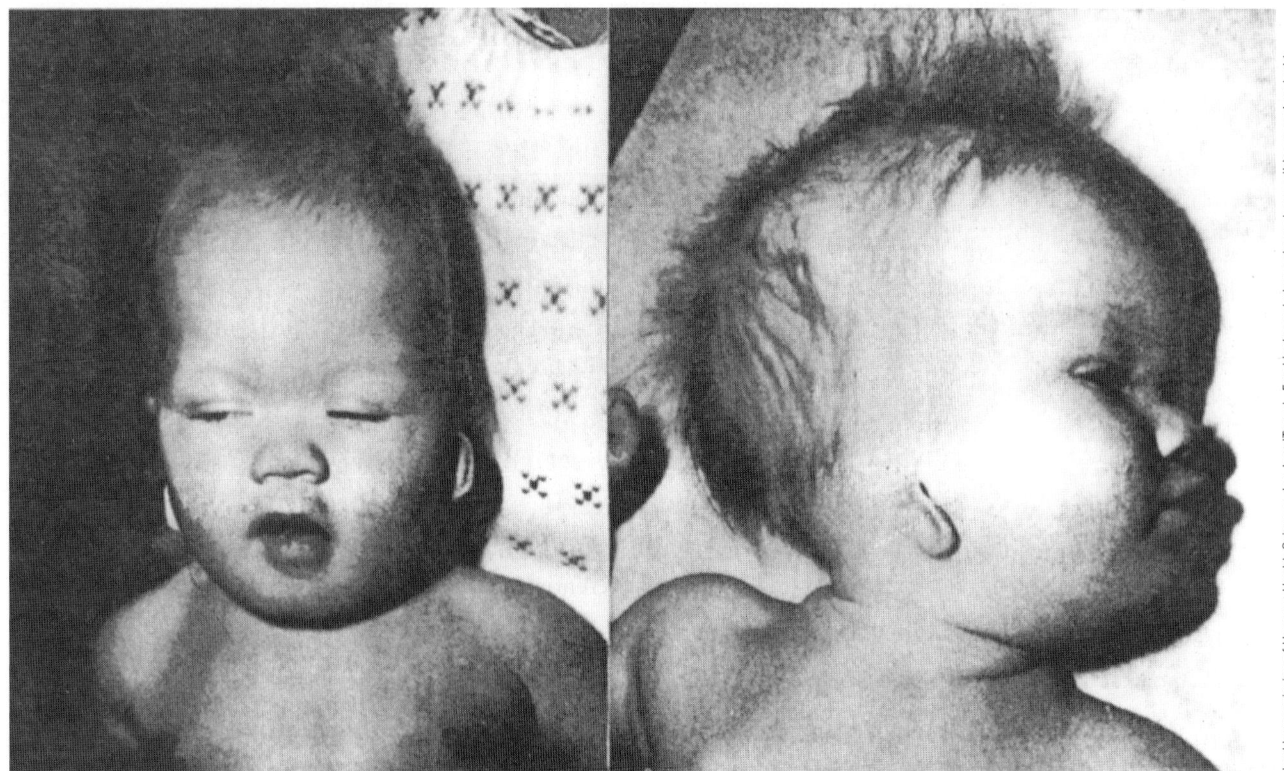



ILLUSTRATION 4.20 ▸ An 8-month-old infant exposed to high levels of retinoic acid *in utero*. Note the high forehead, flat nasal bridge, and malformed ear.

TABLE 4.23 ▸ Risk factors for vitamin D inadequacy during pregnancy

| Vegan diet |
| --- |
| Consumption of small amounts of vitamin D–fortified milk or of raw milk |
| Limited exposure of the skin to the direct rays of the sun |
| Consistent use of sun block |
| Dark skin |
| Obesity |

investigation for they appear to be related to maternal vitamin D deficiency.[183]

***Prevalence of Vitamin D Inadequacy*** Vitamin D inadequacy during pregnancy is common. A study of 206 pregnant women in Toronto found vitamin D deficiency in 35 percent.[181] Of 400 women tested in Pittsburgh, vitamin D deficiency or insufficiency was identified in 83 percent of non-Hispanic Black and 47 percent of non-Hispanic White pregnant women. These high rates of inadequate vitamin D status during pregnancy were mirrored in the vitamin D status of infants.[184] Gene variants that affect vitamin D metabolism may be related to variations in vitamin D status in different racial and ethnic groups.[185]

Obese women appear to be at increased risk for inadequate vitamin D status due to low levels of release of stored vitamin D from fat cells. As many as 61 percent of obese women have been identified as having low serum levels of vitamin D compared to approximately 36 percent in women who are not obese.[184] Vegan women are at risk for poor vitamin D status because vitamin D is naturally present only in animal products (Table 4.23).

***Recommendations for Vitamin D Intake During Pregnancy*** An intake of 15 mcg (600 IU) vitamin D daily from food is officially recommended for pregnancy. (Note: There are 40 mcg vitamin D in one IU vitamin D.) This amount of vitamin D can be obtained by consuming 3 cups of vitamin D–fortified milk a day, or by exposing the skin to sunshine. Two 15-minute sunbathing sessions per week lead to the production of about 1250 mcg (50,000 IU) vitamin D and a low risk of sunburn in most light-skinned people. Individuals with dark skin need two to five times this length of sun exposure to produce that much vitamin D and are at higher risk of vitamin D deficiency. Winter sunlight in northern climates is too weak to produce vitamin D formation in the skin. There is no evidence that vitamin D overdose occurs due to sun exposure.[186]

Several experts have found that more vitamin D than 15 mcg (600 IU) daily during pregnancy is needed to treat vitamin D deficiency.[187] It may take 2000 IU (50 mcg) of vitamin D per day during pregnancy to bring vitamin D serum levels up to the normal range in deficient women. One study employed doses of 4000 IU per day in the second and third trimester of pregnancy and noted positive effects on outcomes and no ill effects related to vitamin D overdose.[188] The Upper Limit for vitamin D intake in pregnancy is 100 mcg (4000 IU) per day. The American College of Obstetrics and Gynecology recommends that 1000 to 2000 IU vitamin D be used daily to correct vitamin D deficiency during pregnancy.[189] Vitamin $D_3$ (cholecalciferol) is the preferred form of supplemental vitamin D because it raises serum levels of vitamin D to a greater extent than does vitamin $D_2$ (ergocalciferol).[190]

Attention should be paid to calcium intake along with vitamin D status. Vitamin D supports the deposition of calcium into fetal bones and a maternal supply of calcium is needed if this is to occur normally. Fetal deposition of calcium in bones represents a critical period during *in utero* development. It is more effective to build fetal bone and ensure an adequate fetal vitamin D status during pregnancy than during the newborn period.[180]

## Calcium

Calcium is primarily needed in pregnancy for fetal skeletal mineralization and maintenance of maternal bone health. Approximately 30 grams of calcium (a little over an ounce) is transferred from the mother to the fetus during pregnancy. Fetal demand for calcium peaks in the third trimester when fetal bones are mineralizing at a high rate.[191]

Calcium metabolism changes meaningfully during pregnancy. Absorption of calcium from food approximately doubles and excretion of calcium in urine decreases. The additional requirement for calcium in the last quarter of pregnancy is approximately 300 mg per day and is partly obtained by increased absorption and by release of calcium from bone.[192] (Calcium is not taken from the teeth, however.[192]) Calcium lost from bones appears to be replaced after pregnancy in women with adequate intakes of calcium and vitamin D.[194]

Calcium needs during pregnancy can be met by drinking 3 cups of milk or calcium-fortified soymilk, or 2 cups of calcium-fortified orange juice plus a cup of milk, or by choosing a sufficient number of other good sources of calcium daily (see Table 1.14).

**Fluoride** Teeth begin to develop *in utero*, so why isn't it recommended that pregnant women consume sufficient fluoride so that the fetus builds cavity-resistant teeth? A limited amount of fluoride is transferred from the mother's blood to the developing enamel of the fetus. Major gains in the fluoride composition of enamel, however, occur in the years after birth when enamel in primary and permanent teeth fully develops and hardens.[195] Children of pregnant women given fluoride supplements during pregnancy have the same rates of dental caries as do children of women who did not receive supplements.[196]

**Iron** Iron status is a leading topic of discussion in prenatal nutrition because the need for iron increases substantially;

TABLE 4.24 ▸ Estimates of the incidence of iron-deficiency anemia in women in developing and developed countries[197,200]

| | % WITH IRON-DEFICIENCY ANEMIA | |
|---|---|---|
| | DEVELOPING COUNTRIES | DEVELOPED COUNTRIES |
| **Nonpregnant** | 30 | 12 |
| **Pregnant** | 50 | 18 |

women require about 1000 mg (1 g) of additional iron for pregnancy:

- 300 mg is used by the fetus and placenta.
- 250 mg is lost at delivery.
- 450 mg is used to increase red blood cell mass.

Maternal iron stores get a boost after delivery when iron liberated during the breakdown of surplus red blood cells is recycled.[198]

*Iron deficiency and iron deficiency anemia* These are the most common nutrient deficiency diseases in the world (Table 4.24).[200] Overall rates of ***iron deficiency*** are lowest in the first trimester (6.9 percent), increase in the second trimester to 14.3 percent, and peak in the third trimester at 28.4 percent.[199] Rates of iron deficiency are higher in low-income women served by the WIC program than those not served, averaging 34 percent by the third trimester.[89] The incidence of iron deficiency is higher in women who have had two or more pregnancies.[200]

*Iron-Deficiency Anemia in Pregnancy* ***Iron-deficiency anemia*** at the beginning of pregnancy increases the risk of preterm delivery and low-birthweight infants by two to three times.[202] It is related to lower scores on intelligence, language, gross motor, and attention tests in affected children at the age of 5 years.[203] The mechanisms underlying these effects appear to be related to decreased oxygen delivery to the placenta and fetus, increased rates of infection, or adverse effects of iron deficiency on brain development.[202] Women with iron deficiency anemia feel tired and weak, find physical activities difficult, and look pale.[199]

A fetus from a well-nourished mother is able to store a 6- to 8-month supply of iron during the last two months *in utero*. Preterm infants are at risk for iron deficiency in infancy because they have less time to accumulate iron in late pregnancy.[204]

**Assessment of Iron Status** Red cell mass increases substantially (30 percent) in pregnancy. However, plasma volume expands more (by about 50 percent). The higher increase in plasma volume compared to red cell mass makes it appear that amounts of hemoglobin, ferritin, and red blood cells have decreased. They have not decreased but, rather, have become diluted by the large increase in plasma volume. Hemoglobin concentration normally decreases until the middle of the second trimester and then rises somewhat in the third. It is not necessary to prevent normal declines in hemoglobin level during pregnancy.[204]

**iron deficiency** A condition marked by depleted iron stores. It is characterized by weakness, fatigue, short attention span, poor appetite, increased susceptibility to infection, and irritability.

**iron-deficiency anemia** A condition often marked by low hemoglobin level. It is characterized by the signs of iron deficiency plus paleness, exhaustion, and a rapid heart rate.

Due to the dilution effects of increased plasma volume, changes in hemoglobin levels tend to be more indicative of plasma volume expansion than of iron status.[202] Low levels of hemoglobin or serum ferritin may be associated with high plasma volume expansion (hypervolemia), and high hemoglobin levels are related to low plasma volume expansion (hypovolemia). Low levels of plasma volume expansion are associated with reduced fetal growth, whereas newborns tend to be larger in women with higher levels of plasma volume expansion.[204]

The Centers for Disease Control and Prevention (CDC) has developed standard hemoglobin levels to be used in the identification of iron-deficiency anemia in pregnant women. These standards (Table 4.25) represent levels below the 5th percentile of hemoglobin values in pregnancy.[205]

By trimester, hemoglobin levels indicative of iron-deficiency anemia are:

- Less than 11.0 g/dL in the first and third trimesters
- Less than 10.5 g/dL in the second trimester

Serum ferritin cut-points indicative of iron-deficiency anemia in pregnancy have also been developed:

| | **Serum Ferritin, ng/mL** |
|---|---|
| Normal | $> 35$ |
| Depleted stores | $< 20$ |
| Iron deficiency | $\leq 15$ |

TABLE 4.25 ▸ CDC's gestational age–specific cutoffs for anemia in pregnancy[205]

| GESTATIONAL WEEKS | HEMOGLOBIN (G/DL) INDICATING ANEMIA[a] |
|---|---|
| 12 | $< 11.0$ |
| 16 | $< 10.6$ |
| 20 | $< 10.5$ |
| 24 | $< 10.5$ |
| 28 | $< 10.7$ |
| 32 | $< 11.0$ |
| 36 | $< 11.4$ |
| 40 | $< 11.9$ |

[a]For women living in high altitudes, hemoglobin values should be increased by 0.2 g/dL for every 1000 feet above 3000 and by 0.3 g/dL for every 1000 feet above 7000. For cigarette smokers, hemoglobin values should be adjusted upward by 0.3 g/dL.[205]

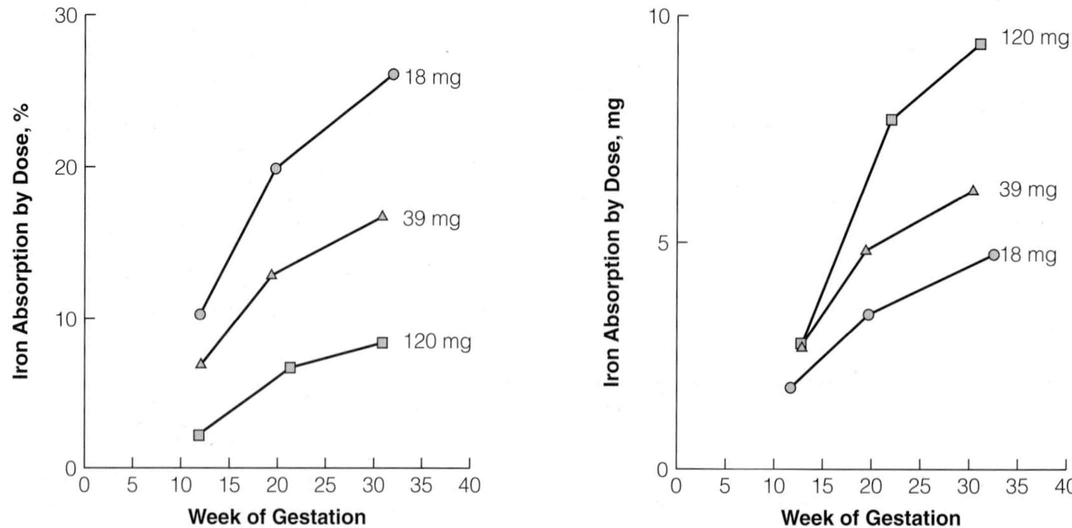


ILLUSTRATION 4.21 ▸ Effect of dose of supplemental iron on iron absorption in women during pregnancy.

SOURCE: Reprinted with permission from Nutrition During Pregnancy: Part I: Weight Gain, Part II: Nutrient Supplements, p. 287, Figure 14–2, 1990 by the National Academy of Sciences, Courtesy of the National Academies Press, Washington, D.C.

Hemoglobin and serum ferritin are the most commonly employed measures of iron status in pregnant women.[205] The diagnosis of iron-deficiency anemia is more complicated than often thought. No single test of iron status is totally accurate because (1) many factors, including infection and inflammation, affect iron status; and (2) each test measures a different aspect of iron status. It is best to base the diagnosis of iron-deficiency anemia on results of several tests.[205] High altitude can influence iron status. The CDC recommends that for women living in high altitudes, hemoglobin values should be increased by 0.2 g/dL for every 1000 feet above 3,000 and by 0.3 g/dL for every 1000 feet above 7,000. For cigarette smokers, hemoglobin values should be adjusted upward by 0.3 g/dL.[207]

Women entering pregnancy with adequate iron stores tend to absorb about 10 percent of total iron ingested; those with low stores absorb more—about 20 percent of the iron consumed. The largest percentage of iron absorption, 40 percent, occurs in women who enter pregnancy with iron-deficiency anemia.[208] Iron absorption from foods and supplements is enhanced in women with low iron stores during pregnancy, and absorption increases as pregnancy progresses.[24] Absorption is highest after the thirtieth week of pregnancy, when the greatest amount of iron transfer to the fetus occurs. Maternal iron depletion in pregnancy decreases fetal iron stores, increases the risk that infants will develop iron-deficiency anemia, and is associated with development of maternal postpartum depression.[209]

**Recommendations for Iron Supplementation in Pregnancy** It is generally recommended in the United States that pregnant women take a 30-mg iron supplement daily. Women with iron-deficiency anemia are often given 60–180 mg of iron per day.[199] The amount of iron absorbed from supplement depends primarily on women's need for iron and the amount of iron in the supplement. The amount of iron absorbed from supplements decreases, and the amount of unabsorbed iron in the intestinal tract increases, as the dose of iron increases (Illustration 4.21).

Iron supplements providing 60 mg or more iron per day regularly expose the intestinal mucosa to free iron radicals. The oxidizing effects of iron radicals cause inflammation and mitochondrial damage in cells.[210] Nausea, cramps, gas, and constipation are associated with the presence of free iron in the intestines, and these side effects increase as doses of supplemental iron increase (Table 4.26). Due to side-effects, acceptance of high levels of iron supplementation by women is often poor.[211] Other concerns about high-dose iron supplements exist. Unused iron supplements, when stored and later found by young children, pose a risk of iron poisoning.[212]

Recommendations for the routine use of iron supplements in all pregnant women, especially high doses of iron, are being reevaluated for two major reasons:

- There is a lack of evidence of benefits to pregnancy outcomes of iron supplement use by women who have adequate iron stores.
- High doses of iron may be harmful due to the effects of excess iron on inflammation, gastrointestinal functions, and plasma volume expansion.

TABLE 4.26 ▸ Increased occurrence of side effects in women by supplemental iron dose[304,305]

| DOSE OF IRON, MG/DAY | SIDE EFFECTS |
|---|---|
| 60 | 32% |
| 120 | 40% |
| 240 | 72% |

- The Upper Limit for iron intake during pregnancy is 45 mg per day, an amount that is exceeded by many iron supplements used during pregnancy.[213–216]

Iron supplements are important for women who are deficient in iron but do not appear to benefit women with adequate iron stores.[213] More women and infants would benefit from healthy diets, adequate iron intake, and sufficient iron stores prior to and early in pregnancy than benefit from "catching up" on iron during pregnancy.[214]

***Recommended Intake of Iron during Pregnancy*** The increased need for iron can be met by intakes that lead to an additional 3.7 mg absorbed iron per day on average throughout pregnancy. This is a large increase, especially considering that nonpregnant women consuming the DRI for iron (18 mg) absorb only around 1.8 mg of iron daily. Given an ongoing need for 1.8 mg of absorbed iron a day, and the additional need of 3.7 mg of iron daily for pregnancy, the total need for absorbed iron during pregnancy is 5.5 mg daily. Assuming 20 percent of iron consumed is absorbed, average iron consumption of 27 mg per day (the RDA for iron for pregnancy) will meet the iron needs of pregnancy. Absorption of iron from foods is facilitated by the consumption of heme sources of iron from meats, and adequate vitamin C intake.[217]

**Iodine** Iodine is required in pregnancy by the mother and fetus for thyroid function and energy production, and for fetal brain development.[218] Deficiency of iodine early in pregnancy can lead to ***hypothyroidism*** in the offspring. Hypothyroidism in infants is endemic in parts of southern and eastern Europe, Asia, Africa, and Latin America.[219] The incidence of infant hypothyroidism has been found to decrease by over 70 percent when at-risk women in developing countries are given iodine supplements before or in the first half of pregnancy. Rates of infant deaths are also substantially improved, as is the psychomotor development of the offspring.[220] Iodine supplementation in the second half of pregnancy did not improve infant outcomes.[219] Countries instituting iodized salt programs have achieved substantially lower rates of iodine deficiency during pregnancy than before the programs.[221]

About half of pregnant women in the United States consume less than the recommended 220 mcg of iodine daily, and 7 percent have low urinary iodine levels.[222] The most reliable source of iodine is iodized salt. One teaspoon contains 400 mcg iodine. Fish, shellfish, seaweed, and some types of tea provide iodine. Women who consume iodized salt are not likely to need supplemental iodine.[224] Kelp and seaweed should not be used as a source of iodine because they vary too much in iodine content.[223]

Iodine can also be provided by supplements. The American Thyroid Association recommends that prenatal supplements contain 150 mcg of iodine,[223] and about half of prenatal vitamin and mineral supplements contain some amount of iodine. The iodine content in prenatal supplements has been found to differ from labeled amounts by 50 percent or more, and the difference is particularly large if kelp is used as the source of iodine. The recommended form of iodine for supplements is potassium iodide (which contains 76 percent iodine).[225] Usual iodine intake should not exceed 1100 mcg daily during pregnancy.

**Sodium** Sodium plays a critical role in maintaining the body's water balance. Requirements for it increase markedly during pregnancy due to plasma volume expansion. But the need for increased amounts of sodium in pregnancy hasn't always been appreciated. Thirty years ago in the United States, it was accepted practice to put all pregnant women on low-sodium diets. It was then thought that sodium increased water retention and blood pressure, and that sodium restriction would prevent edema and high blood pressure. We now know this isn't accurate and that inadequate sodium intake can complicate the course and outcome of pregnancy. Sodium restriction during pregnancy may exhaust sodium conservation mechanisms and lead to excessive sodium loss.[226]

Sodium restriction is not indicated in normal pregnancy or for the control of edema or high blood pressure that develops in pregnancy. Women should be advised to consume salt "to taste" unless contradicted by a medical condition related to salt intake.[227]

## Bioactive Components of Food

Foods contain thousands of biologically active substances that are not considered essential nutrients but nonetheless influence health. These food substances are generally referred to as ***bioactive food components*** and include hundreds of phytochemicals (plant chemicals) that may influence maternal health. Antioxidant pigments in plant foods and caffeine are two primary examples of bioactive food components that have been investigated for effects on maternal and newborn health. Many of the beneficial effects of antioxidant consumption in foods are not found when the antioxidants are taken as supplements, implying that multiple c onstituents of food rather than isolated nutrients are responsible for health effects.[228]

Normal pregnancy is a pro-oxidative state and is accompanied by an increased requirement for antioxidants. Many plant pigments act as antioxidants and help protect fetal DNA from damage due to exposure to oxygen and other oxidizing chemicals produced in the body. Antioxidants also reduce maternal tissue damage associated with inflammation

**hypothyroidism** A condition characterized by growth impairment, intellectual disabilities, and deafness when caused by inadequate maternal intake of iodine during pregnancy. Used to be called *cretinism*.

**bioactive food components** Constituents in foods or dietary supplements other than those needed to meet basic human nutritional needs that are responsible for changes in health status.

and oxidation. Vitamins C and E (also found in plant foods) likewise perform important antioxidant roles during pregnancy.[229] High intakes during pregnancy of foods rich in vitamin E, for example, appear to reduce the risk of asthma in children. Children born to women consuming diets providing 26 mg of vitamin E daily on average are less likely to develop wheezing and asthma during early childhood than are children born to women who consume 14 mg of vitamin E daily.[230] It is suggested that vitamin E intake from food during pregnancy may reduce asthma by decreasing lung inflammation in the offspring.[231]

Foods rich in antioxidants often advertise that fact by their color. Red, orange, dark green, deep yellow, bright white, and blue-purple fruits and vegetables generally provide good amounts of antioxidants. Many of these same foods are rich in vitamin C. Women who are pregnant should consume at least 5 cups of vegetables and fruits daily.

**Coffee/Caffeine** Caffeine has long been suspected of causing adverse effects in pregnant women because it increases heart rate, acts as a diuretic, and stimulates the central nervous system. It easily passes from maternal to fetal blood and lingers in the fetus longer than in maternal blood because the fetus excretes it more slowly.[232] Coffee is by far the largest contributor to caffeine intake in most people (see Table 2.4 in Chapter 2).[233] Pregnant women consume on average 144 mg caffeine from coffee per day in pregnancy.[233]

Although it is sometimes recommended that pregnant women do not drink coffee during pregnancy or limit intake to a cup a day, evidence supporting either recommendation is weak. Most recent reports on caffeine intake and health in general indicate benefits of moderate consumption.[235] Consumption of less than 4 cups of coffee per day is not related to congenital malformations, spontaneous abortions, the duration of pregnancy, or known to have harmful effects on fetal or childhood growth and development.[236,237] Reducing caffeine intake during pregnancy doesn't appear to improve pregnancy outcomes, either.[238,239]

Research results related to the effects of coffee and caffeine intake on pregnancy outcome indicate that a reappraisal of the 1980 FDA recommendation to limit coffee intake during pregnancy would be appropriate. The FDA's position on coffee intake during pregnancy was based on animal studies that utilized extremely high doses of caffeine.[240] Moderate amounts of coffee intake, such as 3 cups daily, do not appear to pose a risk to pregnant women or to pregnancy outcomes.[241,242]

### The Need for Water

The large increase in water need during pregnancy is generally met by increased levels of thirst. On average, women consume about 9 cups of fluid daily during pregnancy.[243] Women who engage in physical activity in hot and humid climates should drink enough to keep urine light-colored and normal in volume. Water, diluted fruit juice, iced tea, and other unsweetened beverages are good choices for staying hydrated.

## Factors Affecting Dietary Intake During Pregnancy

LO 4.7 Identify three factors that influence dietary intake during pregnancy that are not related to food availability.

Several important factors beyond food availability and personal resources influence the type of foods women consume during pregnancy. These factors are important to take into account when working with individual pregnant women or while planning, implementing, and evaluating programs for them.

### Effect of Taste and Smell Changes on Dietary Intake During Pregnancy

No inner voice directs women to consume foods that provide needed nutrients during pregnancy. Pregnant women may, however, develop food preferences and aversions due to changes in the sense of taste and smell, and they may experience ***pica***.

Changes in the way certain foods taste, and the odor of foods and other substances, affect two out of three women during pregnancy. If asked to recall, many previously pregnant women could tell you which foods tasted really good to them, and which odors made them feel queasy even to think about. Increased preference for foods such as sweets, fruits, salty foods, and dairy products are common.[244] The smell of meat being cooked, coffee, perfume, cigarette smoke, and gasoline are common nasal offenders and may stimulate episodes of nausea.[245] The biological bases for such changes are not known, but they are suspected of being related to hormonal changes of pregnancy.

**Pica** Classified as an eating disorder, pica affects over half of pregnant women in some locations of the southern part of the United States. It is more common in non-Hispanic Black Americans than in other groups, and it is common enough to be considered a normal behavior in some countries. Historically, one type of pica—***geophagia***—was thought to provide women with additional minerals and to ease gastrointestinal upsets. The cause of pica remains a mystery and beneficial effects from the practice of pica have not been documented.[246]

Nonfood items most commonly craved and

**pica** An eating disorder characterized by the compulsion to eat substances that are not food.

**geophagia** Compulsive consumption of clay or dirt.

consumed by pregnant women with pica include ice or freezer frost (***pagophagia***), laundry starch or cornstarch (***amylophagia***), baking soda and powder, and clay or dirt (geophagia). Women experiencing pica are more likely to be iron deficient than those who don't, and iron-deficiency anemia is especially common among pregnant women who compulsively consume ice or freezer frost.[247] It is not clear, however, whether iron deficiency leads to pica or if pica leads to iron deficiency.

Pica does not appear to be related to newborn weight or preterm delivery. It can, however, complicate control of gestational diabetes if starch is eaten, and it has caused lead poisoning, intestinal obstruction, and parasitic infestation of the gastrointestinal tract.[247] Women with amylophagia sometimes accept powdered milk as an alternative to laundry starch or cornstarch, and treating anemia often stops the craving for ice or freezer frost.

TABLE 4.27 ▸ Basics of a good diet for normal pregnancy

| GOOD PREGNANCY DIETS: |
| --- |
| 1. Provide sufficient calories to support appropriate rates of weight gain. |
| 2. Follow the ChooseMyPlate food group recommendations. |
| 3. Provide all essential nutrients at recommended levels of intake from the diet. |
| 4. Include 600 mcg folate, of which 400 mcg is folic acid, daily. |
| 5. Provide sufficient dietary fiber (28 g/day). |
| 6. Include 9 cups fluid daily. |
| 7. Include salt "to taste." |
| 8. Exclude alcohol. |
| 9. Are satisfying and enjoyable. |

## Cultural Considerations

People tend to be attached to existing food preferences, many of which may have deep cultural roots. Dietary recommendations will differ, for example, for Native Alaskans accustomed to a diet based on wild game; for Cambodians, Vietnamese, and Somalis who may think no meal is complete without rice; and for lactose-intolerant individuals.

The belief that consumption of certain foods "marks" the baby is common in many cultures. People may think, for example, that a woman who loves mangos and eats lots of them during pregnancy may have a baby born with a "mango-shaped" birthmark. Some cultures would hold that the baby will also have learned to love mangos because its mother ate them often while pregnant. Other people believe, for example, that beets and beet juice are good sources of iron (they are not) and will increase consumption of them during pregnancy.

Dietary recommendations that are not consistent with a person's usual dietary practices and beliefs, or that are not viewed as acceptable or even preferred by the woman, are least likely to be effective. For best results, dietary adjustments recommended for each individual pregnant woman should take into account her usual practices and preferences.

# Healthy Dietary Patterns for Pregnancy

LO4.8 Develop a one-day diet for pregnancy based on ChooseMyPlate.gov food intake recommendations for pregnancy.

Healthy dietary patterns for women during pregnancy are described in terms of calories and nutrient intake, and by food choices. Such diets have a number of characteristics in common (Table 4.27). Healthy dietary patterns emphasize the consumption of whole grains and whole grain products, low-fat dairy products, legumes, vegetables, fruits, fish and seafood, poultry, nuts, and vegetable oils.[248] For nutrient adequacy, healthy dietary patterns for pregnant women should include foods fortified with vitamin D, iron, and folic acid.

Adequacy of caloric intake during pregnancy is generally based on rate of weight gain, but for nutrients it is based on the DRIs (Table 4.28). Nutrient intakes during pregnancy should approximate those given in the DRI table, and food intake should correspond to the types and quantity of foods recommended in ChooseMyPlate guidance materials. Food plans produced by ChooseMyPlate are based on the selection of food types and amounts that provide adequate amounts of essential nutrients in ways that conform to the recommendations of the 2015 Dietary Guidelines and the RDAs for nutrient intake during pregnancy. They adhere to the general advice given in ChooseMyPlate about healthful diets: "Make half your plate vegetables and fruits."

An example of a ChooseMyPlate one-day food intake plan is shown for a woman named Matty (Table 4.29). Based on her physical activity level (30–60 minutes per day), her prepregnancy weight and height, and the fact that she was in the second trimester of pregnancy, it was calculated that she has a total calorie need of 2600 calories. Table 4.30 shows recommended amounts of food from the food groups that correspond to various levels of calorie need during pregnancy. Although it is difficult for any one menu to match the preferences and food availability situation of every person, the food plan generated by ChooseMyPlate gives women a clear idea of the types and amounts of foods that are recommended for pregnancy.

A good deal of additional information is

**pagophagia** Compulsive consumption of ice or freezer frost.

**amylophagia** Compulsive consumption of laundry starch or cornstarch.

TABLE 4.28 ▸ Recommended Dietary Allowances and Upper Limits for pregnant and nonpregnant women aged 19–30 years*

| | PREGNANT | NONPREGNANT | UPPER LIMIT (UL) |
|---|---|---|---|
| **Energy, kcal** | | | |
| 2nd trimester | +350 | 2403 | — |
| 3rd trimester | +452 | | |
| Protein, gm | 71 | 46 | — |
| Linoleic acid, g | 13 | 12 | — |
| Alpha-linolenic acid, g | 1.4 | 1.1 | — |
| Vitamin A, mcg | 770 | 700 | 3000 |
| Vitamin C, mg | 85 | 75 | 2000 |
| Vitamin D, mcg[a] | 15 | 15 | 100 |
| Vitamin E, mg | 15 | 15 | 1000[c] |
| Vitamin K, mcg | 90 | 90 | — |
| Thiamin, mg | 1.4 | 1.1 | — |
| Riboflavin, mg | 1.4 | 1.1 | — |
| Niacin, mg | 18 | 14 | 35[c] |
| Vitamin $B_6$ | 1.9 | 1.3 | 100 |
| Folate, mcg[b] | 600 | 400 | 1000[c,d] |
| Vitamin $B_{12}$, mcg | 2.6 | 2.4 | — |
| Pantothenic acid, mcg | 6 | 5 | — |
| Biotin, mcg | 30 | 30 | — |
| Choline, g | 450 | 425 | 3.5 |
| Calcium, mg | 1000 | 1000 | 2500 |
| Chromium, mcg | 30 | 25 | — |
| Copper, mcg | 1000 | 900 | 10,000 |
| Fluoride, mg | 3 | 3 | 10 |
| Iodine, mcg | 220 | 150 | 1100 |
| Iron, mg | 27 | 18 | 45 |
| Magnesium, mg | 350 | 310 | 350[c] |
| Manganese, mg | 2 | 1.8 | 11 |
| Molybdenum, mcg | 50 | 45 | 2000 |
| Phosphorus, mg | 700 | 700 | 3500 |
| Selenium, mcg | 60 | 55 | 400 |
| Zinc, mg | 11 | 8 | 40 |

*DRIs for females < 19 and < 30 years are listed inside the front covers of this book.

[a]1 mcg = 40 IU vitamin D; DRI applies in the absence of adequate sunlight.

[b]As Dietary Folate Equivalent (DFE). 1 DFE = 1 mcg food folate = 0.6 mcg folic acid from fortified food or supplement consumed with food = 0.5 mcg of a supplement taken on an empty stomach.

[c]UL applies to intake from supplements or synthetic form only.

[d]Applies to intake of folic acid.

available from the ChooseMyPlate.gov website. Information available includes details on the nutrient composition of meal plans generated or for those based on an individual's dietary intake, food sources of nutrients, tips for vegetarian diets, physical activity tips, and a dietary intake tracking system. It can also be used to help plan and implement a weight loss program after pregnancy.

## Vegetarian Diets in Pregnancy

Nutrient needs in pregnancy may be met by many different types of diets, including those that omit animal products[119,249] (Table 4.31). Diets of pregnant vegetarians are sometimes low in vitamins $B_{12}$ and D, calcium, iron, zinc, and the omega-3 fatty acids eicosapentaenoic and docosahexaenoic acids due to the exclusion of animal foods. Vitamin $B_{12}$ deficiency during pregnancy may not become apparent until after delivery. Two cases of neurological impairment and growth failure due to maternal $B_{12}$ deficiency were identified in 4- to 8-month-old infants in Georgia in 2001. Both infants were born to women who followed a vegetarian diet during pregnancy.[250]

Protein intake is generally adequate in the vegetarian diet, but it may be low in vegans. Protein needs are met by vegetarians who regularly consume a variety of plant sources of protein and meet energy needs. In pregnant women who consume no animal products, the variety of plant protein sources needs to include complementary sources of protein daily. Protein sources that complement each other, or provide a complete source of protein, include legumes (such as lentils, chickpeas, black-eyed peas, black beans, and lima beans) and grains (corn, rice, bulgur, and barley, for example). Protein requirements in vegetarians whose main source of protein is cereals and legumes may be 30 percent higher than for non-vegetarians due to the low digestibility of protein in these foods.[251]

Availability of vegetarian food products in large grocery and organic-food stores has expanded substantially.[252] Vegetarians can now select veggie burgers, meat analog entrees, meals-in-a-cup, and frozen desserts from food-store shelves. Fortified juice, soymilks, breakfast cereal, and meat substitutes are available and can contribute substantially to vegetarians' intake of vitamins $B_{12}$ and D and calcium (Table 4.32). DHA derived from algae can be used to provide a source of this omega-3 fatty acid in diets of vegetarian pregnant women who do not consume fish or seafood.[251]

Computerized nutrient analysis of several days of usual food intake may be especially helpful for the evaluation of vegan diets and other special diets that exclude groups of food. Maternal dietary pattern evaluation and assessment of rate of weight gain, provide objective information on the quality of the dietary pattern and the adequacy of energy intake, and indicate what types of changes are needed. See Case Study 4.1, Vegan Dietary Patterns During Pregnancy.

## Dietary Supplements during Pregnancy

Dietary supplements used by pregnant women primarily consist of vitamins, minerals, and/or herbs. Multivitamin and mineral supplements are often recommended for women who are pregnant in the United States, and many women make the decision to use nutrient and herbal

**TABLE 4.29** A ChooseMyPlate generated one-day food intake plan for Matty

| CALORIES | ALLOWANCE | | |
|---|---|---|---|
| **Total Calories**<br>• Empty Calories* | **2600 per day**<br>• ≤ 362 per day | | |
| **FOOD GROUP** | **FOOD GROUP AMOUNT** | **"WHAT COUNTS AS . . ."** | **TIPS** |
| GRAINS | 9 OUNCE(S) PER DAY | 1 OUNCE OF GRAINS | TIPS |
| • Whole Grains | • ≥ 4½ oz per day | • 1 slice of bread (1 ounce)<br>• ½ cup cooked pasta, rice, or cereal<br>• 1 ounce uncooked pasta or rice<br>• 1 tortilla (6 inch diameter)<br>• 1 pancake (5 inch diameter)<br>• 1 ounce ready-to-eat cereal (about 1 cup cereal flakes)<br>See more Grain examples | • Eat at least half of all grains as whole grains.<br>• Substitute whole-grain choices for refined grains in breakfast cereals, breads, crackers, rice, and pasta.<br>• Check product labels—Is a grain with "whole" before its name listed first on the ingredients list? |
| VEGETABLES | 3½ CUP(S) PER DAY | 1 CUP OF VEGETABLES | TIPS |
| • Dark green<br>• Red and orange<br>• Beans and peas<br>• Starchy<br>• Other | • 2½ cup(s) per week<br>• 7 cup(s) per week<br>• 2½ cup(s) per week<br>• 7 cup(s) per week<br>• 5½ cup(s) per week | • 1 cup raw or cooked vegetables<br>• 1 cup 100% vegetable juice<br>• 2 cups leafy salad greens<br>See more Vegetable examples | • Include vegetables in meals and in snacks. Fresh, frozen, and canned vegetables all count.<br>• Add dark-green, red, and orange vegetables to main and side dishes. Use dark leafy greens to make salads.<br>• Beans and peas are a great source of fiber. Add beans or peas to salads, soups, side dishes, or serve as a main dish. |
| FRUITS | 2 CUP(S) PER DAY | 1 CUP OF FRUIT | TIPS |
| | | • 1 cup raw or cooked fruit<br>• 1 cup 100% fruit juice<br>• ½ cup dried fruit<br>See more Fruit examples | • Select fresh, frozen, canned, and dried fruit more often than juice; select 100% fruit juice when choosing juice.<br>• Enjoy a wide variety of fruits, and maximize taste and freshness, by adapting your choices to what's in season.<br>• Use fruit as snacks, salads, or desserts. |
| DAIRY | 3 CUP(S) PER DAY | 1 CUP OF DAIRY | TIPS |
| | | • 1 cup milk<br>• 1 cup fortified soymilk (soy beverage)<br>• 1 cup yogurt<br>• 1½ oz natural cheese (e.g. Cheddar)<br>• 2 oz processed cheese (e.g. American)<br>See more Dairy examples | • Drink fat-free (skim) or low-fat (1%) milk.<br>• Choose fat-free or low-fat milk or yogurt more often than cheese.<br>• When selecting cheese, choose low-fat or reduced-fat versions. |
| PROTEIN FOODS | 6½ OZ PER DAY | 1 OZ OF PROTEIN FOODS | TIPS |
| • Seafood | • 10 oz per week | • 1 oz lean meat, poultry, seafood<br>• 1 egg<br>• 1 Tablespoon peanut butter<br>• ½ oz nuts or seeds<br>• ¼ cup cooked beans or peas<br>See more Protein Food examples | • Eat a variety of foods from the Protein Foods group each week.<br>• Eat seafood in place of meat or poultry twice a week.<br>• Select lean meat and poultry. Trim or drain fat from meat and remove poultry skin. |
| OILS | 8 TSP PER DAY | 1 TSP OF OIL | TIPS |
| | | • 1 tsp vegetable oil (e.g., canola, corn, olive, soybean)<br>• 1½ tsp mayonnaise<br>• 2 tsp tub margarine<br>• 2 tsp French dressing<br>See more Oil examples | • Choose soft margarines with zero *trans* fats made from liquid vegetable oil, rather than stick margarine or butter.<br>• Use vegetable oils (olive, canola, corn, soybean, peanut, safflower, sunflower) rather than solid fats (butter, shortening).<br>• Replace solid fats with oils, rather than adding oil to the diet. Oils are a concentrated source of calories, so use oils in small amounts. |

*Calories from food components such as added sugars and solid fats that provide little nutritional value. Empty calories are part of Total Calories.

SOURCE: ChooseMyPlate.gov

TABLE 4.30 ▸ Recommended amounts of food from the food groups that correspond to various levels of calorie need during pregnancy, and amounts of food in each food group that count as a cup, ounce (oz), or teaspoon (tsp)[a]

| CALORIE NEED | GRAINS | VEGETABLES | FRUITS | DAIRY | PROTEIN FOODS | OILS |
|---|---|---|---|---|---|---|
| 2000 | 6 oz | 2½ cup | 2 cup | 3 cup | 5½ oz | 6 tsp |
| 2200 | 7 oz | 3 cup | 2 cup | 3 cup | 6 oz | 6 tsp |
| 2400 | 8 oz | 3 cup | 2 cup | 3 cup | 6½ oz | 7 tsp |
| 2600 | 9 oz | 3½ cup | 2 cup | 3 cup | 6½ oz | 8 tsp |

| FOOD GROUP | EQUIVALENTS |
|---|---|
| Grains, 1 oz (make half of your servings whole grain) | 1 slice bread<br>½ cup cooked pasta, cereal, rice<br>1 tortilla (6″)<br>1 pancake (5″)<br>1 oz ready-to-eat cereal |
| Vegetables, 1 cup (vary your veggies, choose colourful ones) | 1 cup raw or cooked vegetables<br>1 cup 100% vegetable juice<br>2 cup leafy salad greens |
| Fruit, 1 cup | 1 cup raw or cooked fruit<br>1 cup 100% fruit juice<br>½ cup dried fruit<br>1 large banana (8″–9″)<br>1 large grapefruit, peach, pear, orange, mango<br>3 medium plums |

[a]SOURCE: ChooseMyPlate.gov, accessed May 20, 2015.

supplements on their own.[253] Some women report feeling reassured by a prescription for a vitamin and mineral supplement and may question the competence of clinicians who don't provide one.[254] However, there is little evidence supporting the safety and effectiveness of many of the dietary supplements available on the market and used by pregnant women. The American College of Obstetrics and Gynecology and the Institute of Medicine do not recommend the routine use of multivitamin and mineral supplements during pregnancy, but rather, recommend they be used if indicated by need.[48,255]

**Multivitamin and Mineral Prenatal Supplements [D]** With the possible exception of iron, nutrient needs during pregnancy should be met by the consumption of a well-balanced and adequate diet.[48,255] This approach to

TABLE 4.31 ▸ Vegetarian food guide adapted for pregnant women[251,299]

| FOOD GROUP | SERVINGS PER DAY | FOOD GROUP | SERVINGS PER DAY |
|---|---|---|---|
| **A. Grains**<br>Whole-grain bread, 1 slice<br>Cooked grains, ½ cup<br>Fortified cold cereal, 1 oz<br>Fortified cooked cereal, ½ cup<br>Corn, ½ cup<br>Pasta, ½ cup<br>Tortilla, 1 small<br>Crackers, 4 small | 6–11 | Cow's milk, 1 cup<br>Cheese, 1 oz<br>Yogurt, ½ cup<br>Fortified soymilk, 1 cup | |
| | | **C. Vegetables**<br>Cooked vegetables, ½ cup<br>Raw vegetables, 1 cup<br>Vegetable juice, ½ cup | 4 |
| **B. Legumes, Nuts, Seeds, Dairy**<br>Dried beans, cooked, ½ cup<br>Peas, ½ cup<br>Soy products, ½ cup or 2–3 oz<br>Soynuts, ¼ cup<br>Nut and seed butter, 2 Tbsp<br>Nuts and seeds, ¼ cup<br>Eggs, 1 | 5–7 | **D. Fruits**<br>Medium-sized fruit, 1<br>Cut-up raw or cooked, ½ cup<br>Fruit juice, ½ cup<br>Dried fruit, ¼ cup | 2 |
| | | **E. Fats, Oils, and Sweets**<br>Mayonnaise, oil, margarine, 1 Tbsp<br>Honey, syrup, jams, jellies, sugar, 1 Tbsp | 2 + depending on caloric need |

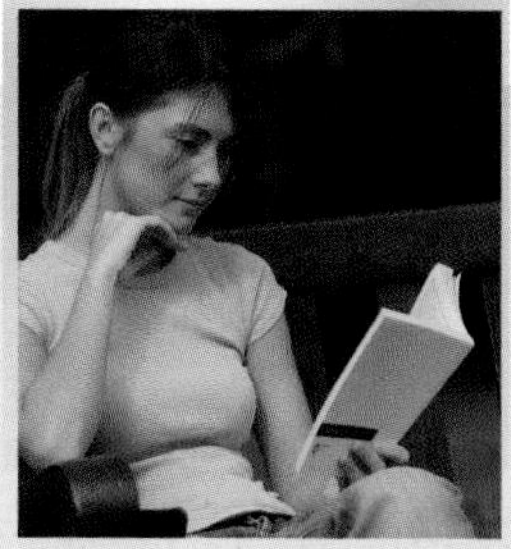
Chrisstockphoto/Alamy

# CASE STUDY 4.1

## Vegan Dietary Patterns During Pregnancy

Ms. Lederman, a healthy 32-year-old woman entering her thirteenth week of pregnancy, asks her doctor for a referral to a dietitian to discuss her vegan diet. She receives the referral, and while making an appointment with the nutrition consulting service, she is asked to record her food intake for 3 days prior to the appointment. Ms. Lederman follows the instructions she was given and carefully completes a 3-day food record. Prior to the appointment, she sends her food record to the dietitian she will be seeing.

During the appointment, the dietitian learns that Ms. Lederman started pregnancy at normal weight, has gained 3 pounds so far in pregnancy, has no history of iron or another nutrient deficiency, and is experiencing a normal course of pregnancy. Ms. Lederman has been a vegan since the age of 16, and although she believes it is good for her health, she worries that her baby may not be getting the nutrients she or he needs. Ms. Lederman wears sunscreen whenever she goes outside, so she makes little or no vitamin D in her skin. She makes sure to combine plant sources of protein (usually dried beans and grains), so she'll consume complete sources of protein every day.

Results of the dietary analysis performed by the dietitian showed the following average calorie and nutrient intake levels:

Kcal: 2237
Protein, g: 71
Linoleic acid (n-6 fatty acids), g: 15.2
Alpha-linolenic acid (n-3 fatty acids), g: 0.54
Vitamin $B_{12}$, mcg: 2.1
Vitamin D, mcg: 3 (120 IU)
Zinc, mg: 15

### Questions

1. Is Ms. Lederman consuming enough protein?
2. Based on the information presented, which nutrients are consumed in amounts that are below the DRI standard for pregnancy?
3. Suggest three types of food Ms. Lederman could consume to bring up her intake of the nutrients identified in question 2.

meeting nutrient needs should be considered first because foods provide antioxidants, fiber, and other beneficial bioactive substances. Healthy diets also provide adequate amounts of protein, health-promoting sources of dietary fat, and nutrient-rich sources of carbohydrates.[119]

Multivitamin and mineral prenatal supplements may benefit women who:

- Do not ordinarily consume an adequate diet
- Have a multifetal pregnancy

TABLE 4.32 ▸ Levels of key nutrients in fortified and other vegetarian foods[a]

| | KEY NUTRIENTS | | | |
|---|---|---|---|---|
| | VITAMIN $B_{12}$ | VITAMIN D | CALCIUM | DHA |
| RDA for adults: | 2.4 mcg | 5 mcg | 1000 mg | 300 mg[b] |
| Rice Dream, 1 cup | 1.5 mcg | 5 mcg | 1000 mg | — |
| Soy milk, 1 cup | 2.6 mcg | 3 mcg | 300 mg | — |
| Meat analogs, 1 serv. | 0–1.4 mcg | — | — | — |
| Tofu w/calcium sulfate, ½ cup | — | — | 130 mg | — |
| Fully fortified breakfast cereal, 1 cup | 6 mcg | 2.5 mcg | 1000 mg | — |
| Other breakfast cereals, ¾ cup | 1.5 mcg | 1 mcg | 0–100 mg | — |
| Nutritional yeast, 2 Tbsp | 7.8 mcg | — | — | — |
| Algae, 1 capsule | — | — | — | 180 mg |
| DHA-fortified fruit juice, 1 cup | — | — | — | 32 mg |
| Collard greens, 1 cup | — | — | 357 | — |
| Kale, 1 cup | — | — | 180 | — |
| Turnip greens, 1 cup | — | — | 107 | — |

[a]Check out product labels for product-specific information on nutrient content.

[b]DRIs for DHA are yet to be established. The figure given in the table is from Harris et al., 2009.[146]

- Are vegans
- Have iron deficiency anemia
- Have a diagnosed nutrient deficiency or a therapeutic need for a specific nutrient[48,256]

Standard prenatal multivitamin and mineral supplements taken before and during pregnancy appear to benefit women in need of them. Prenatal vitamin and mineral supplements use by low-income pregnant women has been found to decrease the risk of preterm, low birthweight, and certain congenital malformations.[257,258]

About 95 percent of all pregnant women and 75 percent of women in WIC take a vitamin and mineral supplement regularly during pregnancy.[256,259] Supplements available by prescription only generally include those that contain over 1 mg folic acid. They contain an amazing array of nutrients, from vitamins and minerals to seaweed, borage, and don guai. Some of the prenatal supplements sold over the Internet contain ingredients that are not considered safe for use in pregnancy, and others provide unreasonably high levels of vitamins or minerals (Table 4.33).

According to national surveys and other sources, nutrients most likely to be lacking in the diets of women before pregnancy include fiber, choline, vitamin D, vitamin E, calcium, magnesium, iron, potassium, and EPA + DHA.[124,222] (Data are not available on the vitamin and mineral content of the diets of a representative sample of U.S. pregnant women.) Nutrients and nutrient amounts provided by general prenatal supplements should address these potential nutrient gaps at level that approximate the RDAs. Supplement use should be accompanied by nutritional counseling that helps women and their families select and consume foods that add up to a healthful diet.

Over 200 prescription and nonprescription prenatal vitamin and mineral supplements are available on the market[259] making it difficult to separate one from the others. The Office of Dietary Supplements has developed a database that helps with this. It can be used to identify which nutrients and how much of those nutrients are labeled as being contained in a particular brand of supplement. This site can also be used to search for dietary supplements that have been recalled by the FDA. The database can be accessed through the Office of Dietary Supplements homepage.

**Herbal Remedies and Pregnancy** Herbs are generally regarded by the public and by some health professionals as helpful, safe, and gentle. It is estimated that in the eastern United States, 45 percent of pregnant women use herbal products during pregnancy. Women may not report use of herbs to their health care provider based on concerns about the provider's knowledge about herbs or a bias against them.[260]

The active ingredients of herbal products are often similar to those in medications that may not be approved for use in pregnancy.[261] About one-third of commonly used herbal supplements have been deemed unsafe for use by pregnant women (Table 4.34).[262] Women who use herbs should be provided with respectful counseling about effectiveness and safety, and directed toward reliable sources of information about them.[260]

Advice to use herbal remedies during pregnancy appears to be based primarily on their traditional use in different societies. This strategy for assessing the safety of herbs doesn't always work. Some herbs considered safe based on traditional use have been found to produce malformations in animal studies.[263] Others, such as blue cohosh, which

**TABLE 4.33** Range of daily dose levels of nutrients in 12 prenatal supplements and comparison with recommended intake levels during pregnancy and mean intakes of nutrients for women age 20–29 years[a]

| NUTRIENT | RANGE IN AMOUNTS | RDA | MEAN INTAKE, 20- TO 29-YEAR-OLD WOMEN | UL |
|---|---|---|---|---|
| Vitamin A | 3000–8000 IU | 2564 IU | 593 mcg | 9990 IU |
| Vitamin E | 4–60 IU | 22 IU | 98.0 mg | 1490 IU |
| Vitamin $B_6$ | 2.6–25 mg | 1.9 mg | 2.0 mg | 100 mg |
| Folate | 800–1000 mcg | 600 mcg | 543 mcg | 1000 mcg |
| Vitamin $B_{12}$ | 4–100 mcg | 2.6 mcg | 4.6 mcg | — |
| Vitamin C | 60–120 mg | 85 mg | 83 mg | 2000 mg |
| Vitamin D | 400–610 IU | 200 IU | 148 IU | 2000 IU |
| Calcium | 68–1300 mg | 1000 mg | 908 mg | 2500 mg |
| Magnesium | 20–200 mg | 350 mg | 266 mg | 350 mg |
| Iron | 21–51 mg | 27 mg | 13.8 mg | 45 mg |
| Iodine | 0–290 mcg | 220 mcg | 200 mcg | 1100 mcg |
| Zinc | 15–30 mg | 11 mg | 10.0 mg | 40 mg |
| DHA/DHA1EPA | 0–440 mg | — | 80 mg | — |

[a]Prenatal nutrient supplement content determined from company website information, 5/09. U.S. population-wide information on average nutrient intake of pregnant women is unavailable, so data for women age 20 to 29 are used.[133] RDAs listed are for 19- to 30-year-old pregnant women, and Tolerable Upper Intake Levels (ULs) for pregnant women age 19–50 years. Table revised by Judith E. Brown, May 2015.

TABLE 4.34 ▸ Herbs to avoid in pregnancy[263,264]

| | |
|---|---|
| Aloe vera | Ergot |
| Anise | Feverfew |
| Black cohosh | Ginkgo |
| Black haw | Ginseng |
| Blue cohosh | Juniper |
| Borage | Kava |
| Buckthorn | Licorice |
| Comfrey | Pennyroyal |
| Cotton root | Raspberry leaf |
| Dandelion leaf | Saw palmetto |
| Ephedra, ma huang | Senna |

was previously thought to safely induce uterine contractions, may increase the risk of heart failure in the baby.[264] Ginseng, one of the most commonly used herb in the world, has been found to cause malformations in rat embryos,[254] and ginkgo may promote excessive bleeding.[265] Peppermint tea and ginger root, taken for nausea, appear to be safe.[263] Ginger, given in oral doses of 1 gram daily for 4 days, has been found to decrease the severity of nausea and vomiting during pregnancy in a majority of women. Ginger use in this study involving 70 women was not related to complications of pregnancy or poor pregnancy outcomes.[266]

Manufacturers of herbal remedies do not have to prove they are safe for use by pregnant women. However, the FDA stipulates that claims related to pregnancy should not be made for herbal supplements.[262]

# Food Safety During Pregnancy

LO 4.9 Describe two reasons why pregnant women and their fetuses are particularly vulnerable to certain foodborne illnessess.

Certain foodborne illnesses can be devastating during pregnancy. Increased progesterone levels that normally occur decrease pregnant women's ability to resist infectious diseases, so they are more susceptible to the effects of foodborne infections.[267] One particularly important foodborne illness is caused by ***Listeria monocytogenes***. The placenta does not protect the fetus from listeria infection in the mother. Listeriosis during pregnancy is associated with spontaneous abortion and stillbirth in one-third of fetuses and mild infection in mothers. To prevent this foodborne infection, pregnant women should not eat raw or smoked fish, oysters, unpasteurized or soft cheeses, raw or undercooked meat, or unpasteurized milk. Luncheon meats, hot dogs, and other processed meats should be stored correctly, and foods such as hot dogs heated thoroughly (Table 4.35).[267]

TABLE 4.35 ▸ Food safety precautions issued for pregnant women[267]

- Don't eat raw or undercooked fish, smoked fish/seafood, or rare or undercooked meat.
- Don't consume fish high in mercury content.
- Don't consume unpasteurized dairy products (includes soft cheeses made from unpasteurized milk).
- Don't eat raw or undercooked eggs or egg products, cookie dough, or other batters.
- Don't drink unpasteurized juices.
- Don't eat grocery store or deli salads (e.g., potato salad, chicken salad, and ham salad).
- Don't eat raw sprouts.
- Heat deli meats such as hot dogs, pate, and luncheon meats to 165°F before eating.

The protozoan ***Toxoplasma gondii*** also causes serious effects in pregnant women and their fetuses. This protozoan can be transferred from mother to fetus and cause mental retardation, blindness, seizures, and death. Sources of *T. gondii* include raw and undercooked meats, the surface of fruits and vegetables, and cat litter. Cats that eat wild animals and undercooked meats can become infected and transfer the infection through the air and via stools left in their litter boxes.[267]

# Assessment of Nutritional Status During Pregnancy

LO 4.10 Identify the basic components of a nutritional assessment of pregnant women.

A comprehensive approach to nutrition assessment in pregnancy includes an evaluation of dietary intake, weight status, biomarkers of nutrient status, food preferences and resources, previous pregnancy and health history, and dietary supplement use.[268] In this section, we highlight two of these components: assessment of dietary intake and nutrition biomarkers.

## Dietary Assessment During Pregnancy

Routine assessment of dietary practices is recommended for all pregnant women to determine the need for an improved diet or vitamin and mineral supplements.[48] Dietary assessment in pregnancy should cover usual dietary intake, dietary supplement use, and weight-gain progress. For

***L. monocytogenes*, or listeria** A foodborne bacterial infection that can lead to preterm delivery and stillbirth in pregnant women. Listeria infection is commonly associated with the ingestion of soft cheeses, unpasteurized milk, ready-to-eat deli meats, and hot dogs.

***T. Gondii*, or toxoplasmosis** A parasitic infection that can impair fetal brain development. The source of the infection is often hands contaminated with soil or the contents of a cat litter box; or raw or partially cooked pork, lamb, or venison.

best results, several days of accurately recorded, usual intake should be used for each assessment.

Several levels of dietary assessment can be undertaken. Which assessment level is best primarily depends on the skill level of the health professional responsible for interpreting the results. Results of food-based assessments are rather straightforward to interpret, whereas computerized assessments of levels of nutrient intake are more complex.

Computerized analysis, given accurate records and entry of dietary intake and a high-quality nutrient database, provides results useful for estimating the quantity of calories and nutrients consumed. Detailed knowledge of dietary intake is particularly useful for women at risk of nutrient inadequacies or excesses, and for women with conditions such as gestational diabetes, food intolerances, and multifetal pregnancy.

## Nutrition Biomarker Assessment

Nutrition assessment of pregnant women usually includes laboratory tests of iron status, and will include tests to determine the status of other nutrients as indicated. Due to the normal physiological changes occurring during pregnancy, such as hemodilution that affects blood nutrient concentrations, assessment of nutrition biomarkers should employ standards developed for pregnancy.[269] Blood nutrient concentrations change with time during pregnancy, so no one value per nutrient for all of pregnancy accurately reflects status.

Studies reporting reference values for nutrition biomarkers during pregnancy are beginning to appear in the scientific literature (Table 4.36). The concentrations listed by week of gestation consists of values from the 2.5 percentile to the 97.5 percentile of the distribution of values within a sample of well-nourished women with healthy, uncomplicated pregnancies. These values are assumed to reflect normal ranges of nutrition biomarker concentrations during pregnancy and may change as new analysis techniques and data become available. The biomarker levels are intended to assist clinicians in distinguishing between physiological changes and pathological states during pregnancy.[269]

TABLE 4.36 ▸ Reference values for nutrition biomarkers during normal pregnancy in healthy women[a,181,205,218,269]

| NUTRIENT | WEEKS GESTATION | REFERENCE VALUES |
|---|---|---|
| Calcium, mmol/L | 7–17 | 2.18–2.53 |
| | 24–28 | 2.04–2.40 |
| | 34–38 | 2.04–2.41 |
| Chloride, mmol/L | 7–17 | 100–107 |
| | 24–28 | 99–108 |
| | 34–38 | 97–109 |
| Ferritin, μg/L | 7–17 | 7.1–106.4 |
| | 24–28 | 3.8–49.8 |
| | 34–38 | 4.8–43.5 |
| Iodine, urinary, μg/L | 0–40 | 150–249 |
| Iron, μmol/L | 7–17 | 8.7–37.0 |
| | 24–28 | 8.0–50.0 |
| | 34–38 | 7.6–34.5 |
| Magnesium, mmol/L | 7–17 | 0.70–0.96 |
| | 24–28 | 0.63–0.91 |
| | 34–38 | 0.57–0.87 |
| Potassium, mmol/L | 7–17 | 3.24–4.86 |
| | 24–28 | 3.27–4.62 |
| | 34–38 | 3.32–5.09 |
| Sodium, mmol/L | 7–17 | 133.2–140.5 |
| | 24–28 | 129.2–139.3 |
| | 34–38 | 127.0–140.2 |
| Transferrin, g/L | 7–17 | 1.92–3.85 |
| | 24–28 | 2.72–4.36 |
| | 34–38 | 2.88–5.12 |
| Triglycerides, mmol/L | 7–17 | 0.55–3.08 |
| | 24–28 | 1.09–3.63 |
| | 34–38 | 1.62–5.12 |
| Vitamin D, nmol/L (25-hydroxyvitamin D) | 0–40 | ≥ 80 (optimum)<br>< 35 (deficient) |

[a]See Appendix A for a table of factors used to convert SI units to conventional units. Nutrition biomarkers considered to be in the normal range vary based on percentile cut-points used. The 5th to 95th percentiles are sometimes used and not the 2.5 to 97.5 percentiles reported in this table. Reference values and blood nutrient concentrations considered "normal" or "abnormal" during pregnancy change based on advances in knowledge. The symbol mg means "micrograms," sometimes abbreviated as mcg.

# Exercise and Pregnancy Outcome

LO 4.11 Identify three health benefits to women of regular exercise during pregnancy.

There is no evidence that moderate or vigorous exercise undertaken by healthy women consuming high-quality diets and gaining appropriate amounts of weight is harmful to mother or fetus. The bulk of evidence indicates that exercise during pregnancy benefits both the mother and her fetus and is encouraged.[270] Women who exercise regularly during pregnancy tend to feel healthier, have an enhanced sense of well-being, and somewhat shorter labors than is the case for women who do not exercise.[271] Women who exercise regularly during pregnancy reduce their risk of developing gestational diabetes, pregnancy-induced hypertension, low back pain, excessive weight gain, and blood clots.[272]

Exercise during pregnancy can reduce fetal growth in women who are poorly nourished and gain little weight in pregnancy. It is also important for women to avoid dehydration by drinking plenty of fluids while exercising and not to become overheated during physical activity.[273]

Is it safe to begin an exercise program during pregnancy? For most women, the answer is yes.[274] Beginning

TABLE 4.37 ▸ Target heart rates for healthy pregnant women[275]

| AGE, YEARS | HEART RATE |
|---|---|
| < 20 | 140–155 |
| 20–29 | 135–150 |
| 30–39 | 130–145 |
| 40+ | 125–140 |

an exercise program during pregnancy may improve fetal growth. This effect was shown in a study involving nonexercising pregnant women who began to exercise at 8 weeks of pregnancy. Women participated in three to five weight-bearing exercise sessions a week until delivery. Placenta function was better, and newborn weight and length greater, in exercising women compared to women who did not exercise.[275]

### Exercise Recommendations for Pregnant Women

Exercise recommendations for pregnant women are similar to those for other healthy women. Pregnant women should exercise three to five times a week for 20–30 minutes at a heart rate that achieves 60–70 percent $VO_2$ max (Table 4.37). Exercise should begin with about five minutes of warm-up movements and end with the same length of cool-down activities. Recommended types of exercise include walking, cycling, swimming, jogging, and dancing. Better left until after pregnancy are activities such as water and snow skiing, surfing, mountain climbing, scuba diving, and horseback riding. Switching to non–weight-bearing exercises is advised toward the end of pregnancy.[271]

## Common Health Problems During Pregnancy

**LO 4.12** Assess three common health problems during pregnancy and the evidence of the effectiveness of dietary interventions for their treatment or amelioration.

Some of the physiological changes that occur in pregnancy are accompanied by side effects that can dull the bliss of expecting a child by making women feel physically miserable. Common ailments of pregnancy, such as nausea and vomiting, heartburn, and constipation, are generally more amenable to prevention than to treatment, but often can be relieved through dietary measures.

### Nausea and Vomiting

Nausea occurs in about 8 in 10 pregnancies, and vomiting in 5 of 10.[276] Symptoms of nausea generally begin around week 5 of gestation and generally disappear by week 12. The conditions are so common that they are considered a normal part of pregnancy. In 20 percent of pregnant women, nausea and vomiting continue throughout pregnancy. If not severe or prolonged, the presence of nausea and vomiting during pregnancy is associated with a reduced risk of miscarriage of greater than 60 percent. The causes of nausea and vomiting are not yet clear, but they are thought to be related to increased levels of human chorionic gonadotropin, progesterone, estrogen, and other hormones early in pregnancy.[277]

In the past, the nausea and vomiting of pregnancy was called *morning sickness,* because it was thought to occur mostly after waking up. It actually occurs at all times of day—a mere 17 percent of women experience nausea and vomiting only in the morning.[278] Iron supplements may aggravate nausea and vomiting when taken in the first trimester of pregnancy.[211]

**Hyperemesis Gravidarum** Between 1 and 2 percent of pregnant women with nausea and vomiting develop *hyperemesis gravidarum* (more commonly called hyperemesis).[278] Hyperemesis is characterized by severe nausea and vomiting that last throughout much of pregnancy. It can be debilitating. In addition to the mother feeling very sick, frequent vomiting can lead to weight loss, electrolyte imbalances, and dehydration. Women with hyperemesis who gain weight normally during pregnancy (about 30 pounds total) are not at increased risk of delivering small infants, but women who gain less (21–22 pounds) are.[279]

**Management of Nausea and Vomiting** Many approaches to the treatment of nausea and vomiting are used in clinical practice, but only a few are considered safe and effective. Dietary interventions represent a safe method, primarily because the short- and long-term safety of many drugs and herbal remedies early in pregnancy is unclear.[280] Here are some general recommendations for women experiencing nausea and vomiting:

- Continue to gain weight.
- Separate liquid and solid food intake.
- Avoid odors and foods that trigger nausea.
- Select foods that are well tolerated.

Many women find that hard-boiled eggs, potato chips, popcorn, yogurt, crackers, and other high-carbohydrate foods are well tolerated. Personal support and understanding are important components of counseling women with nausea and vomiting. Care should be taken to individualize dietary advice based on each woman's food preferences and tolerances. Women with hyperemesis may require rehydration therapy to restore fluids and electrolyte balance.[276]

Periodically, articles will appear in the popular press claiming that nausea and vomiting are caused by certain foods, and that women should avoid them to protect their fetus from harmful substances in the foods. Not too long ago it was claimed that bitter-tasting vegetables, for example, should be avoided. When put to the test, this notion was found to be groundless.[281] Theoretical claims that certain foods elicit nausea and vomiting in order to protect the fetus from harmful effects of the food should be considered unreliable until proven in scientific studies.

***Dietary Supplements for the Treatment of Nausea and Vomiting*** Three types of dietary supplements have been found to decrease the symptoms of nausea and vomiting in pregnancy:

- Vitamin $B_6$ (pyridoxine) supplements given in a 10–25 mg dose every 8 hours reduce the severity of nausea in many women.[277] The upper limit for vitamin $B_6$ intake during pregnancy is 100 mg per day.
- Diclegis (also called Dilectin) is a prescription medication that combines vitamin $B_6$ with doxylamine, effectively reduces nausea and vomiting of pregnancy.[281]
- Ginger in doses of 550–1050 mg a day for 4 days, decrease nausea and vomiting in some women.[277]

Additional research is needed before a definitive statement can be made regarding the safety of high doses of ginger use during pregnancy.[277]

### Heartburn

Pregnancy is accompanied by relaxation of gastrointestinal tract muscles. This effect is attributed primarily to progesterone. Relaxation of the muscular valve known as the cardiac or lower esophageal sphincter at the top of the stomach is thought to be the principal reason for the 40–80 percent incidence of heartburn in women during pregnancy. The loose upper valve may allow stomach contents to be pushed back into the esophagus.[277,283]

**Management of Heartburn** Dietary advice for the prevention and management of heartburn includes:

- Ingest small meals frequently.
- Do not go to bed with a full stomach.
- Avoid foods that seem to make heartburn worse.
- Consume adequate fiber (25–30 g/d).
- Elevate your head and upper body during sleep.[277]

Antacid tablets, which act locally in the stomach, are often recommended in limited amounts, but sodium bicarbonate (baking soda) and heartburn pills usually are not.[283] Although these approaches appear to work for many women, they have not been tested for effectiveness or safety. Approaches to decreasing heartburn should be individualized.[277]

### Constipation

Relaxed gastrointestinal muscle tone is thought to be primarily responsible for the increased incidence of constipation and hemorrhoids in pregnancy. One way to prevent these maladies is to consume approximately 30 grams of dietary fiber daily. (Table 1.5 in Chapter 1 lists food sources of dietary fiber.) Laxative pills are not recommended for use by pregnant women, but soluble fiber in products such as Metamucil, Citrucel, and Perdiem are considered safe and effective for the prevention and treatment of constipation.[283] Women should drink a cup or more of water along with the fiber supplement.

## Model Nutrition Programs for Risk Reduction in Pregnancy

LO 4.13 Describe the nutrition services components of a model nutrition program during pregnancy.

Two programs that have been shown to substantially improve pregnancy outcomes are the intervention program offered by the Montreal Diet Dispensary (MDD) and the Supplemental Nutrition Program for Women, Infants, and Children (WIC).

### The Montreal Diet Dispensary

The Montreal Diet Dispensary (MDD) has served low-income, high-risk pregnant females with nutritional assessment and intervention services since the early 1900s. Part of the rationale for the WIC program in the United States was based on the successes of the MDD program. The core program is located in a large, comfortable house (see Illustration 4.22) in urban Montreal. Clients are warmly welcomed into a nonthreatening, relaxed setting.

Developed as an adjunct to routine prenatal care, the MDD intervention strategy has four major components:

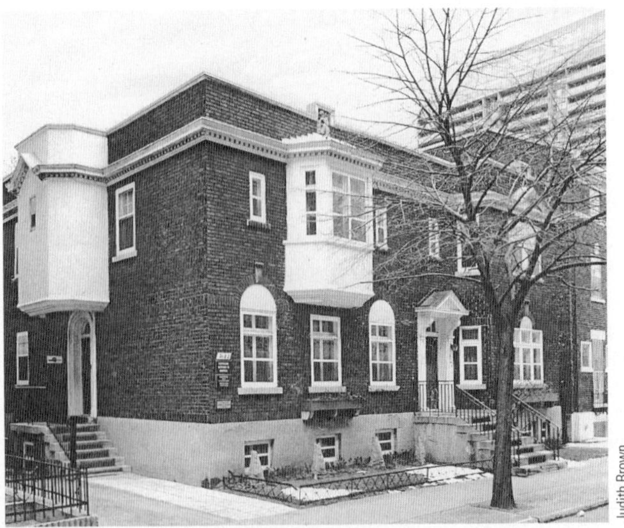
Judith Brown

ILLUSTRATION 4.22 ▸ The Montreal Diet Dispensary.
Photo provided by Marie Paul Duquette, Director of the Montreal Diet Dispensary.

1. Assess the usual dietary intake and risk profile of each pregnant woman, including calories, protein, and selected vitamin and mineral adequacy; also assess stress level.
2. Determine individual nutritional rehabilitation needs based on results of the assessment.
3. Teach clients the importance of optimal nutrition and about changes that should be made through practical examples.
4. Provide regular follow-up and supervision.

The MDD dietitians are carefully trained and hold the interests of their clients first in their hearts. They treat clients with respect, openness, and affection; they also address client needs, such as transportation or emergency food or housing. Staff interactions with clients are nonjudgmental in nature and include positive feedback and praise for dietary changes and other successes of clients.

The initial client visit to the MDD takes about 75 minutes, and follow-up visits are scheduled at 2-week intervals for 40 minutes each. Women are identified as undernourished if their protein intake falls below that recommended for pregnancy, and an additional protein allowance is added to the diet. Women who are underweight are given an additional daily allowance of 20 grams protein and 200 calories for each additional pound of weight gain needed to achieve a maximum of 2 pounds per week. Women identified as being under excessive stress (such as having a partner in jail, being homeless, or being abused) receive an additional allowance of protein and calories and lots of positive attention. Food supplements, including milk and eggs, and vitamin supplements are provided to women who need them.

**Impact of MDD Services** Multiple studies have shown that women receiving MDD services have higher-birthweight infants, fewer low-birthweight infants, and infants with lower rates of perinatal mortality than is the case for similar women not receiving MDD services.[284,285]

The program is cost-effective in relation to savings on newborn critical care, and programs based on MDD services have spread across Canada. Expenditures per client average $450. The program is supported by a number of foundations, provincial and federal programs, and other contributions.[286] It is shaping the delivery of nutrition services to low-income women and families across Canada and beyond.

## The WIC Program

The WIC program represents an outstanding example of a successful public program intended to serve the nutritional needs of low-income women and families. It is cited as a model program in several other chapters and is described in Chapter 1.

In operation since 1974, WIC provides nutritional assessment, education and counseling, food supplements, and access to health services to over 6 million participants. WIC serves low-income pregnant, postpartum, and breastfeeding women, and children up to 5 years of age who are at nutritional risk. Supplemental food provided to women includes milk, yogurt, vegetables, fruits, whole grain products, ready-to-eat cereals, dried beans, fruit juice, and cheese. Some programs offer vouchers for farmer's markets.[287]

Participation in WIC is related to reduced rates of iron-deficiency anemia in pregnancy, higher-birthweight infants, decreased low-birthweight infants, and lower rates of iron-deficiency anemia in women after delivery. For each dollar invested in WIC, approximately $3 in health care costs is saved.

## KEY POINTS

1. Nutritional status before and during pregnancy can modify the health of women during pregnancy, as well as the current and future health of infants.
2. Many aspects of nutritional status, such as dietary intake, supplement use, and weight change, influence the course and outcome of pregnancy.
3. Improved maternal nutrition could help improve the health status of U.S. newborns.
4. A woman's body prepares in advance for upcoming physiological events related to placental growth and fetal growth and development (such as proliferation of cells in organs and tissues of the placenta and fetus, and rapid increases in fetal weight). Consequently, nutritional needs must be met *prior* to the physiological changes.
5. Functions of the placenta include hormone and enzyme production, nutrient and gas exchange between mother and fetus, and removal of waste products from the fetus.
6. The placenta does *not* block all harmful substances from reaching the fetus.
7. The fetus is not a parasite; it depends on the mother's nutrient intake to meet its nutritional needs.
8. Periods of rapid growth and development of fetal organs and tissues occur during specific times throughout pregnancy. Essential nutrients must be available in required amounts during these times

for fetal growth and development to proceed optimally.

9. The risk of heart disease, diabetes, hypertension, and other health problems during adulthood may be influenced by maternal nutrition during pregnancy.
10. Variations in fetal growth and development are generally *not* due to genetic causes but rather to environmental factors such as energy, nutrient, and oxygen availability, and to conditions that interfere with genetically programmed growth, development, and nutrient utilization.
11. Energy and nutrient availability is considered the major intrauterine environmental factor that alters expression of fetal genes. This phenomenon represents the major mechanism that underlies the relationship between maternal nutrition and later disease risk.
12. Pregnancy weight gain affects birthweight and long-term health outcomes. Weight gain recommendations are based on prepregnancy weight status.
13. Excessive weight gain is related to postpartum weight retention and the risk of obesity.
14. High-quality vegetarian and vegan diets promote a healthy course and outcome of pregnancy.
15. Pregnant women are advised to consume at least 2–4 oz. servings of low-mercury fish per week.
16. Caloric adequacy during pregnancy can be estimated by weight gain.
17. ChooseMyPlate dietary recommendations for pregnancy are appropriate and recommended for use by pregnant women.
18. Key nutrients of particular importance during pregnancy based on intake levels in nonpregnant women of childbearing age are folic acid (in specific target groups such as Mexican-Americans), fiber, choline, vitamin D, vitamin E, calcium, magnesium, iron, potassium, and EPA + DHA. Antioxidants and other bioactive compounds in plant foods also play key roles in promoting and maintaining maternal and fetal health.
19. Not all pregnant women need a multivitamin and mineral supplement during pregnancy. Food should provide calories and nutrients needed during pregnancy.
20. In general, exercise is beneficial to the course and outcome of pregnancy. Pregnant women in general are encouraged to exercise regularly.
21. Certain foodborne illnesses in pregnant women can threaten fetal survival.
22. Some of the common discomforts of pregnancy, such as nausea and vomiting and constipation, can be ameliorated by nutritional measures.

## REVIEW QUESTIONS

1. ____ Which of the following statements is incorrect?
   a. Rates of preterm delivery and low birthweight in the United States are trending downward but remain higher in non-Hispanic Black American women and infants than in other groups.
   b. Reductions in the proportion of infants born small, early, or both would clearly decrease infant mortality.
   c. The international ranking of the United States for infant mortality rate has been improving since the beginning of the twenty-first century.
   d. National health objectives for pregnant women and newborns focus on the reduction of low birthweight, preterm delivery, and infant mortality.

The next four questions pertain to the following case:

Tony was born at 35 weeks of pregnancy and weighed 2075 grams. His waist circumference was low relative to his weight and length. Tony was hospitalized for an infection at 4 months of age.

2. Tony was born preterm.
   ____ True ____ False
3. How much did Tony weigh in pounds and ounces?
   ____ lbs ____
4. Tony was proportionately small for gestational age.
   ____ True ____ False
5. Tony was hospitalized during the perinatal period.
   ____ True ____ False
6. ____ Which of the following physiological changes in pregnancy is abnormal?
   a. Plasma volume increases 30 percent
   b. Edema
   c. Increased concentrations of cholesterol, LDL cholesterol, triglycerides, HDL cholesterol
   d. Relaxed gastrointestinal tract muscle tone
7. ____ Which of the following statements about "critical periods" of growth and development is true?
   a. Critical periods are defined as specific time periods early in pregnancy when toxins that may harm fetal growth and development are able to pass through the placenta to the fetus.
   b. It is possible to reverse ill effects of adverse nutrition exposures on fetal growth and development by eliminating the adverse nutritional exposure later.

c. The most intense period of fetal tissue and organ growth and development is in the third trimester of pregnancy.

d. Critical periods of growth and development are characterized by hyperplasia, or an increase in cell multiplication.

The next two questions refer to this situation:

Assume a woman with a singleton pregnancy weighed 154 pounds prior to pregnancy and is 5′7″ tall.

8. ____ What was her prepregnancy BMI?

a. 24.1 kg/m$^2$

b. 33.2 kg/m$^2$

c. 19.7 kg/m$^2$

d. 45 kg/m$^2$

9. ____ What would be the recommended range of total weight for her pregnancy in pounds (lb) and kilograms (kg)?

a. 28–40 lb, 12.7–18.2 kg

b. 25–35 lb, 11.4–15.9 kg

c. 15–20 lb, 6.8–9.1 kg

d. 22–27 lb, 10–12.3 kg

10. The fetus is able to modify gene functions in response to exposure to adverse conditions that threaten its immediate chances of survival.

____ True ____ False

11. Changes in gene functions related to inadequate fetal supply of glucose *in utero* tend to decrease the risk that offspring will become obese in adulthood.

____ True ____ False

12. Famine during pregnancy is associated with pSGA at birth and increased risk of heart disease, stroke, and type 2 diabetes in adult offspring.

____ True ____ False

13. Exposure to famine during prepregnancy has been repeatedly found to increase the risk of schizophrenia in offspring.

____ True ____ False

14. Famine during pregnancy in women who were well nourished prior to pregnancy does not adversely affect pregnancy outcomes.

____ True ____ False

15. Iron needs increase during pregnancy primarily due to the loss of iron that occurs with bleeding after delivery.

____ True ____ False

16. The need for DHA increases during pregnancy because DHA is a major structural component of phospholipids in cell membranes of the central nervous system.

____ True ____ False

17. The need for iron decreases during pregnancy because women do not menstruate during pregnancy.

____ True ____ False

18. Meeting vitamin D requirements during pregnancy is particularly important due to the role of vitamin D in fetal bone formation.

____ True ____ False

19. The need for folate increase during pregnancy due to its functions as a cofactor in the replication of DNA, gene expression, and amino acid metabolism.

____ True ____ False

20. ____ A number of factors influence diet during pregnancy beyond food availability. Which of the following factors does *not* commonly modify dietary intake during pregnancy even when food is easily available?

a. Culturally based food preferences

b. Changes in the senses of taste and smell

c. Lack of appetite

d. Beliefs about the nutrient content and effects of specific foods on pregnancy outcome

21. A one-day diet for a woman in her first trimester of pregnancy who has an estimated need for 2000 calories a day would include the food group amounts of 6 ounces of grain products, 2½ cups of vegetables, 2 cups of fruit, 2 cups of milk, 5 ounces of protein foods, and 6 tsp of oil.

____ True ____ False

22. ____ Which of the following is not a basic component of a prenatal nutrition assessment?

a. Evaluation of a 7-day food intake record

b. Evaluation of biomarkers of nutrient status

c. Evaluation of dietary intake

d. Assessment of food preferences and resources

Use the conversion factors listed in the "Conventional Units to SI Units" table in Appendix A to convert the following conventional unit measures to SI units.

23. 52 ng/mL vitamin D (25 hydoxyvitamin D) = ____

24. 86 ng/mL ferritin = ____

25. 402 ng/mL red cell folate = ____

26. Exercise during pregnancy is associated with a lower risk of preterm delivery.

____ True ____ False

27. Women who did not exercise prior to pregnancy should not start exercising during pregnancy.

____ True ____ False

28. Pregnant women are more susceptible to the effects of foodborne infections in part because decreased progesterone levels decrease resistance to infectious diseases.

____ True ____ False

29. ____ Which of the following foods should women *not* consume during pregnancy?
    a. Fish
    b. Broccoli
    c. Raw sprouts
    d. Pasteurized juices
30. One likely effective dietary intervention for women with nausea and vomiting is separation of solid food and liquid food intake.
    ____ True ____ False
31. The frequent ingestion of small meals does *not* appear to help relieve heartburn during pregnancy.
    ____ True ____ False
32. Nutrition programs that tend to improve pregnancy outcomes include the services of nutrition assessment and counseling based on the results of the assessment.
    ___ True ____ False
33. Nutrition programs that tend to improve pregnancy outcomes include the routine provision of a multivitamin and mineral supplement to women.
    ____ True ____ False

**Visit www.cengagebrain.com to access MindTap, a complete digital course that includes additional resources.**

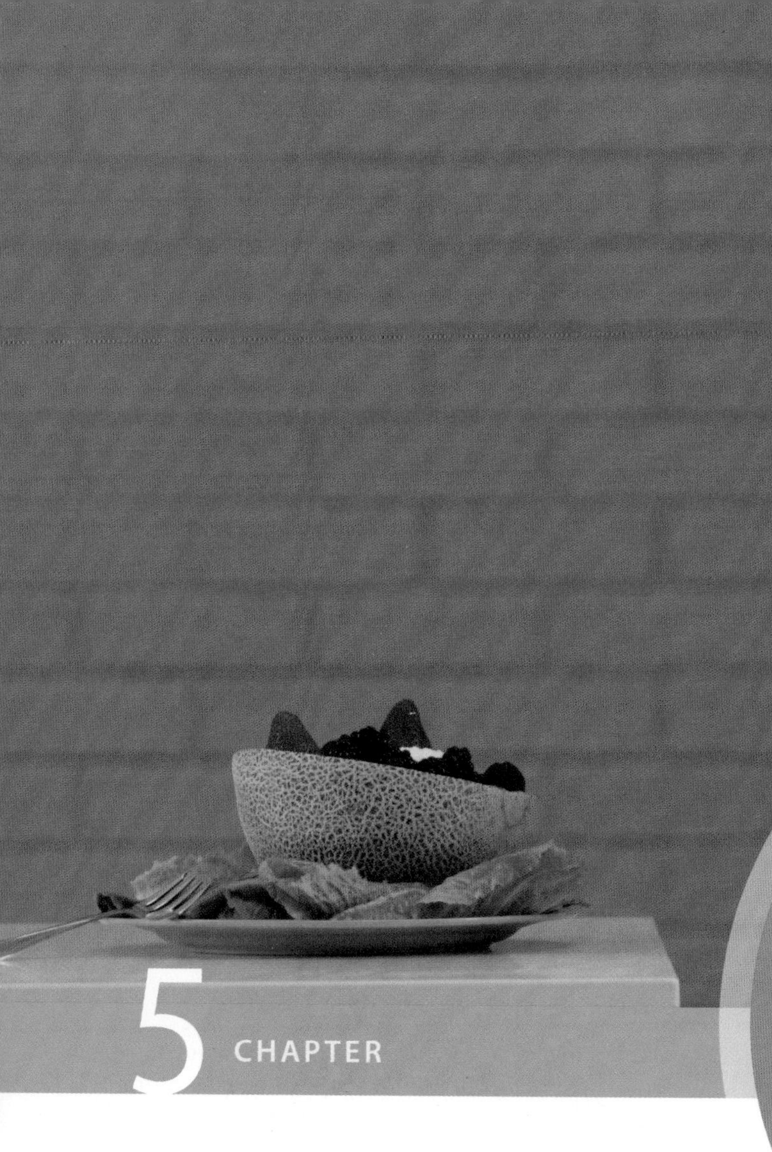

5 CHAPTER

# Nutrition During Pregnancy: *Conditions and Interventions*

***Prepared by***
**Judith E. Brown**

## LEARNING OBJECTIVES

After studying the materials in this chapter, you should be able to:

**5.1** Cite three specific examples of nutrition-related recommendations intended for women who enter pregnancy obese.

**5.2** Distinguish the different types of hypertensive disorders that occur during pregnancy, and connect two components of nutrition care recommended for women with each type.

**5.3** Connect the different, major types of disorders in carbohydrate metabolism that occur during pregnancy and the key components of the nutritional management of each type.

**5.4** Explain three differences in nutrient needs and cite two specific considerations for delivery of effective nutritional care for women with multifetal pregnancy.

**5.5** Identify the components of nutritional care for women with HIV during pregnancy.

**5.6** Identify two primary components of the nutritional care of women with eating disorders during pregnancy.

**5.7** Summarize the consequences of excess alcohol intake during pregnancy, and list four factors that affect relationship between alcohol intake and the outcome of pregnancy.

**5.8** Distinguish three ways in which energy and nutrient needs differ between adults and adolescents during pregnancy.

# Introduction

Almost all healthy women expect that their pregnancies will proceed normally and that they will be rewarded at delivery with a healthy newborn. For the vast majority of pregnancies, this expectation is fulfilled. For other women, however, the path to a healthy newborn entails overcoming certain health challenges. This chapter addresses a number of health conditions and the role of nutrition in their etiology and management. The specific conditions consist of obesity, hypertensive disorders of pregnancy, diabetes in pregnancy, multifetal pregnancy, HIV/AIDS, eating disorders, fetal alcohol spectrum disorders, and adolescent pregnancy.

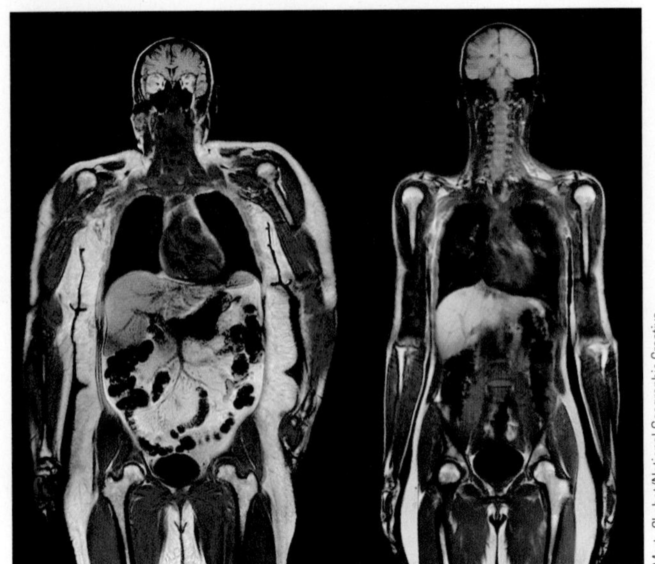

Marty Chobot/National Geographic Creative

ILLUSTRATION 5.1 ▸ The MRI (magnetic resonance image) on the left shows visceral and subcutaneous fat in an obese woman with a high waist circumference. The image on the right is of a normal weight woman with a normal waist circumference.

# Obesity and Pregnancy

**LO 5.1** Cite three specific examples of nutrition-related recommendations intended for women who enter pregnancy obese.

Obesity before and during pregnancy often produces unfavorable genetic, hormonal, and metabolic conditions that affect maternal health, fetal growth and development, and subsequent health of the mother and child.[1] It is associated with a higher incidence of preterm delivery, gestational diabetes, and hypertensive disorders of pregnancy (Table 5.1), and with the delivery of large-for-gestational age newborns.[2] Children born to obese women are more likely to become obese during childhood, and both mother and child have an increased risk of developing type 2 diabetes later in life.[3-5] The increased risk of these disorders is associated with unfavorable metabolic changes related to excessive body fat, such as:

- Increased blood glucose levels
- High C-reactive protein levels (a key marker of inflammation)
- Increased blood concentration of insulin
- Insulin resistance
- Increased blood pressure
- High blood levels of total cholesterol, LDL-cholesterol, and triglycerides
- Low levels of HDL-cholesterol[6,7]

Approximately 70 percent of obese persons and 23 percent of normal-weight individuals have two or more of these metabolic abnormalities that increase disease risk.[8]

Metabolic effects associated with obesity are closely related to the presence of high amounts of visceral fat (also called intra-abdominal fat). Visceral fat lies beneath skin and muscles of the abdomen, and around internal organs (Illustration 5.1). It is much more metabolically active than subcutaneous fat (fat that lies beneath the skin) and is more strongly related to disease risk. Metabolic processes initiated by visceral fat produce chronic inflammation, free-radical generation, and oxidative stress.[9] These disruptions promote the development of insulin resistance, elevated blood glucose, insulin, triglyceride concentrations, and increased blood pressure.[7] These changes, in

TABLE 5.1 ▸ Pregnancy outcomes related to prepregnancy weight status[5]

| WEIGHT STATUS | UNDERWEIGHT | NORMAL | OVERWEIGHT | OBESE | VERY OBESE | EXTREMELY OBESE |
|---|---|---|---|---|---|---|
| BMI, kg/m$^2$ | 18.5 | 18.5–24.9 | 25–29.9 | 30–34.9 | 35–39.9 | .40 |
| Preterm | 11.6% | 8.1% | 8.4% | 10.6% | 8.9% | 12.4% |
| Gestational diabetes | 3.5% | 3.8% | 4.7% | 7.0% | 9.6% | 11.0% |
| Preexisting diabetes | 0% | 0.8% | 1.7% | 2.4% | 6.9% | 9.7% |
| Hypertensive disorder | 5.8% | 9.1% | 13.3% | 20.7% | 23.3% | 31.7% |

turn, increase the risk of gestational diabetes, hypertensive disorders, and other clinical conditions during pregnancy. Normal-weight and overweight individuals with excessive visceral fat deposits are also at increased risk of metabolic abnormalities and diseases associated with them.[9]

The prevalence of disorders such as gestational diabetes and hypertension during pregnancy are increasing due to increased rates of obesity. Approximately one-third of women 20–39 years old in the United States are obese now compared to 10 percent in 1980.[11,12]

## Nutritional Recommendations and Interventions for Obesity During Pregnancy

Obesity is a disease and not a life choice, and many factors are related to its development. Obese women may struggle with reducing food intake due to the presence of genetic predispositions, which modify the metabolic processes that regulate appetite and satiety.[13,14] Many clinical approaches to treating obesity are ineffective or in need of innovation and personalization, and effective treatment options are often unavailable or inaccessible.[15]

Women who enter pregnancy obese are more likely to gain too much weight during pregnancy compared with normal weight women, and to retain more of the weight gained after pregnancy.[16,] Nutrition and other health care services that address weight gain in obese women should be provided in the same nonjudgmental, respectful, and nondiscriminatory manner as for other groups of women.[15] Many nutrition recommendations for pregnancy in obese women, including meeting nutrient needs through consumption of a variety of basic foods, participating in physical activities of choice, and maintaining appropriate rates of weight gain, are the same as those for women of other sizes.[15] Intervention programs should be aimed at reducing excessive weight gain among obese women during pregnancy. These intervention programs are more likely to have meaningful success in improving rate of weight gain and infant outcomes if they include development of individualized plans for food intake and physical activity, behavioral change goal setting, follow-up, and modification of the plan over time to meet the person's needs.[17,18]

Weight loss during pregnancy in obese women appears to decrease the risk of large-for-gestational-age but increases the risk of small-for-gestational-age infant outcomes and lowers the duration of pregnancy.[2,19] Weight loss during pregnancy is not recommended.[20]

**Pregnancy After Bariatric Surgery** The use of bariatric surgery for weight loss has increased dramatically over the past 10 years. About half of individuals who undergo this surgery are women of childbearing age.[21]

Women lose weight rapidly after bariatric surgery due to limited food intake, fat malabsorption, decreased appetite, and the presence of ***dumping syndrome***, a common side effect of the surgery.[25] Nausea, vomiting, and other symptoms of dumping syndrome may persist into pregnancy. The rapid weight loss and limited food and nutrient intake lead to depletion of tissue stores of many nutrients. Thiamin deficiency can develop within 20 days after the surgery,[22] and deficiencies of vitamins D and $B_{12}$, iron, calcium, and folate are common.[23] Vitamin and mineral supplementation and monitoring of nutrient biomarkers are routine components of care for individuals undergoing weight-loss surgery. It is recommended that pregnancy be postponed for a year or two after bariatric surgery, when body weight is stable and nutrient stores have been established.[24]

Maternal and neonatal health outcomes in women who have had bariatric surgery tend to be acceptable as long as adequate maternal nutrition is maintained.[25] Maternal complications such as ***gestational diabetes***, preeclampsia, and large-for-gestational-age newborns, are less frequent in obese women who had weight-loss surgery and lost some weight before pregnancy compared to obese women who did neither.[2,23]

**Nutrition Care for Pregnant Women Post-Bariatric Surgery** Nutrition care services are recommended for pregnant women with a history of bariatric surgery. These services should include assessment of dietary intake, supplement use, nutrient biomarker status, weight gain, physical activity, and gastrointestinal symptoms.[27] Nutrition interventions are then implemented as needed to solve nutrition-related problems identified.[24]

Nutrient deficiencies and supplementation requirements will vary during pregnancy based on the type of bariatric surgery performed.[22] Roux-en-Y bypass and biliopancreatic diversion surgery severely restrict food intake and are associated with greater weight loss and nutrient deficits than is *lap band* (vertical banded gastroplasty) surgery.[23] Lap band surgery involves placement of a band around the top of the stomach. The band limits the size of the stomach and restricts the amount of food that can be consumed. The lap band is sometimes adjusted during pregnancy to help regulate food intake and weight gain.[24]

Women with a history of bariatric surgery generally qualify as "at risk" for gestational diabetes, and blood glucose assessment will be ordered. Many women will experience dumping syndrome if given the 75-gram glucose load for blood glucose testing. Alternatives to this test, such as fasting glucose levels or home blood glucose values, should be used instead of the oral glucose load.[21,23]

**dumping syndrome**
A condition characterized by weakness, dizziness, flushing, nausea, and palpitation immediately or shortly after eating and produced by abnormally rapid emptying of the stomach, especially in individuals who have had part of the stomach removed.

**gestational diabetes**
Carbohydrate intolerance with onset of, or first recognition in, pregnancy.

# Hypertensive Disorders of Pregnancy

LO 5.2 Distinguish the different types of hypertensive disorders that occur during pregnancy, and connect two components of nutrition care recommended for women with each type.

Hypertensive disorders of pregnancy are a worldwide, leading cause of maternal mortality. They affect 5–10 percent of pregnancies and contribute significantly to stillbirths, fetal and newborn deaths, and other adverse outcomes of pregnancy.[28,29] The causes of most cases of hypertension during pregnancy remain unknown, and cures for these disorders remain elusive. Both environmental factors and inherited genetic traits transferred from mothers and fathers are thought to be involved in the development of preeclampsia.[30] Four types of hypertensive disorders in pregnancy have been identified and are described in Table 5.2.

## Hypertensive Disorders of Pregnancy, Oxidative Stress, and Nutrition

All forms of hypertension in pregnancy (as well as other disorders such as diabetes) are related to chronic inflammation, ***oxidative stress***, and damage to the ***endothelium*** of blood vessels.[30,31] Over time, oxidative stress within the endothelium leads to endothelial dysfunction. Consequences of endothelial dysfunction include restriction of placental blood flow, an increased tendency of blood to clot, and plaque formation. Pregnant women with hypertensive disorders may benefit from healthy dietary patterns and lifestyles that lower inflammation and oxidative stress (Table 5.3).

## Chronic Hypertension

The incidence of chronic hypertension—or that diagnosed prior to pregnancy or before 20 weeks after conception—is around 3 percent and is increasing over time, along with rises in obesity and age of childbearing.[32] Most women with chronic hypertension have good pregnancy outcomes. As a group, however, approximately 20 percent will develop preeclampsia versus 4 percent of the general population of pregnant women. Rates of preterm delivery, fetal growth retardation, ***placenta abruption***, and Cesarean delivery are higher in women with chronic hypertension than other women.[29] The condition is more likely to occur in Non-Hispanic Black Americans, obese women, women over 35 years of age, and women who experienced high blood pressure in a previous pregnancy.[33] Adjustments in the types of anti-hypertension medications prescribed (if any) prior to and during pregnancy are usually made because certain medications interfere with embryonic and fetal growth and development.[32]

**oxidative stress** A condition that occurs when cells are exposed to more oxidizing molecules (such as free radicals) than to antioxidant molecules that neutralize them and help repair cell damage. Over time, oxidative stress causes damage to lipids, DNA, cells, and tissues.

**endothelium** The layer of cells lining the inside of blood vessels.

**placenta abruption** The separation of the placenta from its attachment to the uterus wall before the baby is delivered. Also called abruptio placenta. Consequences of this condition range from mild to severe for the mother and fetus depending on blood loss, extent of fetal distress, gestational age of the fetus, and other factors.

TABLE 5.2 Definitions and features of hypertensive disorders of pregnancy*[,29]

**Chronic Hypertension**

Hypertension that is present before pregnancy or diagnosed before 20 weeks of pregnancy. Hypertension is defined as blood pressure ≥140 mm Hg systolic or ≥90 mm Hg diastolic blood pressure. Hypertension first diagnosed during pregnancy that does not resolve after pregnancy is also classified as chronic hypertension.

**Gestational Hypertension**

This condition exists when elevated blood pressure levels are detected for the first time after mid-pregnancy. It is accompanied by proteinuria or the onset of new symptoms. If blood pressure returns to normal within 10 days postpartum, the condition is considered to be transient hypertension of pregnancy. If it remains elevated, then the woman is considered to have chronic hypertension. Women with gestational hypertension are at lower risk for poor pregnancy outcomes than are women with preeclampsia.

**Preeclampsia–Eclampsia**

A pregnancy-specific syndrome that usually occurs after 20 weeks gestation (but that may occur earlier) in previously normotensive women. It is determined by increased blood pressure during pregnancy to ≥140 mm Hg systolic or ≥90 mm Hg diastolic and is accompanied by proteinuria. In the absence of proteinuria, the disease is highly suspected when increased blood pressure is accompanied by headache, blurred vision, abdominal pain, low platelet count, and abnormal liver enzyme values.

- Proteinuria is defined as the urinary excretion of ≥ 0.3 grams of protein in a 24-hour urine specimen. This usually correlates well with readings of ≥ 30 mg/dL protein, or ≥ 2 on dipstick readings taken in samples from women free of urinary tract infection. In the absence of urinary tract infection, proteinuria is a manifestation of kidney damage.
- Eclampsia is defined as the occurrence of seizures that cannot be attributed to other causes in women with preeclampsia.

**Chronic Hypertension with Superimposed Preeclampsia**

This disorder is characterized by the development of proteinuria during pregnancy in women with chronic hypertension. In women with hypertension and proteinuria before 20 weeks of pregnancy, it is indicated by a sudden increase in proteinuria, blood pressure, or abnormal platelet or liver enzyme levels.

*Blood pressure values used to determine status should be based on two or more measurements of blood pressure in relaxed settings.

TABLE 5.3 ▸ Dietary and other environmental exposures that increase or decrease chronic inflammation and oxidative stress[40,54,55]

**1. Decrease**
- Regular intake of colorful fruits and vegetables, dried beans, and whole-grain products
- Vitamin D sufficiency
- Physical activity

**2. Increase**
- Frequent intake of processed and high-fat meats
- Frequent consumption of soft drinks, other high-sugar beverages
- Physical inactivity
- High levels of body fat, especially visceral fat
- Smoking

**Nutritional Interventions for Women with Chronic Hypertension in Pregnancy** Preconceptional and pregnancy diets of women with hypertension should be carefully monitored with the aim of achieving healthy dietary pattern. Weight-gain recommendations are the same as for other pregnant women.

It has been recommended that women with hypertension that was managed successfully with the help of a reduced salt or sodium diet before pregnancy continue that approach during pregnancy.[34] Inadequate sodium intake during pregnancy can impair fetal growth so the restriction in salt intake should not be excessive.[35]

## Gestational Hypertension

Gestational hypertension is hypertension that first occurs during pregnancy. The effects of gestational hypertension on the course and outcome of pregnancy are often benign. However, women developing gestational hypertension are at increased risk for developing preeclampsia later in pregnancy or during the first week postpartum, and chronic hypertension later in life.[29,36] The treatment for gestational hypertension is similar to that for chronic hypertension.

## Preeclampsia–Eclampsia

Preeclampsia-eclampsia occurs in 4 percent of first pregnancies and 1.7 percent of subsequent ones. A history of preeclampsia-eclampsia increases the risk that it will occur in subsequent pregnancies.[37] It represents a syndrome characterized by:

- Oxidative stress, inadequate antioxidant defenses, inflammation, and endothelial dysfunction
- Platelet aggregation and blood coagulation due to deficits in ***prostacyclin*** relative to ***thromboxane***
- Blood vessel spasms and constriction, restricted blood flow
- Increased blood pressure
- Insulin resistance
- Adverse maternal immune system responses to the placenta
- Elevated blood levels of triglycerides, free fatty acids, and cholesterol[31,36]

Virtually all maternal organs can be affected in preeclampsia. Organs most affected by small blood clots, vasoconstriction, and reduced blood flow are the placenta and the mother's kidney, liver, and brain.[36] Many of the metabolic abnormalities observed in preeclampsia are present before it is diagnosed and are the same as those for cardiovascular disease.[38] Occurrence of preeclampsia during pregnancy doubles the risk of cardiovascular disease development within 5 to 15 years.[37] Women with preeclampsia are at increased risk of developing gestational diabetes, type 2 diabetes, and hypertension later in life.[39] About 15 percent of women with gestational diabetes and 30 percent of those with type 2 diabetes prior to pregnancy will develop preeclampsia.[40]

Signs and symptoms of preeclampsia range from mild to severe (Table 5.4), as do the health consequences (Table 5.5). The cause of preeclampsia is unknown but appears to

**prostacyclin** A potent inhibitor of platelet aggregation and a powerful vasodilator and blood pressure reducer derived from n-3 fatty acids.

**thromboxane** The parent of a group of thromboxanes derived from the n-6 fatty acid arachidonic acid. Thromboxane increases platelet aggregation and constricts blood vessels, causing blood pressure to increase.

TABLE 5.4 ▸ Signs and symptoms of preeclampsia[30]

- Hypertension
- Increased urinary protein
- Decreased plasma volume expansion (hemoglobin levels > 13 g/dL)
- Low urine output
- Persistent and severe headaches
- Sensitivity of the eyes to bright light
- Blurred vision
- Abdominal pain
- Nausea

TABLE 5.5 ▸ Outcomes related to the existence of preeclampsia during pregnancy[36,41]

**Mother**
- Early delivery by Caesarean section
- Acute renal (kidney) dysfunction
- Increased risk of gestational diabetes, hypertension, and type 2 diabetes later in life
- Placenta abruption

**Newborn**
- Preterm delivery
- Growth restriction
- Respiratory distress syndrome
- Fetal death
- Maternal death

originate from abnormal implantation and vascularization of the placenta, and poor blood flow through the placenta.[36] Abnormal blood flow through the placenta is an important characteristic of preeclampsia because it decreases the delivery of nutrients and gases to the fetus.

Eclampsia can be a life-threatening condition and one that can be difficult to predict. Eclamptic seizures appear to be related to hypertension, the tendency of blood to clot, and spasms of and damage to blood vessels in the brain. It affects about 1 in 2000 pregnancies.[43] The only cure for preeclampsia and eclampsia is delivery of the placenta.[41] Signs and symptoms of preeclampsia and eclampsia generally disappear rapidly after delivery, but they may occur up to 6 weeks postpartum.[42]

**Risk Factors for the Development of Preeclampsia** The roots of preeclampsia lie before and very early in pregnancy, but as yet there is no reliable means of identifying women who will develop it before the condition is established.[44] However, women with insulin resistance, obesity, abnormally high triglyceride levels, or other characteristics listed in Table 5.6 are at increased risk for developing the disease.

Increased rates of preterm delivery and low birthweight in infants born to women with preeclampsia are partly related to clinical decisions to deliver the fetus early in order to treat the disease. Most infants born to women with this disorder are of appropriate weight for gestational age; however, some newborns are large for gestational age (LGA). Variations in birthweight associated with preeclampsia appear to be related to blood pressure levels in individual women.[45]

The risk of developing preeclampsia is higher in women who were born small for gestational age (SGA) than women who were not. It appears that growth restriction *in utero* may impair mechanisms involved in the regulation of blood pressure and increase the probability that high blood pressure will develop with the physiological stresses of pregnancy.[46] The presence of preeclampsia during pregnancy appears to increase the risk of high body mass index, hypertension, and cardiovascular disease in offspring later in life.[47]

**TABLE 5.6** Risk factors for preeclampsia[33,40,50,165]

- First pregnancy (nulliparous)
- Obesity, especially high levels of central body fat
- Underweight
- Mother's smallness at birth
- African American, American Indian ancestry
- History of preeclampsia
- Preexisting diabetes mellitus
- Age over 35 years
- Multifetal pregnancy
- Insulin resistance
- Abnormally high blood triglyceride levels
- Chronic hypertension
- Renal disease
- Poor vitamin D status
- Poor calcium status
- Consumption of a pro-inflammatory, pro-oxidative stress diet

**Vitamin and Mineral Supplementation and the Risk of Preeclampsia** Oxidative stress and a lack of antioxidant defenses appear to play key roles in the development of preeclampsia. Based on this knowledge, it was theorized that therapeutic doses of vitamins C and E (which function as antioxidants) would decrease oxidative stress and the risk of preeclampsia. Results from early studies suggested that this did happen, but later, better-designed clinical trials failed to identify a true relationship between supplemental vitamin C and E intake and preeclampsia. It is now concluded that vitamin C and E supplements should not be used to prevent preeclampsia. It is also concluded that fish oils, folic acid supplements, magnesium supplements, and garlic are ineffective for the prevention of preeclampsia.[48,49]

Supplemental vitamin D and calcium are related to a reduced risk of preeclampsia in women with poor vitamin D status or calcium intake.[50] Children born to calcium-supplemented women have been found to have lower blood pressure than children whose mothers were not supplemented.[51] Use of multivitamin and mineral supplement in the months before and early in pregnancy have been related to reduced risk of preeclampsia in normal-weight women.[52,53]

**Dietary Intake and the Risk of Preeclampsia** Certain patterns of dietary intake during the first 22 weeks of pregnancy have been related to the risk of preeclampsia. Diets characterized by high intake of plant foods that tend to decrease chronic inflammation and oxidative stress have been linked to a decreased risk of preeclampsia compared to diets that regularly include processed meat, sweet drinks, and salty snacks.[54,55]

Prepregnancy and early-pregnancy diets containing relatively high amounts of fiber (over 21 grams a day) have been related to a significant reduction in the risk of preeclampsia. High-fiber diets may modify the risk of preeclampsia by reducing abnormally high blood concentrations of triglycerides and cholesterol that may contribute to the development of oxidative stress.[56]

**Sodium (Salt) Intake and the Risk of Preeclampsia** In the past it was thought that high sodium intakes were related to the development of preeclampsia and that low salt intakes would help prevent it. These clinical assumptions have not been found to be accurate in clinical studies. Salt restriction during pregnancy does not prevent preeclampsia, hypertension, or other complications related to pregnancy. Routine salt restriction is not recommended. Rather, it is recommended that salt consumption during pregnancy remain a matter of personal preference.[57]

**Preeclampsia Case Presentation** Signs, symptoms, severity, and causes of preeclampsia vary from woman to woman.

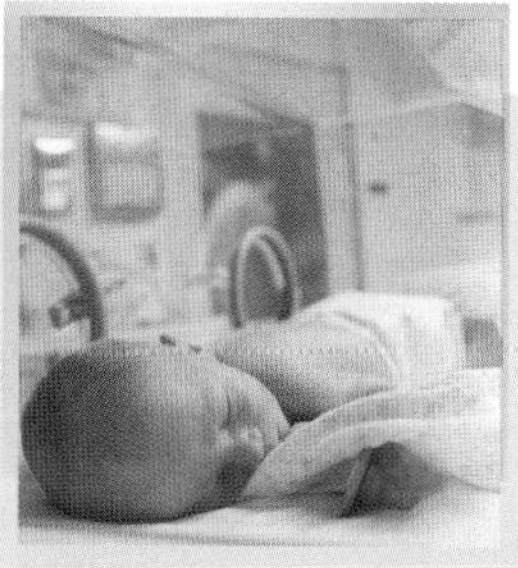
©Cengage Learning

# CASE STUDY 5.1

## A Case of Preeclampsia

Susan is a 19-year-old "meat-and-potatoes" type eater who rarely consumes vegetables, fruits, or dairy products. She likes monosyllabic vegetables (beans, corn, and peas), bananas and oranges, and chocolate milk. She generally consumes one of these vegetables and fruits each day, and always has a glass of chocolate milk. Susan consumes sweetened iced tea throughout the day, and twice a week she eats rice with meat rather than potatoes. She finds this type of diet satisfying and rarely consumes foods other than those mentioned.

Her first 17 weeks of pregnancy were uneventful. At week 18 she was found to have proteinuria. By week 22, her blood pressure had increased to 150/100 mm Hg, and she was diagnosed with preeclampsia. Laboratory studies indicated that her blood glucose level was on the high side of normal and that she was insulin resistant. She was lost to follow-up after her week 22 visit.

A bit overweight prior to pregnancy, Susan did not gain weight and restricted her salt intake after midpregnancy. She believed these actions would help lower her weight and blood pressure. Although she was given a supply of prenatal vitamin and mineral supplements early in pregnancy, she rarely remembered to take them. Her baby, weighing 5 pounds 5 ounces (2380 grams), was delivered by Cesarean section at week 36.

### Questions

1. List three ways in which Susan's dietary intake likely contributes to oxidative stress.
2. Identify two other characteristics of her diet that are contraindicated for women with preeclampsia. Answers should be different than those for question 1.
3. List three health problems Susan is at increased risk of developing due to her history of preeclampsia.

Therefore, appropriate interventions for women presenting differing aspects of the syndrome are best designed on a case-by-case basis. Case Study 5.1 describes the course of preeclampsia in one woman experiencing the condition.

### Nutritional Recommendations and Interventions for Preeclampsia

In the best of circumstances, dietary interventions for preeclampsia would begin prior to pregnancy. This approach might give women the opportunities to decrease body weight and stores of central body fat, become physically fit, and consume a diet that reduces inflammation and oxidative stress. Short of those circumstances, dietary recommendations and interventions should begin in at-risk women as early in pregnancy as possible.

Nutritional and physical activity recommendations that may benefit women at risk of preeclampsia include:

- Adequate calcium and vitamin D status; use of supplemental calcium and vitamin D if needed
- Consumption of five or more servings of colorful vegetables and fruits daily
- Adequate fiber intake (28 grams daily)
- Consumption of the assortment of other basic foods recommended in ChooseMyPlate
- Moderate-intensity physical activity (e.g., brisk walking, swimming, tennis, aerobic dancing) for 30 minutes daily unless medically contraindicated
- Weight gain that follows recommendations based on prepregnancy weight status

Iron supplements, especially if taken in high doses, may aggravate inflammation by increasing the body's free-radical load. Women with preeclampsia should not be given high-dose iron supplements.[58]

# Diabetes in Pregnancy

LO 5.3 Connect the different, major types of disorders in carbohydrate metabolism that occur during pregnancy and the key components of the nutritional management of each type.

Diabetes is a leading complication in pregnancy. It has three main forms:

- Gestational diabetes
- Type 2 diabetes
- Type 1 diabetes[170]

There are other less common forms of diabetes,[170] but this section focuses on gestational diabetes, which is first recognized during pregnancy, preexisting type 2 diabetes during pregnancy, and type 1 diabetes (insulin-dependent diabetes).

Due to placental hormones, growth factors, and other physiological changes, pregnancy exerts a *diabetogenic effect* on maternal carbohydrate utilization. Insulin resistance and requirement increase as pregnancy progresses.

Maintenance of normal blood glucose levels during pregnancy requires that insulin production by beta cells of the pancreas keep up with the increasing need for insulin. A common thread that ties together the three types of diabetes presented here is the absence or lack of beta cell production of insulin and abnormal blood glucose levels that result.[64] Women with diabetes during pregnancy also share an increased risk of developing high blood pressure and preeclampsia during pregnancy.[61] Excellent control of blood glucose levels throughout pregnancy improve maternal and infant outcomes appreciably. Effective nutrition and lifestyle education during pregnancy benefit the health of women and families long after delivery.[62]

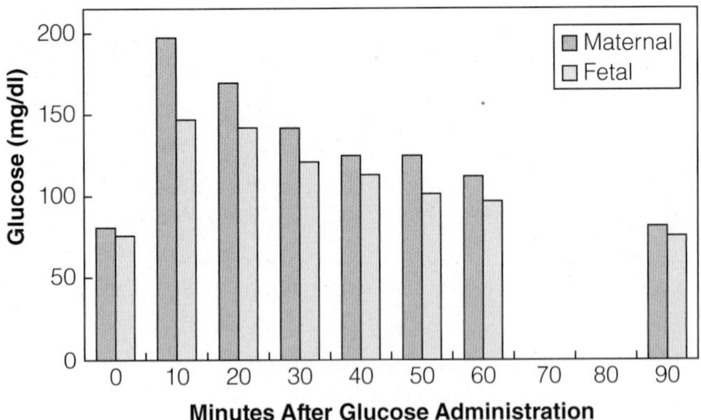


**ILLUSTRATION 5.2** Approximate fetal glucose levels following glucose administration to the mother late in pregnancy.

SOURCE: Graph developed by author from data presented in Walsh, J. M., et al. (2011). The association of maternal and fetal glucose homeostasis with fetal adiposity and birthweight. Eur J Obstet Gynecol Reprod Biol, . 2011;159:, 338–341; Parretti, E., et al. (2001). Third-trimester maternal glucose levels from diurnal profiles in nondiabetic pregnancies: correlation with sonographic parameters of fetal growth. *Diabetes Care, 24*, 1319–1323; and Freinkel N et al. (1970) Metabolic realignments in late pregnancy: a clue to diabetogenesis. Adv Metab Disord. 1970;1:Suppl 1:205.

## Gestational Diabetes

The prevalence of gestational diabetes varies from 2 to 12 percent depending on the population studied.[63] The incidence increases along with obesity and this affect is pronounced among Asian American women whose dietary patterns and lifestyles have become "Westernized."[65,66] Gestational diabetes accounts for 88 percent of all cases of diabetes in pregnancy and is similar in many ways to type 2 diabetes.[64] Women who develop gestational diabetes tend to enter pregnancy with insulin resistance, or a predisposition to insulin resistance, and impaired insulin production, which is expressed due to physiological changes that occur during pregnancy.[66]

**Risks Related to Gestational Diabetes** Potential consequences of gestational diabetes include an increased risk of spontaneous abortion, stillbirth, ***congenital anomalies***, and neonatal death (Table 5.7). High maternal blood glucose levels reach the fetus (Illustration 5.2) and cause the fetus to increase insulin production to lower glucose levels. The higher the level of blood glucose received, the larger the fetal output of insulin.[61] High insulin levels increase glucose uptake into fetal cells and the conversion of glucose to triglycerides. These changes increase the fetus's synthesis of fat as well as muscle tissue, and may program metabolic adaptations that increase the likelihood that insulin resistance, type 2 diabetes, high blood pressure, and obesity will develop later in life. The chances that these disorders will occur increase along with increases in maternal levels of glucose.[67,68]

**TABLE 5.7** Adverse outcomes associated with gestational diabetes[64,96]

**Mother**
- Caesarean delivery
- Shoulder dystocia
- Increased risk for preeclampsia
- Increased risk of type 2 diabetes, hypertension, and obesity later in life
- Increased risk for gestational diabetes in a subsequent pregnancy
- Hypoglycemia
- Maternal death

**Offspring**
- Stillbirth
- Spontaneous abortion
- Congenital anomalies
- Macrosomia (> 10 lb or > 4500 g)
- Stillbirth
- Neonatal hypoglycemia, hypocalcemia, hyperbilirubinemia
- Increased risk of insulin resistance, type 2 diabetes, high blood pressure, and obesity later in life

Effects of high maternal levels of glucose and triglycerides are particularly striking in the Pima Indians of Arizona. Fetal exposure to poorly controlled maternal diabetes incurs a tenfold increase in the risk that children will develop type 2 diabetes. Offspring of diabetic Pima mothers are heavier at birth, have higher body mass index (BMI) throughout childhood, and have 7–20 times greater incidence of type 2 diabetes in early adulthood. Although risks of these conditions increase in offspring of women with poorly controlled diabetes in general, the pronounced effect in Pima Indians is likely due to a strong genetic tendency toward insulin resistance and obesity.[69]

Loss of the placenta at delivery initially restores insulin sensitivity in most women with gestational diabetes. However, a degree of insulin resistance often remains. Close to half of women with gestational diabetes in a previous pregnancy will develop it in a subsequent pregnancy.[70] Women with gestational diabetes who have high BMIs, those who require insulin for the blood glucose control during pregnancy, and women who

**congenital anomalies** Structural, functional, or metabolic abnormalities present at birth. Also called congenital abnormalities.

gain weight after pregnancy are at particularly high risk of developing type 2 diabetes as well as high blood pressure later in life.[71]

**Risk Factors for Gestational Diabetes** Both gestational and type 2 diabetes and are linked to multiple genetic factors and their environmental triggers, such as excess body fat, unhealthy dietary patterns, and low physical activity levels.[59,72,73] A specific variant of the GIP gene involved in the stimulation of insulin production after a meal has been shown to be related to the development of gestational diabetes. Women with two copies of this variant produce less insulin after a meal than other women.[74] Dietary patterns low in fiber, vegetables, nuts, legumes, whole grains, and other foods represented in healthy dietary patterns; and high in added sugars and processed meats are associated with a 24–46 percent increased risk of gestational diabetes development compared to the risk for women consuming a healthy dietary pattern.[73] Results of a large prospective study indicate that the risk for gestational diabetes decreases 26 percent for each 10 grams of fiber consumed daily from plant sources.[75] Some women who develop gestational diabetes have no identified risk for the disease.[76] Risk factors for gestational diabetes are outlined in Table 5.8.

**Diagnosis of Gestational Diabetes** Updated recommendations for the diagnosis of gestational diabetes are available.[60,77] These standards, adopted by the American Diabetes Association and other groups, recommend a two-step approach for testing for gestational diabetes:

1. Pregnant women should be screened at the first prenatal visit for preexisting diabetes by the standard criteria used for individuals who are not pregnant. One positive, confirmed result for any of the following criteria would form the basis of a diagnosis of diabetes:
   - Hemoglobin A1c (A1c) ≥ 6.5%
   - Fasting plasma glucose ≥ 126 mg/dL (7.0 mmol/L)
   - 2-hour glucose ≥ 200 mg/dL (11.1 mmol/L) after a 75-gram oral glucose load
   - Classic symptoms of hyperglycemia present
   - A random plasma glucose level ≥ 200 mg/dL (11.1 mmol/L)
2. All pregnant women without diabetes should be tested for gestational diabetes by a 75-gram, 2-hour oral glucose tolerance test (OGTT) preformed between 24 and 28 weeks of gestation. Women with one elevated plasma glucose level based on the following cut-off points, receive a diagnosis of gestational diabetes:
   - Fasting plasma glucose level ≥ 92 mg/dL (5.1 mmol/L)
   - 1-hour plasma glucose level ≥ 180 mg/dL (10.0 mmol/L)
   - 2-hour plasma glucose levels ≥ 153 mg/dL (8.5 mmol/L)

TABLE 5.8 ▸ Risk factors for gestational diabetes[66,73,78]

- Obesity, especially high levels of central body fat
- Weight gain between pregnancies
- Age over 35 years
- Native American, Hispanic, Asian ancestry
- Genetic traits (GIP variant)
- Strong family history of type 2 diabetes
- History of delivery of a macrosomic newborn (> 4500 g or > 10 lb)
- Chronic hypertension
- Mother was SGA at birth
- History of gestational diabetes in a previous pregnancy
- Physical inactivity
- Polycystic ovary syndrome
- Multifetal pregnancy
- Consumption of Western-type diet (low fiber intake, low vegetable and fruit intake, regular intake of sugars and high-glycemic index foods, red and processed meats)

The ideal approach for screening and diagnosis of gestational diabetes is not known with certainty.[78]

Standards and practices related to gestational diabetes have changed. The 50-gram oral glucose screening test is being used less in practice than in the past. Ingestion of 150 grams or more of carbohydrate 3 days prior to a OGTT does not affect the results of the test and is no longer recommended.[80,81] The use of ***hemoglobin A1c*** for monitoring blood glucose levels is not recommended for diabetes management because the values don't reflect current blood glucose levels.[78] Urinary glucose cannot be used to diagnose or monitor gestational diabetes because the results do not accurately reflect blood glucose levels.[82] However, multiple, positive identifications of glucosuria by urine test strip may indicate undiagnosed gestational diabetes and the need to test further using a 2-hour, 75-gram oral glucose tolerance test.[78]

**Management of Gestational Diabetes** A team approach to caring for women with diabetes in pregnancy is advised. Such teams often consist of an obstetrician, a registered dietitian who is also a certified diabetes educator, a nurse educator, and an endocrinologist. The mainstay of treatment is medical nutrition therapy that begins with attempts to normalize blood glucose levels with diet and exercise.[78,83] Dietary and physical activity changes been shown to effectively normalize blood glucose levels and to decrease the risk of adverse perinatal outcomes in some women (Table 5.9).[78] It can also be noted from the

**hemoglobin A1c** A form of hemoglobin used to identify blood glucose levels over the lifetime of a red blood cell (120 days). Glucose molecules in blood will attach to hemoglobin (and stay attached). The amount of glucose that attaches to hemoglobin is proportional to levels of glucose in the blood. The normal range of hemoglobin A1c is 4–5.9 percent. Also called glycosylated hemoglobin and glycated hemoglobin.

TABLE 5.9 ▸ Comparison of outcomes of unrecognized and diet-treated gestational diabetes[166]

| | GESTATIONAL DIABETES | | |
|---|---|---|---|
| OUTCOME | UNRECOGNIZED | DIET-TREATED | CONTROLS |
| LGA (> 90th percentile) | 44% | 9% | 5% |
| Macrosomia (> 4500 g) | 44% | 15% | 8% |
| Shoulder dystocia | 25% | 3% | 3% |
| Birth trauma | 25% | 0% | 0% |

results that a higher proportion of large newborns occurs even with nutrition therapy, but that the incidence is substantially less than in women with untreated gestational diabetes.

Blood glucose levels can be brought down by low calorie intake. This approach can lead to an elevation of blood ***ketone*** levels if calorie intakes are decreased to < 1500 daily, or less than 33 percent below calorie need.[81,84] Ketones accumulate in blood if insufficient glucose is available for energy formation and fat is primarily used to meet energy needs. High blood concentrations of beta-hydroxybutyrate (the most common type of ketone body) during pregnancy has been related to decreased mental development in 2-year-olds. The potentially deleterious effects of high blood ketone levels on fetal development exclude very low-calorie diets as a blood glucose control method during pregnancy.[85] Modest calorie restriction may be useful for blood glucose and weight gain control in women with gestational diabetes who are overweight or obese and gaining weight too rapidly. Women with diabetes who are underweight or normal weight are encouraged to gain within the IOM guidelines, and overweight and obese women at the low end of their weight gain ranges.[81,84] Weight gain during pregnancy is less predictive of birthweight for infants of women with diabetes than other women primarily due to the influence of blood glucose levels on fetal growth.[84]

The oral medication metformin is generally used for the management of blood glucose levels during gestational diabetes in the second half of pregnancy when diet and exercise aren't adequately controlling blood glucose levels.[81] Metformin (glucophage) suppresses glucose production by the liver, increases tissue uptake of glucose, and improves insulin sensitivity.[86] Insulin will be used if needed. No two women with gestational diabetes share the same history, risks, needs, and response to treatment (Case Study 5.2).

**Exercise Benefits and Recommendations** In women with gestational diabetes, insulin resistance and blood glucose levels are decreased by regular aerobic exercise such as brisk walking, jogging, biking, golfing, hiking, swimming, and strength exercises.[87] Exercising on a recumbent bicycle at a moderately intense pace for 45 minutes three times a week, and weight lifting with the arms 3 days a week for 20 minutes per session for 6 weeks, have been found to normalize blood glucose levels in some women.[88] Other studies have shown that regular exercise, such as 30 minutes a day of brisk walking, decreases the risk of poor pregnancy outcomes in women with gestational diabetes compared to women with gestational diabetes who are physically inactive.[66] Since exercise lowers blood glucose levels, care needs to be taken to monitor blood glucose levels before, during, and after exercise, and to adjust dietary intake and medications appropriately to guard against hypoglycemia.[62] Levels of exercise undertaken should make women become slightly sweaty but not overheated, dehydrated, or exhausted.[88]

**Nutritional Management of Women with Gestational Diabetes** For most women, blood glucose levels can be successfully managed by diet and exercise.[62,78] Diet and exercise–controlled management of gestational diabetes is often preferred because it eliminates the need for women to use insulin injections (which they tend to dislike), is not related to increased appetite and weight gain associated with insulin use, and may foster longer-term healthy diet and exercise patterns. Metformin or insulin will generally be added to diet and lifestyle efforts if targeted blood glucose levels are not obtained within several weeks.[64]

The following are components of the nutritional management of women with gestational diabetes:

- Assessing dietary habits and exercise habits
- Developing an individualized, culturally appropriate, and acceptable dietary pattern and exercise plan for blood glucose control
- Monitoring weight gain, dietary intake
- Interpreting blood glucose and urinary ketone results
- Ensuring follow-up during pregnancy and postpartum[88]

Executive summary of the American Dietetic Association's recommendations for evidence-based practice guidelines for gestational diabetes. Available at www.adaevidencelibrary.com/topic.cfm?cat=3731, accessed 6/09.

***The Dietary Pattern Plan*** There is no one-size-fits-all dietary intake plan that meets the needs of all pregnant women with gestational diabetes.[90] In general, dietary patterns developed for women with gestational diabetes emphasize the following:

- Whole-grain breads and cereals, vegetables, fruits, and high-fiber foods
- Minimally processed, nutrient-dense foods consumed in appropriate portion sizes
- Limited intake of sugars and foods and beverages that contain them
- Low-glycemic index and high-fiber foods
- Unsaturated fats
- Three regular meals and snacks daily[81,84,87,90]

**ketones** Metabolic byproducts of the breakdown of fatty acids in energy formation. Beta-hydroxybutyric acid, acetoacetic acid, and acetone are the major ketones, or "ketone bodies."

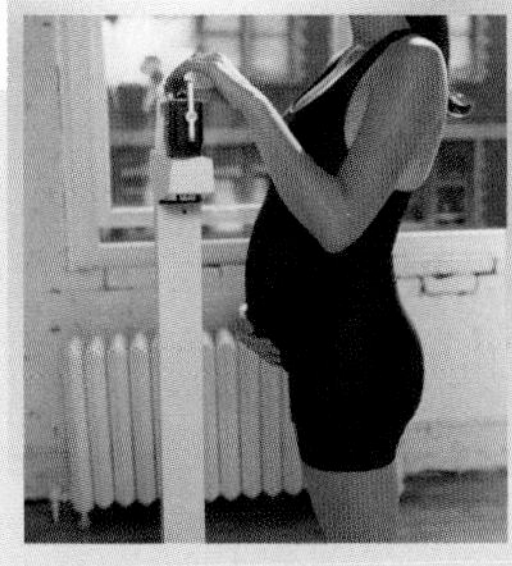

Duncan Smith/Getty Images

# CASE STUDY 5.2

## Elizabeth's Story: Gestational Diabetes

Elizabeth is a 36-year-old who entered pregnancy with a BMI of 23.5 kg/m². She began receiving prenatal care at 32 weeks gestation and was screened for gestational diabetes the next day. Results of her oral glucose tolerance test revealed the following blood glucose levels:

Fasting: 90 mg/dL
1-hour: 195 mg/dL
2-hour: 163 mg/dL

Elizabeth's health care provider advised her to consume a no-sugar, low-carbohydrate diet and to keep her weight gain low throughout the rest of pregnancy. She delivered a large infant (4750 grams) at 39 weeks gestation.

### Questions

1. Did Elizabeth have gestational diabetes?
2. Was she insulin resistant?
3. What's the most likely reason Elizabeth delivered an abnormally large newborn?
4. What was wrong with the dietary advice Elizabeth was given?
5. List three components of appropriate dietary advice for women with gestational diabetes.

Diets are cooperatively planned around a calculated level of caloric need. These initial estimates of caloric need are intended to meet both maternal and fetal need for energy while limiting increases in blood glucose levels. They are based on the pregnant woman's weight status and weight gain goals for pregnancy (Table 5.10).

Women's allotment of calories is generally spread across three meals and several snacks, including a low-carbohydrate bedtime snack to help prevent nighttime hypoglycemia. Proportions of daily calorie intake generally assigned to meals and snacks are:

- 10–20 percent for breakfast
- 20–30 percent for lunch
- 30–40 percent for dinner
- 30 percent for snacks[85]

Caloric levels and meal and snack plans are considered to be starting points and often require modifications after results of blood glucose home monitoring tests are known.

There is no single distribution of calories from carbohydrate, protein, and fat that works best for blood glucose control in diabetes. The American Diabetes Association (ADA) recommends that individuals with diabetes adhere to a calorie distribution from the energy nutrients that meet blood glucose and other goals of treatment, as well as personal preferences. Diets of pregnant women should provide at least 175 grams of carbohydrate daily as recommended by the Institute of Medicine. It is common for women with gestational diabetes to consume about 45 percent of calories from carbohydrates (around 270 grams) daily.[91] Women with genetic traits that lead to increased insulin resistance and blood glucose levels when intake of sugars and high-glycemic index sources of carbohydrates such as white rice, potatoes, white bread, and sugar-sweetened beverages are consumed often benefit from reducing intake of these types of foods (Illustration 5.3).[92] Table 5.11 provides an example meal plan for a pregnant woman with gestational diabetes that meets nutrient needs and includes low-glycemic-index carbohydrate foods and beverages.

TABLE 5.10 ▸ Estimating levels of caloric need in women with gestational diabetes[84]

| CURRENT WEIGHT STATUS | BMI, KG/M² | CALORIES PER KG BODY WEIGHT, KCAL/KG |
|---|---|---|
| Underweight | ≤ 18.5 | 35–40 |
| Normal weight | 18.5–24.9 | 30–35 |
| Overweight | 25–29.9 | 25–30 |
| Obese | ≥ 30 | 23–25 |

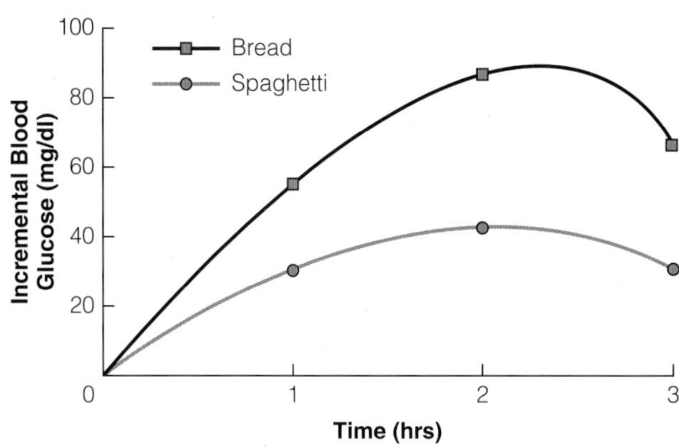


ILLUSTRATION 5.3 ▸ Blood glucose levels after a meal containing white bread (GI = 70) or spaghetti (GI = 48) is consumed by individuals with diabetes.

SOURCE: Graph developed by author from data presented in Riccardi, G., et al. (1999). Diabetes: Nutrition in Prevention and Management, *Nutr Metab Cardiovasc Dis*, *9*, 33–36; Wolever, T. M. S., et al. (1987). The glycemic index: Similarity of values derived in insulin-dependent and non–insulin-dependent diabetic patients. *J Am Col Nutr*, *6*, 295–305; and Jenkins, D. J. A., et al. (1988). Starchy foods and glycemic index. *Diabetes Care*, *11*, 149–159.

TABLE 5.11 ▸ Example of a one-day meal plan that provides 44% of total calories from carbohydrate for a woman with gestational diabetes

| 2400-CALORIE MEAL PLAN | | |
|---|---|---|
| | CARBOHYDRATES, G | CALORIES |
| **Breakfast** | | |
| Complete Wheat Bran Flakes, ¾ cup | 23 | 90 |
| 2% milk, ½ cup | 6 | 61 |
| Egg, 1 | 1 | 74 |
| Black coffee, tea | | |
| **Morning Snack** | | |
| Peanuts, 2 oz | 10 | 326 |
| Carrot, 1 | 7 | 31 |
| Graham crackers, 4 small or 1 sheet | 11 | 59 |
| **Lunch** | | |
| Beef or chicken burrito, 1 | 33 | 255 |
| Salsa, ½ cup | 7 | 33 |
| Black beans, 1 cup | 40 | 228 |
| Apple, 1 | 21 | 81 |
| Black coffee, tea, water, or diet soda | | |
| **Midday Snack** | | |
| Banana, ½ | 28 | 55 |
| 2% milk, 1 cup | 12 | 121 |
| **Dinner** | | |
| Lean pork chop, 4 oz | 0 | 263 |
| Pinto beans, 1 cup | 22 | 116 |
| Corn bread, 1 oz | 12 | 92 |
| Margarine, 1 tsp | 1 | 33 |
| Garden salad, 2 cup | 0 | 10 |
| Feta cheese, 1 oz | 1 | 74 |
| Salad dressing, 2 Tbsp | 3 | 104 |
| Black coffee, tea, water, or diet soda | | |
| **Bedtime Snack** | | |
| Peanut butter, 2 Tbsp | 12 | 190 |
| Rice cake, 1 | 8 | 35 |
| 2% milk, 1 cup | 12 | 121 |
| **Total:** | 270 g | 2442 |

SOURCE: Developed by Judith Brown.

**Postpartum Follow-Up** About 15 percent of women with gestational diabetes will remain glucose intolerant postpartum, and 10–15 percent will develop type 2 diabetes within 2–5 years. Most women who managed their gestational diabetes with diet and exercise will not require monitoring of blood glucose levels after pregnancy. Women requiring insulin for glucose management should be tested for fasting and 2-hour postprandial blood glucose values before hospital discharge. A 75-gram oral glucose tolerance test is recommended 6–12 weeks postpartum in women who were diagnosed with gestational diabetes during pregnancy but tested negative for glucose intolerance postpartum. Negative results should be followed by repeated glucose testing yearly.[60]

**Prevention of Gestational Diabetes** Reducing overweight and obesity, increasing physical activity, and decreasing insulin resistance prior to pregnancy are important components of reducing the risk of gestational diabetes.[93] Women who exercise regularly before and during pregnancy are less insulin resistant late in pregnancy and have a lower risk of developing gestational diabetes in pregnancy.[95] The risk of type 2 diabetes after pregnancy can be reduced substantially by healthful eating, aerobic and resistance exercise, and maintenance of normal weight.[64,94]

## Type 2 Diabetes in Pregnancy

More women are entering pregnancy with type 2 diabetes than in the past largely due to increasing rates of obesity.[96] Care for women with type 2 diabetes in pregnancy should be individualized and follow evidence-based protocols. The primary goal of management is maintenance of blood glucose levels within the normal range. This can be challenging because insulin requirements change throughout pregnancy and requires that women be closely monitored and that care providers remain alert and ready to modify care plans.[71,96] Medical nutrition therapy is a major part of the management of type 2 diabetes during pregnancy, and should be undertaken by an experienced registered dietitian in concert with other members of the clinical team and the woman.[84]

## Management of Type 2 Diabetes in Pregnancy

Women with type 2 diabetes are at risk of developing abnormally high and low blood glucose levels. Hypoglycemia and hyperglycemia pose threats to maternal and fetal health and should be avoided.[97] Hypoglycemia early in pregnancy is associated with spontaneous abortion and congenital anomalies. It is more likely to occur in the first trimester of pregnancy when insulin requirement may decrease due to nausea and vomiting, weight loss, and other conditions, than later in pregnancy.[96,97] Sustained blood glucose levels over 200 mg/dL (11.1 mmol/L) during pregnancy can result in high blood ketone levels and diabetic acidosis due to the lack of insulin and uptake of glucose by cells.[82] Diabetic acidosis is associated with fetal mortality and decreased intelligence and fine motor skills in offspring.[96]

Routine testing for urinary ketones is not recommended.[62] Use of urinary dipsticks for ketone testing is somewhat questionable. Many types of strips do not detect beta-hydroxybutyric acid that accounts for about 80 percent of urinary ketones.[82] Assessment of urinary ketone levels are sometimes used in practice to estimate the adequacy of calorie and carbohydrate intake.[84,87] When

TABLE 5.12 The American Diabetes Association recommendations for the management of type 2 diabetes in pregnancy[64]

- Plan pregnancy, achieve good blood glucose control prior to pregnancy
- Replace oral medications for diabetes with insulin before conception
- Self-monitor blood glucose levels
- Achieve blood glucose goals during pregnancy:
  - Pre-meal, bedtime, overweight: 60–99 mg/dL (3.3–5.4 mmol/L)[a]
  - Post-prandial (post-meal): 100–129 mg/dL (5.6–7.1 mmol/L)
  - Average, daily glucose level: < 110 mg.dL (6.1 mmol/L)
  - Average A1c: < 6.0% (if it can be achieved without significant hypoglycemia)
  - Minimize episodes of hypoglycemia
  - Time meals to correspond with insulin use and blood glucose levels
- Nutritional management
  - Aim for pregnancy weight gains toward the lower end of the Institute of Medicine's recommended pregnancy weight gain range by prepregnancy BMI.
  - Monitor weight gain, adjust energy intake based on rate of gain, physical activity level, and fetal growth pattern
  - Develop a personalized daily food plan based on food preferences, calorie need, and a healthy dietary pattern
  - Include around 175 grams carbohydrate in the food plan.
  - With input from the woman on effects of various carbohydrate foods on her blood glucose level, distribute carbohydrate intake across meals and snacks to control glucose and ketone levels
  - Include 28 grams of fiber daily from whole grains, vegetables, and fruits in the food plan
  - Encourage consumption of unsaturated fats
  - Monitor dietary intake and adjust dietary pattern as needed

[a]You can convert mg/dL to millimoles per liter, or mmol/L, by multiplying mg/dL by 0.0555.

interpreting results of urinary ketone tests, it should be kept in mind that 10–20 percent of pregnant women spill ketones after an overnight fast.[88] This means the severity and consistency of positive findings for urinary ketones should be considered. Assessment of blood ketone level during illness, weight loss, or bouts of hyperglycemia has been recommended. High ketone levels during pregnancy should be prevented to the extent possible.[62,98] Table 5.12 summarizes ADA recommendations for the medical and nutritional management of type 2 diabetes during pregnancy.

Women with type 2 diabetes should be followed closely after delivery due to changes in insulin need, and to facilitate weight loss and achievement of normal weight status when needed.

## Type 1 Diabetes During Pregnancy

Women with type 1 diabetes have deficient insulin output and must rely on insulin injections or an insulin pump to meet their need for insulin. Type 1 diabetes represents a potentially more hazardous condition to mother and fetus than do most cases of gestational or type 2 diabetes due to the increased risk of kidney disease, hypertension, preclampsia, and other complications of pregnancy. Newborns of women with this type of diabetes are at increased risk of mortality, of being SGA or LGA, and of experiencing hypoglycemia and other problems within 12 hours after birth. Hypoglycemia occurs in about half of ***macrosomic*** infants.[67] Coming into pregnancy with this type of diabetes increases the risk of congenital malformations of the pelvis, central nervous system, and heart in offspring (by 2–9 percent). Good control of blood glucose levels before and during pregnancy reduces the risk of malformations and macrosomia substantially.[99]

Blood glucose control from the beginning of pregnancy is also important because the fetal growth trajectory is largely determined in the first half of pregnancy. Exposure to high amounts of glucose and insulin when the fetal growth trajectory is being established may set the "metabolic stage" for fetal accumulation of muscle and fat later in pregnancy.[100] Even relatively low elevations in blood glucose levels can meaningfully increase birthweight.[101]

### Nutritional Management of Type 1 Diabetes in Pregnancy

Primary goals for the nutritional management of type 1 diabetes in pregnancy are continual control of blood glucose levels, calorie and nutrient adequacy of dietary intake, achievement of recommended amounts of weight gain, and a healthy mother and newborn. Careful home monitoring of glucose levels and adjustments in dietary intake, exercise, and insulin dose based on the results are key events that increase the likelihood of reaching these goals. Monitoring ketone levels is particularly important in women with type 1 diabetes because they are more prone to developing ketosis than are women with gestational or type 2 diabetes.[97,102] Inclusion of ample amounts of dietary

**macrosomia** A newborn with an excessive birth weight (macro = big, somia = body). Newborn macrosomia has been defined in several different ways, including birth weight of 4000–4500 grams (8 lb 13 oz to 9 lb 15 oz) or greater than the 90th percentile of weight for gestational age.

fiber (25–35 g per day) reduces insulin requirements in many women with type 1 diabetes in pregnancy.[103]

Availability of new types of insulin, the insulin pump for subcutaneous insulin infusion, and self-monitoring technology is revolutionizing the care of type 1 diabetes during pregnancy.[78] An artificial pancreas that utilizes a closed-loop insulin delivery system with continuous glucose monitoring and insulin pump has been developed and may become available for use in the future. The device appears to effectively assist in the control of blood glucose levels in individuals with type 1 diabetes.[104]

# Multifetal Pregnancies

**LO 5.4** Explain three differences in nutrient needs and cite two specific considerations for delivery of effective nutritional care for women with multifetal pregnancy.

Rates of multifetal pregnancy in the United States have increased markedly since 1980 (Illustration 5.4). Twin births, which accounted for 1 in 53 births in 1980, constituted 1 in 30 births in 2013. Rates of triplet and higher order multiple births (referred to as triplet + births) increased from 1 in 2701 to 1 in 837 births.[105] The leading reason for the increased prevalence of multifetal pregnancies in the United States and other developed countries is the use of ***assisted reproductive technology***.[106] Rates of triplet + pregnancies are headed downward due to improved assisted reproductive technologies that reduce the number of embryos transferred to the womb and therefore higher-order multifetal pregnancies.[108]

The progressively older ages at which U.S. women are bearing children also contribute to rising rates of multifetal pregnancies. The chances of a spontaneous multifetal pregnancy increase with age after about 35 years. Rates of spontaneous multifetal pregnancy also increase with increasing weight status. For example, the rate of twin pregnancy is about two times higher in obese than in underweight women.[107]

**assisted reproductive technology (ART)** An umbrella term for fertility treatments such as *in vitro* fertilization (IVF, a technique in which egg cells are fertilized by sperm outside the woman's body), artificial insemination, and hormone treatments.

Upward trends in low birthweight and preterm delivery in the United States over recent years have been strongly influenced by the upsurge in multiple births. Only 3 percent of newborns are from multifetal pregnancies, yet they account for disproportionally high percentages of all low-birthweight newborns, preterm births, and infant deaths.[109,110]

## Background Information about Multiple Fetuses

The most common type of multifetal pregnancies, those with twin fetuses, come in two types and with several levels of risk. Twins are dizygotic (DZ) if two eggs were fertilized, and monozygotic (MZ) if one egg was. Monozygotic twins result when the fertilized and rapidly dividing egg splits in two within days after conception. The term *identical* is often used to describe MZ twins, and *fraternal* denotes DZ twins. These terms are misleading and outdated, and cannot be used to accurately distinguish twin type. The preferred terms are *monozygotic* and *dizygotic*. About 70 percent of twins are DZ, and 30 percent are MZ.[111]

Monozygotic twins are always the same sex, whereas DZ twins are the same sex half the time. Monozygotic twins are genetically identical in almost all ways, but they are seldom absolutely identical. Genetic differences in pairs of MZ twins can result from chromosome abnormalities in one twin, unequal genetic expression of maternally and paternally derived genes, and environmental effects on gene expression. Rates of MZ twins are remarkably stable across population groups and do not appear to be influenced by heredity.[112]

Dizygotic twins represent individuals with differing genetic fingerprints. The incidence of DZ twin pregnancies is influenced both by inherited and environmental factors. Rates of DZ twins vary among racial groups and by country. Rates tend to decrease in populations during famine and to increase when food availability and nutritional status improve.[113] Periconceptional vitamin and mineral supplement use has also been related to an increased incidence of DZ twin pregnancy.[114]

Twins vary in the number of placentas; some are born having used the

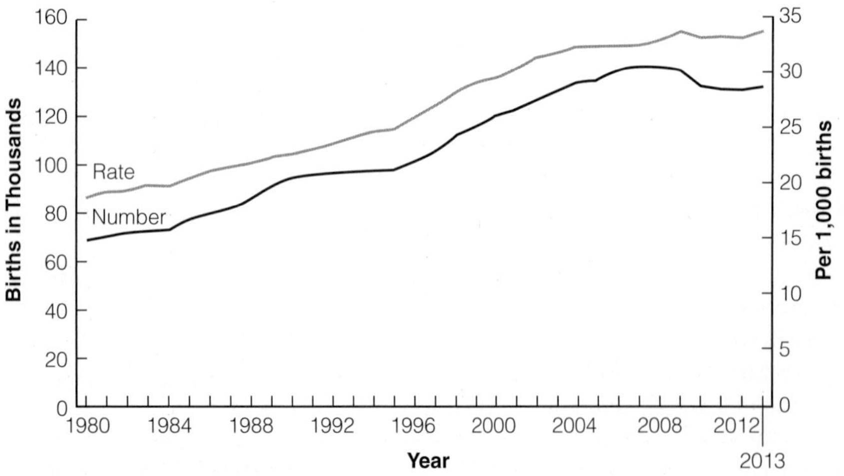

ILLUSTRATION 5.4 ▸ Number and rate of twin births in the United States, 1980–2013.

SOURCE: www.cdc.gov/nchs/data/databriefs/db80_fig1.png, and www.cdc.gov/nchs/data/nvsr/nvsr64/nvsr64_01.pdf.

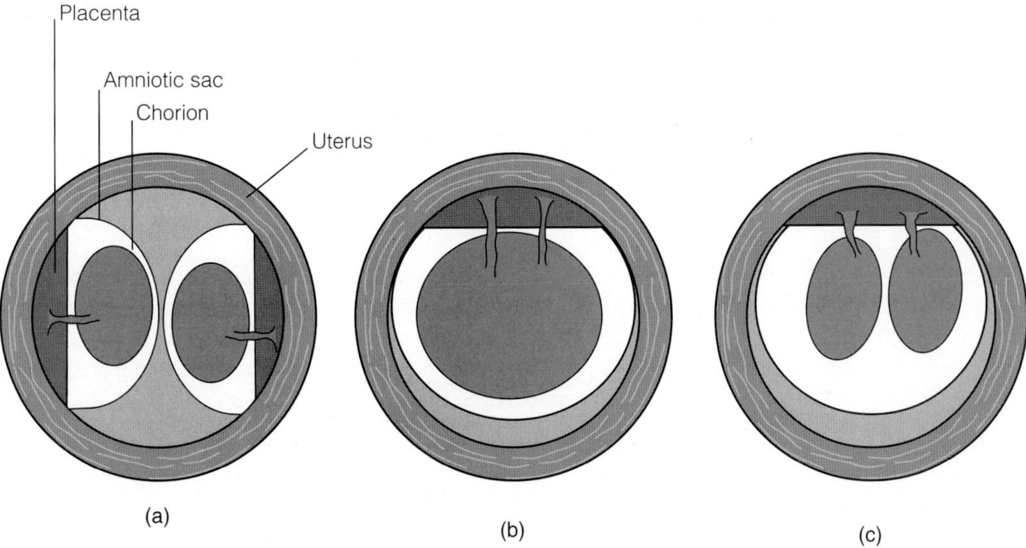


ILLUSTRATION 5.5 Variations in amniotic sacs, chorions, and placentas in twin pregnancy. Drawing (a) shows twins with two amniotic sacs, two chorions, and two placentas. Drawing (b) represents twins sharing one amniotic sac, chorion, and placenta. Drawing (c) shows twins with two amniotic sacs, one chorion, and two placentas that have grown into one.

SOURCE: Schematic representations drawn by the author with the help of Scott Strachan, 2009.

same placenta, but more commonly each fetus has its own. Twins may share a common amniotic sac and one of the membranes around the sac (the chorion), or have separate amniotic sacs and membranes (Illustration 5.5). Twins at highest risk of death, malformations, growth retardation, short gestation, and other serious problems are those that share the same amniotic sac and chorion, and to a lesser degree, MZ twins in general.[115] Determining twin type is not always an easy task during or after pregnancy. Definitive diagnoses of tough cases can be made through DNA analysis.[115]

***In Utero* Growth of Twins and Triplets** Fetal growth patterns of twins and triplets are different compared to singleton fetuses (Illustration 5.6). Rates of weight gain for each group of fetuses are the same until about 28 weeks of gestation. Rates of weight gain begin to decline in twin and triplet fetuses after that point, however, and remain lower until delivery. Variations in birthweight of twin and triplet newborns appear to be related to factors that affect fetal growth after 25 weeks of pregnancy.[115]

***The Vanishing Twin Phenomenon*** The disappearance of embryos within 13 weeks of conception is not unusual. It has been estimated that 6–12 percent of pregnancies begin as twins, but that only about 3 percent result in the birth of twins. Most fetal losses occur silently by absorption into the uterus within the first 8 weeks after conception. The prognosis for continued viability of a pregnancy associated with a vanishing twin tends to be good.[116]

## Risks Associated with Multifetal Pregnancy

Singleton pregnancy is the biological norm for humans, so it may be expected that multifetal pregnancy would be accompanied by increasing health risks (Table 5.13). Multifetal pregnancies present substantial risks to both mother and fetuses, and the risks increase as the number of fetuses increases (Table 5.14).[109] Newborns from twin

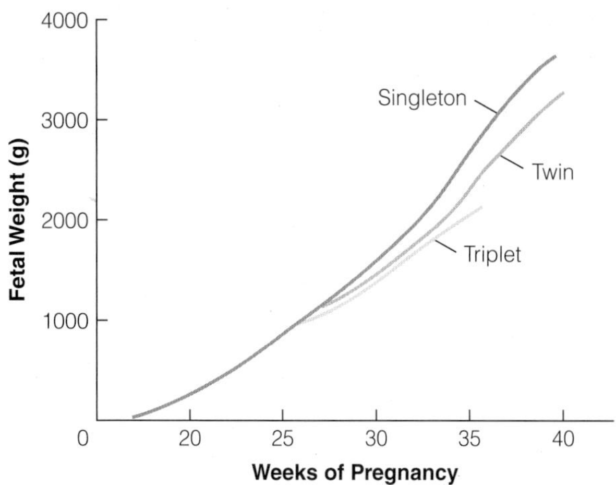


ILLUSTRATION 5.6 Mean fetal weight gain in singleton, twin, and triplet fetuses during pregnancy.

SOURCE: Graph derived by author from data presented in Kramer, M., et al. (2001). A new and improved population-based Canadian reference for birth weight for gestational age. *Pediatrics, 108*, e35; Kuno, A., et al. (1999). Comparison of fetal growth in singleton, twin, and triplet pregnancies. *Hum Reprod, 14*, 1352–1360; and Naeye, R. L., et al. (1966). Intrauterine growth of twins as estimated from liveborn birth-weight data. *Pediatrics, 37*, 409–416.

TABLE 5.13 ▸ Risks to mother and fetuses associated with multifetal pregnancy[106,110]

**Pregnant Women**
- Preeclampsia
- Iron-deficiency anemia
- Gestational diabetes
- Hyperemesis gravidarum
- Placenta previa
- Kidney disease
- Fetal loss
- Preterm delivery
- Cesarean delivery

**Newborns**
- Neonatal death
- Congenital abnormalities
- Respiratory distress syndrome
- Intraventricular hemorrhage
- Cerebral palsy
- Low birthweight

TABLE 5.15 ▸ Median birthweight for gestational age at delivery of twins

| GESTATIONAL AGE, WEEKS | BIRTHWEIGHT |
|---|---|
| 28 | 995 g (2.2 lb) |
| 29 | 1145 g (2.6 lb) |
| 30 | 1300 g (2.9 lb) |
| 31 | 1445 g (3.2 lb) |
| 32 | 1580 g (3.5 lb) |
| 33 | 1750 g (3.9 lb) |
| 34 | 1905 g (4.3 lb) |
| 35 | 2165 g (4.8 lb) |
| 36 | 2275 g (5.1 lb) |
| 37 | 2430 g (5.4 lb) |
| 38 | 2565 g (5.7 lb) |
| 39 | 2680 g (6.0 lb) |
| 40 | 2810 g (6.3 lb) |
| 41 | 2685 g (6.0 lb) |

SOURCE: Data presented in table assembled from Cohen, S. B. et al. (1997). New birthweight nomograms for twin gestation on the basis of accurate gestational age. *Am J Obstet Gynecol, 177*, 1101–1104.

pregnancies at lowest risk of death in the perinatal period weigh between 3000 and 3500 grams (6.7–7.8 lb) at birth and are born at 37–39 weeks gestation. Triplets tend to do best when they weigh over 2000 grams (4.5 lb) and are born at 34–35 weeks gestation.[117]

Unfortunately, these outcomes do not represent the usual. Median weights of twins born at 37, 38, and 39 weeks gestation fall below the 3000- to 3500-gram range (Table 5.15). However, the 3000- to 3500-gram birthweight range for twins, and the 2000-gram mark for triplet newborns, can serve as goals for the provision of nutrition services.

**Interventions and Services for Risk Reduction** Special multidisciplinary programs that offer women with multifetal pregnancy a consistent, main provider of care; preterm prevention education; increased attention to nutritional needs; and intensive follow-up achieve better pregnancy outcomes than does routine prenatal care.[118] Rates of very low birthweight (≤ 1500 g or ≤ 3.3 lb) have been reported to be substantially lower (6 percent versus 26 percent), neonatal intensive care admissions three times lower (13 percent versus 38 percent), and perinatal mortality strikingly lower (1 percent versus 8 percent) among women who receive such services.[119] Interventions offered by the Montreal Diet Dispensary, which focuses on improving the nutritional status and well-being of the pregnant women served, have been shown to substantially reduce poor outcomes compared to those for similar women not receiving the services. Improvements include a 27 percent reduction in the rate of low birthweight, a 47 percent decline in very low birthweight, a 32 percent lower rate of preterm delivery, and a 79 percent drop in mortality during the first 7 days after birth.[120]

TABLE 5.14 ▸ Average birthweight and gestational age at delivery, and low-birthweight rates, of singleton, twin, and triplet newborns[107,118]

| | MEAN BIRTHWEIGHT | MEAN GESTATIONAL AGE | LOW-BIRTHWEIGHT RATE |
|---|---|---|---|
| Singletons | 3440 g (7.7 lb) | 39–40 weeks | 6% |
| Twins | 2400 g (5.4 lb) | 37 weeks | 54% |
| Triplets | 1800 g (4.0 lb) | 33–34 weeks | 90% |

## Nutrition and the Outcome of Multifetal Pregnancy

Nutritional factors are suspected of playing a major role in the course and outcome of multifetal pregnancy, but much remains to be learned. Of the nutritional factors that influence multifetal pregnancy, weight gain during twin pregnancy has been studied most.

**Weight Gain in Multifetal Pregnancy** As with singleton pregnancy, weight gain in multifetal pregnancy is linearly related to birthweight, and weight gains associated with newborn weight vary based on prepregnancy weight status (Table 5.16).[121] The Institute of Medicine makes these

TABLE 5.16 ▸ Prepregnancy weight status and weight-gain relationships in twin pregnancy[167]

| PREPREGNANCY WEIGHT STATUS | WEIGHT GAIN RELATED TO BIRTHWEIGHTS OF > 2500 G (5.5 LB) |
|---|---|
| Underweight | 44.2 lb (20.1 kg) |
| Normal weight | 40.9 lb (18.6 kg) |
| Overweight | 37.8 lb (17.2 kg) |
| Obese | 37.2 lb (16.9 kg) |
| Very obese | 29.2 lb (13.3 kg) |

provisional recommendations for weight gain during twin pregnancy:

- Normal-weight women should gain 37–54 pounds (17–25 kg).
- Overweight women should gain 31–50 pounds (14–23 kg).
- Obese women should gain 25–42 pounds (11–19 kg).

These gains are associated with the birth of infants weighing ≥ 5.5 pounds (≥ 2.5 kg) on average, at 37–42 weeks gestation. The report did not identify a recommended range of weight gain for underweight women with twins.[122] It would be reasonable to conclude that they should gain a somewhat higher range of weight than normal-weight women.

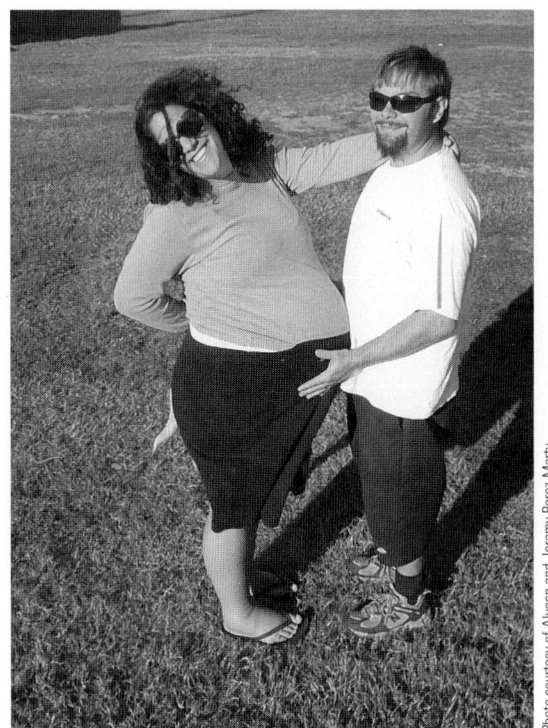
Photo courtesy of Alyeen and Jeremy Perez-Marty

ILLUSTRATION 5.7 ▸ The woman pregnant with twins shown in this photo labeled it, "My poor feet!" The leg and ankle swelling are an expected and normal part of a healthy twin pregnancy.

***Rate of Weight Gain in Twin Pregnancy*** A positive rate of weight gain in the first half of twin pregnancy is strongly associated with increased birthweight.[123] On the other hand, weight loss after 28 weeks of pregnancy increases the risk of preterm delivery threefold.[124] Weight gain should be continually positive and add up to about 5–7 pounds (2.3–3.2 kg) in the first trimester and then 1–2 pounds per week (0.5–0.9 kg) in the second and third trimesters based on prepregnancy weight status.

***Weight Gain in Triplet Pregnancy*** Several studies have examined the relationship between weight gain and birthweight in women with triplets. The general result is that weight gains of about 50 pounds (22.7 kg) correspond to healthy-sized triplets. Rates of gain related to a total weight gain of 50 pounds in women who will average 33–34 weeks of gestation are 1.5 pounds (0.7 kg) per week or more, starting as early in pregnancy as possible.[123]

## Dietary Intake in Twin Pregnancy

Ensuring "adequate nutrition" is widely acknowledged to be a key component of prenatal care for women with multifetal pregnancy. However, it is not clear what constitutes adequate nutrition. Energy and nutrient needs clearly increase during multifetal pregnancy due to increased levels of maternal blood volume, extracellular fluid, and uterine, placental, and fetal growth. The normally high expansion in extracellular volume and its side effect of leg and ankle edema can be seen in the healthy woman with a twin pregnancy (Illustration 5.7). Increases in energy and nutrient needs place demands on the mother in terms of the nutritional costs of building and maintaining these tissues. Although their newborns are smaller, women with twins still produce around 11.2 pounds (5 kg) of fetal weight, and women with triplets 13.4 pounds (5.4 kg) or more.

Evidence of higher caloric need for tissue maintenance and growth in multifetal than in singleton pregnancy comes from studies that show increased weight gain and a quicker onset of starvation metabolism in women expecting more than one newborn. Reduced rates of twin deliveries, as well as the higher incidence of twins in overweight and obese women, imply that energy status is an important factor in multifetal pregnancy.[123] Whereas it is obvious that energy and nutrient needs are higher in multifetal than singleton pregnancy, levels of energy balance and nutrient intake associated with optimal outcomes of multifetal pregnancy have not been quantified.

Results of a large prospective study indicate that women with twins enter pregnancy with higher average caloric intakes (2030 versus 1789 calories per day) and consume an average of 265 calories more per day during pregnancy

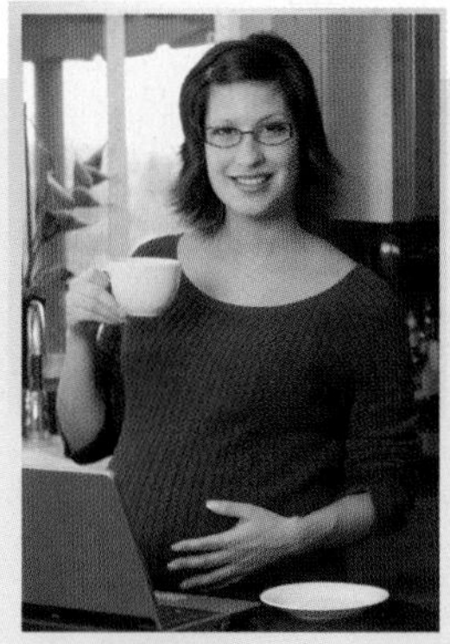
David Buffington/Getty Images

# CASE STUDY 5.3

## Twin Pregnancy and the Nutrition Care Process

This case study involves use of the American Dietetic Association's Nutrition Care Process.

At 37 years of age, Señora Mendez was in her 23rd week of pregnancy and expecting her second child. Or so she thought, until an ultrasound scan detected twins. Her prepregnancy weight was 142 pounds (64.5 kg) and her BMI 23 kg/m$^2$. Señora Mendez's weight-gain progress has been poor due to nausea and vomiting experienced in the first half of pregnancy. Otherwise, Sra. Mendez was experiencing a normal pregnancy for women expecting twins. Concerns about her weight-gain progress and the nutritional needs of women with twin gestation prompted her certified–nurse-midwife to prescribe a prenatal vitamin and mineral supplement and to refer her to a registered dietitian/certified diabetes educator.

A nutritional assessment completed during week 25 of pregnancy identified that Sra. Mendez had gained 14 pounds since conception, and that her typical dietary intake excluded food sources of EPA and DHA. Her plasma 25-hydroxyvitamin D level was below 24 nmol/L, indicating low vitamin D status. No other nutrition-related problems were identified.

### Questions

1. Assume Sra. Mendez will deliver toward the end of week 37 and is now in the beginning of week 25. How many pounds (or kilograms) should be set as a goal for weekly weight gain if a total pregnancy gain at the midpoint of the provisionally recommended range for weight gain in twin pregnancy is to be achieved?
2. State three appropriate nutrition diagnoses for this case.
3. Name one potential nutrition intervention that would address each of the nutrition diagnoses stated.
4. Cite a nutrition-related indicator that could be used to monitor and evaluate each of the nutrition interventions stated.

than women with singleton pregnancy. Nutrient intakes during pregnancy are also higher in women bearing twins than with singleton pregnancy.[107]

Several studies have concluded that the need for specific nutrients is increased during multifetal pregnancy. The need for essential fatty acids (linoleic and alpha-linolenic acid) appears to be increased in multifetal pregnancy. Poor essential fatty acid status is related to neurologic abnormalities and vision impairments in twin offspring.[125] Requirements for iron and calcium have also been found to be increased based on the magnitude of physiological changes that take place in multifetal pregnancy. Levels of essential fatty acids, iron, or calcium required by women to meet these increased needs are unknown, however.[123] Case Study 5.3 addresses a twin pregnancy, and requires use of the American Academy of Nutrition and Dietetics Nutrition Care Process.

**Vitamin and Mineral Supplements and Multifetal Pregnancy** Benefits and hazards of multivitamin and mineral supplement use in multifetal pregnancy have not been reported. Consequently, the extent to which they may be required is unknown. Levels of nutrient intake exceeding the DRI Tolerable Upper Intake Levels should be avoided.

### Nutritional Recommendations for Women with Multifetal Pregnancy

Due to the lack of study results, nutritional recommendations for women with multifetal pregnancy are largely based on logical assumptions and theories (Table 5.17). It is reasoned, for example, that caloric needs for twin pregnancy can be extrapolated from weight gain. Theoretically, to achieve a 40-pound (18.2 kg) weight gain, or 10 pounds (4.5 kg) more than in singleton pregnancy, women with twins would need to consume approximately 35,000 cal more during pregnancy than do women with singleton pregnancies. This increase would amount to about 150 cal per day above the level for singleton pregnancy, or an average of 450 cal more per day than prepregnancy. To achieve higher rates of gain, underweight women may need a higher level of intake, and overweight and obese women lower levels. Energy needs will also vary by energy expenditure levels. As for singleton pregnancy, adequacy of calorie intake can often be estimated by weight-gain progress.[123]

Food-intake recommendations for women with multifetal pregnancy are primarily estimated based on assumptions related to caloric and nutrient needs. Women with multifetal pregnancy likely benefit from dietary patterns

TABLE 5.17 ▸ Best practice recommendations for nutrition during multifetal pregnancy[123,168]

**Weight Gain**

Twin pregnancy

- Overall gain of 35–45 lb (15.9–20.5 kg): Underweight women should gain at the upper end of this range, and overweight and obese women at the lower end.
- First trimester: 4–6 lb (1.8–2.7 kg)
- Second and third trimesters: 1.5 lb (0.7 kg) per week

Triplet pregnancy

- Overall gain of approximately 50 lb (22.7 kg)
- Gain of 1.5 lb (0.7 kg) per week through pregnancy

**Daily Food Intake**

Twin pregnancy (2400–2800 calories a day)

- Grains, primarily whole: 8–10 oz
- Vegetables: 3–3.5 cup
- Fruits: 2–2.5 cup
- Fish, poultry, beans: 6.5–7 oz
- Milk: 3 cup
- Oil: 7–8 tsp
- Extra calorie allowance: 362–426

Triplet pregnancy

- Food intake from the basic food groups should be consumed at a level that promotes targeted weight gain.

**Caloric Intake**

Twin pregnancy

- 450 calories above prepregnancy intake; the amount should be consistent with targeted weight-gain progress.

Triplet pregnancy

- Caloric intake levels should promote targeted weight-gain progress.

**Nutrient Intake**

Twin and triplet pregnancy

- RDA levels or somewhat more than these levels.
- Intakes should be lower than ULs.

**Vitamin and Mineral Supplements**

Twin and triplet pregnancy

- Use vitamin and mineral supplements as needed.

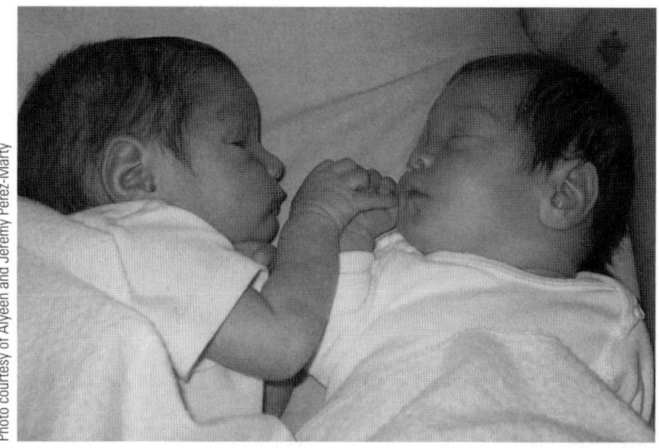

Photo courtesy of Alyeen and Jeremy Perez-Marty

ILLUSTRATION 5.8 ▸ The outcome of a healthy twin pregnancy: Isa weighed 6 pounds, 8 ounces (2912 g) and Manu, 6 pounds, 7 ounces (2884 g). The twins were delivered by a scheduled Caesarean section at 38 weeks, 4 days, and were above average weight for their gestational age.

selected from the ChooseMyPlate groups and nutrient intakes that somewhat exceed the RDAs/AIs.

Although twin pregnancies are higher-risk than singleton pregnancies, outcomes of twin pregnancy can be excellent (Illustration 5.8). Their mother remained in good health during pregnancy while consuming the type of diet and supplements and gaining weight as recommended by her health care providers.

**Recommendations from the Popular Press** Websites, books, and pamphlets are available that provide ample amounts of scientifically unsupported "guesses" about food and nutrient requirements of women with multifetal pregnancy. Even if presented with steely resolution, any advice that strays from current scientifically based wisdom about nutritional needs of women during pregnancy should be sidestepped.

# HIV/AIDS During Pregnancy

**LO 5.5** Identify the components of nutritional care for women with HIV during pregnancy

The world first became aware of acquired immunodeficiency syndrome (AIDS) in the summer of 1981. It was caused by a microbe, the human immunodeficiency virus (HIV). Since then, over 100,000 women of childbearing age in the United States have been diagnosed with AIDS.[126] Currently, 38 million people worldwide live with HIV, but rates of transmission and infection are declining due to increased availability of HIV drugs and positive behavioral changes.[127,128] Transmission of the virus during pregnancy and delivery is a major route to the spread of the infection. Approximately 20 percent of children with HIV/AIDS are infected during pregnancy or delivery, and 14–21 percent during breastfeeding.[126] New drug therapy regimes implemented during and after pregnancy in the past 10 years have shown it is possible to reduce transmission from mother to infant to 1.1 percent.[129] In developing countries where there is not enough money or aid to purchase or obtain the drugs, transmission rates can be substantially reduced by giving the mother a relatively short course of a specific anti-HIV drug before delivery.[130]

The future outlook for the control of HIV/AIDS is improving. Care for individuals with HIV now primarily involves the prevention and management of metabolic disorders related to the virus and the therapies utilized.[131]

## Consequences of HIV/AIDS During Pregnancy

Disease processes such as compromised immune system functions related to HIV/AIDS progress during pregnancy, but it does not appear that the infection itself is related to adverse pregnancy outcomes. Although adverse pregnancy outcomes such as preterm delivery, fetal growth retardation, and low birthweight tend to be higher in women with HIV/AIDS, differences are most closely related to poverty, poor food availability, compromised health status, and the coexistence of other infections.[126]

## Nutritional Factors and HIV/AIDS During Pregnancy

HIV/AIDS is related to poor nutritional status that further compromises the body's ability to fight infections. The disease can lead to nutrient losses and fat malabsorption due to diarrhea, and inflammatory responses to the infection cause the loss of lean muscle mass. Loss of calcium from bones and decreased bone density is a common finding in individuals with HIV/AIDS.[132] Drugs used to treat HIV/AIDS and metabolic processes related to the diseases are associated with increased insulin resistance and the accumulation of central body fat.[133] Nutritional needs increase the most during the later stages of HIV/AIDS as diarrhea, wasting, and reductions in CD4 counts (a measure of white blood cells that help the body fight infection) increase.[134]

The compromised immune status of women with HIV/AIDS, and further decreases in immune response during pregnancy, mean that women with the disease are at high risk of developing foodborne infections during pregnancy. Risk of infection originating from foods can be decreased if raw or uncooked meats and seafood and unpasteurized milk products and honey are not consumed. Safe food-handling practices at home can also reduce the risk of foodborne infection.[132]

## Nutritional Management of Women with HIV/AIDS During Pregnancy

Two major reports that address the nutritional care and needs of women with HIV/AIDS during pregnancy are available.[134,135] The overriding message in the reports is that sound nutrition status is a basic element of health and important for individuals with HIV. Guidelines for nutritional assessment and care for women with HIV during pregnancy are summarized in Table 5.18.

High doses of vitamin and mineral supplementations are not recommended for pregnant women with HIV. Several studies have found that high doses of certain vitamins and minerals can increase viral replication and shedding of the virus in genital secretions. High doses of vitamins A and D, and iron in particular, should not be used. Until more in known, dose levels of vitamin and mineral supplements should adhere to recommended nutrient intake levels identified in the RDAs.[134]

**TABLE 5.18** Nutrition recommendations for pregnant women with HIV[134,135]

**Nutrition Assessment**

- Dietary assessment
  - adequacy of calorie and nutrient intake
  - food security, maternal access to food
  - food and water food safety
  - food taboos
  - dietary supplement use
- Anthropometric assessment
  - Height, weight, weight gain during pregnancy
  - Estimate BMI prior to or early in pregnancy
  - Estimate body composition
- Biochemical assessment
  - Screen for iron deficiency
  - Test for gestational diabetes in women with BMI ≥ 25 mg/kg$^2$ (2-hr, 75 g OGTT around 24 weeks)
  - Test for clinically suspected nutrient deficiencies (vitamin D, vitamin C, etc.)
- Clinical assessment
  - Screen for nausea, vomiting, diarrhea, oral lesions etc. that might affect dietary intake or nutritional status (each prenatal visit)
- Nutrition interventions
  - Intervene to modify unhealthful dietary pattern
  - Facilitate access to food assistance programs
  - Counsel/assist in ensuring adequate intake of calories, essential fatty acids
  - Intervene to modify inappropriate patterns of weight gain
  - Treatment of iron deficiency with high iron foods, adequate vitamin C intake, and iron (not to exceed 27 mg/day)
  - Address food and water safety concerns

# Eating Disorders in Pregnancy

LO 5.6 Identify two primary components of the nutritional care of women with eating disorders during pregnancy.

Eating disorders represent relatively rare conditions in pregnancy because many women with such disorders are subfertile or infertile. Such disorders can have far-reaching effects on both mother and fetus, however, when they do occur. The eating disorder most commonly observed among pregnant women in the United States is bulimia nervosa, a condition marked by both severe food restriction and bingeing and purging.[136] It is estimated that 1–3 percent of adolescents and young women in the United States have this condition.[137] Women with bulimia nervosa exhibit poorly controlled eating patterns marked by recurrent episodes of binge eating. To prevent weight gain, women will induce vomiting, use laxatives, exercise intensely, or fast after binges. Self-worth in women with bulimia nervosa is usually closely tied to their weight and shape. A history of sexual abuse is common among women with this eating disorder, as well as in women with anorexia nervosa.[137]

Women with anorexia nervosa may occasionally ovulate and become pregnant. To women with anorexia nervosa, body weight is of utmost importance, and they are generally fully dedicated to achieving and maintaining extreme thinness.[138] Adolescents and women with this condition may refuse to eat, even when ravenously hungry, limit their food choices to low-calorie foods, and exercise excessively.[137]

Eating disorder symptoms often subside during the second and third trimesters of pregnancy, but they rarely vanish altogether. Symptoms tend to return after delivery, sometimes to a more severe extent than was the case prior to pregnancy.[139] Information on eating disorders in non-pregnant individuals is included in Chapter 15.

## Consequences of Eating Disorders in Pregnancy

Women with eating disorders during pregnancy are at higher risk for spontaneous abortion, hypertension, preterm labor, anemia, genitourinary tract infection, and difficult deliveries than are women without an eating disorder. Pregnancy weight gain is variable but often below the recommended amounts, and newborns tend to be smaller and to experience higher rates of neonatal complications.[136,140]

## Treatment of Women with Eating Disorders During Pregnancy

It is recommended that pregnant women with eating disorders be referred to an eating disorders clinic or specialist. Most large communities have special clinics and programs for women with eating disorders, and they commonly use a team approach to problem solving around the eating disorder. Nutritionists or dietitians often participate in these services because they are knowledgeable about the woman's individual nutritional needs and those of pregnancy. Health professionals serving women with eating disorders in pregnancy can facilitate open communication and behavioral change by gently encouraging women to talk about their eating disorder, fears, and concerns.[139]

## Nutritional Interventions for Women with Eating Disorders During Pregnancy

Behavioral changes required for improvements in nutritional status and weight gain in women with eating disorders are most likely to work when the changes are considered acceptable to the women with the disorder. Frequently, the health professional presents the types of changes that need to be made and explains why, and then works with the woman to develop specific plans accomplishing these changes.

The term *pregorexia* is emerging in clinical practice as an unofficial term for women with restrictive eating behaviors during pregnancy. The term refers to women with eating disorders who fail to gain weight during pregnancy and are at high risk of intrauterine growth retardation and early delivery. In order to stress the importance of eating right and gaining weight, some dietitians will supply the women with *ketosticks* and ask them to check their urine several times a day. It is explained that when test results are positive for ketones, not enough calories and food are being consumed. It is intended that, faced with positive results about an inadequate food intake, women will eat more.[141]

It can be very difficult to normalize food intake and eating behavior in women with eating disorders. Some women will gain weight quickly and exceed recommendation while others will struggle to gain any weight al all.[138]

# Fetal Alcohol Spectrum Disorders

LO 5.7 Summarize the consequences of excess alcohol intake during pregnancy, and list four factors that affect relationship between alcohol intake and the outcome of pregnancy.

Alcohol consumed by a woman easily crosses the placenta to the fetus. Because the fetus has yet to fully develop enzymes that break it down, alcohol lingers in the fetal circulation. This situation, combined with the fact that the fetus is smaller and has far less blood than the mother does, increases the harmful effects of alcohol on the fetus as compared to the mother.[142]

Fetal exposure to alcohol during pregnancy is a leading, preventable cause of birth defects, intellectual disability,

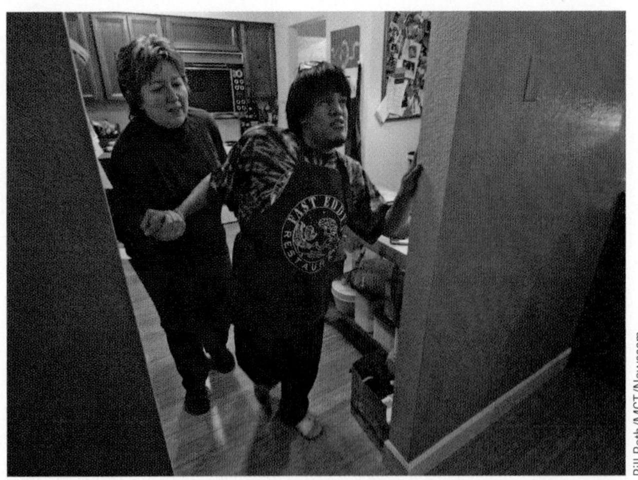
Bill Roth/MCT/Newscom

ILLUSTRATION 5.9 ▸ A 20-year-old with fetal alcohol syndrome being helped by his adoptive mother. He was born to a woman who drank heavily throughout pregnancy and experiences physical, behavioral, and intellectual problems associated with the severe form of fetal alcohol spectrum disorder.

and developmental disorders in children and adults. Approximately 12 percent of women in the United States consume alcohol once a month during pregnancy, and 2 percent consume 5 or more drinks on at least one occasion.[143] It is estimated that 2.4–4.6 percent of Americans have symptoms related to alcohol consumption during pregnancy.[145]

The term *fetal alcohol spectrum disorders* (FASD) is used to describe the range of affects of fetal alcohol exposure on development and physical growth. Three distinct subtypes of outcomes included in FASDs have been defined by the Centers for Disease Control and Prevention (CDC):[146]

- *Fetal alcohol syndrome (FAS).* The most severe form of the fetal alcohol spectrum disorders. It is generally characterized by abnormal facial features (flat mid-face, abnormally shaped ears, presence of a smooth ridge between nose and lips, for example), growth problems, central nervous system abnormalities, and problems with social skills, learning, memory, attention span, communication, vision, or hearing (Illustration 5.9).
- *Alcohol-related neurodevelopmental disorder (ARND).* A less severe form of the fetal alcohol spectrum disorders not characterized by overt physical features. It can be characterized by intellectual disabilities and problems with behavior, learning, coping, impulse control, and attention.
- *Alcohol-related birth defects (ARBD).* A fetal alcohol spectrum disorder characterized by abnormalities of the heart, kidneys, bones, or of hearing. A mix of these characteristics can be present.

Fetal alcohol spectrum disorder. www.cdc//gov/ncbdd/fasd/index.html, accessed Jan 18 2012.

Some fetuses exposed to alcohol during pregnancy develop characteristic signs of fetal alcohol exposure and some do not. Consequently, it is concluded that women and fetuses vary in their susceptibility to the harmful affects of alcohol. Factors that account for differences is susceptibility appear to involve environmental and genetic factors.[144,147] It appears that adequacy of folate intake, maternal diet quality, and interactions between alcohol and nutrient availability may contribute to susceptibility differences related to alcohol exposure during pregnancy.[147]

Adverse outcomes related to alcohol exposure in utero vary from none (20 percent) to mild, moderate, and severe outcomes depending on the timing of alcohol exposure, the amount of alcohol consumed, the health status and lifestyle of the mother, and genetic susceptibility to alcohol affects. The most common outcomes related to fetal alcohol exposure involve behavioral and intellectual impairments.[148] It is estimated that 44 percent of children diagnosed with a FASD have central nervous system impairments that result in behavioral and intellectual disabilities. Children affected by fetal alcohol exposure tend to be growth restricted (27 percent versus 13 percent in the general population), and 17 percent (versus 1.1 percent in the general population) have facial features characteristic of FAS. Consumption of four or more drinks a day throughout pregnancy is associated with FASD in 80 percent of children.[148] Drinking, especially binge drinking (consumption of five or more drinks at a time), in the first trimester of pregnancy appears to be strongly related to FASDs outcomes.[142,148]

**Recommendations Concerning Alcohol Intake during Pregnancy** It is recommended that women do not drink alcohol while pregnant.[151] However, this recommendation is evolving as more is learned about the effects of alcohol intake on fetal growth and development. There is no firm evidence that consumption of a small amount of alcohol during pregnancy, such as a drink or two per week, is harmful.[141,152] Some experts suggest that the effects of consumption of small amounts of alcohol during pregnancy on the fetus have been overstated in the past, potentially causing undue fear and concern in women. Although women should be advised that the safest approach is to not drink during pregnancy, care should be taken to present this information in an objective and balanced manner.[153]

# Nutrition and Adolescent Pregnancy

LO 5.8 Distinguish three ways in which energy and nutrient needs differ between adults and adolescents during pregnancy.

Rates of teen birth have declined by 63 percent over the past 20 years and reached a record low in 2013 of 26.5 births/1000 females aged 15–19 years.[171] Rates of teen

TABLE 5.19 ▸ Risks associated with adolescent pregnancy[156,157,169]

- Low birthweight
- Perinatal death
- Caesarean delivery
- Cephalopelvic disproportion (head too large for birth canal)
- Preeclampsia
- Iron-deficiency anemia
- Delayed, reduced educational achievement
- Poverty
- Poor diet quality

pregnancy in the United States, however, continue to be among the highest reported for developed countries.[154] Adolescents are at higher risk for a number of clinical complications and other unfavorable outcomes compared to adult women (Table 5.19).

The extent to which increased rates of poor outcomes in pregnant teens are associated with biological immaturity or with lifestyle factors such as drug use, smoking, and poor dietary intakes is unclear. Age-related differences in outcome diminish substantially when potentially harmful lifestyle factors are taken into account, diminishing the theory that biological immaturity accounts for the differences. Iron deficiency, vitamin D insufficiency, and poor diet quality have been identified in 30–60 percent of pregnant adolescents.[155-157]

Very young adolescents becoming pregnant within a few years after the onset of menstruation may be at risk due to biological immaturity. They tend to have shorter gestations and a higher likelihood of ***cephalopelvic disproportion***. Poorly nourished, growing adolescent mothers may compete with the fetus for calories and nutrients—and win.[158]

## Growth During Adolescent Pregnancy

Young teens who are growing when pregnancy occurs continue to gain height and weight during pregnancy—but at the expense of fetal growth. Teens who continue to grow during pregnancy give birth to infants that weigh, on average, 155 grams less than infants of adult women, even if they gain more weight than adults do.[149] Rates of spontaneous abortion, preterm birth, and low birthweight are also higher in growing than in nongrowing adolescents.[159] Growing adolescents gain more maternal fat tissue during the last trimester of pregnancy and retain more weight postpartum than do nongrowing teens. Growing teens experience a surge in blood leptin levels during the last trimester, which may decrease maternal use of fat stores and increase utilization of glucose by the mother. Increased use of glucose by the mother appears to decrease energy availability to the fetus.[161]

## Obesity, Excess Weight Gain, and Adolescent Pregnancy

Increasing rates of overweight and obesity among adolescents appear to be placing additional teens at risk of poor pregnancy outcomes. Adolescents entering pregnancy overweight or obese are at increased risk for Cesarean delivery, hypertensive disorders of pregnancy, gestational diabetes, and the delivery of excessively large newborns.[162] In obese adolescents, weight gains during pregnancy that exceed those recommended are related to decreased placental growth and the birth of infants disproportionately small for gestational age.[19 More] research is needed to determine why this happens.

## Nutritional Recommendations for Pregnant Adolescents

Recommendations for pregnant adolescents are basically the same as for older pregnant women, with a few exceptions. Recommendations for weight gain and protein intake are the same, but young adolescents may need more calories to support their own growth as well as that of the fetus. Caloric need should be met by a nutrient-dense diet and lead to rates of weight gain that follow those recommended. Pregnant adolescents have a higher requirement for calcium. The RDA for pregnant teens for calcium is 1300 mg per day, or 300 mg higher than for adult pregnant women. This increased need can be met by the consumption of 4 daily servings of milk and milk products, combined with a varied, basic diet. Since calcium and vitamin D are both needed in adequate amounts for the teen's and the fetus's bone formation, sufficient intake of both nutrients is seen as particularly important during teen pregnancy.[163]

The importance of lifestyle and other environmental factors to pregnancy outcome in teens emphasizes the need for special, comprehensive teen pregnancy health care programs. Nutrition counseling is an important component of the multidisciplinary services that should be offered to pregnant adolescents. Nutrition services that include individualized nutrition assessment, intervention, education, guidance on weight gain, and follow-up enhance birthweight outcomes. Additional specialized services that focus on the psychosocial needs of pregnant adolescents, support/discussion groups, and home visits also contribute to improved maternal and infant outcomes for adolescents.[164] Because most pregnant adolescents have low income, referral to appropriate food and nutrition programs and other assistance related to health care, housing, and education should be core components of services.

## Evidence-Based Practice

The clinical nutritional management of the conditions covered in this chapter, as well as other complications during pregnancy, are not always evidence based due to the lack of knowledge or availability of qualified nutrition professionals. Such practices are a problem

**cephalopelvic disproportion** A mismatch between the size of the fetal head and size of the maternal pelvis, resulting in "failure to progress" in labor for mechanical reasons.

when they burden women and families with costs, call for dietary changes not known to work, or potentially cause harm. Practices not based on evidence that likely pose little risk or burden and may potentially be of help should nonetheless be carefully evaluated. Outdated practices often linger far too long, at the expense of missed opportunities for real improvements.

Use of practices not supported by scientific evidence should always be questioned and confirmed to represent "best practice" insofar as that can be determined. To know what best practice is requires vigilant attention to scientific developments related to the nutritional management of clinical conditions during pregnancy.

## KEY POINTS

1. Maternal diet, weight status, and physical activity levels influence the development of healthy pregnancy outcomes and a number of conditions that adversely affect the course and outcome of pregnancy.
2. Nutritional interventions for a number of complications of pregnancy can benefit maternal and infant health outcomes.
3. Oxidative stress and endothelial dysfunction appear to be related to the development and progression of hypertensive disorders of pregnancy. Oxidative stress occurs when the body's exposure to oxidizing agents is greater than its supply of antioxidants.
4. Excess body fat, low levels of physical activity, *trans* fats, lack of antioxidants, and elevated blood glucose increase oxidative stress. It is lowered by weight loss in overweight individuals, increased levels of exercise, normal blood glucose levels, and sufficient intake of antioxidants from foods such as vegetables, fruits, and whole grains.
5. Nutritional management of gestational diabetes focuses on individually based dietary and exercise plans that help maintain blood glucose levels within the normal range and that foster maternal health and appropriate weight gain.
6. There is no set range of percent of calories from the macronutrients that works best for all women with diabetes during pregnancy.
7. Multifetal pregnancies are classified as "high risk" because of above-average rates of complications and less-than-optimal pregnancy outcomes. Energy, nutrient, and weight-gain needs are somewhat higher in multifetal than singleton pregnancies.
8. Pregnant women with HIV/AIDS may benefit from nutrition interventions that conserve lean muscle and bone mass, correct nutrient deficiencies, and lead to healthful dietary intake and weight gain in pregnancy. Individuals with HIV should not be given high dose levels of vitamin and mineral supplements.
9. Foodborne illnesses can severely affect people with HIV/AIDS, making food safety a priority concern.
10. Women with eating disorders should be closely monitored during pregnancy by an interdisciplinary, experienced clinical team to facilitate appropriate dietary intake, weight gain, and long-term eating habits and weight status.
11. High levels of alcohol intake during pregnancy, especially in the first trimester, are associated with a broad range of intellectual, behavioral, and physical disorders in offspring. Three distinct "fetal alcohol spectrum disorders" have been defined. It is recommended that women do not drink alcohol-containing beverages during pregnancy.
12. Growing adolescents are at risk of poor pregnancy outcomes. Pregnancy outcomes of adolescents who are not growing primarily depend on the health status of the teen. Dietary quality and weight status are important components of the health status of adolescents and influence the course and outcome of their pregnancies.
13. Nutritional interventions during pregnancy should be based on scientific evidence that supports their safety, effectiveness, and affordability.

## REVIEW QUESTIONS

1. Obesity prior to pregnancy is associated with metabolic disorders that promote the development of hypertensive disorders of pregnancy and gestational diabetes.

   _____True _____False

2. Bariatric surgery prior to pregnancy decreases the risk of gestational diabetes and preeclampsia during pregnancy.

   _____True _____False

3. Chronic inflammation and oxidative stress occur in preeclampsia but not in other hypertensive disorders of pregnancy.

   _____True _____False

4. Supplementation with vitamins C and E before and early in pregnancy is associated with a decreased risk of preeclampsia during pregnancy.

   _____True _____False

5. Salt restriction during pregnancy decreases the incidence of all forms of hypertension during pregnancy and is recommended for all pregnant women.

   _____True _____False

6. Gestational diabetes is associated with high blood triglyceride levels.

   _____True _____False

7. It is recommended that women with diabetes gain 5 pounds (2.3 kg) less during pregnancy than the IOM-recommended, lower limit of their weight gain range based on prepregnancy BMI.

   _____True _____False

8. ___ Assume Minh, who weighed 123 pounds and was 5′4″ tall prior to pregnancy, is diagnosed with gestational diabetes at 25 weeks of gestation. She is referred to a registered dietitian for medical nutrition therapy. Which of the following statements of advice would be appropriate for the dietitian state related to Minh's dietary intake?

   a. Eat only carbohydrates that are not white.

   b. Reduce salt intake to a minimum.

   c. Reduce calorie intake to less than 1900 calories per day.

   d. Distribute carbohydrate intake across meals and snacks.

9. In women with type 1 diabetes during pregnancy, high blood levels of ketones can indicate either low or high blood glucose levels.

   _____True _____False

10. The American Diabetes Association recommends that women with diabetes during pregnancy monitor urine glucose and ketone levels daily.

    _____True _____False

11. It is estimated that women with twin pregnancy need 150 calories more each day than do women with singleton pregnancy.

    _____True _____False

12. Women with HIV/AIDS who are well nourished prior to pregnancy tend to have better pregnancy outcomes than do poorly nourished women.

    _____True _____False

13. Supplementation with vitamin A and iron is recommended for women with HIV during pregnancy.

    _____True _____False

14. Women with anorexia nervosa cannot conceive because they do not ovulate.

    _____True _____False

15. Iron and vitamin C status may be compromised in many pregnant adolescents.

    _____True _____False

16. Time-tested clinical assumptions about appropriate dietary therapies during pregnancy tend to work as well in practice as do evidence-based therapies.

    _____True _____False

**Visit www.cengagebrain.com to access MindTap, a complete digital course that includes additional resources.**

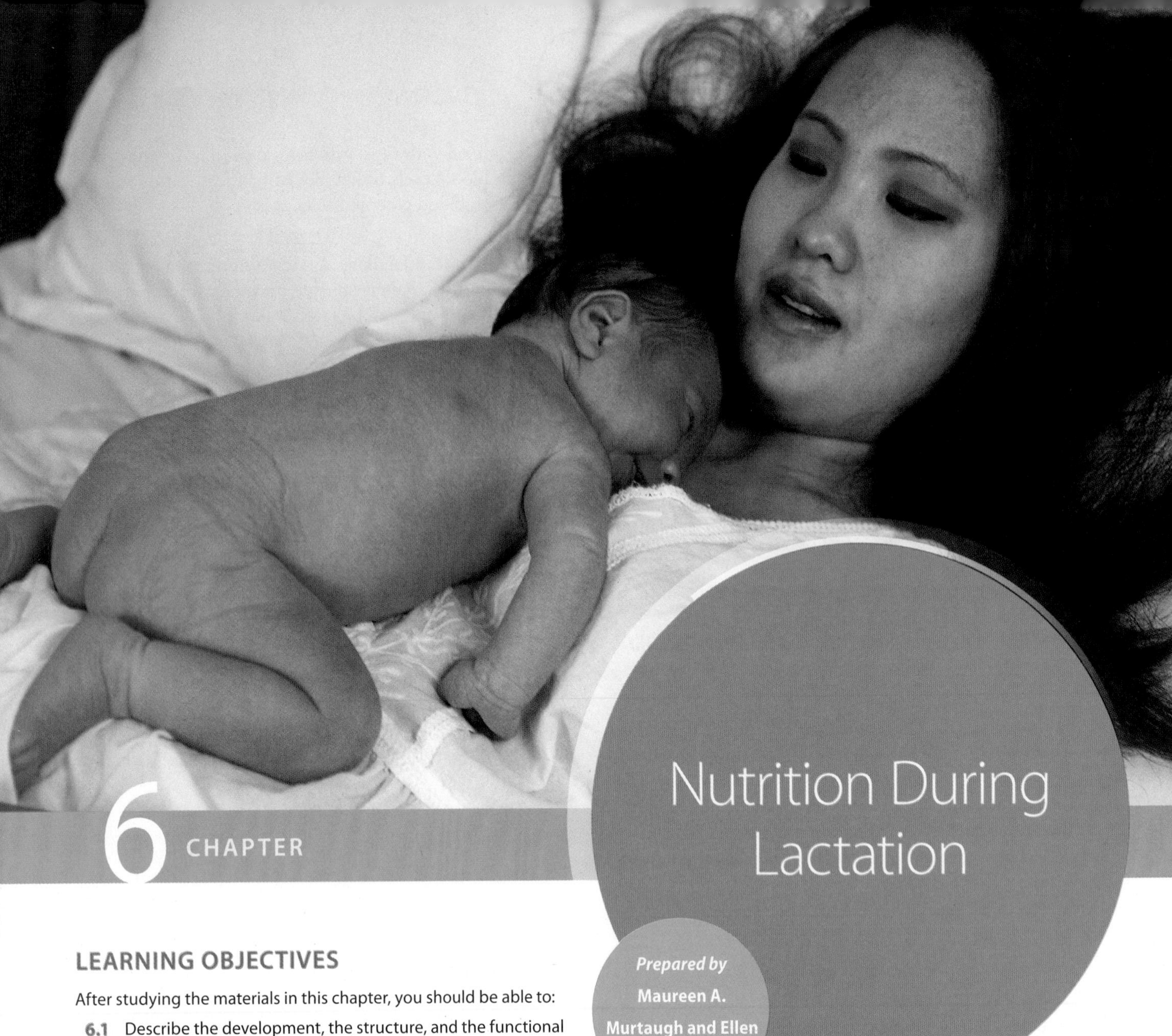

6 CHAPTER

# Nutrition During Lactation

*Prepared by* **Maureen A. Murtaugh and Ellen Lechtenberg**

## LEARNING OBJECTIVES

After studying the materials in this chapter, you should be able to:

**6.1** Describe the development, the structure, and the functional components of the mammary gland. Describe the key hormonal influences on development and function.

**6.2** Identify similarities and differences in nutrients levels between colostrum and mature human milk, and between mature human milk, whole cow's milk, and human milk substitutes (infant formula).

**6.3** Summarize the benefits of breastfeeding for mothers and their babies in a manner that could be included in breastfeeding education for expecting mothers, their partners, and family members.

**6.4** Generate an education plan for new mothers that includes the answers to common questions about milk supply, including what is typical milk production, what is the relationship between infant demand and maternal supply, and the influence of the size of the breast, feeding frequency, pumping, and breast surgeries on milk production.

**6.5** Describe maternal steps to prepare the breast, and the basic position of the infant at the breast.

**6.6** Describe infant behaviors that indicate readiness to feed, and vitamin supplement recommendations for breastfeeding infants.

**6.7** First, identify the professional and government sources of nutrient recommendations for healthy women for diet and supplements. Second, list common nutrition diagnoses for breastfeeding women, coupled with nutrition intervention and appropriate parameters for monitoring.

**6.8** Identify at least two breastfeeding promotion programs that have demonstrated effectiveness at increasing breastfeeding initiation and duration.

**6.9** Summarize factors known to be associated with higher and lower rates of breastfeeding, and the gap between current rates and the Breastfeeding Goals for the United States.

# Introduction

The health care system, the workplace, and the community can either hinder or facilitate the initiation and continuation of breastfeeding. Health programs can play a significant role in increasing and supporting sustained breastfeeding rates to optimize maternal and infant nutrition. Health care professionals who wish to manage and promote breastfeeding should understand the physiology of lactation, the composition of human milk, and the benefits to mothers and infants. Helping women achieve or maintain appropriate nutritional status to optimize breastfeeding requires consideration of energy and nutrient needs, weight goals, effects of exercise during breastfeeding, and vitamin and mineral supplement needs.

The benefits of breastfeeding to mothers and infants are well established. Federal breastfeeding promotion efforts and greater understanding of the advantages of breastfeeding have contributed to the resurgence of breastfeeding in the United States since the 1970s. Nevertheless, racial and ethnic disparities in breastfeeding initiation rates remain. In the last decade gains were realized in both initiation and duration of breastfeeding, but there is still a long way to go to reach exclusive breastfeeding for 4–6 months and continued breastfeeding for at least a year to optimize health for women and children.

Multilevel (health care system, community, workplace, and family) support is critical for women who suffer from common breastfeeding challenges and medical conditions and their infants. Human milk is the preferred food for healthy and premature and sick newborns. It is rarely necessary to discontinue breastfeeding to manage medical problems or medication use. However, adequately experienced and informed health care professionals are needed to provide support for successful breastfeeding. Common breastfeeding conditions and interventions are discussed in Chapter 7.

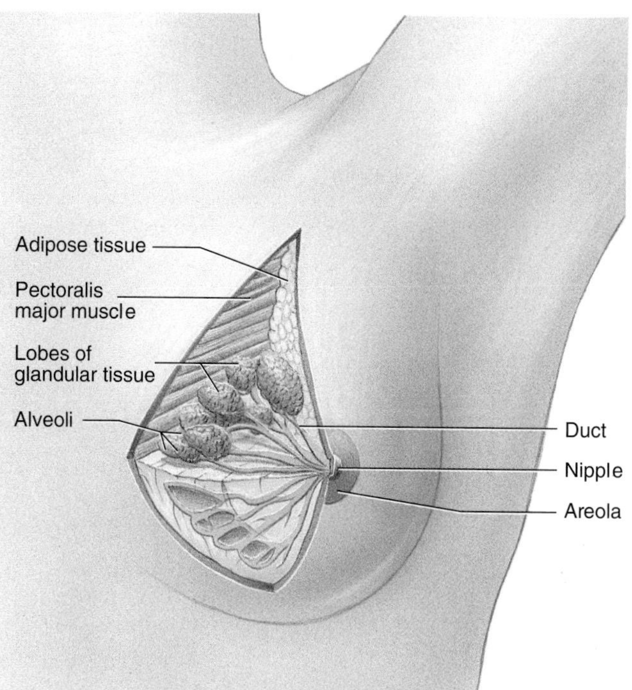


ILLUSTRATION 6.1 ▸ Breast of a lactating female.
This cutaway view shows the mammary glands and ducts.


# Lactation Physiology

LO 6.1 Describe the development, the structure, and the functional components of the mammary gland. Describe the key hormonal influences on development and function.

## Functional Units of the Mammary Gland

The functional units of the ***mammary gland*** are the ***alveoli*** (Illustration 6.1). Each alveolus is composed of a cluster of cells (***secretory cells***) with a duct in the center, whose job it is to secrete milk. The ducts are arranged like branches of a tree, each smaller duct leading to six to ten larger collecting ducts. These branchlike collecting ducts lead to the nipple. ***Myoepithelial cells*** surround the secretory cells. Myoepithelial cells can contract under the influence of ***oxytocin*** and cause milk to be ejected into the ducts.

## Mammary Gland Development

During puberty, the ovaries mature and the release of estrogen and progesterone increases (Table 6.1). The cyclic release of these two hormones governs pubertal breast development (Illustration 6.2). The mammary gland develops its lobular structure (***lobes***) under the cyclic production of progesterone and is usually complete within 12 to 18 months after menarche. As the ductal system matures, cells that can secrete milk develop, the nipple grows, and its pigmentation changes. Fibrous and fatty tissues increase around the ducts.

In pregnancy, the luteal and placental hormones (placental lactogen and chorionic gonadotropin) allow further preparation for breastfeeding

**Mammary gland** The source of milk for offspring, also commonly called the breast. The presence of mammary glands is a characteristic of mammals.

**Alveoli** A rounded or oblong-shaped cavity present in the breast.

**Secretory cells** Cells in the acinus (milk gland) that are responsible for secreting milk components into the ducts.

**Myoepithelial cells** Specialized cells that line the alveoli and that can contract to cause milk to be secreted into the duct.

**Oxytocin** A hormone produced during letdown that causes milk to be ejected into the ducts.

**Lobes** Rounded structures of the mammary gland.

TABLE 6.1 ▸ Hormones contributing to breast development and lactation

| HORMONE | ROLE IN LACTATION | STAGE OF LACTATION |
|---|---|---|
| Estrogen | Ductal growth | Mammary gland differentiation with menstruation |
| Progesterone | Alveolar development | After onset of menses and during pregnancy |
| Human growth hormone | Development of terminal end buds | Mammary gland development |
| Human placental lactogen | Alveolar development | Pregnancy |
| Prolactin | Alveolar development and milk secretion | Pregnancy and breastfeeding (from the third trimester of pregnancy to weaning) |
| Oxytocin | Letdown: ejection of milk from myoepithelial cells | From the onset of milk secretion to weaning |



(Illustration 6.2). Estrogen stimulates development of the glands that will make milk. Progesterone allows the tubules to elongate and the cells that line the tubules (epithelial cells) to duplicate.

## Lactogenesis

Breast milk production, or ***lactogenesis***, is classically described as occurring in three stages.[1] The first stage, or lactogenesis I, begins during the last trimester of pregnancy: the second and third stages (lactogenesis II and III) occur after birth. Lactogenesis may be impacted by premature delivery, method of delivery, maternal obesity, diabetes, and other factors. These may explain why mothers who deliver prematurely are often unable to develop a full milk supply (25–35 ounces per day).

- *Lactogenesis I.* During the first stage of milk production, milk begins to form, and the lactose and protein content of milk increase. This stage extends through the first few days postpartum.
- *Lactogenesis II.* This stage begins 2–5 days postpartum and is marked by increased blood flow to the mammary gland. Clinically, it is considered the onset of copious milk secretion, or "when milk comes in." Significant changes in both the milk composition and the quantity of milk that can be produced occur over the first 10 days of the baby's life. Delayed lactogenesis II is associated with failure to sustain breastfeeding.[2]
- *Lactogenesis III.* This stage of breast milk production begins about 10 days after birth and is the stage in which the milk composition becomes stable.[3]

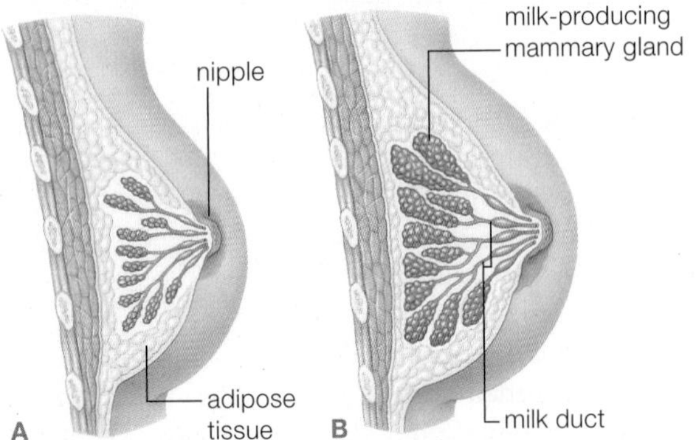


ILLUSTRATION 6.2 ▸ Breast of a mature woman, before pregnancy and during lactation.



## Hormonal Control of Lactation

Prolactin and oxytocin are necessary for establishing and maintaining a milk supply (Table 6.1). ***Prolactin*** is a hormone that stimulates milk production. Suckling is a major stimulator of prolactin secretion: prolactin levels double with suckling.[4] Stress, sleep, and sexual intercourse also stimulate prolactin levels. To allow the mother's body to prepare for milk production during the last three months of pregnancy without making milk, prolactin activity is suppressed by a prolactin-inhibiting factor that is released by the hypothalamus. The actual level of prolactin in the blood is not related to the amount of milk made, but prolactin is necessary for milk synthesis to occur.[5]

Oxytocin release is also stimulated by suckling or nipple stimulation. Its main role is in letdown, or the ejection of milk from the milk gland (***acinus***) into the milk ducts. Women may experience tingling or sometimes sharp shooting pain that lasts about a minute and corresponds with contractions in the milk ducts. Oxytocin also acts on the uterus during and after delivery, causing it to contract, seal blood vessels, and shrink its size.

## Secretion of Milk

Although the process of milk production is complex, understanding the basic mechanisms of milk secretion is important to understanding how factors such as nutritional status, supplementation, medications, and disease may affect breastfeeding or milk composition. The secretory

**Lactogenesis** Another term for human milk production.

**Prolactin** A hormone necessary for milk production.

**Acinus** Small sacs lined by cells that produce milk.

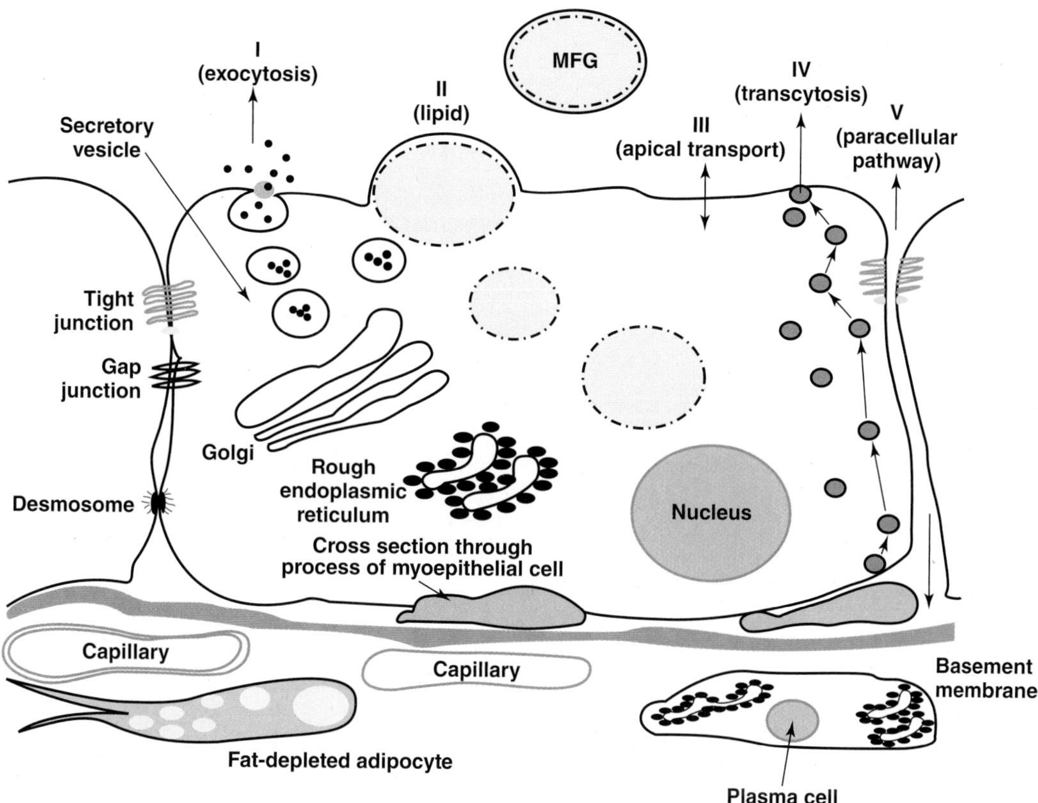


ILLUSTRATION 6.3 ▸ Cellular mechanisms for milk synthesis and secretion.

cell in the breast uses several pathways for milk secretion (Illustration 6.3).[6] Some components like lactose are made in the secretory cells and secreted into ducts (exocytosis). Other components are made in the cell and secreted either with or without protein carriers. Milk fat comes from triglycerides from the mother's blood and from new fatty acids produced in the breast. These fats are made soluble in milk by addition of a protein carrier to form milk-fat globules.[7] The milk-fat globules are then secreted into the ducts. Other components originate in the mothers blood and are then secreted (pinocytosis-exocytosis). For example, immunoglobulin A and other plasma proteins are captured from the mother's blood and taken into the alveolar cells.[6] These proteins are then secreted into the milk ducts. Passive diffusion allows water, sodium, potassium, and chloride to pass through alveolar cell membranes in either direction. Other plasma components and leukocytes pass directly between cells (paracellular pathway).

### The Letdown Reflex

The letdown reflex stimulates milk release from the breast. The stimuli from the infant suckling are passed through nerves to the hypothalamus, which responds by promoting oxytocin release from the posterior pituitary gland (Illustration 6.4). The oxytocin causes contraction of the myoepithelial cells surrounding the secretory cells. As a result, milk is released through the ducts, making it available to the infant. Other stimuli, such as hearing a baby cry, sexual arousal, and thinking about nursing, can also cause letdown, and milk will leak from the breasts.

## Human Milk Composition

LO 6.2 Identify similarities and differences in nutrients levels between colostrum and mature human milk, and between mature human milk, whole cow's milk, and human milk substitutes (infant formula).

> "Thus, [our understanding of] the complexity of milk as a system designed to deliver nutrients and nonnutritive messages to the neonate has increased."
>
> —R. G. Jensen, *Handbook of Milk Composition*[7]

Human milk is an elegantly designed natural resource. It is the only food needed by the majority of healthy infants for approximately the first 6 months. The composition of milk is designed not only to nurture, but also to protect infants from infectious and chronic diseases such as celiac disease, inflammatory bowel disease, diabetes, and leukemia.[4,7]

Human milk composition is changeable over a single feeding, over a day, according to the age of the infant or gestation at delivery, with the presence of infection in the breast, with menses, with maternal nutritional status, and by geographical location.

As our ability to measure and identify novel components increases, we recognize that the composition of human milk is complex. Hundreds of components of human milk have been identified, and their nutritive and non-nutritive roles are under investigation.[8] The basic nutrient composition of colostrum and mature milk is provided in Table 6.2.[9] Composition of mature milk with human milk substitutes is provided in Table 6.3. International standards for human milk substitutes are set by the Codex Alimentarius Commission of the Food and Agriculture Organization of the United Nations (FAO) and the World Health Organization.[10] The composition of specific products vary across brand and with time. Their composition can be found on websites maintained by the producers of these products.

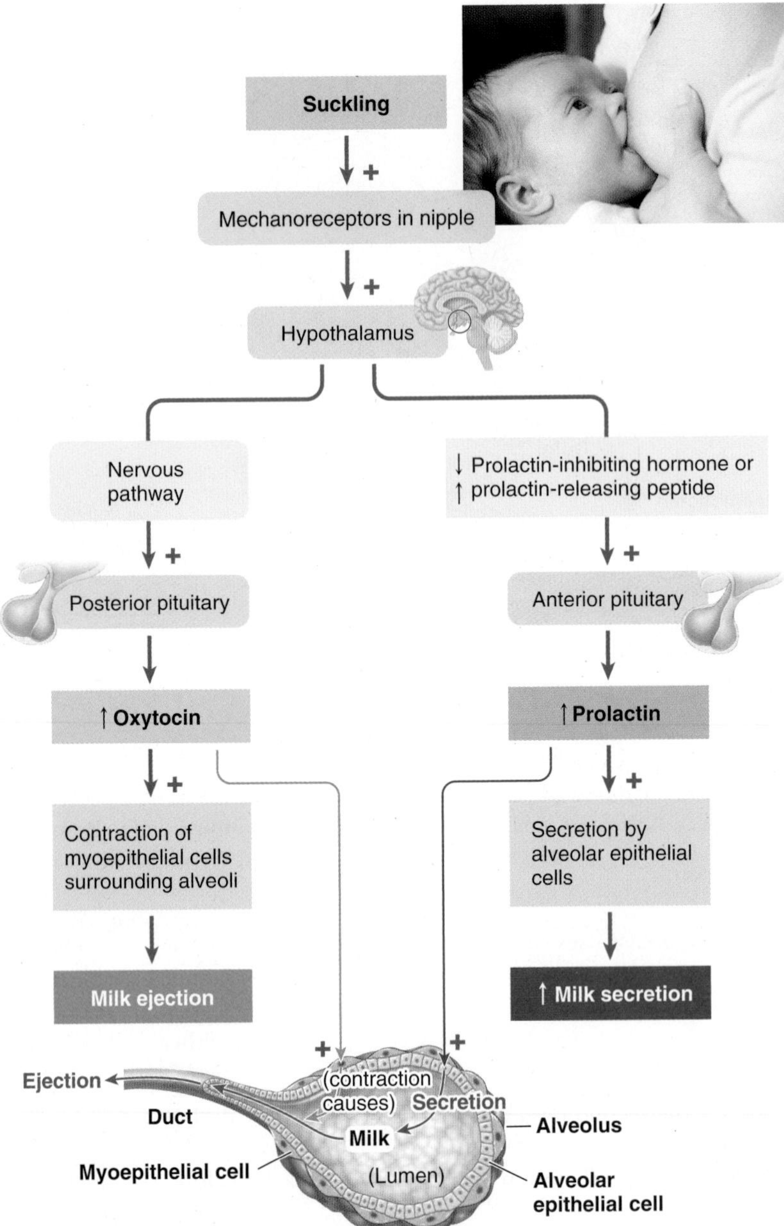


ILLUSTRATION 6.4 ▸ The letdown reflex.

An infant suckling at the breast stimulates the pituitary to release the hormones prolactin and oxytocin.



## Colostrum

The first milk, ***colostrum***, is a thick, often yellow fluid produced during lactogenesis II (days 1–3 after infant birth). Infants may drink only 2 to 10 mL (1.5–2 tsp) of colostrum per feeding in the first 2–3 days. Colostrum provides about 580–700 kcal/L and is higher in protein and lower in carbohydrate and fat than mature milk (produced 2 weeks after infant birth). Secretory immunoglobulin A and lactoferrin are the primary proteins present in colostrum, while other proteins present in mature milk are not present. The concentration of mononuclear cells (a specific type of white blood cell from the mother that provides immune protection) is highest in colostrum. Colostrum has higher concentrations of nutrients including sodium, potassium, vitamin E,[11] carotenoids, and chloride than more mature milk.

## Water

Breast milk is ***isotonic*** with plasma. This biological design of milk means that babies do not need water or other fluids to maintain hydration, even in hot weather.[12] As a major component of human milk, water allows suspension of the milk sugars, proteins, immunoglobulin A, sodium, potassium, citrate, magnesium, calcium, chloride, and water-soluble vitamins.

## Energy

Human milk provides approximately 0.65 kcal/mL, although the energy content varies with its fat (and, to a lesser degree, protein and carbohydrate) composition. Breastfed infants consume fewer calories than infants fed human milk substitute (HMS).[13,14] It is not known whether this difference in energy

**Colostrum** The milk produced in the first 2–3 days after the baby is born. Colostrum is higher in protein and lower in lactose than milk produced after a milk supply is established.

**Isotonic** Similar salt concentration as the blood.

TABLE 6.2 Compositions of 100 mL colostrum (days 1–5 postpartum) and mature milk (day 15 postpartum)

| CONTENTS | COLOSTRUM | MATURE MILK |
|---|---|---|
| Calories (kcal) | 55 | 67 |
| Fat (g) | 2.9 | 4.2 |
| Lactose (g) | 5.3 | 7.0 |
| Total protein (g) | 2.0 | 1.1 |
| Secretory IgA | 0.5[a] | 0.1 |
| Lactoferrin | 0.5 | 0.2 |
| Casein | 0.5 | 0.4 |
| Calcium (mg) | 28 | 30 |
| Sodium (mg) | 48 | 15 |
| Vitamin A (μg retinol equivalents) | 151 | 75 |
| Vitamin $B_1$ (μg) | 2 | 14 |
| Vitamin $B_2$ (μg) | 30 | 40 |
| Vitamin C (μg) | 6 | 5 |

[a] Concentration is considerably higher at 1–3 days postpartum than at days 4 and 5.

SOURCE: Adapted from Prentice A. Constituents of human milk. *Food and Nutrition Bulletin* 17(4), The United Nations University Press. December 1996.[9]

intake of breastfed infants has to do with the composition of human milk versus human milk substitutes, the inability to see the volume of feedings when providing human milk, the differences in the suckling at the breast compared to an artificial nipple, or other factors. Infants who are breastfed are thinner for their weight at 8–11 months than infants fed HMS, but these differences disappear by 12–23 months of age and few differences are notable by 5 years of age.[15]

## Lipids

Lipids are the second largest component of breast milk by concentration (3–5 percent in mature milk). Lipids provide half of the energy of human milk.[7] Human milk fat is low at the beginning of a feeding in foremilk, and higher at the end in the hindmilk that follows.

**Effect of Maternal Diet on Fat Composition** Although the amount of human milk fat does not vary according to maternal diet,[16] the fatty acid profile of human milk reflects variation in the mother's dietary fatty acid intake during pregnancy and postpartum.[17] When a mother is losing weight, the fatty acid profile of her mobilized fat stores is reflected in the milk.[18] When mothers eat very low-fat diets with adequate calories from carbohydrate and protein, more medium-chain fatty acids are synthesized in the breast.

Fat content may vary considerably from mother to mother and may vary diurnally as well as within a feeding. Overall, the energy ranges from 20.9 to 26.2 calories per ounce. Fat values in foremilk range from 39.7–46.7 percent energy (17.9–23.6 kcal/oz) and hindmilk from 60.7–80.1 percent energy (23.5–33.2 kcal/oz).[19]

**DHA** Milk DHA levels are influenced by maternal lipid nutrition.[16,20] DHA is essential for retinal development and accumulates during the last months of pregnancy. The advantages of human milk seem particularly important to premature infants born before 37 weeks, perhaps because the concentrations of DHA are higher in the milk of mothers delivering preterm infants as compared to full-term infants.[21] Among term infants a Norwegian study suggests that cod liver oil supplementation during pregnancy was associated with higher IQ scores at 4 years of age in breastfed versus HMS-fed infants.[22] Cod liver oil contains high levels of DHA as well as high levels of vitamin A and vitamin D, so it should be used with caution.

***Trans* Fatty Acids** *Trans* fatty acids stemming from the mother's diet are present in human milk.[23] *Trans* fat concentrations used to be similar in American and Canadian women, but lower in the milk of women from European and African countries. The reduction of *trans* fatty acids from food products in Canada has led to progressively lower levels of *trans* fat in human milk.[24] A similar reduction is expected in the United States since the Federal Drug Administration ban on trans fats in 2013.

**Cholesterol** Cholesterol, an essential component of all cell membranes, is needed for growth and replication of cells. Cholesterol concentration ranges from 6.5–18.5 mg/100 mL[25] and varies between women, and from day to day within women.[25,26] Breastfed infants have higher intakes of cholesterol and higher levels of serum cholesterol than infants fed HMS.[27]

## Protein

The protein content of mature human milk is relatively low (0.8–1.0 percent) compared to other mammalian milks, such as cow's milk (Table 6.3). The concentration of proteins synthesized in the breast are more affected by the age of the infant (time since delivery) than maternal intake and maternal serum proteins. Proteins synthesized by the breast are more variable because hormones that regulate gene expression and guide protein synthesis change with time.[28] Despite the relatively low concentration, human milk proteins have important nutritive and non-nutritive value. Proteins and their digestive products, such as peptides, exhibit a variety of antiviral and antimicrobial effects.[29]. Enzymes present in human milk might also provide protection by facilitating actions that prevent inflammation.

**Casein** Casein is the major class of protein in mature milk from women who deliver either at term or preterm.[30] Casein, calcium phosphate, and other ions such as magnesium and citrate appear as an aggregate and are the source of milk's white appearance.[28,31] Casein's digestive products, casein phosphopeptides, keep calcium in soluble form and facilitate its absorption.

TABLE 6.3 ▸ Human and cow's milk and human milk substitute (HMS, or infant formula) composition

| NUTRIENT | UNITS | HUMAN MILK (1 FL OZ) | WHOLE COW'S MILK (1 FL OZ) | NESTLE GOOD START (1 FL OZ) |
|---|---|---|---|---|
| Water | g | 26.95 | 26.94 | 26.69 |
| Energy | kcal | 22 | 19 | 20 |
| Energy | kj | 90 | 78 | 84 |
| Protein | g | 0.32 | 0.96 | 0.44 |
| Total lipids (fat) | g | 1.35 | 0.99 | 1.03 |
| Carbohydrate | g | 2.12 | 1.46 | 2.25 |
| Fiber, total dietary | g | 0.0 | 0.0 | 0 |
| Sugars, total | g | 2.12 | 1.60 | 1.52 |
| **Minerals** | | | | |
| Calcium, Ca | mg | 10 | 34 | 13 |
| Iron, Fe | mg | 0.01 | 0.01 | 0.3 |
| Magnesium, Mg | mg | 1 | 3 | 2 |
| Phosphorus, P | mg | 4 | 26 | 7 |
| Potassium, K | mg | 16 | 40 | 22 |
| Sodium, Na | mg | 5 | 13 | 5 |
| Zinc, Zn | mg | 0.05 | 0.11 | 0.16 |
| Copper, Cu | mg | 0.016 | 0.008 | 0.016 |
| Manganese, Mn | mg | 0.008 | 0.001 | 0.003 |
| Selenium, Se | mcg | 0.6 | 1.1 | 0.4 |
| **Vitamins** | | | | |
| Vitamin C, total ascorbic acid | mg | 1.5 | 0.0 | 1.8 |
| Thiamin | mg | 0.004 | 0.014 | 0.02 |
| Riboflavin | mg | 0.011 | 0.052 | 0.028 |
| Niacin | mg | 0.055 | 0.027 | 0.211 |
| Pantothenic acid | mg | 0.069 | 0.114 | |
| Vitamin $B_6$ | mg | 0.003 | 0.011 | 0.015 |
| Folate, DFE | mcg_DFE | 2 | 2 | 5 |
| Vitamin $B_{12}$ | mcg | 0.02 | 0.14 | 0.07 |
| Vitamin A, RAE | mcg_RAE | 19 | 14 | 18 |
| Vitamin E (alpha tocopherol) | mg | 0.02 | 0.02 | 0.3 |
| Vitamin D | IU | 1 | 16 | 13 |
| Vitamin K (phylloquinone) | mcg | 0.1 | 0.1 | 1.6 |
| **Lipids** | g | 0.619 | 0.569 | 0.448 |
| Saturated fatty acids, total | g | 0.000 | 0.023 | 0.00 |
| 4:0 | g | 0.000 | 0.023 | 0.00 |
| 6:0 | g | 0.000 | 0.023 | 0.00 |
| 8:0 | g | 0.000 | 0.023 | 0.015 |
| 10:0 | g | 0.019 | 0.023 | 0.012 |
| 12:0 | g | 0.079 | 0.023 | 0.104 |
| 14:0 | g | 0.099 | 0.091 | 0.043 |
| 16:0 | g | 0.283 | 0.000 | 0.238 |
| 18:0 | g | 0.090 | 0.253 | 0.037 |
| Monounsaturated fatty acids, total | g | 0.511 | 0.000 | 0.329 |
| Polyunsaturated fatty acids, total | g | 0.153 | 0.000 | 0.226 |
| Cholesterol | mg | 4 | 0.000 | 1 |

| NUTRIENT | UNITS | HUMAN MILK (1 FL OZ) | WHOLE COW'S MILK (1 FL OZ) | NESTLE GOOD START (1 FL OZ) |
|---|---|---|---|---|
| **Amino acids** | | | | |
| Tryptophan | g | 0.005 | 0.022 | |
| Threonine | g | 0.014 | 0.043 | |
| Isoleucine | g | 0.017 | 0.049 | |
| Leucine | g | 0.029 | 0.079 | |
| Lysine | g | 0.021 | 0.042 | |
| Methionine | g | 0.006 | 0.022 | |
| Cystine | g | 0.006 | 0.005 | |
| Phenylalanine | g | 0.014 | 0.044 | |
| Tyrosine | g | 0.016 | 0.045 | |
| Valine | g | 0.019 | 0.057 | |
| Arginine | g | 0.013 | 0.022 | |
| Histidine | g | 0.007 | 0.022 | |
| Alanine | g | 0.011 | 0.031 | |
| Aspartic acid | g | 0.025 | 0.071 | |
| Glutamic acid | g | 0.052 | 0.193 | |
| Glycine | g | 0.008 | 0.022 | |
| Proline | g | 0.025 | 0.102 | |
| Serine | g | 0.013 | 0.032 | |

SOURCE: *US Department of Agriculture, Agricultural Research Service. 2014. USDA National Nutrient Database for Standard Reference, Release. Nutrient Data Laboratory Home Page, http://www.ars.usda.gov/nutrientdata.

**Whey Proteins** Whey proteins are the proteins that remain soluble in water after casein is precipitated from milk by acid or enzymes. Whey proteins include milk and serum proteins, enzymes, and immunoglobulins, among others. Several mineral-, hormone-, or vitamin-binding proteins are also identified as components of whey proteins. These include lactoferrin, which carries iron in a form that is easy to absorb and can inhibit bacterial growth. The enzymes present in whey proteins aid in digestion and protection against bacteria.

**Nonprotein Nitrogen** Nonprotein nitrogen provides 20–25 percent of the nitrogen in milk.[9] Urea accounts for 30–50 percent of nonprotein nitrogen, and nucleotides for 20 percent, depending on the stage of lactation and the diet of the mother. Some of this nitrogen is available for the infant to use for producing nonessential amino acids. Some of the nonprotein nitrogen is used to produce other proteins with biological roles such as hormones, growth factors, free amino acids, nucleic acids, nucleotides, and carnitine. The role of individual nucleotides in human milk is under investigation; however, nucleotides appear to play important roles in growth and disease resistance.

## Milk Carbohydrates

Lactose is the dominant carbohydrate in human milk. Other carbohydrates—including monosaccharides (such as glucose), polysaccharides, oligosaccharides, and protein-bound carbohydrates—are also present.[32] Lactose enhances calcium absorption. As the second largest carbohydrate component, oligosaccharides contribute calories at low ***osmolality***, stimulate the growth of *bifidus* bacteria in the gut, and inhibit the growth of *E. coli* and other potentially harmful bacteria.

**Oligosaccharides** Oligosaccharides are medium-length carbohydrates containing lactose on one end. Oligosaccharides can be free, or bound to proteins as glycoproteins, or bound to lipids as glycolipids, or they can bind to other structures. The conjugated and unconjugated oligosaccharides are classified as glycans. Over 130 different oligosaccharides are present as functional ingredients of human milk.[33,34] Oligosaccharides in human milk prevent the binding of pathogenic microorganisms to the surface receptors of their target cell, thereby preventing infection. Accordingly, oligosaccharides in human milk can be considered part of the innate immune protection provided by breastfeeding.[35]

## Fat-Soluble Vitamins

**Vitamin A** Colostrum has approximately twice the concentration of vitamin A as mature milk does. Some of the vitamin A in human milk is in the form of beta-carotene. Its presence is responsible for the characteristic yellow

**Osmolality** A measure of the concentration of particles in solution.

color of colostrum. In mature milk, vitamin A is present at 75 μg/dL or 280 IU/dL.[36] These levels are adequate to meet infant needs. Although milk levels are influenced by maternal dietary intake, a Cochrane review of clinical trials of vitamin A supplementation failed to demonstrate mortality or morbidity benefit to women or their infant.[37]

**Vitamin D** When maternal dietary intake of vitamin D is adequate, transport of Vitamin D into human milk appears to be adequate to meet infant needs.[38] Most vitamin D in human milk is in the form of 25-OH$_2$ vitamin D and vitamin D$_3$. Maternal exposure to sunlight has been reported to increase the vitamin D$_3$ level in milk tenfold.[38,39] It is yet unknown how much maternal vitamin D supplement is needed to ensure adequate maternal and infant vitamin D status when sunlight exposure is insufficient.[40]

**Vitamin E** It is believed that level of total tocopherols in human milk is related to the milk's fat content (40 μg of vitamin E per gram of lipid[41]). Alpha-tocopherol concentration decreases from colostrum to transitional milk and to mature milk[11], whereas beta and gamma tocopherols remain stable throughout each stage of lactation. The level of vitamin E present in human milk is adequate to meet the needs of full-term infants for muscle and red blood cell integrity. The levels of vitamin E in preterm milk are not considered adequate to meet the needs of preterm infants.[42,43]

**Vitamin K** Vitamin K is present in human milk at levels of 2.3 μg/dL.[41] Approximately 5 percent of breastfed infants are at risk for vitamin K deficiency based on vitamin K–dependent clotting factors. There are cases of vitamin K deficiency among exclusively breastfed infants who did not receive vitamin K at birth.

## Water-Soluble Vitamins

Most water-soluble vitamins in human milk are responsive to the content of the maternal diet or vitamin status (thiamin, riboflavin, vitamin B$_6$, vitamin B$_{12}$, and choline).[44] Milk of well-nourished women in the United States provides these nutrients in quantities meeting the estimated needs for their infants.[45] Rarely, B$_{12}$ deficiency resulting in long-term neurological deficits has been reported in infants whose mothers had poor vitamin B$_{12}$ status relating to vegan diet or pernicious anemia.[46] Folate is bound to whey proteins in human milk; therefore, its content in milk is less influenced by maternal intake of these vitamins than are the other water-soluble vitamins.

## Minerals in Human Milk

The minerals in human milk contribute substantially to the osmolality of human milk. ***Monovalent ion*** secretion is managed closely by the alveolar cells, in balance with lactose, to maintain the isosmotic composition of human milk.

Mineral content in milk is related to the growth rate of the offspring. The mineral content of human milk is much lower than the concentration in cow's milk and the milk of other animals whose offspring grow faster. With the exception of magnesium, the concentration of minerals decreases over the first 4 months postpartum. This decline in the mineral content of milk during the period of rapid growth is not what one would expect, but infant growth is well supported.[47] The lower mineral concentration of human milk is easier for the kidneys to handle. This reduced load on the kidneys is considered a significant benefit of human milk.

**Bioavailability** An important feature of several of the minerals (magnesium, calcium, iron, zinc) in human milk is the packaging that makes them highly available (bioavailable) to the infant.[48] Packaging minerals so that the infant can use them efficiently also reduces the burden to the mother because less of the mineral is needed in the milk. For example, zinc is 49 percent available from human milk, but only 10 percent available from cow's milk and cow's milk–based HMS.[49] Exclusively breastfed infants have little risk of anemia,[50] despite the seemingly low concentration of iron in human milk, but duration of breastfeeding can affect the risk of anemia. One study suggests that infants who are exclusively breastfed for 6.5 months are less likely to be anemic than those nursed exclusively for 5.5 months.[51]

**Zinc** Human milk zinc is bound to protein and is highly available, in comparison to cow's milk and cow's milk–based HMS. Both the zinc intake (per kg) and the zinc requirements of infants decline after the first few months.[52] Human milk zinc levels are maintained even in the face of low maternal zinc intake.[53] Rare cases of zinc deficiency, which appears as dermatitis or intractable diaper rash, have been noted in exclusively breastfed infants, however.[49] A defect in the mammary gland uptake of zinc has been described as the cause of low milk concentration when maternal serum zinc concentrations are normal. In these cases, infants respond to zinc supplementation.

**Trace Minerals** Trace minerals (copper, selenium, chromium, manganese, molybdenum, nickel, and fluorine) are present in the human body in small concentrations and are essential for growth and development. Less is known about trace minerals and infant health than about other nutrients. In general, however, the levels of trace minerals in human milk are not altered by the mother's diet or supplement use, excepting fluoride. The DRI for fluoride is 0.1 mg daily for infants less than 6 months of age.[54] Fluoride provided in community water is safe for breastfeeding women and their infants. Most infants who live in

**Monovalent ion** An atom with an electrical charge of +1 or −1.

areas with fluoridated water do not need an additional supplement.[55–57] When bottled water is the primary source, water with fluoride added should be purchased.

### Taste of Human Milk

> "... too full o' th' milk of human kindness to catch the nearest way."
>
> —Shakespeare's *Macbeth*, Act I, Scene V

This line from Shakespeare reflects the centuries-old belief that a breastfeeding woman's diet influences the composition of her milk and has a long-lasting influence on the child. The flavor of human milk is an important taste experience for newborn infants, but flavor is often ignored when the benefits of human milk or its composition are considered. Human milk is slightly sweet[58] and it carries the flavors of compounds ingested, such as mint, garlic, vanilla, and alcohol.[59]

The transfer of flavor compounds appears to occur selectively and in relatively low amounts.[60] Infant responses to flavors in milk seem to depend on the length of time since the mother consumed the food, and the amount and frequency of the flavor that the mother consumed (new versus repeated exposure). Infants seem more interested in their mother's milk when flavors are new to them. Infants nursed at the breast longer if a flavor (garlic) was new to them than if the mother had taken garlic tablets for several days.[61] Thus, exposing infants to a variety of flavors in human milk may contribute to their interest in and consumption of human milk as well as their acceptance of new flavors in solid foods.[62] As well, the longer an infant was exclusively breastfeed the more she preferred an umami solution at 6 months.[63] Thus breastfeeding duration may influence flavour preference at the onset of complementary feeding.

## Benefits of Breastfeeding

**LO 6.3** Summarize the benefits of breastfeeding for mothers and their babies in a manner that could be included in breastfeeding education for expecting mothers, their partners, and family members.

### Breastfeeding Benefits for Mothers

Breastfeeding women experience hormonal, physical, and psychosocial benefits.[64] Breastfeeding immediately increases levels of oxytocin, a hormone that stimulates uterine contractions, minimizes maternal postpartum blood loss, and helps the uterus to return to nonpregnant size.

After the birth, the return of fertility (through monthly ovulation) is delayed in most women during breastfeeding, particularly with exclusive breastfeeding. This delay in ovulation results in longer intervals between pregnancies. Breastfeeding alone, however, is not as effective as other available birth control methods. Consequently, many health care professionals in the United States do not promote breastfeeding as an option for birth control.

Many women experience psychological benefits, including increased self-confidence and facilitated bonding with their infants.[65] Many still consider faster return to prepregnancy weight a benefit of breastfeeding; however, women may lose or gain weight while nursing. The impact of breastfeeding on maternal weight is discussed in more detail later in this chapter. In addition to these short-term benefits, women who nurse at a younger age and for longer duration may have lower risk of breast and ovarian cancer[64] and rheumatoid arthritis.[66]

### Breastfeeding Benefits for Infants

> "Breastfeeding—the main source of active and passive immunity in the vulnerable early months and years of life—is considered to be the most effective preventive means of reducing the death rate of children under five."[767]
>
> —Labbok, M. H., Clark, D., and Goldman, A. S. Breastfeeding: maintaining an irreplaceable immunological resource. *Nature Reviews Immunology.* 2004; 4(Jul):565–572.

**Nutritional Benefits** The value of the composition of human milk is widely recognized. Companies that make HMS often use human milk as the standard, recognizing the many unique properties of human milk:

- With its dynamic composition and the appropriate balance of nutrients, human milk provides optimal nutrition to the infant.
- The balance of nutrients in human milk matches human infant requirements for growth and development closely; no other animal milk or HMS meets infant needs as well.
- Human milk is isosmotic (of similar ion concentration; in this case, human milk and plasma are of similar ion concentration) and therefore meets the requirements for infants without other forms of food or water.
- The relatively low protein content of breast milk compared to cow's milk meets the infant's needs without overloading the immature kidneys with nitrogen.
- Whey protein in human milk forms a soft, easily digestible curd.

- Human milk provides generous amounts of lipids in the form of essential fatty acids, saturated fatty acids, medium-chain triglycerides, and cholesterol.
- Long-chain polyunsaturated fatty acids, especially docosahexaenoic acid (DHA), which promotes optimal development of the central nervous system, are present in human milk but are present in only some of the HMS marketed in the United States.
- Minerals in breast milk are largely protein bound and balanced to enhance their availability and meet infant needs with minimal demand on maternal reserves.

**Immunological Benefits** One of the most important realizations about breastfeeding in the last few decades is that human milk provides protection against infection. Cells (T- and B-lymphocytes), secretory immunoglobins (sIgA, sIgG, sIgM, sIgE, sIgD), histocompatibility antigens, T-cell products, many nonspecific factors (e.g., complement, bifidus factor), carrier proteins (lactoferrin, transferring, vitamin $B_{12}$-binding protein, and corticoid-binding protein), and enzymes (lysozyme, lipoprotein lipase, leukocyte enzymes) are components of milk that confer immunological benefits.

Cellular components in human milk (***macrophages, neutrophils, T- and B-lymphocytes***, and ***epithelial cells***) are especially high in colostrum but are also present for months in mature human milk in lower concentrations. The function of macrophages in human milk includes phagocytosis of fungi and bacteria, killing of bacteria, and production of the complement proteins, lysozyme, and lactoferrin and immunoglobin A and G.[4]

Leukocyte function appears to offer more protection to the breast than to immunocompetence of the infant. Neutrophils, however, appear to be activated and contribute to phagocytosis at the mucosa of the infant's gastrointestinal tract.[68] Both T- and B-lymphocytes provide the infant with protection against organisms in the gastrointestinal tract. This protection may extend beyond acute infection to allergy, necrotizing enterocolitis, tuberculosis, and neonatal meningitis.[4]

Immunoglobins are transported from maternal plasma across secretory epithelium to become secretory immunoglobins. The predominant (90 percent) immunoglobulin in human milk, ***secretory immunoglobin A (sIgA)***, also appears to be most important in terms of the protection conferred to the infant. Immunoglobins sIgA and sIgM protect the infant by blocking colonization with pathogens and limiting the number of antigens that cross the mucosal barrier. sIgA protects against enteroviruses, cytomegalovirus, herpes simplex virus, respiratory syncytial virus, rubella, retrovirus, and rotavirus[4] and sIgM protects against cytomegalovirus, respiratory syncytial virus, and rubella.

Bifidus factor is a growth factor (probably a carbohydrate) that supports growth of *Lactobacillus bifidus. Lactobacillus* is a probiotic bacterium that stimulates antibody production and enhances phagocytosis of antigens.[4]

Lysozyme protects against enterobacteria and other gram-positive bacteria. Lysozyme is secreted by neutrophils and macrophages.

Binding proteins in human milk bind iron and vitamin $B_{12}$, making the nutrients unavailable for pathogens to grow in the infant's gastrointestinal tract. Such factors are also responsible for some of the differences in intestinal flora (natural bacteria of the gastrointestinal tract) of breastfed infants versus HMS-fed infants.

Individual fatty acids and other milk components (oligosaccharides, gangliosides, and glycoconjugates) resulting from digestion of human milk are antimicrobial.[68,69] The digestive products of triacylglycerides and the lipid globule appear to protect against *Escherichia coli* 0157:H7, *Campylobacter jejuni, Listeria monocytogenes*, and *Clostridium perfringens*.[70] Monoacylglycerides are able to lyse enveloped viruses, bacteria, and protozoa. Glycoconjugates (glycoproteins, glycolipids, glycoaminoglycans, and oligosaccharides) may bind pathogens directly, thus preventing infection. Nucleotides are reported to increase resistance to *Staphylococcus aureus* and *Candida albicans* and may increase response to vaccine antigens.[71]

Growth factors and hormones in human milk, such as insulin, enhance the maturation of the infant's gastrointestinal tract. These substances also help to protect the infant, especially neonates, against viral and bacterial pathogens.

**Lower Infant Mortality** In the developing world, improving breastfeeding practices could prevent more than 1 million deaths annually. This protection of lives is at the center of the World Health Organization's (WHO) and UNICEF's joint effort, called the Global Strategy for Infant and Young Child Feeding, to remind the international community of the impact of feeding practices (including breastfeeding) on children's health outcomes.[72]

Breastfeeding to any duration and to any extent reduces the risk of sudden infant death syndrome (SIDS).[73] A meta-analysis of 18 studies demonstrated a 60 percent reduction in risk of SIDS with any level of breastfeeding, although the influence was greater with exclusive breastfeeding and

**Macrophages** A white blood cell that acts mainly through phagocytosis.

**Neutrophils** Class of white blood cells that are involved in the protection against infection.

**T-lymphocyte** A white blood cell that is active in fighting infection. (May also be called T-cell; the t in T-cell stands for thymus.) These cells coordinate the immune system by secreting hormones that act on other cells.

**B-lymphocytes** White blood cells that are responsible for producing immunoglobulins.

**Epithelial cells** Cells that line the surface of the body.

**Secretory immunoglobin A** A protein found in secretions that protect the body's mucosal surfaces from infections. The mode of action may be by reducing the binding of a microorganism with cells lining the digestive tract. It is present in human colostrum but not transferred across the placenta.

greater duration. This analysis suggests that breastfeeding was an independent factor associated with reduction in risk. These results are consistent with the American Academy of Pediatrics' recommendation of breastfeeding exclusively for 4 to 6 months where no contraindications are present.[74]

**Fewer Acute Illnesses** Breastfeeding reduces infant illness in countries with high infant illness (***morbidity***) and death (***mortality***) rates, poor sanitation, and questionable water supplies. Even in the United States and other developed nations, where modern health care systems, safe water, and proper sanitation are commonplace, there is a clear relationship between breastfeeding and reduced rates of illness in infants. Exclusive breastfeeding for 4 months is associated with reduced gastrointestinal illness with effects lasting for 2 months after weaning.[74] Ear infections are 23 percent lower, with a reduction in risk of 50 percent for infants breastfed longer than 3 months. The risk of hospitalization for lower respiratory infections is 72 percent lower among infants exclusively breastfeed for more than 4 months when compared to infants fed HMS. These results support the current public health recommendations for breastfeeding.

**Reductions in Chronic Illness** In addition to the lower rate of acute illnesses in breastfed children, breastfeeding also seems to protect against chronic childhood diseases including celiac disease, inflammatory bowel disease, diabetes, and leukemia.[73] Risk of asthma, atopic dermatitis, and eczema is reduced among infants with a family history who are breastfed for 3 to 4 months.[64,75,76]

**Breastfeeding and Childhood Weight** Considerable attention has been paid to the role of breastfeeding in preventing obesity, but this relationship is still a topic of active investigation. Breastfed infants typically are leaner than HMS-fed infants at one year of age without any difference in activity level or development.[76,77] Several potential mechanisms have been identified for the modest reduction in obesity in children who were breastfed, including metabolic programming, possibly related to leptin, ghrelin, and other neurometabolic messengers delivered in human milk.[81,78] Other contributors could include learned self-regulation of energy intake and other characteristics of the families or parents, such as healthy lifestyle. Accordingly, the influence of breastfeeding usually disappears by age 5.

**Cognitive Benefits** Breastfeeding, and especially duration of breastfeeding, is associated with cognitive benefits, assessed by intelligence quotient (IQ).[74] The increases in cognitive ability associated with breastfeeding are significant even after adjusting for family environment.[79] A recent randomized study comparing breastfed infants to those fed cows' milk and soy milk–based HMS found all groups scored within normal ranges, but breastfed infants scored slightly higher. In addition, higher IQ of infants breastfed for six months appears to be more prevalent among infants born small for gestational age (11 points) than among infants born appropriate weight for age (3 points)[80,81] The differences in ***cognitive function*** are also greater in premature infants fed human milk than in those fed HMS.[85,82] Recognition that the fatty acid composition of milk plays an important role in neuropsychological development bolsters the credibility of psychological or cognitive benefits from breastfeeding.

**Analgesic Effects** Breastfeeding seems to work as an analgesic in infants. Breastfeeding during venipuncture seems to reduce infant pain as well as a 30 percent glucose solution followed by pacifier use.[82] Breastfeeding may be used to comfort infants during minor invasive procedures.[83]

### Benefits

The economic cost of not breastfeeding is staggering. A decrease in medical care for breastfed infants is the primary socioeconomic benefit of breastfeeding. A 2001 study estimated that the United States could have saved $13 billion and 911 lives, mostly infants, if 90 percent of infants were breastfed.[84] This estimate was based on the breastfeeding-related reduction in necrotizing enterocolitis, otitis media, gastroenteritis, hospitalization for lower respiratory tract infections, atopic dermatitis, sudden infant death syndrome, childhood asthma, childhood leukemia, type 1 diabetes mellitus, and childhood obesity. In Louisiana alone, the estimate of savings was in excess of $216 million and 18 lives if 90 percent of infants in that state were breastfed.[85] Companies benefit through lower medical costs and greater employee productivity. A $1 investment in creating a lactation support program provides two to three times the return.[86]

# Breast Milk Supply and Demand

**LO 6.4** Generate an education plan for new mothers that includes the answers to common questions about milk supply, including what is typical milk production, what is the relationship between infant demand and maternal supply, and the influence of the size of the breast, feeding frequency, pumping, and breast surgeries on milk production.

### Can Women Make Enough Milk?

Typical milk production averages approximately 600 mL (240 mL = 1 cup, or 8 oz) in the first month postpartum and continues to increase

**Morbidity** The rate of illnesses in a population.

**Mortality** Rate of death.

**Cognitive function** The process of thinking.

to approximately 750–800 mL per day by 4–5 months postpartum.[14,87] Milk production can range from 450–1200 mL per day in women who are nursing one infant.[14] Infant weight, the caloric density of milk, and the infant's age contribute significantly to the infant demand for milk. Milk increases to meet the demand of twins, triplets, or infants and toddlers suckling simultaneously; it can also be increased by pumping the milk.

Traditionally, factors such as how vigorously an infant nurses, how much time the infant is at the breast, and how many times he or she nurses in a day were thought to control milk production. We now know that milk synthesis (rate of accumulation of milk in the breast) is related to infant demand.[88-90] That is, the removal of milk from the breast seems to be the signal to make more milk, and most women are able to increase their milk production to meet infant demand.[91]

An average of 24 percent of milk is left in the breast after feeding.[92] Thus, the short-term milk storage of the breast does not seem to be a limiting factor to infant milk intake. The average rate of synthesis in a day is only 64 percent of the highest rate of milk synthesis, suggesting that milk synthesis could be increased considerably. Comparisons of milk production between mothers of singletons and twins show that the breasts have the capacity to synthesize much more than a singleton infant usually drinks.

## Does the Size of the Breast Limit a Woman's Ability to Nurse Her Infant?

The size of a woman's breast does not determine the amount of milk production tissue (clusters of alveoli containing secretory cells that produce the milk).[89] Much of the variation in breast size is due to the amount of fat in the breast. The size of the breast does limit storage because of limitations in the expansion of the ducts. Daily milk production is not related to the total milk storage capacity within the breast, however.[92] This means that women with small breasts can produce the same amount of milk as women with large breasts, although the latter woman may be able to feed her infant less frequently to deliver the same volume of milk compared with a woman with smaller breasts.

## Is Feeding Frequency Related to the Amount of Milk a Woman Can Make?

Feeding frequency is not consistently related to milk production. The rate of milk synthesis is highly variable between breasts and between feedings.[93] However, the amount of milk produced in 24 hours and the total milk withdrawn in that 24-hour period are highly related.[92] Milk synthesis is able to quickly respond to infant demand.

The breast responds to the degree of emptying during a feeding, and this response is a link between maternal milk supply and infant demand. Daly proposed that the breast responds to the infant's need by measuring how completely the infant empties the breast.[92,93] For example, if a lot of milk is left in the breast, then milk synthesis will be low to prevent engorgement; if the breast is fully emptied, synthesis will be high to replenish the milk supply.

Exact mechanisms of milk supply and demand are not well understood, but they seem to be related to a protein called feedback inhibitor of lactation (FIL).[93] FIL is an active whey protein that inhibits milk secretion. This protein inhibits all milk components equally according to their concentration in milk. Therefore, this protein seems to affect milk quantity only, not milk composition.

## Can Women Pump or Express Enough Milk?

Pumping or expressing milk may be needed for many reasons, including maternal or infant illness or separation. Women can express milk using several different methods: manually, hand pumps, commercial electric pumps, or hospital-grade electric pumps. A pump that allows mothers to pump both breasts at the same time (10 minutes per session) can save time over single pumping (20 minutes per session).[94] Electric pumps are efficient and may increase prolactin more than hand expression or hand pumping.[94] Insufficient milk production is a common problem among women who express milk. Researchers working with women who pumped their breasts report that 8 to 12 or more milk expressions per day were necessary to stimulate an adequate production of milk. The optimal number of expressions in a 24-hour period is likely to differ for women according to how well they empty the breast and the storage capacity of the breast. Women who are able to establish an adequate volume of milk (500 mL per day) in the first 2 weeks postpartum are more likely to still have enough milk for their infant at 4–5 weeks postpartum. This recommendation is consistent with the advice to nurse the infant (or pump) early and often to build a good milk supply. See the section in Chapter 7, "Human Milk Collection and Storage," for information on storage of milk.

## Can Women Breastfeed after Breast Reduction or Augmentation Surgery?

Information regarding breastfeeding rates after breast surgery is scarce. Accumulating evidence does suggest that women who undergo breast reduction surgery may be at risk for unsuccessful lactation, as evidenced by lower breastfeeding rates and duration and greater perception of insufficient milk supply than among women without prior breast surgery. Almost all (91.8 percent) women with prior breast reduction surgery reported problems with breastfeeding.[95,96] The type of surgery, including the location and amount of breast tissue removed and the damage to remaining tissue, appears to be an important determinant of ability to breastfeed. Women may choose to have an incision around the lower part of the breast to avoid damage to the ductal system caused by incision in the midst

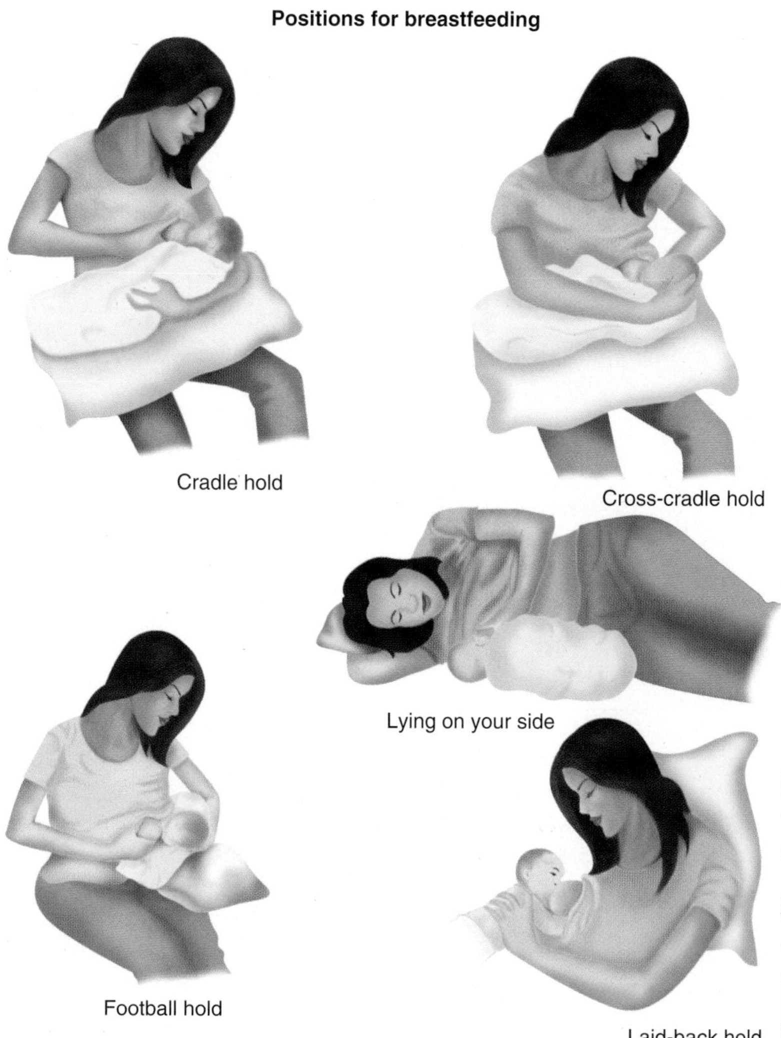



ILLUSTRATION 6.5 ▸ Breastfeeding Positioning

of the breast. Women with periareolar (around the nipple) incisions experience greater difficulties with breastfeeding because of damage to the ductal system.[97] After augmentation surgery, compression of the ducts in the breast may lead to poor milk production. Lactation consultants recommend that the surgery date, type, and incision used, as well as prior breastfeeding experience, be ascertained. Infants should be closely followed to prompt intervention when needed.

Breast implants are not a contraindication to breastfeeding. Nearly a million women in the United States have breast implants containing silicone. Early reports introduced concern of esophageal dysfunction in children of women who had silicone implants, but more recent research found no evidence to support such claims, and silicone concentrations in milk from women with implants are not elevated and, in fact, are lower than those in formula and cow's milk.[98] It is possible that immunological responses could cause unfavorable effects; however, there is no evidence suggesting direct toxicity to the infant. Therefore, the most likely influence on breastfeeding is similar to the effects of saline implants: compression of ducts leading to poor milk production.

# The Breastfeeding Process

LO 6.5 Describe maternal steps to prepare the breast, and the basic position of the infant at the breast.

## Preparing the Breast for Breastfeeding

Breasts and nipples begin to be sore in the first trimester of pregnancy, but the tenderness usually subsides by the end of the first trimester. Enlargement of the breast and nipple are evident by the end of the first trimester and continue through pregnancy. By the third trimester, Montgomery glands, sebaceous glands that produce oils to lubricate the nipple and areola, become pronounced and the nipples darken. Gentle massage is recommended by the La Leche League to get women accustomed to handing their breasts and to prepare them for expressing milk. Women with flat or inverted nipples may be instructed on the Hoffman technique to break up adhesions. The thumbs are placed opposite each other at the base of the nipple and thumbs are simultaneously pressed in and away from each other. This procedure is repeated with the position of the thumbs varied around the nipple. Women should understand that breasts may leak milk prior to delivery. Anecdotal reports include milk leaking as early as 20 weeks of pregnancy.

## Breastfeeding Positioning

Proper positioning of the infant at the breast is important to breastfeeding success. Mothers need to learn from health professionals experienced in optimal positioning, because improper positioning causes pain and possible damage to nipple and breast tissue. The mother may need to use cushions, pillows, or a footstool to be comfortable and positioned well to nurse the infant (Illustration 6.5).

## Presenting the Breast to the Suckling Infant

Women use their hand to shape and position the breast so that the infant can easily latch. The grasp should allow the infant to place a sufficient amount of the areola into his or her mouth. For palmar grasp, the mother places her thumb above the areola, and remaining fingers are placed under the breast to form a C or *V*. A scissor grasp, placement of her thumb and index finger above the areola with the remaining three fingers below, may also be used. It is important to note that the nipple is not tipped upward when the breast is presented to the infant to avoid improper latch-on and nipple abrasion.

Once the mother is comfortable, she should hold the baby so the mouth is directly in front of the nipple and stimulate the oral search reflex by touching the baby's bottom lip with her nipple. Then the infant will open his or her mouth wide and should be brought to the breast with the nipple centered in the mouth (Illustration 6.6). This process is called *latching on*. Infants who are properly attached at the breast have all or most of the areola in their mouth. If the mother pulls down the infant's lower lip, she should see the tongue lying around the lower gum line. The baby's nose should be close to the breast, with breathing unrestricted. The mother should hear swallowing, but not smacking, clicking, or slurping. Women who consistently have pain when the infant is suckling should consult a professional trained in lactation to correct the attachment position.[99] Infants who are positioned correctly at the breast start to suckle almost immediately, change from quick short sucks to slow deep sucks, and remain relaxed.

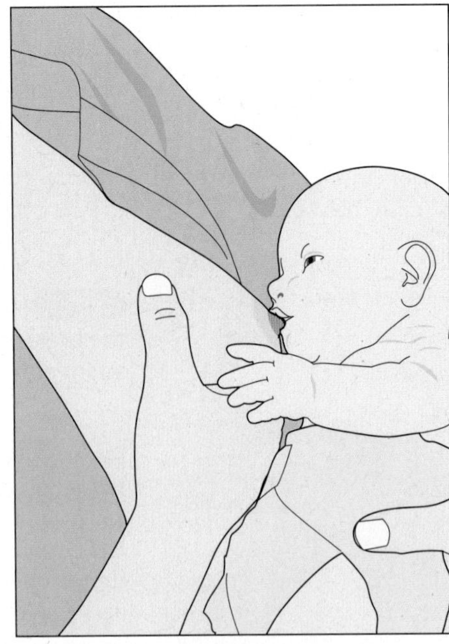

**a.** Touching the baby's bottom lip with the nipple stimulates the oral search reflex.

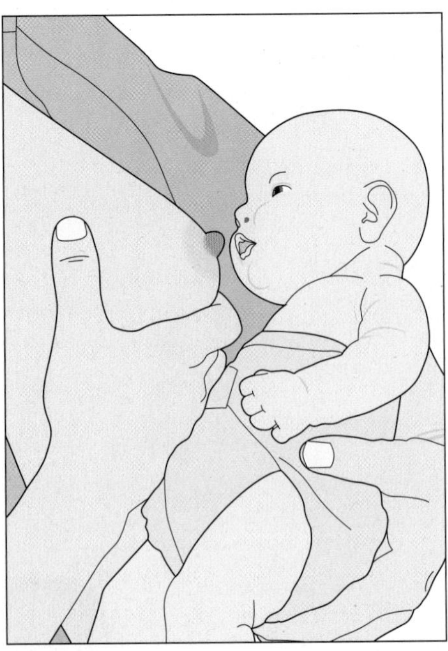

**b.** The infant opens his mouth wide.

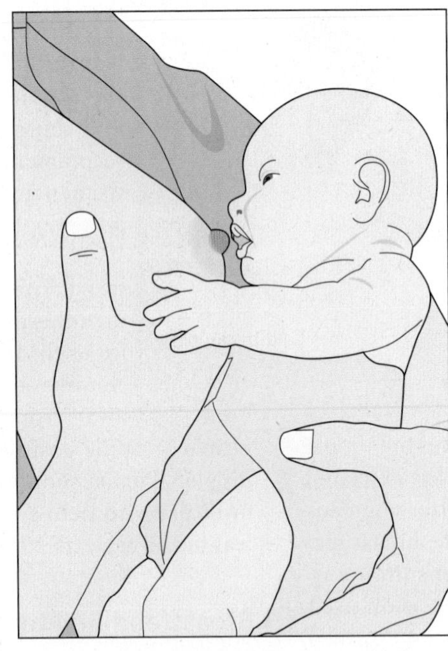

**c.** The infant is brought to the breast with the nipple centered in his mouth.

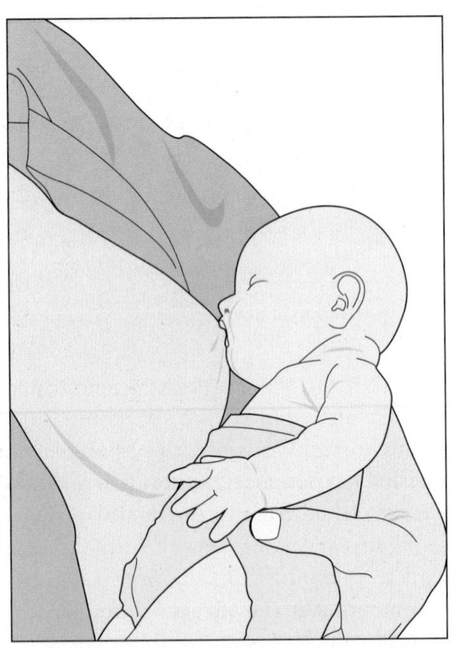

**d.** The infant is properly latched at the breast and has all of the areola in his mouth.



ILLUSTRATION 6.6 ▸ Attachment

# The Breastfeeding Infant

LO 6.6 Describe infant behaviors that indicate readiness to feed, and vitamin supplement recommendations for breastfeeding infants.

## Infant Reflexes

Healthy-term infants are born with several reflexes that enable them to nourish themselves. Observations show that 18-week-old fetuses start sucking. By 34 weeks' gestation, the suck has adequate pace and rhythm to be nutritive. The gag reflex is the reflex that prevents taking food and fluids into the lungs. This reflex is developed by 28 weeks' gestation. These reflexes allow term infants to suck and swallow in a coordinated pattern that protects the airways.

Two other reflexes describe the infant's ability to position herself to breastfeed. The *oral search reflex* is described as the infant opening his or her mouth wide in proximity to

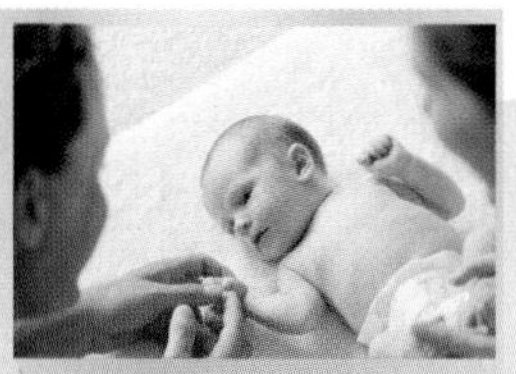
Kaz Mori/The Image Bank/Getty Images

# CASE STUDY 6.1

## Breastfeeding and Adequate Nourishment

Molly G. is a 24-year-old office manager and part-time aerobics instructor who has delivered vaginally, without complications, a healthy, full-term son, Daniel. With a birthweight of 3200 grams (7 lb), Daniel is the first child for Molly and her husband. Molly is 162 cm (5 ft 4 in) tall with a prepregancy weight of 56.8 kg (125 lb). She gained 25 kg (55 lb) during her uncomplicated pregnancy and has been a lacto-ovo vegetarian for 5 years. After a 12-hour stay in a birthing center, Molly and her husband bring Daniel home.

At 4 days postpartum, Molly, her husband, and her mother-in-law bring the baby to the health care center for his first follow-up visit. Molly and her husband are very concerned about whether their son is getting adequate nourishment, so the dietitian is called to see the family. During nutrition assessment, the following information is documented. Daniel weighs 3,000 grams (6 lb 6 oz). The parents report that Daniel nurses vigorously about every 1½ to 2 hours and never sleeps for more than a couple of hours. Molly says that her milk "came in" on the second postpartum day and that she feels like all she does is nurse. Her nipples are tender, but not uncomfortably sore. She reports that Daniel has at least six to eight wet diapers and two to three very loose stools each day. She wonders if she has enough milk and worries about how she will ever return to work in 2 months. She also wants to lose the excess weight she gained during the pregnancy and is eager to return to her aerobics classes. Her husband and mother-in-law are supportive, but they worry about the baby.

The dietitian's nutrition assessment of the infant concludes that Daniel is a healthy infant with no nutritional problems. The family is referred to their pediatrician for further follow-up.

### Questions

1. What factors put Molly at high risk for early termination of breastfeeding?
2. What factors indicate that Daniel is getting adequate nourishment?
3. What concerns do you have about Molly's diet? What advice would you give her about her weight-loss plans and eagerness to return to exercise? Do Molly or Daniel need any vitamin/mineral supplements?
4. If Molly lived in your community, what resources would be available for help and support for breastfeeding mothers?
5. What steps can Molly take to continue successful breastfeeding when she returns to work in 2 months?

(Answers are located in the Instructor's Manual for the 6th edition of *Nutrition Through the Life Cycle.*)

the breast while thrusting the tongue forward. The *rooting reflex* results in the infant turning to the side when stimulated on the side of the upper or lower lip. Infants come forward, open their mouth, and extend the tongue when the center of either the upper or lower lip is stimulated.

The presence of these reflexes is important to the success of breastfeeding. However, successful nursing also requires appropriate positioning of the infant at the breast and adequate maternal letdown and milk production. Appropriate positioning and maternal assessment of infant nursing behaviors must be learned. Support from lactation consultants and/or other health care professionals who are trained in lactation may be necessary.

## Mechanics of Breastfeeding

During feeding, suction created within the baby's mouth causes the mother's nipple and areola to elongate and form a teat. The baby's jaw moves her tongue toward the areola, compressing it and causing milk to travel from the milk ducts to the infant's mouth. The baby then raises the anterior portion of the tongue to complete the process. Afterward, the baby depresses and retracts the posterior portion of her tongue in peristaltic motions, forming a groove in the tongue that channels milk to the back of the oral cavity. This backward movement of the tongue creates a negative pressure, allowing milk to be delivered into the baby's mouth. Receptors in the back of the oral cavity are stimulated and initiate the swallowing reflex. A correctly placed nipple does not move in the baby's mouth during suckling.

## Identifying Hunger and Satiety

When infants are hungry, they begin to bring their hands to their mouth, suck on them, and start moving their head from side to side with their mouth open (rooting reflex). Infants should be fed when these signs of hunger are displayed rather than waiting for crying, a late sign of hunger. Recognizing early hunger behaviors and initiating feeding before the infant becomes very upset helps mothers and infants who have difficulty nursing.

Nutritive and non-nutritive sucks are different. Feedings begin with non-nutritive sucking. The infant sucks quickly and not particularly rhythmically. Nutritive sucking is slower and more rhythmic as the infant begins to suck and swallow. A mother can hear the infant suck in a quiet room.

Infants should be allowed to nurse as long as they want at one breast. Infants who are fed for shorter periods from both breasts can get larger amounts of foremilk. The high lactose content of foremilk can cause diarrhea.[99,100] Allowing the infant to nurse at one breast until satisfied creates a pattern that assures that the infant gets both foremilk and hindmilk. Infants who fall asleep before they empty the breast can be kept awake by gently tickling the feet, rubbing the head, and talking to the baby.

The higher fat content of hindmilk may help in signaling satiety. Infants will stop nursing when full. If they are still hungry, after burping, they can be offered the other breast.

## Feeding Frequency

Stomach emptying occurs in about 1½ hours for breastfed infants. Ten to 12 feedings per day are normal for newborn infants. Different feeding patterns can meet infant needs. In one study, infants who did not feed from midnight through early morning consumed more in the other feedings, particularly in the morning. Milk intake and weight gain of these infants in the first 4 months of life were similar to those of infants whose feedings were distributed over 24 hours.[101]

## Identifying Breastfeeding Malnutrition

A normal newborn weight loss of up to 7 percent can occur in the first 5 days, but no further weight loss should occur[74]. Malnourished infants become sleepy and nonresponsive, and they have a weak cry and few wet diapers. By the fifth to seventh day postpartum, infants who are getting adequate nourishment (8–12 feedings per day) have wet diapers approximately six times a day and have three to four soft, yellowish stools per day. Their urine is pale yellow and dilute, while stools are loose and seedy (some small particles are present in the stool). Infants who are slow gainers and not malnourished are alert, bright, responsive, and develop normally. In contrast, infants who are failing to thrive are apathetic, hard to arouse, and have a weak cry. They have few wet diapers, and their urine is concentrated. Their stools are infrequent.

Mothers of slow-gaining infants in particular should be advised to let the infant nurse at one breast until it is empty or the infant stops nursing, rather than switching breasts after a specific amount of time. This regimen assures that the infant gets hindmilk with a higher fat and calorie content.

## Tooth Decay

Human milk has infection-fighting components that inhibit the formation of dental caries. Nevertheless, caries can occur in children who are breastfed.[102,103] Frequent nursing at night after 1 year of age is a risk factor for dental caries. Nevertheless, the prevention of dental caries is not justification for advising early weaning. Rather, the mother should be instructed on the prevention and treatment of early childhood dental caries. All children should be seen by a qualified dentist 6 months after the first tooth erupts or by 12 months of age. Mothers are the primary source of bacteria that cause early childhood caries. Therefore, mothers or primary caregivers should be given information on oral hygiene, diet, fluoride, caries removal, and prevention of caries.

Breastfed babies may have straighter teeth due to the development of a well-rounded dental arch.[103,104] A well-rounded arch may also help prevent sleep apnea later in life.

## Vitamin Supplements for Breastfeeding Infants

All infants, whether they are fed human milk or HMS, are vulnerable to vitamin K–deficiency bleeding (VKDB). All infants in the United States receive a vitamin K supplement (0.5–1.0 mg by injection) at birth because it is known to decrease the risk of VKDB.[105,25]

Exclusively breastfed infants should be given a supplement of 400 IU of vitamin D per day beginning in the first 2 months of life.[106,107] A minimum intake of 600 IU of vitamin D supplementation should be achieved by age 1 and maintained.[108]

Routine fluoride supplements are not needed by breastfed infants during the first 6 months of life.[74] After 6 months, the decision to supplement with fluoride should be made based on individual situations. If the water, food, and toothpaste contains less than 0.3 ppm fluoride, then supplemental fluoride is recommended. When supplementation is indicated for breastfed infants, maternal supplementation may be the best route.

Breastfed infants born at term do not need iron-fortified HMS or supplements be-cause they rarely experience iron deficiency.[74] The excess iron in HMS might bind with lactoferrin in human milk, resulting in a loss of the protective activity of lactoferrin.

# Maternal Diet

LO 6.7 First, identify the professional and government sources of nutrient recommendations for healthy women for diet and supplements. Second, list common nutrition diagnoses for breastfeeding women, coupled with nutrition intervention and appropriate parameters for monitoring.

The U.S. Dietary Guidelines recommendations on healthy eating patterns (presented in Chapter 1) have been adapted for pregnant and breastfeeding women. The Dietary Guidelines indicate that moderate weight reduction can be achieved by the breastfeeding mother without compromising the weight gain of the nursing infant by consuming a healthy variety of foods.[109]

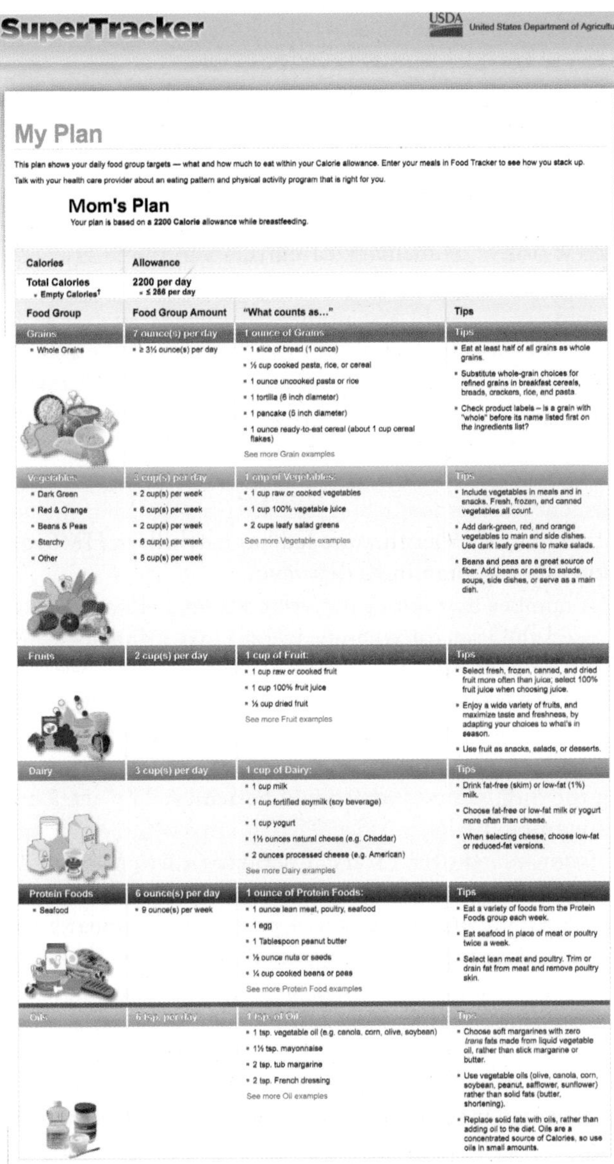

SuperTracker — USDA United States Department of Agriculture

**My Plan**

This plan shows your daily food group targets — what and how much to eat within your Calorie allowance. Enter your meals in Food Tracker to see how you stack up.

Talk with your health care provider about an eating pattern and physical activity program that is right for you.

**Mom's Plan**

Your plan is based on a **2200 Calorie** allowance while breastfeeding.

| Calories | Allowance | | |
|---|---|---|---|
| **Total Calories**<br>• Empty Calories† | **2200 per day**<br>• ≤ 266 per day | | |
| **Food Group** | **Food Group Amount** | **"What counts as..."** | **Tips** |
| **Grains** | **7 ounce(s) per day** | **1 ounce of Grains** | **Tips** |
| • Whole Grains | • ≥ 3½ ounce(s) per day | • 1 slice of bread (1 ounce)<br>• ½ cup cooked pasta, rice, or cereal<br>• 1 ounce uncooked pasta or rice<br>• 1 tortilla (6 inch diameter)<br>• 1 pancake (5 inch diameter)<br>• 1 ounce ready-to-eat cereal (about 1 cup cereal flakes)<br>See more Grain examples | • Eat at least half of all grains as whole grains.<br>• Substitute whole-grain choices for refined grains in breakfast cereals, breads, crackers, rice, and pasta.<br>• Check product labels – is a grain with "whole" before its name listed first on the ingredients list? |
| **Vegetables** | **3 cup(s) per day** | **1 cup of Vegetables:** | **Tips** |
| • Dark Green<br>• Red & Orange<br>• Beans & Peas<br>• Starchy<br>• Other | • 2 cup(s) per week<br>• 6 cup(s) per week<br>• 2 cup(s) per week<br>• 6 cup(s) per week<br>• 5 cup(s) per week | • 1 cup raw or cooked vegetables<br>• 1 cup 100% vegetable juice<br>• 2 cups leafy salad greens<br>See more Vegetable examples | • Include vegetables in meals and in snacks. Fresh, frozen, and canned vegetables all count.<br>• Add dark-green, red, and orange vegetables to main and side dishes. Use dark leafy greens to make salads.<br>• Beans and peas are a great source of fiber. Add beans or peas to salads, soups, side dishes, or serve as a main dish. |
| **Fruits** | **2 cup(s) per day** | **1 cup of Fruit:** | **Tips** |
| | | • 1 cup raw or cooked fruit<br>• 1 cup 100% fruit juice<br>• ½ cup dried fruit<br>See more Fruit examples | • Select fresh, frozen, canned, and dried fruit more often than juice; select 100% fruit juice when choosing juice.<br>• Enjoy a wide variety of fruits, and maximize taste and freshness, by adapting your choices to what's in season.<br>• Use fruit as snacks, salads, or desserts. |
| **Dairy** | **3 cup(s) per day** | **1 cup of Dairy:** | **Tips** |
| | | • 1 cup milk<br>• 1 cup fortified soymilk (soy beverage)<br>• 1 cup yogurt<br>• 1½ ounces natural cheese (e.g. Cheddar)<br>• 2 ounces processed cheese (e.g. American)<br>See more Dairy examples | • Drink fat-free (skim) or low-fat (1%) milk.<br>• Choose fat-free or low-fat milk or yogurt more often than cheese.<br>• When selecting cheese, choose low-fat or reduced-fat versions. |
| **Protein Foods** | **6 ounce(s) per day** | **1 ounce of Protein Foods:** | **Tips** |
| • Seafood | • 9 ounce(s) per week | • 1 ounce lean meat, poultry, seafood<br>• 1 egg<br>• 1 Tablespoon peanut butter<br>• ½ ounce nuts or seeds<br>• ¼ cup cooked beans or peas<br>See more Protein Food examples | • Eat a variety of foods from the Protein Foods group each week.<br>• Eat seafood in place of meat or poultry twice a week.<br>• Select lean meat and poultry. Trim or drain fat from meat and remove poultry skin. |
| **Oils** | **6 tsp. per day** | **1 tsp. of Oil** | **Tips** |
| | | • 1 tsp. vegetable oil (e.g. canola, corn, olive, soybean)<br>• 1½ tsp. mayonnaise<br>• 2 tsp. tub margarine<br>• 2 tsp. French dressing<br>See more Oil examples | • Choose soft margarines with zero *trans* fats made from liquid vegetable oil, rather than stick margarine or butter.<br>• Use vegetable oils (olive, canola, corn, soybean, peanut, safflower, sunflower) rather than solid fats (butter, shortening).<br>• Replace solid fats with oils, rather than adding oil to the diet. Oils are a concentrated source of Calories, so use oils in small amounts. |

† Calories from food components such as added sugars and solid fats that provide little nutritional value. Empty Calories are part of Total Calories.

ILLUSTRATION 6.7 ▸ Daily Food Plan for Moms menu planning resource.



Diets formed around healthy dietary patterns for pregnant and breastfeeding women provide a healthy assortment of nutrients at specified caloric levels appropriate for the stage of breastfeeding (www.choosemyplate.gov/pregnancy-breastfeeding.html; see Illustration 6.7).

## Nutrition Assessment of Breastfeeding Women

Nutrition assessment for adults is outlined in Table 2.10. Assessment for breastfeeding women includes similar parameters, with a focus on commonly encountered problems, delineated in Table 6.4. Attention should be paid to appropriate maternal energy intake to achieve or maintain ideal or healthy target maternal body weight. Specific foods that may be related to infant colic may need to be avoided among women whose infants exhibit symptoms. A careful history of food and supplement use, as well as physical activity, and pertinent medical and breast health history are obtained. Common diagnoses include altered maternal weight status, concern for inadequate milk supply, and need for $B_{12}$ supplement for vegan dietary pattern.

TABLE 6.4 ▸ Summary of the components of the four steps of the Nutrition Care Process for Breastfeeding Women (Academy of Nutrition and Dietetics)

**Step 1. Nutrition Assessment for Breastfeeding Women**

- Food and nutrient intake
  - Diet history
- Knowledge/attitudes/beliefs
  - Foods that may increase risk of infant colic
  - Adequate energy intake for return to prepregnant weight
- Medications, herbs, and supplements
  - Check for safety and compatibility with breastfeeding (see more on herbs and medications in Chapter 7)
  - Need for supplements based on inadequate intake, missing food groups, or vegan dietary pattern
- Nutrition-related behaviors
  - Excessive dieting or calorie restriction
- Physical activity
  - Return to physical activity after adequate recovery from delivery
- Biochemical data, medical tests, and procedures
  - Gradual return to nonpregnant, nonlactating values
- Anthropometric measures
  - BMI to return to prepregnant or ideal levels
- Client history
  - Medical history, treatments (beast surgeries), use of alternative/complementary medicine, social history

**Step 2. Common Nutrition Diagnoses for Breastfeeding Women**

- Altered maternal BMI
  - Obesity, underweight, or related to rate of weight loss
- Nutrient inadequacy or excess
  - Vegan
  - Lactose intolerance
- Perceived or real inadequate milk production
- Behavioral-environmental
  - Knowledge deficit
  - Need/qualify for WIC services

**Step 3. Common Nutrition Interventions for Breastfeeding Women**

- Alter energy intake to achieve ideal weight or weight goal
- Reinforce principles of milk production, early signs of infant hunger, and signs of adequate infant milk intake
- Recommend vitamin $B_{12}$ for vegans or other supplements if intake is inadequate

**Step 4. Common Nutrition Monitoring and Evaluation Plan Components**

- Weight change/BMI
- Infant growth
- $B_{12}$ status

Knowledge deficit relating to dieting and breastfeeding and qualifications for WIC services are also common. Nutrition intervention may include a plan for adjusting energy intake to promote appropriate maternal weight change, education regarding milk production mechanisms and appropriate maternal feeding and/or pumping to achieve appropriate supply, and/or alternate food sources or supplement recommendations for nutrient deficiency or inadequate intake of nutrients such as calcium or vitamin $B_{12}$. A plan for monitoring maternal weight change, infant growth (adequate milk supply), or nutrient status rounds out the nutrition assessment process.

## Energy and Nutrient Needs

The DRIs for normal-weight lactating women assume that the energy spent for milk production is 500 cal per day in the first 6 months and 400 cal afterward.[110,111] The 2005 DRI is 330 additional kcal to support 0.8 kg per month weight loss (170 cal per day) for the first 6 months and 400 kcal per day afterward. With mobilization of approximately 170 kcal per day, net energy needs were estimated at approximately 450 kcal per day.

We now understand that women use several mechanisms to meet the energy needs of lactation. Adjustments in energy intake and energy expenditure must be balanced to meet those needs. Goldberg et al.[112] found that women increased food intake (56 percent of the need for milk production) and decreased physical activity (44 percent of the energy need for milk production) to meet the increase in energy needs for lactation. Doubly labeled water studies suggest that the components of energy expenditure vary greatly, and measurements of dietary intake can be unreliable. Therefore, a single recommendation for energy for lactating women could never address all of the individual ways that women meet their energy needs. Assessment of adequacy of energy intake of breastfeeding women should always be made within the context of the mother's overall nutritional status and weight changes and the adequacy of the infant's growth.

## Maternal Energy Balance and Milk Composition

The composition of breast milk depends on maternal nutritional status. Protein–calorie malnutrition results in an energy deficit that reduces the volume of milk produced but does not usually compromise the composition of the milk. Several studies show that milk production is maintained when there is a modest level of negative calorie balance. Animal models first identified a potential threshold effect of energy restriction. Baboons fed 60 percent of their voluntary intake significantly reduced milk production.[113] Yet, baboons fed 80 percent of their usual intake maintained milk production. Randomized studies such as the one performed on baboons cannot ethically be done with humans. However, a series of human studies on weight loss during breastfeeding (discussed below) support a threshold effect of energy limitations on lactation.

## Weight Loss During Breastfeeding

Current DRIs are written assuming a weight loss of 0.8 kg/month.[111] In addition, mechanisms that favor use of maternal fat stores and delivery of nutrients to the breast seem to occur during lactation. Despite these mechanisms that should favor weight loss in breastfeeding women, loss by 12 months postpartum is on average less than the amount needed to return to prepregnancy weight.[114] A 2015 study reported that nearly a third of women who were of normal body weight prior to pregnancy were overweight or obese at a year postpartum.[114] Postpartum weight management programs for breastfeeding women that include an energy-restricted diet appear to be the most effective approach to promoting weight loss.[115]

A number of small studies in the United States have addressed the issue of whether weight loss influences milk production. Strode et al.[116] first observed women who voluntarily reduced their energy intake to 68 percent of their estimated needs for 7 days. No differences in infant intake or milk composition were observed. In the week following the diet, women who consumed fewer than 1500 cal tended to experience a decrease in milk volume. Women who consumed over 1500 cal per day experienced no decrease.[116] In addition, 22 health postpartum women who participated in a 10-week weight-loss program that reduced energy intake by 23 percent maintained milk production.[117] The women lost an average of about a pound a week during the 10 weeks.

Studies of weight loss during lactation also suggest that modest energy restriction (500 cal per day) can be accomplished without large decreases in the quality of the maternal diet, but that the macronutrient content of the diet may influence maternal weight loss and fat content of the milk differentially. Maternal reduction of energy intake through lowered intake of sugary and high-fat foods resulted in similar micronutrient intakes to women who did not decrease intake, with the exceptions of calcium and vitamin D.[118] None of the women consumed adequate vitamins C or E. Therefore, careful attention to consumption of (1) calcium- and vitamin D–rich foods such as low-fat and fat-free dairy products, and (2) fruits, vegetables, and whole grains is needed. A small recent study challenges conventional wisdom that suggests that diet does not substantively alter human milk composition. When the women consumed a high-fat diet (55 percent fat, 30 percent carbohydrate, 15 percent protein), they had similar milk volume and similar protein and carbohydrate content of milk, but a greater energy deficit through higher milk-fat content milk than when they consumed a high-carbohydrate diet (60 percent carbohydrate, 15 percent protein, 25 percent fat).[119]

## Exercise and Breastfeeding

Studies[120] examining the effect of increasing energy expenditure on weight and lactation suggest that it is safe, but does not promote weight loss as compared to diet or a combination of diet and exercise.[115,120] The available evidence suggests that modest energy restriction combined with increases in activity may be effective at helping women to lose weight, while improving their metabolic profile and increasing fat losses.

## Vitamin and Mineral Supplements

A 1991 Institute of Medicine report, *Nutrition during Lactation,* stated that well-nourished breastfeeding women do not need routine vitamin or mineral supplementation.[87] Instead, supplementation should target specific nutritional needs of individual women. Supplementation strategies should take into account how nutrients are secreted into human milk and the potential for nutrient–nutrient interactions in mothers and their infants. For example, women who avoid dairy products completely should use calcium (1200 mg) and vitamin D (10 $\mu$g) supplements.

## Vitamin and Mineral Intakes

Vitamin and mineral intakes that do not meet recommended levels (of folate, thiamin, vitamin A, calcium, iron, and zinc) have been reported for lactating women.[36,108,121] However, these reports of inadequate intake have not often been followed by reports of deficits in nutritional status of the mother–infant pair. Nor is there a recommendation for vitamin and mineral supplements for all breastfeeding women. A careful balance is needed between concern over inadequate maternal dietary intake and causing women not to breastfeed because they do not have an optimal diet.

## Functional Foods

Concern has been expressed about possible ill effects of high intakes of fortified foods in addition to supplements. Although this is an important issue, studies to date have not identified adverse reactions related to fortified-food consumption and RDA levels of nutrients in supplements.

## Fluids

There is no evidence that increasing fluid intake will increase milk production or that a short-term fluid deficit results in a decrease in milk production. Fluid demands rise during breastfeeding, however, so women should drink fluids to thirst. Once a mother and her infant have the nursing routine down, she may find it convenient to have something to drink while she nurses. Although many women want to know how many glasses to drink per day, the amount needed varies depending on climate, milk production, body size, and other factors. Therefore, women are advised to drink enough fluids to keep their urine pale yellow. The current RDI for water for lactating women is 3.8 L.[121]

## Vegetarian Diets

A vegetarian dietary pattern can be chosen by breastfeeding women without compromise to their nutritional status or their infant. The goal is to adequately nourish the mother and child, not to force women to use supplements and/or products that are not part of their normal eating patterns. Incorporation of soy products, vegetarian diets of various sorts, and other alternative diet choices can be followed as long as they meet maternal nutritional needs. Vegans who do not consume dairy products and eggs, however, may need to plan carefully to consume adequate amounts of calories, protein, calcium, vitamin D, vitamin $B_{12}$, iron, and zinc. Vegetarians' intakes of protein are generally adequate as long as energy intake is adequate. Breastfeeding women who consume no animal products should use plant foods with bioavailable $B_{12}$ from sources such as yeasts, seaweed, and fortified soy products. Women who are unable to get adequate $B_{12}$ from foods should take a vitamin $B_{12}$ supplement because human milk may be low in vitamin $B_{12}$ even when mothers do not exhibit deficiency symptoms. See Chapter 7 for information on the use of herbals during breastfeeding.

## Infant Colic

Infant colic is defined as crying for more than three hours a day when the cause is not a medical problem. It is widely believed that components of maternal diet are related to infant colic. Information is growing to support this idea.[122,123] An observational trial suggested that a mother's consumption of cow's milk, onions, cabbage, broccoli, and chocolate were associated with greater likelihood of colic in the infant.[122] A randomized trial assessing maternal avoidance of cow's milk, eggs, peanuts, tree nuts, wheat, soy, and fish resulted in a reduction in colic symptoms of their infants in the first 6 weeks of life.[123] Women should be encouraged to exclude only those foods that seem to cause problems and to be careful to replace nutrients that might be lost by avoiding classes of foods. For example, excluding dairy foods may limit calcium and vitamin D intake.

Probiotics have been proposed as a treatment or potential prevention for colic. Differences in gut microbiota of infants with and without colic[124] suggested promise for probiotics as treatment or prevention.[124] However, a meta-analysis concluded that *l. retueri might* be effective as a treatment for colic in breastfed infants.[125] The group found insufficient evidence to suggest that probiotics are useful to prevent crying in formula fed infants or to prevent colic. Further research will be revealing.

# Public Food and Nutrition Programs

LO 6.8 Identify at least two breastfeeding promotion programs that have demonstrated effectiveness at increasing breastfeeding initiation and duration.

In 1989, Congress mandated (Public Law 101–147) a specific portion of each state's WIC budget allocation to be used exclusively for the promotion and support of breastfeeding. This law authorized the use of WIC administrative funds to purchase breastfeeding aids such as breast pumps. Through this legislation, each state has a breastfeeding coordinator and a plan to coordinate operations with local agency programs for breastfeeding promotion.

The USDA Food and Nutrition Information Center supports a WIC Works website (http://lovingsupport.nal.usda.gov/wic-staff) to serve health and nutrition professionals working in the WIC program. The website includes links to training materials on breastfeeding promotion and information on how to share resources and recommendations. In participating states, the Farmers Market Nutrition Program provides checks to WIC participants so that they can purchase locally grown fruits and vegetables (http://www.health.ny.gov/prevention/nutrition/fmnp/).

# Optimal Duration, Influential Factors, and U.S. Goals for Breastfeeding

LO 6.9 Summarize factors known to be associated with higher and lower rates of breastfeeding, and the gap between current rates and the Breastfeeding Goals for the United States.

> "During the twentieth century, infant feeding practices have undergone dramatic changes that reflect shifts in values and attitudes in the U.S. society as a whole. They have tended to occur first among those women at the forefront of changes in dominant social values and among those with resources (whether it is time, energy or money) to permit adoption of new feeding practices."
>
> —Institute of Medicine, Subcommittee on Nutrition During Lactation, 1991[87]

## Optimal Breastfeeding Duration

The health of mother–child pair should be the primary criteria to determine the optimal duration of breastfeeding—and not simply whether the cultural environment makes such duration practical. The consensus among expert groups,[64,74] the World Health Organization and the U.S. Surgeon General, recommends human milk feeding exclusively for 6 months. Infants who are breastfed for 6 months experience fewer ill-nesses from gastrointestinal infection than do infants who are given HMS and breast milk at 3 or 4 months of age. Deficits in growth have not been demonstrated among infants in developing or developed countries who are exclusively breastfed for 6 months or longer. Breastfeeding can prevent intestinal blood loss in infants—a factor that should be considered when determining its optimal duration. Infants fed cow's milk before the age of 6 months suffer nutritionally significant losses of iron via intestinal blood.[126] Through 1 year, breastfed infants suffer fewer acute infections than formula-fed infants do, a finding that supports breastfeeding beyond the introduction of solids.

## Breastfeeding Goals for the United States

Healthy People 2020 has a vision of "A society in which all people live long, healthy lives."[127] The breastfeeding

TABLE 6.5 ▸ Healthy People 2020 objectives on breastfeeding

| MATERNAL CHILD HEALTH OBJECTIVE | BASELINE (YEAR MEASURED) % | 2020 TARGET % |
|---|---|---|
| Increase the proportion of infants who are breastfed: | (2006 births) | |
| Ever | 74.0 | 81.9 |
| At 6 months | 43.5 | 60.6 |
| At 1 year | 22.7 | 34.1 |
| Exclusively through 3 months | 33.6 | 46.2 |
| Exclusively through 6 months | 14.1 | 25.5 |
| Increase the proportion of employers who have worksite lactation support programs | 25.0 (2009) | 38.0 |
| Reduce the proportion of breastfed newborns who receive formula supplementation within the first 2 days of life | 24.2 (2006 births) | 14.2 |
| Increase the proportion of live births that occur in facilities that provide recommended care for lactating mothers and their babies | 2.9 (2009) | 8.1 |

SOURCE: http://www.usbreastfeeding.org/LegislationPolicy/FederalPolicies Initiatives/ and CDC National Immunization surveys 2010 and 2011, Provisional Data, 2009 births. http://www.cdc.gov/breastfeeding /data/NIS_data /index.htm141

**Actions for Mothers and Their Families:**

1. Give mothers the support they need to breastfeed their babies.
2. Develop programs to educate fathers and grandmothers about breastfeeding.

**Actions for Communities:**

3. Strengthen programs that provide mother-to-mother support and peer counseling.
4. Use community-based organizations to promote and support breastfeeding.
5. Create a national campaign to promote breastfeeding.
6. Ensure that the marketing of infant formula is conducted in a way that minimizes its negative impacts on exclusive breastfeeding.

**Actions for Health Care:**

7. Ensure that maternity care practices around the United States are fully supportive of breastfeeding.
8. Develop systems to guarantee continuity of skilled support for lactation between hospitals and health care settings in the community.
9. Provide education and training in breastfeeding for all health professionals who care for women and children.
10. Include basic support for breastfeeding as a standard of care for midwives, obstetricians, family physicians, nurse practitioners, and pediatricians.
11. Ensure access to services provided by International Board Certified Lactation Consultants.
12. Identify and address obstacles to greater availability of safe banked donor milk for fragile infants.

**Actions for Employment:**

13. Work toward establishing paid maternity leave for all employed mothers.
14. Ensure that employers establish and maintain comprehensive, high-quality lactation support programs for their employees.
15. Expand the use of programs in the workplace that allow lactating mothers to have direct access to their babies.
16. Ensure that all child care providers accommodate the needs of breastfeeding mothers and infants.

**Actions for Research and Surveillance:**

17. Increase funding of high-quality research on breastfeeding.
18. Strengthen existing capacity and develop future capacity for conducting research on breastfeeding.
19. Develop a national monitoring system to improve the tracking of breastfeeding rates as well as the policies and environmental factors that affect breastfeeding.

**Action for Public Health Infrastructure:**

20. Improve national leadership on the promotion and support of breastfeeding.

ILLUSTRATION 6.8 ▸ Levels of support needed for increasing breastfeeding.

objectives continue to focus on increasing both the proportion of infants ever breastfed as well as the duration of breastfeeding (Table 6.5). Additionally, new objectives are set to increase worksite lactation programs, reduce formula supplementation in the first 2 days of life, and increase the number of births in facilities providing recommended care for breastfeeding mothers and their babies.

## The Surgeon General's Call to Action to Support Breastfeeding

The 2011 Surgeon General's Call to Action to Support Breastfeeding recognizes the levels of support needed for increasing breastfeeding (Illustration 6.8) and the key barriers to breastfeeding (Illustration 6.9). Twenty specific actions to increase support for breastfeeding are identified. These actions recognize that support is needed at the individual and family level, by communities, health care providers, employers, through research and surveillance, and in public health infrastructure. Key barriers are organized into seven domains: (1) Lack of Knowledge; (2) Social Norms; (3) Poor Family and Social Support; (4) Lactation Problems; (5) Embarrassment; (6) Employment and Child Care; and (7) Barriers Related to Health Services.

## Breastfeeding Rates in the United States

Breastfeeding duration has changed markedly over the last century. In the early 1900s, almost all infants in the United States were breastfed. As safe human milk substitutes (HMSs) became widely available, breastfeeding rates steadily declined, reaching levels below 30 percent in the 1950s and 1960s, and then rose dramatically in the 1970s.[133] In the early 1980s, levels peaked above 60 percent, declined until the early 1990s, and then began rising again through the 2000s.[134] The 2014 Breastfeeding Report Card suggests that breastfeeding rates continue to rise (http://www.cdc.gov/breastfeeding/data/nis_data/rates-any-exclusive-bf-socio-dem-2011.htm).

**Lack of Knowledge**

While breastfeeding is considered a natural skill, some mothers may need education and guidance. Providing accurate information can help prepare mothers for breastfeeding.

**Lactation Problems**

Without good support, many women have problems with breastfeeding. Most of these are avoidable if identified and treated early, and need not pose a threat to continued breastfeeding.

**Poor Family and Social Support**

Fathers, grandmothers, and other family members strongly influence mothers' decisions about starting, continuing, and accommodating breastfeeding.

**Social Norms**

Many people see breastfeeding as an alternative rather the routine way to feed infants.

**Embarrassment**

The popular culture's sexualization of breasts compels some women to conceal breastfeeding. Improving support for women to breastfeed can help them better accommodate the demands of everyday life while protecting their infants' health.

**Employment and Child Care**

Employed mothers typically find that (1) returning to work and (2) lack of maternity leave are significant barriers to breastfeeding.

**Health Services**

Health care systems and health care providers can improve mothers' breastfeeding experiences by pursuing and obtaining the training and education opportunities they need in order to fully support their patients.

ILLUSTRATION 6.9 ▸ Key barriers to breastfeeding.

**TABLE 6.6** Provisional breastfeeding rates by sociodemographic factors, among children born in 2011 (percent +/– half 95% confidence interval)[1]

| | ANY BREASTFEEDING | | | | EXCLUSIVE BREASTFEEDING[2] | |
|---|---|---|---|---|---|---|
| SOCIO-DEMOGRAPHIC FACTORS | N | EVER BREASTFED % ± HALF 95% CI | BREASTFED AT 6 MONTHS % ± HALF 95% CI | BREASTFED AT 12 MONTHS % ± HALF 95% CI | N | EXCLUSIVE BREASTFEEDING THROUGH 6 MONTHS % ± HALF 95% CI |
| **US National** | 14,456 | 79.2±1.2 | 49.4±1.5 | 26.7±1.3 | 14131 | 18.8±1.2 |
| **Race/Ethnicity** | | | | | | |
| Hispanic | 2801 | 83.8±2.4 | 48.4±3.8 | 24.8±3.3 | 2756 | 17.1±2.9 |
| Non-Hispanic White | 8382 | 81.1±1.4 | 52.3±1.8 | 28.4±1.6 | 8162 | 20.3±1.4 |
| Non-Hispanic Black | 1414 | 61.6±4.1 | 35.0±3.9 | 16.4±3.3 | 1386 | 13.7±3.2 |
| Non-Hispanic Asian | 648 | 90.9±3.0 | 71.2±7.1 | 47.3±7.8 | 634 | 26.6±7.0 |
| Non-Hispanic Hawaiian/Pacific Islander | 67 | 75.0±21.7 | 49.8±22.0 | 25.7±16.4 | 67 | 21.0±17.5 |
| Non-Hispanic American Indian/ Alaska Native | 221 | 77.1±8.3 | 37.3±11.8 | 25.0±9.7 | 216 | 15.6±7.4 |
| 2 or more races | 923 | 75.0±5.3 | 48.4±5.8 | 29.3±5.0 | 910 | 19.6±4.3 |
| **Maternal Education** | | | | | | |
| Less than high school | 1582 | 69.1±3.7 | 34.4±4.0 | 19.7±3.4 | 1555 | 13.5±3.1 |
| High school graduate | 2622 | 69.2±2.8 | 38.2±3.2 | 19.6±2.8 | 2573 | 15.8±2.6 |
| Some college or technical school | 3859 | 81.0±2.3 | 46.1±2.9 | 23.6±2.6 | 3776 | 16.5±2.3 |
| College graduate | 6393 | 91.2±1.1 | 68.3±2.1 | 38.1±2.2 | 6227 | 25.5±1.9 |
| **Maternal Age** | | | | | | |
| Under 20 | 201 | 66.9±10.6 | 19.4±8.2 | 13.1±7.1 | 201 | 5.6±5.0 |
| 20–29 | 5559 | 73.6±2.1 | 39.1±2.4 | 18.8±2.0 | 5458 | 15.2±1.7 |
| 30 or older | 8696 | 84.2±1.3 | 58.8±1.9 | 33.6±1.9 | 8472 | 22.2±1.7 |
| **Poverty Income Ratio[3]** | | | | | | |
| Less than 100 | 3690 | 70.5±2.5 | 37.8±2.9 | 20.3±2.5 | 3627 | 14.2±2.2 |
| 100–199 | 2919 | 77.9±2.6 | 45.5±3.1 | 24.7±2.7 | 2843 | 18.0±2.5 |
| 200–399 | 3732 | 85.8±1.9 | 57.7±2.9 | 32.1±2.7 | 3633 | 22.0±2.4 |
| 400–599 | 2237 | 87.1±2.2 | 61.9±3.4 | 34.9±3.5 | 2200 | 25.2±3.3 |
| 600 or greater | 1878 | 90.6±2.2 | 67.9±4.0 | 33.5±4.4 | 1828 | 23.1±3.8 |
| **Marital Status[4]** | | | | | | |
| Married | 10371 | 86.7±1.2 | 60.1±1.8 | 33.3±1.7 | 10102 | 22.6±1.5 |
| Unmarried | 4085 | 67.1±2.4 | 32.1±2.6 | 16.1±2.2 | 4029 | 12.7±1.9 |

[1]Breastfeeding rates presented in this table are based on dual-frame (landline and cellular telephone) samples from 2012 and 2013 National Immunization Survey. See survey methods for details on study design.

[2]Exclusive breastfeeding is defined as ONLY breast milk — NO solids, no water, and no other liquids.

[3]Poverty Income Ratio = Ratio of self-reported family income to the federal poverty threshold value depending on the number of people in the household.

[4]Unmarried includes never married, widowed, separated, divorced.

Adapted from: Centers for Disease Control and Prevention. Rates of Any and Exclusive Breastfeeding Rates by Sociodemographics—2011 Birth, CDC National Immunization Survey. Atlanta, GA. Available at http://www.cdc.gov/breastfeeding/data/nis_data/rates-any-exclusive-bf-socio-dem-2011.htm. Accessed 4/3/2015.[142]

TABLE 6.7 ▸ Supportive Hospital Practices

**Supportive Hospital Practices**

Birth facility policies and practices that create a supportive environment for breastfeeding begin prenatally and continue through discharge, and include:

- **Skin-to-skin contact**—Doctors and midwives place newborns skin-to-skin with their mothers immediately after birth, with no bedding or clothing between them, allowing enough uninterrupted time (at least 30 minutes) for mother and baby to start breastfeeding well.
- **Teaching about breastfeeding**—Hospital staff teach mothers and babies how to breastfeed and to recognize and respond to important feeding cues.
- **Early and frequent breastfeeding**—Hospital staff help mothers and babies start breastfeeding as soon as possible after birth, with many opportunities to practice throughout the hospital stay. Pacifiers are saved for medical procedures.
- **Exclusive breastfeeding**—Hospital staff only disrupt breastfeeding with supplementary feedings in cases of rare medical complications.
- **Rooming-in**—Hospital staff encourage mothers and babies to room together and teach families the benefits of this kind of close contact, including better quality and quantity of sleep for both and more opportunities to practice breastfeeding.
- **Active follow-up after discharge**—Hospital staff schedule in-person breastfeeding follow-up visits for mothers and babies after they go home to check-up on breastfeeding, help resolve any feeding problems, and connect families to community breastfeeding resources.

SOURCE: Division of Nutrition, Physical Activity, and Obesity, National Center for Chronic Disease Prevention and Health Promotion http://www.cdc.gov/breastfeeding/data/mpinc/maternity-care-practices.htm

Gaps in breastfeeding remain—geographically, among racial groups, by age, educational groups, marital status, and income level[133] (Table 6.6). However, breastfeeding rates in Alaska, California, Connecticut, Hawaii, Idaho, Iowa, Minnesota, Montana, Nebraska, New Hampshire, North Dakota, Oregon, Utah, Vermont, Washington, Wisconsin, and Wyoming already meet or exceed the 2020 target of 81.99 percent. Some of the lowest rates persist among southern states, including Alabama, Delaware, Louisiana, Mississippi, and West Virginia. Breastfeeding varies substantially by racial groups, highest among Asian and Hispanic or Latina and lowest among Black or African American. Breastfeeding initiation and duration increases with the age and education of the mother. Married women breastfeed more often than unmarried women and breastfeeding rates rise with income level.

The CDC monitors maternity practices and policies related to breastfeeding support in hospitals and birthing centers with the Maternity Practices in Infant Nutrition and Care (mPINC) survey. This survey monitors supportive practices (Table 6.7). Data are reported at the national, state, and individual facility data showing strengths and areas needing improvement at each level. For example, the number of births in hospitals providing recommended breastfeeding care increased to 7.79 percent in 2011, from 2 percent in 2008. Still, nearly 20 percent of infants received formula by 2 days of age, and only seven state's childcare regulations supports onsite breastfeeding.

# Breastfeeding Promotion, Facilitation, and Support

LO 6.8 Identify at least two breastfeeding promotion programs that have demonstrated effectiveness at increasing breastfeeding initiation and duration.

> "Significant steps must be taken to increase breastfeeding rates in the United States and to close the wide racial and ethnic gaps in breastfeeding. This goal can only be achieved by supporting breastfeeding in the family, community, workplace, health care sector, and society."
>
> —Health and Human Services Blueprint for Action on Breastfeeding, 2000[135]

## Prenatal Breastfeeding Education and Support

Culturally competent prenatal breastfeeding education that is given frequently in person can have a significant positive influence on breastfeeding rates.[136,137] Early in pregnancy, women need information on what to expect in the hospital or birthing center and practical tips for initiating breastfeeding (Table 6.8). Because fathers,[138] grandmothers,[139] ***doulas***, friends, and social networks[137] all have a powerful influence on infant feeding decisions, it is important to include these key people as often as possible in breastfeeding promotion efforts. Several key points are shown in Table 6.9.[107,126,129]

## Breastfeeding Support for Individuals

Peer counselors and peer group discussions with at least one or two women who have successfully breastfed is a successful way to promote breastfeeding.[142] Exposure to mothers nursing their babies increases a woman's level of comfort with breastfeeding

**Doula** An individual who surrounds, interacts with, and aids the mother at any time within the period that includes pregnancy, birth, and lactation; may be a relative, friend, or neighbor and is usually but not necessarily female. One who gives psychological encouragement and physical assistance to a new mother.[1]

TABLE 6.8 ▸ The Best Start three-step breastfeeding counseling strategy[136,129]

1. Ask open-ended questions to identify the woman's concerns.
   - Dietitian: "What have you heard about breastfeeding?"
   - Client: "I hear it's best for my baby, but all my friends say it really hurts!"
2. Affirm her feelings by reassuring her that these feelings are normal.
   - Dietitian: "You know, most women worry about whether it will hurt."
3. Educate by clarifying how other women like her have dealt with her concerns. Avoid overeducating or giving the impression that breastfeeding is hard to master.
   - Dietitian: "Did you know that it is not supposed to be painful, and if you are having discomfort, there are people who can help make it better?"



and provides a forum for informal discussion with family and friends. Social media is an important vehicle for breastfeeding information that has not yet been utilized to its full potential.[143] Discussion of an individual's personal experience can be an effective way to help women see and believe that others like her share her concerns.

All new mothers need support for breastfeeding. However, low-income women often lack the support, knowledge, and confidence to interpret the abundant and pervasive mixed messages on infant feeding practices. Consider the strikingly different context for pregnancy, birth, and parenting for low-income women and their more affluent counterparts.

**Profile of a Low-income Pregnant Woman** She says she wants to do what is best for her baby and, in fact, knows the breast is best. However, she is afraid breastfeeding will cause her baby to be too "clingy." She feels uncomfortable about nursing around family, her employer, and co-workers, much less in public. She is certainly not up for the pain she has heard breastfeeding causes. To make things more difficult, in the hospital, she is separated from her baby soon after delivery and is given little assistance for getting started. She is sent home from the hospital with free samples of formula.

TABLE 6.9 ▸ Key teaching points prior to birth

**In the hospital or birthing center, mothers should:**

Request early first feeding and skin to skin contact
Practice frequent, exclusive breastfeeding
Ask to be taught swallowing indicators
Learn indicators of sufficient intake
Ask for help if it hurts
Know sources for help
Understand postpartum rest and recovery needs
Avoid supplements unless medically indicated

SOURCE: Adapted from S. Page-Goertz and S. McCamman, Breast-feeding Success: You Can Make the Difference. *The Perinatal Nutrition Report,* 4 (Winter 1998).[152]

**Profile of an Affluent Pregnant Woman** The affluent expectant mother has friends who have breastfed and have helped build her confidence that she can breastfeed successfully. She may have been able to choose her birth setting and select a hospital with knowledgeable staff who allow mother and baby to stay together around the clock. Because she knows there may be bumps in the road getting started, she seeks out support from friends, a lactation consultant, or the doctor after discharge. At home, she has a supportive husband who is proud of her for offering the best for their baby. When she returns to work, she knows she can still pump during the day and breastfeed at night to keep that special closeness with her baby even after returning to work.[116,129,135,140,141,144]

## Role of the Health Care System in Supporting Breastfeeding

In 2002, the WHO and UNICEF came together to try to revitalize the international community in breastfeeding promotion with the Global Strategy for Infant and Young Child Feeding.[72] This report builds on the ***Innocenti Declaration*** and the Baby Friendly Hospital Initiative by recognizing the importance of breastfeeding in all children, including those in difficult circumstances such as emergency situations, low-birth-weight infants, and infants of mothers with HIV. The initiative includes the following:

- A call on governments to develop and implement policy on infant and child feeding within the context of the national policy for nutrition, child, and reproductive health as well as poverty reduction
- Access to skilled support for initiation and maintenance of breastfeeding exclusively for 6 months and with safe complementary foods for up to 2 years or beyond
- Empowerment of health care professionals to provide breastfeeding support and extend their services into the community
- Review of progress in implementation of the International Code of Marketing of Breast Milk Substitutes (Table 6.10)[145] and consideration of new measures to protect families from commercial interests and influence
- Enactment of legislation to protect the breastfeeding rights of working women in accordance with international labor standards

This report provides an important framework for

**Innocenti Declaration** On the Protection, Promotion, and Support of Breastfeeding: Policy statement adopted by participants at the World Health Organization UNICEF policymakers' meeting on breastfeeding, a global initiative held in Italy in 1990. The policy established exclusive breastfeeding from birth to 4–6 months of age as a global goal for optimal maternal and child health.

TABLE 6.10 ▸ World Health Organization's international/ UNICEF code on the marketing of breast milk substitutes

- No advertising of breast milk substitutes
- No free samples or supplies
- No promotion of products through health care facilities
- No company sales representative to advise mothers
- No gifts or personal samples to health workers
- No gifts or pictures idealizing formula feeding, including pictures of infants, on the labels of the infant milk containers
- Information to health workers should be scientific and factual
- All information on artificial feeding, including labels, should explain the benefits of breastfeeding and the costs and hazards associated with formula feeding
- Unsuitable products should not be promoted for babies
- Manufacturers and distributors should comply with the Code's provisions even if countries have not adopted laws or other measures

SOURCE: Adapted from "World Health Organization International Code of Marketing of Breast-milk Substitutes. Geneva, Switzerland: 1981.[155]

acceleration of support of appropriate feeding for infants and children worldwide by linking resources and intervention areas available in many sectors.

Health care providers and facilities exert tremendous influence over the mother–infant dyad, with the power to promote and model optimal breastfeeding practices during prenatal care, at delivery, and after discharge. The importance of the health care system in breastfeeding success is evident by the inclusion of process indicators for breastfeeding in the Healthy People 2020 objectives.[126,]

## Lactation Support in Hospitals and Birthing Centers

Hospital policies and routines significantly affect critical early experience with breastfeeding, with effects extending far beyond the short stay.[156,146] Table 6.11 provides examples of practices that influence this pivotal initiation experience. As in prenatal care settings, the distribution of infant formula coupons and free samples of formula in hospital discharge packs is discouraged because of the detrimental effects of this practice on breastfeeding success, particularly among vulnerable groups such as new mothers and low-income women. Model policies for hospitals and physicians are available from the U.S. Breastfeeding Committee (www.usbreastfeeding.org) and the Academy of Breastfeeding Medicine (www.bfmed.org).

In an effort to promote, protect, and support breastfeeding in hospitals and birthing centers worldwide, the World Health Organization (WHO) and UNICEF established the Baby-Friendly Hospital Initiative (BFHI) in 1992 (www.babyfriendlyusa.org).[147] This initiative focuses on 10 evidence-based components of hospital care that impact on breastfeeding success (Table 6.11). The Baby-Friendly Hospital Initiative is responsible for an increase in breastfeeding rates. The Baby-Friendly USA program that designates facilities within the United States who meet the guidelines likely contributed to the rapid increase in number of infants in the United States born in hospitals providing recommended breastfeeding care.[140]

Successful maternal education program examples are highlighted in *The CDC Guide to Breastfeeding Interventions*.[144] These include health insurance plans that provide breastfeeding education for their members, BFHI programs offering patients infant-feeding classes, and health departments offering training programs for persons who provide breastfeeding education.

## Model U.S. Baby-Friendly Hospital Programs

Across the United States, several states have taken BFHI and developed programs to increase breastfeeding initiation rates and breastfeeding duration. Twenty-nine states are participating in the Best Feeds program.

Kaiser Permanente has made a commitment to the Partnership for a Healthier America (PHA) to have all maternity facilities in their system implement the Baby-Friendly Hospital Ten Steps.[141] The number of BFHI-designated hospitals increased from 20 in 2008 to 56 in 2012 (Hardy, 2014). The highest standards of breastfeeding have been achieved in its 28 maternity hospitals with an increase in breastfeeding rate from 57 percent in 2010 to 63 percent in 2012.

The State of California has also been working to increase breastfeeding rates by implementing other programs. The Paid Family Leave program is an insurance program that replaces income for workers who take time to

TABLE 6.11 ▸ 10 steps to successful breastfeeding

1. Have a written breastfeeding policy that is routinely communicated to all health care staff.
2. Train all health care staff in the skills necessary to implement this policy.
3. Inform all pregnant women about the benefits and management of breastfeeding.
4. Help mothers initiate breastfeeding within half one hour of birth.
5. Show mothers how to breastfeed and how to maintain lactation, even if they are separated from their infants.
6. Give infants no food or drink other than breast milk, unless medically indicated.
7. Practice rooming-in, allow mothers and infants to remain together 24 hours a day.
8. Encourage breastfeeding on demand.
9. Give no artificial pacifiers or artificial nipples to breastfeeding infants.
10. Foster the establishment of breastfeeding support groups and refer mothers to them on discharge from the hospital or birth center.

SOURCE: Baby-Friendly USA, www.babyfriendlyusa.org/about-us/baby-friendly-hospital-initiative/the-ten-steps.

care for a child. Women who participated in this program had double the breastfeeding duration when compared to women who did not participate. Increasing awareness of this program is a current statewide effort.

New York conducted a statewide survey of 138 hospitals assessing how hospitals were doing with meeting the Ten Steps was also part of the survey. Over half of the hospitals surveyed reported having interest in implementing Baby-Friendly Hospital protocols. Exclusive breastfeeding was more likely when a hospital supported immediate breastfeeding initiation.

The environment for the delivery of prenatal care is an important barrier or facilitator of breastfeeding. It should provide positive messages about breastfeeding, such as posters that promote breastfeeding and magazines and literature in the waiting room; there should be no advertisements or promotions of formula. Patient education materials that include formula advertising, samples, and business reply cards for free formula[153] are in direct violation of the World Health Organization's International Code on the Marketing of Breast Milk Substitutes (see Table 6.10). Women who have been exposed to materials and products from formula companies prenatally are more likely to stop breastfeeding in the first 2 weeks. Use of these materials provides a subtle message that infant formula is equivalent to breast milk.

Evidence stemming from focus groups intended to inform a national campaign to promote breastfeeding in the United States suggests that breastfeeding is a learned skill.[154] The process associated with success is called *confident commitment*. The components are (1) confidence in the process of breastfeeding, (2) confidence in the ability to breastfeed, and (3) commitment to making breastfeeding work despite obstacles. Mothers who achieved confident commitment before birth were successful when faced with common challenges of breastfeeding. In contrast, among mothers without "confident commitment," the decision to breastfeed weakened with challenges.

Although not all women will choose to breastfeed, the goal of prenatal breastfeeding education is to empower every woman with sufficient knowledge to make an informed decision about how to feed her baby. Some professionals view breastfeeding as a personal choice rather than a public health issue and voice concern that breastfeeding promotional efforts may cause women who choose HMS feeding to feel guilty. On the other hand, some women who formula-feed report feeling angry about not getting enough breastfeeding information during their pregnancy.[136129] In recognition of the benefits of breastfeeding and the important role of health professionals in promoting and supporting breastfeeding, the leading health and professional organizations in the United States that provide perinatal care have established policies in support of breastfeeding as the preferred infant feeding method.[107,126]

## Lactation Support after Discharge

Breastfeeding support is essential in the first few weeks after delivery, as lactation is being established.[135] Younger women and women with lower socioeconomic status are more likely to stop breastfeeding by 4 weeks postpartum and cite sore nipples, inadequate milk supply, feeling that the infant is not satisfied, and infant problems as reasons for stopping.[148]

A pediatrician, nurse, or other knowledgeable health care practitioner should see all breastfeeding mothers and their newborns, either on a home visit or in the office, when the newborn is 2 to 4 days of age. Breastfeeding should be observed and evaluated for evidence of successful breastfeeding behavior. This is also an important time to revisit the major concerns the mother identified during pregnancy, as well as discuss any new concerns. Mothers should be armed with information on sources of trained, skilled, and available help in the community, such as ***lactation consultants***, peer counselors, the WIC program, or ***La Leche League***, should questions or complications arise.[130] Follow-up telephone calls, as necessary, provide additional support to mothers who are not fully confident in their ability to breastfeed successfully.

## The Workplace

One of the important barriers to breastfeeding includes lack of on-site day care, insufficiently paid maternity leave, rigid work schedules, and employers who lack knowledge about breastfeeding. Current law ensures a woman's right to breastfeed her infant anywhere on federal property that she and her child are authorized to be. Still in process is further legislation to require that women cannot be fired or discriminated against if they breastfeed or express milk during their own lunchtime or break time, to provide a tax credit for employers who provide lactation services, and to develop minimum standards for breast pump safety.

Breastfeeding duration is adversely affected by employment.[149,150] Return

**Lactation consultant** Health care professional whose scope of practice is focused on providing education and management to prevent and solve breastfeeding problems and to encourage a social environment that effectively supports the breastfeeding mother–infant dyad. Those who successfully complete the International Board of Lactation Consultant Examiners (IBLCE) certification process are entitled to use the IBCLC (International Board Certified Lactation Consultant) after their names (www.iblee.org).

**La Leche League** International, nonprofit, nonsectarian organization dedicated to providing education, information, support, and encouragement to women who want to breastfeed. Founded in 1956 by seven women who had learned about successful breastfeeding while nursing their own babies, it currently has approximately 7,100 accredited lay leaders to facilitate more than 3,000 monthly mother-to-mother breastfeeding support group meetings around the world (www.lalecheleague.org).

to work before 3 months post-partum is associated with a lower likelihood of meeting ones' breastfeeding intentions.[143,150] Breastfeeding duration appears to be reduced by longer hours of work and shorter maternity leave.[151] A Los Angeles–area WIC program provided electric pumps upon request to participants and found a 5.5 times greater chance that women did not request formula at 6 months if they received an electric pump when requested than if they did not, suggesting that breastfeeding was more successful after return to work when a breast pump was available.[152] A lactation program (including an employee's choice of a class on the benefits of breastfeeding), services of a lactation consultant, and a private room in the workplace with equipment for pumping resulted in longer duration even among mothers working full time.[151] The inclusion of a Healthy People 2020 goal to increase worksite support of breastfeeding highlights its importance to improving duration of breastfeeding.

Studies indicate that women who continue to breastfeed once they return to work miss less time from work because of baby-related illnesses and have shorter absences when they do miss work, compared with women who do not breastfeed.[153] Worksite programs that support breastfeeding facilitate the continuation of breastfeeding after mothers return to their jobs and offer additional advantages to employers: employee morale and loyalty, image as family-friendly, recruiting for personnel, and retention of employees after childbirth all improved.[154]

TABLE 6.12 ▸ Important elements of worksite lactation support programs

- Prenatal lactation education tailored for working women
- Corporate policies providing information for all employees on the benefits of breastfeeding and on why their breastfeeding co-workers need support
- Education for personnel about the services available to support breastfeeding women
- Adequate breaks, flexible work hours, job sharing, and part-time work
- Private "Mother's Rooms" for expressing milk in a secure and relaxing environment
- Access to hospital-grade, autocycling breast pumps at the workplace
- Small refrigerators for the safe storage of breast milk
- Subsidization or purchase of individually owned portable breast pumps for employees
- Access to lactation professional on-site or by phone to give breastfeeding education, counseling, and support during pregnancy, after delivery, and when the mother returns to work
- Coordination with on-site or near-site child care programs so the infant can be breastfed during the day
- Support groups for working mothers with children

SOURCE: U.S. Department of Health and Human Services. HHS Blueprint for Action on Breastfeeding. Washington, DC: U.S. Department of Health and Human Services, Office on Women's Health, 2000.[58]

National breastfeeding promotion includes Breastfeeding (http://mchb.hrsa.gov/pregnancyandbeyond/breastfeeding/), which provides resources for employers and employees consistent with federal law. Key elements of worksite lactation support programs are presented in Table 6.12.

Women planning to return to work have several choices. Breast milk can be expressed during the day into sterile containers, refrigerated or frozen, and then used for subsequent bottle feedings when the mother is at work. (See Chapter 7 for storage guidelines.) With on-site childcare, it is possible to breastfeed during breaks and lunch hours. Another possibility is to train the body to produce milk only when the mother is home during the evenings and during the night. To accomplish this, a woman should omit one feeding at a time during the periods of the day when she will not be feeding or expressing milk. This will help her to reduce her milk supply without experiencing engorgement. She gradually weans to the feedings at the appropriate time of the day. This method works because removal of milk is the stimuli for milk production. Generally, at least two feedings per day are needed for women to continue making milk. Unless a mother is returning to work immediately after delivery, a bottle should not be introduced before lactation is well established, which is usually at least 4 weeks. Information about hospital-grade breast pumps is readily available on the Internet.

## The Business Case for Breastfeeding

The Office of Women's Health has created a program called the Business Case for breastfeeding (http://www.womenshealth.gov/breastfeeding/employer-solutions/business-case.html) to educate employers about the value of supporting breastfeeding in the workplace. The kit provides a sample policy for supporting breastfeeding employees, a breastfeeding program assessment form, and templates for flyers and feedback, as well as a resource guide so that employers and employees can understand their responsibilities according to federal law.

## The Community

To increase breastfeeding rates in a community, it is important to identify community attitudes and obstacles to breastfeeding, and to solicit the support for breastfeeding from community leadership. Establishment of a multidisciplinary breastfeeding task force with representatives from physicians, hospitals and birthing centers, public health, home visitors, La Leche League, government, industry, school boards, and journalists can be an effective vehicle for assessing community breastfeeding support needs and sponsoring collaborative efforts to overcoming community obstacles to breastfeeding.[137] Barriers to breastfeeding may include lack of access to reliable and culturally appropriate sources of information and social support, cultural perception of bottle feeding as the norm, aggressive marketing of breast milk substitutes, and laws that prohibit breastfeeding in public. Public outrage in response to a 2006 image of an infant feeding at a woman's breast on the front of a magazine about babies demonstrates that breastfeeding is not perceived as a cultural norm.

### Public Health Support of Breastfeeding

In the past decade, legislative efforts at both the federal and state level have been made to protect a woman's right to breastfeed (Table 6.13). States vary widely in not only whether there is legislation relating to breastfeeding, but also the depth and breadth of the legislation (http://www.usbreastfeeding.org/p/cm/ld/fid=7). Legislation is used to protect a woman's right to breastfeed, to consider breastfeeding in family law situations, to regulate breast pumps, and to provide incentives to employers who provide breastfeeding support. Legislation addresses issues such as a woman's right to breastfeed in public and on federal property, express milk at work, and be exempt from jury duty. In 2010, Section 4207 of the Patient Protection and Affordable Care Act amended the Fair Labor Standards Act. The amendment requires employers to provide reasonable break time and a private, non-bathroom place for nursing mothers to express breast milk during the workday, for one year after the child's birth.

TABLE 6.13 ▸ Landmark U.S. breastfeeding policy statements and conferences

- Report of the Surgeon General's Workshop on Breastfeeding and Human Lactation[162]
- Follow-up Report: Surgeon General's Workshop on Breastfeeding and Human Lactation[169]
- Healthy People 2010 Breastfeeding Goals for the Nation[141]
- DHHS Maternal and Child Health Bureau National Workshop: Call to Action: Better Nutrition for Mothers, Children, and Families. Washington, DC: National Center for Education in Maternal and Child Health[170]
- Second Follow-up Report: Surgeon General's Workshop on Breastfeeding and Human Lactation[171]
- National Breastfeeding Policy Conference. Presented by the UCLA Center for Healthier Children, Families and Communities, Breastfeeding Resource Program, in cooperation with the U.S. Department of Health and Human Services, Health Resources and Services Administration, Maternal and Child Health Bureau, and the Centers for Disease Control and Prevention.[172]
- Healthy People 2010 Breastfeeding Goals for the Nation[141]
- DHHS Blueprint for Action on Breastfeeding[58]
- US Breastfeeding Committee Strategic Plan[173]
- The Surgeon General's Call to Action to Support Breastfeeding, 2011[174]
- Healthy People 2020 Breastfeeding Goals for the Nation[140]



Many HHS agencies have breastfeeding initiatives. The Title V Maternal and Child Health programs of the Health Resources and Services Administration provide substantial support services, training, and research for breastfeeding (www.mchb.hrsa.gov). The Centers for Disease Control and Prevention play a major role in supporting breastfeeding nationally through applied research, program evaluation, and surveillance (www.cdc.gov).

## Model Breastfeeding Promotion Programs

**LO 6.8** Identify at least two public health breastfeeding promotion programs that have demonstrated effectiveness at increasing breastfeeding initiation and duration.

### WIC National Breastfeeding Promotion Project—Loving Support Makes Breastfeeding Work

The WIC has always supported breastfeeding, but in 1995 it began to reposition breastfeeding as a way for a family to establish a special relationship with their child from the very onset of his or her life using a social marketing campaign called Best Start.[132,155] The campaign slogan, "Loving Support Makes Breastfeeding Work," capitalizes on the concept that everyone is important to women's breastfeeding success—family, friends, doctors, and the community. Campaign materials and a counseling program were developed to help mothers work through individual barriers and constraints to breastfeeding. The key messages are (1) helping women feel comfortable with breastfeeding, (2) tips on how breastfeeding can work around a busy schedule, and (3) the involvement of family and friends to make breastfeeding a success. Since 1997, the Loving Support Makes Breastfeeding Work campaign has expanded to 72 state agencies, Indian tribal organizations, and territories participating at various levels.[156,157]

This program has been implemented at the state level with positive outcomes, including better initiation and duration of breastfeeding.[158] Building on the idea that fathers are important, a father-to-father breastfeeding promotion program in Texas resulted in increased breastfeeding rates at WIC clinics using peer dads.[156] Increased breastfeeding support from relatives and friends was also documented from data collected in a mail survey.

Federal regulations as part of the 2009 appropriations contained provisions to expand the scope of WIC activities to encourage its participants to breastfeed. A national program called Loving Support to Grow and Glow in WIC provided training for local agencies.

### Wellstart International

Wellstart International is an independent, nonprofit organization headquartered in San Diego, California, that is dedicated to supporting the health and nutrition of mothers and infants worldwide through the promotion of breastfeeding. Wellstart focuses on the development of local leadership and teamwork by providing education and technical assistance to perinatal health care providers and educators around the world, enabling them to promote maternal and child health in their own settings through the support of breastfeeding. Wellstart faculty and staff offer in-depth clinical and programmatic expertise and both domestic and international experience to hospitals, clinics, and university schools of medicine, nursing, and nutrition, as well as to a wide variety of governmental and nongovernmental health and population agencies. Wellstart is a designated World Health Organization Collaborating Center on Breastfeeding promotion, with international and domestic efforts actively taking place.

The combined approach of community outreach activities, combined with the use of Information, Education, and Communication (IEC) materials targeting key behaviors, and coordination and referral to trained service providers, produced significant behavior changes at the local, regional, and national levels.[156] Increases in breastfeeding initiation, exclusive breastfeeding duration, and reductions in water, herbal tea, and pacifier use were among the positive changes.

On a global level, we must do everything we can "to increase women's confidence in their ability to breastfeed. Such empowerment involves the removal of constraints and influence that manipulate perceptions and behavior towards breastfeeding, often by subtle and indirect means. Furthermore, obstacles to breastfeeding within the health system, the workplace, and the community must be eliminated." These words are from the WHO/UNICEF Innocenti Declaration on the Protection Promotion and Support of Breastfeeding (1990).[159] As we have seen, breastfeeding is best for the vast majority of infants and is physiologically possible for the vast majority of women. The challenge is to overcome barriers and provide support systems at the local, national, and international level so that the initiation and duration of breastfeeding continue to increase.

## KEY POINTS

1. With rare exceptions, human milk is the optimal food for infants, exclusively for 6 months and with supplemental foods for a year or longer. Benefits to infants include protection from iron deficiency, better gains in cognitive ability, fewer acute respiratory and gastrointestinal illnesses, and lower risk of sudden infant death syndrome, celiac disease, inflammatory bowel disease, neuroblastoma, allergies, and asthma.
2. A thorough understanding of the anatomy and physiology of lactation is key to enabling health care providers in providing effective lactation support.
3. Maternal benefits of breastfeeding include minimization of postpartum blood loss, delayed fertility, greater self-confidence and bonding with the baby, and reduced risk of ovarian and breast cancers.
4. Newborns who are getting adequate human milk have about six wet diapers and three to four soft, yellowish stools per day by 5–7 days postpartum. Even slow gainers are alert, bright, and responsive, whereas infants who are failing to thrive are apathetic, hard to arouse, and have a weak cry.
5. Removal of milk from the breast is the stimulus for making more milk. Most women can make enough milk for their infant, although storage capacity (breast size) differences may determine how often the infant feeds in 24 hours.
6. Breastfed infants should be supplemented with vitamin K at birth and with 400 IU of vitamin D per day beginning at 2 months. In areas where water is not fluoridated, infant supplementation after the age of 6 months may be the best choice.
7. Breastfeeding women can lose modest amounts of weight while breastfeeding by choosing a diet following a healthy dietary pattern. Breastfeeding women need an additional 330 calories per day in the first 6 months, and 400 cal thereafter. Energy intake should be adjusted for activity level and achievement and maintenance of healthy weight.
8. Maternal diet does not significantly alter the protein, carbohydrate, and major mineral composition of breast milk, but it does affect the fatty acid profile, amounts of some vitamins, and some, but not all, trace minerals. For a majority of nutrients, the quality of the milk is preserved over the quantity of milk when maternal diet is inadequate.
9. Maternal diet may be associated with infant colic. Avoidance of cow's milk and cow's-milk products, eggs, peanuts, tree nuts, wheat, soy, and fish have been associated with a reduction in infant colic symptoms in the first 6 weeks of life.

10. Successful breastfeeding is possible for women who follow vegetarian diets. Careful attention to vitamin $B_{12}$ supplementation is important for women who are vegan.

11. Support for breastfeeding women from husbands, mothers, sisters, health care providers, communities, employers, and policy makers is critical to breastfeeding success and impacts breastfeeding rates in the community.

## REVIEW QUESTIONS

1. The composition of human milk changes
   a. over the time of day, but stays constant through a single feeding, and over time from birth.
   b. over the time from birth, but stays constant through a single feeding and over the day.
   c. over a single feeding, and across the day, but stays constant over time from birth.
   d. over the time of day, within a single feeding, and over the time since birth.
2. Colostrum differs from mature human milk in the following ways:
   a. It is higher in protein mononuclear cells and is thick and yellow in color.
   b. It is higher in protein, but lower in sodium, potassium, and chloride, and is yellow in color.
   c. It is lower in protein, but higher in fat, sodium, potassium, and chloride, and is bluish in color.
   d. It is lower in protein, higher in carbohydrates, and similar in sodium, potassium, and chloride.
3. The benefits of breastfeeding include
   a. hormonal, physical, and psychological benefits for the mother, but no differences for the infant.
   b. no hormonal physical, or psychological benefits for the mother, but the infant gets heightened protection from infections and several chronic diseases.
   c. hormonal, physical, and psychological benefits for the mother, and the infant gets heightened protection from infections and several chronic diseases.
   d. no hormonal benefits, but decreased breast cancer in the mother, and the infant gets heightened protection from infections and several chronic diseases.
4. The best way to increase human milk production is to
   a. reduce fat in the mothers' diet.
   b. remove milk from the breast and feed frequently.
   c. feed the infant at both breasts in a single feeding.
   d. use a pump to express milk at the beginning of a feeding.
5. Nipple pain is common in breastfeeding. Women should be counseled to
   a. get used to it; it will eventually go away.
   b. use antibiotic creams to prevent mastitis.
   c. see a lactation consultant for proper positioning of the infant at the breast.
   d. use a pump instead of having the infant at the breast until the pain goes away.
6. When counseling a healthy woman about what to eat during breastfeeding, the best advice is:
   a. Eat and drink whatever you want; it doesn't change the milk composition or hurt the baby as long as you take a multivitamin.
   b. Eat a variety of foods, following a healthy eating pattern for moms.
   c. Avoid chocolate, mint, tomatoes, onions, and cabbage because they cause colic in the baby.
   d. Avoid wheat, milk, eggs, and nuts to prevent allergies in the infant.
7. Which of the following is true about maternal weight loss while breastfeeding?
   a. Women should not try to lose weight while breastfeeding because it changes the milk composition.
   b. Women should not try to lose weight while breastfeeding because milk production will suffer.
   c. Women can try to lose weight while breastfeeding as long as it is modest (500 kcal/day deficit).
   d. Women can try to lose as much weight as they want while breastfeeding because ketones in breast milk are not harmful to the baby.
8. A vegan breastfeeding woman should be advised to
   a. continue her vegan diet, if she chooses, while making sure that her intake of vitamin $B_{12}$ and other nutrients is adequate from food and/or supplements.
   b. continue her vegan diet with no concerns about adequate nutrients in her milk.

c. become a lacto-ovo vegetarian to ensure adequate calcium and vitamin D intake.

d. begin adding meat and other iron-rich foods to her diet to ensure her milk has adequate iron.

9. Fear of inadequate milk supply is a contributor to early breastfeeding cessation. What would be key components of breastfeeding advice to give to a new mother in the early postpartum period to help her develop confidence in her milk supply?

   a. Buy an infant scale and weigh the infant before and after each feeding.

   b. Feed the infant every four hours even if the infant doesn't seem hungry, and if the infant has about six wet diapers a day, she is eating adequately.

   c. Feed the infant when she displays early signs of hunger, and if the infant has about six wet diapers and about three stools daily, she is eating adequately.

   d. Nurse the infant at both breasts at each feeding and offer a formula supplement if the infant still seems hungry.

10. Describe the stages of lactogenesis, including the time frame of breastfeeding, where it occurs, major milk composition changes (if any), and milk production changes.

11. Describe four of the nutritional benefits of human milk to the infant.

Visit www.cengagebrain.com to access MindTap, a complete digital course that includes additional resources.

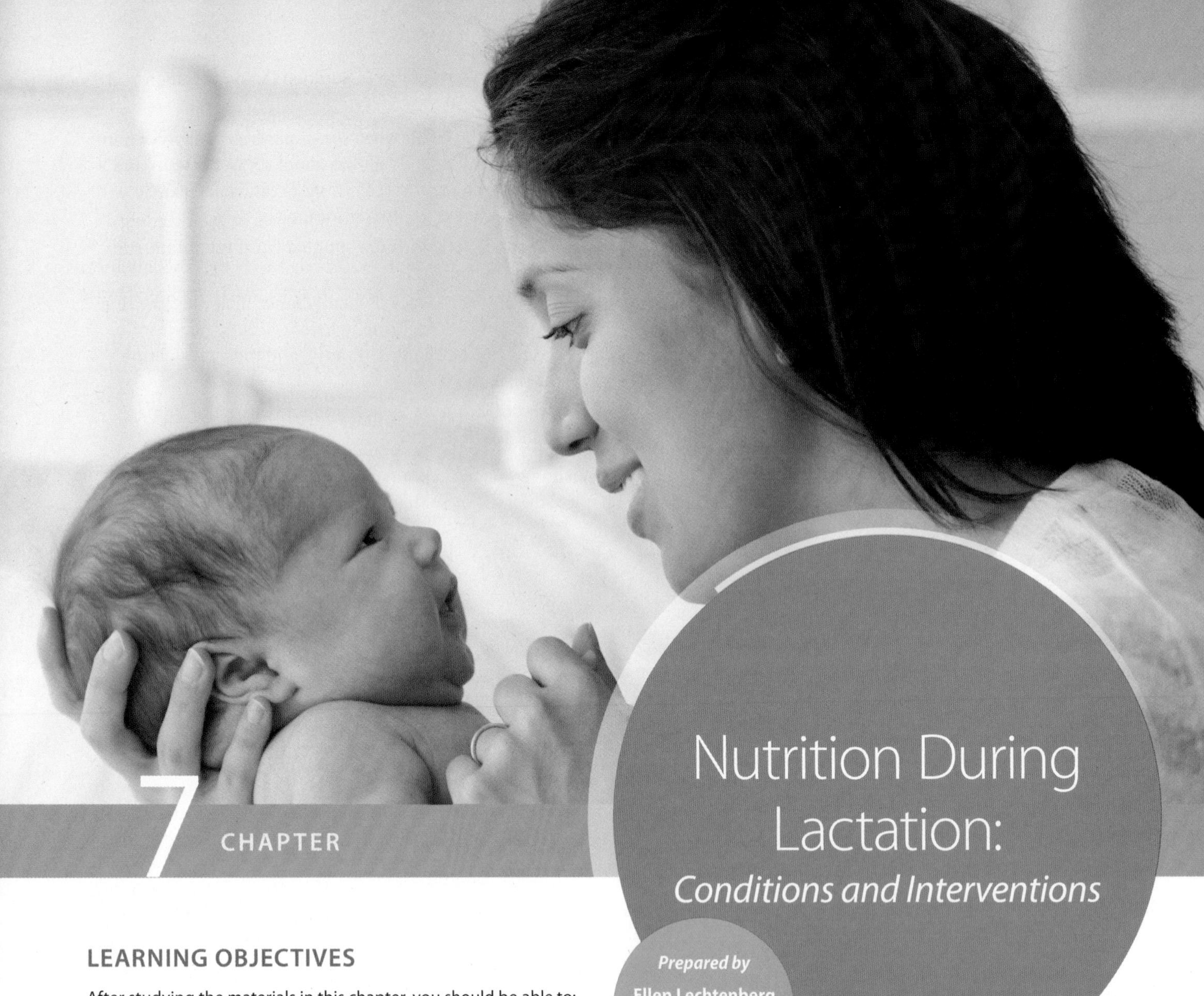

7 CHAPTER

# Nutrition During Lactation: *Conditions and Interventions*

*Prepared by*
**Ellen Lechtenberg and Maureen A. Murtaugh**

## LEARNING OBJECTIVES

After studying the materials in this chapter, you should be able to:

**7.1** List at least five common breastfeeding conditions.

**7.2** Associate positive and negative impacts of maternal medications on mother's breast milk.

**7.3** List two examples of herbal galactogogues used during lactation.

**7.4** Describe the impact of alcohol on mother's milk.

**7.5** Explain causes of hyperbilirubinemia and ways to prevent kernicterus.

**7.6** Identify ways health professionals can help the mother of multiples face the challenges of breastfeeding.

**7.7** Distinguish between food allergy and food intolerance.

**7.8** Identify at least three factors that contribute to increased readmission rates for late-preterm infants.

**7.9** List three benefits of mother's breast milk for premature infants.

**7.10** Demonstrate knowledge of medical contraindications to breastfeeding.

**7.11** List three guidelines for storage of human milk for home use.

**7.12** Analyze one of the model programs for breastfeeding promotion in the United States.

Ariel Skelley/Getty Images

# Introduction

The key to successful breastfeeding management is for the mother–infant breastfeeding pair to receive informed, consistent, and individualized support from health care professionals both in the hospital and after discharge. The vast majority of women do not experience significant problems with breastfeeding. Many of the more common problems that do arise can be prevented through prenatal breastfeeding education and a positive, supportive breastfeeding initiation period.

This chapter discusses prevention and treatment of common breastfeeding conditions. Issues related to maternal use of medications, herbal remedies, drugs of abuse, and environmental contaminants are addressed. The chapter presents important considerations for breastfeeding multiples, preterm infants, and infants with medical problems. It provides information on the safe collection and storage of human milk and milk banks. The chapter concludes with case studies providing examples of management of challenging breastfeeding problems and with examples of model programs promoting support for breastfeeding in the health care system that others should model themselves after.

# Common Breastfeeding Conditions

LO 7.1 List at least five common breastfeeding conditions.

## Sore Nipples

Early, mild nipple discomfort is common among women initiating breastfeeding. In most women, the discomfort is transient and usually subsides by the end of the first week. It is, however, not uncommon for some women to experience nipple pain lasting a month postpartum.[2] Severe nipple pain, the presence of nipple cracks or fissures, pain that persists throughout a feeding, or pain that is not improved by the end of the first week should not be considered normal and requires a detailed evaluation.[3] Painful nipples and nipple trauma can lead women to become discouraged and depressed with breastfeeding. As many as one third of women who experience nipple pain and trauma switch to bottle feeding within the first 6–8 weeks postpartum.[2,3,7] Nipple pain is the second reason mothers list for discontinuation of breastfeeding and the top reason mothers stop breastfeeding in the hospital.[2] The first reason for discontinuation of breastfeeding is perceived low milk supply.

The best prevention of nipple pain and soreness is proper positioning of the baby on the breast. In order to feed effectively, the baby needs to draw the breast deeply into the mouth, so that the mother's nipple approximates to the junction of the hard and soft palate.[4] This enables the baby to use its tongue smoothly and rhythmically against the under surface of the breast and remove milk from the ducts. With a good latch, the mother's nipple is so far back in the baby's mouth that it is beyond the reach of the compression wave of the tongue, so no pain is caused, and no damage is done. If a woman is experiencing pain, a lactation consultant or a health care professional well trained in lactation should observe the mother nursing her baby. The lactation consultant can determine whether the pain is simply related to breastfeeding a new baby, or if a problem exists.

The main causes of persistent nipple pain are trauma from poor positioning of the infant at the breast, poor latch, improper release of suction after a feed, infection (thrush or *staphylococcus aureus*), pumping with too much suction or incorrect breast flange size, a disorganized or dysfunctional suck, and dermatologic abnormalities.[3] Nipple damage can occur even prior to discharge from the hospital.[2,5] Breast care and cleaning rituals can also contribute to nipple soreness. Proper cleaning of the lactating breast involves only daily washing with warm water. Soaps and other cleansing products can irritate the nipple, and some creams and lotions can cause an allergic reaction and skin irritation. Plastic-backed breast pads used to prevent milk leakage can trap moisture and inhibit airflow to the nipple.[3]

Women can take simple steps to manage nipple pain. Recommended strategies include letting breasts air-dry after nursing, rubbing expressed milk or an all-purpose ointment (not petroleum-based) on nipples, and using warm compresses on sore nipples.[2,3] The common belief that limiting the frequency or duration of feedings will prevent or heal sore nipples is not substantiated by the literature.[5] Use of a pump to express milk can help to maintain supply if the nipples are so sore that the mother cannot nurse.[4] However, the suction on the breast pump should be adjusted carefully. High suction can make nipples sore and red and even cause blisters.

## Flat or Inverted Nipples

Some women have flat or inverted nipples, which do not extend very far into the baby's mouth. This should not impact breastfeeding if the latch is correct. If the baby is struggling with latch, instruct the mother to roll her nipple between her fingers or use a breast pump prior to feeding to help draw out the nipple.

## Letdown Failure

> "After she latches on, take deep, long breaths—think yoga not Lamaze when you nurse. As you exhale, visualize the milk letting down through your breasts into the baby's mouth."
>
> —C. Martin and N. F. Krebs[6]

Letdown failure is not common,[6] but because letdown is necessary to successful breastfeeding, it is important to address the matter. Stress may inhibit oxytocin, as well as alcohol and distractions. Oxytocin nasal spray can be prescribed by a physician for letdown failure. The synthetic oxytocin is sprayed into the nose and stimulates letdown, but it can only be used for a few days to help women get through a tough time. Other methods should be used at the same time to stimulate letdown. Prolonged letdown failure will cause lactation suppression.[7] Martin and Krebs[6] recommend a number of techniques to help women relax and enhance letdown:

- Play soothing music that the mother can focus on while nursing.
- Have the partner rub his knuckles down her spine.
- Try different nursing positions.
- Get out of the house. Most babies enjoy a walk.
- Arrange for some time alone (a few hours).
- Decrease number of caffeinated beverages and increase water consumption for a few weeks.

## Hyperactive Letdown

Hyperactive letdown can also be a problem, especially among first-time mothers. When letdown is overactive, milk streams from the breast as feeding begins. Milk may also leak from the breast that the infant is not being nursed from. The milk streams quickly, and the infant may be overwhelmed by the volume. The infant may choke, cough, or gulp to keep up with the flow. When the infant gulps, the infant may take in air, develop gas pain, and then become fussy.

Management includes removing the infant from the breast when letdown occurs and waiting for the milk flow to slow down before putting the infant back to the breast.[7] The mother can also express the milk until the flow slows. (Expressed milk can be frozen for later use.) Expressing milk also allows infants to get hindmilk and prevents gas and colic that may result from a large volume of relatively low-fat milk.

## Hyperlactation

Hyperlactation occurs when the milk volume being produced by the mother far exceeds the intake of the baby. A hyperactive letdown may be a sign of overproduction. Other signs include breasts that are not drained completely during a feeding, chronic plugged ducts, leaking in between feedings, and pain with letdown or deep in the breast. Symptoms in the baby include those already mentioned with hyperactive letdown, as well as spitting up, poor weight gain due to the high volume of low-fat milk, or good initial weight gain followed by poor weight gain. During the feeding, the baby may have difficulty maintaining latch and may also arch back off of the breast.[8] Other symptoms in the baby may include excessive gas and green, frothy explosive stools due to rapid transit time. These symptoms often lead the mother to incorrectly limit her intake of milk or other foods, believing the symptoms are caused by an allergy instead of a foremilk/hindmilk imbalance. If intake of high volume of low-fat foremilk continues over time, the baby may develop colitis.

Management in the mother is to reduce production. This can be done by having the baby nurse on only one side during feedings and having the mother express milk on the other side only for comfort. Cabbage leaves or cold compresses may also be used to decrease production.

## Engorgement

Engorgement occurs when breasts are overfilled with milk. This is common during the first week of the birth and in first-time mothers.[9] Engorgement occurs when the supply-and-demand process is not yet established, and the milk is abundant. It also occurs with infrequent or ineffective removal of milk from the breast because of mother–infant separation, a sleepy baby, sore nipples, or improper breastfeeding technique.[3] The best way to prevent engorgement is to nurse the infant frequently. (Newborn infants will often nurse every hour and a half.) If the infant is not available to nurse, expressing milk every few hours will prevent engorgement while helping to build and maintain a milk supply.

The peak time for engorgement varies among women and can occur any time from day 2 through day 14, but is most common on days 2–3. Engorgement can result in discomfort, difficulty in establishing milk flow, and difficulty in latch-on.[7,9] Severe engorgement inhibits milk flow because the swollen tissue is compressing the milk ducts—not because the mother is failing to experience the letdown or milk ejection reflex. Once engorgement occurs, there are several simple treatments to help ease the discomfort. It is important for the mother to express milk until her breasts are no longer hard before putting the infant to breast. This will make it more comfortable for her and easier for her baby to latch on. The use of hand expression or an electric breast pump can help establish milk flow and soften the breast to make it easier for the infant to attach properly and further extract milk. Women can use analgesics to reduce pain from engorgement. A warm shower or warm compresses with massage before feedings may be helpful to relieve pressure and trigger milk flow. Application of cold compresses or gel packs between feedings helps to reduce pain and swelling.[3,8]

**Cabbage Leaves** Many believe that cabbage leaves (either cool or at room temperature) reduce discomfort and swelling associated with engorgement, although it is not known how the effects are mediated. In randomized trials, cabbage leaves and gel packs were equally effective in the treatment of engorgement, as were cabbage extract and a placebo cream.[9] The Academy of Breastfeeding medicine suggest these treatments may help discomfort but not actually relieve engorgement.[10] Raw cabbage leaves are applied directly to the breast until they wilt, which is approximately 20 minutes.

TABLE 7.1 ▸ Common breast problems and their symptoms

| CHARACTERISTICS | ENGORGEMENT | PLUGGED DUCTS | MASTITIS | BREAST ABSCESS |
|---|---|---|---|---|
| Cause | Incomplete and/or inefficient milk emptying from baby or pump | Infrequent breast feeding/ pumping, incorrect flange size (pumping) | Unresolved plugged duct | Unresolved mastitis |
| Onset | Gradual, immediately postpartum | Gradual, after feedings | Sudden, after 10 days | Sudden, after 10 days |
| Breast Symptoms | Generalized swelling and hot area with pain in both breasts | Swelling may shift, little or no heat with mild focused pain in one breast | Localized pain and red, hot, swollen area usually on breast | Localized pain and, red, hot, swollen area on affected breast, tender lump |
| Temperature | <38.4° C (101° F) | No fever <38.4° C | Fever (>38.4°) | Fever (>38.4°) |
| Other Symptoms | Feels well | Feels well | Flu-like | Flu-like |
| Treatment | Increase frequency of breastfeeding or pumping<br>Cold compresses, anti-inflammatory for pain, use heat, massage, and pumping before feeding as needed | Continue breast feeding, be sure to empty the breast, evaluate flange size<br>Anti-inflammatory for pain<br>Use warm compresses | Frequent pumping<br>Anti-inflammatory for pain<br>May need antibiotics | Doctor required to drain the abscess<br>Anti-inflammatory for pain<br>Antibiotics |

SOURCE: http://women.webmd.com/blocked-milk-ducts-and-breast-feeding, http://www.nbci.ca/index.php?option=com_content&view=article&id=7:blocked-ducts-a-mastitis&catid=5:information&Itemid=17 Breastfeeding: A Guide for the Medical Professions, 7th Ed. by R.A. Lawrence and R.M. Lawrence, Table C16.1, ©2011

## Plugged Duct

An obstructed, or *plugged*, duct is a localized blockage of milk resulting from milk stasis (milk remaining in the ducts).[3] The mother may feel a painful knot in one breast but usually does not have a fever or other signs of illness. Treatment for plugged ducts is gentle massage, warm compresses, and complete emptying of the breast.[3,6] Women should consider changing nursing positions to facilitate emptying of the breast. For example, if the woman is nursing while lying down, she may try a sitting position, or she may switch the position of holding the infant (see Illustration 6.5 in Chapter 6). If the woman is pumping, the flange size should be assessed. In most cases, using a larger size flange will improve efficiency of pumping. When plugging occurs repeatedly, a gentle manual massage before nursing often results in the plug being expelled. Consider use of lecithin for chronic plugged ducts. Lecithin is a phospholipid used as an emulsifier to keep fat dispersed and suspended in water instead of building up in the ducts. One tablespoon per day of oral granular lecithin has been reported an effective therapy. If not resolved, plugged ducts lead to mastitis.[11]

## Mastitis

Mastitis is an inflammation of the breast most commonly found in breastfeeding women. It can be infective or non-infective. It occurs in about 1–33 percent of breastfeeding women. This range is large and depends on breastfeeding duration.[8,11] Mastitis can occur any time during lactation. The higher percentages of mastitis occur 2–3 weeks after birth with the majority of cases occurring within the first 12 weeks.[3,11] Some women get mastitis after having cracked or sore nipples, and some get it without any noticeable problem on the surface of the breast. Missing a feeding or the infant sleeping through the night may precipitate engorgement, plugged ducts, and then mastitis. Restriction from a tight bra or clothing may also increase risk of developing mastitis. Symptoms of mastitis are similar to those of a plugged duct (Table 7.1). In both conditions, there is a tender, hot, enlarged, hard, wedge-shaped area in the breast, and often an area of redness on the surface of the breast. Cases of mastitis are usually accompanied by a fever and flu-like symptoms.

It is important for the mother to continue nursing through mastitis. Effective milk removal is the most important management step in mastitis. If nursing is too painful, the mother should express milk from the breast by hand or pump. The techniques used to minimize pain from engorgement may also be used for mastitis. Ibuprofen is commonly recommended to help with the pain and inflammation.[12] Adequate rest, fluids, and nutrition are also important. In mild cases of mastitis or when symptoms have been present for less than 24 hours, efficient milk emptying via frequent nursing or pumping may be sufficient to resolve the mastitis. If symptoms do not improve within 24 hours, antibiotics should be started.[12] In a randomized trial, half of 55 women treated only with antibiotics had breast abscess, recurrent mastitis, or symptoms lasting longer than 2 weeks, compared to only 2 of 55 who also emptied their breasts (breasts can be emptied by feeding the baby or pumping).[14]

Significant delays in seeking treatment for mastitis are associated with the development of abscess and recurrent

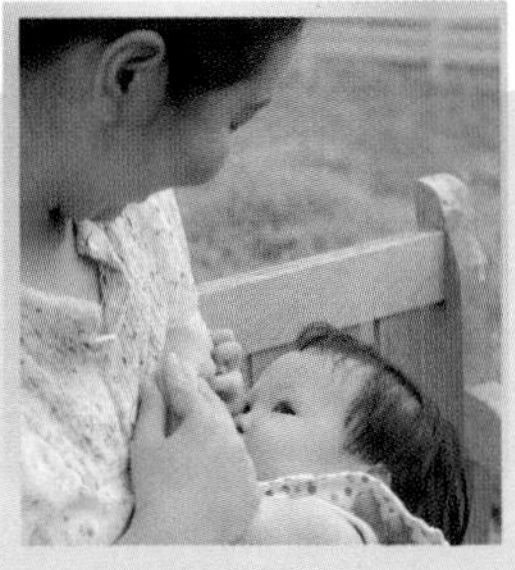
parinyabinsuk/Shutterstock.com

# CASE STUDY 7.1

## Chronic Mastitis

This was an unremarkable first pregnancy for 29-year-old Barbara Ann. Barbara Ann has reported experiencing "a little" breast enlargement during her pregnancy.

Her infant is first put to the breast at 2 hours postpartum, and the infant latches well according to mom, and suckles vigorously. The infant nurses every 2 hours over the first 3–4 days postpartum. Barbara Ann's breasts became noticeably fuller during the third postpartum day, and by the fourth postpartum day they are painfully engorged. In addition, Barbara Ann reports painful, burning, cracked nipples. The engorgement makes it difficult for her baby to latch at the breast. The baby becomes irritable, and Barbara Ann experiences a significant amount of pain. A lactation consultant gives Barbara Ann guidelines for engorgement management.

On day 5, the engorgement is still causing discomfort. Barbara Ann's nipples have become more cracked and painful. The lactation consultant notes that the infant's latch has become shallow and tight, probably in an attempt to control the flow of milk. However, the infant shows all the signs of adequate intake, including 10 very wet and 5 soiled diapers during the 24 hours prior to the consultation.

By day 7 postpartum, Barbara Ann has mastitis. She is treated with a 7-day course of dicloxacillin. A lactation consultant assists her in achieving a proper infant latch.

By day 14, Barbara Ann is feeling much better. The mastitis has resolved, and her nipples are healing. She still has tenderness during infant feedings and a healing crack on the right side. Her breasts are still uncomfortably full and are occasionally swollen and tender.

At 3 weeks postpartum, Barbara Ann develops an inflamed area on the right breast that remains red and tender despite applying warmth and massage to the area. The lactation consultant helps Barbara Ann to position the infant in a way that allows drainage of the inflamed area and recommends she pump the affected side to relieve the discomfort. The crack on the right nipple has improved, but is still not completely healed. Barbara Ann continues to show signs of oversupply, such as breasts feeling uncomfortably full, even after feeding, and excessive milk leakage between feedings. The lactation consultant provides Barbara Ann with techniques to decrease her overproduction.

After 10 days of persistent burning pain in the nipple area, Barbara Ann is treated with fluconazole for a yeast infection. Seven days after starting the fluconazole, a topical nystatin ointment is prescribed for her nipples and an oral suspension for her infant.

At 7 weeks postpartum, Barbara Ann calls the lactation consultant to report another flare-up of mastitis. Her health care provider prescribes a 10-day course of dicloxacillin. Barbara Ann is still treating her nipples with nystatin ointment. At 8 weeks postpartum her mastitis resolved; her nipple pain is still present, but improving. Barbara Ann is nursing the infant on one side only per feeding and reports that the infant latches better when she is in a more reclined position.

SOURCE: Adapted from: Anonymous. Case management of a breastfeeding mother with persistent oversupply and recurrent breast infections. *J Hum Lact*, 2000, 16:221–5.

### Questions

1. Name the causes of engorgement.
2. List at least two possible nutrition diagnoses for this case.
3. Identify at least one nutrition intervention for each diagnosis listed.
4. Name potential indicators for each intervention listed.

mastitis.[3] Abrupt weaning is not recommended and increases risk of abscess development (see also Case Study 7.1). Vertical transmission of human immunodeficiency virus (HIV) from mother to child increases during mastitis infection. The World Health Organization recommends HIV positive mothers avoid breastfeeding on the affected side until the infection resolves.[8]

## Low Milk Supply

Real or perceived insufficient milk supply is the most common reason for cessation of breastfeeding.[2] Low milk supply is usually caused by the mother not breastfeeding or pumping often enough or inefficient emptying of the breast caused by a poor latch or incorrect flange size while pumping. Stress may also contribute to a low milk supply.[13] The mother may wish to use a ***galactogogue***, which is a drug or herb used to increase milk supply. Galactogogues should be used only after evaluating maternal causes for low supply and when increasing breastfeeding and/or pumping has not been successful. According to the Academy of Breastfeeding Medicine, caution should be used when recommending galactogogues due to potentially serious side effects.[15] Encourage the mother to nurse or pump using a hospital-grade electric breast pump every 2–3 hours during the day and once at night. If the baby is not nursing effectively, the mother may need to pump

**galactogogue** A medicine or herbal substance taken with the belief to increase milk supply. It may also be taken to help with breastmilk initiation and maintenance.[15]

after breastfeeding to improve her supply. Make sure her diet is adequate and her fluid intake is appropriate. Encourage resting and relaxation techniques. Review current medication and hormonal contraceptives. Estrogen is known to inhibit lactation. Progesterone-only birth control pills have been used without problems on milk supply.[16]

Common medications used as galactogogues are Metoclopramide (Reglan) and Domperidone (Motilium). Metoclopramide is the most commonly used medication in the United States for improving milk supply.[15] It is prescribed by a physician, who should also follow the mother for potential side effects. The usual dose is 10 mg taken 3–4 times per day for 14 days with a taper over 4–5 days. Metoclopramide may cause fatigue and drowsiness as well as diarrhea. Increased depression, anxiety, confusion, dizziness, or headache may also occur. A black box warning by the FDA has been issued warning regarding long-term or high-dose use of Methoclopramide. Tardive dyskinesia (involuntary and repetitive movements of the body) has been linked to Methoclopramide use even when the drug is discontinued. Side effects should be reported to the prescribing physician. It may be necessary for the mother with these side effects to discontinue use of the medication. Domperidone is commonly used outside the United States. It has been approved for use in most countries in the developed world. In September 2011, the FDA granted Domperidone orphan drug status and approved its use for breastfeeding mothers with low milk supply. Side effects are not common. Domperidone has been shown to be safe and effective in improving milk production in a randomized control study.[15] Both medications increase prolactin levels through dopamine receptors.

Fenugreek (*Trigonella foenum-graceum*), goat's-rue (*Galega officinalis*), and milk thistle (*Silybum marianum*)/ blessed thistle (*Cnicus benedictus*) are common herbal galactogogues.[15] It is important to inform the mother that most herbal or natural galactogogues have not been evaluated scientifically and are not regulated by the U.S. Food and Drug Administration. Galactogogues are used in the short-term (1–3 weeks). Studies are lacking on potential side effects of longer-term use. These products are discussed further in the "Herbal Remedies" section of this chapter.

# Maternal Medications

**LO 7.2** Associate positive and negative impacts of medications on mother's breast milk.

> "It is equally inappropriate to discontinue breastfeeding when it is not medically necessary to do so as it is to continue breastfeeding while taking contraindicated drugs."
>
> —R. A. Lawrence[18]

The single most common medical issue health care provider's face in managing breastfeeding patients is maternal medication use.[18] Ninety to 99 percent of breastfeeding women receive some type of medication during their first week postpartum.[19] Most medications taken by nursing mothers are excreted in breast milk. These include both over-the-counter medications and prescription drugs. Unfortunately, data on drug safety may not be readily available to women and health care providers.[20] Some mothers who discontinue breastfeeding prematurely reported concern about the use of medications as a major reason.[19] Recommending that a mother discontinue breastfeeding to take a medication is almost never required and should only be done as a last resort. For most maternal conditions, required drug therapy choices are available that will not cause harm to the infant.[19,21]

Two key questions to address in the analysis of the risk of an infant's exposure to a drug excreted in breast milk are: How much of the drug is excreted in milk, and at the level of excretion, what is the risk of adverse effects?[22,23] Among the numerous variables to examine to answer these questions are:

- The pharmacokinetic properties of the drug
- Time-averaged breast ***milk/plasma ratio*** of the drug
- The drug ***exposure index***
- The infant's ability to absorb, detoxify, and excrete the agent
- The dose, strength, and duration of dosing
- The infant's age, feeding pattern, total diet, and health[18,22]

Additional considerations are the well-established interethnic and racial differences in drug responsiveness, exposure of the infant to the drug during pregnancy, whether the drug can be safely given to the infant directly,[18] and the relative infant dose.[19] The ultimate test of drug safety is the measurement of the infant's plasma drug concentration and any side effects from the drug on the infant.[22] Carefully controlled studies on large enough samples to validate the results are rare but have increased during the last decade. Use of the risk–benefit algorithm for assessment of drug use in breastfeeding may also be helpful.

**milk-to-plasma drug concentration ratio (M/P ratio)** The ratio of the concentration of drug in milk to the concentration of drug in maternal plasma.[19] Since the ratio varies over time, a time-averaged ratio provides more meaningful information than data obtained at a single time point. It is helpful in understanding the mechanisms of drug transfer and should not be viewed as a predictor of risk to the infant, as it is the concentration of the drug in milk, and not the M/P ratio, that is critical to the calculation of infant dose and assessment of risk.[19,23,24]

**exposure index** The average infant milk intake per kilogram body weight per day × (M/P ratio ÷ Rate of drug clearance) × 100. It is indicative of the amount of the drug in the breast milk that the infant ingests and is expressed as a percentage of the therapeutic (or equivalent) dose for the infant.[14]

**TABLE 7.2** ▸ Resources on drugs, medications, and contaminants in human milk

- Sachs, H. C., and the AAP Committee on Drugs. Clinical Report: The Transfer of Drugs and Therapeutics Into Human Milk: An Update on Selected Topics. Pediatrics 2013:132:e796-e809.[24]
- http://pediatrics.aappublications.org/content/108/3/776.full.pdf+html
- Briggs, G. G., Freeman, R. K., and Yaffe, S. J. *Drugs in Pregnancy and Lactation*, 9th ed. Baltimore, MD: Williams and Wilkins, 2011.[21]
- Hale, T. W. *Medications and Mothers' Milk*, 15th ed. Amarillo, TX: Pharmasoft Medical Publishing, 2014.[19] Dr. Hale will answer questions from health professionals posed on the Pharmasoft website: www.iBreastfeeding.com.
- *Breastfeeding and Maternal Medication: Recommendations for Drugs in the Eleventh WHO Model List of Essential Drugs.*[30] UNICEF World Health Organization, 2003. www.who.int/child-adolescent-health/New_Publications/NUTRITION/BF_Maternal_Medication.pdf.
- Blumenthal, M., Busse, W., Goldberg, A., et al., eds. *The Complete German Commission E Monographs: Therapeutic Guide to Herbal Medicines.* Boston: Integrative Medicine Communications, 1998.[31]
- The Breastfeeding and Human Lactation Center, University of Rochester. This service is available for complex medication questions (9:30 a.m. to 4 p.m. EST, Monday to Friday, at 585-275-0088).
- HerbMed (www.herbmed.org): an interactive, electronic herbal database with links to scientific publications.
- Humphrey, S. *The Nursing Mother's Herbal.* MN: Fairview Press, 2003.
- TOXNET: National Library of Medicine Drug and Lactation database, containing summaries of published literature on the effects of over 400 drugs on lactation.
- REPROTOX: An online proprietary reproductive toxicology database, http://reprotox.org.



Fortunately, numerous resources (Table 7.2) based on a thorough evaluation of available evidence can assist the health care provider and mother in identifying which drugs are safe and which are not. The American Academy of Pediatrics (AAP) Committee on Drugs publishes guidelines for practitioners.[24–26] These guidelines provide a list of drugs divided into the following seven categories according to risk factors in relationship to breastfeeding:

1. Cytotoxic drugs that may interfere with the cellular metabolism of the nursing infant
2. Drugs of abuse for which adverse effects on the infant during breastfeeding have been reported
3. Radioactive compounds that require temporary cessation of breastfeeding
4. Drugs for which the effect on nursing infants is unknown, but may be of concern
5. Drugs that have been associated with significant effect on some nursing infants and should be given to nursing mothers with caution
6. Maternal medications usually compatible with breastfeeding
7. Food and environmental agents having no effect on breastfeeding

The list, which is updated periodically, includes only those drugs about which there is published information. Other useful monographs and review articles provide additional information on a wide array of medications.[19–22, 26]

The Breastfeeding and Human Lactation Study Center at the University of Rochester (see Table 7.2) continually updates its database of more than 3,000 references on drugs, medications, and contaminants in human milk and is a resource for complex questions on the risks to the breastfed infant. The TOXNET LactMed database is available online (http://toxnet.nlm.nih.gov/). There are also textbooks with information on drugs and breastfeeding. "Medications and Mother's Milk" by Thomas Hale (see Table 7.2) is updated regularly. It includes information on prescription and over-the-counter medications as well as common herbal remedies.[19] The *Physician's Desk Reference (PDR)* is not a good source for information about drugs and breastfeeding because the information is derived directly from pharmaceutical companies whose first concern is avoiding liability. When there are no studies that prove beyond a doubt that a drug is safe for nursing mothers, the drug companies must advise against use while breastfeeding—even if what is known about the drug suggests that there is little cause for concern.

Medications contraindicated during breastfeeding include antineoplastic agents, radioactive isotopes, drugs of abuse and drugs that suppress lactation.[18,19, and 24] Fortunately, safer alternative medications can be recommended as a substitute for most other drugs with known adverse effects on infants. Specific knowledge about a medication's safety during breastfeeding will allow proper treatment and avoid unnecessary maternal anxiety and undue risk. For example, many cold remedies, antihistamines, and decongestants are listed as usually compatible with breastfeeding, but they may suppress lactation. In a study of women who took a single 60 mg dose of Sudafed (pseudoephedrine), 24-hour milk production was decreased by 24 percent.[19] This medication should be avoided in mothers with marginal or low production. The mother taking such medications should closely monitor milk production.

Many women have questions on the safety of oral contraceptive use during lactation. There is currently no evidence of harm, but few women have been studied. There is evidence that combined oral contraceptives that contain both estrogen and progesterone may reduce the volume of breast milk.[19,27] The American College of Obstetricians and Gynecologists (ACOG) and the World Health Organization recommend against using combined oral contraceptives in the first 6 weeks postpartum. If lactation is well established at 6 weeks, ACOG recommends monitoring the infant's nutritional status if combined oral contraceptives are initiated.[27] WHO does not recommend using combined oral contraceptives from 6 weeks to 6 months unless other forms of contraceptives are not available. The La Leche League International recommends avoiding combined oral contraceptives in breastfeeding because other forms on contraception are available.[27] Progestin-only oral contraceptives and implants are safe and effective during lactation.[19,28] Implants that deliver orally active steroids should only be used after 6 weeks postpartum to avoid transferring of steroids to the newborn.[28] The Depo-Provera shot is also recommended at 6 weeks postpartum.[19]

If a drug or surgery is elective, a mother may be able to delay it until the baby is weaned. If a breastfeeding mother needs a specific medication, and the hazards to the infant are minimal, she should be instructed to take the medication after breastfeeding, at the lowest effective dose, and for the shortest duration.[18,29] Other important steps can be taken to further minimize the effects (Table 7.3). It is also sometimes possible to choose alternative routes for administration of a medication to reduce exposure. For example, prescribing an inhalant instead of a drug taken by mouth, or a topical application rather than oral dosing, reduces infant exposure. If a drug is to be taken for diagnostic testing (such as a radioactive agent) or procedure, a mother may need to withhold breastfeeding for a short period of time, pumping and discarding her milk during that time period. The mother can plan ahead in these cases and pump prior to the procedure or surgery. She can freeze her expressed milk for use while breastfeeding is withheld. Discontinuing breastfeeding due to maternal medications is a last resort but may be necessary for the health and well-being of the mother (for example, if she needs chemotherapy or radioactive treatment). Any decision to limit a mother's breastfeeding must be justified by the fact that the risk to her baby clearly outweighs the benefits of breastfeeding.

**TABLE 7.3** ▸ Minimizing the effect of maternal medication[18]

1. *Avoid long-acting forms*: Accumulation in the infant is a genuine concern because the infant may have more difficulty excreting a long-acting form of a drug, which usually requires detoxification in the liver.
2. *Schedule doses carefully*: Check usual absorption rates and peak blood levels of the drug, and schedule the doses so that the least amount possible gets into the milk. In order to minimize milk levels of most drugs, the safest time for a mother to take the drug is usually immediately after her infant nurses.
3. *Evaluate the infant*: Watch for any unusual signs or symptoms, such as changes in feeding pattern or sleeping habits, fussiness, or rash.
4. *Choose the drug that produces the least amount in the milk.*



## Herbal Remedies

**LO 7.3** List two examples of herbal galactogogues used during lactation.

Numerous herbs have been used in folk and traditional systems of healing to affect the flow of milk (Table 7.4), or to treat mastitis, infant colic, and thrush.[31–34] However, scientific information about herb use during lactation, particularly from recent studies, is sparse. The limited pertinent safety data are based on traditional use, animal studies, and knowledge of the pharmacologic activities of the products' constituents. The 2011 Academy of Breastfeeding Medicine Protocol on use of galactogogues has shifted the attitude of

**TABLE 7.4** ▸ Herbs traditionally used to affect milk production*[32,33]

| **Herbs to Promote Milk Flow** |
|---|
| Anise |
| Astralagus |
| Milk thistle |
| Caraway |
| Celery root and seed |
| Chaste tree berry (chasteberry) or monk's pepper |
| Fennel |
| Fenugreek |
| Goat's-rue |
| Hollyhock |
| Hibiscus flower |
| Lemongrass |
| Marshmallow |
| Stinging nettle |
| Raspberry |
| Rauwolfia |
| Verbena |
| **Herbs that Reduce Milk Flow** |
| Castor bean |
| Jasmine flower |
| Fresh parsley |
| Sage |

SOURCE: Journal of Pharmaceutical Sciences, M. L. Hardy. Copyright © 2000 by the American Pharmacists Association. Reproduced with permission of John Wiley & Sons, Inc.

*Many traditional galactogogues are not currently considered appropriate during lactation (see Table 7.5).

TABLE 7.5 ▸ Medicinal herbs considered not appropriate for use during pregnancy or lactation[18,36,42]

| | | | |
|---|---|---|---|
| Agnus castus | Coltsfoot | Hawthorne | Pokeroot |
| Alkanet | Comfrey | Heliotropium | Poplar |
| Aloes | Cornsilk | Hops | Prickly ash |
| Angelica | Cottonroot | Horehound, black | Pulsatilla |
| Apricot kernel | Crotalaria | Horehound, white | Queen's delight |
| Aristolchia | Darniana | Horsetail | Ragwort |
| Asafoetida | Devil's claw | Hydrocotlye | Red clover |
| Avens | Dogbane | Jamaica dogwood | Roman chaparral |
| Basil | Dong quai | Joe-pye weed | Sassafras |
| Bladderwrack | Echinacea | Juniper | Senna |
| Blue flag | Ephedra (ma huang) | Kava kava | Shepherd's purse |
| Bogbean | Eucalyptus | Licorice | Skullcap |
| Boldo | Eupatorium | Liferoot | Skunk cabbage |
| Bonese | Euphorbia | Lobelia | Squill |
| Borage | Fennel | Male fern | St. John's Wort |
| Broom | Feverfew | Mandrake | Stephania |
| Buchu | Foxglove | Mate | Stillingia |
| Buckthorn | Frangula | Meadowsweet | Tansy |
| Bugleweed | Fucus | Melilot | Tonka bean |
| Burdock | Gentian | Mistletoe | Uva-ursi |
| Calamus | German chamomile | Motherwort | Valerian root |
| Calendula | Germander | Myrrh | Vervain |
| Cascara | Ginkgo biloba | Nettle | Wild carrot |
| Cayenne pepper | Ginseng, eleuthero | Osha | Willow |
| Chamomile | Ginseng, panax | Passionflower | Wormwood |
| Chasteberry | Golden seal | Pennyroyal | Yarrow |
| Chinese rhubarb | Ground ivy | Petasites | Yellow dock |
| Cohosh, black | Groundsel | Plantain | Yohimbine |
| Cohosh, blue | Guarana | Pleurisy root | |

*Exclusion from this list should not be a recommendation for safety.



galactogogue use to one of more caution as more significant side effects have been documented for some of them.[15] Medicinal herbs should be viewed as drugs, with evaluation of both their pharmacological and toxicological potential.[1,9,35]

A mother may perceive herbs as natural and therefore safe and even preferable to conventional over-the-counter medicines or prescription drugs. However, the risks of using some herbal remedies may outweigh the potential benefits. The same risk factors that apply to drugs also apply to herbs. *Medications and Mother's Milk* (2014) contains a systematic lactation risk analysis of numerous herbal remedies. Many herbs are far from benign, and many are contraindicated during lactation (Table 7.5). Because little is known about the amount secreted in human milk or the effects on preterm or term infants, herbs that are central nervous system stimulants, herbs that destroy cells (cytotoxic), or herbs that are laxatives, hepatotoxic, carcinogenic, mutogenic, or contain potentially toxic essential oils are not recommended during lactation.[32,36]

The toxic effects of herbs are often not due to the herb itself, but are caused by products containing misidentified plants or contaminants such as heavy metals, synthetic drugs, microbial toxins, and toxic botanicals.[37] ***Medicinal herbs*** in the United States are regulated as dietary supplements and are not tested for safety or efficacy.

Herbal teas that are safe for the infant and mother during lactation are presented in Table 7.6. Lawrence[18] recommends using only herbal teas "that are prepared carefully, using only herbs for essence (e.g., Celestial Seasonings brand tea) and avoiding heavy doses of herbs with active principles." Careful attention should also be given to preparation, avoiding long steeping times.

Some culinary herbs may lead to problems when used extensively. In lactation and herbal texts, sage has a folk reputation for lowering milk supply,[32] as does parsley and peppermint, especially if the oil is taken by mouth in large doses.[38] Consumed on occasion, however, in small amounts as part of a reasonably varied diet, peppermint, parsley, sage, and other culinary herbs currently have no documented negative effect on lactation.

Although various herbal oils, gels, ointments, or creams are often suggested for use on the nipples, any substance applied to the breast or nipples could easily be ingested by the nursing child. The use of herbal oils is not recommended.[38] In one infant,

**medicinal herbs** Plants used to prevent or remedy illness.[34]

TABLE 7.6 ▸ Herbal teas generally regarded as safe during lactation[18]

| TEA | USE | COMMON USES |
|---|---|---|
| Rose hips | vitamin C | Boost the immune system |
| Raspberry | flavoring | Tone the uterus, increase milk production, decrease nausea and ease labor pain |
| Red bush tea | beverage | |
| Orange spice | flavoring | |
| Peppermint | flavoring (limit duration use) | Relieve nausea, morning sickness and flatulence |
| Chicory | caffeine-free coffee substitute | General health, constipation, improving bowel function |

SOURCE: Based on data from Breastfeeding: A Guide for the Medical Professions, 7th ed. St Louis: Mosby, Inc., 2011.and from "Herbal Tea and Pregnancy, American Pregnancy Association, from http://www.americanpregnancy.org/pregnancyhealth/herbaltea.html.

severe breathing difficulties were documented after the mother used menthol, a significant component of peppermint oil, on her nipples.[39]

Although health care practitioners may wish otherwise, some mothers may refuse prescription drugs and insist on using herbal alternatives. It is estimated that 15–43 percent of breastfeeding mothers use herbal products.[34] If a mother is consuming a large amount of any herbal product, its contents should be checked. Important information to obtain on the product includes its name, a list of all ingredients, the names of the plants or other components (include the plants' Latin names, if possible), details of the preparation, and the amount consumed.[38] Reliable sources of herbal information[30,31,40,41] (Table 7.2) or the regional poison-control center may be able to identify potentially harmful pharmacological and toxicological ingredients.

In balancing the risks and benefits in a given situation, consideration should be given to the benefits of continued breastfeeding to the baby and the mother. It is also important to consider the varied nature of lactation: Newborns face different risks than do older babies or toddlers because of immaturity; infants consume varying amounts of human milk; mothers may be looking forward to many months of lactation yet need or desire the benefits of medicinal herbs. A few of the widely used herbs in the United States are discussed next.

## Specific Herbs Used in the United States

**Echinacea** Echinacea is used for the common cold and to enhance the immune system. Insufficient reliable data are available on its entry into breast milk and effects on the infant. It is available in many forms; the tincture form contains 15–90 percent alcohol.[36] Gastrointestinal distress in some women has been reported. Consumption of echinacea during lactation is not recommended.[42]

**Ginseng Root** Ginseng root, widely believed to increase capacity for mental work and physical activity and to reduce stress, contains dozens of steroid-like glycosides, sterols, coumarins, flavonoids, and polysaccharides.[18] It is reported to have estrogen-like effects in some women, with breast pain common with extended use and mammary swelling also reported. While there has been considerable animal experimentation with ginseng root, human data are not extensive. There is no information on transfer to human milk.[36] The lack of standardized preparations, information on dosage, and accurate recording of side effects is a problem. Because of the reported breast effects and occasional reports of vaginal bleeding, the use of ginseng during lactation may not be advisable.[5,28]

**St. John's Wort** St. John's wort is widely used in the United States and Europe as a mood stabilizer and antidepressant. It has been shown to have fewer side effects in trials compared to prescription antidepressants.[19] Although the plant contains at least 10 classes of biologically active compounds, hypericin and hyperforin, and their metabolites pseudohypericin and adhyperforin, seem to be the most important for their neuropharmocologic properties.[43] There is growing evidence that hyperforin may be the key constituent responsible for the antidepressant property of this herb. Composition of St. John's wort preparations may vary based on climate and other variables related to growth, harvesting, and processing. Many products available in the United States and Canada may be of poor quality and contain little or no St. John's wort. The mother taking St. John's wort should only purchase from reputable sources. Large doses decrease prolactin levels, which could potentially reduce breast milk supply.[18] There are also concerns about the numerous potential herb–drug interactions because of the ability of St. John's wort to induce the metabolic activity of cytochrome P450 (CYP), particularly for drugs used to treat human immunodeficiency virus (HIV).[43]

There is limited information on the excretion of active components in breast milk and effect on the infant. In a study of five mothers who were taking 300 mg of St. John's wort three times daily, hyperforin was excreted into breast milk at very low levels and the relative infant doses were 0.9–2.5 percent. This level of infant exposure to hyperforin through milk is comparable to levels reported in most studies assessing antidepressants or neuroleptics. No side effects were seen in the mothers or infants.[43]

A recent clinical trial compared 33 breastfeeding women taking St. John's wort with 101 disease-matched controls and 33 age- and parity-matched controls. No differences between groups were found in maternal adverse side effects, maternal report of decreased milk production or in infant weight in the first year. In the group taking St. John's wort, five of the infants reported colic, drowsiness, or lethargy, compared with only one infant in each of the control groups.[44] The symptoms were not severe, and specific medical treatment of the affected infants was not required. St. John's wort may be a reasonable choice for treatment of postpartum depression using high-quality products.[19] Mothers who are breastfeeding while taking St. John's wort should be alert to changes in infant behavior and should be closely supervised by a pediatrician. If the mother is taking other medications or herbal supplements, she should be informed that drug–herb interactions are possible.

**Fenugreek** This spice is used as an artificial flavor for maple syrup, in teas, poultices, and ointments, and as an ingredient in East Indian cooking. It is also the most commonly used herbal galactogogue. While there is limited scientific evidence to back this claim, there are anecdotal reports of its successful use to increase milk supply. In one account of 1200 women taking fenugreek, almost all reported an increase in milk production within 24 to 72 hours.[45] Rare maternal adverse effects include diarrhea; a maple-like aroma in urine, breast milk, or sweat; and exacerbation of asthmatic symptoms.[46] This herb is derived from a plant in the same family as peanuts and chickpeas and has potential for allergy in sensitive infants. There are reports of colic, abdominal upset, and diarrhea among babies whose mothers took fenugreek.[36] Transfer into milk is assumed because the infant's urine smells of maple syrup. The usual dosage (2–3 capsules three times daily or 1 cup of tea three times a day) is considered compatible with breastfeeding.[46]

**Goat's-Rue** This is a widely used galactogogue in Europe and South America and is becoming increasingly popular in the United States. In the 1900s, cows fed goat's-rue were observed to have increased milk supply. No controlled human studies have been done. Only one side effect has been reported, according to the Academy of Breastfeeding Medicine. "Maternal ingestion of a lactation tea containing extracts of liquorice, fennel, anise, and goat's-rue was linked to drowsiness, hypotonia, lethargy, emesis, and poor suckling in two breastfed neonates. An infection work-up was negative, and symptoms and signs resolved on discontinuation of the tea and a 2-day break from breastfeeding."[15] No other side effects have been reported. The usual dose is 1 teaspoon dried leaves steeped in 8 ounces of water for 10 minutes and used as a tea, with 1 cup taken three times per day.

**Milk Thistle/Blessed Thistle** Blessed thistle has been used in Europe and has become increasingly popular in the United States. It is often combined with fenugreek. There have been no randomized controlled studies done on this galactogogue. It is taken as a tea two to three times per day. The tea is usually prepared by simmering 1 teaspoon of crushed seeds in 8 ounces of water. It is also available in capsules.

Many mothers may be taking herbal products for low milk supply. There are many other commonly used herbal galactogogues (see Table 7.4). Keep in mind that there are few human studies done on most of these products. These studies often are not well-designed and/or well-controlled.[34] Safety, proper dosing, and intended and unintended effects may be unknown.[11]

# Alcohol and Other Drugs and Exposures

**LO 7.4** Describe the impact of alcohol on mother's milk.

> "Avoid prescribing or proscribing it [alcohol] and . . . assist the mother in appropriately adjusting her alcohol consumption in both timing and volume."
>
> —R. A. Lawrence[18]

## Alcohol

The harmful effects of alcohol consumption during pregnancy are well documented, and drinking during pregnancy is clearly not recommended. In the past, recommendations on alcohol consumption during lactation were ambiguous and somewhat controversial. Recommendations ranged from using alcohol as a galactogogue to complete avoidance. The AAP policy statement on "Breastfeeding and the Use of Human Milk" states, "Alcohol is not a galactogogue; it may blunt prolactin response to suckling and negatively affect infant motor development. Ingestion of alcohol should be minimized."[47] Alcohol consumed by the mother passes quickly into her breast milk, and the effects on the breastfeeding baby are directly related to the amount the mother consumes.[48,49]

The level of alcohol in breast milk matches the maternal plasma levels at the time of the infant feeding. Peak maternal plasma and breast milk levels are reached 30–60 minutes after alcohol consumption and approximately 60–90 minutes when taken with food.[18,48] As the alcohol clears from a mother's blood, it clears from her milk. It takes a 120-pound woman about 2–3 hours to eliminate from her body the alcohol in one serving of beer or wine

TABLE 7.7 ▶ Alcohol and breastfeeding: Time (h:min) until zero level in milk is reached for women at different body weights[50]

| MATERNAL BODY WEIGHT | | TIME ALCOHOL REMAINS | | |
|---|---|---|---|---|
| LB | (KG) | 1 DRINK | 2 DRINK | 3 DRINK |
| 100 | (45.4) | 2:42 | 5:25 | 8:08 |
| 120 | (54.4) | 2:30 | 5:00 | 7:30 |
| 140 | (63.5) | 2:19 | 4:38 | 6:58 |
| 160 | (72.6) | 2:10 | 4:20 | 6:30 |
| 180 | (81.6) | 2:01 | 4:03 | 6:05 |

NOTE: Time is calculated from beginning of drinking. Assumptions made: alcohol metabolism is constant at 15 mg/dl; height of the women is 162.56 cm (5 feet, 4 inches). 1 drink 5 12 oz of 5% beer or 5 oz of 11% wine or 1.5 oz of 40% liquor. Example: For a 100-lb woman who consumed 2 drinks in 1 h, it would take 5 h 25 min for there to be no alcohol in her breast milk, but for a 180-lb woman drinking the same amount, it would take 4 h 3 min.

SOURCE: Haastrup, M. B., Potteg, A., and Damkier, P. Alcohol and Breastfeeding. Basic & Clinical Pharmacology & Toxicology 2014; 114: 168–173.

(Table 7.7).[50] The common practice of pumping the breasts and then discarding the milk immediately after drinking alcohol does not hasten the disappearance of alcohol from the milk, as the newly produced milk will still contain alcohol as long as the mother has measurable blood alcohol levels.[48]

In many cultures, folklore passed down for generations encourages the use of alcohol as a galactogogue that facilitates milk letdown and rectifies milk insufficiency, as well as sedating and calming the "fussy" infant.[51] In contrast to this folklore, there is now strong evidence of a negative dose-related impact of alcohol on milk supply and the milk letdown reflex. In 2005, a study[51] found that during the immediate hours after alcohol consumption by lactating women, the hormonal milieu underlying lactation performance is disrupted. Oxytocin levels significantly decrease, whereas prolactin levels increase significantly. The diminished oxytocin response was significantly related to decreases in milk yield and milk ejection (letdown). The oxytocin release is blocked by alcohol.[18] In contrast, changes in prolactin were related to self-reported feelings of drunkenness. Recommending alcohol to women as an aid to lactation may be counterproductive; mothers may feel more relaxed, but the hormonal disruption diminishes the infant's milk supply.

Maternal alcohol consumption affects the odor of breast milk and the volume consumed by the infant within a half-hour to an hour after consumption.[8] Breast-fed infants consumed, on average, 20 percent less breast milk during the 3- to 4-hour period following their mothers' consumption of an alcoholic beverage (0.3 g ethanol/kg).[48,52] Compensatory increases in intake were then observed during the 8–16 hours after exposure when mothers refrained from drinking.[52]

Recent studies on the impact of maternal alcohol ingestion during lactation on infant sleep patterns and psychomotor development have raised concerns about regular consumption of alcohol while lactating. In one study, 11 of 13 breastfed infants had a reduction of more than 40 percent in active sleep after consuming their mothers' expressed breast milk flavored with alcohol (32 mg) on one testing day and expressed breast milk alone on the other.[53] All infants spent significantly less total time sleeping after consumption of the breast milk with alcohol (56.8 minutes with alcohol compared to 78.2 minutes without). A follow-up study replicated this finding and showed that infants can compensate for this deficit by increasing the amount of time spent in active (rapid eye movement) sleep during the 20.5 hours after the sleep-deficit period.[54] The investigators concluded that short-term exposure to small amounts of alcohol in breast milk produces distinctive changes in the infant's sleep–wake patterning. Since both the observed reduced milk consumption and the infant sleep deficits occur only when breastfeeding follows after the mother's alcohol consumption, a nursing woman who drinks occasionally can limit her infant's exposure to alcohol by planning in relation to her drinking and breastfeeding prior to drinking alcoholic beverages and using previously expressed human milk.[55]

Epidemiologic data on the effects of moderate drinking throughout the lactation period on the human infant are limited. In a study of 400 infants born to members of a health insurance plan, no differences in the infant's cognitive development scores were found at 1 year of age between infants whose mothers consumed alcohol while nursing and those that did not. However, Bayley Psychomotor Development Index scores at 1 year of age were slightly lower among infants who were exposed to any alcohol through breast milk than among those who were not exposed.[56] Since current research does not show that occasional use (one to two drinks) of alcohol is harmful to the baby, La Leche League continues to support the opinion that the occasional use of alcohol in limited amounts is compatible with breastfeeding.[57] The American Academy of Pediatrics places alcohol in the category "Maternal Medication Usually Compatible with Breastfeeding."[24,25] It lists possible side effects if consumed in large amounts, including drowsiness, deep sleep, weakness, and abnormal weight gain in the infant. The Institute of Medicine Subcommittee on Nutrition During Lactation recommends that lactating women be advised that if alcohol is consumed, intake should be limited to "no more than 0.5 grams of alcohol per kilogram of maternal body weight per day."[58] For a 60-kilogram (132-pound) woman, 0.5 grams of alcohol per kilogram of body weight corresponds to approximately 2 to 2.5 ounces of liquor, 8 ounces of table wine, or 2 cans of beer.[47,59] Many feel that nursing mothers are already placed under too many restrictions and may be discouraged from initiating or continuing to breastfeed if alcohol is prohibited because they feel they will face too many limitations.

If a mother does choose to have a drink or two, she can wait for the alcohol to clear her system before nursing according to the times given in Table 7.7. She can plan ahead and have alcohol-free expressed milk stored for the occasion. If she becomes engorged, she can pump her breasts as a means of comfort, and discard her alcohol-containing milk. Drinking water, resting, or pumping and discarding breast milk will not hasten the removal of alcohol from the milk, as the alcohol content of milk matches the maternal plasma alcohol levels. Mothers who are intoxicated should not breastfeed until they are completely sober. Drinking more than two alcoholic drinks daily has been associated with decreased breastfeeding duration after 6 months by more than double compared to women who consumed less.[34]

## Nicotine (Smoking Cigarettes)

Regardless of feeding choice (breast or bottle), the health risks for infants posed by having a mother who smokes are many, including otitis media, exacerbations of asthma, respiratory infections, and gastrointestinal dysregulation such as colic and acid reflux.[60] It is not ideal to smoke and breastfeed, but it is worse to smoke and not breastfeed. It is estimated that between 5 and 20 percent of breastfeeding mothers smoke.[18]

Well-documented data provide clear evidence that children of smoking mothers do better if breastfed in regard to general health, respiratory illness, and risk of sudden infant death syndrome (SIDS) [18,47] than if bottle fed. Unfortunately, women who smoke cigarettes are less likely to breastfeed than nonsmokers, are less likely to seek help with breastfeeding difficulties than nonsmokers, and are at increased risk for stopping breastfeeding by 3 months.[61] While lower milk output has been reported among smoking mothers,[61,62] it is unknown which components of cigarette smoke are responsible for the reduced milk production, and several studies provide evidence that smoking does not necessarily hinder breastfeeding.[61] Lower fat content in breast milk has been reported. Breastfeeding infants whose mothers smoke show poorer growth. The reasons for this are not clear.[15] The AAP Breastfeeding Policy Statement lists "smoking as a risk factor for low milk supply and poor weight gain"[47] Changes in the odor and flavor of the breast milk might affect breast milk intake in the breastfed infant.[15,62] Mennella et al. found that sleep patterns were affected by smoking. They documented a dose-response effect with the greatest impact on sleep disruptions in the infants receiving the largest dose of nicotine via human milk.[63]

Substantial epidemiological evidence suggests that social and behavioral factors and not physiological factors are largely responsible for the lower rates of breastfeeding found among smokers.[61] Some women believe that smoking is a barrier to breastfeeding; they do not believe they could, or should, adhere to the kinds of healthy practices they think are required of mothers to breastfeed.

Nicotine levels in breast milk of women who smoke are between 1.5 and 3.0 times higher than the level in the mother's blood, [24,61,63] and the mean 24-hour nicotine concentrations in breast milk rise as cigarette consumption increases. There is no evidence to document whether this amount of nicotine presents a health risk to the nursing infant, and because breastfeeding and smoking may be less detrimental to the child than bottle feeding and smoking, the AAP Committee on Drugs removed nicotine (and thus smoking) from its 2001 list of drugs of abuse with adverse effects on the infant during breastfeeding.[24]

Dahlstrom et al.[64] estimated that the dose of nicotine in breastfeeding infants was 1 μg per kilogram per feeding, based on data on nicotine concentrations in breast milk within 30 minutes after smoking. Women who smoke 10–20 cigarettes per day have 0.4–0.5 mg of nicotine/L in their milk. The authors indicated preterm infants and neonates receive larger dose of nicotine from breast milk compared to larger and older infants due to their lower body weight.[64] With gradual intake over a day's time, the infant can metabolize nicotine in the liver and excrete the chemical in the kidney. Numerous studies of nicotine and cotinine concentrations in the nursing mother and her infant confirm that although bottle-fed infants born to smoking mothers and raised in a smoking environment have significant levels of nicotine and metabolites in their urine, breastfed infants have higher levels.[62]

Tobacco smoking also increases the exposure of infants to organochloride pesticides, PCBs, and hexachlorobenzene through breast milk and second-hand smoke.[65,66] Women should be counseled not to smoke while nursing or in the infant's presence. Mothers who are not willing to stop smoking should cut down, consider low-nicotine cigarettes, and delay feedings as long as possible after smoking. The half-life of nicotine is 95 minutes.

When used as directed, smoking cessation aids that replace nicotine do not appear to pose any more problems for the breastfeeding infant than maternal smoking does.[61,] Since transdermal nicotine (nicotine patch) provides a steady level of nicotine in plasma and thus in breast milk, the mother cannot control the level of nicotine in breast milk except by changing the strength of the patch. As the mother progresses through to lower patch strengths during smoking cessation therapy, the transfer of nicotine to the infant via milk decreases by as much as 70 percent.[61] Mothers who use nicotine replacement therapy intermittently (gum, nasal spray, or inhalation) might minimize the nicotine in their milk by prolonging the duration between nicotine administration and breastfeeding.[65]

A relative new trend to provide nicotine is use of electronic cigarettes (e-cigarettes). These products are becoming increasingly popular in adolescents and young adults. They are also being used by cigarette smokers who are looking for less harmful nicotine alternatives.[67] Baeza-Loya et al. reported that e-cigarettes are more popular online than alternative tobacco products. One reason for this popularity is the perception that e-cigarettes are a safer smoking alternative because they don't have as many substances found in regular tobacco products. Research is needed to determine the impact of e-cigarettes on breastfeeding. Much knowledge is currently available on nicotine and breastfeeding. Any nicotine exposure during lactation should be discouraged, whether from traditional tobacco products or from e-cigarettes.

## Marijuana

Marijuana is a commonly used drug. Delta-9-tetrhydrocannabinol (THC), an active ingredient in marijuana, transfers and concentrates in breast milk and is absorbed and metabolized by the nursing infant. One study showed that 1 hour after ingestion, there was an eightfold accumulation of THC in the breast milk compared to the maternal plasma level.[15,19] There is evidence from animal studies of structural changes in the brain cells of newborn animals nursed by mothers whose milk contained THC. Impairment of deoxyribonucleic acid (DNA) and ribonucleic acid (RNA) formation and neurotransmitter systems essential for proper growth and development has been described.[68] Significant absorption and metabolism has been shown in studies.[19] In one study following breastfeeding mothers and their infants for 12 months, marijuana exposure via the mother's milk during the first month postpartum appeared to be associated with a decrease in infant motor development at 1 year of age.[69] Concerns about marijuana use during lactation include the amount of the drug the infant ingests while nursing and the amount inhaled from the environment. Exposure in infants to marijuana via breast milk will provide positive urine tests for up to 2–3 weeks.[19] The possible effect on DNA and RNA metabolism should discourage any maternal use, especially since brain cell development is still taking place in the first months of life. Many states have legalized use of THC for medicinal purposes and some states have legalized any use of this product. Despite being legal drug in many states, the American Academy of Pediatrics classifies THC as a drug of abuse that is contraindicated during lactation.[24]

## Caffeine

Although caffeine ingestion is a frequent concern of breastfeeding mothers, moderate intake causes no problems for most breastfeeding mothers and babies. A dose of caffeine equivalent to a cup of coffee results in breast milk levels of 1 percent of the level in maternal plasma and, consequently, low levels in the infant.[18] However, because the infant's ability to metabolize caffeine does not fully develop until 3–4 months of age, caffeine does accumulate in the infant. Within 15 minutes of consumption, caffeine is detectable in breastmilk. Caffeine levels peak around 1 hour after consumption.[70] Cases of caffeine excess in breastfed infants have been documented.[71] Symptoms, which include infants being wakeful, hyperactive, and fussy, did not require hospitalization and disappeared over a week's time after caffeine was removed from the maternal diet. No long-term effects of caffeine exposure during lactation have been documented.[70]

While most breastfed infants can tolerate a maternal caffeine intake equivalent to 3 cups of coffee per day, some babies may be more sensitive than others. If a mother suspects her baby is reacting to caffeine, she may try avoiding caffeine from all sources (coffee, tea, soft drinks, over-the-counter medications, chocolate) for 2–3 weeks.[57]

## Other Drugs of Abuse

Amphetamines, cocaine, heroin, and phencyclidine hydrochloride (angel dust, PCP) are classified by the AAP[24] as drugs of abuse that are contraindicated during lactation. The AAP guidelines strongly state that these compounds and all other drugs of abuse are hazardous not only to the nursing infant but also to the mother's physical and emotional health. In addition to their adverse pharmacological effects on the mother and infant, street drugs lack standardization and may be contaminated with other active ingredients, bacteria, heavy metals, or pesticides.[59] The Academy of Breastfeeding Medicine has developed a clinical protocol addressing specific drugs and lactation in the *Clinical Protocol 21: Guidelines for Breastfeeding the Drug Dependent Woman.*

## Environmental Exposures

> "The advantages of breastfeeding far outweigh the potential risks from environmental pollutants. Taking into account breastfeeding's short- and long-term health benefits for infants and mothers, the World Health Organization (WHO) recommends breastfeeding in all but extreme circumstances."
>
> —World Health[72]

There is now unambiguous evidence that breast milk accumulates and harbors potentially toxic environmental

TABLE 7.8 ▸ Steps a breastfeeding mother can take to reduce exposure to environmental chemicals

1. Avoid smoking cigarettes and drinking alcohol. Some studies have found levels of contaminants are higher in those who smoke and drink alcoholic beverages.
2. Be aware in purchasing homes that some houses or apartments, especially those built before 1978, might have lead-based paints.
3. In general, eat a variety of foods low in animal fats; remove skin and excess fat from meats and poultry. Avoiding high-fat dairy products may reduce the potential burden of fat-soluble contaminants. Avoid processed foods made from ground meat and animal parts such as sausage and hot dogs.
4. Increase consumption of grains, fruits, and vegetables. Thoroughly wash and peel fruits and vegetables to help eliminate the hazard of pesticide residues on the skin. When available, eat food grown without fertilizer or pesticide application. Eat organically grown food, if available.
5. Avoid fish that may have high mercury levels, such as swordfish, shark, tuna, king mackerel, tilefish, and locally caught fish from areas with fish advisories.
6. Limit exposure to chemicals such as solvents found in paints, non–water-based glues, furniture strippers, nail polish, and gasoline fumes.
7. If you work with solvents (in the workplace or at home), postpone breastfeeding for several hours after exposure.
8. Run tap water through a home filter before drinking. Filters can reduce levels of common tap water pollutants.
9. Remove the plastic cover of dry-cleaned clothing. Air out the garments in a room with open windows, or hang dry-cleaning outside for 12–24 hours.
10. Attempt to avoid occupational exposure to chemical contaminants in the workplace, and seek improved chemical safety standards for all employees, especially pregnant and lactating women. Workers should be diligent in following their workplace's safety recommendations.
11. Alert other family members to be sensitive to contaminant residue they may inadvertently bring into the home. It is possible, for example, to carry PCBs home on clothes, body, or tools. If this is the case, the individual should shower and change clothing before leaving work and keep and launder work clothes separate from other clothing.
12. Review additional suggestions for avoiding chemical exposures in and around the home from the report from the Environmental Working Group (see www.ewg.org/reports/mothersmilk/part5.php).

SOURCE: Reprinted from Pediatric Nursing with permission of the publisher, Jannetti Publications, Inc., East Holly Avenue, Box 56, Pitman, NJ 08071–0056; (856) 256–2300; FAX (856) 589–7463; www.pediatricnursing.net. For a sample copy of the journal, please contact the publisher.

pollutants.[66,72–75] Persistent organohalogens, including ***persistent organic pollutants (POPs)***, heavy metals, and volatile solvents, are among the toxic chemicals most often found in breast milk. A woman comes in contact with environmental chemicals as a matter of course in daily life,[74] through air pollution, drinking water, and diet. A woman also comes in contact with a wide range of environmental chemicals in the home that have the potential to appear in her breast milk, such as household cleaning and personal care products, paints, furniture strippers, and pesticides. Exposure to environmental chemicals can also be occupational.

While the presence of low levels of environmental chemicals in most human milk samples is well documented, the significance of the presence of these contaminants on the well-being of the mother and the infant is unknown. Several studies[66,72–76] address concerns about potential impact on duration of lactation, neurodevelopmental and immunologic outcomes, and carcinogenic effects. While the body of research is growing, huge gaps in the current knowledge of any ill effects remain. In fact, other factors in breast milk may have a protective effect on normal neurologic development and immunologic outcomes.[63,66] At this time, there are no established "normal" or "abnormal" levels in breast milk for clinical interpretation, and breast milk is not routinely tested for environmental exposures.[66,75,76]

Unless the mother has a high level of occupational exposures, extreme dietary exposures (e.g., from fish in contaminated waters), or unusual residential exposures to hazardous or toxic chemicals, breastfeeding remains overwhelmingly the preferred choice compared with breast milk substitutes.[76,78–80] The World Health Organization,[79] the American Academy of Pediatrics,[80] the Centers for Disease Control and Prevention,[78] and other major health organizations overwhelmingly support the importance of breastfeeding even in a contaminated world. The benefits of breastfeeding, which include high levels of antioxidants, may prove to be essential to compensate for and outweigh the risk of toxic effects from the environment.

Women should be advised about how to reduce exposures that may affect breast milk quality rather than abandoning breastfeeding for artificial methods (Table 7.8). Women should avoid fish such as swordfish and shark or freshwater fish from waters reported as contaminated by local health agencies and limit exposure to chemicals such as pesticides and solvents found in paints, non–water-based glues, furniture strippers, nail polish, and gas fumes.

**persistent organic pollutants (POPs)** A family of chemicals manufactured either for a specific purpose (e.g., pesticides or flame retardants in electrical equipment or furniture) or produced as byproducts of incinerated waste. The POP family includes dioxins, polychlorinated biphenyuls (PCBs), polybrominated didphenyl ether (PBDE), and organochlorine pesticides.

# Neonatal Jaundice and Kernicterus

LO7.5 Explain causes of hyperbilirubinemia and ways to prevent kernicterus.

"The AAP discourages the interruption of breastfeeding in healthy term newborns and encourages continued and frequent breastfeeding (at least eight to twelve times every 24 hours)."

—American Academy of Pediatrics[81]

Neonatal jaundice is a yellow discoloring of the skin caused by too much bilirubin in the blood (***hyperbilirubinemia***). It is a common and usually benign condition that resolves on its own or with minimal intervention. At least 40 percent of healthy full-term[82] and 80 percent of preterm infants will become visibly jaundiced[83] with their serum bilirubin levels exceeding 5–7 mg/dL (85–199 μmol/L).[84] If hyperbilirubinemia does not resolve and becomes sufficiently severe, the elevated bilirubin levels can cause permanent neurological damage.[82–86]

In recent years, the overall incidence of infant jaundice has risen,[85] and hyperbilirubinemia is the most frequent cause for hospital readmission during the first 2 weeks of life in the United States.[87] More infants are becoming jaundiced, and their jaundice is more severe. The Joint Commission on Accreditation of Healthcare Organizations (JCAHO),[88] the Centers for Disease Control, and the American Academy of Pediatrics[81] have all noted the increasing rates and the need for prevention, early detection, and prompt treatment. Risk factors for the development of severe hyperbilirubinemia have been identified (see Table 7.9). Higher rates of breastfeeding in conjunction with shorter postpartum hospital stays is the leading explanation for the higher prevalence of neonatal jaundice.[85,89]

TABLE 7.9 ▸ Severe hyperbilirubinemia risk factors[82]

| |
|---|
| **Maternal** |
| Diabetes |
| Rh Sensitization |
| Previous child with phototherapy |
| Race–East Asian or Mediterranean |
| **Infant** |
| Premature or late-preterm |
| High total serum bilirubin(TSB) levels at discharge |
| Poor breastfeeding in exclusive breastfed infant |
| Blood group incompatibility, e.g., ABO |
| Hemolytic disease, e.g., Glucose-6-phosphate dehydrogenase deficiency (G6PD) |

SOURCE: AAP/Pediatrics, ABM Protocol #22, and CDC

It is important for all health professionals to understand the causes of, risk factors for, and early signs of hyperbilirubinemia. Preventing toxicity from excessive jaundice and protecting and ensuring successful breastfeeding require an understanding of the normal and abnormal patterns and mechanisms of jaundice in the newborn period, particularly the mechanisms related to human milk intake.[90]

## Bilirubin Metabolism

Bilirubin is a byproduct of the normal physiologic degradation of hemoglobin. Most hemoglobin in the neonate is derived from fetal erythrocytes. Since higher levels of hemoglobin are necessary *in utero* to carry the oxygen delivered to the fetus by the placenta, the normal full-term infant has a hematocrit of 50–60 percent. As soon as the infant is born and begins to breathe room air, the need for high levels of hemoglobin is gone, and excess erythrocytes are destroyed. The released hemoglobin is broken down by the reticuloendothelial system; bilirubin, an insoluble byproduct of the breakdown of hemoglobin, is released into the circulation bound to albumin or another transport protein. The insoluble form of bilirubin is removed from circulation by the liver, which conjugates bilirubin to a water-soluble form and excretes it via the bile to the stool. The balance between liver cell uptake of bilirubin, the rate of bilirubin production, and the rate of bilirubin reabsorption through the intestines determines the total serum bilirubin (TSB) level.

Before birth, the maternal liver is responsible for metabolism and clearance of fetal bilirubin. After birth, unique developmental factors that control the production, conjugation, and excretion of bilirubin predispose the neonate to hyperbilirubinemia:[11,85,91,92]

- Bilirubin production in the neonate is double that of an adult because of breakdown of fetal erythrocytes.
- Uptake of insoluble bilirubin by the liver is limited because of a reduction in the concentration of ligandin, a bilirubin-binding protein in the liver cell.
- Conjugation to a water-soluble form is limited in the liver because of deficient activity of uridine diphosphoglucuronosyl transferase (UDPGT), a liver enzyme responsible for bilirubin conjugation.
- Excretion of bilirubin is delayed because of an enzyme present in the intestine of the newborn, beta glucuronidase, which converts conjugated bilirubin back into its unconjugated state, which is reabsorbed.

## Physiologic Versus Pathologic Newborn Jaundice

After the first 24 hours, rising bilirubin levels in healthy term infants are reflective of the physiological

**hyperbilirubinemia** Elevated blood levels of bilirubin, a yellow pigment that is a byproduct of the breakdown of fetal hemoglobin.

breakdown of fetal hemoglobin, the increased resorption of the bilirubin from the intestines, and the limited ability of the newborn's immature liver to process large amounts of bilirubin as effectively as a mature liver. Neonates tend to produce more bilirubin than they can eliminate. Prematurity magnifies this imbalance. Retention of unconjugated bilirubin by the newborn is known as normal newborn jaundice or physiologic jaundice of the newborn.[90] Excessive bilirubin is deposited in various tissues, including the skin, muscles, and mucous membranes of the body, causing the skin to take on a yellowish color. In healthy newborns, this condition is temporary and usually resolves within a few days without treatment. In the typical newborn population, bilirubin levels rise steadily in the first 3–4 days of life and peak around the fifth day of life, and then decline. Bilirubin levels of healthy preterm infants peak later (day 6 to day 7) and take longer to resolve. Bilirubin levels in physiologic jaundice are usually less than 12 mg of bilirubin per dL of blood of infants of White or Black mothers, and average 10–14 mg in infants of Asian ancestry, including Chinese, Japanese, and Korean, and Native Americans.[93] Levels in White and Black mothers also peak earlier than in Asian or Native American mothers.[94]

In contrast to physiologic jaundice of the newborn, pathologic jaundice begins earlier (sometime it is observed before 24 hours of age), rises faster, and lasts longer. A TSB greater than 8 mg/dL in the first 24 hours should be investigated for pathologic origin. Causes of pathologic jaundice include the following:[84]

- Hemolytic disease (immune disorders, Rh isoimmunization, ABO, or minor blood type incompatibility)
- Erythrocyte disorders (glucose-6-phosphate-dehudrogenase deficiency, hereditary spherocytosis)
- Extravasation of blood (cephalohematoma, subgaleal hemorrhage, bruising)
- Inborn errors of metabolism/conjugation defects (galactosemia, Crigler-Najjar syndrome types I and II, Gilbert's syndrome, Lucey-Driscoll syndrome)
- Hypothyroidism
- Polycythemia
- Macrosomic infant of diabetic mother
- Intestinal obstruction; delayed passage of meconium
- Sepsis

In most cases of pathological jaundice, frequent breastfeeding (8–12 times every 24 hours) can continue during diagnosis and treatment of pathological jaundice.[82,89] An advantage of colostrum and mature human milk is stimulation of bowel movements, speeding elimination of bilirubin. However, in jaundice caused by galactosemia, breastfeeding is contraindicated.[11,18]

Since bilirubin is a cell toxin, concern arises when TSB elevates to levels with the potential to cause permanent damage. The brain and brain cells, if destroyed by bilirubin deposits, do not regenerate.[85] ***Bilirubin encephalopathy***, or ***kernicterus***, has a mortality rate of 50 percent, and survivors usually are burdened with severe problems including cerebral palsy, hearing loss, paralysis of upward gaze, intellectual, and other handicaps.[74] While full-scale kernicterus is rare, there has been an increase in reported cases in the last two decades.[85,86,87] There is also concern that mild effects of bilirubin on the brain may be manifested clinically in later life with symptoms such as incoordination, excessive contractions of muscles (hypertonicity), and mental retardation, or perhaps learning disabilities.[18,86,87]

## Hyperbilirubinemia and Breastfeeding

Jaundice in the breastfed infant has been divided into types, early or late, based on the age of onset (Table 7.10). It is important to differentiate between the two to establish effective prevention and treatment. Early onset of elevated unconjugated bilirubin unexplained by other pathologic factors is associated with inadequate feeding and is called *breastfeeding jaundice* or, more precisely, *breast-nonfeeding jaundice*.[90] Late onset (after day 5) prolonged elevation of unconjugated bilirubin associated with the ingestion of breast milk is called breast milk jaundice.[90,95]

**Breast-Nonfeeding Jaundice** The optimally breastfed infant initiates breastfeeding in the first hours, followed by at least 8–12 breastfeeds per day for the first 1–2 weeks without any water or other food supplementation, and with good positioning that assures effective milk transfer to the infant, and weight loss of less than 8 percent of birthweight.[88,89] Differences in bilirubin levels between adequately breastfed infants and formula-fed infants have not been found to be significant.[90] In contrast, infants who nurse infrequently or inefficiently ingest fewer calories and lose more weight than formula-fed infants are at risk for elevated bilirubin levels.[82] Suboptimal breastfeeding can delay passage of meconium and reduce fecal weight, increasing the hepatic circulation of bilirubin. In addition, reduced milk intake produces a state of partial starvation in the infant, which further increases the intestinal absorption of bilirubin.[87,96] Delay in initiation of breastfeeding beyond the first hour of life, and administration of water to infants either before initiation of breastfeeding or in addition to breastfeeding, significantly reduce the frequency of breastfeeding and increase bilirubin concentrations. Excessive hyperbilirubinemia causes lethargy and poor feeding in some infants, further reducing breastfeeding frequency and duration and milk production, feeding a vicious cycle of increasing bilirubin levels.

**bilirubin Encephalopathy or Kernicterus** The chronic and permanent clinical sequelae that are the end result of very high untreated bilirubin levels. Excessive bilirubin in the system is deposited in the brain, causing toxicity to the basal ganglia and various brainstem nuclei.[82]

TABLE 7.10 ▸ Comparison of breast-nonfeeding jaundice and breastmilk jaundice associated with hyperbilirubinemia while breastfeeding

| | BREAST-NONFEEDING JAUNDICE | BREASTMILK JAUNDICE |
|---|---|---|
| Peak | Peaks 2–5 days of age | Peaks second & third week of age |
| Resolves | 1–2 weeks after birth | Progressively declines 3–12 weeks after birth |
| Incidence | More common with first child; approximately 60% of U.S. newborns become clinically jaundiced | All children of a given mother, Approximately 50% of breastfed infants may have mild to moderate jaundice |
| Feeding | Infrequent feeds, poor milk transfer, Receiving water or dextrose water | Adequate feeding frequency (8–12 times/24 hr, good milk transfer, no supplements |
| Supply | Low milk supply | Good milk supply |
| Stools | Stools delayed and inadequate | Normal stooling |
| Treatment | None or phototherapy, rarely exchange transfusion | None or phototherapy, Temporarily discontinue breastfeeding |
| Associations | Low Apgar scores, water or dextrose water supplement, late-preterm, and prematurity | Previous sibling requiring phototherapy |

SOURCE: Adapted from Breastfeeding: A Guide for the Medical Profession, 7th ed., by R. A. Lawrence and R. M. Lawrence, Table 14.4 2011.

It is now well established that early-onset breastfeeding jaundice results from reduced volume of milk transfer to the infant, limiting caloric intake and producing a state of partial starvation and weight loss equivalent of the adult disorder known as starvation jaundice.[82] Lawrence outlines treatment guidelines (Table 7.11) aimed at treating the actual cause—that is, failed breastfeeding or inadequate stooling or underfeeding.[18] The goal is to evaluate the breastfeeding for frequency, length of suckling, and apparent supply of milk, and then adjust the breastfeeding to solve the problem.[96] If stooling is an issue, the infant should be stimulated to stool. If starvation is the problem, the infant should receive temporary supplemental feeding by cup or bottle while the milk supply is being increased by better breastfeeding techniques.

TABLE 7.11 ▸ Prevention and management of early jaundice while breastfeeding infant, 35 weeks gestation

1. Initiate breastfeeding early, preferably within the first hour after birth. Nurse infant 8–12 times per day for the first several days.
2. Monitor stooling pattern, wet diapers, and baby weight.
3. Optimize breastfeeding management from the beginning.
4. Exclusive breastfeeding is recommended. Avoid supplementation with glucose water, water, or formula supplements. This delays the establishment of breastfeeding and may increase risk of breastfeeding-nonfeeding jaundice. Supplements including expressed breast milk should be limited and used only in the presence of inadequate intake with weight loss, inadequate milk transfer, inadequate milk production, and dehydration.
5. Provide adequate breastfeeding support and educate mother on feeding cues and to respond to early feeding cues. Crying is a late hunger cue may contribute to poor breastfeeding.
6. Identify at risk mothers and babies prior to discharge.
7. Breastfeeding should be continued and encouraged during phototherapy.
8. If temporary interruption of breastfeeding is needed, mother should protect milk production with electric pump.

SOURCE: Based on Subcommittee on Hyperbilirubinemia, "Management of Hyperbilirubinemia in the Newborn Infant 35 or More Weeks of Gestation," *Pediatrics*, 114(1), 2004, 297–316.

Early discharge of infants from the hospital at less than 72 hours of life has raised concerns about the ability to evaluate breastfeeding and the opportunity to evaluate infants for jaundice.[81,85,89,92] Formal observation of breastfeeding with evaluation of effectiveness of breastfeeding and milk transfer at regular intervals throughout the first days of life can identify breastfeeding problems sufficiently early to ensure correction of problems. The American Academy of Pediatrics strongly recommends that all breastfed infants be evaluated by a trained observer within 2–3 days after discharge from the hospital.[81] Particular attention must be paid to infants who are less than 38 weeks gestation and infants at moderate or high risk for severe hyperbilirubinemia (Table 7.10).[81,92]

**Breast Milk Jaundice Syndrome** In contrast to physiological newborn jaundice, which peaks around day 5 and then begins to drop, breast milk jaundice syndrome becomes apparent after the third day, and bilirubin levels may peak any time from the seventh to the tenth day, with untreated cases being reported to peak as late as the fifteenth day.[18] In breast milk jaundice syndrome, no correlation exists with weight loss or gain, and stools are normal. Initially, breast milk jaundice syndrome was thought to be an unusual and distinct type of newborn jaundice affecting 1 percent of all breastfed neonates. More recent research reports demonstrated that at least one-third of all breastfed infants are clinically jaundiced in the third week of life and that two-thirds have significant unconjugated hyperbilirubinemia in the third week, in contrast to the absence of hyperbilirubinemia in the third week in full-term artificially fed infants.[11,95] What was once believed to be a clinical disorder is now recognized as a normally occurring extension of physiologic jaundice of the newborn.[94,95] However, at this time there is insufficient evidence to support the popular theory that breast milk jaundice may provide protective effects for newborns by the antioxidant effects of bilirubin, compensating for the relative deficiency of endogenous antioxidants in newborns.[90]

The cause of breast milk jaundice syndrome is believed to be a combination of factors: a substance in most mothers' milk that increases intestinal absorption of bilirubin and individual variations in the infant's ability to process bilirubin.[11,18,90] To treat severe elevations in unconjugated bilirubin in breast milk jaundice syndrome, the AAP Clinical Practice Guidelines for Hyperbilirubinemia[82] are applied with the goal of promptly lowering TSB bilirubin levels substantially to limits set for the infant's age and level of risk. To establish the diagnosis of breast milk jaundice firmly when the bilirubin level is above 16 mg/dL for more than 24 hours, a short, temporary interruption of breastfeeding (12–24 hours) while monitoring bilirubin levels is recommended.[18,90]

The belief that severe hyperbilirubinemia in breastfed infants cannot result in kernicterus is erroneous and dangerous; 98 percent of the 105 cases of kernicterus in the U.S. Kernicterus Registry were breastfed infants.[96] Kernicterus, while rare, can develop in otherwise healthy full-term breastfed newborns or breastfed infants with sepsis. Breastfed infants need to be followed closely, supported effectively, and evaluated appropriately in order to avoid rare cases of severe hyperbilirubinemia and kernicterus.[81]

**Interrelationships between Breast-Nonfeeding Jaundice and Breast Milk Jaundice Syndrome** While breast-nonfeeding jaundice and breast milk jaundice are two separate entities, they can have an interactive effect on each other. Infants with breast milk jaundice who manifest higher levels of bilirubin in the second and third weeks of life, often over 15 mg/dL, have been noted to have had relatively high serum bilirubin concentrations during the first 3–5 days of life due to breast-nonfeeding jaundice, hemolysis, or unknown etiology.[95] Gartner postulates that these early, elevated bilirubin levels may produce an enlarged bilirubin pool. Then the ingestion of mature milk and a consequent enhancement of the enterohepatic circulation may enlarge the pool even further.[95]

## Prevention and Treatment for Severe Jaundice

The American Academy of Pediatrics guidelines for the management of hyperbilirubinemia in healthy term newborns include a detailed algorithm for the management of jaundice in the newborn nursery and guidelines for initiating phototherapy.[81] Phototherapy involves placing the newborn under special fluorescent lights that, like sunlight, assist in removing jaundice from the skin. The light is absorbed by the bilirubin, changing it to a water-soluble product, which can then be eliminated without having to be conjugated by the liver.

Historically, treatment for jaundice in American hospitals involved phototherapy and discontinuing breastfeeding either permanently or until the bilirubin levels were acceptable. In addition, many health professionals believed that newborn infants would become dehydrated if they were not supplemented with water or formula during the first days of breastfeeding. Recent research shows these practices are counterproductive.[82,90] The benefits of early and frequent breastfeeding in the first days of life for prevention of hyperbilirubinemia through maintaining hydration and stimulating the passage of stool are now well documented. The passage of stool in the newborn is important because there are 450 mg of bilirubin in the intestinal tract ***meconium*** of the average newborn.[18] To avoid reabsorption of bilirubin from the gut into the serum, passing meconium in the stool is critical. The current AAP hyperbilirubinemia management guidelines encourage continued and frequent breastfeeding (at least 8–12 feedings every 24 hours) in healthy term newborns, and recommends against routine supplementation of nondehydrated breastfed infants with water or dextrose water, as this practice will not prevent hyperbilirubinemia or decrease total serum bilirubin levels.[82]

## Information for Parents

Health professionals should convey a balanced approach when communicating with parents about jaundice. Parents need to know that most breastfed infants will become jaundiced and that the overwhelming majority of cases will be benign. Only a small fraction of these infants are at risk for developing extreme hyperbilirubinemia and kernicterus. However, parents also need to fully understand the serious consequences of extremely elevated bilirubin levels and should have their infant evaluated by a health professional if jaundice develops. Health professionals need to understand that feelings of guilt are common among mothers of jaundiced infants as many mothers feel that they caused the jaundice by breastfeeding.[97] By providing accurate information and encouragement to breastfeed, health professionals have great impact on whether a mother continues breastfeeding after her experience with neonatal jaundice.

**meconium** Dark green mucilaginous material in the intestine of the full-term fetus.

## Breastfeeding Multiples

LO 7.6 Identify ways health professionals can help the mother of multiples face the challenges of breastfeeding.

Since 1980, the birthrate of twins has increased by 59 percent, and the birthrate of higher-order multiples (triplets and more) has increased by over 400 percent. In the United States multiples currently represent over 3 percent of live births. The benefits of breastfeeding to mother and infant are multiplied with twins and higher-order multiples, who often are born at risk.[99] History and numerous case reports[100–102] provide ample evidence that an individual mother can provide adequate nourishment for more than one infant. In seventeenth-century France, wet nurses in foundling homes fed three to six infants, who were often of differing ages with different daily requirements.[18,103] Breastfeeding initiation rates of nearly 70 percent have been reported by surveys of members of Mothers of Super Twins (MOST), Parents of Multiple Births Association (POMBA) of Canada, and *Double Talk*, a newsletter for parents of multiples. Some mothers of triplets and quadruplets have fully breastfed their babies.[11,101]

Frequency and effectiveness of breastfeeding are the keys to building a plentiful milk supply. The more often a baby nurses, the more milk there will be.[18,99] Mothers who exclusively breastfeed twins or triplets can produce 2 to 3 liters/day, although this involves nursing an average of 15 or more times per day.[104] The main obstacle to nursing multiples is not usually the milk supply, but time and fatigue of the mother. Parents of twins and higher-order multiples need support in four major areas: organization, feeding, individualized time for each baby and stress management.[99]

Mothers of twins or higher-order multiples often face special challenges in the establishment of lactation after birth. Approximately 60 percent of twins and 90 percent of higher-order multiples in the United States are born at less than 37 weeks' gestation, and premature multiples often experience medical complications that potentially interfere with breastfeeding.[106] Breastfeeding initiation may take place in the neonatal intensive care unit, usually because of prematurity and low birthweight. Mothers of multiples may be coping with the effects of a more physically demanding pregnancy and birth or complications of pregnancy. Mothers may experience exaggerated postpartum sleep deprivation related to round-the-clock care of two or more newborns, concern for sick newborns, or staggered infant discharge, which results in time divided between infants at home and in the hospital. In addition, every aspect of breastfeeding management is affected by the dynamics that multiple newborns create.[18,99] In a recent study, breastfeeding initiation rates as high as 73 percent were found among full-term multiples compared with initiation rates of only 57 percent in preterm multiples. Breastfeeding duration was also lower in preterm multiples than in term multiples (12 weeks versus 24 weeks).[11,106]

Health care professionals can help the mothers of multiples face the many challenges of breastfeeding by offering consistent, informed, individualized care and support in the hospital and after discharge.[104] Knowledgeable care providers can help parents distinguish among multiples-specific issues, normal variations in an individual infant's breastfeeding abilities and patterns, and actual breastfeeding problems. Mothers need information on when and how to initiate simultaneous feedings, practical tips for managing night-time nursing and fatigue, and how to evaluate whether their babies are getting ample nourishment.[99] Parents need to be informed of resources for parenting multiples and for receiving support for breastfeeding in their community A well-defined plan for the health care of the lactating woman that includes screening for nutritional problems and providing dietary guidance is also important.[58] Mothers should be encouraged to drink to satisfy their thirst, to eat nutritious foods, and to sleep when the babies sleep. As in singleton nursing, women nursing multiples should be encouraged to obtain their nutrients from a well-balanced, varied diet rather than from vitamin/mineral supplements.

## Infant Allergies

LO 7.7 Distinguish between food allergy and food intolerance.

Protection from ***allergic diseases*** is one of the most important benefits of breastfeeding. There are numerous studies in this area being done at the present time. Many studies have shown exclusive breastfeeding for at least 4 months can protect against ectopic dermatitis and wheezing illnesses in children for the first 10 years of life.[16,107–109] Other studies have shown no effect on allergy.[16] Elimination of major food allergens from the diet of breastfeeding mothers of infants at high risk for atopic disease was previously recommended to delay or prevent some food allergies and atopic dermatitis. However, recent expert reviews concluded that there is no strong evidence to support this recommendation.[107,109,110,111] Studies continue on the role of maternal diet restrictions while breastfeeding high-risk infants. The National Institute of Allergy and Infectious Diseases released guidelines in 2010 for diagnosing and managing food allergies. They discussed inadequacies in many of the published literature and studies. They do not recommend avoidance of food allergens during lactation. The committee encouraged exclusive breastfeeding for at least 4 months.[18,110,111] A recent well-controlled study confirmed that the presence of food proteins in human milk is common, but this can be highly variable among women consuming the same challenge (dose) food.[110] A number of other studiesmeasuringproteinsin

**allergic diseases** Conditions resulting from hypersensitivity to a physical or chemical agent.

human milk following challenge doses of eggs, cow's milk, gluten, and wheat protein also found variable response among women.[108,109,110]

## Food Allergy (Hypersensitivity)

A ***food allergy***, or ***hypersensitivity***, is an abnormal or exaggerated immunologic response, usually immunoglobulin E (IgE) mediated, to a specific food protein. The development of infant food allergies is influenced by genetic risk for allergy, duration of breastfeeding, time for introduction of other foods, maternal cigarette smoking during pregnancy and parental smoking, air pollution, exposure to infectious disease, and by maternal diet and immune systems.[108] Several mechanisms (Table 7.12) are thought to contribute to the protective effect of breastfeeding.

Common pediatric food allergens include:

- Cow's milk
- Wheat
- Eggs
- Peanuts
- Soybeans
- Tree nuts (e.g., almonds, Brazil nuts, walnuts, hazelnuts)

Infants with a positive family history of allergies should be exclusively breastfed for at least 4–6 months with continuance of breastfeeding for as long as possible.[18,25,108]

## Food Intolerance

Although infants may have sensitivities to certain foods, there is no scientific basis for the concern about gassy foods, such as cabbage or legumes, causing gas in the breastfed baby. In mothers, the normal intestinal flora produces gas from the action on fiber in the intestinal tract. Neither the fiber nor the gas is absorbed from the intestinal tract, and neither enters the mother's milk. Likewise, the acid content of the maternal diet does not affect the breast milk because it does not change the pH of the maternal plasma.

It is common for the mother who is breastfeeding her child with colic to believe her child's symptoms are caused by a ***food intolerance***. However, the role of diet in infantile colic, which affects up to 28 percent of infants in the first months of life,[112] is controversial. While breastfeeding is not protective against infantile colic, several studies report a reduction in persistent crying after elimination of cow's milk and other food proteins from the maternal diet. In a recent randomized, controlled trial, a low-allergen maternal diet was associated with a reduction in distressed behavior among breastfed infants with colic.[112] The mothers excluded cow's milk, eggs, peanuts, tree nuts, wheat, soy, and fish from their diet.

Characteristic essential oils in foods such as garlic and spices may pass into the milk, and an occasional infant objects to their presence. Studies by Mennella and Beauchamp confirm that the diet of lactating women alters the sensory qualities of her milk.[113,114] Extensive clinical experience also suggests that some infants are sensitive to certain foods in the mother's diet. According to Lawrence, garlic, onions, cabbage, turnips, broccoli, beans, rhubarb, apricots, or prunes may be bothersome to some infants, making them colicky for 24 hours.[18] In the summer, a heavy diet of melon, peaches, and other fresh fruits may cause colic and diarrhea in the infant. Red pepper has been reported to cause dermatitis in the breastfed infant within an hour of milk ingestion.[115] Contrary to popular belief, chocolate rarely causes problems and can be consumed in moderation without causing colic, diarrhea, or constipation in most infants.[18]

If a mother suspects that her baby reacts to a specific food, it may be helpful for her to keep a record of foods eaten, along with notes on the baby's symptoms or behavior. If highly allergic or sensitive, infants may react to foods their mothers have eaten within minutes, although symptoms generally show up between 4 and 24 hours after exposure. While symptoms will improve in most infants after the offending food has been removed from the mother's diet for 5–7 days, it may take 2 weeks to totally eliminate all traces of the offending substance from both the mother and baby[116] (see Case Study 7.2).

**TABLE 7.12** Possible reasons for allergy-preventive effects of breastfeeding[101, 102]

- Low content of allergens
- Transfer of maternal immunity
- Long-chain fatty acids and IGA in breast milk protect against inflammation and infections
- Regulation of infant immunity
- Influence on gut microbial flora



# Late-Preterm Infants

**LO 7.8** Identify as least three factors that contribute to increased readmission rates for late-preterm infants.

Infants born between 34 and 37 weeks are considered late-preterm. They account for as high as 75 percent of all preterm singleton births.[117] These infants too often are treated as full-term; they often have subtle immaturity that makes establishing breastfeeding difficult and places the

**food allergy (hypersensitivity)** Abnormal or exaggerated immunologic response, usually immunoglobulin E (IgE) mediated, to a specific food protein.

**food intolerance** An adverse reaction involving digestion or metabolism but not the immune system.

# CASE STUDY 7.2

## Breastfeeding Premature Infants

Bryan Mullennix/Photodisc/Getty Images

Thirty-five-year-old Stacey delivers twin boys at 30 weeks' gestation: baby Andrew is 2 pounds, 9 ounces, and 13.5 inches long; baby Mark is 1 pound, 13 ounces, and 14 inches long. Stacey had a difficult pregnancy that included severe nausea and vomiting, heartburn, preeclampsia, and preterm labor.

Stacey is very committed to breastfeeding and was able to use a hospital-grade electronic breast pump approximately 6 hours after delivery. She pumps every 2–3 hours or 8–9 times daily in order to establish her milk supply. At the end of the first week, Stacey is pumping about 14–16 ounces/day per baby, and by 3½ weeks she is pumping 4–5 ounces per breast at each pumping. Stacey wakes at night to pump when she is full. She has placed the pumping equipment by the bed and become adept at pumping, getting out of bed only to put the milk in the refrigerator. At 2 weeks postpartum, Stacey experiences a plugged duct and has difficulty emptying the right breast for 2 days.

The twin boys have suffered the usual preterm difficulties with breathing, apnea, and bradycardia. Initially the twins are tube-fed. As their condition improves, baby Andrew is first put to breast 3 weeks after his birth, and baby Mark several weeks later. Baby Mark has more difficulty learning to latch on and suck and is growing more slowly than is his brother. Multiple interventions are used to achieve breastfeeding success. On advice from a lactation consultant, Stacey uses a nipple shield to help baby Mark latch on. In response to slow weight gain in baby Mark, the lactation consultant recommends that the baby receive hindmilk, which is often higher in fat and calories.

Mark and Andrew are released from the hospital a day after their due date. Stacey continues using the nipple shield for several weeks with Mark, trying without the nipple shield every few days. After 3 weeks at home, baby Mark is able to latch on without the nipple shield. The twins are breastfed and also receive up to 3 bottles of fortified expressed breast milk or premature infant formula per day for the first 2 months at home. The babies take feedings equally well from bottle or breast.

### Questions

1. How often should the mother be pumping to establish and maintain a full milk supply?
2. List at least two possible nutrition diagnoses for this case.
3. Identify at least one nutrition intervention for each diagnosis listed.
4. Name potential indicators for each intervention listed.

(Answers are located in the Instructor's Manual for the 6th edition of *Nutrition Through the Life Cycle.*)

infant at risk for insufficient milk intake, hypoglycemia, jaundice, and poor weight gain.[16,118] Late-preterm infants have higher rates of readmission during the neonatal period compared to term infants.[118,119] Infants may have cardiorespiratory instability, especially in upright position; poor temperature control; lower glycogen and fat stores to prevent hypoglycemia; and an immature immune system. In addition, the suck–swallow coordination may be poorly coordinated and result in poor latch-on and milk transfer.

The main emphasis in postpartum care should be on building and maintaining the milk supply and feeding the infant. Milk production relies on adequate suckling stimulation. Late-preterm infants may not be able to stimulate the breast enough to produce an adequate milk supply.[118] If an infant is not sucking vigorously or the suckling ability is weak, mothers of late-preterm infants should pump after each feeding attempt, or at least every 3 hours, to build the milk supply. A specific feeding plan, including the plan to wake a sleepy infant every 2–4 hours, is recommended to avoid the late-preterm breastfeeding cascade

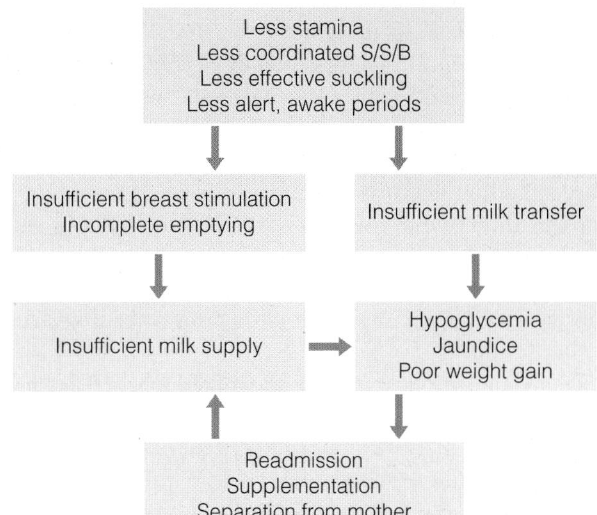


ILLUSTRATION 7.1 ▸ Later preterm infant breastfeeding cascade.

SOURCE: Reprinted with permission from SLACK Incorporated: Wight, N. E. (2003). "Breastfeeding the Borderline (Near Term) Preterm Infant." *Pediatric Annals*, 32 (5), 329–336.

(Illustration 7.1). Mothers and their late-preterm infants should have a feeding assessment by a trained lactation professional who can provide intervention for positioning, potential suck problems, and other breastfeeding issues. Weighing an infant before and after feedings may be useful to determine milk transfer. Discharge planning should include follow-up care, home visits, and lactation counseling as needed. Close follow-up should be continued until the infant is gaining weight and the mother is comfortable.[118]

# Human Milk and Preterm Infants

LO 7.9 List three benefits of mother's breast milk for premature infants.

> "The potent benefits of human milk are such that all preterm infants should receive human milk. Mother's own milk, fresh or frozen, should be the primary diet, and it should be fortified appropriately for the infant born weighing less than 1.5 kg."
>
> —American Academy of Pediatrics[47]

The benefits of breastfeeding may be most visible among preterm infants who are born immature and without adequate stores of nutrients. The nutritional benefits include ease of protein digestion, fat absorption, and improved lactose digestion.[120–123] The known health and developmental benefits include better visual acuity, greater motor and mental development at 1.5 years of age, greater verbal intelligence quotient at 7–8 years of age, and a lower incidence of serious infectious disease, including necrotizing enterocolitis and sepsis, even among infants who also receive some human milk substitutes.[122–124] Nosocomial infection rates may also be decreased by as much as 50 percent in premature infants who receive at least 50 percent of their daily feedings from mother's milk.[124]

The composition of milk from women who deliver preterm infants is higher in protein, slightly lower in lactose, and higher in energy content (58–70 kcal/100 mL) compared to the milk of women who deliver full-term infants (approximately 62 kcal/100 mL). Once growth is established, the nutritional needs of the preterm infant exceed the content of human milk for protein, calcium, phosphorus, magnesium, sodium, copper, zinc, riboflavin, pyridoxine, folic acid, and vitamins C, D, E, and K.[25] Lower weight and length gains and poorer bone mineralization has been reported for preterm infants fed human milk without fortification.[125] Human milk fortifiers are available that provide additional protein, minerals, and vitamins.[25] Infants who receive fortified human milk do not need additional supplementation unless a specific nutritional problem is identified. The health benefits, particularly reduction in sepsis and necrotizing enterocolitis, outweigh the slightly lower rate of weight gain and length gain observed among preterm infants fed fortified human milk compared to those who receive a human milk substitute for premature infants.[125]

Early feeding seems to be important for preterm infants (when medically appropriate). Early feeding may be important to the ability to digest[121] and to the development of the infant's digestive system.[126] Often, milk must be expressed and stored for preterm infants. Establishing a milk supply is important to the mother's ability to maintain a milk supply that will meet her infant's demands after several weeks (see "Can Women Make Enough Milk?" in Chapter 6). A woman who is pumping less than 750 mL of milk by 2 weeks may need additional support to establish a milk supply that will meet her infant's needs beyond the first month.

Despite the health benefits of feeding human milk to preterm infants, the incidence and duration of breastfeeding of preterm infants in the United States is about 30 percent lower than rates for full-term infants.[123] The challenges of feeding low-birthweight infants include provision of adequate calorie and nutrient intake, establishing and maintaining an adequate milk supply, and transitioning from gavage feeding to feeding from the breast.[123] Strategies to improve breastfeeding rates in this vulnerable population include providing the parents with information necessary to make an informed decision to breastfeed; assisting the mother with the establishment and maintenance of a milk supply; ensuring correct breast milk management (storage and handling) techniques; providing skin-to-skin (kangaroo) care and opportunities for nonnutritive sucking at the breast; managing the transition to the breast; measuring milk transfer; preparing the infant and family for discharge; and providing appropriate follow-up care.[127] A nipple shield may be a useful to help the preterm infant maintain latch and breastfed easier. A nipple shield is a thin, soft silicone breastfeeding device that does not impact nipple stimulation. Counseling mothers of very low-birthweight infants on the benefits of breast milk and providing breastfeeding support increases breastfeeding initiation and breast milk feeding without increasing maternal anxiety and stress.[128]

In addition to improving breast milk supply, skin-to-skin contact provides protection to the premature infant in the NICU. The lactating mother produces specific antibodies in her milk against pathogens in the infant's environment through the enteromammary system.[16]

# Medical Contraindications to Breastfeeding

LO 7.10 Demonstrate knowledge of medical contraindications to breastfeeding.

Few medical problems in the mother or baby are absolute contraindications to breastfeeding (Table 7.13). There are very few infectious pathogens that pose a risk to the newborn that outweighs the potential benefits of breastfeeding.[129] Even infants with metabolic disorders such as phenylketonuria can continue to breastfeed in combination with a specialized formula to meet calorie and protein needs. When mothers or infants have medical or other problems that cause a poor suck or other feeding problems, early identification and appropriate support from a lactation consultant is necessary for successful breastfeeding. In some cases, pumping milk may be necessary to maintain a supply of milk while problems with the infant suck are addressed and corrected. Whenever a medical situation presents a potential risk for breastfeeding infants, the theoretical risk must be carefully measured against the projected benefits of breastfeeding.[130]

TABLE 7.13 When should a mother avoid breastfeeding?

Health professionals agree that human milk provides the most complete form of nutrition for infants, including premature and sick newborns. However, there are rare exceptions when human milk is not recommended. Under certain circumstances, a physician will need to make a case-by-case assessment to determine whether a woman's environmental exposure or her own medical condition warrants her to interrupt or stop breastfeeding.

**Breastfeeding is NOT advisable if one or more of the following conditions is true:**

1. An infant diagnosed with galactosemia, a rare genetic metabolic disorder
2. The infant whose mother:
   - Has been infected with the human immunodeficiency virus (HIV)
   - Is taking antiretroviral medications
   - Has untreated, active tuberculosis
   - Is infected with human T-cell lymphotropic virus type I or type II
   - Is using or is dependent on an illicit drug
   - Is taking prescribed cancer chemotherapy agents, such as antimetabolites that interfere with DNA replication and cell division
   - Is undergoing radiation therapies; however, such nuclear medicine therapies require only a temporary interruption in breastfeeding

For additional information, visit American Academy of Pediatrics' Breastfeeding and the Use of Human Milk, or read: American Academy of Pediatrics Committee on Drugs. (2001) "The Transfer of Drugs and Other Chemicals into Human Milk," *Pediatrics*, 108, 776–789. Available online at http://pediatrics.aappublications.org/cgi/content/full/108/3/776

SOURCE: From cdc.gov/breastfeeding/diseases

## Breastfeeding and HIV Infection

Every year, approximately 750,000 children worldwide become infected with ***HIV***, mostly through mother-to-child transmission during pregnancy, delivery, or breastfeeding.[131] The transmission of HIV type 1 from mother to child through breastfeeding is well documented. Reports of transmission rates range between 5 percent and 20 percent, with prolonged breastfeeding doubling the rate to 35–40 percent.[131] Factors contributing to these variable rates include strain of HIV, maternal illness, immune status and viral load, duration of breastfeeding (timing of transmission), primary infection of the mother during the breastfeeding period, exclusive breastfeeding versus mixed feeding, mastitis, maternal vitamin deficiencies (A, C, E, or B vitamins), and the availability of antiretroviral therapy.[129–133]

In developed countries, where safe and affordable breast milk substitutes are available, HIV-infected women should be counseled strongly not to breastfeed.[134] The U.S. Department of Health and Human Services' Blueprint for Action on Breastfeeding states that "HIV-infected women in the United States should not breastfeed or provide their breast milk for the nutrition of their own or other infants because of the risk of HIV transmission to the child" (p. 12).[78]

The choice for women with HIV in developing countries differs. In most cases, breast milk substitutes are not affordable to families or to government-sponsored public health programs, and they pose a serious health risk to infants both with and without HIV.[131,133] In 2010, the World Health Organization updated recommendations regarding breastfeeding and HIV. In 2007, it had recommended children of HIV-infected mothers be exclusively breastfed until 6 months of age. The revised guidelines now recommend all infants be exclusively breastfed for the first 6 months of life, at which time solid foods may be introduced. Breastfeeding is recommended for at least the first 12 months of life. It is common in many undeveloped countries for mothers to breastfeed their children for at least 24 months. In the new guidelines, the importance of antiretroviral therapy is stressed to reduce HIV transmission via breast milk. Replacement feeding is not recommended in the new guidelines unless it is "acceptable, feasible, affordable, sustainable and safe (AFASS)."[135] In certain populations, the benefits of breastfeeding may outweigh the risks of HIV transmission. Breastfeeding is thought to be responsible for about 300,000 HIV infections per year, while UNICEF estimates that not breastfeeding is responsible for 1.5 million child deaths per year.[136] Recent studies have provided strong evidence that breastfeeding does not pose any mortality or other health risks to the HIV-infected mother.[136]

Exclusive breastfeeding by the HIV-infected mother has been shown

**HIV** Human immunodeficiency virus.

to reduce risk of transmission in the early months when compared to partial breastfeeding or mixed feeding.[137] Use of antiretroviral can be significant to reduce transmission risk through breastfeeding. Authorities in each country should make recommendations regarding breastfeeding and antiretroviral therapy to prevent HIV transmission.[137]

Detailed instructions on counseling HIV-infected women are available from WHO. All women should be encouraged to know their HIV status and seek early prenatal care. Women need to be aware of the risks of HIV transmission during pregnancy and lactation.

# Human Milk Collection and Storage

LO 7.11 List three guidelines for storage of human milk for home use.

> "Human milk is the most appropriate food for infants, and is also used as medical therapy for older children and adults with certain medical conditions. Human milk has a long history and proven track record both as nutrition and therapy."
>
> —Human Milk Banking Association of North America

The appropriate collection and storage of human milk is important whether the milk is for the mother's own infant or to be donated. All of the collection containers used should be cleaned by dishwasher or sterilized by boiling. Hand pumps, electric handheld pumps, hospital-grade electric breast pumps, and manual expression can be used to extract the milk. The American Academy of Breastfeeding Medicine has published evidence-based guidelines for the collection and storage of human milk for home and human milk banking.[138] The Human Milk Banking Association of North America has published "Best Practice for Expressing, Storing and Handling Human Milk in Hospitals, Homes and Child Care Settings."[138] Table 7.14 presents current recommendations for milk storage for home use.

How much volume should the mother be pumping? Volumes vary according to initiation and frequency of pumping. Prematurity and stress also impact production, as discussed earlier. The pumping frequency in the early days after delivery correlates to production goals. The mother who pumps 8–10 times per day on days 2 and 3 post-delivery is more likely to achieve production goals than the mother who doesn't initiate pumping until day 3 and only pumps 3–4 times per day. The mother should begin pumping 6 hours after delivery, if possible. Typical volumes to produce the first few days are 1–10cc/pumping. By days 5–8, those volumes should increase to 1½–2½ ounces, and by days 10–14, the mother should be producing 2½–4 ounces/day. A full milk supply is considered 25–35 ounces per day.[140–141]

## Milk Banking

> "If mother's own milk is unavailable despite significant lactation support, pasteurized donor milk should be used."
>
> —American Academy of Pediatrics[42]

Human Milk banks in North America (HMBANA) adhere to national guidelines for quality control of screening and testing of donors and pasteurize all milk before distribution. HMBANA member milk banks are nonprofit organizations. Fresh human milk from unscreened donors is not recommended because of the risk of transmission of infectious agents.

Human milk banks provide human milk to infants who cannot be breastfed by their mother. Premature and sick infants are most likely to receive banked milk. A woman can donate milk once or on a continuing basis if her supply exceeds the demands of her infant. There is a long history of providing human milk to infants by persons other than the biological mother.[142] Wet nurses were the main source of human milk until the early 1900s for infants not fed by their biological mothers. Milk banks began in Europe and followed in the United States. Some neonatal intensive care units had informal milk banks until the 1980s. As a result of the human immunodeficiency virus, the resurgence of tuberculosis, and risks related to donors who might abuse drugs, human milk banks are now scarce in North America, but because of recognition of the importance of human milk, demand is increasing. There are 18 HMBANA member banks currently open in the United States and Canada with several more in the process of becoming a milk bank.[143] A network of milk banks meets and shares information through the Human Milk Banking Association of North America (HMBANA). A copy of the association's guidelines for milk storage is available for a fee. Millions of ounces are distributed annually in North America.

Human milk donors are chosen by their health profile. Women are carefully screened before they can donate extra milk to milk banks. Milk banks that belong to the Milk Banking Association of North America require telephone screening, a written health and lifestyle history, and

TABLE 7.14 ▸ Storage duration of fresh human milk for use with healthy full-term infants

| LOCATION | TEMPERATURE | DURATION | COMMENTS |
|---|---|---|---|
| **Countertop, table** | Room temperature (up to 77°F or 25°C) | 6–8 hours | Containers should be covered and kept as cool as possible; covering the container with a cool towel may keep milk cooler. |
| **Insulated cooler bag** | 5°–39°F or –15°–4°C | 24 hours | Keep ice packs in contact with milk containers at all times, limit opening cooler bag. |
| **Refrigerator** | 39°F or 4°C | 5 days | Store milk in the back of the main body of the refrigerator. |
| | | **Freezer** | |
| **Freezer compartment of a refrigerator** | 5°F or –15°C | 2 weeks | Store milk toward the back of the freezer, where temperature is most constant. Milk stored for longer durations in the ranges listed is safe, but some of the lipids in the milk undergo degradation resulting in lower quality. |
| **Freezer compartment of refrigerator with separate doors** | 0°F or –18°C | 3–6 months | |
| **Chest or upright deep freezer** | –4°F or –20°C | 6–12 months | |

SOURCE: Based on Academy of Breastfeeding Medicine. (2004). *Protocol Number #8: Human Milk Storage Information for Home Use for Healthy Full-Term Infants*. Princeton Junction, NJ: Academy of Breastfeeding Medicine.

verification of the health of the mother and baby by the health care provider of each. Blood samples are tested for hepatitis B, hepatitis C, HIV, HTLV, and syphilis by the milk bank. Women are not accepted if they are acutely ill, have had a blood transfusion or an organ transplant within a year, drink more than 2 ounces of liquor daily, regularly use medications or megavitamins, smoke, or use street drugs. Additionally, women who eat no animal products must take vitamin supplements with $B_{12}$ to be eligible to donate.

Human milk is carefully pasteurized to kill any potential pathogens while preserving the nutrients and active immune properties of the milk. The North American Human Milk Banking Association communicates closely with the Food and Drug Administration to follow guidelines for use of human tissues and fluids. Human milk for milk banks is stored frozen to preserve the immunologic and nutritional components. Rigid plastic (polypropylene) containers are recommended for keeping the milk composition stable. White blood cells stick to glass, but not to plastic containers.[144]

A prescription from a physician or a hospital is needed to order milk for an infant from one of the North American Milk Banking Association milk banks. Costs are approximately $3.50 per ounce before shipping charges.[146] Some insurance companies and Medicaid programs cover the fees when it is demonstrated that donor milk is the most appropriate therapy for a specific patient.

A new way to share milk began in 2004 with the development of the website Human Milk 4 Human Babies (www.hm4hb.com). Since that time, additional Internet opportunities have become available to share unpasteurized human milk. Milk sharing continues to grow in popularity. There are many concerns with stranger-to-stranger milk sharing. These concerns include unregulated, untested human milk with potential for infectious agents in the milk, and the potential for harmful medications to be present in the milk. These medications may be prescriptions, over-the-counter, and/or recreational drugs. Additional concerns involve potential for contamination in pumping and cleaning breast pump practices and possible bioactive factor changes due to thaw/freeze cycles.[144] A study by Keim et al. purchased several containers of human milk and assessed bacterial counts as well as infectious contents. They reported that most Internet samples would have failed HMBANA criteria for feeding. The samples were frequently contaminated with overall high bacterial growth. Time-in-transit were predictive of bacteria counts. None of the Internet samples were HIV positive; however, 21 percent were cytomegalovirus DNA-positive. This is concerning, as many mothers seeking to purchase milk for medically fragile infants.[143] The American Academy of Pediatrics, the Center for Disease Control and Prevention, and The FDA do not support milk sharing or unpasteurized donor milk.

Prolacta, the first commercial for-profit milk bank, was established in 2006. This company has several specialized products for the NICU population including human milk fortification.[145]

# Model Programs

LO 7.12 Analyze one of the model programs for breastfeeding promotion in the United States.

## Breastfeeding Promotion in Physicians' Office Practices (BPPOP)

The American Academy of Pediatrics (AAP) receives funding support from the Maternal and Child Health Bureau (MCHB), USDHHS, and the AAP Friends of the Children Fund for this innovative program designed to boost breastfeeding promotion and support in underserved populations. Initiated in 1997, BPPOP's original mission was to improve the ability of AAP members to support new mothers and their breastfeeding infants and to encourage pediatricians to collaborate with others to develop breastfeeding promotion programs. Pediatricians enrolling in the program received a resource kit of educational materials and other strategies to more effectively promote, support, and manage breastfeeding with all families in their practice. In addition, pediatricians were provided technical assistance by telephone and email regarding breastfeeding concerns from AAP staff and were encouraged to participate in community and regional collaborative action groups. After over 700 pediatricians nationwide joined the program, BPPOP was expanded in 2002 (BPPOP II) to include obstetricians, family physicians, and other health care providers and to specifically target office practices working with racially and ethnically diverse populations. A speaker's kit and materials targeting underserved populations were added to the resource kit, along with the newest strategies and opportunities for multidisciplinary networking for community breastfeeding promotion. Physicians joining the program complete a self-assessment questionnaire at the beginning and end of the program and measure the impact of breastfeeding promotion efforts by tracking the breastfeeding initiation and duration rates within their practices.

BPPOP II concluded in 2004. Gaps in the program were identified—including the need for focused training related to breastfeeding support and management. It also became evident that this training should occur well before physicians are in practice, preferably in residency and medical school. To address this shortcoming, the BPPOP program entered its third phase (BPPOP III) in 2008. This phase aimed, to educate pediatric, obstetric/gynecologic, and family medicine residents. A pilot-tested breastfeeding residency curriculum was tested at 14 residency programs throughout the United States. The American Academy of Pediatrics (AAP) has finalized this breastfeeding residency curriculum. Implementation strategies and use of the curriculum are available through the AAP.

## The Rush Mothers' Milk Club

The Rush Mothers' Milk Club at Rush Presbyterian–St. Luke's Medical Center is an evidence-based program of breastfeeding interventions for the neonatal intensive-care unit (NICU).[133] The program uses a team approach to feeding very low-birthweight infants their own mothers' milk (OMM). The infants' mothers work in partnership with neonatologists, neonatal nurse practitioners, bedside nurses, and other health care professionals to ensure that the latest research is applied to an infant's OMM feeding plan. Interventions to sustain lactation for program participants have evolved from the evidence about barriers to providing OMM to NICU infants. They include preventing and treating low milk volume, achieving adequate infant growth on OMM feedings, and making the transition to at-breast feedings in the NICU and post-discharge periods. Additionally, research about the effectiveness of peer support to sustain lactation has been incorporated into the program.[146]

Major program components include: (1) providing information for mothers to make an informed decision, (2) providing access to a hospital-grade electric breast pump, (3) providing skin-to-skin care and suckling at the empty breast as practice for the newborn, (4) babies feeding at the breast as soon as they are able to suck and swallow effectively, and (5) nursery staff helping the mother prepare for breastfeeding after discharge (www.rush.edu/patients/children/publications/notes/preemies.html). The club serves as a place for mothers to discuss their goals and concerns about breastfeeding. Mothers learn the value of their milk to their high-risk baby from the Special Care Nursery Staff and from the Rush Mothers' Milk Club. The mothers learn to measure the amount of fat and calories in their own milk and learn to capture the highest-calorie portion of milk, which is usually produced during the last 10 minutes of pumping. To create a bond between the mother and baby, mothers are encouraged to use the breast pumps at the baby's bedside. Family members and friends are also encouraged to participate in the weekly Mothers' Milk Club meetings to learn the importance of breastfeeding to the high-risk infant.

The success of the Rush Mothers' Milk Club is measured by its breastfeeding initiation rates. Between 95 and 97 percent of all mothers who deliver high-risk infants at Rush Presbyterian–St. Luke's Medical Center begin to nurse, compared with national rates for high-risk infants of only 30–40 percent. A group of low-income African American mothers who delivered babies below 1500 grams had OMM initiation rates of 63.4 percent, the highest reported rates for this population in the nation.[149] The program has evidence that these high rates of initiation are due to two primary interventions: the clarity of the message that the mothers received about the importance of OMM from health care providers and their immediate access to electric breast pump rental.

## KEY POINTS

1. The majority of mothers and infants do not experience significant problems with breastfeeding. Many of the more common problems can be prevented through prenatal breastfeeding education and from informed, consistent, and individualized care and support from health professionals, both in the hospital and after discharge.
2. Most medications (prescription or over-the-counter) and herbal supplements taken by the mother are excreted in her breast milk and should not be ingested until the risks to the infant are established. For most maternal conditions, required drug therapy choices are available that will not cause harm to the breastfeeding infant; recommending that a mother discontinue breastfeeding to take a medication is rarely required.
3. The level of alcohol in breast milk matches the maternal plasma alcohol levels at the time of the infant feeding; a nursing woman who drinks occasionally can limit her infant's exposure to alcohol by timing breastfeeding in relation to her drinking.
4. Maternal smoking presents significant health risks for infants and children. Data show that children of smoking mothers who are breastfed have better general health, and decreased respiratory illness and risk of sudden infant death syndrome, compared to children of smoking mothers who were not breastfed.
5. While low levels of environmental pollutants are present in most human milk, their impact on the well-being of the mother and infant is unknown. The World Health Organization and other scientific groups state that the advantages of breastfeeding far outweigh the potential risks from environmental pollutants and recommend breastfeeding in all but extreme circumstances.
6. A thorough understanding of the normal and abnormal patterns and mechanisms of jaundice (hyperbilirubinemia) in the newborn period is important for all health professionals to prevent toxicity from excessive jaundice and for protecting and ensuring successful breastfeeding. Early and frequent breastfeeding (at least 8–12 times in 24 hours) in the first days of life helps prevent hyperbilirubinemia through maintaining infant hydration and stimulating the passage of stool. The AAP recommends against routine supplementation of nondehydrated breastfed infants with water or dextrose water, as this practice will not prevent jaundice.
7. Twins and other multiples can be successfully breastfed without supplementation.
8. Exclusive breastfeeding for at least 4 months is recommended to protect against ectopic dermatitis and wheezing illnesses in at-risk children up to age 10. If there is no history of allergy to a specific food in the mother's or father's family, avoiding a food because it is a potential allergen is an unnecessary precaution.
9. Human milk is the preferred food for all premature and sick newborns, with rare exceptions.
10. In developed countries, where safe and affordable breast milk substitutes are available, HIV-infected women should be counseled strongly not to breastfeed to prevent mother-to-child transmission of HIV through breast milk.
11. Health professionals should provide breastfeeding mothers with current evidence-based guidelines for the collection (through hand pumps, electric handheld pumps, hospital-grade electric breast pumps, or manual expression) and storage of human milk for home use or human milk banking.
12. In most situations, the medical problems of the mother or infant can be managed without discontinuing breastfeeding. Any medical decision to limit breastfeeding must be justified by the fact that the risk to the infant clearly outweighs the benefits of breastfeeding.

## REVIEW QUESTIONS

1. List three common causes of persistent nipple pain.
2. Signs of a hyperactive letdown are:
   a. Milk streams quickly
   b. Infant may be overwhelmed by the volume
   c. Infant may choke, cough, or gulp
   d. All of the above
3. List three reasons a breastfeeding mother may develop mastitis.
4. Before a mother uses galactogogues to improve supply, she should be pumping with a hospital-grade electric pump every 2–3 hours during the day and once at night or she should be pumping after each feeding.

   _____ True _____ False

5. The alcohol level in breast milk matches maternal plasma levels.

   _____ True _____ False

6. Smoking can lower milk production and decrease fat content.

   _____ True _____ False

7. The main obstacle to nursing multiples is milk supply.

   _____ True _____ False

8. List at least three major risk factors for developing severe hyperbilirubinemia.

9. Preterm infants have higher readmission rates because of:
   a. Hypoglycemia
   b. Suck–swallow coordination
   c. Hypothermia
   d. All of the above

10. Marijuana is excreted into breast milk at what ratio compared to maternal plasma levels?
    a. Twofold
    b. Fourfold
    c. Sixfold
    d. Eightfold

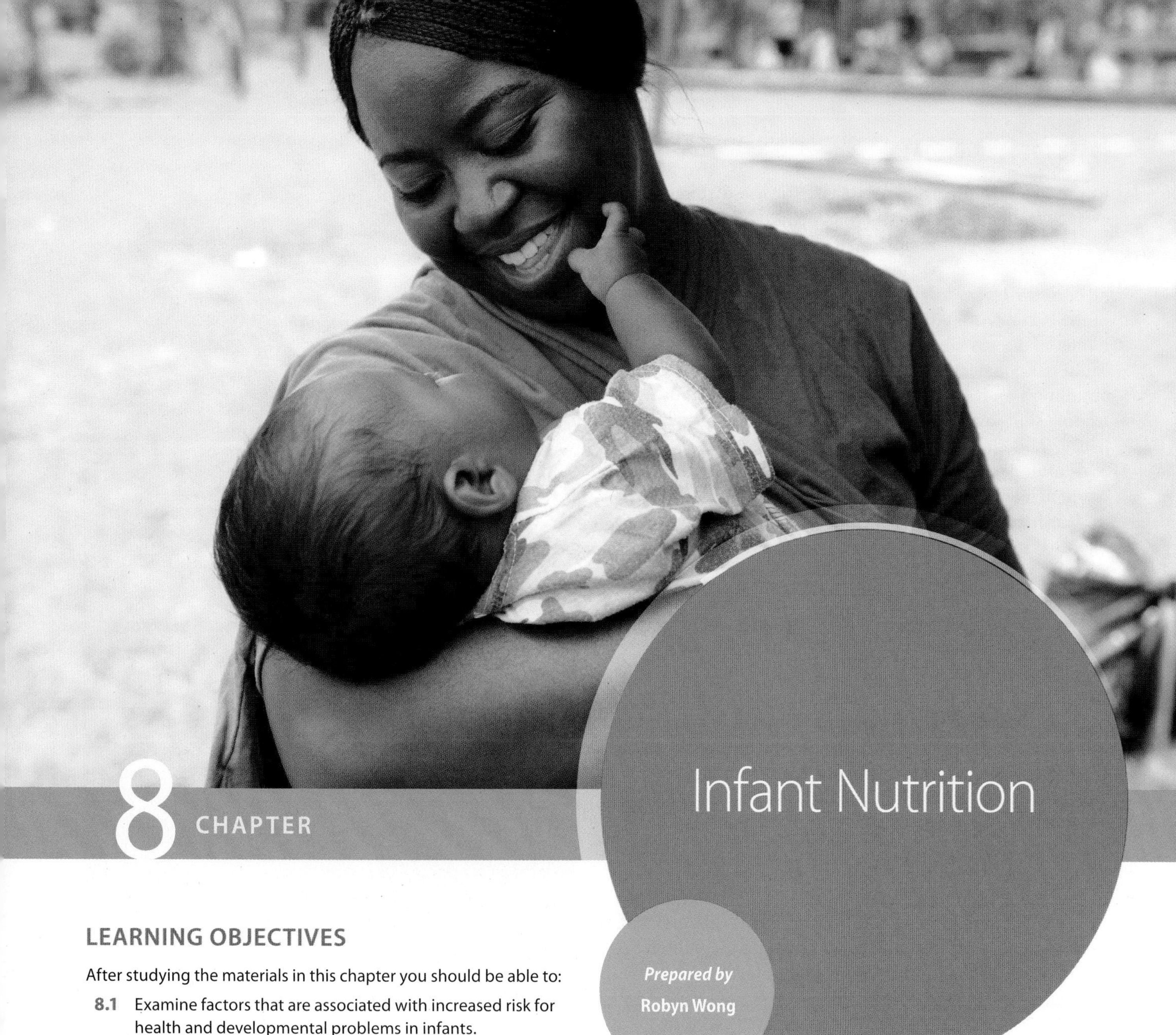

# 8 CHAPTER

# Infant Nutrition

*Prepared by*
**Robyn Wong**

## LEARNING OBJECTIVES

After studying the materials in this chapter you should be able to:

**8.1** Examine factors that are associated with increased risk for health and developmental problems in infants.

**8.2** Describe guidelines and tools that can be used to identify appropriate energy and nutrient needs of infants.

**8.3** Describe how to assess adequate growth in infants.

**8.4** Discuss how feeding and food choices that parents make for their infants can affect later health status.

**8.5** Identify infant developmental milestones related to feeding.

**8.6** Describe how providers and families can access nutrition guidance for infants.

**8.7** Identify how nutrition problems and concerns impact overall infant health and development.

**8.8** Cite examples of nutritional interventions that can reduce risk for nutrition and health problems in infancy.

CDC/Lt. Cmdr. Gary Brunette

# Introduction

Rapid growth during the first year of life differentiates infancy from all other ages.[1] From birth to 6 months of age, growth occurs most rapidly than at any other period in the life cycle.[2] Adequate nutrition is required for normal development of the brain. Infancy is a critical period for formation of the brain. During this time, the foundation for cognitive, motor, and socio-emotional skill development is established. These developmental skills will continue to progress through childhood and adulthood.[3] This is also the period when feeding skills and healthful eating patterns are being established. This chapter is about healthy ***full-term infants*** born at or after 37 weeks of gestation.[4] These infants are expected to achieve normal patterns of growth and development in their first year. Infants generally double their birth weight by 4 to 6 months of age; and triple their birth weight at one year of age (Illustration 8.1).[5] Their birth length will double at the end of the first year. Head circumference is reflective of brain growth, and the weight of the newborn brain will double by 1 year of age.[5]

This chapter discusses how nutrition is an important component in the complex development of infants. Both biological and environmental factors interact during infant growth and development. Models about the interaction of biological and environmental factors are often incomplete. They are not always adequate for describing complex interactions, such as how mealtime stimulates language development and how food preferences develop during infancy.

The Healthy People 2020 objectives focus on infant health target reductions in infant mortality, preterm birth rates, incidence of spina bifida and neural tube defects, fetal alcohol syndrome, and other birth defects.[6] Table 8.1 shows some of the infant-related 2020 objectives that are tracked by public health indicators.

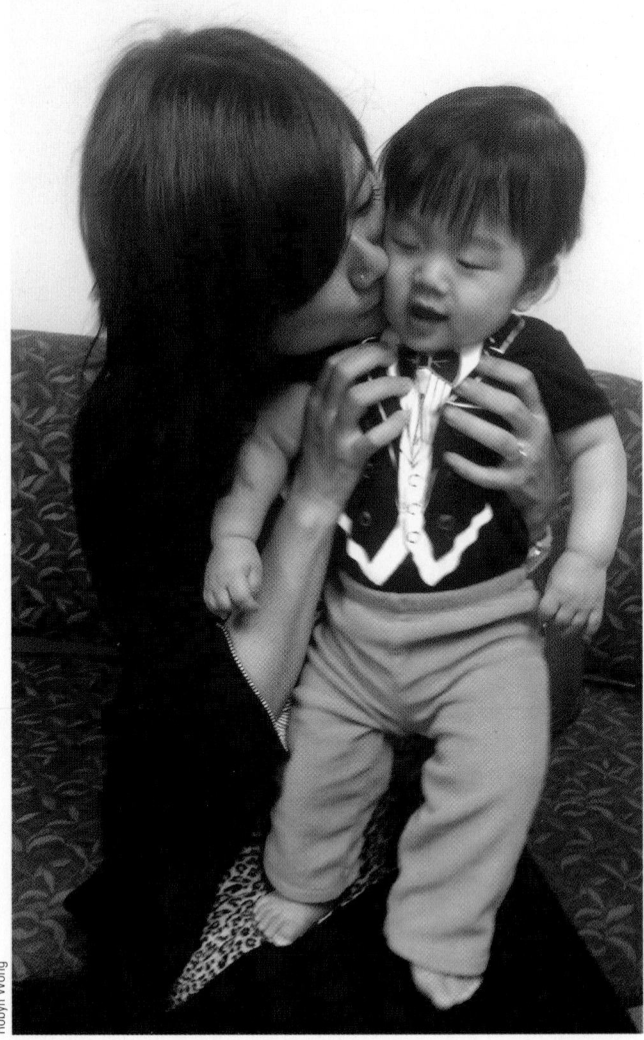

Robyn Wong

ILLUSTRATION 8.1 ▸ A former very low birthweight infant growing and gaining well in his first year.

# Assessing Newborn Health

LO 8.1 Examine factors that are associated with increased risk for health and developmental problems in infants.

## Birthweight and Gestational Age as Outcome Measures

The birthweight of a newborn is one of the indicators of the infant's health status. Full-term infants, born at 37–42 weeks gestation, usually weigh between 2500–3800 grams (5.5–8.5 pounds). There were over 3.9 million births in the United States in 2013, and 89 percent of these newborns were born full term.[7] Full-term infants with normal birth weights are generally healthy, and less likely to require intensive care. Premature or ***preterm infants*** are born before 37 weeks gestation and are classified by their gestational age and birth weight. Low-birthweight (LBW) infants weigh less than 2500 grams; very low-birthweight (VLBW) infants weigh less than 1500 grams. Extremely low-birthweight (ELBW) infants weigh less than 1000 grams. Birthweight and the length of gestation are two of the most important predictors of an infant's survival and later health.[8] Very preterm and very low-birthweight infants are at much greater risk of death and disability than infants born at term or with birth weights over 2500 grams.[8]

## Infant Mortality

Infant mortality is one of the key indicators of the health of a nation. It is associated with numerous factors including maternal health, quality and access to medical care, socioeconomic conditions, and public health practices.[8] The leading causes of infant mortality in the United States in 2011 were

**full-term infants** Infants born at or after 37 weeks gestation.

**preterm infants** Infants born before 37 weeks of gestation.

TABLE 8.1 ▸ United States 2020 Healthy People Objectives related to infants

| SELECTED GOALS IN MATERNAL, INFANT, AND CHILD HEALTH | BASELINE | TARGET |
|---|---|---|
| Reduce all infant deaths within 1 year | 6.7 infant deaths per 1000 live births | 10 percent improvement |
| Reduce preterm births | 12.7 percent of live births preterm | 10 percent improvement |
| Increase the proportion of infants who are put to sleep on their backs | 69.0 percent of infants were put to sleep on their backs | 10 percent improvement |
| Reduce the proportion of breastfed newborns who receive formula supplementation within the first 2 days of life | 24.2 percent of breastfed newborns | 10 percent improvement |
| Increase the proportion of infants who are ever breastfed | 74.0 percent of infants | 81.9 percent |
| Increase appropriate newborn blood-spot screening and follow-up testing | 98.3 percent of screen-positive infants | 100% |

SOURCE: Healthy People.gov topics and objectives, Maternal, Infant and Child Health, online access http://www.healthypeople.gov/2020/topicsobjectives2020

congenital malformations, prematurity/low birthweight, sudden infant death (SIDS), maternal complications, and unintended injuries.[9]

In 2010, the U.S. ***infant mortality rate*** was 6.1 deaths per 1,000 live births. This ranked the United States 26th in infant mortality among the 29 countries in the Organization for Economic Cooperation and Development (OECD).[10] This low ranking has been attributed to the very high incidence of preterm births; 9.8 percent of births in the United States in 2010 were preterm—the highest rate among the 29 OECD countries.[10]

## Combating Infant Mortality

Over the past two decades in the United States, much of the efforts to reduce infant mortality have focused on preventing preterm and low-birthweight deliveries.[8] Successful efforts contributing to a decline in this rate include improved access to specialized care for mothers and infants.[11,12]

This is a multifaceted problem, however, also affected by:

- Socioeconomic level
- Access and availability of quality health care
- Medical interventions such as caesarean section and induction of labor
- Teen pregnancy
- Increased incidence of multiple births
- Large differences in rates among racial/ethnic groups

### Health Outcomes of High-Risk and At-Risk Infants

Medicaid and the Child Health Initiatives Program (CHIP) provide health care coverage and contribute to improved access to quality health care for high-risk and at-risk infants.[13] The Early Periodic Screening, Detection, and Treatment Program ***(EPSDT)*** is a major source of preventive and routine health care for infants and children in low-income families. Immunizations in infancy are another example of a public health prevention-focused program. Bright Futures is a collaborative project of the U.S. Department of Health and Human Services and the American Academy of Pediatrics (AAP). The goal of Bright Futures is to improve the health, education, and well-being of infants, children, adolescents, and their families.[14] This project has developed exemplary health supervision guidelines, tools and materials for practitioners working with the pediatric population. *Bright Futures Nutrition* is an excellent publication and series of tools and materials which focus on improving the nutritional health of infants, children, adolescents, and children with special health care needs.[15]

## Newborn Growth Assessment

Newborn health status is assessed by various indicators of growth and development taken right after birth. Indicators include gestational age, birthweight, length, and head circumference. The designation "small for gestational age" (SGA) indicates that the newborn's weight, length, or head circumference plots below the 10th percentile on the growth chart. When all three measurements fall below the 10th percentile, the infant is symmetrically small for gestational age. Measurements above the 90th percentile are considered large for gestational age (LGA) and more often are noted in infants of diabetic mothers. Appropriate for gestational age (AGA) infants have birth measurements that plot between the 10th and the 89th percentile. SGA, AGA, and LGA are indicators of the infant's size at birth. Another indicator, ***intrauterine growth restriction (IUGR)***, is a medical diagnosis identified antenatally. The etiology of IUGR may be associated with genetic factors, congenital anomalies, infection, multiple gestation, maternal nutrition, environmental toxins, placental factors and maternal vascular disease such as diabetes, chronic hypertension, advanced maternal age, and morbid obesity. IUGR is a significant factor in perinatal morbidity and mortality.[16]

**infant mortality** Death that occurs within the first year of life.

**infant mortality rate** The number of infant deaths for every 1000 live births.

**EPSDT** The Early Periodic Screening, Detection, and Treatment Program is a part of Medicaid and provides routine checkups for low-income families.

**intrauterine growth retardation (IUGR)** Fetal undergrowth from any cause, resulting in a disproportionality in weight, length, or weight-for-length percentiles for gestational age. Sometimes called *intrauterine growth restriction.*

## Normal Physical Growth and Development

There is now evidence that the rate and progression of early growth is a major risk factor for development of certain chronic diseases including coronary heart disease and type 2 diabetes.[17] Monitoring infants' nutritional status requires an understanding of their overall development. Full-term newborns have a wider range of abilities than previously recognized; for example, they hear and move in response to familiar sounds, such as their mother's voice.[18] States of arousal describe sleep and awake states in infants, and affect the way they respond at any given time. They provide a framework for parents and caregivers to observe, understand, and interact with their infants. For infants, states of arousal allow them to control the type and amount of input they receive from their environments. These states include quiet sleep, active sleep, drowsy, quiet alert, active alert and crying.[19]

Organs and organ systems developed in utero continue to increase in size and complexity during infancy. The newborn's central nervous system is immature; the neurons in the brain are less organized compared to those of the older infant.[20] As a result, the newborn gives inconsistent or subtle cues of hunger and other needs, compared to the cues given at a later age. The fact that newborns can ***root***, ***suckle***, and coordinate sucking, swallowing, and breathing within hours of birth shows that feeding is directed by reflexes and the central nervous system.[18,21] Newborn reflexes are protective. These ***reflexes*** later fade as they are replaced by more purposeful movements during the first few months of life (see Table 8.2.).[18,21,22]

## Motor Development

Motor development reflects an infant's ability to control voluntary muscle movement. There are several models for describing infant development, but none provides a complete description and explanation of the rapid advances in motor skills achieved during infancy.[18,21] Illustration 8.2 depicts motor development during the first 15 months.[18]

It is a great source of pride for parents when their baby first rolls over or sits up. The development of muscle control and coordination progresses from top down; initiating with head control and ending with lower leg coordination and walking.[22] Muscle development also progresses centrally to peripherally; meaning that the infant learns to control the shoulder and arm muscles before muscles in the hands.[22,23] Motor development influences both the ability of the infant to feed and the amount of energy expended in the activity. An example of how motor development affects feeding is the ability to sit in a high chair. When an infant has achieved head and trunk control, sitting balance, and fading of certain reflexes such as tongue thrust, oral feeding can be initiated.[23] As motor skills continue to progress, daily energy needs increase because of higher energy expenditure. Infants who are crawling or starting to walk will expend more energy in physical activity than younger infants who are not yet rolling over.

## Critical Periods

The concept of critical period is based on a fixed time period when certain behaviors emerge. Piaget's stages of cognitive development and Erickson's psychological stages of development are examples of theories of development stating that there are time periods or windows of development, when certain skills must be learned in order for subsequent learning to occur.[21] A critical period for the development of oral feeding skills may explain some later feeding problems in infancy.[23] In a

**root reflex** Action that occurs if one cheek is touched, resulting in the infant's head turning toward that cheek and the infant opening his mouth.

**suckle** A reflexive movement of the tongue moving forward and backward; earliest feeding skill.

**reflex** An automatic (unlearned) response that is triggered by a specific stimulus.

TABLE 8.2 ▸ Major reflexes found in newborns

| NAME | RESPONSE | SIGNIFICANCE |
|---|---|---|
| Babinski | Baby's toes fan out when the sole of the foot is stroked. | Perhaps a remnant of evolution from heel to toe |
| Blink | Baby's eyes close in response to bright light or loud noise. | Protects the eyes |
| Moro | Baby throws arms out and then inward (as if embracing). | May help a baby cling to the mother in response to loud noise or when baby's head falls |
| Palmar | Baby grasps an object placed in the palm of his or her hand. | Precursor to voluntary grasping |
| Rooting | When a baby's cheek is stroked, baby turns head toward the cheek that was stroked and opens mouth. | Helps a baby find the nipple |
| Stepping | Baby is held upright by an adult and is then moved. | Precursor to voluntary walking forward; begins to step rhythmically |
| Sucking | Baby sucks when an object is placed in mouth. | Permits feeding |
| Withdrawal | Baby withdraws foot when the sole is pricked with a pin. | Protects a baby from unpleasant stimulation |

SOURCE: From KAIL/CAVANAUGH. Human Development, 2nd ed.

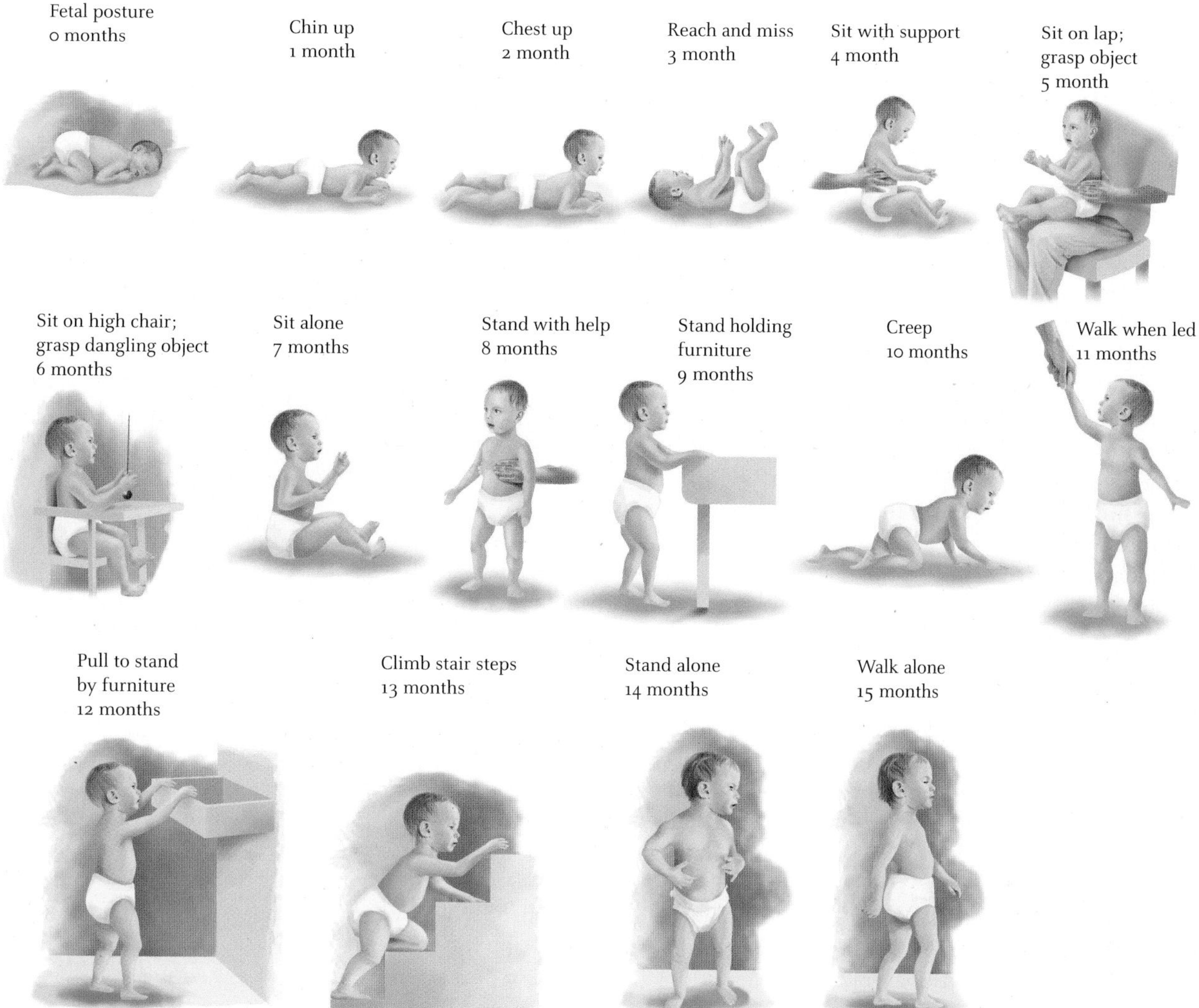


**ILLUSTRATION 8.2** ▸ Gross motor skills.

Based on Shirley, 1931, and Bayley, 1969.

SOURCE: From KAIL/CAVANAUGH. Human Development, 2E.



healthy newborn, the mouth is a source of oral pleasure and exploring, an important form of early learning. An infant on prolonged respiratory support may not associate oral sensations and stimulation with pleasure, but instead with discomfort. The critical period for developing positive associations with oral sensations, stimulation, and feeding may have adversely been affected. After discharge, this infant may become a reluctant feeder and have difficulty learning to enjoy eating and mealtimes. Feeding issues that may occur in preterm infants and infants with special health care needs will be discussed in Chapter 9.

## Cognitive Development

Risk factors for poor cognitive, motor, and socio-emotional development include: severe, acute malnutrition (very low weight for length), chronic undernutrition (intrauterine growth retardation and linear growth retardation or stunting), iron deficiency anemia, and iodine deficiency.[3] The baby's interactions with the environment stimulate the developing brain, which is now seen as structuring the nervous system in the long term (see Illustration 8.3 on p. 230).[3] Research has shown that access to adequate energy and protein alone may not be sufficient for maximizing brain maturation without simultaneously providing psycho-social stimulation.[24]

Improving the nutritional status of infants can positively affect their environment-related experiences and stimulation. Undernourished infants may frequently be ill and subsequently irritable, fussy, tired, and withdrawn. Caregivers may experience more difficulty when feeding these infants. A decrease in their activity level may occur and alter their ability to explore their environment and interact with their caregivers, and poor brain development may result.[3]

## Digestive System Development

"Now good digestion wait on appetite, and health on both."

—William Shakespeare, *Macbeth*

A healthy digestive system is necessary to support adequate nutrition. Parents may worry about gastrointestinal problems, in part because of misinformation about nutrition in infancy.[25] An infant passing soft, loose stools may be thought to have diarrhea if parents do not know that these are typical stools for breastfed infants. Parents may feel that their infant's gastrointestinal discomfort may affect and interfere with weight gain, even though growth has been progressing well. It takes up to 6 months for the infant gastrointestinal tract to mature, and the time required is variable among infants.[14,26]

During the third trimester, the fetus swallows amniotic fluid, and this stimulates the lining of the intestine to grow and mature. At birth, the healthy newborn's digestive system is sufficiently mature to digest fats, protein, and simple sugars and to absorb fats and amino acids. Although healthy newborns do not have the same levels of digestive enzymes or rate of gastric emptying as older infants, the gut is functional at birth.[26] After birth and through early infancy, the coordination of peristalsis within the gastrointestinal tract improves.

Infants may have conditions that reflect the immaturity of the gut, such as colic, *gastroesophageal reflux (GER)*, unexplained diarrhea, and constipation.[27] Such conditions do not usually interfere with the ability of the intestinal villi to absorb nutrients, and typically do not hinder growth.[27] Many factors influence the rate of food passage through the colon and the gastrointestinal discomfort seen in infants. These include:

- ***Osmolarity*** of foods or liquids (which affects how much water is drawn into the intestine)
- Bacterial flora in the colon
- Water and fluid balance in the body

## Parenting

"A babe in the house is a well-spring of pleasure."

—Martin Farquhar Tupper, *On Education*

Even though the newborn is able to breastfeed or bottle feed soon after birth, skills of new parents develop slowly. The parents' ability to recognize and respond to infant cues of hunger and satiety improves over time. Table 8.3 highlights some of the hunger and satiety cues observed at varying ages during the first year of life. New parents are also

**gastroesophageal reflux (GER)** Movement of the stomach contents backward into the esophagus due to stomach muscle contractions. The condition may require treatment depending on its duration and degree.

**osmolarity** Measure of the number of particles in a solution, which predicts the tendency of the particles to move from high to low concentration. Osmolarity is a factor in many systems, such as in fluid and electrolyte balance.

**TABLE 8.3** Infant hunger and satiety cues

| INFANT'S APPROXIMATE AGE | HUNGER CUES | SATIETY (FULLNESS) CUES |
|---|---|---|
| Birth through 5 months | • Wakes and tosses<br>• Sucks on fist<br>• Cries or fusses<br>• Opens mouth while feeding to indicate wanting more | • Seals lips together<br>• Turns head away<br>• Decreases or stops sucking<br>• Spits out the nipple or falls asleep when full |
| 4 through 6 months | • Cries or fusses<br>• Smiles, gazes at caregiver or coos during feeding to indicate wanting more<br>• Moves head toward spoon or tries to swipe food towards mouth | • Decreases rate of sucking or stops sucking when full<br>• Spits out the nipple<br>• Turns head away<br>• May be distracted or pay more attention to surroundings |
| 5 through 9 months | • Reaches for spoon or food<br>• Points to food | • Eating slows down<br>• Pushes food away |
| 8 through 11 months | • Reaches for food<br>• Points to food<br>• Gets excited when food is presented | • Eating slows down<br>• Clenches mouth shut or pushes food away |
| 10 through 12 months | • Expresses desire for specific food with words or sounds | • Expresses desire for specific food with words or sounds<br>• Shakes head to say "no more" |

SOURCE: Infant Nutrition and Feeding: A Guide for Use in the WIC and CSF Programs. United States Department of Agriculture, Food and Nutrition Service, Special Supplemental Program for Women, Infants and Children (WIC), 2009.

learning about the temperament of their infants. Infant temperament related to feeding includes emotionality, activity, attention span and persistence, reaction to food, and soothability.[28] Infants also have variable eating styles, which can be seen in their reaction to foods, predictability of appetite, and distractability at mealtime. The infant's temperament and eating style might be related to potential feeding problems and risk for obesity in childhood.[23,28]

A healthy parent–infant feeding relationship involves responsive parenting.

Parental skills that support healthful feeding and eating in infancy include:

- Responding early and appropriately to the infant's hunger and satiety cues
- Recognizing the infant's developmental abilities and feeding skills
- Balancing the infant's need for assistance with encouragement of age-appropriate feeding skills
- Allowing the infant to initiate and guide feeding interactions[15]

# Energy and Nutrient Needs

LO 8.2 Describe guidelines and tools that can be used to identify appropriate energy and nutrient needs of infants.

Well-researched nutrient and energy recommendations have been established by the Food and Nutrition Board, Institute of Medicine, and the National Academies of Sciences. The DRIs have identified age-specific recommendations for energy and for macro and micronutrients for healthy infants from 0 to 6 months and from 7 to 12 months of age. The American Academy of Pediatrics (AAP) and the Academy of Nutrition and Dietetics provide guidelines and position papers related to infant health, nutrition and feeding.

The 2014 Dietary Guidelines for Americans provide recommendations for healthful eating and physical activity for individuals starting at 2 years of age. These guidelines do not provide recommendations for infants.[29]

## Energy Needs

The energy needs of infants are higher per kilogram of body weight than at any other time of life. The range in energy requirements for individual infants is broad, ranging from 80 to 120 calories per kg of body weight.[30] The average energy needs of infants in the first 6 months of life is 108 cal per kg body weight, based on growth in breastfed infants. From 6 to 12 months of age, the average energy need is 98 cal/kg.[30] Factors that account for the range of energy needs of infants include the following:

- Weight
- Growth rate
- Sleep/wake cycle
- Temperature and climate
- Physical activity
- Metabolic response to food
- Health status and recovery from illness

## Protein Needs

The recommended protein intake for infants from birth to 6 months of age is 1.52 grams per kilogram body weight, and 1.2 grams per kilogram from 7 to 12 months of age.[30] Protein requirements of infants are affected by age, growth, illness, and adequacy of other nutrients in the diet.[31] Essential amino acids requirements for healthy infants remain the same throughout the first year of life.[30]

Infants from birth to 6 months of age who are breastfed or who consume appropriate amounts of infant formula will obtain adequate protein. Infants may exceed protein recommendations if they consume excessive formula or if protein sources such as infant cereal are added to bottles of formula. Excessive or inadequate protein intake can result with incorrect mixing of formula.

## Fat Needs

Fat is an essential component in the diets of infants. It provides essential fatty acids, is a concentrated source of energy, and facilitates the absorption of fat-soluble vitamins. Fat is especially important in infancy and early childhood because it is essential for neurological development and brain function.[32]

Infants are at higher risk for essential fatty acid deficiency related to their rapid growth rate and higher requirements for polyunsaturated fatty acids. They also have limited stores of body fat.[33] Restrictions of fat and dietary cholesterol are not recommended in infancy.

The Adequate Intake for fat is 31 grams for infants 0–6 months of age and 30 grams for infants 7–12 months of age.[30] Fat contributes approximately half of the calories in breast milk[2,34] and 40 to 50 percent of calories in infant formulas.[35] The percentage of fat in the diet will decrease as the infant accepts complementary foods, since most of these foods are low in fat.

Infants use fats to supply energy to the liver, brain, and muscles, including the heart. The fact that infants have high energy needs compared to those of older children means that infants use fats more regularly for generating energy. Young infants cannot tolerate fasting for long because it quickly uses up both carbohydrate and fat energy sources. This effect of fasting explains in part why young infants cannot sleep through the night.

Fats in food provide the essential fatty acids, linoleic acid (LA) and alpha-linolenic acid (ALA), and polyunsaturated fatty acids, including docohexaenoic acid (DHA) and arachidonic acid (ARA). Essential fatty acids are substrates for hormones, steroids, endocrine, and neuroactive compounds. DHA is a major fatty acid in brain and retinal phospholipids.[32]

## Metabolic Rate, Energy, Fats, and Protein—How Do They All Tie Together?

The metabolic rate of infants is the highest of any period after birth.[14] The higher rate is primarily related to infants' rapid growth rate and high proportion of muscle. The usual body fuel for metabolism is glucose. When sufficient glucose is available, growth will typically progress. When glucose from carbohydrates is limited, amino acids will be converted into glucose for generating energy and are less available for growth. The conversion of amino acids into glucose is a more dynamic process in infants in comparison to adults. The breakdown of amino acids for use as energy occurs during illness in adults, but it can occur daily in fast-growing infants. Circulating amino acids in the blood from ingested foods will be used for glucose production, and if these are not sufficient, the body will release amino acids from muscles. This process of breaking down body protein to generate energy is known as catabolism. If catabolism continues for an extended duration, it can contribute to growth faltering in infants.

## Other Nutrient and Non-Nutrient Needs

**Fluoride** Fluoride is a naturally occurring mineral compound that can contribute to the prevention and reduction of dental caries. When ingested during the time that teeth are developing the fluoride will be deposited on tooth surfaces. The maximum reduction in dental caries will be achieved when fluoride is provided systemically while teeth are developing and topically after teeth are present in the mouth. Fluoride helps to reduce tooth decay by decreasing the solubility of tooth enamel, decreasing the production of acid by oral bacteria, and by supporting further remineralization. Dental caries are the most common chronic disease of childhood.[36]

Infants can obtain fluoride from fluoridated water, bottled water with added fluoride, and from fluoride supplements. Fluoride content in breast milk is low.[37]

Water fluoridation has been shown to reduce caries in primary teeth of children by as much as 60 percent.[38] In 2012, 74.6 percent of the U.S. population on public water systems had access to fluoridated water.[39] Community water fluoridation is one of the objectives in Healthy People 2020, with desired outcome that 79.6 percent of people on public water systems receive water that has the optimal level of fluoride recommended for preventing tooth decay.[6]

The DRI for fluoride is 0.1 mg daily for infants less than 6 months of age, and 0.5 mg daily for infants 7–12 months old.[40] Most infants who live in areas with fluoridated water do not need additional fluoride. Supplemental fluoride is recommended for breastfed and formula-fed infants residing in communities where fluoride concentration in the water is low; beginning at 6 months of age.[36]

**Vitamin D** Vitamin D is a key nutrient in the diets of infants. It has an essential role in bone mineralization and calcium and phosphorus homeostasis, and regulates genes associated with immune response and cellular growth.[41] There are two forms: vitamin $D_2$ (ergocalciferol), which is from plants and fungi, and vitamin $D_3$ (cholecalciferol), which is synthesized in the skin during exposure to sunlight. Vitamin $D_3$ also is found in fatty fish like salmon and mackerel. The Adequate Intake (AI) for vitamin D is 400 international units (IU) for infants. Breast milk is low in vitamin D at 22 IU per liter.[42] Standard infant formulas are manufactured to contain 400 IU per liter.

The AAP recommends that all breastfed and partially breastfed infants receive 400 IU of vitamin D daily. Formula-fed infants who are consuming less than one liter of infant formula daily should receive 400 IU of vitamin D daily.[43] Vitamin D needs during lactation are discussed in Chapter 6.

**Sodium** Sodium is a major component of extracellular fluid and an important regulator of fluid balance. The Adequate Intake (AI) for sodium is 120 mg for 0- to 6-month-old infants and 370 mg for 7- to 12-month-old infants. The sodium content in breast milk was used as the basis for establishing sodium requirements for infants. Infant formula is supplemented with sodium to match the amount contained in breast milk.[44] Generally, infants do not have difficulty with maintenance of body fluids and electrolytes, even though they may not show thirst as a separate signal from hunger. Young infants do not sweat as much as older children, so losses from sweating are not usually problematic. Illnesses such as diarrhea or vomiting cause the loss of fluid and sodium and increase the risk of dehydration. Infants do not need salt added to foods to maintain adequate sodium intake.

**Iron** Infants are at risk for iron deficiency because of rapid growth in the first year. From 4 to 12 months of age, an infant's blood volume will double.[45] Those with lower iron stores at birth or low intakes of dietary iron are also at risk. Iron deficiency anemia in infancy is associated with short- and long-term consequences, including poor cognitive and motor development. These infants have been reported with socio-emotional impairments including being more wary, hesitant, solemn, unhappy, and more closely keeping with their mothers.[46] Newborns at risk for iron deficiency include infants of diabetic mothers, growth-restricted (IUGR) newborns, and preterm infants.[47]

Young infants have iron levels that reflect their mother's health during late pregnancy and delivery. Infants born at term generally have adequate iron stores that will last through 4–6 months of age.[45] According to the Institute of Medicine, healthy-term infants 0–6 months of age need 0.27 mg of iron each day. This AI recommendation was based on the iron content of breast milk, and the average breast milk intake of infants at this age. The RDA for older infants 7–12 months of age increases to 11 mg daily related to depletion of their iron stores 4–6 months after birth.[48] To assure that preterm, full term, and older infants have sufficient iron regardless of the method of feeding, the AAP recommends initiation of supplemental iron for exclusively breastfed infants starting at 4 months of age.[49]

**Lead** Although lead is not a nutrient, it can be associated with iron and calcium status during infancy. Children's blood lead levels increase most rapidly at 6–12 months of age, and peak at 18–24 months of age.[50] Elevated blood lead levels have a neurotoxic effect on infants and young children, and are associated with intellectual and behavioral functioning impairments.[51] There is a negative correlation between blood lead levels and blood calcium and iron levels.

Infants may inadvertently be exposed to environmental sources of lead. Lead may be a contaminant in water from lead pipes, particularly if the house was built before 1950. Older homes may contain lead-based paints that taste sweet to infants. The American Academy of Pediatrics recommends screening children at risk beginning at 9–12 months of age.[53]

# Growth Assessment

LO 8.3 Describe how to assess adequate growth in infants.

Physical growth is defined as the increase in the mass of body tissues that occurs in genetically determined rates, patterns, and ages as a healthy infant grows into adulthood.[5] Adequate nutrition and physical activity are needed to achieve optimal growth and maturation. In most normal, healthy infants, growth and maturation progress with few, if any, problems.[5]

Frequent measurements of weight, length, and head circumference during infancy will facilitate early identification of potential problems such as slow or excessive weight gain or slow linear growth. There is a wide range of appropriate growth patterns in infancy. Healthy infants may have brief periods when their weight gain is slower or more rapid than at other times. Slight variations in growth rate may result from illness, inappropriate feeding routine, or family disruption. The overall growth pattern is important, and each assessment is compared to the overall health assessment.

Accurate growth measurements and interpretation of growth rates are important components in evaluating an infant's nutritional status. Use of calibrated infant scales, recumbent measuring boards, and non-stretch head circumference tapes improves measurement accuracy.

Standardized methods should be utilized when measuring growth; these require practice and consistency. Equipment used to measure infants differs from equipment for measuring older children. The scale bed must be long enough to allow the infant to lie down or sit. Length is measured with the infant lying down with head and feet touching the measuring board at right angles. Positioning the baby quickly and carefully is a skill needed for accurate measurement of recumbent length. Clothing, hair ornaments, and excessive movement of the infant while on the scale will affect measurement accuracy. Illustration 8.4 shows weight, length and head circumference measurements obtained with recommended measuring equipment.

## Interpretation of Growth Data

A comparison of the WHO growth charts and the CDC growth charts is shown in Table 8.4. Both sets of growth charts show:

- Weight for age
- Length for age
- Weight for length
- Head circumference for age

The 2006 WHO growth charts include charts for the age range of 0–24 months for each gender.[54] The WHO growth charts are based on longitudinal and cross-sectional data of infants who were exclusively or predominantly breastfed, and living in urban, middle-class communities in Brazil, Ghana, Oman, Norway, India, and Davis, California. These growth charts show how infants and children should grow under ideal conditions and environments. The European Society for Pediatric Gastroeneterology, Hepatology and Nutrition reported that the patterns of linear growth were remarkably

TABLE 8.4 Accurately measuring growth in infants

**To Avoid Measurement Errors**

- Use measuring equipment that was recently calibrated.
- Confirm that the scale is on zero before starting.
- Weigh the infant nude or wearing a dry diaper.
- Confirm the position of the infant for length measurements:
  - Head position—the infant's eyes are looking straight up and the head is in midline, touching the head board.
  - Neither hips nor knees are bent.
  - Heel is measured with foot flat against the foot board.
- Head circumference measure is at the widest part of the head.

**SUBSTAGES DURING THE SENSORIMOTOR STAGE OF DEVELOPMENT**

| Substage | Age (months) | Accomplishment | Example |
|---|---|---|---|
| 1 | 0–1 | Reflexes become coordinated. | Sucking a nipple |
| 2 | 1–4 | Primary circular reactions appear—an infant's first learned reactions to the world. | Thumb sucking |
| 3 | 4–8 | Secondary circular reactions emerge, allowing infants to explore the world of objects. | Shaking a toy to hear a rattle |
| 4 | 8–12 | Means–end sequencing of schemes is seen, marking the onset of intentional behavior. | Moving an obstacle to reach a toy |
| 5 | 12–18 | Tertiary circular reactions develop, allowing children to experiment. | Shaking different toys to hear the sounds they make |
| 6 | 18–24 | Symbolic processing is revealed in language, gestures, and pretend play. | Eating pretend food with a pretend fork |

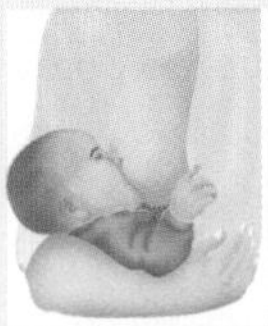

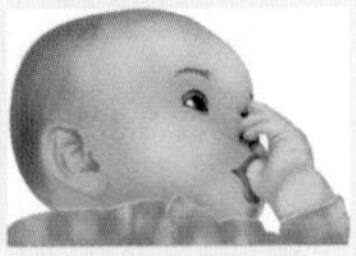

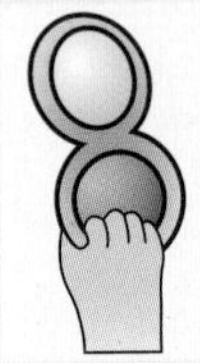

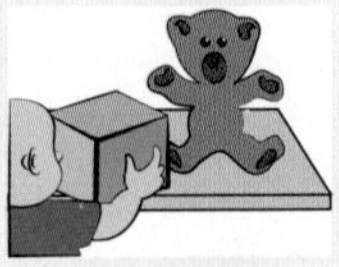

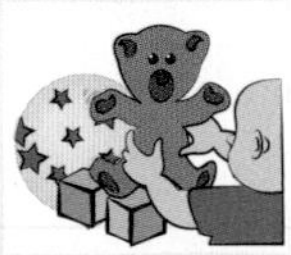

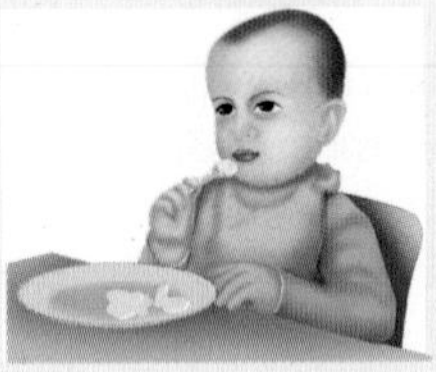

ILLUSTRATION 8.3 ▸ *Sensorimotor* stage of development.

SOURCE: From KAIL/CAVANAUGH. Human Development, 2E.



Robyn Wong

Robyn Wong

Robyn Wong

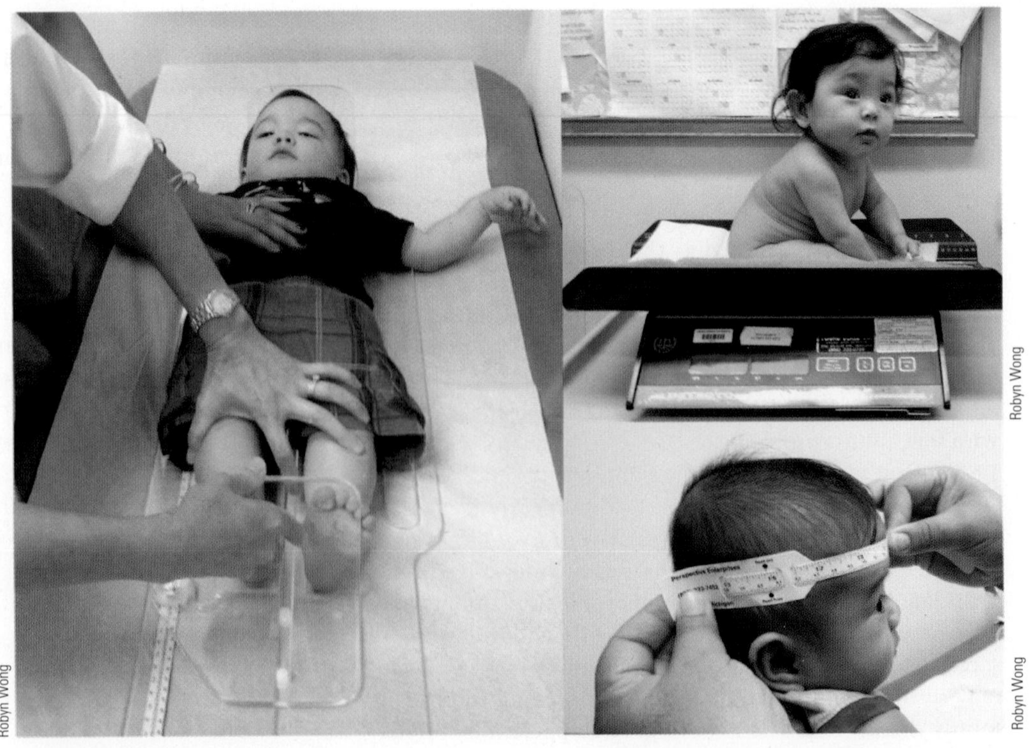

ILLUSTRATION 8.4 ▸ Infant measurements taken with recumbent length board, digital scale and head circumference tape.

TABLE 8.5 ▸ Comparing infant growth in CDC and WHO growth charts

| BASIS | CDC 2000 | WHO 2011 |
|---|---|---|
| Geography and sample size | U.S. selected sites with 5,000 measurements | Worldwide six selected sites with 19,000 measurements |
| Concept | Descriptive reference reflecting past: "How infants have grown" | Prescriptive optimal standard: "How infants should grow" |
| Feeding Method | 66% formula fed and 33% breastfed for 3 months | All breastfed at least 4 months |
| Time covered | Birth to 36 months | Birth to 24 months |
| Low weight for age in 12 months | Higher prevalence | Lower prevalence |
| High weight for length up to 12 months | Higher prevalence | Lower prevalence |



consistent between the different countries and ethnic groups.[55] In late 2010, the CDC and the AAP recommend use of the WHO growth charts for 0- to 24-month-old infants and children (Table 8.5). Sample WHO growth charts with plotted infant measurements are found in Chapter 9.

Warning signs of growth difficulties include: no increase in weight or length; and a continued decline or rapid increase in weight, length, or head circumference percentile.[15] Head circumference increases are reflective of brain growth.[5] Atypical rates of head circumference growth (notable slowing or rapid increase) will warrant close follow-up by the infant's primary care physician.

# Feeding in Early Infancy

**LO 8.4** Discuss how feeding and food choices that parents make for their infants can affect later health status.

"Food is the first enjoyment of life."

—Lin Yutan, *The Importance of Living*

## Breast Milk and Formula

The AAP and the Academy of Nutrition and Dietetics (AND) recommend that optimal nutrition for infants be provided by exclusive breastfeeding for the first 6 months of life and continuation of breastfeeding for the second 6 months.[56,57] Breastfeeding is a key public health strategy for improving infant health and reducing morbidity and mortality in the first 12 months.[15]

The benefits of breastfeeding and composition of breast milk are well described in Chapter 6. Nutrient recommendations for young infants were established based on intakes of exclusively breastfed infants. No additional fluids or foods are needed for infants prior to 6 months of age.[58]

Infant formulas are manufactured to closely resemble human milk; however, there are numerous components that cannot be replicated in commercial formula. Examples include immunoglobulins, lactoferrin, and lysozyme. See Chapter 6 to review the benefits of breastfeeding and breast milk. Table 8.6 provides a comparison of the various types of infant formula and indications for their use.[57] In the United States the manufacture of infant formula is closely regulated by the Food and Drug Administration through the Infant Formula Act of 1980 and its amendments in 1986. In 2014, the FDA updated these quality control and safety regulations to include manufacturer testing of formula products for nutrient composition and presence of any harmful pathogens, and demonstration that their products support normal physical growth in infants.[59] There are frequent changes made in formula composition and product lines by manufacturers. There are standard cow-milk based and soy-based infant formulas, and types such as "organic," "***hypoallergenic***," "for spit up or reflux," "reduced lactose," and "follow-up." Table 8.6 lists different types of infant formulas and indications for their use.[60]

Growth and health status of an infant are better indicators of dietary adequacy than the volume of breast milk or formula alone. It is optimal for infants to continue breastfeeding through the first year of life. If breastfeeding is discontinued prior to one year of age, infants will need to be transitioned to infant formula. Formula-fed infants need to remain on formula through the first year of life. Routine formulas for full-term infants provide 20 calories per ounce when prepared as directed. Premature post-discharge formulas provide higher energy typically at 22 or 24 calories per ounce. Some health providers recommend further increasing the caloric density of formula for some infants, such as those with volume restrictions or increased energy needs.

**sensorimotor** An early learning system in which the infant's senses and motor skills provide input to the central nervous system.

**hypoallergenic** Foods or products that have a low risk of promoting food or other allergies.

TABLE 8.6 ▸ Infant formulas: Types and indications for use

| FORMULA TYPE | INDICATIONS FOR USE | PRODUCT EXAMPLES |
|---|---|---|
| Standard cow milk–based formula | Healthy term infants 0–12 months of age<br>Most commonly used formula | Bright Beginnings<br>Enfamil Premium<br>Similac Advance<br>Generic store brands |
| Symptoms of intolerance | Term infants with fussiness or spit up<br>Contains partially hydrolyzed protein and reduced lactose<br>Some have added rice starch | Enfamil Gentlease<br>Similac Sensitive<br>Enfamil AR<br>Similac for Spit-Up |
| Partially hydrolyzed protein | Not considered hypoallergenic<br>Not for use with allergic condition or disease<br>Can be considered for spitting up or fussiness | Gerber Good Start<br>Enfamil Gentlease<br>Similac Total Comfort |
| Soy-based | Vegetarian diet<br>Galactosemia<br>Hereditary lactase deficiency<br><br>Not recommended for preterm infants | Bright Beginnings Soy<br>Enfamil Prosobee<br>Good Start Soy<br>Similac Isomil<br>Generic store brands |
| Premature post discharge | For preterm infants transitioning home<br>Higher in energy, protein and micronutrients than standard term formula<br>Usual concentration: 22 cal/oz but can be mixed to higher concentrations | Bright Beginnings Neocare<br>Enfamil Enfacare<br>Similac Neosure |
| Extensively hydrolyzed protein | Hypoallergenic<br>Intolerance to cow milk protein, soy protein<br>Significant malabsorption | Nutramigen<br>Pregestimil<br>Similac Alimentum |
| Amino Acid based | Extreme protein hypersensitivity | Elecare<br>Neocate Infant<br>Pur Amino |

SOURCE: Adapted from Corkins MR (ed.) Pediatric Nutrition Support Handbook, American Society for Parenteral and Enteral Nutrition, 2011.



### Cow Milk

The American Academy of Pediatrics and the Academy of Nutrition and Dietetics Pediatric Practice Group recommend that whole cow milk, skim milk, and reduced-fat milk not be used in infancy.[61,62] Iron-deficiency anemia has been linked to early introduction of whole cow's milk. Low iron availability may result from gastrointestinal blood loss or the lack of other iron-rich foods.[61]

## Development of Infant Feeding Skills

LO 8.5 Identify infant developmental milestones related to feeding.

Infants are born with reflexes that will prepare them to feed successfully. As noted earlier, these reflexes include rooting, sucking, gagging, swallowing, and grasping. To successfully feed, infants need to coordinate sucking, swallowing, and breathing.[18] Infants are also born with food-intake regulation mechanisms that develop over time. In early infancy, self-regulation of feeding is mediated by the pleasure of the sensation of fullness. Inherent preferences are in place for a sweet taste, which is also a pleasurable sensation. After the first 4 to 6 weeks, reflexes fade and infants learn to purposely signal wants and needs. However, it is not until much later—about age 3—that children can verbalize that they are hungry. In between reflexes fading and advancing verbal skills, children's appetites and food intakes are regulated by biological and environmental factors interacting with one another.

Table 8.7 lists infant developmental milestones and indicators of readiness for feeding. The interaction of biological and environmental factors prevails here, too. Depression in a caregiver may be an underestimated or overlooked variable in an infant's progression in feeding skills. Maternal depression may bring about a lower level of interaction between the parent and infant during feeding, reducing the number or volume of feedings and increasing the risk of slower weight gain.[34] Media influences and changes in social practices also affect how babies are fed. Examples are cultural and ethnic perceptions of breastfeeding and the availability of quality child care for infants.

TABLE 8.7 ▸ Sequence of development and feeding skills in healthy, full-term infants

| BABY'S AGE | APPROXIMATE MOUTH PATTERNS | DEVELOPMENTAL SKILLS HAND & BODY CONTROL | BABY CAN: |
|---|---|---|---|
| Birth –5 months | • Sucking/swallowing reflex<br>• Tongue thrust reflex<br>• Poor lip closure | • Poor control of head, neck, and trunk | • Swallow liquids but pushes most solid objects from the mouth |
| 4–6 months | • Draw in lower lip as spoon is removed from mouth<br>• Up and down movement<br>• Immediately transfer food from front to back of tongue to swallow | • Sit with support<br>• Good head control<br>• Use whole hand to grasp objects (palmar grasp) | • Take in a spoonful of pureed or strained food and swallows it without choking<br>• Control the position of food in the mouth |
| 5–9 months | • Up and down munching movement<br>• Position food between jaws for chewing | • Begin to sit alone, unsupported<br>• Begin to use thumb and index finger to pick up objects (pincer grasp) | • Begin to eat mashed foods<br>• Eat from a spoon easily |
| 8–11 months | • Complete side-to-side tongue movement<br>• Begin to curve lips around rim of cup | • Sit alone easily | • Begin to eat ground or finely chopped foods<br>• Begin to feed self with fingers<br>• Drink from a cup (with assistance) |
| 10–11 months | • Rotary chewing (grinding) | • Begin to put spoon in mouth<br>• Begin to hold cup | • Eat chopped foods, small pieces of soft, cooked foods |

SOURCE: Infant Nutrition and Feeding: A Guide for Use in the WIC and CSF Programs. United States Department of Agriculture, Food and Nutrition Service, Special Supplemental Program for Women, Infants and Children (WIC), 2009.



Several models help assess infant readiness for solid food and spoon feeding. The developmental model is based on identifying infant signs such as movement of the tongue from side to side, good head and trunk control, and ability to sit well with some support. Most infants adapt to a variety of feeding regimens, and various feeding practices can be healthy for them. The parents' ability to read the infant's cues of hunger, satiation, tiredness, disinterest, and discomfort influence feeding-skill progression. The cues infants give may include:

- Watching the food being prepared and anticipation of eating
- Tight fists or reaching for the spoon as a sign of hunger
- Showing displeasure if the feeding pace is too slow or if the feeder temporarily stops
- Starting to play with the food or spoon as satiety sets in
- Slowing the pace of eating, or turning away from food when wanting the feeding to end
- Refusing or spitting out food when they have had enough to eat

Infants will display positive and pleasurable signs of satisfaction and satiety during successful feeding experiences. If over time an infant associates eating with discomfort—for example, from gastroesophageal reflux or constipation—this infant might be seen as irritable or difficult to feed. Parental frustration could occur. If this cycle is not replaced by a more positive association of eating and pleasure, the feeding difficulty in infancy may later be characterized by pickiness, food refusals, and difficult mealtime behavior in an older child.[22]

Bright Futures Nutrition has developed "Nutrition Questionnaire for Infants," a tool to help identify potential areas of concern.[15] The questionnaire is completed by parents and can provide helpful information about the infant-parent feeding experience and dietary intake. Sample questions include:

- How would you describe feeding time with your baby? (always pleasant, usually pleasant, sometimes pleasant, never pleasant)
- How do you know when your baby is hungry or has had enough to eat?

## Introduction of Complementary Foods

The goals of infant feeding are to meet all nutritional needs, to enhance mother-infant bonding, to assist the infant in initiating the transition from a primarily liquid diet to a predominantly solid food diet in childhood, and to establish routines of eating in moderation.[1] Complementary foods are solid foods and fluids other than breast milk and formula.

The purpose of introducing complementary foods is to provide additional energy and nutrients because breast milk alone will no longer provide adequate intakes of energy and most micronutrients after 6 months

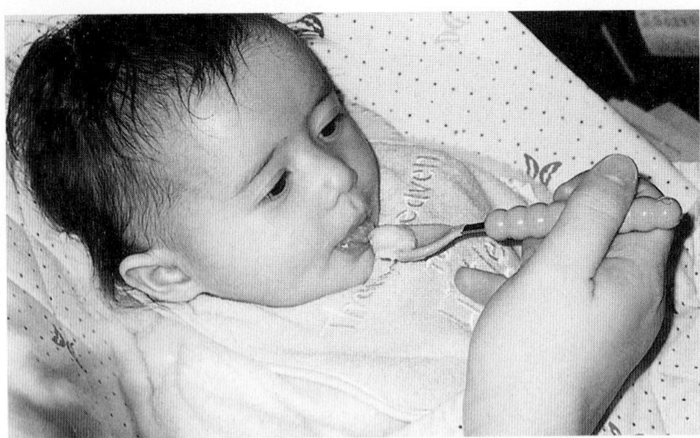

ILLUSTRATION 8.5 ▸ Infant showing readiness for next spoonful of food.

Janet Sugarman Isaacs

of age.[58] Watching a baby learn how to eat from a spoon is fun for new parents (Illustration 8.5). If the baby has achieved the developmental milestones in Table 8.7, it may take him only a few days of practice to start spoon-feeding and to learn to consume 1 tablespoon of semisoft food as a meal. Spoon-feeding is really two new experiences for a baby: a spoon is not soft and warm in the mouth like the breast, and whatever food is selected does not provide the same oral sensation as breast milk or formula. Initially, the baby may try to suck the food from the spoon, and some of the food may spill out of the mouth.

Babies respond strongly to new tastes or smells, regardless of the first food. Recommendations for introducing complementary foods to infants include the following:

- Time the first spoon-feeding experiences when the baby is not overly tired or hungry, but active and alert.
- Use a small spoon with a shallow bowl. The temperature of the spoon needs to be considered if it readily conducts heat or cold.
- Allow the baby time to open his or her mouth and extend the tongue toward the food. If the baby cannot extend the tongue farther out than the lower lip, the baby is not ready for spoon-feeding.
- Place the bowl of the spoon on the tongue with slight downward pressure toward the front of the mouth. Touching the back of the tongue may elicit a gag response.
- The spoon should be almost level. It is not a good practice to scrape the food off the spoon with the baby's gums by tilting the spoon handle up too high. The baby's chin should be slightly down to protect the airway.
- The pace of the feeding should be based on the infant's ability to swallow the food. Rushing will increase the risk of choking or an unpleasant feeding experience.
- First meals may be small in volume—only five or six baby spoons—and last about 10 minutes, based on the baby's interest.

After mastering the new skill of eating from a spoon, babies quickly teach their parents how to feed them by providing cues related to their desired rate of feeding.

## The Importance of Infant Feeding Position

Positioning of infants for feedings at breast or with a bottle and when eating from a spoon are important because improper positioning may be associated with choking and discomfort while eating.[23] Unsafe feeding positions, such as propping a bottle or placing the baby on a pillow, increase the risk for choking, overfeeding, and ear infections. The recommended sleeping position for young infants is lying on the back without elevating the head on a pillow. This position, however, is unsafe and not recommended for feeding.[15,22] The semi-upright position can be achieved with use of a car seat or infant carrier.

Effective positioning at mealtimes will facilitate successful infant feeding. The infant can better control his head and trunk when in a seated position with good support for his back and feet. The parent or caregiver offering the spoon can sit directly in front of the infant and make eye contact during the feeding.[22,23] A high chair is an appropriate feeding chair when the infant can sit without assistance. The infant should be kept in a sitting position with the hips and legs at 90 degrees.

Some healthy infants show resistance or refusal of complementary foods. These early feeding experiences may be of concern if they persist and contribute to inadequate intakes and slow growth.[62] Case Study 8.1 discusses challenges when a child shows resistance to eating.

## Preparing for Drinking from a Cup

The process of ***weaning*** starts in infancy, and usually is completed in toddlerhood. The American Academy of Pedodontics and the AAP recommend that parents should be encouraged to have their infants drink from a cup as they approach 1 year of age, and that they are weaned from the bottle between 12 to 18 months of age.[64] Infants who are exclusively breastfed through the first year can readily transition to the cup when weaning is desired.

Infants who are not exclusively breastfed, or are breastfed for less than 12 months, need to have fluids from a bottle because their skills in cup drinking are not yet sufficient to meet their fluid needs. Developmental readiness for a cup begins at 6 to 8 months.[23] Eight-month-old infants enjoy trying to mimic drinking from open cups that they see at home. The ability to elevate the tongue and control the liquid emerges later, at closer to a year. The 10- to 12-month-old infant enjoys drinking from a held cup and trying to hold his own cup, even though the main feeding method is the breast or bottle.

Infants are likely to consume a decreased total

**weaning** Discontinuation of breastfeeding or bottle feeding and substitution of food for breast milk or infant formula.

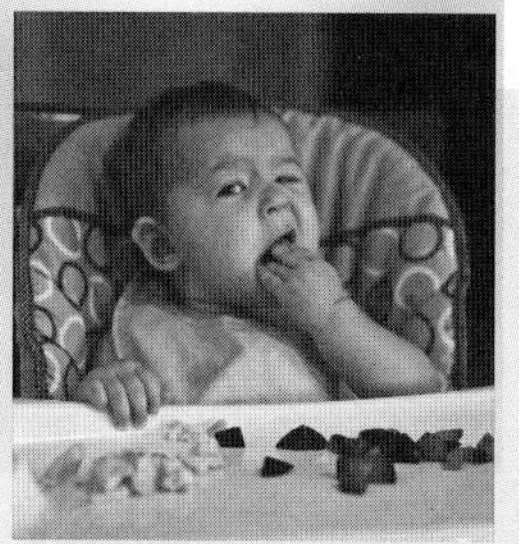



## CASE STUDY 8.1

### Baby Samantha Will Not Eat

Samantha is a healthy 8-month-old girl who lives with her mother, Kathy, her father, and her older sister, who is almost 3 years old. Both parents now work full-time, and both children attend day care full-time. Kathy nursed Samantha exclusively before she returned to work and built up a supply of frozen breast milk. She nurses her twice per day now, early in the morning and before Samantha goes to sleep. Samantha gets breast milk offered in bottles at day care. Samantha is reported by the day care staff to be a good baby. However, when Kathy picks her up after work, Samantha wants to be held and will not sit in her high chair or eat dinner. She cries if she is not held. Samantha's sister wants to eat as soon at they get home. Kathy has so much to do at home after work that she finds it difficult to hold Samantha. Kathy thinks that Samantha must be hungry and that she would be less irritable if she ate her dinner.

#### *Questions*

1. What signs is baby Samantha giving to show that she needs to be comforted rather than fed?
2. How might Kathy change her routine to give baby Samantha more attention and meet the needs of her older daughter?
3. At 8 months, is Samantha too young to overeat due to unmet emotional needs?
4. Should Kathy stop or continue breastfeeding to improve Samantha's eating?

amount of energy from breast milk or infant formula if served in a cup, because they are less efficient in their oral-motor skills. The infant who is weaned too soon may plateau in weight because of decreased total energy intake. At first the typical portion size of fluid from a cup is 1–2 ounces. The drop in total fluids consumed may result in constipation. Changing from a bottle to a covered "sippy" cup with a small spout is not the same developmental step as weaning to an open cup (Illustration 8.6).[23] The oral skills needed in controlling liquids with the tongue are more advanced with an open cup. The skills learned in drinking from an open cup also encourage speech development.

## Food Texture and Development

> "They say fingers were made before forks and hands before knives."
>
> —Jonathan Swift

Weaning is not complete until the energy intake from breast milk or formula is provided by other foods and fluids. Infants progress from swallowing only fluids to eating pureed foods at 6 months of age.[14, 23] Before that, they can only move liquids from the front to the back of the mouth, and not from side to side. At 6–8 months of age, infants are ready for foods with a soft, lumpy texture to elicit munching and jaw movements; these movements simulate chewing. By 8–10 months, infants are able to chew and swallow soft mashed foods without choking. It is important to offer infants foods that do not require much chewing, because infants do not develop mature chewing skills until they are toddlers.

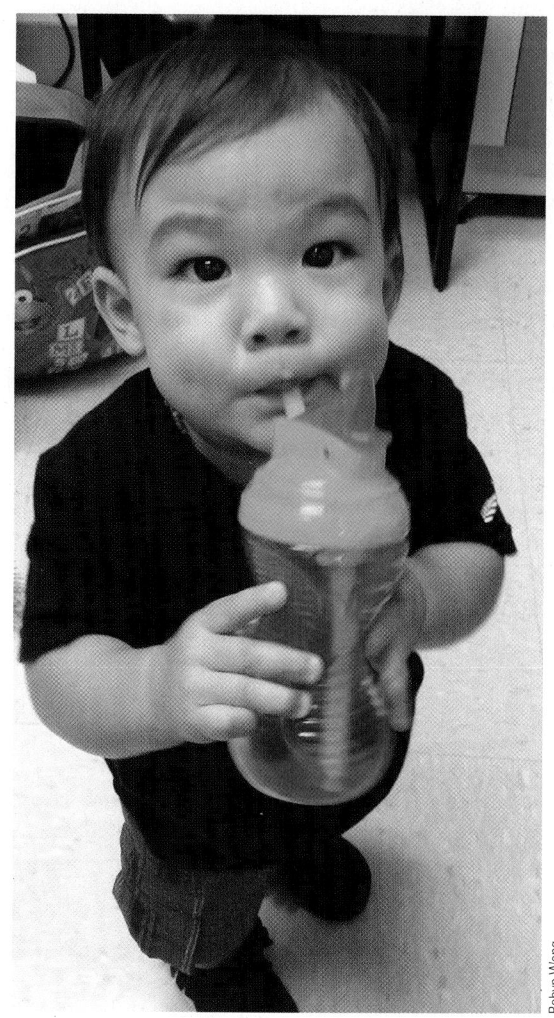



ILLUSTRATION 8.6 ▸ Infant drinking water with a straw.

## Complementary Feeding

The introduction of solid and semi-solid foods to complement the infant's diet of breast milk or formula generally begins at approximately 6 months of age. Infant cereal, mixed with breast milk, formula, or water is commonly the first food introduced to infants. Single-ingredient foods are recommended, and all solid foods are fed by spoon. Addition of infant cereal or baby foods to bottles of formula or use of a "feeder" instead of a spoon is not recommended.

Some parents add baby foods because they think this will make the baby sleep longer. This practice is neither recommended nor effective for most infants. This common belief may result in introduction of baby cereal before the infant has developed the skills to eat from a spoon, and contributes additional, unneeded calories from carbohydrates.

What are considered healthy first foods for infants will vary in different cultures and ethnic groups. Regardless of what foods are offered first, the timing and spacing of new foods can be used to identify any negative reactions. When introducing new foods, select single-ingredient foods. Only one new food is offered over a 3- to 5-day period. Commercially prepared baby foods are not a necessity for infants. Parents and caregivers can make baby foods at home using a blender or food processor, or by mashing foods with a fork. Care must be taken, however, to provide developmentally appropriate textures and to use safe food preparation and storage practices. The addition of salt and sugar to baby food is not recommended. The advantage of home-prepared baby food is that a wider variety of foods may be offered, including foods from the family diet.

Commercially prepared baby foods are frequently selected because of their convenience. Families who pack food for the baby sitter or for day care, or who travel with infants, find these foods easy to store and to use. Parents have numerous choices in selecting baby foods. Selections should be based on the nutritional needs of the infant, and not on the preferences or eating habits of the purchaser. Examples of foods that may reflect purchasers' preference are baby food desserts and snack foods. These are not recommended for most infants.

Jar and plastic containers of baby foods are based on manufacturers' standards, not necessarily on recommended serving sizes for infants. Portion sizes should be based on appetite. Finishing an entire container of baby food may foster overeating if parents do not pay attention to cues from the infant.

Many foods eaten by other family members are appropriate for infants who are 9–12 months of age. Examples are unsweetened applesauce, yogurt, soft-cooked vegetables, soft ripe fruits such as pear, banana and watermelon, mashed potato and sweet potato, cooked hot cereal, and Cheerios.

## Inappropriate and Unsafe Food Choices

New parents may inadvertently select foods for infants based on their own likes and dislikes, rather than on the infant's needs. Such choices are problematic when they increase the risk of choking. Infants accounted for 37.8 percent of all food-related choking episodes. Formula, cow milk, and breast milk were associated with over one third of choking episodes in infants; with mean occurrence age at 4 months of age. Other foods associated with choking in infants were fruits, vegetables, biscuits, cookies, and crackers.[65]

Some foods present a choking risk for infants because their chewing skills are emerging and not well developed. Coarse or inappropriate food textures can obstruct the infant's airway because voluntary coughing and clearing of the throat are skills not yet learned.[22] The AAP policy statement on choking in children recommends that young children should be supervised when eating, and that they not lay down with food in their mouths.[66]

## Fluids

Breast milk and formula will generally provide adequate fluid for healthy infants for the first 6 months. DRIs have established adequate intakes (AI) for water. Newborn to 6-month-old infants need 700 mL of water per day; 7- to 12-month-old infants need 800 mL per day.[67]

Fluid needs during illness are of concern because dehydration is a common response to illness in infancy. The infant has limited ability to signal thirst, especially when sick. Vomiting and diarrhea result in dehydration more rapidly in infants than in older children, with symptoms that are more difficult to interpret.[22] Replacement of electrolytes has been the basis for a variety of over-the-counter fluid replacement products, such as Pedialyte and generic oral rehydration products. These products contain some glucose (dextrose) along with sodium, potassium, and water. The amount of glucose provides significantly fewer calories than that contained in breast milk or formula—usually 3 calories per fluid ounce compared to 20 calories per fluid ounce in breast milk or formula. These rehydration products are intended for short-term use; prolonged use will result in energy and nutrient deficits.

Juice is not needed to meet the fluid needs of infants. Juices and other sugar-containing drinks can promote development of early childhood caries or dental caries.[67] If juice is offered, it is recommended after the age of 6 months, and from a cup, not bottle. Infancy provides a timely opportunity for infants to develop a preference for milk and water.

## How Much Food Is Enough for Infants?

Parental understanding of infant feeding behavior increases as the infant–parent interaction matures from early to late infancy. During early infancy while the sleep/wake cycle of the infant is irregular, it is common for new parents to interpret discomfort as a sign of hunger. The infant's ability to self-calm is a developmental step that plays out differently with different temperaments and parenting styles.[63] Infants who are more sensitive to their environment could seem to be fussy, irritable or frequently hungry. In contrast, infants who sleep through usual household noises and are less reactive to their environment may be fed less often throughout the day. As a result of varying responses to infant temperament, a pattern of excessive, adequate, or inadequate intakes may result. Parent–infant interaction during early feeding can have long-lasting effects on how parents perceive their child's temperament.[68]

In the first few months, the infant's physiological need to suck may easily be confused with hunger by new parents. Typical forward and backward tongue movements with first attempts to eat from a spoon may seem to be a rejection of the food.[23] The infant appears to spit out the food, but this could be a sign of a fading tongue thrust reflex, learning to swallow, and not necessarily a taste preference. The same food that appears to be rejected will be accepted as the infant learns to move the food from the front to the back of the mouth. It may appear to a parent that the infant does not like a food if he or she appears to choke. This choking response is more likely based on the position of the spoon on the tongue.[22,23] The mouth is very sensitive, particularly toward the back. If the bowl of the spoon is too far back, it could trigger a gag reflex, regardless of the taste of the food.[14]

### Influence of Food Preferences on Feeding Behavior

Infants have been exposed to flavors while in utero. The amniotic fluid and breast milk contain compounds reflective of their mothers' diets.[69] Breastfed infants may be exposed to a wider variety of tastes in breast milk than infants offered formula.[70] These early experiences initiate the ongoing process of developing food preferences and food habits throughout the lifespan. Infants have genetic, unlearned preference for sweet and salty tastes, and rejection of sour and bitter tastes.[71]

Food preferences of infants are largely learned, but genetic predisposition toward sweet tastes and against bitter foods may modify food preferences. Food preferences developed in infancy set the stage for lifelong food habits. Twin studies are showing that food preferences, appetite, and feeding skills are more complicated and genetically influenced behaviors than previously understood.[72]

## Nutrition Guidance

**LO8.6** Describe how providers and families access nutrition guidance for infants.

Nutrition guidance materials and resources for parents and caregivers, and health care providers are available from many sources, including the WIC program, *Bright Futures Nutrition*[15] and Zero to Three: National Center for Infants, Toddlers and Families.[73]

The WIC Program has published *Infant Nutrition and Feeding*, a comprehensive and very practical guide for health professionals who provide nutrition services to infants, children, and children with special health care needs.[104] The WIC Program also publishes a variety of infant and child-focused nutrition education materials for families and caregivers.

*Bright Futures Nutrition* provides nutrition and feeding recommendations for parents and caregivers of infants, children, adolescents and children with special health care needs. There are also Bright Futures Nutrition publications for health professional focusing on anticipatory guidance including key age-related issues and discussion points at well child visits.

Zero to Three is a national nonprofit organization that provides parents, professionals, and policy makers with resources, tools, and publications to nurture development in infancy and childhood. There is a featured section on health and nutrition. Table 8.8 identifies some key issues

**TABLE 8.8** Infant feeding recommendations

| TOPICS | NUTRITION EDUCATION SAMPLE CONTENT |
|---|---|
| Appropriate use of infant formula (if not breastfeeding) | Mixing instructions when using infant formula powder or concentrate; safe storage and handling; positioning during feedings; appropriate feeding volumes, frequency and duration of feedings |
| Baby food and sanitation | Recommended serving sizes for infants of different ages, preparation and use of homemade and commercially prepared foods, food safety, and sanitation |
| Prevention of dental caries | Recommendations for bedtime and nap time to avoid sugary liquids pooling in the mouth; identifying foods and fluids that promote dental caries, role of fluoride including water fluoridation and fluoride supplementation |
| Feeding position and mealtime environment | Optimal seating positions for feeding; minimizing mealtime distractions; parental role modeling |
| Signs of hunger and satiety | Identifying infants' signs of hunger and indications of satiety; avoidance of overfeeding |
| Preventing accidents and injury | Checking temperature of baby foods and liquids; use of appropriate car seats, avoidance of foods associated with choking |

related to infant feeding and focused content of nutrition education.

### The Infant's Home Environment

Keeping infants healthy at home includes other lifestyle factors along with nutrition. According to the National Institutes of Health Expert Panel on Cardiovascular Health Risks, infants have lower long-term risks if they are breastfed and not exposed to smoking at home.[74] The AAP recommends that infants not be exposed to screen time from televisions, DVD players, computers, and similar devices at home or in cars.[75] Although early learning may be the goal, parents' voices surpass electronic media as a stimulus for language and communication. The AAP Committee on Sports Medicine policy statement recommends that structured infant exercise programs should not be promoted as therapeutically beneficial for healthy infants.[76] Infants do not have the strength or reflexes to protect themselves, and their bones are more susceptible to trauma than those of older children and adults.

### Supplements for Infants

Specific supplements are recommended for breastfed infants in the United States and Canada, under certain circumstances:

- Fluoride supplementation is recommended starting at 6 months of age for infants residing in communities with low levels of water fluoridation.[36,38]
- Iron supplementation is recommended for exclusively breastfed term infants starting at four months of age at a dose of 1 mg/kg/d, and continued until iron-containing complementary foods are introduced in the diet.[48] Meat as an early complementary food for breastfed infants has been associated with improved iron and zinc status.[1, 77]
- Vitamin $B_{12}$ supplementation may be needed for breastfed vegan infants if the maternal diet is inadequate.[78,79] There are no unfortified plant food that contain significant amounts of the active form of vitamin $B_{12}$.[80] Fermented soy products are not reliable sources of the active form of this vitamin.[80]

### Cross-Cultural Considerations

Cultural practices and values are a major influence on the decision and duration to breastfeed, and on what and how infants are fed. Manufactured baby foods are reflective of the American culture and diet. There is little ethnic diversity in baby foods—no collards or Mexican beans. Some cultures consider meat-based soups and rice soups as typical foods for infants. There are a variety of successful avenues to nourish healthy infants. Knowledge of cultural models for feeding is highly desirable when counseling families and caregivers at this time when infant feeding and family mealtime routines are being established.

Cultural practices that support the development of competence in parents are encouraged. Examples of practices that may reflect cultural caregiving practices are swaddling an infant, or having an infant sleep in the parent's bed or in a room at a certain temperature. Food patterns may also reflect cultural or religious traditions; also, practices based on family traditions may be forms of social support for new parents. Cultural factors may affect the family's willingness to receive assistance from programs such as WIC or Early Intervention.

## Common Nutritional Issues and Concerns

**LO 8.7** Identify how nutrition problems and concerns impact overall infant health and development.

Some problems that may occur during infancy and may be related to nutrition include colic, diarrhea, and constipation. Less frequent problems include formula or feeding intolerance, iron-deficiency anemia, and food allergies. Tooth eruption begins in infancy; this is the opportune time for families to implement preventative measures to reduce their infants' risk of early childhood caries (EEC), also known as dental caries.

### Colic

*Colic* is described as a condition of irritability, and excessive, inconsolable crying in healthy, well-fed infants.[81] It can occur from early infancy up to 4 or 5 months of age, and can have a pattern of onset and duration.[82] The association of colic symptoms, gastrointestinal upset, and infant feeding practices has been studied, but no definitive cause of colic has yet been identified.[83] Research on the use of prebiotics in infancy continues; however, there is limited data on probiotic use in infants with colic, and results to date have been inconsistent. One study reported positive improvement in breastfed infants with colic but this effect was not seen in formula-fed infants.[84] More research is needed before recommending probiotic use for infantile colic.[27]

The frequent response to colic in formula-fed infants is to change to another infant formula. The change, however, may not always alter the pattern of colic. Recommendations to relieve colic may include rocking, swaddling, bathing, or utilizing other ways of calming the infant, positioning the baby well during feedings, or burping more frequently. Other interventions previously discussed in Chapter 7 include elimination of cow milk protein and other food proteins from mothers' diets.[85]

**colic** A condition marked by a sudden onset of irritability, fussiness, or crying in a young infant between 2 weeks and 3 months of age who is otherwise growing and healthy.

## Iron-Deficiency and Iron-Deficiency Anemia

Iron deficiency is the most common micronutrient deficiency throughout the world.[2] Both iron-deficiency anemia (IDA) and iron deficiency without anemia (ID) during infancy are of major significance because of their relationship with neurodevelopment and behavior.[46] Research in infants who have long-term and severe iron-deficiency anemia suggests inadequate iron contributes to long-term learning delays from its role in central nervous system development.[46] Iron deficiency is associated with poor cognitive, motor and socio-emotional development in infancy, and in later childhood with poor cognition and school achievement.[3] Risk factors associated with a higher prevalence of IDA include low birthweight, high cow milk intake, low intake of iron-rich complementary foods, low socioeconomic status, and immigrant status.

In the United States, standard infant formulas contain 12 mg of iron per liter. The Adequate Intake (AI) for iron for infants 0–6 months of age is 0.27 mg daily related to adequate iron stores of term infants. After 6 months of age, the iron recommendation increases, with a RDA established at 11 mg per day. Iron deficiency in infants is less common than iron deficiency in toddlers. Infants who have iron deficiency may have other risk factors to their overall development, such as low birthweight, elevated lead levels, or generalized undernutrition. The AAP iron recommendations in infancy are as follow:[49]

- Iron supplementation is recommended for infants with severe iron deficiency anemia at a dose of 4 to 6 mg/kg/d divided into three doses.
- For mild to moderate iron deficiency, the recommended dosing is 3 mg/kg/d divided into one to two doses.
- When breast milk is the sole source of nutrition, supplemental iron may be prescribed depending on the infant's age, length of gestation, and medical history. Refer to the Supplements for Infants section of this chapter for further information on dosing recommendations.
- Older infants receive iron through iron-fortified baby cereal at 6 months of age.
- For infants who are not breastfed, a usual source of iron for formula-fed babies is iron-fortified infant formula. Iron from this source improves iron status during the first year and is well accepted. The level of iron in iron-fortified formula is 15 mg per liter, or 11.5 mg per quart. The RDA for iron is 0.27 mg for infants up to 6 months and 11 mg for infants 7–12 months old.

## Diarrhea and Constipation

Diarrhea is one of the most common illnesses among children in the United State, and three hundred to five hundred children will die each year from this potentially preventable condition.[86] Approximately 65 percent of the hospitalizations for diarrhea and 8.5 percent of diarrhea-associated deaths occur in the first 12 months of life.[86] Infants with acute diarrhea are at increased risk for dehydration compared to older children because of their higher metabolic rate, smaller fluid reserves, and dependence on others for fluids.[87] Diarrhea is described as the passage of three or more loose, watery stools per day or a stool volume greater than 10 grams per kilogram of body weight in infants.[87,88] The cause of diarrhea during infancy may or may not be identifiable. Diarrhea may result from viral and bacterial infections, food intolerance, or changes in fluid intake.[89] Excessive intake of fruit juice may be a cause of diarrhea in older infants.[90]

The first line of treatment is to continue breastfeeding or feeds of regular strength formula, and to resume an age-appropriate diet, which may include complementary foods. Gut rest is not needed.[87,88] Feeds of an oral rehydration solution are recommended to help replace fluid losses.[87,88] Foods high in simple sugar content are not recommended because the high osmotic load could worsen the diarrhea. Restriction of fat is not recommended; a moderate intake of fat will be beneficial.[91] Vital components of home management of diarrhea are to provide increased volumes of fluids and to maintain adequate energy intakes.[86] Diarrhea can become a serious problem if an infant becomes dehydrated or less responsive; timely medical follow-up is imperative.[86]

Constipation is defined as changes in the frequency, size, consistency, or easy of passing stool.[92] Difficulty with defecation is a common occurrence in infancy and childhood. The problem is often short in duration and of little consequence.[92]

Recommendations for the infant with constipation focus on normal fluid and fiber intake.[93] If formula fed, assess if formula is mixed correctly. Foods with high dietary fiber content are generally not recommended for infants with constipation because many sources, such as whole-wheat crackers or apples with peels, present a choking hazard. The routine use of prebiotics and probiotics in the treatment of childhood constipation is not recommended.

## Early Childhood Caries (ECC)

Early childhood caries are also known as baby bottle caries and baby bottle tooth decay. Feeding practices established in infancy may increase risk of EEC.

Infants have high oral needs, which mean they love to suck and to explore by putting things in their mouths. They derive comfort from sucking and may relax or fall asleep while sucking. The use of a bottle containing formula, juice, or other sweetened liquid to calm a baby or at bedtime will contribute to demineralization of the teeth.[36]

The following preventive measures are recommended by the American Academy of Pediatric Dentistry and the AAP to prevent early childhood caries citation:[36,9]

- Avoid high-frequency consumption of liquids and solid foods containing sugar. In particular, sugar-containing beverages such as juice, soft drinks, sweetened tea, and milk with sugar added from a baby bottle or training cup should be avoided.
- Infants should not be put to sleep with a bottle filled with milk or liquids containing sugars.
- Very frequent breastfeeding should be avoided after the first primary tooth begins to erupt and other dietary carbohydrates are introduced.
- Infants should be weaned from the bottle between 12 and 18 months of age.
- Infants should be seen by a dentist by 12 months of age.
- Brush or wipe emerging baby teeth to promote good oral hygiene.

## Food Allergies

Infants develop their immune systems over a few years, and while breastfeeding, the mothers' immune system may confer immunological-active compounds to the infant.[95] Infants fed breast milk and those fed formula differ in measured antibodies. Infants' gastrointestinal tracts are very sensitive compared to those of older children, so it is difficult to determine what is food intolerance, sensitization, or a true allergy.[96] However, the prevalence of true food allergies is higher in younger than in older children. About 6–8 percent of children under 4 years of age have allergies that started in infancy.[96,97]

An infant may develop a reaction to the protein in a cow's milk–based formula. Often, such a problem follows a gastrointestinal illness. When the infant is well, protein digestion and absorption is of groups of two or three amino acids linked together. After an illness, small patches of irritated or inflamed intestinal lining may allow protein fragments of larger lengths of amino acids to be absorbed. Such fragments are hypothesized to trigger a reaction as if a foreign protein had invaded, setting up a local immune or inflammatory response.[96] This absorption of intact protein fragments is the basis for allergic reactions. Recent type of allergy testing is based on measuring precise fractions of antibodies in response to specific triggers so that a sensitized state can be found before a medical emergency occurs. When an infant has reacted to cow's milk protein, it is likely that soy-based formulas will also cause the same allergic reaction.

The most common allergic reactions are respiratory and skin symptoms, such as wheezing or skin rashes.[95] Although food allergies can start in infancy, they are confirmed by specific laboratory tests after infancy.[97] True allergies can present as an array of reactions building up over time, so that it may take several years for the initiating cause to be identified.

Food intolerances are frequently suspected in infants. Families may consider skin rashes, upper airway congestion, diarrhea, and other forms of gastrointestinal upset to be food allergies, but often they are not.[98] The infant with suspected protein intolerance may be changed to a specialized formula composed of ***hydrolyzed protein***. Such formulas are expensive and have a taste that many older infants reject. With true food allergies, the protein of a hydrolyzed formula is needed because it does not trigger the same response as intact protein fragments do.

The National Institute of Allergy and Infectious Diseases, a part of the National Institutes of Health, released its 2010 guidelines for diagnosing and managing food allergies.[95] These guidelines do not recommend prevention of food allergies by delaying the introduction of or avoiding specific foods thought to cause allergies for most infants. Avoiding and restricting specific foods may decrease nutritional adequacy and reinforce behaviors of rejecting foods and limiting variety. These guidelines recommend breast milk for infants considered at risk for allergies, but do not recommend soy-based infant formula if breast milk is not available. Allergy and intolerance symptoms are more common in response to nonfood items such as grasses and dust, so many different sources of symptoms must be considered.

**Lactose Intolerance** True lactose intolerance is a medical diagnosis that is based on specific gastrointestinal testing for lactase activity. Lactose intolerance is less common during infancy than at older ages in groups that are susceptible to it. Some adults self-identify themselves as lactose intolerant if they have cramps, nausea, and pain, or alternating diarrhea and constipation. Some families apply the term *lactose intolerance* to their infants for these same symptoms. It tends to be overestimated, since it is easy to confuse with colic, and symptoms can appear after a variety of minor illnesses. Gastrointestinal infections may temporarily cause lactose intolerance because the irritated area of the intestine affects the digestion of lactose.[99] The ability to digest lactose generally returns shortly after the illness subsides. ***Lactose*** is present in all dairy products, including cow milk–based infant formulas. Lactose-reduced infant formulas are available; they contain less lactose, and additional carbohydrate is provided by other sources such as modified cornstarch or sucrose. An infant who was fed a reduced-lactose

**hydrolyzed protein formula** Formula that contains enzymatically digested protein, or single amino acids, rather than protein as it naturally occurs in foods.

**lactose** A form of sugar or carbohydrate composed of galactose and glucose.

formula will likely be able to eat dairy products later. Because dairy products are an important source of calcium, gradual introduction of foods with low lactose is recommended for older infants who appeared to be lactose intolerant when younger.

### Vegetarian Diets

Vegetarian diets can support normal growth and development in infants when well planned to meet their nutritional needs in the first year.[78,79] Lacto-ovo vegetarian diets were reported to well meet the nutritional needs of the growing infant.[100] More restrictive vegan and macrobiotic diets may increase the risk for nutrient deficiencies. Vegan diets have not recommended for infants.[20] Lifelong vegetarians were noted to have similar adult height, weight, and BMIs as those who became vegetarians later in life. This suggests that appropriate vegetarian diets in infancy and childhood do not affect final adult height or weight; vegetarian infants grow as well as non-vegetarian infants.[101] Nutrients of concern for infants on vegetarian diets include vitamin $B_{12}$, vitamin D, calcium, iron, zinc, and omega-3 fatty acids.

The DHA content in breast milk is lower in vegetarian mothers than non-vegetarian mothers.[102] DHA is important in infancy because of its role in neurological and visual development.[33] Because of this, DHA-fortified foods are recommended in the maternal diet, or a daily DHA supplement can be provided to these infants. Poorly nourished mothers or those on vegan diets may require supplementation of DHA and multivitamins.[56]

## Nutrition Intervention for Risk Reduction

LO 8.8 Cite examples of nutritional interventions that can reduce risk for nutrition and health problems in infancy.

Early Head Start is a federally funded program that provides early, continuous, intensive, and comprehensive child development and family support services to low-income infants and toddlers and their families (Table 8.9).[103] Early Head Start programs must design and implement nutrition programs, which identify the nutritional needs of each participant and provide meals and snacks that are appropriate for developmental readiness and feeding skills.

### Model Program: Newborn Metabolic Screening

In the United States, newborn infants are screened shortly after birth for metabolic disorders; most commonly phenylketonuria (PKU), congenital ***hypothyroidism***, ***galactosemia***, and sickle cell disease. The panel of screening disorders varies from state to state. Early identification and treatment of these inborn errors of metabolism may help to prevent or reduce adverse consequences of these disorders. Treatment for some of these inborn errors of

**hypothyroidism** Condition in which thyroid hormone is not produced in sufficient quantities, interfering with growth and mental development if untreated in infants.

**galactosemia** A rare genetic condition of carbohydrate metabolism in which a blocked or inactive enzyme does not allow breakdown of galactose, causing serious illness in infancy.

TABLE 8.9 Desired Outcomes for the Infant, and the Role of the Family

| | EDUCATIONAL/ATTITUDINAL | BEHAVIORAL | HEALTH |
|---|---|---|---|
| Desired Outcomes for the Infant | • Has a sense of trust<br>• Bonds with parents<br>• Enjoys eating | • Breastfeeds successfully<br>• Bottle feeds successfully if not breastfeeding<br>• Consumes supplemental foods to support appropriate growth and development | • Develops normal rooting, sucking and swallowing reflexes<br>• Develops fine and gross motor skills<br>• Grows and develops at an appropriate rate<br>• Maintains good health |
| Role of the Family | • Bonds with the infant<br>• Enjoys feeding the infant<br>• Understands the infant's nutrition needs<br>• Acquires a sense of competence in meeting the infant's needs<br>• Understands the importance of a healthy lifestyle, including healthy eating behaviors and regular physical activity, to promote shortterm and longterm health | • Meets the infant's nutrition needs<br>• Responds to the infant's hunger and fullness cues<br>• Holds the infant when breastfeeding or bottle-feeding, and maintains eye contact<br>• Talks to the infant during feeding<br>• Provides a pleasant feeding environment<br>• Uses nutrition programs and food resources if needed<br>• Seeks help when problems occur | • Maintains good health |

Holt K, Wooldridge N, Story M, Sofka D. *Bright Futures Nutrition*, 3rd ed., American Academy of Pediatrics, 2011.

metabolism will require therapeutic diets and use of medical foods, supplements, or medications. Food and nutrient modifications are implemented to avoid or reduce the offending component(s) involved in the affected metabolic pathway. Registered dietitian-nutritionists are members of specialty metabolic teams that provide medical treatment and nutritional management of individuals with inborn errors of metabolism.

## KEY POINTS

1. Infancy is a unique time when feeding skills and eating behaviors are emerging. It is an opportune time for families and caregivers to foster healthy eating and mealtime behaviors.
2. Parents' ability to read their infant's signals of readiness, hunger, and satiety promote successful feeding relationships and development of healthy eating habits.
3. Nutrition assessments in infancy often include a review of dietary intakes of vitamin D, iron, and fluoride. These micronutrients may require supplementation to achieve recommended levels.
4. Rates of linear growth and weight gain occur more rapidly in the first year of life than at any other time in the life cycle. Frequent weight, length, and head circumference measurements are needed to assess adequacy of growth in infancy.
5. Common nutrition problems in the first year such as colic, diarrhea, constipation, regurgitation, and spit-up may be resolved with parental education, dietary interventions, and medical approaches.
6. Infant feeding can embrace varied cultural and parenting styles, ethnic foods, and cultural feeding practices.

## REVIEW QUESTIONS

1. Which is a true statement about limiting nutrients in infancy?
   a. Iron supplementation is initiated when infants are 6 months of age.
   b. Vitamin D supplementation is needed in breastfed infants because the content is low in breast milk.
   c. Low intake of dietary fiber is a common cause of constipation in infants.
   d. Fluoride is not needed until teeth start erupting in late infancy.
2. What is an accurate statement about newborn infants?
   a. The large-for-gestational-age infant is born at or after 42 weeks gestation.
   b. The newborn rooting reflex may interfere with an infant's ability to bottle feed.
   c. Newborn reflexes promote the coordination of feeding and breathing.
   d. The ability to sit is achieved with the help of newborn reflexes.
3. Which meal carries the lowest choking risk for a 9-month-old infant?
   a. Scrambled egg, slice of sausage, buttered toast pieces
   b. Vegetable and chicken dinner, soda cracker, apple slice
   c. Chicken nuggets, mashed potatoes, grapes
   d. Cooked carrot, applesauce, beef and macaroni dinner
4. The digestive system during infancy can be accurately described by which statement?
   a. Gastrointestinal problems frequently interfere with health and growth in young infants.
   b. The GI tract is completely functional for digestion at 9 to 12 months of age.
   c. Infant stools change based on the ability of the intestinal villi to absorb nutrients.
5. Which is a true statement concerning fats?
   a. Infants need a higher percentage of their daily calories from fat than children and adults.
   b. Breast milk is lower in fat than standard infant formulas.
   c. Long-chain fatty acids are not needed for healthy infants in the first year.
   d. Fat restriction can be initiated in the first year for infants who were born at term.
6. What is a disadvantage of feeding a larger volume of formula or breast milk than recommended? ________________ (short answer)
7. Which of the following statements is accurate?
   a. Formula-fed infants are ready for complementary foods at 4 months of age.

b. A delayed introduction of solid foods is recommended for infants with a family history of food allergies.
c. Complementary foods high in iron and zinc are recommended for breastfed infants.
d. Use of commercially prepared baby foods can reduce the risk of food allergy.

8. A 4-month-old infant girl is growing well but not sleeping through the night. Her mother thinks she may be sick because she cries so much. What is a possible explanation for an infant not sleeping through the night?
   a. The infant is ready for the introduction of complementary foods.
   b. A maternal restriction of dairy foods may help reduce gastrointestinal upset.
   c. A change in infant formula will improve feeding tolerance.
   d. Increasing the frequency or duration of breastfeeding will provide more satiety.

9. Describe the relationship between motor development and oral feedings in infancy. ______________
______________________________
______________________________

(short answer) Relate four strategies that parents and caregivers can implement to foster healthy eating behaviors starting in infancy.

Visit www.cengagebrain.com to access MindTap, a complete digital course that includes additional resources.

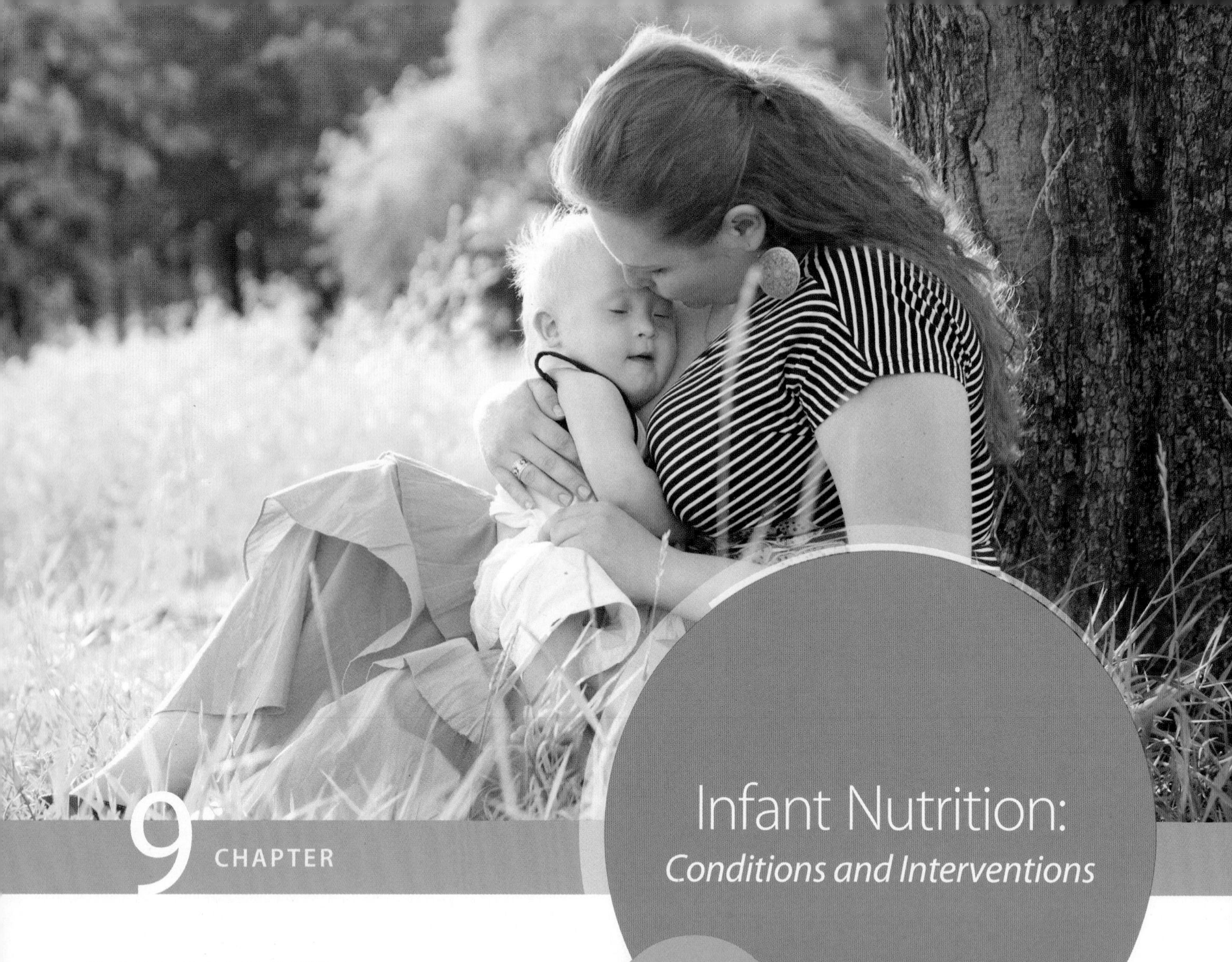

9 CHAPTER

# Infant Nutrition: *Conditions and Interventions*

*Prepared by* **Robyn Wong**

## LEARNING OBJECTIVES

After studying the materials in this chapter, you should be able to:

**9.1** Describe factors that put infants at nutritional risk and how nutritional assessment and interventions address these risks.

**9.2** Compare the energy and nutrition needs of preterm infants, infants with special health care needs, and healthy full-term infants.

**9.3** Identify how growth is tracked and interpreted in infants at risk or with special health care needs.

**9.4** Describe nutrition problems that are more frequently identified in preterm infants and infants with special health care needs.

**9.5** Identify the nutrition problems during infancy after severe preterm birth that are not generally found in infants born full-term.

**9.6** Describe examples of nutrition assessment and interventions for infants with special health care needs and chronic illness.

**9.7** Identify infants with feeding problems and appropriate nutrition services for them.

**9.8** Identify appropriate nutrition intervention strategies for infants who are experiencing problems with linear growth or weight gain.

**9.9** Describe how families of high-risk infants and infants with special health care needs access nutrition resources and services in their communities.

# Introduction

Most infants are born healthy and then achieve normal growth and development in the first year of life. These infants may experience minor illnesses that do not adversely affect their growth, development, and overall health status.

Infants who are born prematurely, or have special health care needs or ***developmental delay***, are at increased risk for compromised nutritional status and altered growth.[1] ***Children and youth with special health care needs (CYSHCN)*** is defined as "those who have or are at risk for a chronic physical, developmental, behavioral, or emotional condition and who also require health and related services of a type or amount beyond that required by children generally."[2] Infants are included in this population.

Up to 40 percent of infants and children with special health care needs were found to be at nutritional risk,[3] while 79 to 90 percent of infants and children from birth to 3 years of age with developmental delays were found to have one or more nutritional risk factors.[4] Indicators of nutritional risk include altered growth, increased or decreased energy needs, drug-nutrient interactions, metabolic disorders, impaired nutrient utilization, poor feeding skills, and use of partial or exclusive enteral or parenteral nutrition.[3] This chapter discusses the some of the common nutritional concerns of preterm infants, infants with special health care needs, and/or developmental delay.

# Infants at Risk

LO 9.1 Describe factors that put infants at nutritional risk and how nutritional assessment and interventions address these risks.

The number of infants requiring nutritional services is increasing in large measure because of advances in perinatal and neonatal intensive care. Increased survival and reduced long-term morbidity in preterm infants have occurred; most notably in ***extremely low-birthweight infants (ELBW)*** (weighing less than 1000 grams at birth) and ***very low-birthweight infants (VLBW)*** (weighing less than 1500 grams at birth).[5] ***Low birth weight infants (LBW)*** weigh less than 2500 grams at birth. Infant mortality is one of the key indicators of the health of a nation, and the overall U.S. infant mortality rate declined 12 percent from 2005 to 2011.[6,7] The infant, neonatal, and post neonatal mortality rate was 6.05 per 1,000 live births.[7]

Health outcome measures provide a more comprehensive view of the impact of preterm birth and illness than infant mortality rates alone. Preterm infants, infants with genetic disorders, malformations, or birth complications have benefited from advances in medical care; however, they are at increased risk for chronic conditions, and need for medical care and services as they grow older. Health outcome measures can be used to assess longitudinal growth, health problems, functional limitations, and utilization of health care and other resources.[8,9] Their nutritional needs are found to differ from those of full-term infants, sometimes well past infancy.[3,4]

Term infants are born at or after 37 weeks gestation. Late preterm infants are born between 34 to 36 6/7 weeks gestation and have higher incidence of temperature instability, respiratory distress, ***hyperbilirubinemia***, hypoglycemia, feeding problems and re-hospitalization than term infants. Late preterm infants may have more difficulty with establishing breastfeeding and have immature gastrointestinal function. More attention is being given to the medical needs and developmental issues of this population of infants.[10,11]

Regardless of what condition is involved, these nutrition questions are helpful:[12]

- How often does your baby feed? How long does a feeding generally take?
- How does your baby behave during a feeding? Pulls away, arches back, looks irritable or calm?
- How does your baby behave after feedings? Satisfied, still hungry, anxious?
- Has your baby had any other fluids from a bottle?
- How many wet diapers and stools does your baby have every day?

In-depth nutrition assessments are completed to determine adequacy of energy and nutrient intakes in supporting optimal growth and development. Such assessments are important for the following infants:

- *Infants born before 34 weeks of gestation.* These infants have very inadequate nutrient stores, increased nutritional demands, and immature organ function and altered feeding patterns.[13]
- *Infants affected by abnormal development in utero.* These include infants with cardiac malformations, exposure to drugs or alcohol, or genetic conditions such as ***Down syndrome.***
- *Infants at risk for chronic health problems.* Risks may come from the treatment needed to save their lives, or from the

**developmental delay** An impairment in the performance of tasks or achieving developmental milestones that an infant or child should achieve by a specific chronological age. The diagnosis is made with testing that assesses cognitive, physical, social and emotional development, communication and adaptive skills.

**children and youth with special health care needs (CYSHCN)** Infants, children and adolescents who have or are at increased risk for a chronic physical, developmental, behavioral, or emotional condition and who also require health and related services of a type or amount beyond that required by children generally

**low-birthweight infant (LBW)** An infant weighing <2500 g at birth.

**extremely low-birthweight infant (ELBW)** An infant weighing <1000 g at birth.

**very low-birthweight infant (VLBW)** An infant weighing <1500 g at birth.

**hyperbilirubinemia** Presence of an excess of bilirubin in the blood.

**Down syndrome** Condition in which three copies of chromosome 21 occur and can be associated with decreased muscle tone, short stature and increased risk for overweight.

home environment. Some examples of conditions that increase nutritional risk are ***seizures***, cystic fibrosis, and fetal alcohol syndrome. Long-term consequences, such as learning, attention, and behavioral problems, may not be known for years.

### Families of Infants with Special Health Care Needs

Every parent's wish is that his or her baby will be healthy. When parents find out their newborn has medical problems, they may grieve for the loss of the perfect child of their dreams. The emotional impact of having a sick newborn may overwhelm many parents, and health care providers need to be sensitive to parents' emotional needs. Coping styles of various family members will vary, even if they are well prepared for the diagnosis. It may take more time for some family members to comprehend how their baby is doing and to adjust to the special needs of their child (Illustration 9.1).

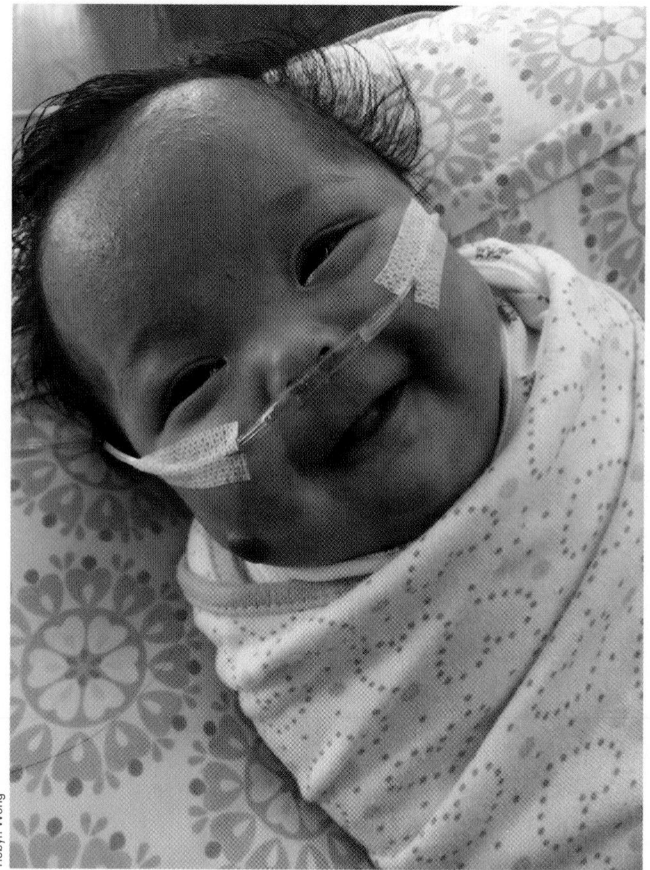

Robyn Wong

ILLUSTRATION 9.1 ▸ Baby girl at home on oxygen.

## Energy and Nutrient Needs of Preterm Infants and Infants with Special Health Care Needs and/or Developmental Delay

LO 9.2 Compare the energy and nutrition needs of preterm infants, infants with special health care needs, and healthy full-term infants.

Nutrient and energy requirements for high-risk infants with health conditions are based on the recommendations for healthy infants.[14] Specific nutrients may be adjusted higher or lower based on the health condition involved. Adjusting the nutrition care plan to changing conditions and close monitoring of growth and development may result in frequently changing recommendations in the first year.

### Energy Needs

When assessing energy needs of infants with special health care requirements, use of the Recommended Daily Allowance (RDA) may not be appropriate, as the RDA is based on only age and gender. The revised Daily Reference Intake (DRI) for energy—the Estimated Energy Requirements (EER)—may be more accurate in predicting the energy needs of infants and children with special health care needs.[15] The EER for infants uses predictive equations that account for total energy expenditure and energy deposition. There are three EER age-group categories in infancy: 0–3 months; 4–6 months; and 7–12 months.[16,17] Energy needs may be the same as, less than, or greater than the EER for age. For infants with cleft lip and/or cleft palate, or phenylketonuria (PKU), use of the DRI for energy will be appropriate. Infants with bronchopulmonary dysplasia often need energy intakes above the EER for age.

Infants with reduced activity and energy expenditure, lower basal energy needs, or slower rates of growth generally need fewer calories than their peers. These infants include those with Down syndrome and spina bifida.[17] Excess energy for these infants may contribute to overweight and adversely affect their growth and development.

Estimated energy requirements can change, related to medication use, activity level, health status, and growth velocity. Additional energy may be indicated in circumstances such as the following:

- Infections
- Fever
- Difficulty breathing
- Temperature regulation
- Recovery from surgery and complications

Infants who are born before 34 weeks of gestation have higher energy needs than late preterm and term infants. The American Academy of Pediatrics advises that premature infants need 105–130 cal/kg, while the European Society for Gastroenterology and Nutrition recommends an energy intake range of 110–135 cal/kg.[18,19] Intakes for recovering premature infants may be even higher, and the range of energy needs can be wide.

**seizures** Condition in which electrical nerve transmission in the brain is disrupted, resulting in periods of loss of function that vary in severity.

### Protein Requirements

As with energy needs, protein requirements of infants with special health care needs may be the same as, less than, or greater than those of other infants. In the first 6 months of life, the DRI for protein is 1.52 grams per kg body weight. It declines to 1.2 g/kg from 7 to 12 months of age. Protein recommendations are sufficient if total calories are high enough to meet energy needs.[18]

Conditions that could slow growth may require protein intakes above the DRI. Higher protein intakes are recommended for preterm infants; for micropreterm infants born before 30 weeks gestation, this recommendation may be as high as 4.5 grams per kilogram body weight.[20] The importance of protein for growing neonates is hard to overemphasize. Protein is needed to develop the structural scaffolding for the brain, and it supports linear growth. It provides the building blocks for signaling molecules including growth factors and neurotransmitters, which have an influential role in cognition.[21] Linear growth in the first year of life, independent of weight gain, influences later cognitive and language development in preterm and term infants.[22,23]

Because of increased catabolism during trauma and surgery, provision of optimal protein is required. This quantity of protein is disease-specific and needs to be individualized.[24] Protein requirements are also higher in infant needing to achieve ***catch-up growth***.[25] Protein recommendations lower than the DRI are unusual in infancy. Some inborn errors of metabolism such as phenylketonuria can affect protein metabolism; treatment may require a restriction or reduction in dietary protein or in certain amino acids. Phenylketonuria (PKU) is an example of an inborn error of metabolism that requires a dietary restriction in protein and monitoring of the blood level of the amino acid phenylalanine.

### Forms of Protein

Many illnesses interfere with the functioning of the gastrointestinal tract and digestion, even for term infants born with intact enzymes for protein digestion. Protein and fat digestion depend on liver and pancreatic enzymes for intestinal absorption. Sick infants may require partially or extensively hydrolyzed protein or amino acid-based formulas. Use of modified protein and amino acids may also be indicated with cow milk protein allergy, multiple food protein intolerance,[26] and in the medical management of inborn errors of nitrogen metabolism.[27]

### Fat

An adequate fat intake is essential to support the rapid growth and development and high-energy requirements in infancy.[28] Compared to children and adults, infants need a higher percentage of their daily calories from fat. Fat provides 45–55 percent of the energy content in human milk.[29] Low-fat diets or restriction of fat are not recommended for infants. Conditions that require limiting fats for infants are very rare. Fats are more difficult for preterm infants to digest and absorb related to a reduced secretion of pancreatic and liver enzymes.[30] Medium-chain triglycerides do not require bile for absorption, and are a routine source of fat in preterm infant formula.

### Vitamins and Minerals

DRIs of vitamins and minerals for infants were established to meet the nutrient requirements of nearly all healthy and well infants. These recommendations are also generally applicable for most infants with special health care needs. Vitamin and mineral requirements may be affected by various health conditions, particularly those involving the gastrointestinal tract. Certain medications may decrease or impair nutrient absorption or increase excretion.[31] The treatment for some inborn errors of metabolism requires micronutrient supplementation well above the DRI for age.[32]

The American Academy of Pediatrics has addressed the higher iron needs of preterm infants, and recommends iron supplementation for preterm infants on breast milk feedings. Preterm infants who are formula fed may need earlier initiation of iron supplementation, and at a higher dose than full-term infants.[33]

Some infants with special health care needs have fluid restrictions that result in a lower feeding volume and reduction in micronutrient intakes. Infants with cystic fibrosis (CF) may continue to have problems with fat malabsorption. Fat-soluble vitamin supplementation at levels above the DRI for age are recommended; there are CF-specific multivitamin supplements available.[34]

Human milk fortifiers are routinely used in neonatal intensive care units to increase the content of specific nutrients and energy content of breast milk, and to meet the high nutritional needs of preterm infants. The key nutrient in human milk fortifiers is protein. An inadequate protein intake in preterm infants will adversely affect their growth and neurocognitive development.[35]

In addition to protein, other key nutrients in human milk fortifiers include calcium, phosphorus, magnesium, sodium, potassium, chloride, zinc, and copper.[35] Iron is contained in some human milk fortifiers. Premature infant formulas provide very similar amounts of macronutrients and micronutrients as fortified breast milk.

## Growth of Infants at Risk or with Special Health Care Needs

LO 9.3 Identify how growth is tracked and interpreted in infants at risk or with special health care needs.

Growth in infancy is usually a reassuring sign that sufficient energy and nutrients are being provided.

**catch-up growth** The accelerated growth of a premature or small infant, or malnourished infant or child that occurs during the first two years of life.

Sometimes slow growth is a symptom of an underlying condition, rather than a sign of inadequate nutrition. For example, some infants who are born with chromosomal disorders may be small for their age although they are consuming adequate nutrients and energy during the first year. Modifications in the usual methods and interpretation of growth are needed in conditions known to influence growth and development:

- Use of specialty growth charts for specific diagnoses such as Down syndrome. A list of specialty growth charts is included in Chapter 13.
- Looking at biochemical indicators of tissue stores of nutrients such as iron and protein, and electrolytes such as potassium and sodium.
- Obtaining additional anthropometric measurements to facilitate assessment of body composition, such as mid-arm circumference and triceps skinfold.
- Close monitoring of head circumference in the first year when the brain is rapidly growing. There is a high risk of growth failure in children with ***developmental disabilities***; this can be seen with slower gains in weight, length, or head circumference.[15]
- Using available evidence-based practice treatment guidelines or published protocols for conditions such as cystic fibrosis and inborn errors of metabolism.
- Assessing medications that may affect weight gain, appetite, or body composition. Side effects of medications can explain rapid changes in weight.

## Growth in Preterm Infants

There are a variety of growth charts used to assess and monitor preterm infants; these were developed based on growth data of different populations of preterm infants. The recently updated Fenton preterm infant growth charts are based on a sample size of almost 4 million infants at birth using population-based surveys in Germany, United States, Italy, Australia, Scotland, and Canada. These growth charts are gender specific and provide weight, length, and head circumference percentiles from 23 to 40 weeks gestation. The Fenton growth data and the WHO growth curves for term infants were smoothed to extend from 40–50 weeks postmenstrual age, which is equivalent of term to 2½ months corrected age.[36] The Olsen intrauterine growth charts are based on a sample size of more than 250,000 infants born in the United States. These charts are also gender specific. They provide intrauterine growth data from 23–50 weeks postmenstrual age.[37] Olsen et al. recently published gender-specific reference curves to track the BMI changes in preterm infants. These BMI curves were developed utilizing data of the same population of racially diverse infants. There have not been tools available to assess appropriate weight for length in preterm infants prior to the release of these BMI curves.[38]

An important consideration when using the Fenton and Olsen preterm growth charts is that they reflect cross-sectional birth data. They are not reflective of the longitudinal postnatal growth actually achieved by preterm infants. Nutrient intakes of very low-birthweight and extremely low-birthweight infants are much lower than intakes received by the fetus in utero. These nutritional deficits often continue throughout the duration of their hospitalization.[39]

There are concepts that impact how growth is assessed regardless of which specific growth chart is being used. The body composition of preterm infants is not the same as that of term infants, in part because these infants have missed part of the third trimester, when accretion of body fat occurs. In addition to low fat stores, they have low stores of glycogen, protein, fat-soluble vitamins, calcium, phosphorus, and trace minerals.[40] Treatment of the infant's medical condition may also affect growth expectations; for instance, fluid accumulation may artificially increase weight.

Extremely low-birthweight infants (weighing under 1000 grams at birth) with higher growth velocity rates during their hospitalization were found to have better neurodevelopmental and growth outcomes at 18–22 months corrected age.[9] As the rate of weight gain increased, the incidence of cerebral palsy, low developmental index scores, and abnormal neurological exam declined. Slower weight gain and head circumference growth velocity were associated with increased likelihood of suboptimal growth, below the 10th percentile at 18–22 months corrected age.

## Corrected Age

***Corrected age*** is calculated by subtracting the infant's gestational age at birth from 40 weeks, which is the length of a full-term pregnancy. The resulting number of weeks is divided by four to obtain months. The result in months is then subtracted from the infant's current age. For example, an infant born at 32 weeks gestation was 8 weeks, or 2 months, early. When she is 3 months old, her corrected age is 1 month. This age of 1 month would be used in plotting her measurements on the growth charts. Illustration 9.2 shows the chronological age and corrected age measurements of a former 32-week gestation girl. She remains small for her corrected age, but her weight is in good proportion to her length, as noted by a weight-for-length at the 10th percentile.

**developmental disabilities** A group of conditions related to impairment in physical, learning, language, or behavioral areas. These conditions have onset in the developmental period, may impact daily functioning, and usually last throughout a person's lifetime.

**corrected age** A term also known as adjusted age; it is used with preterm infants. It is calculated by subtracting the number of weeks born before 40 weeks of gestation from the infant or child's chronological (actual) age.

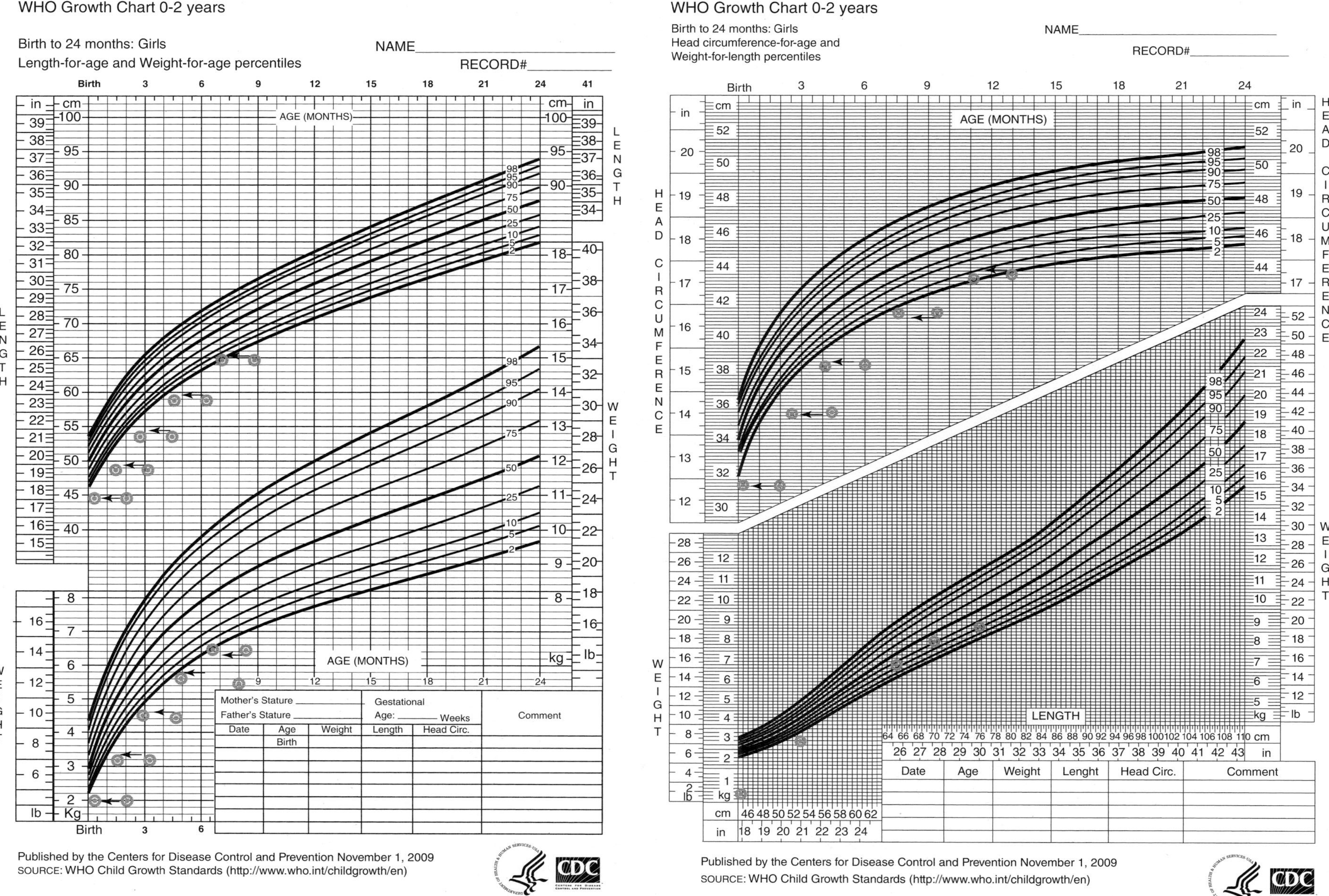


**ILLUSTRATION 9.2** ▸ WHO growth charts showing chronological and corrected age measurements of a girl born at 32 week gestation.

This girl may be smaller than her peers at two years of age, but is currently achieving appropriate growth at a corrected age of 7 months.

## Does Intrauterine Growth Predict Extrauterine Growth?

"Apples don't fall from a pear tree."

—French saying

The answer is yes, no, and maybe. Fetal monitoring during pregnancy and knowledge about the timing and development of fetal organs provide a projection of growth at various gestational ages. However, many factors during and after pregnancy are known to affect growth rate:

- Intrauterine environment, particularly the adequacy of the placenta in delivering nutrients
- The presence of toxins such as viruses, alcohol, or maternal medications
- The depletion of a needed nutrient, such as iron or folic acid
- Fetal-origin errors in cell migration or formation of organs, whether or not a cause is known (various nutrients, such as vitamin A, have been implicated in such errors)

Research shows that some infants were born prematurely due to conditions originating during the intrauterine period.[41] Infants with intrauterine growth retardation (IUGR) are at increased risk for metabolic disturbances related to fatty acid and glucose metabolism.[42] The abnormal fetal growth pattern may persist despite adequate medical and nutrition support after birth.

Other factors associated with IUGR include genetic factors, congenital anomalies, infection, multiple gestation, maternal nutrition, environmental toxins including cigarette smoking, excess alcohol ingestion and illicit drug use, placental factors and maternal vascular disease including diabetes, chronic hypertension, advanced maternal age, and morbid obesity.[43] There are known association between birthweight below the 10th percentile (SGA) and later development of hypertension, hypercholesterolemia, coronary heart disease, impaired glucose tolerance, and diabetes.[43] Illustration 9.3 shows the growth of a male infant who was identified as small for gestational age at birth.

Intrauterine growth may not predict postnatal growth for some infants whose birth removes them from adverse exposure within the intrauterine environment. Examples include uncontrolled maternal diabetes, smoking or drug exposure, maternal phenylketonuria, or maternal seizures treated by medications. In such cases, the rate of growth after birth may improve after delivery and in the first year.

There is evidence that supports a hypothesis called *fetal programming*, or fetal origins of adult disease. This hypothesis proposes that what happens in early life during critical or sensitive periods can have lifetime consequences.[44] Many studies on the outcome of preterm birth, including those on feeding, growth, and types of nutrition, support the fetal programming hypothesis. Preterm birth has been correlated with lifelong impacts on measures such as school performance, dropout rate, adult size, adult chronic diseases, and mental health status.[45,46] Poor head circumference growth in neonates was associated with abnormal neurological exam, abnormal mobility at 5.4 years of age, higher incidence of cerebral palsy, and neurological impairment.[47]

The fetal origins hypothesis can explain why medical treatment may not change the rate of early growth. Preterm birth or its complications may contribute to slow growth early in infancy. Various studies that have measured recovery from early growth problems have found that several factors can overwhelm nutrition benefits.[45,46,47] For example, a study of infants who were short for age and provided with nutritional supplements for two years remained short in stature at 11 and 12 years of age.[46]

More aggressive feeding and nutritional management practices for infants continue to be implemented; however, postnatal growth failure continues.[9,48] Growth outcomes after preterm birth can be impacted by a wide range of medical conditions, such as respiratory problems. Catch-up growth may be achieved during recovery in many infants, resulting in improved growth patterns. Surgery required for cardiac conditions, may alter growth for a brief period of time. Close monitoring over time may identify signs of early catch-up growth, such as an increase in fat stores or length.[49] Rapid rates of growth in preterm infants may increase risk for later chronic conditions, such as cardiovascular disease and diabetes, if the rate of weight gain is excessive.[49,50]

## Interpretation of Growth

An adequate and consistent pattern of weight gain of 20–30 grams per day is needed as preterm infants progress toward discharge.[51] Strong emphasis is placed on growth as a sign of improving health in small and sick infants after discharge, but complications make this difficult to achieve.[52,53] An example of a diagnosis in preterm babies and difficulty in interpretation of growth is the lung condition bronchopulmonary dysplasia (BPD). Rates of growth among infants with BPD are different from those of full-term infants and preterm infants who do not have BPD. While infants with BPD are recovering, their growth pattern is affected for the entire first year of life.[54] The reasons for the slower growth are increased nutritional requirements, changes in endocrine and pulmonary systems, and perhaps interaction among these systems.

Changes in growth rate are associated with the frequency of illness, hospitalizations, and medical history.[49] Conditions acquired as a result of preterm birth that make growth difficult to interpret include symptoms related to intestinal absorption that can temporarily or permanently change nutrient requirements, and ***microcephaly*** (small head size) or ***macrocephaly*** (large head size) compared to other growth indicators, which may be associated with neurological concerns.

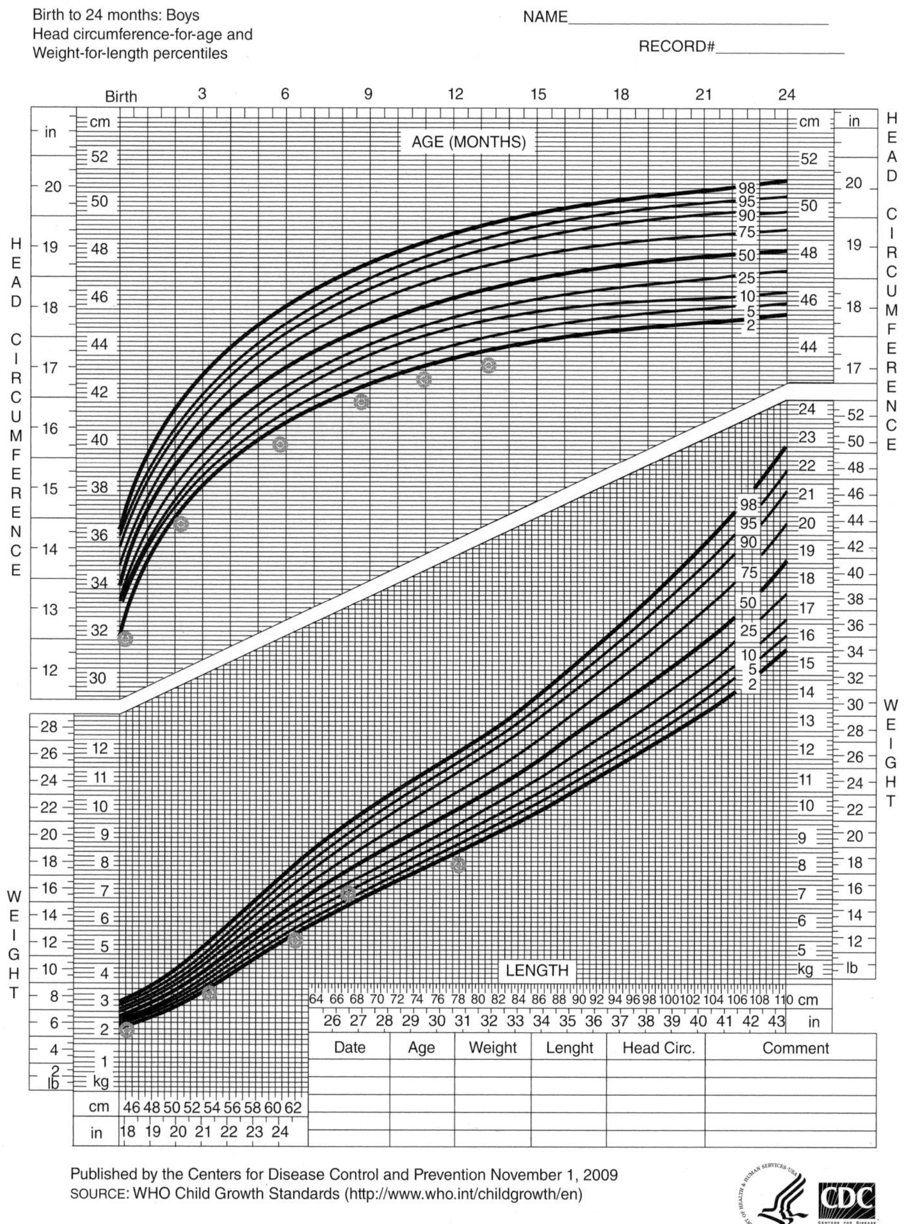


ILLUSTRATION 9.3 WHO growth charts showing head circumference growth and weight-for-length percentiles of a boy born at term. These charts show that his head circumference remains small for his age, and he is underweight.

# Nutrition for Infants with Special Health Care Needs

LO 9.4 Describe nutrition problems that are more frequently identified in preterm infants and infants with special health care needs.

Infants who are small or sick near the time of birth may have major growth and feeding problems. Infancy is such a vulnerable time of life, so health conditions occurring this early can impact growth and development. Over time, most of these problems resolve, although some will persist. Nutrition plays an important part in preventing illness, maintaining health, and treating certain conditions in infancy. Table 9.1 shows potential nutrition problems in infants with special health care needs.

## Nutrition Risks to Development

Infants and children with neurodevelopmental disorders or developmental delays more often have feeding difficulties, and

**microcephaly** Abnormally small head size for age and gender.

**macrocephaly** Abnormally large head size for age and gender.

TABLE 9.1 ▶ Potential nutrition problems in infants with special health care needs

| | |
|---|---|
| **Growth** | Slow rate of weight gain<br>Accelerated rate of weight gain<br>Slow linear growth<br>Disproportionate weight for length |
| **Nutritional Adequacy** | Increased or decreased energy needs<br>Altered nutrient requirements<br>Vitamins, minerals, or cofactors (such as carnitine) required in higher or lower amounts |
| **Feeding** | Disruption of the delivery of nutrients as a result of:<br>• Altered structure or function of the mouth, oral cavity, or gastrointestinal tract<br>• Disrupted interaction or response to cues between the infant and caregiver<br>• Difficulty with achieving or maintaining adequate positioning when feeding<br>• Lengthy duration or increased energy expenditure with feedings |



oral-motor and swallowing problems.[55] They are also at increased risk for other nutrition-related problems including altered growth (failure to thrive, obesity, and growth retardation), drug-nutrient interactions, and the need for ***enteral*** or ***parenteral feedings***.[56] A developmental disability may be related to chromosomal abnormalities, congenital anomalies, inherited metabolic disorders, certain syndromes, or may not be associated with any diagnosed condition.[56] A high percentage—70 to 90 percent—of children with special health care needs were found to have nutrition-related problems.[4] Nutrition diagnoses relating to feeding are varied, and examples include breastfeeding difficulty, swallowing difficulty, and self-feeding difficulty.[57]

Down syndrome is an example of a condition in which developmental delay can be noted in infancy. It has a prevalence of 14.47 per 10,000 live births, or 1 in 691 births.[58] Nutrition diagnoses with infants who have Down syndrome may include swallowing difficulty, self-feeding difficulty, inadequate or excessive energy intake, or suboptimal growth rate. Cardiac and gastrointestinal conditions may be identified in infants with Down syndrome, and their energy and nutrient needs may need to be modified. This is also an example of a chronic condition in which nutritional risk for problems such as overweight could increase over time if prevention and health maintenance are not addressed. Growth requires close monitoring to identify and prevent the onset of overweight. Motor development may progress at a slower rate, and reduced physical activity and energy expenditure can contribute to overweight.

Not all infants with developmental delay have developmental disabilities that continue into childhood. An infant with respiratory problems may experience slower growth, and have higher energy needs related to increased work of breathing. This infant may initially be identified with developmental delay but soon after achieve age appropriate developmental skills. This child would not meet the criteria of having a developmental disability. Other examples are infants from high-risk pregnancies, such as those born large for gestational age as a result of poorly controlled gestational diabetes. Some of these infants require short stays in intensive care units for glucose regulation or poor feeding, while others may have developmental delays that persist. After infancy, when standardized testing and evaluation can be performed, the term developmental delay may be replaced with a more specific medical or developmental diagnosis.[53]

# Severe Preterm Birth and Nutrition

LO 9.5 Identify the nutrition problems during infancy after severe preterm birth that are not generally found in infants born full-term.

Nutrition in early infancy has a key role in immediate neonatal survival, growth, neurodevelopment, as well as a conditioning factor for long-term health.[5,59] Despite advances in the care of very preterm infants, moderate to severe deficits in academic achievement, behavioral and attention problems, and poor executive function have frequently been reported.[60] Provision of adequate energy and nutrients to the very preterm infant requires ***parenteral nutrition support***, followed by slow transition to enteral feeding. Preterm infants have high metabolic rates, and they will use fat stores and protein in tissues and muscles to meet glucose needs if provision of energy is not adequate.

## How Sick Babies Are Fed

The guiding principles for feeding preterm infants are to provide nutrients to approximate the growth rate and composition of growth that would have occurred in utero; to maintain normal concentrations of blood and tissue nutrients; and to achieve appropriate functional development.[61] For preterm infants, breast milk is the desired feeding[62,63] and milk from their own mothers is the optimal enteral feeding choice.[18] Donor breast milk is primarily provided by mothers of term infants. It is pooled, pasteurized, tested for HIV and infections, and frozen when stored. There are established operational guidelines for human milk banks.[64] Donor milk is typically lower in protein than preterm breast milk, which is milk from mothers who delivered prematurely.[18] Mother's own breast milk and donor breast milk will need to be fortified to meet the nutritional needs of very preterm and extremely preterm infants. Higher volumes of mother's

**enteral feeding** Method of delivering nutrients directly to the digestive system, in contrast to methods that bypass the digestive system.

**parenteral feeding** Delivery of nutrients directly into the bloodstream.

**nutrition support** Intravenous nutrition or orally modified formulas needed because of inability to consume a regular diet.

own breast milk were associated with lower incidence and severity of necrotizing enterocolitis (NEC) and late-onset sepsis, and decreased length of stay.[65]

There are gastrointestinal conditions that could interfere with feeding preterm infants and sick neonates such as decreased gut motility, impaired absorption, and gastroesophageal reflux. These conditions, however, do not rule out enteral feeding, which stimulates the secretion of gastrointestinal hormones, gut motility, and maturation.

Feeding methods are selected based on the projected length of time the infant will need to achieve successful bottle or breastfeeding. ***Gavage feedings*** are often needed by preterm infants because coordination of their suck-swallow-breathe pattern does not generally occur until 32–34 weeks postmenstrual age. Gavage feedings are tube feedings originating from the mouth to the stomach (orogastric) or from the nose to the stomach (nasogastric). Other enteral routes include ***gastrostomy*** and *jejunostomy feeding*. These methods are used when enteral nutrition is expected to be needed long term, generally over 3 months.[66]

## Food Safety

Preterm babies have immature immunological systems and are more susceptible to infection. Every effort should be made to ensure their feedings meet food safety requirements. The rate of administering feeds to preterm infants is often much slower than that for full-term infants, and formula or breast milk is at room temperature for a longer period of time. Contamination of feeding equipment increases with time; consequently, hospitals have implemented policies requiring changing of tube feeding assemblies every 4 hours and limiting duration of hang time of continuous feeds to 4 hours.[67] Formula powder is not sterile; liquid concentrates and ready-to-feed formulas are sterile products and are recommended when nutritionally appropriate.[67] Freshly expressed and frozen breast milk are closely tracked and monitored in the NICU to assure that the infant is provided with the correct milk feeding.

## What to Feed Preterm Infants

Term infants achieve mature patterns of sucking and swallowing within days following birth. Preterm infants will begin to display a nutritive suck at approximately 34 weeks; it may be immature in pattern.[68] They will need to remain on tube feedings while oral feeds are initiated and advanced. Prior to 34 weeks, preterm infants can benefit when put to the breast to elicit ***non-nutritive sucking***. Non-nutritive sucking is defined as the act of sucking or suckling with little or no secretion of milk.[69] This can be observed when infants suck on a pacifier, or at breast after a mom has expressed her milk. Non-nutritive sucking has been found to decrease the length of stay in hospitalized preterm infants and facilitate transition from tube to bottle feeding.[70]

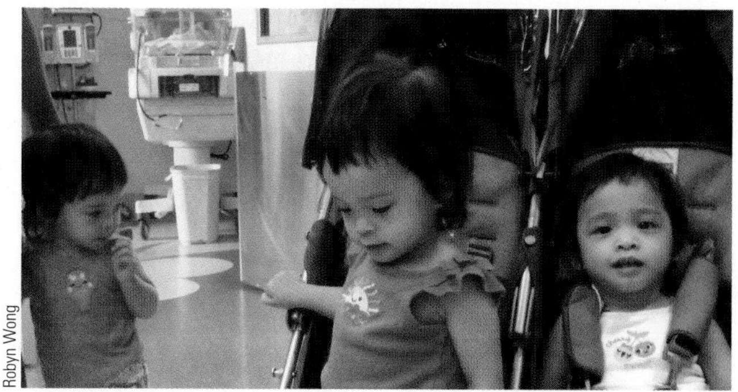

Robyn Wong

**ILLUSTRATION 9.4** Former 29 week gestation VLBW triplets visiting the NICU.

Nutrition problems including impaired growth may be seen in infants with congenital heart disease (Illustration 9.4). The incidence of IUGR is approximately 6 percent among infants with symptomatic heart disease.[71] Case Study 9.2 (later in this chapter) discusses the nutritional concerns of an infant with a cardiac condition.

Breast milk is the recommended source of nutrition when initiating enteral feeds for preterm infants.[62,65] Colostrum and breast milk are produced even when the mother delivers very early, and preterm human milk has increased protein content compared to term milk. The energy content of preterm and term breast milk is comparable at 20 calories per ounce.[69,72] Encouraging new mothers to pump frequently will help to stimulate breast milk production.[72] Barriers to breastfeeding premature and sick newborns are related to their gestational age, developmental readiness, health status, and the practices in the NICU. Pasteurized donor milk is recommended if mother's milk is not available or contraindicated. Use of breast milk and breastfeeding are contraindicated when breast milk contains harmful medications, street drugs, viruses, or other infective agents, or when the infant has galactosemia, an inborn error of metabolism.[69]

When breast milk is not available or contraindicated, preterm infant formulas are available. They contain higher energy and nutrient levels than standard infant formula (Table 9.2). The disadvantage of these formulas, however, is that their use is associated with higher rates of ***necrotizing enterocolitis (NEC)*** in preterm infants.[65] Necrotizing enterocolitis is a very serious condition that affects the intestinal tract of preterm infants. Bacterial infection and inflammation can cause

**gavage feeding** A procedure where a tube is passed through the nose or mouth into the stomach. This is used to feed preterm or newborn infants who are not yet able or have weak or uncoordinated ability to suck and swallow.

**gastrostomy feeding** Form of enteral nutrition support for delivering nutrition by tube placement directly into the stomach, bypassing the mouth through a surgical procedure that creates an opening through the abdominal wall and stomach.

**non-nutritive sucking** The sucking by newborns and young infants on items that do not provide fluid or nutrition.

**necrotizing enterocolitis (NEC)** Condition with inflammation or damage to a section of the intestine, with a grading from mild to severe.

TABLE 9.2 ▸ Selected nutrients in term, premature post-discharge and premature infant formulas per 100 ml

| NUTRIENT | TERM 20 CAL/OZ | POST DISCHARGE 22 CAL/OZ | PREMATURE 24 CAL/OZ |
|---|---|---|---|
| Energy, kcal | 68 | 74 | 80 |
| Protein, g | 1.4 | 2.1 | 2.7 |
| Vitamin A, IU | 203 | 330 | 1014 |
| Vitamin D, IU | 51 | 52 | 122 |
| Vitamin E, IU | 1.0 | 3.0 | 3.3 |
| Thiamin, mcg | 68 | 148 | 203 |
| Riboflavin, mcg | 101 | 148 | 503 |
| Niacin, mcg | 710 | 1480 | 4058 |
| Vitamin $B_6$, mcg | 41 | 74 | 203 |
| Vitamin $B_{12}$, mcg | 0.17 | 0.22 | 0.45 |
| Vitamin C, mg | 6.1 | 11.8 | 30 |
| Folic acid, mcg | 10.1 | 19.2 | 30 |
| Calcium, mg | 53 | 89 | 146 |
| Phosphorus, mg | 28 | 49 | 81 |
| Magnesium, mg | 4.1 | 5.9 | 9.7 |
| Iron, mg | 1.2 | 1.33 | 1.46 |
| Zinc, mg | 0.5 | 0.9 | 1.2 |

Mead Johnson Nutrition, *Pediatric Products Handbook*, ©2014 Mead Johnson & Company, LLC, http://www.meadjohnson.com/pediatrics/us-en/sites/hcp-usa/files/LB6-ProductGuide-REV-10-14-hi.pdf

"Product Category: Similac," http://static.abbottnutrition.com/cms-prod/abbottnutrition.com/img/Similac.pdf

Accessed June 1, 2015.

bowel wall destruction and intestinal perforation and surgical intervention. Overwhelming NEC can result in death.

Preterm infants usually require high calorie feeds that provide 22–24 calories per ounce. Standard infant formulas and unfortified breast milk contain 20 calories per ounce. Higher calorie formulas, such as 26, 28, or sometimes 30 calories per ounce may be needed to support the growth of infants with bronchopulmonary dysplasia or on fluid restrictions. Close nutritional monitoring is needed to evaluate the effectiveness of the feeding plan.

## Preterm Infants and Feeding

The goal of feeding preterm infants is the same as for term infants—to achieve appropriate patterns of linear growth and weight gain and to achieve appropriate feeding skills for their *corrected age*. An infant born 3 months prematurely would at 9 months of age have a corrected age of 6 months. Nutrition and feeding recommendations for 6-month-old infants would be appropriate guidance for this infant and his family.

Feeding skills of preterm infants can be assessed by looking at the following:

- Ability to remain engaged, actively participate in the feeding
- Ability to organize oral-motor functioning, readily accept nipple, and maintain rhythmic sucking
- Ability to coordinate sucking, swallowing, and breathing
- Ability to maintain physiological stability—for example, adequate oxygenation and normal breathing throughout the feeding[73]

Most families enjoy feeding their infants and experience few long-term feeding problems. Infants who were born preterm, however, might be more difficult to feed. Some of the reasons for this include:

- *Lethargy.* Low levels of arousal in preterm infants may reduce duration of effective feeding.
- *Low tolerance of volume.* Abdominal distension may alter breathing and heart rate, so that the infant stops feeding.
- *Stress responses connected to feeding.* "Disorganized feeding" may result from the infant's prior unpleasant oral-tactile experiences while in the NICU—for example suctioning, use of nasogastric and ***orogastric (OG) feedings***, and delayed introduction of non-nutritive sucking or nipple feeding. Oral stimulation and feeding attempts may elicit stress responses rather than pleasure.

Regardless of the associated conditions, certain feeding characteristics of preterm infants are distinct from those of term infants (Table 9.3). The feeding skills of most preterm infants improve over time. Anxiety decreases as parents become more comfortable and adept in caring for their infants at home. The underlying reflexes that associate pleasure with feeding reemerge, and the interactions between the infants and their caregivers will continue to improve (see Case Study 9.1).

**oral-gastric (OG) feeding** A form of enteral nutrition support for delivering nutrition by tube placement from the mouth to the stomach.

TABLE 9.3 ▸ Signs of feeding problems in high-risk infants

**In Early Infancy (Under 6 Months of Age)[1, 55]**

- The infant has an abnormal sucking pattern, which can be arrthymic or disorganized. A weak suck or poor seal around the nipple may contribute to fluid loss; a poor seal allows breast milk or formula to run out of the mouth.
- Lengthy duration of feedings can tire the infant and the caregiver, and increase the infant's energy expenditure.
- Gagging, coughing, choking during the feeding, or noisy breathing after the feeding may suggest problems with swallowing.
- Baby may appear to be hungry all the time because of low nippled volumes, and is unable to nipple higher volumes over time.

**In Later Infancy (Over 6 Months of Age)**

- The baby is not able to maintain adequate head and trunk control while being fed from a spoon.
- The baby drinks from a bottle but does not readily accept baby foods after repeated attempts.
- The baby resists, gags, coughs, or chokes on foods with increased texture.

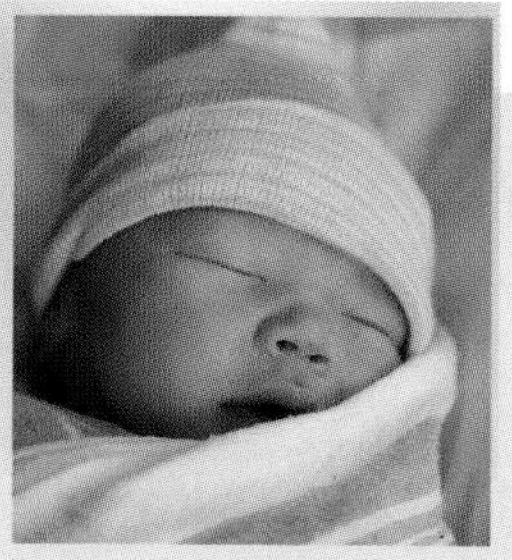
Steven Blandin/Shutterstock.com

# CASE STUDY **9.1**

## Premature Birth in an At-Risk Family

Erica is a former 27-week female, birthweight 1.14 kg, and birth length 38.0 cm; his weight, length, and head circumference measurements were appropriate for age. She was born to a 32-year-old woman with hypercholesterolemia and a pre-pregnant BMI of 18. This was her second pregnancy; she and her husband also have an 20-month-old daughter.

Respiratory support and parenteral feeds of amino acids and dextrose were initiated on the day of delivery. The day after birth, small volumes of mother's own breast milk were introduced via orogastric tube but were discontinued because of suspected intolerance. Breast milk was reintroduced three days later and Erica's mother had a very good milk supply.

There were multiple occurrences of abdominal distension and periods when enteral feeds were put on hold. Erica's tolerance to fortified breast milk feeds slowly improved, and fortified feeds of breast milk were initiated at 18 days of age. Erica received parenteral nutrition for a total of 20 days. She was diagnosed with anemia of prematurity, and received two blood transfusions during her stay.

Throughout this time, Erica's weight and length progressed appropriately. Her head circumference showed minimal growth over a 3-week period. The concentration of her feeds was increased to 26 calories per ounce. Because of suspected gastroesophageal reflux, the volume of her feeds were decreased and feeding concentration increased to 28 calories per ounce. Mom continued to provide breast milk for all of Erica's feedings.

Breastfeeding was initiated when Erica was 33 weeks postmenstrual age. Respiratory support was discontinued at 36 weeks postmenstrual age. At 37 weeks postmenstrual age, she was bottle feeding and breastfeeding well and no longer needed tube feedings.

Erica had a 105-day stay in the NICU. She remained anemic, and iron and multivitamin supplements were continued at discharge. The recommended discharge feeding plan was comprised of ad lib breastfeeding/expressed breast milk and supplemental feeds of 22 calorie post-discharge formula daily. At time of discharge, Erica's weight, length and head circumference were at the 50th percentile on the Fenton growth chart for preterm infant girls. Her mom's milk supply continued to be very adequate; and Erica was breastfeeding well. She was enrolled in the ***Early Intervention Program*** and was achieving appropriate developmental skills for her corrected age. Complementary foods were introduced at 6 months corrected age. At 9 months corrected age she transitioned off supplemental feeds of post-discharge formula to exclusive feeds of breast milk and breastfeeding. Erica continued to meet nutrition and growth goals. At 15 months of age, Erica's corrected age was 12 months and all of her growth measurements were above the 50th percentile for corrected age.

### Questions

1. What effects did Erica's preterm birth have on her nutrition and feedings? On her growth?
2. What are the nutritional issues that need to be monitored after Erica's discharge?
3. What are the signs that Erica can outgrow these problems?

# Infants with Congenital Anomalies and Chronic Illness

**LO 9.6** Describe examples of nutrition assessment and interventions for infants with special health care needs and chronic illness.

Some infants are born at term but require neonatal intensive care because of cardiac, genetic, or chromosomal conditions such as cardiac malformations, central nervous system defects, and chromosomal anomalies. About half of babies in neonatal intensive care units have normal birthweights and experience lower mortality than LBW infants. They tend to have a higher rate of ***congenital anomalies*** (22 percent) and often require rehospitalization.[74] These infants may need more nutrition services and monitoring than healthy-term infants. Spina bifida and ***anencephaly*** are examples of central nervous system anomalies. Since folic acid has been added as a supplement in grains and flours and supplementation has been promoted for women of

**Early Intervention Program** Educational intervention for the development of children from birth up to 3 years of age.

**congenital anomaly** Condition evident in a newborn that is diagnosed at or near birth, usually as a genetic or chronic condition, such as spina bifida or cleft lip and palate.

**anencephaly** Condition initiated early in gestation of the central nervous system in which the brain is not formed correctly, resulting in neonatal death.

childbearing age, the prevalence of spina bifida has declined by 31 percent.[75]

"Children with special health care needs" is defined as children who have or are at increased risk for chronic physical, developmental, behavioral, or emotional condition and who also require health and related services of a type or amount beyond that required of children generally.[2] They would be eligible for a wide range of medical, nutritional, and educational services to maximize their growth and development.[76] Nutrition assessments can identify problems such as inadequate linear growth or weight gain, inadequate energy or nutrient intake, or delayed progression in the infant's diet (see Table 9.1). Major nutritional impacts are exemplified by disorders that involve the gastrointestinal tract. Newborn infants identified with ***congenital diaphragmatic hernia (CDH)*** or ***tracheoesophageal atresia (TEF)*** will need timely surgical intervention, neonatal intensive care, and parenteral nutrition support. CDH is a birth defect attributed to incomplete formation and function of the diaphragm. Abdominal organs can move into the chest and compromise breathing. TEF is associated with an abnormal connection in one or more places of the trachea and esophagus; swallowed fluid can enter the infant's lungs.

The successful medical care and treatment of CDH and TEF have contributed to disease-specific reductions in the infant mortality rate. Both of these conditions affect motility of the gastrointestinal tract. Optimal provision of energy and nutrients are needed to support the infant's growth and transition to oral feeding (Illustration 9.5).

Another example of a congenital anomaly identified in infancy is ***cleft lip with or without cleft palate, or cleft palate.*** A cleft of the palate is associated with increased risk for ineffective feeding because of the difficulty in establishing an effective seal, suck, and swallow. A team approach is needed, as these infants are at risk for hearing, speech, language, and dental problems. Use of special nipples and feeding devices can improve bottle feedings and increase feeding volumes for these infants.

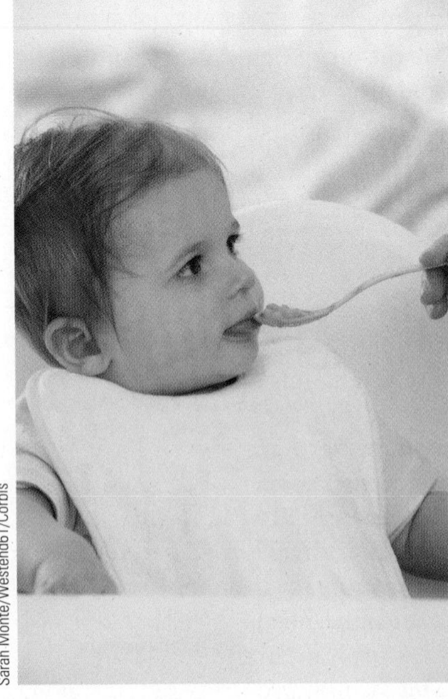

Sarah Monte/Westend61/Corbis

ILLUSTRATION 9.5 ▸ Infant in hospital being encouraged to eat with a spoon.

## Infants with Genetic Disorders

Infants diagnosed with genetic disorders near birth are a small subset of infants with congenital anomalies or chronic conditions. They may also fit into the classification of infants with special health care needs. A result of prenatal genetic testing is that families will learn ahead of time that their baby will have a specific condition at birth.

The number of genetic disorders that can be identified in newborns has been increasing, particularly through expanded newborn infant screening programs across the United States. Expanded newborn screening and follow-up has enabled more newborns to receive timely diagnosis and treatment. Some of these conditions require specific medical treatment and nutritional support, and use of therapeutic formulas known as medical foods. Infants with rare genetic conditions such as ***phenylketonuria*** and ***galactosemia*** will need dietary interventions and restriction of specific compounds. Failure to implement medical protocols and nutritional management can result in irreversible mental retardation, metabolic crises, neurological crises, growth failure, and in some inborn errors, death.[27]

Genetic centers and metabolic clinics are notified when a newborn screening result needs follow-up. Immediate action is taken to contact the family and assure confirmatory work-up. In such circumstances, newborn screening programs and follow-up contribute to timely diagnosis and treatment. For example, an infant with galactosemia, if not picked up by the initial abnormal screening result, is likely to have been hospitalized with possible sepsis or liver problems by the time a second screen is to be collected. If the baby with galactosemia receives timely medical treatment and dietary intervention, recovery is usually rapid. Some of the disorders picked up by newborn screening do not make the infant ill in early infancy, but signs, symptoms, or

**congenital diaphragmatic hernia** Displacement of the intestines up into the lung area due to incomplete formation of the diaphragm *in utero*.

**tracheoesophageal atresia** Incomplete connection between the esophagus and the stomach *in utero*, resulting in a shortened esophagus.

**cleft lip and palate** Condition in which the upper lip and/or palate are not completely formed and in need of surgical correction. The cleft may contribute to feeding problems in early infancy.

**Phenylketonuria** An inherited error in protein metabolism involving phenylalanine and the enzyme phenylalanine hydroxylase.

**Galactosemia** A rare genetic condition of carbohydrate metabolism. It can cause serious illness if not identified and treated shortly after birth.

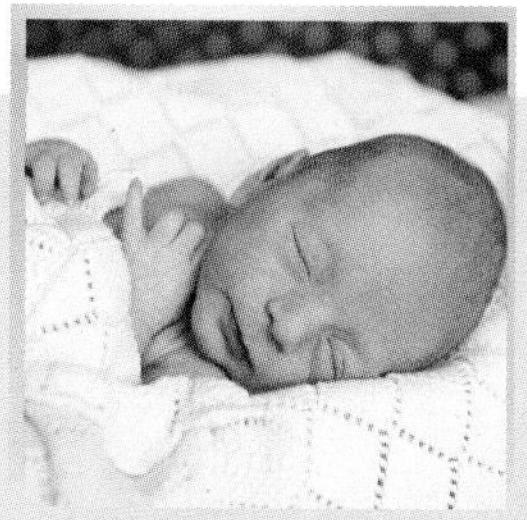
Cheryl E. Davis/Shutterstock.com

# CASE STUDY 9.2

## Noah's Cardiac Condition

Noah is a former late preterm male born at 38 weeks gestation. He weighed 2100 grams and was small for gestational age. His mother's medical history included chronic hypertension, obesity, and gestational diabetes. Noah was diagnosed prenatally with a cardiac condition that could affect his ability to feed.

His mother planned to breastfeed Noah and has been successful at expressing her milk and maintaining her breast milk supply. Noah has a weak suck and tires easily at the breast. He is able to drink small volumes, 1 to 1½ ounces from a bottle. The feedings can last 30 minutes or longer.

At discharge, the family is referred to the WIC program, Supplemental Social Insurance (SSI), and the state Children with Special Health Needs program. Specialty cardiac clinic and local follow-up appointments are made. Feeding difficulties concern the family, and both a lactation consultant and a registered dietitian are involved prior to and after discharge.

Noah nurses frequently, but briefly, due to fatigue. Growth is slower than expected, but the cardiologist does not think Noah's slow weight gain is a result of his cardiac condition. Noah continues to nipple small volumes even after his family implements the recommendations from the lactation consultant. The registered dietitian recommends increasing the caloric density of expressed breast milk with the addition of infant formula powder. The family perceives this recommendation as undermining Noah's mother's effort to nurse him, and is unsure about implementing this change. Noah likes to nurse, however feedings are brief and Noah is not able to obtain the higher fat/higher calorie hindmilk. Over time, his family starts to introduce baby foods from a spoon and his mom continues to breastfeed. Noah's weight gain is progressing slowly; his length and head circumference are progressing along the 10th percentile. Because of his slow weight gain his weight-for-length percentile has fallen to the 3rd percentile.

Noah's family enjoys the interactions during feedings and feels that Noah is doing well for an infant with a cardiac problem. They have not contacted the WIC Program or the Children with Special Health Needs Program. Some people they meet assume that Noah was a premature baby, but his small size is not of concern to his parents.

### Questions

1. How do breastfeeding and feeds of breasts milk benefit Noah?
2. How would you know if Noah's nutritional intake is sufficient?
3. Why might the family not desire services and benefits from the WIC program or Children with Special Health Needs program?
4. What next steps would you recommend to help Noah with his weight gain?

other concerns could present later. It may sometimes be difficult for parents of a well-appearing newborn to learn that a special diet is needed to prevent serious illness or significant consequences in the future. An example of a condition that can be picked up by newborn screening before illness presents is cystic fibrosis.

Other genetic conditions that have nutrition interventions requiring restriction or supplemental levels of nutrients or compounds include:

- Urea cycle disorders requiring protein restriction (e.g., citrullinemia)
- Fat-related disorders requiring restrictions on specific fatty acids (e.g., LCHAD, long-chain hydroxyacyl-CoA dehydrogenase deficiency)
- Carbohydrate-related disorders requiring restrictions of type or timing of carbohydrates (e.g., glycogen-storage disease)
- Disorders sensitive to high-dose vitamins (e.g., $B_{12}$ responsive methylmalonic acidemia; also may require a protein-modified dietary intake)
- Renal genetic disorders managed with a protein-restriction to delay end-stage renal disease (e.g., polycystic kidney disease)

Case Study 9.2 discusses a child with a cardiac condition.

# Feeding Problems

**LO 9.7** Identify infants with feeding problems and appropriate nutrition services for them.

Infants who were born preterm or have chronic health problems may be more irritable and less able to signal their wants and needs compared to healthy infants. Feeding difficulties are reported in 40–45 percent of families with VLBW infants.[3] Children with developmental disabilities have more frequent feeding problems, as high as 70 percent, that may or may not be identified in infancy.[52]

By the time feeding problems require intervention to prevent further growth and developmental problems, families and infants may be frustrated from their feeding experiences. Infants who are difficult to feed are at risk for failure to thrive (FTT), child abuse, and neglect.[52] Infant feeding guidelines for term infants are appropriate for use in most preterm infants using their corrected age. Term infants can be introduced to complementary foods at 6 months of age.[77] An infant born at 32 weeks gestation would be ready for complementary foods at 8 months of age, which is a corrected age of 6 months.

# Nutrition Interventions

**LO 9.8** Identify appropriate nutrition intervention strategies for infants who are experiencing problems with linear growth or weight gain.

When feeding problems are identified in infancy, interventions are required to ensure growth and development (see Table 9.3). Interventions may include any of the following:

- Monitor weight, length, and head circumference more frequently.
- Monitor the infant's fluid and food intakes and assess adequacy of energy and nutrients, while acknowledging that the infant's intake may be variable due to illness, congestion, or medication use.
- Change the frequency, volume, or concentration of feedings as needed to meet energy and nutrient needs.
- Modify the timing of breastfeeding or bottle feedings, meals, and snacks to fit medication or sleep schedules.
- Assess the infant's position during feeding. This may be important if the infant is not able to sit without support.
- Increase the nutrient density of foods or fluids, so that the infant has to expend less energy during feedings.
- Provide parent education and/or support services as needed, so that the feeding environment is positive and low in stress.
- Observe the infant-caregiver interaction during feedings, at home or in a developmental program, to make sure that signs of hunger, satiety, and comfort result in positive feeding experiences.
- Adjust nutrition goals to the developmental abilities of the infant.

# Nutrition Services

**LO 9.9** Describe how families of high-risk infants and infants with special health care needs access nutrition resources and services in their communities.

Infants who were born preterm or with special health care needs may qualify for nutrition-related services and programs. Some of these include:

- Early Intervention Programs funded through the Individuals with Disabilities Education Act (IDEA), Part C
- Early Head Start
- WIC
- State Children with Special Health Care Needs programs

Infants with disabling conditions are eligible for Supplemental Social Insurance (SSI), a federal program within the Social Security Administration.[48] SSI provides the family with financial support and access to health insurance if the family meets income eligibility guidelines.

The following are some examples of how nutrition services may be accessed:

- Specialty clinics, such as cardiac, neurology, pulmonology, metabolic, and high-risk infant follow-up clinics frequently have registered dietitian-nutritionists on the specialty team.
- Specialty formulas, medical foods, or medical nutrition therapy may be provided through contractual agreements, health plan coverage, and enacted state laws.

Every state also has a program funded by the Maternal Child Health Bureau of the U.S. Department of Health and Human Services to identify and advocate for children with special needs, such as the Developmental Disabilities Council.

## KEY POINTS

1. The number of infants at risk for having special health care needs is increasing even though survival rates of preterm infants are improving over decades.
2. Nutrition guidance for preterm infants and infants with special health care needs are adjusted to fit their individual energy and nutrient needs.
3. Infants born extremely preterm will require higher intakes of protein and micronutrients per kilogram body weight than term infants.
4. Growth in infants with special health care needs reflects nutritional intake and other factors such as intrauterine exposure to toxins, developmental delay, and underlying medical condition.

5. Feeding difficulties may be seen more often in infants who required intensive medical care and lengthy hospitalizations.
6. Some inborn errors of metabolism are identified in infancy and require medical treatment and nutrition support, including use of medical foods.

## REVIEW QUESTIONS

1. Why are infant feeding problems more common in extremely low birthweight and very low birthweight infants?
   a. Preterm birth reduces the nutritional composition of mothers' breast milk.
   b. Preterm infants develop the skills for nursing when they reach a postmenstrual age of 40 weeks gestation.
   c. Impaired nutrient absorption and slow gut motility affect tolerance of feedings.
   d. Increased energy needs are difficult to achieve because of the preterm infant's ineffective nippling skills.
2. What factors make nutritional requirements higher for an infant who was born at 28 weeks gestation?
   a. Preterm birth resulted in reduced body fat and nutrient reserves.
   b. Newborn reflexes persist and interfere with oral feeding.
   c. Frequent illness and infection increase nutrient needs.
   d. The immaturity of the gastrointestinal tract increases energy needs.

Questions 3, 4, and 5 concern an infant who was born at 32 weeks gestation and weighed 1200 grams (2 pounds 10 ounces). He is now 3 months old. *Answer true or false for each statement.*

3. Standard infant formula would be appropriate at this time.

   _____ True _____ False
4. This infant has a chronological age of 3 months and a corrected age of 1 month.

   _____ True _____ False
5. This infant's nutritional needs can be met with exclusive feeds of breast milk.

   _____ True _____ False
6. Complementary foods can be introduced in 3 months.

   _____ True _____ False
7. Identify a genetic condition that is not found by maternal or newborn screening.
8. Describe two or more factors other than nutrition that could impact growth of an infant with special health care needs.
9. Describe two other modes of feeding infants in addition to breast and bottle feeding.

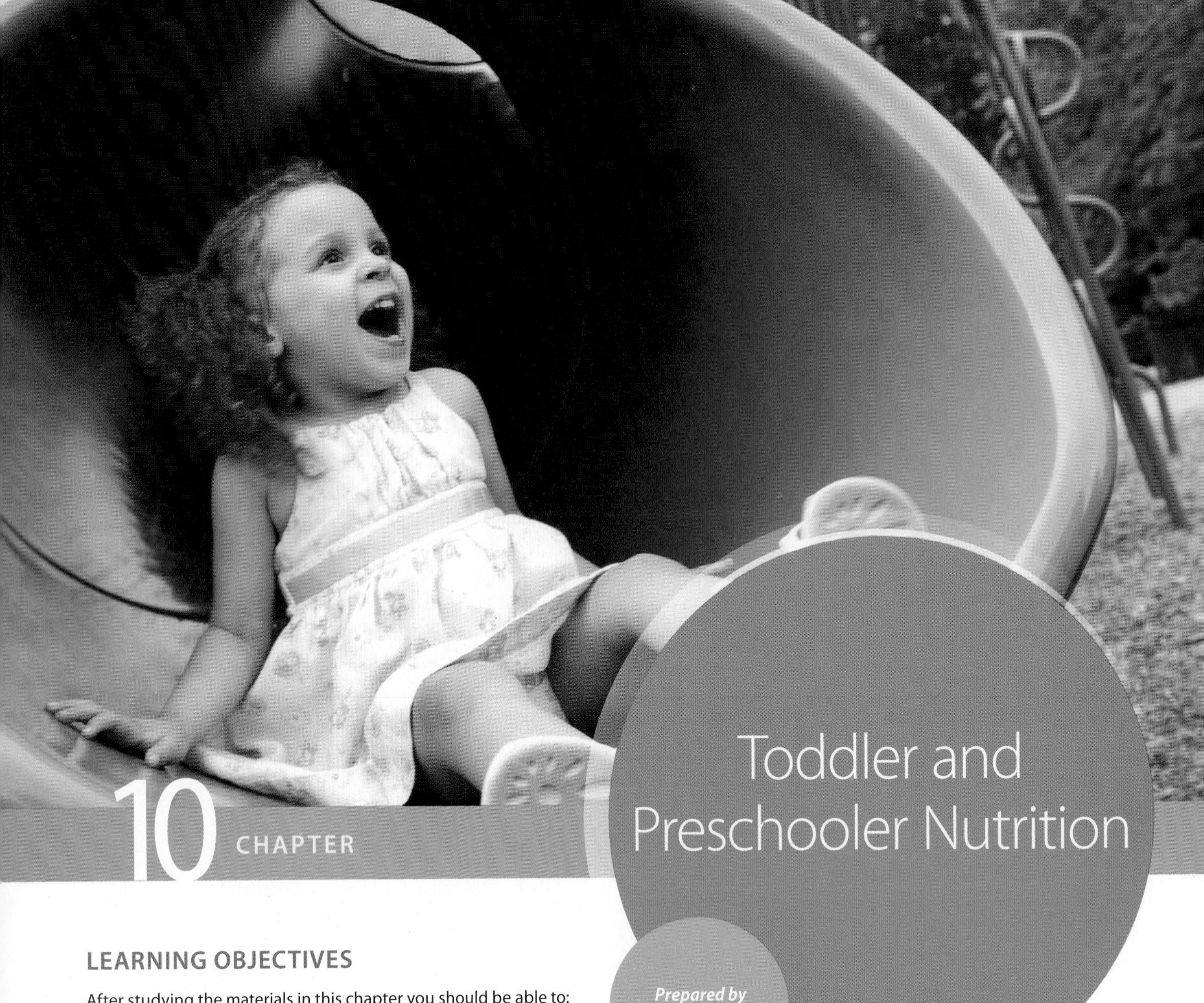

# 10 CHAPTER

# Toddler and Preschooler Nutrition

*Prepared by*
**Ellen K. Bowser**

## LEARNING OBJECTIVES

After studying the materials in this chapter you should be able to:

**10.1** List two Healthy People 2020 objectives related to toddlers and preschool age children.

**10.2** Identify the screening tool used for assessing underweight, overweight, or obesity in young children.

**10.3** Describe two strategies that parents/caretakers can employ to encourage toddlers/preschoolers to accept a variety of foods in their diets.

**10.4** Explain what influences energy needs of young children.

**10.5** Identify one common nutritional problem of young children and describe prevention strategies.

**10.6** Define overweight and obesity in young children.

**10.7** Describe the components of a healthy diet for young children as recommended by health and professional organizations and agencies.

**10.8** Identify the basic premise upon which Bright Futures Nutrition is based.

**10.9** Identify one public food or nutrition program that provides services to young children and describe the program's strategies in improving nutrition of young children.

CDC/PHIL

# Introduction

This chapter describes the growth and development of toddlers and preschool-age children and their relationships to nutrition and the establishment of eating patterns. Growth during the toddler and preschool-age years is slower than in infancy but steady. This slowing of ***growth velocity*** is reflected in a decreased appetite; however, young children need adequate calories and nutrients to meet their nutritional needs. The eating and health habits established at this early stage of life may impact food habits and subsequent health later in life. The development of new skills and increasing independence marks the toddler and preschool stages. Learning about and accepting new foods, developing feeding skills, and establishing healthy food preferences and eating habits are important aspects of this stage of development.

## Definitions of the Life-Cycle Stage

***Toddlers*** are generally defined as children between the ages of 1 and 3 years. This stage of development is characterized by a rapid increase in ***gross*** and ***fine motor skills*** with subsequent increases in independence, exploration of the environment, and language skills. ***Preschool-age children*** are between 3 and 5 years of age. Characteristics of this stage of development include increasing autonomy; experiencing broader social circumstances, such as attending preschool or staying with friends and relatives; increasing language skills; and expanding ability to control behavior.

## Importance of Nutrition

Adequate intake of energy and nutrients is necessary for toddlers and preschool-age children to achieve their full growth and developmental potential. Undernutrition during these years impairs children's cognitive development as well as their ability to explore their environments.[1] Long-term effects of undernutrition, such as failure to thrive and cognitive impairment, may be prevented or reduced with adequate nutrition and environmental support.

# Tracking Toddler and Preschooler Health

**LO 10.1** List two Healthy People 2020 objectives related to toddlers and preschool age children.

The percentage of children living in poverty is a widely used indicator of child well-being, and this rate has increased dramatically with the economic recession of recent years.[2,3] Poverty rates for children under the age of 6 have increased from 20 percent in 2007 to 25 percent in 2013. Approximately 48 percent of U.S. children under the age of 6 are living in poor and near poor families. Children living in poor and low-income homes are more likely to be from African-American and Hispanic populations.[1]

When evaluating young children's nutritional status and offering nutrition education to parents, it is important to consider children's home environments. Establishing healthy eating habits may not be high on a family's priority list when the home environment is one of poverty and food insecurity. Disparities in child health indicators, including those of nutrition status in this age group, exist among races and ethnicities.

## Healthy People 2020

Healthy People 2020—includes a number of objectives that directly relate to toddlers and preschoolers in the topic areas of Food Safety, Nutrition, and Weight Status (NWS), and Physical Activity (PA).[5] The NWS topic area includes objectives related to Healthier Food Access, Healthcare Settings, Weight Status, Food Insecurity, Food and Nutrient Consumption (Table 10.1), and Iron Deficiency. Examples of objectives related to toddlers and preschoolers will be presented in the discussion of specific topics throughout this chapter.

# Normal Growth and Development

**LO 10.2** Identify the screening tool used for assessing underweight, overweight, or obesity in young children.

An infant's birth weight triples in the first 12 months of life, but growth velocity slows thereafter until the adolescent growth spurt. On average, toddlers gain 8 ounces (0.23 kg) per month and 0.4 inches (1 cm) of height per month, while preschoolers gain 4.4 pounds (2 kg) and 2.75 inches (7 cm) per year.[6] This decrease in rate of growth is accompanied by a reduced appetite and food intake in toddlers and preschoolers. A common complaint of parents of children this age is that their children have a much lower appetite and a lower interest in food or eating compared to their appetite and food intake during infancy. Parents need to be reassured that a decrease in appetite is part of normal growth and development for children in this age group.

**growth velocity** The rate of growth over time.

**toddlers** Children between the ages of 1 and 3 years.

**gross motor skills** Development and use of large muscle groups as exhibited by walking alone, running, walking up stairs, riding a tricycle, hopping, and skipping.

**fine motor skills** Development and use of smaller muscle groups demonstrated by stacking objects, scribbling, and copying a circle or square.

**preschool-age children** Children between the ages of 3 and 5 years who are not yet attending kindergarten.

TABLE 10.1 ▸ Healthy People 2020 objectives in the Nutrition and Weight Status (NWS) topic area related to Food and Nutrient Consumption of the population aged 2 years and older[4]

| HEALTHY PEOPLE 2020 OBJECTIVE | | BASELINE | TARGET |
|---|---|---|---|
| NWS-14: | Increase the contribution of fruits to the diets of the population aged 2 years and older | 0.5 cup equivalents of fruits per 1000 calories | 0.9 cup equivalents of fruits per 1000 calories |
| NWS-15.1: | Increase the contribution of total vegetables to the diets of the population aged 2 years and older | 0.8 cup equivalents of total vegetables per 1000 calories | 1.1 cup equivalents per 1000 calories |
| NWS-15.2: | Increase the contribution of dark green vegetables, orange vegetables, and legumes to the diets of the population aged 2 years and older | 0.1 cup equivalents of dark green or orange vegetables or legumes per 1000 calories | 0.3 cup equivalents per 1000 calories |
| NWS-16: | Increase the contribution of whole grains to the diets of the population aged 2 years and older. | 0.3 oz equivalents of whole grains per 1000 calories | 0.6 oz equivalents per 1000 calories |
| Nws-17.1: | Reduce consumption of calories from solid fats in the population aged 2 years and older. | 18.9% of total daily calorie intake | 16.7% |
| NWS-17.2: | Reduce consumption of calories from added sugars in the population aged 2 years and older. | 15.7% of total daily calorie intake | 10.8% |
| NWS-17.3: | Reduce consumption of calories from solid fats and added sugars. | 34.6% of total daily calorie intake | 29.8% |
| NWS-18: | Reduce consumption of saturated fat in the population aged 2 years and older. | 11.3% of total daily calorie intake | 9.5% |
| NWS-19: | Reduce consumption of sodium in the population aged 2 years and older. | 3641 mg | 2300 mg |
| NWS-20: | Increase consumption of calcium in the population aged 2 years and older. | 1118 mg | 1300 mg |

SOURCE: "2020 Topics & Objectives: Nutrition Weight Status," U.S. Department of Health and Human Services, www.healthypeople.gov. Table arranged by Nancy H. Wooldridge.

## Measuring Growth

In monitoring a child's physical growth, it is important for children to be accurately weighed and measured at periodic intervals. Toddlers less than 2 years of age should be weighed without clothing or a diaper. The ***recumbent length*** of toddlers should be measured on a length board with a fixed head board and movable foot board. Proper measurement of recumbent length requires two adults—one at the child's head making sure the crown of the head is placed firmly against the head board, and the other making sure that the child's legs are fully extended and placing the foot board at the child's heels (Illustration 10.1). Preschool-age children should be weighed and measured without shoes and in lightweight clothing. Calibrated scales should be used and a height board should be used for measuring ***stature*** (Illustrations 10.2 and 10.3). It is important that both weight and height be plotted on the appropriate growth charts, such as the WHO and CDC Growth Charts discussed next.

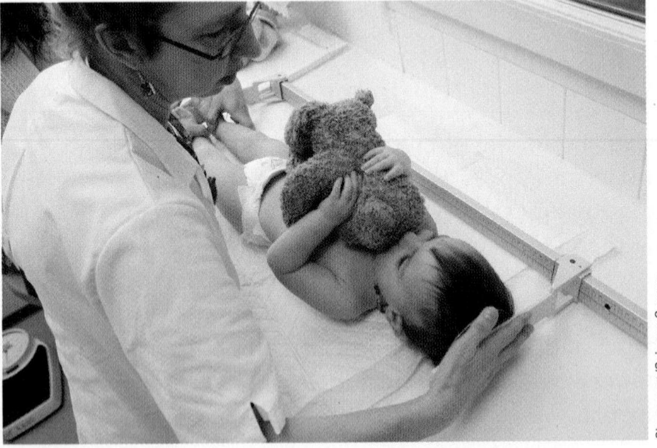

Chassenet/Science Source

ILLUSTRATION 10.1 ▸ easuring the recumbent length of a toddler is a two-person job!

## The WHO and CDC Growth Charts

The Centers for Disease Control and Prevention (CDC) and the American Academy of Pediatrics (AAP) recommend the following charts be used to monitor growth in infants and children: The WHO growth charts be used for children aged birth to younger than 2 years regardless of type of feeding and the 2000 CDC growth charts for children aged 2 until aged 20 years.

**recumbent length** Measurement of length while the child is lying down. Recumbent length is used to measure toddlers <24 months of age and those between 24 and 36 months who are unable to stand unassisted.

**stature** Standing height.

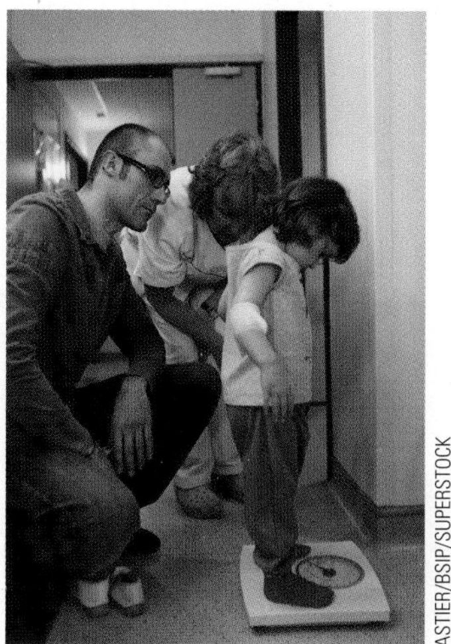


ILLUSTRATION 10.2 ▸ Young child being weighed.

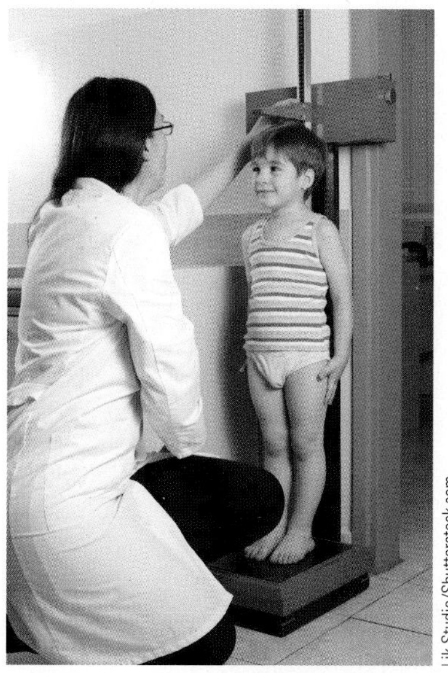


ILLUSTRATION 10.3 ▸ Measuring the stature of a preschool-age child.

The WHO charts were developed as growth standards, which demonstrate how healthy children grow under optimal conditions.[3,4]

The CDC growth charts are based on data from cycles 2 and 3 of the National Health and Examination Survey (NHES) and the National Health and Nutrition Examination Surveys (NHANES) I, II, and III, and they provide a reference for how children in the United States are growing.[7] Charts are gender specific. With these charts, the health care professional can plot and monitor weight-for-age, length- or stature-for-age, head-circumference-for-age, weight-for-length, weight-for-stature, and BMI-for-age. Children's growth usually "tracks" within a fairly steady percentile range. It is important to monitor a child's growth over time and to identify any deviations in growth. It is the pattern of growth that is important to assess rather than any one single measurement. A weight measurement without a length or stature measurement will not indicate how appropriate the weight is for the child's length or stature. There are Internet-based programs and apps for smartphones and tablets available that will compute exact growth percentiles, but tracking and assessing growth curves over time are still essential.

***Body mass index,*** is predictive of body fat for children over 2 years of age, as BMI normative values are not available for children less than 2 years of age.[8] For children 2 years of age or older, a BMI in the 85th percentile or greater but less than the 95th percentile indicates overweight, and a BMI in the 95th percentile or greater indicates obesity.[8] For children less than 2 years of age, a weight-for-length greater than the 95th percentile is considered overweight.[8] A weight-for-length or a BMI for age percentile less than the 5th percentile indicates underweight in all age categories. BMI fluctuates throughout childhood. BMI increases in infancy; it decreases during preschool years, hitting its lowest point at approximately 4–6 years of age; and then it increases into adulthood. Because of this normal fluctuation of BMI, the only way to know whether a child's BMI is within a normal range is to plot BMI-for-age on the appropriate growth curve. In pediatrics, the goal is to strive for a BMI-for-age percentile in the normal range and not a specific BMI value, as is the goal in adults. Healthy People 2020 objective NWS-5.2 is to increase the proportion of primary care physicians who regularly assess BMI for age and sex in their child patients.[3] Growth charts visually aid parents by demonstrating the expected slowing of the growth velocity during the toddler and preschool stage of development. Although the curves for weight-for-age and length- or stature-for-age continue to increase during the toddler and preschool-age years, the slope of the curve is not as steep as it is during the first year of life.

## WHO Growth Standards

In 2006, the World Health Organization (WHO) published growth standards for children from birth to 5 years of age, based on growth data collected over time on healthy breastfed infants and young children in six different countries. The mothers of these children were nonsmokers and the children had adequate diets and were free of infections. WHO growth standards are available for boys and girls from birth to 5 years of age for length/height-for-age, weight-for-age, weight-for-length, weight-for-height, and BMI-for-age (www.who.int/childgrowth or the CDC website at www.cdc.gov/growthcharts/who_charts.htm).[9] Illustration 10.4 shows an example of one of the charts, which depicts the growth of a healthy child.[3,4]

**body mass index** An index that correlates with total body fat content or percent body fat and is an acceptable measure of adiposity or body fatness in children and adults.[8] It is calculated by dividing weight in kilograms by the square of height in meters (kg/m$^2$).

## Common Problems with Measuring and Plotting Growth Data

Incorrectly measured or plotted growth parameters in young children can lead to errors in health status assessment. Standard procedures should be followed, calibrated and appropriate equipment should be used, and plotting should be double checked—including checking the age of the child—to avoid such errors. Choosing the appropriate growth chart based on how the child was measured (recumbent length versus stature) and on the child's gender is as important as using the current growth charts.

# Physiological and Cognitive Development

**LO 10.3** Describe two strategies that parents/caretakers can employ to encourage toddlers/preschoolers to accept a variety of foods in their diets.

## Toddlers

An explosion in the development of new skills occurs during the toddler years. Most children begin to walk independently at about their first birthday. At first the walking is more like a "toddle" with a wide-based gait.[6] After practicing for several months, the toddler achieves greater steadiness and soon will be able to stop, turn, and stoop without falling over. Gross motor skills, such as sitting on a small chair and climbing on furniture, develop rapidly at this age, and with practice, great improvements in balance and agility take place. At about 15 months, children can crawl up stairs; by about 18 months, they can run stiffly. Most toddlers can walk up and down stairs one step at a time by 24 months, and jump in place. At about 30 months, children have advanced to going up stairs by alternating their feet. By 36 months of age, children are ready for tricycles.

Children become increasingly mobile and independent with improvements in gross motor skills. Toddlers are fascinated with these newfound skills, showing a readiness to put the skills into practice and to develop new skills. However, toddlers have no sense of dangerous situations. At this age, children are especially vulnerable to accidental injuries and ingestion of harmful substances. In fact, the leading cause of death among young children is unintentional injuries. Parents and caregivers have to constantly watch over toddlers, preferably in environments made "child-safe."

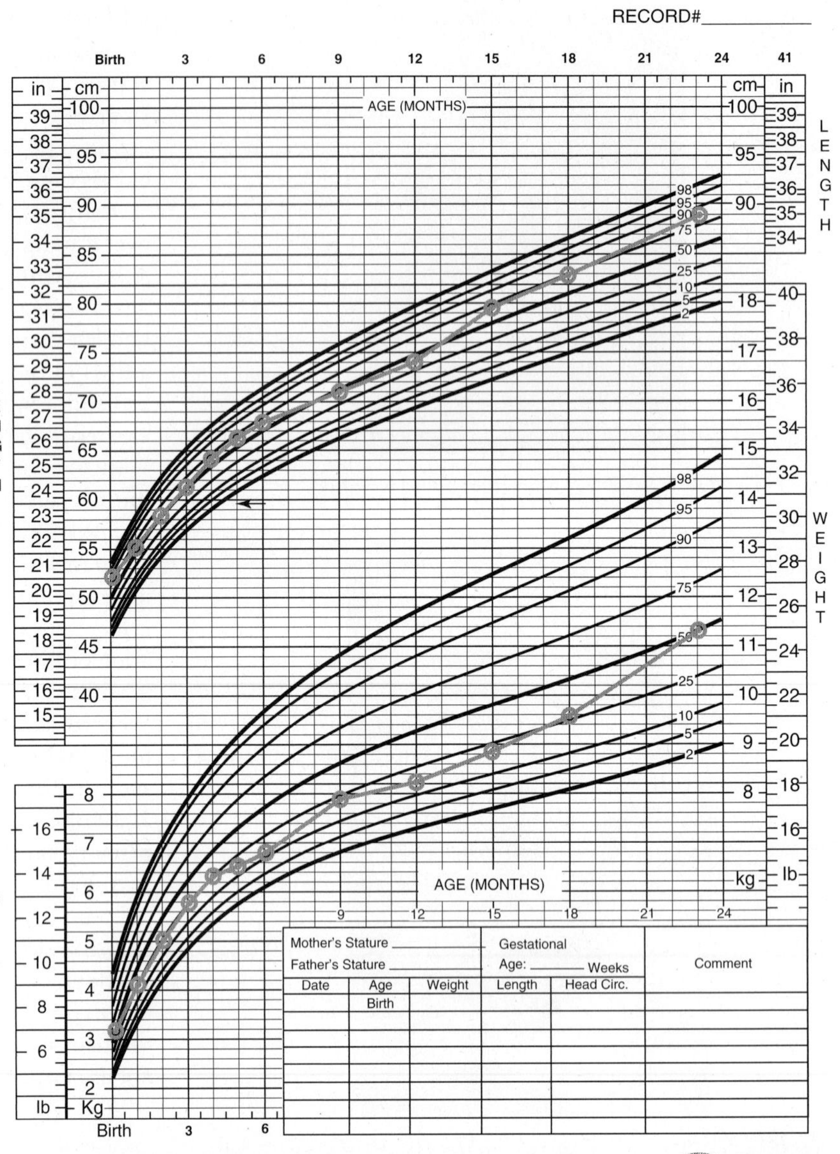


SOURCE: Developed by the National Center for Health Statistics in collaboration with the National Center for Chronic Disease Prevention and Health Promotion (2000). http://www.cdc.gov/growthcharts

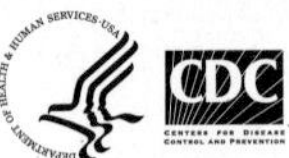


ILLUSTRATION 10.4 ▸ Birth to 24 months: Girls' length-for-age and weight-for-age percentiles.[6]

**Cognitive Development of Toddlers** With toddlers' newly acquired physical skills, exploring the environment accelerates, and exerting their newfound independence becomes very important to them. Toddlers now have the power to control the distance between themselves and their parents. Toddlers often "orbit" around their parents like planets, moving away, looking back, moving farther, and then returning.[6]

From a socialization standpoint, the child moves from being primarily self-centered to being more interactive. The toddler now possesses the ability to explore the environment and to develop new relationships. Fears of certain situations, such as separation, darkness, loud sounds, wind, rain, and lightning, commonly emerge during this period as the child learns to deal with changes in the environment. Children develop rituals in their daily activities in an attempt to deal with these fears.

Social development also involves imitating others, such as parents, caretakers, siblings, and peers, during this time. The child in this stage begins to learn about the family's cultural customs, including those related to meals and food.

Dramatic development of language skills occurs from age 18–24 months. Once a child realizes that words can stand for things, his vocabulary erupts from 10–15 words at 18 months to 100 or more words at 2 years of age. The toddler soon begins combining words to make simple sentences. By 36 months, the child uses three-word sentences.[6]

An important social change for toddlers is increased determination to express their own will. This expression often comes in the form of negativism and the beginning of temper tantrums, which give this stage of development its label of "the terrible twos." With an increase in motor development, coupled with an increasing quest for independence, toddlers try to do more and more things, pushing their capabilities to the limit. Thus, the toddler can easily become frustrated and negative. The child seeks more independence and at the same time needs the parents and caretakers for security and reassurance. Toddler behavior uncannily parallels the same type of behavior commonly seen in adolescents!

**Development of Feeding Skills in Toddlers** Many babies begin to wean from the breast or the bottle at about 9–10 months of age, when their solid food intake increases, and they learn to drink from a cup.[10] Parents need to pay attention to cues of readiness for weaning, such as disinterest in breastfeeding or bottle feeding. The time it takes to wean is variable and depends on both the child and the mother. Weaning will be easier for those babies who adapt well to change. Weaning is a sign of the toddler's growing independence and is usually complete by 12–14 months of age, although the age varies from child to child.

Gross and fine motor development during the toddler years enhances children's ability to chew foods of different textures and to self-feed. Between 12 and 18 months, toddlers are able to move the tongue from side to side (or laterally) and learn to chew food with rotary, rather than just up and down, movements. Toddlers can now handle chopped or soft table food.

At about 12 months, children have a refined pincer grasp that enables them to pick up small objects, such as cooked peas and carrots, and put them into their mouths. Children will be able to use a spoon around this age, but not very well. At 18–24 months, toddlers are able to use the tongue to clean the lips and have well-developed rotary chewing movements. Now the toddler can handle meats, raw fruits and vegetables, and multiple food textures.

A strong need for independence in self-feeding emerges during the toddler age. "I do it!" and "No, no, no!" are commonly heard phrases in households where toddlers reside. As toddlers practice their newfound skills, they become easily distracted. Parents need to realize that their toddler's sometimes-fierce independence is part of normal growth and development and represents an ongoing process of separation from dependency on the parents and caretakers.

Increasing fine motor and visual motor coordination skills allows toddlers to use cups and spoons more effectively. Although skill with a spoon increases during the second year, toddlers prefer to eat with their hands. Initial attempts at self-feeding are inevitably messy (Illustration 10.5), but represent an important stage of development. It is important that parents and caretakers keep distractions, such as television, to a minimum during mealtimes, and allow their toddlers to practice self-feeding skills and to experience new foods and textures. The child derives pleasure in self-feeding and exploring new tastes. Learning to self-feed allows the child to develop mastery of an important part of everyday life.

Adult supervision of eating is imperative due to the high risk of choking on foods at this age. Toddlers should always be seated during meals and snacks, preferably in a high chair or booster seat with the family, and not allowed to "eat on the run." Foods that may cause choking, such as hard candy, popcorn, nuts, whole grapes, and hot dogs, should not be served to children less than 2 years of age.[10]

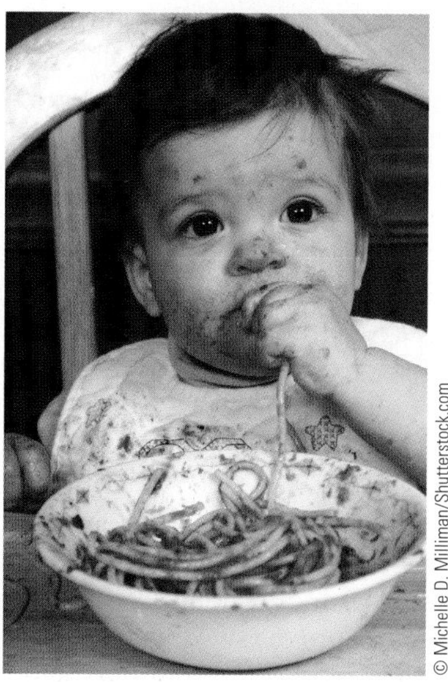


ILLUSTRATION 10.5 ▸ Toddler enjoying mealtime!

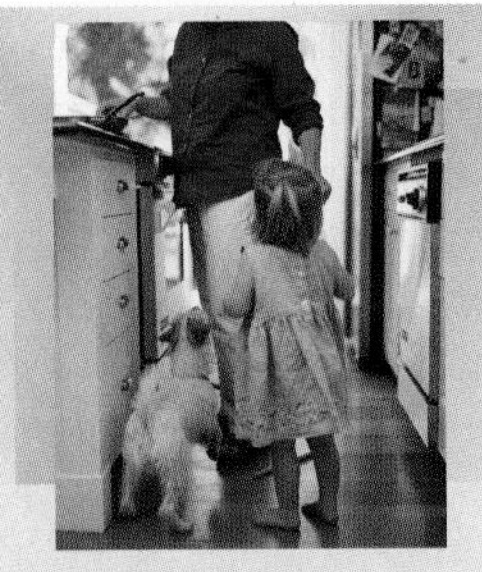
Ryan McVay/Getty Images

# CASE STUDY 10.1

## Meal Time With a Toddler

Josiah, a 22-month-old boy, lives with his mother and grandmother. He is at an early childhood center during the weekdays, and due to his mother's work schedule does not get home until after 6 p.m. most days. His mother and grandmother allow him to walk around the house with apple juice in a sippy cup while they are preparing dinner. He also "demands" snacks such as crackers, slices of cheese, and cookies. When they attempt to put Josiah in his booster chair at the table, he fights with them and yells, "NO chair!" Mother and grandmother often eat quickly in front of the television while feeding Josiah from their plates while he also watches TV. Josiah's mother and grandmother are frustrated and are concerned that he is not eating enough for dinner. The early childhood staff also state that they are having a difficult time with him sitting down at lunch time.

### *Questions*

1. Describe the issues surrounding Josiah's mealtime behaviors.
2. Describe how Josiah's mother and grandmother could introduce new foods into Josiah's diet.
3. What suggestions can you give for between-meal snacks for Josiah?
4. What concerns do you have about giving Josiah unlimited access to apple juice in the sippy cup?
5. How can healthy eating behaviors be developed in Josiah?
6. Should Josiah be encouraged to eat all the food on his plate before he is allowed to get down from his booster chair and play? Why or why not?

**Feeding Behaviors of Toddlers** The toddler's need for rituals, a hallmark of this stage of development, may be linked to the development of food jags. Many toddlers demonstrate strong food preferences and dislikes. They can go through prolonged periods of refusing a particular food or foods they previously liked. The intensity of the refusal or the negative attitude toward a particular food will be influenced by the child's temperament (see the "Temperament Differences" section). To circumvent food jags, parents can serve new foods along with familiar foods. New foods are better accepted if they are served when the child is hungry and if she sees other members of the family eating these foods. Eventually, toddlers' natural curiosity will get the best of them. Toddlers are great imitators, which includes imitating the eating behavior of others.

Mealtime is an opportunity for toddlers to practice newly acquired language and social skills and to develop a positive self-image. It is important for caregivers to offer a variety of foods and textures but not to force a toddler to eat. Battles over food intake should be avoided, as family mealtime should provide an opportunity for parents and caretakers to model healthy eating behaviors for the young child establishing the habit of eating breakfast is also an important part of healthy eating behaviors.

**Appetite and Food Intake of Toddlers** Parents need to be reminded that toddlers naturally have a decreased interest in food because of slowing growth, and a corresponding decrease in appetite. Besides, with all of their newfound gross and fine motor skills, they have places to go and new environments to explore! It is a part of normal growth and development for toddlers to be easily distracted at mealtime.

Toddlers need toddler-sized portions. One rule of thumb for serving size is 1 tablespoon of food per year of age. Applying this rule, a serving for a 2-year-old child would be about 2 tablespoons. It is better to give the child a small portion and allow him to ask for more than to serve large portions. Parents often overestimate portion sizes needed by their young child, which may contribute to labeling the child as a "picky" eater. Because toddlers can't eat a large amount of food at one time, snacks are vital in meeting the child's nutritional needs. It is important, however, that toddlers not be allowed to "graze" throughout the day on sweetened beverages and foods such as cookies and chips. These foods can blunt their limited appetite for basic foods at meal and snack times.

In considering the toddler's need for rituals and limit setting, parents and caretakers need to establish regular but flexible meal and snack times, allowing enough time between meals and snacks for the toddler to get hungry. It is important that toddlers be allowed to control the amount of food eaten by hunger rather than by parental pressure to eat more (Case Study 10.1).

## Preschool-Age Children

Preschool-age children continue to expand their gross and fine motor capabilities. At age 4, the child can hop, jump on one foot, and climb well. The child can ride a tricycle, or a bicycle with training wheels, and can throw a ball overhand.[6]

**Cognitive Development of Preschool-Age Children** Magical thinking and egocentrism characterize the preschool period.[5] Egocentrism does not mean that the child is selfish, but rather, that the child is not able to understand that another individual has a point of view. The child is beginning to interact with a widening circle of adults and peers. During the preschool years, children gradually move from primarily relying on external behavioral limits, such as those demanded by parents and caregivers, to learning to limit behavior internally. This transition is a prerequisite to functioning in a school classroom.[6] Also, during this time, children's play starts to become more cooperative, such as building a tower of blocks together. Toward the end of the preschool years, children move to more organized group play, such as playing tag or "house."

Control is a central issue for preschool children. They will test their parents' limits and still resort to temper tantrums to get their way. Temper tantrums generally peak between the ages of 2 and 4 years.[6] The child's challenge is to separate, and the parent's challenge is to appropriately set limits and at the same time to let go, another parallel with adolescence. Too-tightly controlled limits can undermine the child's sense of initiative and cause him or her to act out, whereas loose limits can cause the child to feel anxious and that no one is in control.

Language develops rapidly during the preschool years and is an important indicator of both cognitive and emotional development. Between ages 2 and 5, children's vocabularies increase from 50 to 100 words to more than 2,000 words, and their language progresses from two- to three-word sentences to complete sentences.[6]

**Development of Feeding Skills in Preschool-Age Children** The preschool-age child can use a fork and a spoon and uses a cup well. Cutting and spreading with a knife may need some refinement. Children should be seated comfortably at the table for all meals and snacks. Eating is not as messy a process during the preschool years as it was during toddlerhood. Spills still do occur, but they are not intentional. Foods that cause choking in young children should be modified to make them safer, such as cutting grapes in half lengthwise and cutting hot dogs in quarters lengthwise and then cutting into small bites. Adult supervision during mealtime is still imperative.

**Feeding Behaviors of Preschool-Age Children** As during the toddler years, parents of preschool-age children need to be reminded that the child's rate of growth continues to be relatively slow, with a relatively small appetite and food intake. Growth occurs in "spurts" during childhood. Appetite and food intake increase in advance of a growth spurt, causing children to add some weight that will be used for the upcoming spurt in height. Therefore, the appetite of a preschool-age child can be quite variable.

Preschool-age children want to be helpful and to please their parents and caretakers. This characteristic makes the preschool years a good time to teach children about foods, food selection, and preparation by involving them in simple food-related activities. For instance, outings to a farmers' market can introduce children to a variety of fresh vegetables and fruit. Allowing children to be involved in meal-related activities (Table 10.2) can be quite instructive.[11] Families of preschool-age children need to continue to be encouraged to eat together (Illustration 10.6).

**Innate Ability to Control Energy Intake** An important principle of nutrition for young children, and one with direct application to child feeding, is children's ability to self-regulate food intake. If allowed to decide when to eat and when to stop eating without outside interference, children eat as much as they need.[12,13] Children have an innate ability to adjust their caloric intake to meet energy needs. The preschool-age child's intake may fluctuate widely from meal to meal and day to day. But over a week's time, the young child's intake remains relatively stable.[14] Parents who try to interfere with the child's ability to self-regulate intake by forcing the child to "clean her plate" or using food as a reward are asking the child to overeat or undereat.

Although children can self-regulate caloric intake, no inborn mechanisms direct them to select and consume a well-balanced diet.[15] Children learn healthful eating habits.[16] Parents give up some control over what their preschool child eats if the child spends more time away

TABLE 10.2 ▸ MyPlate meal preparation activities for young children[11]

| At 2 years: |
|---|
| • Tear lettuce or greens.<br>• Rinse vegetables or fruits.<br>• Snap green beans. |
| **At 3 years:** |
| • Mash potatoes.<br>• Squeeze citrus fruits.<br>• Stir pancake batter. |
| **At 4 years:** |
| • Peel eggs and some fruits, such as oranges and bananas.<br>• Crack eggs.<br>• Help make sandwiches and tossed salads. |
| **At 5 years:** |
| • Measure liquids.<br>• Cut soft fruits with a dull knife.<br>• Use an eggbeater. |

SOURCE: "Picky Eating: Kitchen Activities," U.S. Department of Agriculture, www.choosemyplate.gov.

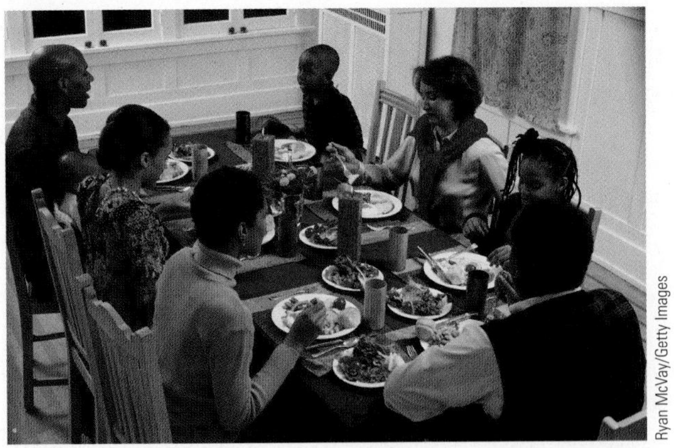

Ryan McVay/Getty Images

ILLUSTRATION 10.6 ▸ Sharing family meals is an important aspect of development in young children.

from home in a child care center or with extended family members. Preschool-age children continue to learn about food and food habits by observing their parents, caretakers, peers, and siblings, and they begin to be influenced by what they see on television and through other forms of media. Their own food habits and food preferences are established at this time.

**Appetite and Food Intake of Preschoolers** Parents of a preschool-age child often describe their child's appetite as "picky." One reason a child may want the same foods all of the time is because familiar foods may be comforting to her. Another reason is that the child may be trying to exert control over this aspect of her life. The child's eating and food selection can easily become a battleground between parent and child and this scenario should be avoided. Some practical suggestions include serving child-sized portions and serving the food in an attractive way. Young children often do not like their foods to touch or to be mixed together, such as in casseroles or salads. They typically do not like strongly flavored vegetables and other foods, or spicy foods, at this young age. Just as with toddlers, parents of preschool-age children should not allow their children to eat and drink indiscriminately between meals and snacks. This behavior often causes a blunted appetite at mealtime. Children should not be forced to stay at the table until they have eaten a certain amount of food as determined by the parent.

### Temperament Differences

> "Better is a dinner of herbs where love is, than a fatted ox and hatred with it."
>
> —Proverbs 15:17

Temperament is defined as the behavioral style of the child, or the "how" of behavior. Three temperamental clusters have been defined: the "easy" child (about 40 percent of children), the "difficult" child (10 percent), and the "slow-to-warm-up" child (15 percent).[17] The remaining children, classified as "intermediate-low" or "intermediate-high," demonstrate a mixture of behaviors but gravitate toward one end of the spectrum.[17]

Children's temperaments affect feeding and mealtime behavior. The "easy" child is regular in function, adapts easily to regular schedules, and tries and accepts new foods readily. The "difficult" child, on the other hand, is characterized by irregularity in function and slow adaptability. This child is more reluctant to accept new foods and can be negative about them. The "slow-to-warm-up" child exhibits slow adaptability and negative responses to many new foods with mild intensity. With repeated exposure to new foods, this child can learn to accept them over time with limited complaining.[17]

The "goodness of fit" between the temperaments of the child and the parent or caretaker can influence feeding and eating experiences.[17] A mismatch can result in conflict over eating and food. Parents and caretakers need to be aware of the child's temperament when attempting to meet nutritional needs. The difficult or slow-to-warm-up child may pose special challenges that need to be addressed by gradually exposing the child to new foods and not hurrying him or her to accept them.[17]

### Food Preference Development, Appetite, and Satiety

Food preference development and regulation of food intake have been studied extensively by Leann Birch and associates.[18,19] It is clear that children's food preferences do determine what foods they consume. Children naturally prefer sweet and slightly salty tastes and generally reject sour and bitter tastes. These preferences appear to be unlearned and present in the newborn period. Children eat foods that are familiar to them, a fact that emphasizes the importance environment plays in the development of food preferences. Children tend to reject new foods initially but may learn to accept a new food with repeated exposure to it. It may take 8–10 exposures to a new food before it is accepted. Children who are raised in an environment where all members of the family eat a variety of foods are more likely to eat a variety of foods. One study showed that 5-year-old girls' fruit and vegetable intakes were related to their parents' fruit and vegetable intakes.[20]

Children also appear to have preferences for foods that are energy dense due to high levels of sugar and fat.[18,19] These preferences may develop because children associate eating energy-dense foods with pleasant feelings of satiety, or because these types of foods may be associated with special social occasions such as birthday parties. The context in which foods are offered to a child influences the child's food preferences. Foods served on a limited basis but used as a reward become highly desirable. Restricting a young child's access to a palatable food may actually promote the desirability and intake of that food.[21] Coercing or forcing children to eat foods can have a long-term negative impact on their preference for these foods.[18–20]

**Media Influence** Young children are also influenced by media. One study of advertisements during programming aimed specifically at toddlers and preschool-age children on three different networks found that more than half of all food advertisements were aimed specifically at children, and the majority of these advertisements were for fast-food chains or sweetened cereals. The ads associated the advertised product with fun and/or excitement and energy. Fast-food ads seemed to focus on building brand recognition through the use of licensed characters, logos, and slogans and were less likely to show food during the ads.[22]

**Appetite, Satiety** Children's energy intake regulation has been studied by giving children ***preloads*** of food or beverage of varying energy content followed by self-selected meals. In one such study, children ages 3–5 years were given either a low-energy preload beverage made with aspartame, or a high-energy preload beverage made with sucrose. Fat and protein content of the preloads did not differ. Children were then allowed to self-select their lunches. Children who had the low-calorie beverage before lunch consumed more calories at lunch, while those who had the higher-calorie beverage consumed fewer calories. These results indicate that young children are able to adjust caloric intake based on caloric need.[19,23] Similar studies were conducted in 2- to 5-year-olds using foods with dietary fat or Olestra, a nonenergy fat substitute. Results indicate that children compensated for the lower level of calories in food when Olestra was substituted for dietary fat.

The preloading protocol just described was also used to study children's responsiveness to caloric content of foods in the presence or absence of common feeding advice from adults. In one group, teachers were trained to minimize their control over how much the children ate. In the other group, teachers were trained to focus the children on external factors to control their intake, such as rewarding the children for finishing the portions served to them or encouraging them to eat because it was "time to eat." Results of this investigation show that when the adults focused the children on external cues for eating, children lost their ability to regulate food intake based on calories. It appears that children's innate ability to regulate caloric intake can be altered by child-feeding practices that focus on external cues rather than the child's own hunger and satiety signals.[23]

The effects of portion size on children's intakes were compared between classes of 3-year-old and 5-year-old children. The children were served a small, medium, or large portion of macaroni and cheese along with standard amounts of other foods in their usual lunchtime setting. Analysis of amount of food eaten showed that portion size did not affect the younger children's intakes; their intakes remained constant despite the amount of food served to them. In contrast, the 5-year-old children's intakes increased significantly with the larger portion sizes. The researchers conclude that by 5 years of age, children are influenced by the size of portions served to them, another external factor that influences intake.[24] A similar study in preschoolers with an average age of 4 years found that doubling an age-appropriate portion size of an entrée increased entrée and total energy intake by 25 percent and 15 percent, respectively.[25] These investigators raise the question of what effect large portion sizes have on overeating and, consequently, on the development of childhood overweight, and their results point to the possible benefits of allowing children to self-select their portion sizes.

Another study of 5-year-old girls and their parents looked at the effects of parents' restriction of palatable foods on their children's consumption of these foods. After a self-selected standard lunch, these 5-year-old girls were given free access to snack foods, such as ice cream, potato chips, fruit-chew candy, and chocolate bars. The daughters of parents who reported restricting access to snack foods indicated to the investigators that they ate "too much" of the snack foods and also reported negative emotions about eating the snack foods. Parents' restriction of foods actually promoted the consumption of these foods by their young daughters and, of even more concern, the daughters reported feeling badly about eating these "forbidden" foods.[26]

A related study found a lower self-concept in 5-year-old girls with high body weight.[27] Daughters of parents who restricted access to food and expressed concern about their daughter's weight status tend to have negative self-evaluations.[26] Mothers in particular seem to have more influence over their young daughters' beliefs about food and dieting.[28] Satter describes the optimal "feeding relationship" as one in which parents and caretakers are responsible for what children are offered to eat and the environment in which the food is served, while children are responsible for how much they eat or even whether they eat at a particular meal or snack.[29] According to Satter, if this feeding relationship is respected, then feeding and potential weight problems can be prevented.[29]

What implications does all this research have on child feeding practices? Based on the results of these studies, it appears that by late preschool age, children are more responsive to external cues than to their innate ability to self-regulate intake (Table 10.3).[19] The importance of appropriate parenting skills in helping children learn to self-regulate food intake and possibly avoid problems with obesity is echoed by a panel of obesity experts.[8,30] Birch's research also reinforces the

**preloads** Beverages or food such as yogurt in which the energy/macronutrient content has been varied by the use of various carbohydrate and fat sources. The preload is given before a meal or snack and subsequent intake is monitored. This study design has been employed by Birch et al. in their studies of appetite, satiety, and food preferences in young children.[19]

TABLE 10.3 ▸ Practical applications of child-feeding research[19]

- Parents should respond appropriately to children's hunger and satiety signals.
- Parents should focus on the long-term goal of developing healthy self-controls of eating in children and should look beyond their concerns regarding composition and quantity of foods children consume or fears that children may eat too much and become overweight.
- Parents should not attempt to control children's food intakes by attaching contingencies ("No dessert until you finish your rutabagas") and coercive practices ("Clean your plate, children in Bangladesh are starving").
- Parents should be cautioned not to severely restrict "junk foods," foods high in fat and sugar, as that may make these foods even more desirable to the child.
- Parental influence should be positively focused on the child developing food preferences and selection patterns of a variety of foods consistent with a healthy diet. Parental modeling of eating a varied diet at family mealtime will have a strong influence on children.
- Children have an unlearned preference for sweet and slightly salty tastes; they tend to dislike bitter, sour, and spicy foods.
- Children tend to be wary of new foods and tastes, and it may take repeated exposures to new foods before these are accepted.
- Children need to be served appropriate child-sized servings of food.
- Child feeding experiences should take place in secure, happy, and positive environments with adult supervision.
- Children should never be forced to eat anything.



important role that parents and caretakers play in modeling healthy eating behaviors for young children.

# Energy and Nutrient Needs

LO 10.4 Explain what influences energy needs of young children.

***Dietary Reference Intakes (DRIs)*** were developed from 1997 through 2010 and are continuingly updated based on science. The series of reports presents a comprehensive set of reference values for nutrient intakes for healthy individuals and populations in the United States and Canada. In the pediatric age range, reference intake values are available for females and males aged 0.0–0.5 year, 0.5–1 year, 1–3, 4–8, and 9–13 years of age. Information about the various DRI publications can be found on the National Academy Press website (www.nap.edu). Published DRI tables are provided on the inside front cover of this book.

## Energy Needs

DRIs have been established for the energy needs of young children.[31] The formula for Estimated Energy Requirements (EER) for children ages 13–36 months is (89 × weight of child [kg] – 100) + 20 (kcal for energy deposition). For example, a healthy 24-month-old girl who weighs 12 kg would have an EER of (89 × 12 kg – 100) + 20 = 988 kilocalories. Beginning at age 3, the DRI equations for estimating energy requirements are based on a child's gender, age, height, weight, and physical activity level (PAL). Categories of activity are defined in terms of walking equivalence (Table 10.4). Energy needs of toddlers and preschool-age children reflect the slowing growth velocity of children in this age group.

## Protein

***Recommended Dietary Allowances (RDAs)*** have been established for protein (Table 10.5).[31] These recommendations are easily met with typical American diets as well as with vegetarian diets. Adequate energy intake to meet an individual child's needs has a protein-sparing effect; that is, with adequate energy intake, protein is used for growth and tissue repair rather than for energy. Ingestion of high-quality protein, such as milk and other animal products, lowers the amount of total protein needed in the diet to provide the essential amino acids.

## Vitamins and Minerals

DRIs for vitamins and minerals have been established for the toddler and preschool-age child (Table 10.6).[32,33] Most children from birth to 5 years are meeting the targeted levels of consumption of most nutrients, except for iron, calcium, and zinc (see the "Recommended vs. Actual Intake" section).

# Common Nutrition Problems

LO 10.5 Identify one common nutritional problem of young children and describe prevention strategies.

## Iron-Deficiency Anemia

Iron deficiency and iron-deficiency ***anemia*** are prevalent nutrition problems among young children in the United States.

**Dietary Reference Intakes (DRIs)** Quantitative estimates of nutrient intakes, used as reference values for assessing the diets of healthy people. DRIs include Recommended Dietary Allowances (RDAs), Adequate Intakes (AI), Tolerable Upper Intake Levels (UL), and Estimated Average Requirements (EAR).

**Recommended Dietary Allowances (RDAs)** The average daily dietary intake levels sufficient to meet the nutrient requirements of nearly all (97–98%) healthy individuals in a population group. RDAs serve as goals for individuals.

**anemia** A reduction below normal in the number of red blood cells per cubic mm in the quantity of hemoglobin, or in the volume of packed red cells per 100 mL of blood. This reduction occurs when the balance between blood loss and blood production is disturbed.

TABLE 10.4 ▸ Estimated energy requirements (in kcals) for reference boys and girls at selected ages and varying physical activity levels (PAL)[31]

| AGE/GENDER | REFERENCE WEIGHT (KG [LBS]) | REFERENCE HEIGHT (M [IN]) | SEDENTARY PAL (KCAL/D) | LOW ACTIVE PAL (KCAL/D) | ACTIVE PAL (KCAL/D) | VERY ACTIVE PAL (KCAL/D) |
|---|---|---|---|---|---|---|
| 3-year-old boy | 14.3 (31.5) | 0.95 (37.4) | 1162 | 1324 | 1485 | 1683 |
| 4-year-old boy | 16.2 (35.7) | 1.02 (40.2) | 1215 | 1390 | 1566 | 1783 |
| 5-year-old boy | 18.4 (40.5) | 1.09 (42.9) | 1275 | 1466 | 1658 | 1894 |
| 3-year-old girl | 13.9 (30.6) | 0.94 (37.0) | 1080 | 1243 | 1395 | 1649 |
| 4-year-old girl | 15.8 (34.8) | 1.01 (39.8) | 1133 | 1310 | 1475 | 1750 |
| 5-year-old girl | 17.9 (39.4) | 1.08 (42.5) | 1189 | 1379 | 1557 | 1854 |

SOURCE: Data from National Academy of Sciences, Institute of Medicine, Food and Nutritional Board.

TABLE 10.5 ▸ Dietary Reference Intakes for protein[31]

| AGE | RDA* G/KG/D |
|---|---|
| 1–3 years | 1.1 g/kg/d or 13 g/day* |
| 4–8 years | 0.95 g/kg/d or 19 g/day* |

SOURCE: From the National Academy of Sciences, Institute of Medicine, Food & Nutritional Board.

*RDA based on average weight for age (reference individual).

TABLE 10.6 ▸ Dietary Reference Intakes for key nutrients for toddlers and preschoolers[32,33]

| | RECOMMENDED DIETARY ALLOWANCES | | |
|---|---|---|---|
| AGE | IRON (MG/D) | ZINC (MG/D) | CALCIUM (MG/D) |
| 1–3 years | 7 | 3 | 700 |
| 4–8 years | 10 | 5 | 1000 |

SOURCE: National Academy of Sciences, Institute of Medicine, Food and Nutritional Board.

A rapid growth rate coupled with frequently inadequate intake of dietary iron places toddlers, especially 9- to 18-month-olds, at the highest risk for iron deficiency.[34] According to the National Health and Nutrition Examination Survey (NHANES), 15.9 percent of toddlers aged 1–2 years and 5.3 percent of children aged 3–4 years were iron deficient from 2005–2008.[4] Iron-deficiency anemia is more common among low-income children and among African American and Mexican American children.[1] The full impact of this nutrition problem is profound. Iron-deficiency anemia in young children appears to cause long-term delays in cognitive development and behavioral disturbances.[1,10,34] Healthy People 2020 objective NWS-21 is to reduce iron deficiency in young children to 14.3 percent for 1- to 2-year-olds (a 10 percent improvement) and 4.3 percent for 3- to 4-year-olds (a 1 percentage point improvement).[4]

Iron deficiency can be defined as absent bone marrow iron stores, an increase in hemoglobin concentration of <1.0 g/dL after treatment with iron, or other abnormal lab values, such as serum ferritin concentration, the storage form of iron (Table 10.7).[34] The definition of iron-deficiency anemia is less than the 5th percentile of the distribution of ***hemoglobin*** concentration or ***hematocrit*** in a healthy reference population. Age- and sex-specific cutoff values for anemia are derived from NHANES III data. For children 1–2 years old, the diagnosis of anemia would be made if the hemoglobin concentration is <11.0 g/dL and hematocrit <32.9 percent. For children ages 2–5 years, a hemoglobin value <11.1 g/dL or hematocrit <33.0 percent is diagnostic of iron-deficiency anemia. Not all anemias are due to iron deficiency. Other causes of anemia include other nutritional deficiencies (such as folate or vitamin $B_{12}$), chronic inflammation, or recent or current infection.[34]

**Preventing Iron Deficiency** The Centers for Disease Control recommends that children 1–5 years of age drink no more than 24 ounces of cow's milk, goat's milk, or soy milk each day because of the low iron content of these milks. Larger intakes of these milks may displace high-iron foods. For detecting iron deficiency, it is recommended that children at high risk for iron deficiency, such as low-income children and migrant and recently arrived refugee children, be tested for iron deficiency between the ages of 9 and 12 months, 6 months later, and then annually from ages 2–5 years. For children who are not at high risk for iron deficiency, selective screening of children at risk only is recommended by the CDC.[34] Children at risk include those who have a low-iron diet, consume more than 24 ounces of milk per day, have limited access to food because of poverty or neglect, and who have special health care needs, such as an inborn error of metabolism or chronic illness. The American Academy of

**hemoglobin** A protein that is the oxygen-carrying component of red blood cells. A decrease in hemoglobin concentration in red blood cells is a late indicator of iron deficiency.

**hematocrit** An indicator of the proportion of whole blood occupied by red blood cells. A decrease in hematocrit is a late indicator of iron deficiency.

TABLE 10.7 ▸ Evidenced-Based Recommendations for Diet and Nutrition (for cardiovascular health)[65]

| CHILD-1 (CARDIOVASCULAR HEALTH INTEGRATED LIFESTYLE DIET FOR CHILDREN WITH RISK FACTORS) | |
|---|---|
| **12 to 24 months** | Transition to reduced-fat unflavored cow's milk<br>Limit/avoid sugar-sweetened beverage intake, encourage water<br>Transition to table food with:<br>• Total fat 30% of daily kcal/Estimated Energy Requirement (EER)<br>• Saturated fat 8%–10% of daily kcal/EER<br>• Avoiding *trans* fat as much as possible<br>• Monounsaturated and polyunsaturated fat up to 20% of daily kcal/EER<br>• Cholesterol <300 mg/d |
| **2 to 10 years** | Primary beverage fat-free unflavored milk<br>Limit/avoid sugar-sweetened beverages, encourage water<br>Fat content:<br>• Total fat 25%–30% of daily kcal/EER<br>• Saturated fat 8%–10% of daily kcal/EER<br>• Avoid *trans* fats as much as possible<br>• Monounsaturated and polyunsaturated fat up to 20% of daily kcal/EER<br>• Cholesterol <300 mg/d<br>Encourage high dietary fiber intake from foods |
| **CHILD-2-LDL (DIETARY MANAGEMENT OF ELEVATED LDL CHOLESTEROL)** | |
| **2 to 21 years** | Refer to a registered dietitian for family medical nutrition therapy<br>25%–30% of calories from fat<br><7% of calories from saturated fat<br>≈10% from monounsaturated fat<br><200 mg/d of cholesterol<br>Avoid *trans* fats as much as possible |
| **CHILD-2-TG (DIETARY MANAGEMENT OF ELEVATED TRIGLYCERIDES OR NON-HDL CHOLESTEROL)** | |
| **2 to 21 years** | Refer to a registered dietitian for family medical nutrition therapy<br>25%–30% of calories from fat<br>≤7% of calories from saturated fat<br>≈10% from monounsaturated fat<br><200 mg/d of cholesterol<br>Avoid *trans* fats as much as possible<br>Decrease sugar intake<br>• Replace simple with complex carbohydrates<br>• No sugar-sweetened beverages<br>Increase dietary fish to increase omega-3 fatty acids |

SOURCE: *Pediatrics,* 128, (December), Supplement 5, Nutrition and Diet section, pp. S220–S222, and Table 9–8, page S243.

Pediatrics recommendations support universal screening for iron deficiency and iron-deficiency anemia at about 12 months of age.[35]

**Nutrition Intervention for Iron-Deficiency Anemia**
Treatment of iron-deficiency anemia includes supplementation with iron drops at a dose of 3 mg/kg per day, counseling of parents or caretakers about diets that prevent iron deficiency, and repeat screening in 4 weeks. Dietary recommendations include increased consumption of lean meat, fish, and poultry and the inclusion of sources of vitamin C at meal time to increase the absorption of nonmeat sources of iron.[10,35] An increase of >1 g/dL in hemoglobin concentration, or >3 percent in hematocrit, within 4 weeks of initiation of treatment confirms the diagnosis of iron deficiency. If the anemia is responsive to treatment, dietary counseling should be reinforced, and the iron treatment should be continued for two months.

At that time, the hemoglobin and hematocrit should be rechecked, and the child should be reassessed in 6 months. If the hemoglobin and hematocrit do not increase after 4 weeks of iron treatment, further diagnostic tests are needed. Iron status will not improve with iron supplements if the cause of the anemia is not directly related to a need for iron.[34]

## Dental Caries

Approximately one in three children aged 3–5 years had decay in at least one primary or permanent tooth in 1999–2004.[4] During this same time period, 23.8 percent of children aged 3–5 years had at least one primary tooth with untreated dental decay. This issue occurs across all ethnic and racial groups although it appears to be more prevalent in Non-White children. Recent NHANES data show that untreated tooth decay in primary teeth among children aged 2–8 was twice as high for Hispanic and Non-Hispanic black children compared with Non-Hispanic white children in 2011–2012.[36]

Healthy People 2020 Oral Health (OH) objectives 1.1 and 2.1 focus on reducing the proportion of children and adolescents who have dental caries experience and with untreated dental decay in their primary teeth.[4] A primary cause of dental decay is habitual use of a bottle or a no-spill training cup with milk or fruit juice at bedtime or throughout the day. Prolonged exposure of the teeth to these fluids can produce ***early childhood caries (ECC)***, formerly called *nursing bottle caries* or *baby bottle tooth decay*.[36] Upper front teeth are most severely affected by decay, which is where fluids pool when toddlers fall asleep while drinking from a bottle. Toddlers with baby-bottle tooth decay are at increased risk for caries in the permanent teeth as the conditions that lead to ECC (poor diet and poor oral health habits) often continue into childhood.[36] Food sources of carbohydrates such as milk and fruit juice can have direct effects on dental caries development because *Streptococcus mutans,* the main type of bacteria that cause tooth decay, use carbohydrates for food. Bacteria present in the mouth excrete acid that causes the tooth decay.[37] Consequently, the more often and longer teeth are exposed to carbohydrates, the more the environment in the mouth is conducive to the development of tooth decay.[10] Foods containing carbohydrates that stick to the surface of the teeth, such as sticky candy like caramel, are strong caries promoters. Rinsing the mouth with water or brushing teeth to get rid of the carbohydrate stuck to teeth reduces caries formation. Young children allowed to "graze" or indiscriminately eat or drink throughout the day likely expose their teeth to carbohydrates for a longer period of time, which encourages bacteria proliferation and tooth decay. Crunchy sweet foods such as carrot sticks and apple slices, when age-appropriate, are good choices for snacks because they are less likely to promote tooth decay than are sticky candies.

**Fluoride** Children need a source of fluoride in the diet, preferably from fluoridated water and the use of fluoridated toothpaste. If the water supply is not adequately fluoridated, a fluoride supplement is recommended. The American Dental Association, the American Academy of Pediatrics, and the American Academy of Pediatric Dentistry have devised a fluoride supplementation schedule, which is based on the child's age and the fluoride content of the local water supply.[37,38] Children ages 6 months to 3 years need 0.25 mg of fluoride per day if their local water supply has <0.3 ppm of fluoride. Children 3–6 years of age need 0.5 mg fluoride per day if their water supply has <0.3 ppm, but only 0.25 mg fluoride per day if the local water has 0.3–0.6 ppm of fluoride.[37,38] Excessive fluoride supplementation, consumption of toothpaste with fluoride, and natural water supplies high in fluoride can cause ***fluorosis***.

Although otherwise harmless, fluorosis produces permanent staining of the enamel of teeth, particularly permanent teeth. Because of the risk of fluorosis, fluoride supplements are only available by prescription. Few foods contain much fluoride, but fluoridated water used in beverages and food preparation does provide fluoride.

## Constipation

Constipation, or hard and dry stools associated with painful bowel movements, is a common problem of young children. Sometimes *stool holding* develops when the child does not completely empty the rectum, which can lead to chronic overdistension so that eventually the child is retaining a large fecal mass.[39] Then having a bowel movement can become painful to the child, which leads to more stool holding, and a vicious cycle ensues. A pediatrician should manage the treatment of stool holding.

Diets providing adequate total or dietary fiber for age Table 10.10 and appropriate amounts of fluid guard against constipation. Some of the best food sources of dietary fiber for toddlers and preschoolers are whole-grain breads and cereals, legumes, and fruits and vegetables appropriate for age. Too much fiber should be avoided, however. Young children easily develop diarrhea from high amounts of fiber, and high-fiber foods may displace other energy-dense foods and may decrease the bioavailability of some minerals, such as iron and calcium.

## Elevated Blood Lead Levels

According to NHANES 1999–2002 data, approximately 1.6 percent of children 1–5 years of age had high blood lead levels, exceeding 10 mcg/dL, which

**early childhood caries (ECC)** The presence of one or more decayed (noncavitated or cavitated lesions), missing (due to caries), or filled tooth surfaces in any primary tooth in a child 71 months of age or younger.[36]

**fluorosis** Permanent white or brownish staining of the enamel of teeth caused by excessive ingestion of fluoride before teeth have erupted.[37]

was the highest prevalence of all age groups.[40] A further reduction was seen in the NHANES 2005–2008 data when 0.9 percent of children aged 1–5 years were found to have elevated blood lead levels.[5] Healthy People 2020 Environmental Health (EH) objective 8.1 is to eliminate blood lead levels ≥10 mcg/dL, in young children and objective EH-8.2 is to reduce the mean blood lead levels in children aged 1–5 years from 1.5 mcg/dL in 2005–2008 to a target of 1.4 mcg/dL.[5] The major sources of lead exposure for young children are airborne lead, which has decreased in recent decades with the elimination of lead from gasoline and with the enforcement of industrial emissions standards, and leaded chips and dust, mainly from deteriorating lead paint.[41] Young children are particularly at risk for developing high levels of lead because, in exploring their environment, they enjoy putting things into their mouths. Depending on their surroundings, some of these objects may be high in lead. Damage caused by lead exposure may begin during pregnancy as lead is transported across the placenta to the fetus. Blood lead levels peak at about 2 years of age.[41] There are racial, ethnic, and socioeconomic disparities in children with high lead levels, with higher rates found in children living in poverty, children of minority groups, and recent immigrants.[41,42]

High blood lead levels affect the functioning of many tissues in the body, including the brain, blood, and kidneys. Low-level exposure to lead is associated with decreases in IQ and impaired motor, behavioral, and physical abilities.[41,43] Elevated blood lead levels may decrease growth in young children.[44] Historically, a blood lead level of 10 mcg/dL prompted action. However, some more recent research indicates that the physical and mental development of children may be affected by blood lead levels <10 mcg/dL, and no safe level of blood lead in children has been established.[41,45]

About 25 percent of children still live in housing with deteriorated lead-based paint.[41] Children living in housing built before 1978 are at increased risk of high lead levels because lead-based paint may have been used on these houses.[45] Lead-based paint chips taste sweet, tempting children to consume them. As the age of housing decreases nationally, so does the incidence of high lead levels in children.[5] Lead can enter the food supply through lead-soldered water pipes, contaminated water supplies, and from certain canned goods from other countries that contain lead-solder seals. Nonfood items containing lead include contaminated dirt and lead weights. Some parental occupations can be a source of lead. In these cases, parents should remove work clothing at work and wash work clothes separately. Other sources of lead include ceramic glazes and pewter used in some folk remedies and hobbies.[41]

The CDC published guidelines for screening children for lead poisoning in 1997, which was endorsed by the American Academy of Pediatrics (AAP).[46,41,47] The AAP advocates for a shift in focus from case identification and management to primary prevention. The CDC's recommendation includes a reference value of the 97.5th percentile of the NHANES generated blood lead levels distribution in children 1–5 years old (currently 5 mcg/dL) be used to identify those children with elevated blood lead levels.[47]

Federal policy requires lead screening of children who are enrolled in Medicaid.[10,41,46,47] Most local and state health departments have established recommendations for targeted screening based on the risk factors in the community. When indicated, lead screening should be obtained at 9–12 months of age and again around 24 months of age, when blood lead levels peak. Besides the age of the housing, other risk factors for high blood lead levels include living in poverty and having a sibling or playmate who has had high blood lead levels.

**Nutritional Considerations** Some of the risk factors for elevated blood lead levels are also the same risk factors for iron-deficiency anemia, such as young age, poor nutrition, and low socioeconomic status.[43] Iron-deficiency anemia is associated with pica, the ingestion of nonfood items, such as paint chips, which is a risk factor for lead ingestion. Some studies suggest that adequate iron intake may decrease lead absorption, which reinforces the benefits of treating iron-deficiency anemia in young children.[43] Some studies suggest that vitamin C may increase lead excretion. Although the evidence is not strong enough to recommend for or against vitamin C supplementation for children with elevated blood lead levels, it is important for young children to have sources of vitamin C in their diets for the prevention of iron deficiency.[34,43] There is good evidence that dietary calcium competitively decreases lead absorption, but there is no clinical evidence that supplementing calcium beyond the adequate intake for age has a clinical effect on elevated blood lead levels.[43] Although animal and epidemiological studies point to an association between dietary fat intake and elevated blood lead levels, low-fat diets are not recommended for the treatment of elevated blood lead levels in young children. No clinical data exist showing the benefits, and fat is an important source of calories for young children.[41,43] To summarize, eliminating sources of lead in the child's environment is the most important step toward eliminating elevated blood lead levels in children. In addition, preventing iron deficiency and promoting a well-balanced diet that includes good sources of calcium and vitamin C help to prevent this problem in young children.

## Food Security

Healthy People 2020 NWS-12 objective is to eliminate very low ***food security*** among children.[5] In 2010, food insecurity was reported in 14.5 percent of households. Food insecurity is more likely to exist in households with children, particularly those headed by single women

**food security** Access at all times to a sufficient supply of safe, nutritious foods.

or single men, in households near or below the federal poverty line, and Black and Hispanic households.[48] Fifty-nine percent of households experiencing food insecurity reported participating in one or more of the three largest federal food and nutrition assistance programs.[48]

Food security is particularly important for young children because of their high nutrient needs for growth and development. Young children are a vulnerable group because they must depend on their parents and caretakers to supply them with adequate access to food. It appears that children who are hungry and have multiple experiences with food insufficiency are more likely to exhibit behavioral, emotional, and academic problems as compared to other children who do not experience hunger repeatedly.[49]

### Food Safety

Young children are especially vulnerable to foodborne illnesses because they can become ill from smaller doses of organisms. Key foodborne pathogens include *Campylobacter* species and *Salmonella* species, which are the most frequently reported foodborne illnesses in the United States, and the pathogen *E. coli 0157:H7,* which is the most commonly identified Shiga toxin–producing *E. coli* (STEC) in North America.[50] The highest rate of *Campylobacter* species infections is seen in children under age 1.[50] *Campylobacter* is transmitted by handling raw poultry, eating undercooked poultry, drinking raw milk or nonchlorinated water, or handling infected animal or human feces.[50] The most common cause of *Salmonella* food poisoning is consumption of foods containing undercooked or raw eggs, such as raw cookie dough containing eggs. Children younger than 10 years of age account for a disproportionate percent of cases of *E. coli*-related illness. It is a serious disease and can cause bloody diarrhea and ***hemolytic uremic syndrome (HUS),*** which can be fatal. Outbreaks of *E. coli* have been associated with ingestion of contaminated, undercooked hamburger meat, unpasteurized apple cider and juice, and unpasteurized milk. Employing proper food storage and preparation techniques at home, in child care centers, and in retail food establishments is essential for decreasing the incidence of foodborne illnesses in young children. Contamination of food products can occur at any point along the way from production to consumption. Therefore, risk reduction and controls can be targeted at various steps in food processing. One food safety education program, called FightBAC,™ was developed by the Partnership for Food Safety Education, a public/private partnership of industry, state and consumer organizations, and government agencies, including the CDC and EPA. FightBAC has four food-safety practice messages:[51]

- Clean: Wash hands and surfaces often.
- Separate: Don't cross-contaminate.
- Cook: Cook to proper temperatures.
- Chill: Refrigerate promptly.

The Dietary Guidelines for Americans include a recommendation for following food safety principles when preparing and eating foods to reduce the risk of foodborne illnesses.[52]

The AAP endorses the consumption of only pasteurized milk and milk products for pregnant women, infants, and children and a ban on the sale of raw or unpasteurized milk and milk products through out the United States. This ban includes the sale of certain raw milk cheeses, such as fresh cheeses, soft cheeses, and soft-ripened cheeses.[50]

## Prevention of Nutrition-Related Disorders

LO 10.6 Define overweight and obesity in young children.

The prevalence of ***overweight*** and ***obesity*** among children, adolescents, and adults in the United States has increased and represents a major public health problem. High-energy, high-fat diets, coupled with sedentary lifestyles, are thought to be major contributors to the increase in weight. Cardiovascular disease, a major cause of death and morbidity in the United States today, is also thought to be influenced by diets and sedentary lifestyles. Food habits, preferences, and behaviors established during the toddler and preschool ages logically influence dietary habits later in life and subsequent health status. Behaviors associated with risk factors for cardiovascular disease, including dietary habits, physical activity behaviors, and the use of tobacco, can be acquired in childhood.[53] The American Heart Association strongly advocates that primary prevention of atherosclerotic disease begin in childhood.[53] Families are encouraged to adopt dietary and exercise patterns that promote a healthy lifestyle.

### Overweight and Obesity in Toddlers and Preschoolers

Overweight and obesity continue to remain an issue in the toddler and preschool population; however, NHANES 2010–2011 data reported that the prevalence of obesity among children aged 2–5 years decreased significantly from 13.9 percent in 2003–2004 to 8.4 percent in 2011–2012.[54] No significant difference in prevalence of overweight and obesity was found between male

**hemolytic uremic syndrome (HUS)** A serious, sometimes fatal complication associated with illness caused by *E. coli 0157:H7,* which occurs primarily in children under the age of 10 years. HUS is characterized by renal failure, hemolytic anemia, and a severe decrease in platelet count.[50] Clean: Wash hands and surfaces often.

**overweight** Body mass index-for-age between the 85th and 94th percentiles.[8,55]

**obesity** BMI-for-age greater than or equal to the 95th percentile.[8,55]

and female children, but differences do exist by race/ethnicity. Obesity rates were lowest in Non-Hispanic Asian children (8 percent) compared to Non-Hispanic Whites (14 percent), Non-Hispanic Blacks (20 percent), and Hispanics (22 percent).[54]

Obesity is a multifaceted problem that is difficult to treat, making prevention the preferred approach. The American Medical Association (AMA) in collaboration with the Department of Health and Human Services (DHHS) convened a multidisciplinary committee of experts to develop evidence-based recommendations on the assessment, prevention, and treatment of child and youth overweight and obesity. The expert committee's work culminated in the publication of four articles: a summary report and three separate articles on the topics of assessment, prevention, and treatment, which were endorsed by 12 professional organizations including the American Academy of Pediatrics (AAP), the Academy of Nutrition and Dietetics (formerly the American Dietetic Association), and the American Heart Association (AHA).[8,30,55,56]

## Assessment of Overweight and Obesity

Body mass index-for-age percentile is recommended as the screening tool for assessment of pediatric overweight and obesity. A BMI-for-age percentile of 85th to 94th is defined as *overweight,* and a BMI-for-age ≥95th is defined as *obesity.*[8,55] BMI normative values are not available for children less than 2 years of age. For these young children, a weight-for-length >95th percentile is considered to be overweight.[8]

During the preschool years, a decrease in body mass index (BMI), or weight-for-height squared [wt(kg)/ht(m)$^2$], is a normal part of growth and development. BMI usually reaches its lowest point at approximately 4–6 years of age and then increases gradually in the period called ***BMI rebound.***[57] Early BMI rebound in children increases the risk of adult obesity.[58]

Other essential components of assessment include (1) evaluation of the child's medical risk, including parental obesity, family medical history, and evaluation of weight-related problems such as sleep and respiratory problems, and (2) behavior risk assessment, including dietary and physical activity behaviors.[8,55] Another aspect of the behavioral assessment is evaluation of the child's and/or family's attitudes toward and capacity to change some behaviors.[8,55]

## Prevention of Overweight and Obesity

All children should be targeted for prevention of overweight and obesity from birth by instituting lifestyle behaviors that prevent obesity.[8,30] The expert panel has identified the following target behaviors in the prevention of pediatric overweight and obesity based on available evidence and on analysis of available data and expertise:[8,30]

- Limiting sugar-sweetened beverages
- Encouraging consumption of recommended amounts of fruits and vegetables
- Limiting television and other screen time by allowing a maximum of 2 hours of screen time per day and removing televisions and other screens from children's bedrooms
- Eating breakfast every day
- Limiting eating out at restaurants, especially fast-food restaurants
- Limiting portion sizes
- Eating a diet rich in calcium
- Eating a diet high in fiber (see Table 10.10 for fiber recommendations)
- Eating a diet that follows the Dietary Reference Intakes for macronutrients (carbohydrates, protein, and fat)
- Promoting moderate to vigorous physical activity for at least 60 minutes each day
- Limiting energy-dense foods

Parenting techniques, such as finding reasons to praise the child's behavior but never using food as a reward, foster the development of healthy eating behaviors in children and help children to self-regulate food intake (see the "Food Preference Development, Appetite, and Satiety" section).

## Treatment of Overweight and Obesity Expert Committee: Recommendations

The goal of overweight and obesity treatment is the improvement of long-term physical health through permanent healthy lifestyle habits and behavior modification.[8,56] Improvement is measured by a decrease in BMI-for-age percentile, but this is difficult to see in the short-term. Weight measurements on a regular basis can be used to measure progress in the short-term. Maintaining weight while gaining height can be the best treatment for obese children between the ages of 2 and 5. This approach allows the obese child to "grow into his or her weight" and to lower BMI. If weight loss does occur, it should not exceed 1 pound per month in children this age, whether they fall into the overweight or obese category.[8,56]

The expert committee recommends a staged approach to pediatric overweight and obesity treatment (Illustration 10.7).

### Stage 1: Prevention Plus

This stage focuses on the behaviors identified in the prevention section. The health care provider can identify dietary and

**BMI rebound** A normal increase in body mass index that occurs after BMI declines and reaches its lowest point at 4–6 years of age.[57]

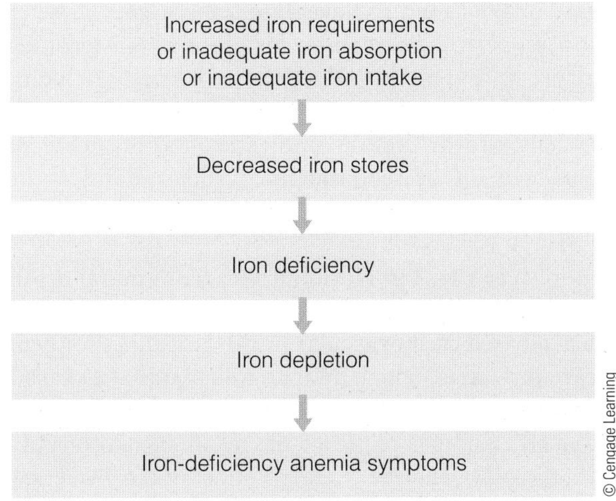


ILLUSTRATION 10.7 ▸ Progression of iron deficiency.

physical activity behaviors in the individual child and family that would be appropriate to target and, using motivational interviewing techniques, can assist the family in making appropriate changes. Targeted behaviors can be achieved in steps, with the ultimate goal being an improvement in BMI-for-age percentile. This stage involves more frequent follow-up based on the individual child and family's needs.[8,56]

**Stage 2: Structured Weight Management (SWM)** This stage of treatment is more structured and requires more frequent follow-up. Some of the elements of the Structured Weight Management Plan include a planned diet or daily eating plan, further reduction of screen time to less than 1 hour per day, and planned supervised physical activity or active play for 60 minutes per day. This stage includes monitoring behavior through the use of logs and planned reinforcement for achieving targeted behaviors. A registered dietitian or a clinician who has received additional training is required to work with the child and her family on an eating plan. Staff members also need to be trained in motivational interviewing. Depending on the family, a counselor may need to be involved to address parenting skills or to help resolve family issues that may be barriers to healthy lifestyle behaviors. Monthly visits are recommended, some of which may be group sessions.[8,56]

**Stage 3: Comprehensive Multidisciplinary Intervention** In this stage, the intensity of behavior change is increased and a multidisciplinary team, including a registered dietitian, an exercise specialist, a behavioral counselor, and the primary care provider, is needed to maximize support for behavior change. Weekly visits are recommended for a minimum of 8–12 weeks, some of which may be group visits. This stage is a structured program in behavior modification that includes, at a minimum, food monitoring, short-term diet resulting in a negative energy balance, and physical activity goal setting. Parents are involved in behavior modification for their child and in parental training for improving the home environment. There is a systematic evaluation of body measurements, diet, and physical activity at specified time intervals.

**Stage 4: Tertiary Care Intervention** This stage is offered to severely obese adolescents who have failed other interventions. This stage is not appropriate for the obese toddler or preschool-age child.[8,56]

## Dietary Guidelines for Americans 2010

The Dietary Guidelines for Americans 2010 emphasize the importance of maintaining appropriate calorie balance during each stage of life, including childhood, to manage weight and support the principles of pediatric weight management endorsed by the expert committee. Reducing weight at this young age is tricky because sufficient nutrients must be provided for children to reach their full height potential and to remain healthy.

## Nutrition and Prevention of Cardiovascular Disease in Toddlers and Preschoolers

***Heart disease*** is the number-one cause of death in the United States today. A leading risk factor for cardiovascular disease, which includes diseases of the heart and blood vessels, is elevated levels of ***LDL cholesterol***. Children with ***familial hyperlipidemias*** and obese children can have high levels of LDL cholesterol. High intakes of saturated fat, ***trans fatty acids***, and, to a lesser extent, dietary cholesterol elevate LDL cholesterol levels in children and adults alike. Other nutrition-related risk factors for cardiovascular disease include high triglyceride levels and high body mass index.[53] Fatty streaks, which can be precursors to the buildup of fat deposits in blood vessels, have been found in the arteries of young children. Some experts believe that these streaks can represent the beginning of ***atherosclerosis*** and cardiovascular disease.[53] Guidelines for promoting cardiovascular health and risk reduction in children have been published by several professional organizations and health agencies.

**heart disease** The leading cause of death and a common cause of illness and disability in the United States. Coronary heart disease is the principal form of heart disease and is caused by buildup of cholesterol deposits in the coronary arteries, which feed the heart.

**LDL cholesterol** Low-density lipoprotein cholesterol, the lipid most associated with atherosclerotic disease. Diets high in saturated fat, *trans* fatty acids, and dietary cholesterol have been shown to increase LDL cholesterol levels.

**familial hyperlipidemia** A condition that runs in families and results in high levels of serum cholesterol and other lipids.

***trans* fatty acids** Fatty acids that have unusual shapes resulting from the hydrogenation of polyunsaturated fatty acids. *Trans* fatty acids also occur naturally in small amounts in foods such as dairy products and beef.

**atherosclerosis** A type of hardening of the arteries in which cholesterol is deposited in the arteries. These deposits narrow the coronary arteries and may reduce the flow of blood to the heart.

The American Heart Association (AHA) has published guidelines for the primary prevention of atherosclerotic cardiovascular disease beginning in childhood.[53] In these guidelines, the AHA recommends that all children be screened for risk factors of developing future cardiovascular disease. Furthermore, the AHA recommends that all children have an overall healthy eating pattern while maintaining an appropriate body weight, desirable lipid profile, and desirable blood pressure. Avoidance of smoking is encouraged as well as daily physical activity and the reduction of sedentary time.[53] Like the obesity expert panel, the AHA has also published strategies for implementing the recommended guidelines that employ behavior change theory and motivational interviewing.[59] The AHA has published dietary recommendations for children, which have been endorsed by the American Academy of Pediatrics (AAP) and which are consistent with the U.S. Dietary Guidelines (see the "Dietary Guidelines" section on pages 293–294).[52,60,61] The recommended diet includes fruits and vegetables, whole-grain breads and cereals, the use of nonfat or low-fat dairy products, and two servings of fish weekly. The use of vegetable oils and soft margarines low in saturated fat and *trans* fatty acids instead of butter or most other animal fats is recommended. The recommendations also include reducing intake of sugar-sweetened beverages and foods and reducing salt intake.[60–62] For children ages 2–3 years, 30–35 percent of total energy from fat is recommended. For children 4 years of age or older, the recommendation is 25–35 percent of total energy from fat.[60,61] A *trans* fatty acid intake <1 percent of total calories is also recommended.[60,61] Studies have shown that such dietary restrictions are safe and effective for reducing risk factors in childhood without negatively impacting growth.[63]

According to the new DRIs,[31] the acceptable macronutrient distribution ranges (AMDRs) for fat are 30–40 percent for children 1–3 years and 25–35 percent for children 4–18 years. No specific recommendations for total fat per day in the diets of young children have been made. Adequate intake levels for the essential fatty acids, linoleic acid and alpha-linolenic acid, have been determined.[31]

The AAP endorses the population approach to a healthful diet for all children older than 2 years of age. Children with a positive family history of dyslipidemia or premature cardiovascular disease should be screened for high lipid levels. The individual approach to screening with a fasting lipid profile is also recommended for children whose family history is not known and for those children with other cardiovascular risk factors such as overweight/obesity, hypertension, or diabetes mellitus. Screening for these children should take place after 2 years of age, but not later than 10 years of age.[64]

Dietary recommendations are different for children who are at increased risk of developing premature cardiovascular disease or are found to have high lipid levels. These children need periodic screening for blood cholesterol levels and close follow-up. If LDL cholesterol levels are high, restriction of total calories from saturated fat to less than 7 percent and of dietary cholesterol to no more than 200 mg per day is recommended. These children need to be closely monitored by a physician and registered dietitian.[53]

More recently, the National Heart, Lung, and Blood Institute (NHLBI) convened a panel of experts to develop evidence-based cardiovascular health guidelines for pediatric care providers, which address all major cardiovascular risk factors simultaneously.[65] For the most part, this expert panel's findings reinforce the recommendations of the AHA, the AAP, and the Dietary Guidelines for Americans. The panel recommends a Cardiovascular Health Integrated Lifestyle Diet (CHILD-1) for children with identified dyslipidemia and other risk factors such as overweight and obesity as well as for children with a positive family history of early cardiovascular disease or risk factors such as obesity or primary hypertension. This panel recommends universal lipid screening between the ages of 9 and 11 years, as this has been determined to be a stable time for lipid assessment. Further dietary restrictions are recommended for children who have elevated LDL Cholesterol levels (CHILD-2-LDL) and elevated triglyercides (CHILD-2-TG) (see Table 10.7).[65]

## Vitamin and Mineral Supplements

Children who consume a variety of basic foods can meet all of their nutrient needs without vitamin or mineral supplements. Eating a diet of a variety of foods is the preferred way to get needed nutrients because foods contain many other substances, such as phytochemicals, in addition to nutrients that benefit health.

The AAP recommends vitamin and mineral supplementation for children who are at high risk of developing or have one or more nutrient deficiencies.[38] Children at risk of nutrient deficiency according to the AAP include those

1. With anorexia or an inadequate appetite or who follow fad diets
2. With chronic disease
3. From deprived families or who suffer from parental neglect or abuse
4. Who participate in a dietary program for managing obesity
5. Who consume a vegetarian diet without adequate intake of dairy products
6. With failure to thrive

Despite these recommendations, survey data indicate that young children are major users of supplements.[66,67] HANES 2003–2006 showed 39 percent of children ages

1–3 years and 43 percent ages 4–8 years have used one or more dietary supplements.[67] The most common type of supplement used by children was multivitamins and multiminerals.[67] Children most likely to receive supplements were underweight or at risk for underweight.[67] Considering characteristics of families who give their children supplements, such as a greater household income, the children most likely to receive a supplement are those at low risk of developing nutrient deficiencies—in other words, children who would most likely benefit from supplements are less likely to receive them.

If given to children, vitamin and mineral supplement doses should not exceed the DRI for age. Parents and caretakers should be warned against giving high amounts of vitamins and minerals to children, particularly vitamins A (retinol) and D. The ***Tolerable Upper Intake Levels*** shown in the DRI tables should serve as a guide to excessive levels of nutrient intake from fortified foods and supplements.

### Herbal Supplements

The use of herbal remedies for various disorders is increasing in the United States today, as is the use of complementary and alternative medicine practices in general. Parents and caretakers who take herbs are likely to give these products to their children. In one survey with a 59.4 percent response rate, participants of the Special Supplemental Nutrition Program for Women, Infants, and Children (WIC) in the states of Kansas and Wisconsin indicated herbal use by caregivers, children, or both in nearly half of the returned surveys. Herb use was statistically greater among Hispanic children than Non-Hispanic children, 48.4 percent versus 31.4 percent respectively. Of the 1363 children reported to use herbs, 820 of them were younger than 5 years of age.[68]

Few definitive studies exist on the effectiveness of these substances in preventing disease and promoting health in adults, much less in children. In spite of the lack of scientific evidence, anecdotal reports of benefits abound. However, some reports have linked herbal preparations to adverse effects.[69] Information on herb use should be obtained during the nutrition assessment of a child to rule out herbs as a source of health problems. Currently, herbal supplements are not regulated and using the products can lead to uncertain results. Children given various herbs are the "test subjects" in these uncontrolled studies. Parents should be advised of the potential risks of herbal therapies and the need for close monitoring of their child if they choose to give herbs to their child. The National Institutes of Health's (NIH) National Center for Complementary and Alternative Medicine (NCCAM) website (www.nccam.nih.gov) provides reports on the known safety and effectiveness of various herbal remedies and alternative medical practices.

## Dietary and Physical Activity Recommendations

LO 10.7 Describe the components of a healthy diet for young children as recommended by health and professional organizations and agencies.

"... Children ages 2 to 11 years should achieve optimal physical and cognitive development, attain a healthy weight, enjoy food, and reduce the risk of chronic disease through appropriate eating habits and participation in regular physical activity."[70]

—The American Dietetic Association (now The Academy of Nutrition and Dietetics)

Taking into consideration the energy and nutrient needs of young children and the common nutritional problems and concerns of this age group, it is easy to understand the importance of dietary recommendations for toddlers and preschoolers. A primary recommendation is that young children eat a variety of foods. This recommendation is more easily achieved if healthful food preferences and eating habits are acquired during the early years. Food preferences in conjunction with food availability form the foundation of the child's diet. Limited food selection, therefore, will influence the adequacy of the child's diet by decreasing variety. Parents and caretakers cannot expect a child to "do as I say, but not as I do." Nutrition education aimed at the adults in the child's life becomes as important as nutrition education directed at the child, if not more so.

Dietary recommendations have been developed and disseminated by the federal government and professional organizations. Two sets of guidelines for young children's diets are available: the Dietary Guidelines for Americans and MyPlate.[11,52] Recommendations for energy and nutrient intake are represented in the DRIs.

### Dietary Guidelines for Americans 2010

The Dietary Guidelines for Americans 2010 (discussed in Chapter 1) include some key recommendations for specific population groups, including children. The guidelines emphasize that children should be offered

**Tolerable Upper Intake Levels**
Highest level of daily nutrient intake that is likely to pose no risk of adverse health effects to almost all individuals in the general population; gives levels of intake that may result in adverse effects if exceeded on a regular basis.

TABLE 10.8 ▸ Tips for offering a variety of foods[11]

- Mix it up. Change your typical foods. Try something new with your family. Here are just a few ideas: fresh pineapple, green peppers, low-fat cheese, canned salmon, or a whole-wheat pita with hummus.
- Let your child choose a new vegetable to add to soup. Only an adult should heat and stir hot soup.
- Add different ingredients to your typical salads. Try adding mango, Swiss chard, or tuna to your green salad.
- Vary the cereals, types of bread, and sandwich fillings you buy week to week.
- Add fruit to your preschooler's breakfast by using it to top cereal.
- Put rinsed and cut fruits and vegetables, in a bag or bowl, on a shelf in your refrigerator where your child can see them.

SOURCE: "Develop Healthy Eating Habits: Offer a Variety of Foods," U.S. Department of Agriculture, www.choosemyplate.gov

a variety of foods, including grain products (at least half of which should be whole grains), vegetables (especially dark-green and red and orange vegetables) and whole fruits, and low-fat dairy products (Table 10.8).[52]

The guidelines also recommend reducing the amount of sugar-sweetened beverages and added sugar in children's diets. Children 2–8 years should drink 2 cups per day of fat-free or low-fat milk or equivalent milk products. With regard to fats, the guidelines recommend keeping total fat intake between 30 and 40 percent of calories for children 1–3 years of age and between 25 and 35 percent of calories for children and adolescents 4–18 years of age. Fat is an important source of calories, fat-soluble vitamins, and essential fatty acids for young children. Most fats in children's diets should come from sources of polyunsaturated and monounsaturated fatty acids, such as fish, nuts, and vegetable oils. Some fish may contain higher levels of mercury that may harm a young child's developing nervous system. The Food and Drug Administration (FDA) and the Environmental Protection Agency (EPA) advise that young children should eat fish and shellfish that are lower in mercury. Fish that are highest in mercury are tilefish from the Gulf of Mexico, shark, swordfish, and king mackerel. Draft Updated Advise from the FDA and EPA recommend these fish be avoided in young children.[70] Information about the mercury content of fish in a specific area can be obtained from the FDA (www.fda.gov).

The guidelines also recommend that beans, lean meats, and poultry be added as appropriate for the child. Foods high in solid fats and added sugar (SoFAS), such as candy, cookies, and cakes, should be limited in children's diets. The Dietary Guidelines also emphasize the importance of parents modeling this type of diet for their children, or encouraging them "to do as I say and as I do." The guidelines emphasize the importance of physical activity. Parents are advised to encourage their children, ages 6 years and older, to engage in at least 60 minutes of physical activity on most (preferably all) days of the week and to limit the time spent in sedentary activities, such as watching TV and playing computer and video games, that replace physical activity.[52] Although no specific quantitative recommendation for physical activity has been set for children 2–5 years of age, young children should play actively several times each day.[52] It is important that parents model for their children a lifestyle that includes a varied diet and regular physical activity. As mentioned previously, the American Heart Association dietary recommendations are consistent with the U.S. Dietary Guidelines. The AHA places special emphasis on adequate intake of omega-3 fatty acids and recommends introducing and regularly serving fish as an entrée to children. The recommendations also emphasize physical activity and balancing intake with physical activity.[53,60,61]

## MyPlate

The USDA has developed MyPlate, which replaces the MyPyramid and MyPyramid for Kids, as an education tool for consumers to employ the Dietary Guidelines for Americans.[11,52] The color-coded MyPlate icon, which is depicted in Chapter 1, encourages the consumption of a variety of foods from five food groups, using a place setting (a familiar mealtime visual), and is based on the Dietary Guidelines for Americans 2010 (Illustration 10.8).[52] Selected messages of ChooseMyPlate.gov, a website that provides practical information for building healthier diets, include making half the plate fruits and vegetables, making at least half of grains whole grains, switching to fat-free or low-fat milk, choosing foods lower in sodium, and drinking water instead of sugary drinks (Table 10.9).[11] Age-appropriate physical activity is also encouraged (Illustration 10.9).

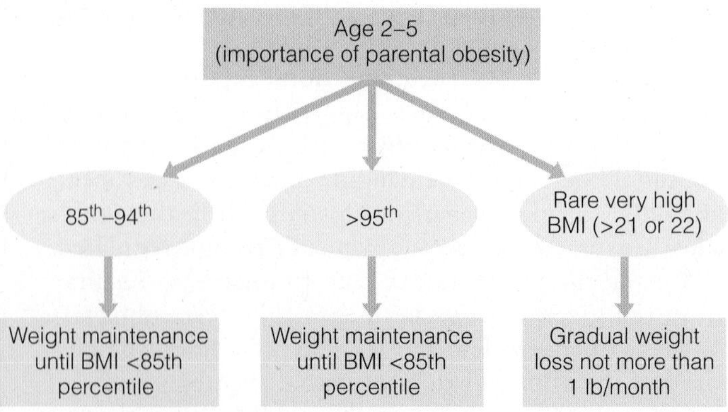


ILLUSTRATION 10.8 ▸ Suggested weight changes in staged treatment of pediatric obesity.

SOURCE: Based on data from Spear, B.A., et al. (2007). "Recommendations for treatment of child and adolescent overweight and obesity." *Pediatrics*, 120:S254–S288.

TABLE 10.9 ▸ MyPlate—Individual plan for a 4-year-old boy who is physically active for at least 60 minutes every day[11]

| CALORIES | ALLOWANCE | | |
|---|---|---|---|
| **Total Calories**<br>• Empty Calories* | **1600 per day**<br>• ≤121 per day | | |
| **FOOD GROUP** | **FOOD GROUP AMOUNT** | **"WHAT COUNTS AS . . ."** | **TIPS** |
| **Grains**<br>• Whole Grains | **5 oz per day**<br>• ≥3 oz per day | **1 oz of grains**<br>• 1 slice of bread (1 oz)<br>• ½ cup cooked pasta, rice, or cereal<br>• 1 oz uncooked pasta or rice<br>• 1 tortilla (6-in. diameter)<br>• 1 pancake (5-in. diameter)<br>• 1 oz ready-to-eat cereal (about 1 cup cereal flakes) | **Tips**<br>• Eat at least half of all grains as whole grains.<br>• Substitute whole-grain choices for refined grains in breakfast cereals, breads, crackers, rice, and pasta.<br>• Check product labels—is a grain with "whole" before its name listed first on the ingredients list? |
| **Vegetables**<br>• Dark Green<br>• Red & Orange<br>• Beans & Peas<br>• Starchy<br>• Other | **2 cup(s) per day**<br>• 1½ cup(s) per week<br>• 4 cup(s) per week<br>• 1 cup(s) per week<br>• 4 cup(s) per week<br>• 3½ cup(s) per week | **1 cup of vegetables**<br>• 1 cup raw or cooked vegetables<br>• 1 cup 100% vegetable juice<br>• 2 cups leafy salad greens | **Tips**<br>• Include vegetables in meals and in snacks. Fresh, frozen, and canned vegetables all count.<br>• Add dark-green, red, and orange vegetables to main and side dishes.<br>• Use dark leafy greens to make salads.<br>• Beans and peas are a great source of fiber. Add beans or peas to salads, soups, side dishes, or serve as a main dish. |
| **Fruits** | **1½ cup(s) per day** | **1 cup of fruit**<br>• 1 cup raw or cooked fruit<br>• 1 cup 100% fruit juice<br>• ½ cup dried fruit | **Tips**<br>• Select fresh, frozen, canned, and dried fruit more often than juice; select 100% fruit juice when choosing juice.<br>• Enjoy a wide variety of fruits, and maximize taste and freshness, by adapting your choices to what's in season.<br>• Use fruit as snacks, salads, or desserts. |
| **Dairy** | **2½ cup(s) per day** | **1 cup of dairy**<br>• 1 cup milk<br>• 1 cup fortified soymilk (soy beverage)<br>• 1 cup yogurt<br>• 1½ oz natural cheese (e.g. Cheddar)<br>• 2 ozs processed cheese (e.g. American) | **Tips**<br>• Drink fat-free (skim) or low-fat (1%) milk.<br>• Choose fat-free or low-fat milk or yogurt more often than cheese.<br>• When selecting cheese, choose low-fat or reduced-fat versions. |
| **Protein Foods**<br>• Seafood | **5 oz per day**<br>• 8 oz per week | **1 oz of protein foods**<br>• 1 oz lean meat, poultry, seafood<br>• 1 egg<br>• 1 Tablespoon peanut butter<br>• ½ oz nuts or seeds<br>• ¼ cup cooked beans or peas | **Tips**<br>• Eat a variety of foods from the Protein Foods group each week.<br>• Eat seafood in place of meat or poultry twice a week.<br>• Select lean meat and poultry. Trim or drain fat from meat and remove poultry skin. |
| **Oils** | **5 tsp per day** | **1 tsp of oil**<br>• 1 tsp vegetable oil (e.g. canola, corn, olive, soybean)<br>• 1½ tsp mayonnaise<br>• 2 tsp tub margarine<br>• 2 tsp French dressing | **Tips**<br>• Choose soft margarines with zero *trans* fats made from liquid vegetable oil, rather than stick margarine or butter.<br>• Use vegetable oils (olive, canola, corn, soybean, peanut, safflower, sunflower) rather than solid fats (butter, shortening).<br>• Replace solid fats with oils, rather than adding oil to the diet. Oils are a concentrated source of calories, so use oils in small amounts. |

*Calories from food components such as added sugars and solid fats that provide little nutritional value. Empty Calories are part of Total Calories.

SOURCE: http://www.choosemyplate.gov/

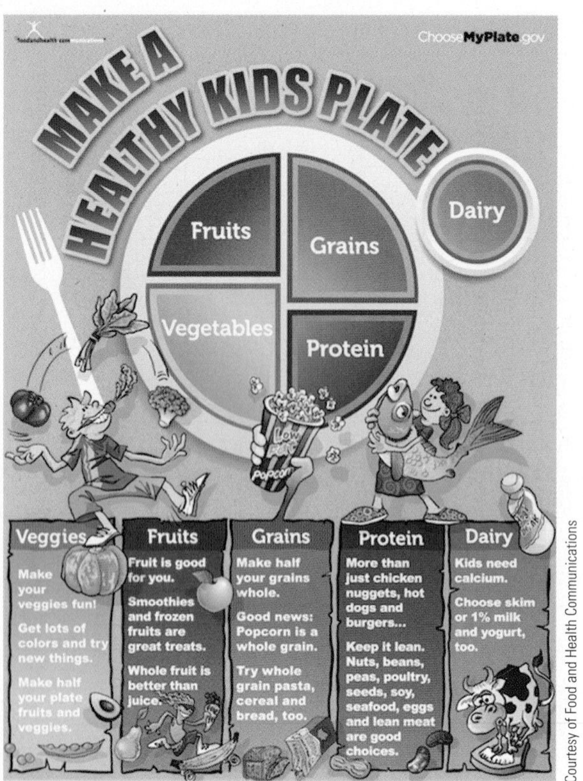


ILLUSTRATION 10.9 ▸ MyPlate for kids.[11]

## Recommendations for Intake of Iron, Fiber, Fat, and Calcium

Adequate iron intake is necessary to prevent iron deficiency and iron-deficiency anemia in toddlers and preschoolers. Appropriate fiber intake is needed to prevent constipation and may provide long-term disease prevention. Fat is an important source of calories, essential fatty acids, and fat-soluble vitamins in young children's diets. Adequate calcium intake is important for children to achieve peak bone mass.

**Iron** Adequate iron intake is important in this age group to prevent iron deficiency. Good sources of dietary iron can be found in Chapter 1, Table 1.14. Meats, which are good sources of iron, can be ground or chopped to make them easier for toddlers to chew. Fortified breakfast cereals and dried beans and peas are also good sources of iron.

"Toddler" milks, or iron-fortified commercial formulas for toddlers, are available. Healthy children who consume a variety of foods, and whose milk intake is less than 24 ounces daily, obtain adequate iron without these special products. Other commercial beverages being marketed to parents include formulas that were originally designed for children with illnesses or who had to be fed complete nutrition through a feeding tube. Such special products are expensive and are unnecessary for healthy children. It would be better for parents of healthy children to spend their food dollars on a variety of healthy foods rather than on these special products.

TABLE 10.10 ▸ Adequate intake of total fiber for children[31]

| | |
|---|---|
| 1–3 years of age | 19 g/day of total fiber |
| 4–8 years of age | 25 g/day of total fiber |

SOURCE: Data from National Academy Press. Table created by Nancy H. Wooldridge.

**Fiber** Ample dietary fiber intake has been associated with the prevention of heart disease, certain cancers, diabetes, and hypertension in adults. Whether fiber helps prevent these problems as young children become adults is not known, but it is clear that fiber in a child's diet helps prevent constipation and is part of a healthy diet (Table 10.10).[31] Excessive fiber (defined as the child's age plus 15 grams) can be detrimental, however, because high-fiber diets have the potential of reducing the energy density of the diet, which could impact growth.[72] High-fiber diets could also impact the bioavailabilty of some minerals, such as iron and calcium.

Total fiber is the sum of dietary fiber and functional fiber. Earlier recommendations were based on dietary fiber alone. Including fruits, vegetables, and whole-grain breads and cereal products in the diet can increase the dietary fiber intake of children. Those who meet the recommendation consume more breads and cereals, fruits, vegetables, legumes, nuts, and seeds than those who do not. Children with adequate fiber intake tend to have lower intakes of fat and cholesterol, and higher intakes of vitamins A and E, folate, magnesium, and iron, than do those children who have low dietary fiber intakes.[72,73]

**Fat** An appropriate amount of fat in a young child's diet can be achieved by employing the principles of the Dietary Guidelines for Americans and MyPlate that promote a diet of whole-grain breads and cereals, beans and peas, fruits and vegetables, low-fat dairy products after 2 years of age, and lean meats.[11,52] Foods high in fat are used sparingly, especially foods high in saturated fat and *trans* fatty acids. However, an appropriate amount of dietary fat is necessary to meet children's needs for energy, essential fatty acids, and fat-soluble vitamins. As discussed in Chapter 1, good sources of the essential fatty acid linoleic acid are peanut, canola, corn, safflower, and other vegetable oils. Flaxseed, soy, and canola oils are good sources of the essential fatty acid alpha-linolenic acid.

## Fat Soluble Vitamins

It is important to include sources of fat-soluble vitamins in the diets of young children. Good sources of vitamin A include whole eggs and dairy products. Sources of vitamin D include exposure to sunlight and vitamin D–fortified milk. The American Academy of Pediatrics recommends a daily intake of 400 IU of vitamin D for all healthy children, while the DRIs for vitamin D were increased to 600 IUs for children 1–8 years of age with the revision of the DRIs for calcium and vitamin D in 2010.[32,73] Corn, soybean, and safflower oils are excellent sources of vitamin E. Vitamin K is widely distributed in both animal and plant foods.

TABLE 10.11 ▸ Mean percentages of total calories from carbohydrate, protein, total fat, saturated fatty acids, and cholesterol intake[79]

| 2–5 YEARS OF AGE | CARBOHYDRATE (%) | PROTEIN (%) | TOTAL FAT (%) | SATURATED FATTY ACIDS (%) | CHOLESTEROL (MG/D) |
|---|---|---|---|---|---|
| Males | 56.0 | 14.0 | 31.0 | 11.0 | 170 |
| Females | 55.0 | 15.0 | 32.0 | 12.0 | 178 |

SOURCE: Data from www.ars.usda.gov. Table created by Nancy H. Wooldridge.

**Calcium** Adequate calcium intake in childhood affects peak bone mass. A high peak bone mass is thought to be protective against osteoporosis and fractures later in life.[74] However, many children do not consume adequate calcium.[52] The DRIs for calcium intake is 700 mg/day for children ages 1–3 years and 1000 mg/day for children ages 4–8 years.[32] An important aspect of adequate calcium intake in toddlers and preschoolers is the development of eating patterns that will lead to adequate calcium intake later in childhood.[74]

Dairy products are good sources of calcium, as are canned fish with soft bones such as sardines, dark green leafy vegetables such as kale and bok choy, tofu made with calcium, and calcium-fortified foods and beverages such as calcium-fortified orange juice (Table 1.14). Nonfat and low-fat dairy products are low in saturated fat while still serving as a good source of calcium.

**Fluids** Healthy toddlers and preschoolers will consume enough fluid through beverages, foods, and sips and glasses of water to meet their needs. Fluid requirements increase with fever, vomiting, diarrhea, and when children are in hot, dry, or humid environments.

Consumption of milk has decreased among young children since the late 1970s, but consumption of carbonated soft drinks has increased by about the same amount. According to food consumption surveys, young children consume large amounts of sweetened beverages, including fruit juice, soft drinks, and sweetened iced tea, to the detriment of the overall nutritional balance of their diet and oral health. Consumption of sugar-sweetened beverages and 100 percent fruit juice begins at a young age and has increased in recent years.[75,76] Approximately 50 percent of children ages 2–5 years consume soft drinks.[77,78] Sugar-sweetened beverages contribute 10–15 percent of total calorie intake for children.[75] Children with high consumption of regular soft drinks (more than 9 ounces per day) consume more calories and less milk and fruit juice than those with lower consumptions of regular soft drinks. Water is a good and underused "thirst quencher" for toddlers and preschoolers, as long as milk (2 cups) is part of their regular diet and fruit juice consumption is less than 4–6 ounces, as recommended by the American Academy of Pediatrics.[79] Parents and caretakers can offer children water to drink between meals and snacks.

## Recommended Versus Actual Food Intake

Ongoing national surveys examine food and nutrient intakes of Americans, including young children. The report "What We Eat in America" (WWEIA), a joint project of the U.S. Department of Agriculture (USDA) and the U.S. Department of Health and Human Services (DHHS), is the dietary intake component of the NHANES. In these national surveys, dietary data for children younger than 6 years of age is provided by an adult caretaker.[80]

According to the most recent WWEIA report, which utilizes data from NHANES 2009–2010 and the USDA's Continuing Survey of Food Intakes by Individuals (CSFII),[80] young children meet their energy needs, and more than enough protein and fat (Table 10.11). Toddlers who participated in the Feeding Infants and Toddlers Study 2008 (FITS) met or exceeded estimated energy requirements.[80] The total fat intake of 31 percent of males and 32 percent of females of total calories is within the target range for children this age. Two- to five-year-olds have mean sodium intakes of 2331 mg per day for boys and about 2283 mg per day for girls, with the sodium intake recommendation at 2300 mg per day.[52,79]

In a longitudinal study of the nutrient and food intakes of preschool children ages 24–60 months, mean intakes of zinc, folic acid, and vitamins D and E were consistently below the recommended levels.[81] Low intakes of zinc, vitamin E, and iron were found in toddlers ages 12–18 months, a time of dietary transition.[80,82] Vitamin E intakes less than the estimated average requirement were found in toddlers and preschoolers who participated in the Feeding Infants and Toddlers Study 2008 (FITS).[80] The means for nutrient intakes often hide problems at the extremes, however. They fail to indicate the percentage of children with low nutrient intakes of less than 66 percent of the recommended levels, and children with high nutrient intakes that exceed the Tolerable Upper Intake Levels.

The diets of children who ate fast food were found to be higher in total energy, total fat, total carbohydrate, added sugars, and sugar-sweetened beverages, and to have less fiber, less milk, and fewer fruits and nonstarchy vegetables than the diets of children who did not eat fast food.[83] Using this same data set, it was found that 11 percent of children ages 2–3 years and 12 percent of children ages 4–5 years consumed greater than 25 percent of total energy from added sugar. Increased added sugar consumption was associated with decreased nutrient and food-group intakes and increased percentage of children not meeting the DRIs.[84] Children's portions sizes have remained constant over the years except for meat portions, which have decreased. This stability in portion sizes of young children over time reinforces the hypothesis that young children are capable of self-regulating energy intake. Portion sizes were positively related to both bodyweight percentiles and energy intake.

It seems that young children self-regulate energy intake by adjusting portion size.[85]

## Cross-Cultural Considerations

When working with families from different cultures, it is important to learn as much as possible about the culture's food-related beliefs and practices. Ask the parents and caretakers about their experiences with food, including foods used for special occasions. It is also helpful to know whether foods are used for home remedies or to promote certain aspects of health. Cultural beliefs influence many child feeding practices, such as what foods are best for young children, which cause digestive upsets, or which help relieve illnesses. It is important for the health care provider to build on the cultural practices of the family and to reinforce the positive practices while attempting to affect change that could be more beneficial to the young child. For example, peanut or polyunsaturated oils can be recommended to Chinese Americans for stir-frying instead of the more traditional lard or chicken fat.

## Vegetarian Diets

Young children can grow and develop normally on vegetarian or vegan diets, as long as their dietary patterns are intelligently planned. Vegetarian diets are rich in fruits, vegetables, and whole grains, the consumption of which is encouraged for the general population. However, young children in particular need some energy-dense foods to reduce the total amount of food required. The amount of vegetarian foods needed to meet nutrient needs may be more food than young children can eat. Young children need to eat several times a day to meet their energy needs because their stomachs cannot hold a lot of food at one time.

Children who are fed ***vegan*** and ***macrobiotic diets*** tend to have lower rates of growth, although still within normal ranges, during the first 5 years of life compared to children given a mixed diet.[86] Strict vegan diets, which exclude all foods of animal origin, may be deficient in vitamins $B_{12}$ and D, zinc, and omega-3 fatty acids, and may also be low in calcium, unless fortified foods are consumed. Protein needs are usually met if the diet is adequate in energy and a variety of foods are included.[87] Children on vegan diets should receive vitamin $B_{12}$ supplements or consume fortified breakfast cereals, textured soy protein, or soy milk fortified with vitamin $B_{12}$. The vitamin $B_{12}$ status of children following vegetarian and vegan diets should be monitored on a regular basis, as vitamin $B_{12}$–deficiency may cause vitamin $B_{12}$–deficiency anemia, leading to fatigue, pale skin and shortness of breath. Iron-deficiency anemia is an infrequent problem among children consuming a vegetarian diet.

Vitamin D adequacy can be achieved through diet or by sun exposure. Good sources of vitamin D for children include fortified soy milk, fortified breakfast cereals, and fortified margarines. Zinc is found in foods of animal origin. Plant sources of zinc include legumes, nuts, and whole grains. Vegetable products are also lacking in omega-3 fatty acids. Therefore, including a source of these fatty acids, such as canola or soybean oils, is advisable.[87] Foods containing phytates, such as unrefined cereals, may interfere with calcium absorption; if the child's diet contains a lot of unrefined cereals, higher calcium intakes may be needed.[87] Good sources of calcium for children on strict vegetarian diets include calcium-fortified soy milk, calcium-fortified orange juice and breads, tofu processed with calcium, blackstrap molasses, sesame seeds, tahini (sesame butter), almond and almond butter, and certain vegetables, such as broccoli and kale.[10] Calcium in vegetables such as spinach, Swiss chard, beet greens, and rhubarb is not well absorbed because insoluble calcium oxalate is formed with the high amounts of oxalate in these vegetables. Supplements may be necessary for some children with inadequate intakes that are not remedied by dietary means.

Guidelines for vegetarian eating practices for young children include:[10]

- Provide three meals and two to three snacks per day. Avoid serving bran and excessive intake of bulky foods, such as raw fruits and vegetables.
- Encourage eating nutrient-dense foods such as cheese, avocado, soy cheese, hummus, nut butters, tahini, and tofu.
- Provide an omega-3 fatty acid source, such as canola oil, soybean oil, tofu, soybeans, walnuts, and wheat germ.
- Avoid excessive restriction of dietary fat.
- Ensure an adequate intake of calcium, zinc, iron, and vitamins $B_{12}$ and D.

## Child Care Nutrition Standards

> ". . . child-care programs should achieve recommended benchmarks for meeting children's nutrition needs in a safe, sanitary, and supportive environment that promotes optimal growth and development."[88]
>
> —The American Dietetic Association (now The Academy of Nutrition and Dietetics)

An estimated 23 million children in the United States require child care while their parents work, making foods children eat away from home a major contribution to their overall intake. Nutrition

**vegan diet** The most restrictive of vegetarian diets, allowing only plant foods.

**macrobiotic diet** This diet falls between semivegetarian and vegan diets and includes foods such as brown rice, other grains, vegetables, fish, dried beans, spices, and fruits.

standards for child care services exist and specify minimum requirements for amounts and types of foods to include in meals and snacks, as well as food-service safety procedures.[88,89] These standards also address nutrition learning experiences and education for children, staff, and parents as well as the physical and emotional environment in which meals and snacks are served. It is recommended that children in part-day programs (4–7 hours per day) receive food that provides at least one-third of their daily energy and nutrient needs in at least one meal and two snacks or two meals and one snack. A child in a full-day program (8 hours or more) should receive foods that meet one-half to two-thirds of the child's daily needs based on the DRIs in at least two meals and two snacks or three snacks and one meal. Food should be offered at intervals of not less than 2 hours and not more than 3 hours and should be consistent with the Dietary Guidelines for Americans.[52] Healthy People 2020 Nutrition and Weight Status objective NWS-1 is to increase the number of states with nutrition standards for foods and beverages provided to preschool children in child care and Physical Activity objective PA-9 is to increase the number of states with licensing regulations for physical activity in child care.[5]

### Physical Activity Recommendations

Physical activity is an important component of a healthy lifestyle. Physical activity helps to maintain energy balance while strengthening muscles. Inactivity is thought to be a major contributor to the increasing prevalence of obesity. The Dietary Guidelines for Americans 2010 recommend that children engage in active play several times a day.[52] Some suggested activities for preschoolers from MyPlate[11] include:

Outdoor Activities:

- Games in the yard or park
- Family walks after dinner
- Walking the dog together
- Freestyle dance
- Playing catch
- Family bike rides on the weekend

Indoor Activities:

- Follow the leader
- Playing with a dog
- Hide and seek
- Ring around the rosie
- Simon says
- Walking around the shopping mall or museum

This advice is reinforced by the American Academy of Pediatrics (AAP).[90] The AAP suggests that toddlers, under the supervision of an adult caregiver, engage in activities such as walking in the neighborhood, park, or zoo and free play outdoors. For the preschool-age child, the AAP lists appropriate activities as running, swimming, tumbling, throwing, and catching, under adult supervision. No television viewing is recommended for children less than 2 years of age, while screen time should be limited to less than 2 hours per day for all other age groups. Removing screens from children's bedrooms is also recommended.[30] Parents are encouraged to set a good example for their children by being physically active themselves and limiting the amount of time that the family spends watching TV and playing computer and video games.

## Nutrition Intervention for Risk Reduction

LO 10.8 Identify the basic premise upon which Bright Futures Nutrition is based.

### Nutrition Assessment

Components of a nutrition assessment include a food/nutrition-related history, pertinent biochemical measurements, anthropometric measurements such as weight, height, body mass index percentile, and a medical history (Table 10.12). Based on this information, the nutrition professional can identify any nutrition diagnoses, design a nutrition intervention plan with family input, and make a plan for monitoring and evaluation (see Table 2.10 for the four steps of the Nutrition Care Process).

TABLE 10.12 Normal values of biochemical nutritional parameters[38,64]

| TEST IRON STATUS | NORMAL VALUES |
|---|---|
| Hematocrit, % | 39 |
| Hemoglobin, g/dL | 14 |
| Serum ferritin, ng/mL | >15 |
| Serum iron, mcg/dL | >60 |
| Serum total iron binding capacity, mcg/dL | 350–400 |
| Serum transferring [revert to original] saturation, % | >16 |
| Serum transferrin, mg/dL | 170–250 |
| Erythrocyte prtoporphyrin, mcg/dL red blood cells | >70 |
| **Lead screening** | |
| Blood lead levels | <10 mcg/dL |
| **Dyslipidemia screen** | |
| Total cholesterol | <170 mg/dL |
| LDL cholesterol | <110 mg/dL |

Refer to page A-4 of the Appendix for a table for converting Conventional Units shown in the table to SI units.

## Model Program

*Bright Futures: Nutrition* is an example of a model program for nutrition intervention for risk reduction.[10] This guide is a component of the larger project "Bright Futures Guidelines for Health Supervision of Infants, Children, and Adolescents."[92]

The purpose of the Bright Futures program is to foster trusting relationships between the child, health professionals, the family, and the community to promote optimal health for the child.[92] Bright Futures guidelines are developmentally based and address the physical, mental, cognitive, and social development of infants, children, adolescents, and their families.

Many different user-friendly materials and tools are available from this program to assist in the implementation of the guidelines. In addition to the "Bright Futures Guidelines for Health Supervision," implementation guides have been published for oral health, general nutrition, physical activity, mental health, and families.

*Bright Futures: Nutrition* is based on the premise that optimal nutrition for children should be approached from the perspective of the development of the child and put in the context of the environment in which the child lives.[10] It emphasizes the development of healthy eating and physical activity behaviors. Nutrition supervision guidelines are given for each age group, and within each broad age group, interview questions, screening, and assessment; tips for anticipatory guidance are also provided. The program information includes a section on frequently asked questions and resources for families for each broad age group. For example, by utilizing the guidelines, health care providers will be able to provide anticipatory guidance to parents of toddlers for the proper advancements of toddler diets based on growth and development. The implementation guide also addresses special issues and concerns related to pediatric nutrition, including oral health, vegetarian eating practices, iron-deficiency anemia, pediatric undernutrition, and obesity. The *Bright Futures: Nutrition* guidelines are a valuable resource for anyone who is interested in promoting healthy eating and physical activity behaviors in children. Ordering information for Bright Futures materials is available on the program's website (https://brightfutures.aap.org).

# Public Food and Nutrition Programs

**LO 10.9** Identify one public food or nutrition program that provides services to young children and describe the program's strategies in improving the nutrition of young children.

Young children and their families can benefit from a number of federally sponsored food and nutrition programs. Four example programs are presented here.

## WIC

The Special Supplemental Nutrition Program for Women, Infants, and Children (WIC),[93] previously described in Chapter 8, is administered by the Food and Nutrition Service of the U.S. Department of Agriculture (USDA). It is one of the most successful federally funded nutrition programs in the United States. In April 2012, there were 9.7 million mothers, infants, and children enrolled in the WIC program.[94] Participation in WIC services improves the growth, iron status, and quality of dietary intake of nutritionally at-risk infants and children up to age 5 years.[93]

As in infancy, children must live in a low-income household, 185 percent or less of the federal poverty level, and be at "nutrition risk" to be eligible for WIC services. "Nutrition risk" means a child has a medical or dietary-based condition that places the child at increased risk. Such conditions include iron-deficiency anemia, underweight, overweight, or a chronic illness such as cystic fibrosis, or consumption of an inadequate diet.[92] Children receive nutrition assistance, education, and follow-up services by specially trained registered dietitians and nutritionists. WIC recipients are provided with supplemental food, in the form of vouchers, checks, or electronic benefits transfer (EBT) cards that allow them to obtain specific types of food from participating retail stores at no charge. Revisions in the WIC food packages to coincide with the Dietary Guidelines for Americans include low-fat or nonfat milk, whole-grain bread and cereals, and the substitution of soy milk and tofu for milk and cheese.[95]

## WIC's Farmers' Market Nutrition Program

The Farmers' Market Nutrition Program (FMNP) is a special seasonal program for WIC participants. This program provides vouchers for the purchase of locally grown produce at farmers' markets. The program is designed to help low-income families increase their consumption of fresh fruits and vegetables. In FY 2011, 1.9 million WIC participants received FMNP benefits.[96]

## Head Start and Early Head Start

Administered by the U.S. Department of Health and Human Services, Head Start and Early Head Start are comprehensive child development programs, serving children from birth to 5 years of age, pregnant women, and their families. Over one million U.S. children participate in this program. The overall goal is to increase the readiness for school of children from economically disadvantaged families. A range of individualized, culturally appropriate services are provided through Head Start and related agencies, including educational, health, nutritional, social, and other services.[97] More specific information about Early Head Start can be found in Chapters 8 and 9.

## Supplemental Nutrition Assistance Program

The Supplemental Nutrition Assistance Program (SNAP), administered by the USDA, is designed to help adults in low-income households buy food, thereby improving food security and nutrition of participants. In FY 2013 about 47.6 million individuals living in 23 million households received assistance in the United States.[98] The monetary amount of food vouchers provided to an eligible household depends on the number of people in it and the income of the household. Income eligibility criteria for this and a number of other federal programs can be found at the USDA's Food and Nutrition Service website (http://www.fns.usda.gov/snap/supplemental-nutrition-assistance-program-snap). The average monthly amount of benefits received through SNAP in 2013 was $133 per individual, enough to help families and individuals pay for a portion of the food they need. Each state must develop a nutrition education plan for SNAP recipients based on federal guidance.[98] Participation in SNAP is associated with increased intakes of a number of nutrients and a decrease in food insecurity by roughly 30 percent.[96,98,99]

# KEY POINTS

1. Periodic and accurate measurements of a young child's growth are important indicators of the child's nutritional status. Adequate and appropriate growth is the ultimate outcome indicator of adequate nutrition and health.
2. The types of foods offered to children and methods of feeding are based on an individual child's growth and development.
3. Food habits are learned behaviors.
4. Common nutritional problems such as iron-deficiency anemia, dental caries, and constipation in a healthy child can be addressed through adjustments in the child's diet.
5. The risk for overweight and obesity are increasing even among young children in the United States.
6. The U.S. Dietary Guidelines recommend that children eat a variety of foods and increase physical activity.
7. MyPlate reinforces eating a variety of foods and increasing physical activity.
8. Surveys of food intake indicate that most children meet their nutritional needs, but that their intakes exceed recommendations for energy and saturated fat.
9. A well-planned vegetarian diet can meet the needs of a growing child.
10. Public food and nutrition programs are important resources for many young children in the United States.

# REVIEW QUESTIONS

1. Which of the following growth parameters is used as a screening tool for assessing underweight and overweight or obesity in young children?
   a. Weight-for-age percentile
   b. Length- or stature-for-age percentile
   c. Body mass index-for-age percentile
   d. Actual body mass index (weight in kg/height in meters$^2$)
   e. Actual weight in kg
2. Which of the following strategies would be appropriate for parents to use in teaching their young child healthy eating behaviors?
   a. Give a dessert as a reward for eating fruits and vegetables.
   b. Expect the child to eat foods that parents will not eat themselves.
   c. Coax the child to eat, especially new foods.
   d. Serve child-sized portions or allow the child to self-serve portions.
   e. Make the child stay at the table until she has cleaned her plate.
3. Obesity is defined as:
   a. Weight-for-age percentile ≥85th to 94th
   b. Weight-for-age percentile ≥95th
   c. Weight-for-length percentile ≥95th
   d. BMI-for-age percentile ≥85th to 94th
   e. BMI-for-age percentile ≥95th
4. Which of the following statements regarding fat in children's diets is correct?
   a. Dietary fat is an important source of calories in a young child's diet.
   b. The amount of saturated fat is not restricted in a young child's diet.
   c. The amount of *trans* fatty acids is not restricted in a young child's diet.
   d. Restricting fat in a young child's diet has been shown to decrease growth.
   e. Dietary fat recommendations are the same for children regardless of cardiovascular disease risk.

5. True or false: According to food consumption surveys, young children exceed estimated needs for calories.
6. Which of the following would be the best choice for a between-meal snack for a preschooler? Choose the one best answer.
   a. 100 percent fruit juice
   b. Raisins
   c. Fortified gummy bears
   d. Peanut butter crackers
   e. Oatmeal cookies
7. Several health and professional organizations and agencies, such as the American Academy of Pediatrics, the American Heart Association, and the USDA, have published similar recommendations for a healthy diet for young children. Briefly describe the food components of such a diet.
8. Describe the role of physical activity in a healthy lifestyle for young children. Give examples of appropriate activities for children.

Visit www.cengagebrain.com to access MindTap, a complete digital course that includes additional resources.

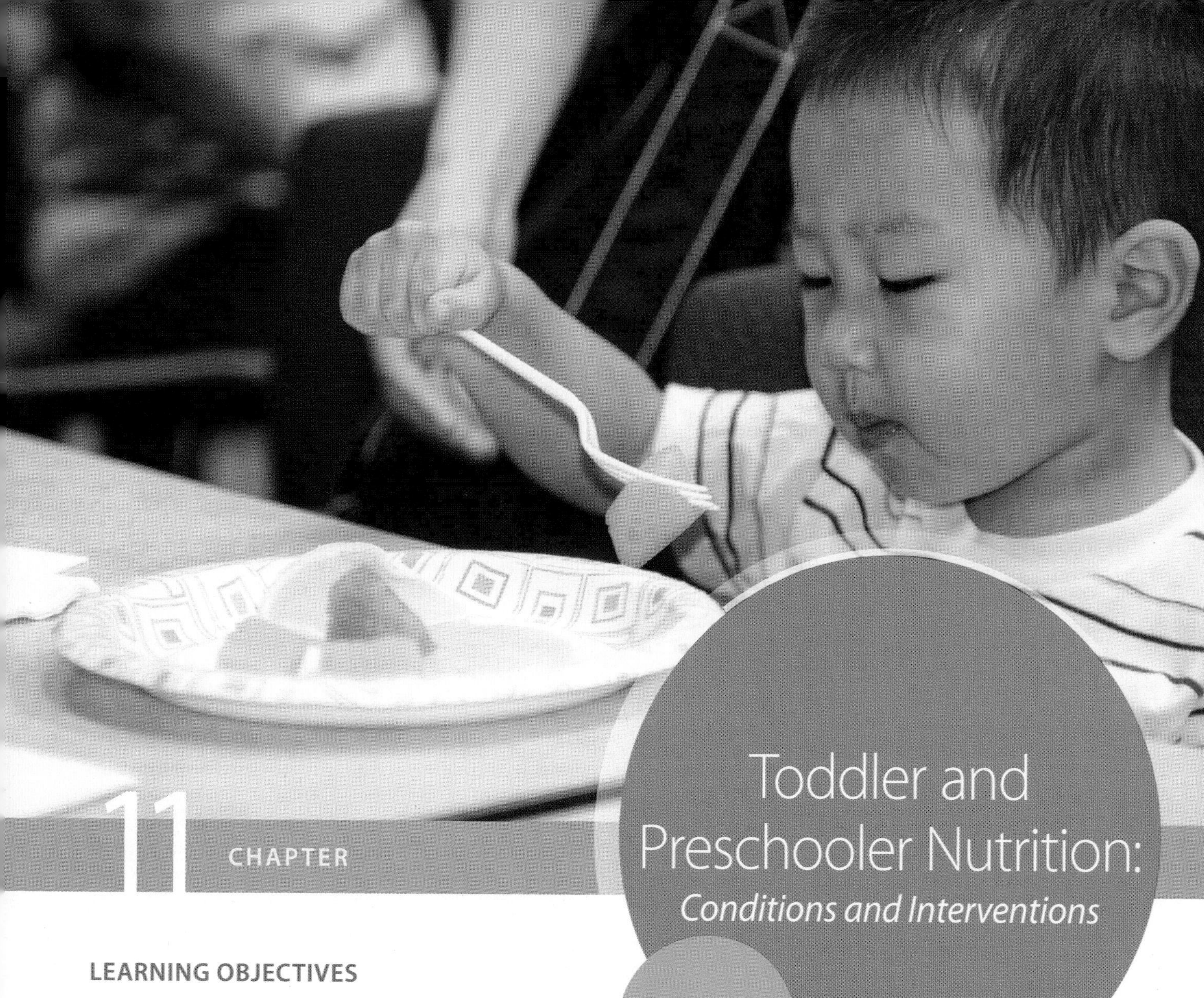

11 CHAPTER

# Toddler and Preschooler Nutrition: *Conditions and Interventions*

*Prepared by*
**Ellen K. Bowser**

## LEARNING OBJECTIVES

After studying the materials in this chapter you should be able to:

**11.1** Differentiate the similarities and differences in young children with and without special health care needs.

**11.2** Identify the more common nutrition problems in young children with special health care needs that result from chronic health conditions.

**11.3** Recognize approaches for completing a growth assessment in young children with special health care needs.

**11.4** Describe how feeding difficulties in preschoolers and toddlers are included in nutrition assessments and interventions.

**11.5** Identify conditions in young children with special needs in which nutrition services are a part of medical management.

**11.6** Review food allergy and intolerance consequences for young children.

**11.7** Compare use of dietary and herbal remedies in young children with and without special health care needs.

**11.8** Explain how families access community and regional resources that provide nutrition services for toddlers and preschoolers with chronic health problems.

CDC/PHIL

# Introduction

Most toddlers and preschoolers are healthy and develop as expected. Most are not referred to nutrition services unless their low-income families participate in the WIC program. This chapter discusses children who do not fit the typical pattern, ***children with special health care needs*** associated with a ***chronic condition*** or disability, or children who are at risk. Nutritionists with pediatric experience spend most of their time with these children and their families. This chapter covers nutrition needs and services for young children with autism spectrum disorder (ASD), food allergies, breathing or ***pulmonary*** problems, feeding and growth problems, developmental delays, and those at risk for needing nutritional intervention.

This chapter demonstrates how nutrition assessments, diagnoses, and interventions complement medical diagnoses and medical treatment. Sources for diagnoses are more important in clinical nutrition services than in nutrition services delivered in public health settings, but are essential for quality health care. Healthy People 2020 objectives (Table 10.1) include children with special health care needs, especially in those objectives concerning access to health care and reducing health care disparities.[1] Some objectives are not appropriate because children with specific conditions may have different energy needs or key nutrient requirements than their healthy peers. Similarly, the 2010 U.S. Dietary Guidelines are based on a healthy population and are not adapted for children with special health care needs.[2]

# Who Are Children with Special Health Care Needs?

**LO 11.1** Differentiate the similarities and differences in young children with and without special health care needs.

The child who does not see, hear, or walk, or does not reach the appropriate developmental milestones may be recognized as having a chronic condition. It can be difficult and expensive, however, to identify other children with special health care needs. Some already have a medical diagnosis, but others may not. Nutrition services are needed regardless, although the type of nutrition assessment and interventions differ. Most children start school at age 5 or 6 years, but children at risk, or who have special needs, may attend well before that, as soon as the need is identified. The earlier special educational, nutritional, and health care interventions are started, the better for the overall child's development. Criteria used for identifying disabilities in adults do not fit children, as these criteria are related to a person's ability to work or perform household chores.[3] *Chronic condition* and *disability* mean the same thing in referring to toddlers and preschoolers. Prevalence estimates for disabilities range from 5 percent to 31 percent of children.[4,5]

The 2009–2010 National Survey of Children with Special Health Needs reported a range of 5–13.2 percent of children ages 0–5 having special health needs.[4] Nutritional problems are common in children with disabilities and up to 90 percent of children with disabilities have some type of nutrition problem.[6]

Nutrition services are provided to toddlers and preschoolers who carry forward medical and nutrition diagnoses from infancy. The majority of infants are healthy, so this group of infants who become children with special health care needs is only a small percentage of the population. What is rapidly growing is that portion of healthy-appearing toddlers and preschoolers who are at risk for health or developmental problems. The availability of services for toddlers and preschoolers who are at risk for nutritional or developmental delays has been positively impacted by parent advocacy groups and professional organizations who have identified the value of early intervention services.

Although the importance of identifying problems early to start therapy has been recognized for a long time, the American Academy of Pediatrics (AAP) and developmental pediatricians have intensified efforts to screen all toddlers in primary care offices.[7,8] Nutrition-related problems also can be identified in primary care offices when developmental screening is conducted. This is because feeding is a developmental milestone for toddlers, so many health care providers, such as speech-language therapists and occupational therapists, work with families when children have feeding problems. Nutritionists work as a part of a multidisciplinary team with such providers.

What is important is that toddlers and children are entitled to the same services as older people with chronic illnesses are, with additional help. They are covered by the Americans with Disabilities Act, the Social Security Disability Program, the Supplemental Social Security Insurance (SSI) Program, and services for families without health insurance coverage.[3,9] Additional help comes from educational regulations ensuring that all children with disabilities have a free, appropriate public education. Nutrition services are funded within education regulations in the Individuals with Disabilities Education Act (IDEA).[9]

Parents of a typical child choose and pay for day care or a preschool program. For a child with special health care needs, day care or educational programs are selected based on nutrition and other types of

**children with special health care needs** A general term for infants and children with, or at risk for, physical or developmental disabilities or chronic medical conditions from genetic or metabolic disorders, birth defects, premature births, trauma, infection, or prenatal exposure to drugs.

**chronic condition** Disorder of health or development that is the usual state for an individual and unlikely to change, although secondary conditions may result over time.

**pulmonary** Related to the lungs and their movement of air for exchange of carbon dioxide and oxygen.

TABLE 11.1 ▸ Educational, medical, and nutrition problems for one toddler and one preschooler

| "BILL," AN 18-MONTH-OLD BOY (BORN AT 30 WEEKS OF GESTATION) | | |
|---|---|---|
| EDUCATION PROBLEMS | MEDICAL PROBLEMS | NUTRITION PROBLEMS |
| 25% delay in motor, social, and cognitive skills documented, meeting eligibility for services under The Infants and Toddlers with Disabilities Program (Part C) of the Individuals with Disabilities Education Act (IDEA) | Diagnosed, treated seizures, short stature | Self-restricted energy and nutrient intake due to prolonged use of infant formula fed in a bottle, with acceptance of only pureed foods from a spoon |
| "SUE," A 4-YEAR-OLD WITH AUTISM SPECTRUM DISORDER | | |
| EDUCATION PROBLEMS | MEDICAL PROBLEMS | NUTRITION PROBLEMS |
| Speech and language impairment, banging and hitting behaviors (emotional disturbance), meeting eligibility for the Individuals with Disabilities Education Act (IDEA) | Sleep disruption, complaints about gastrointestinal pain 2 times/week, in diagnostic testing | Dietary analysis of food and nutrient intake shows food refusals resulting in excessive liquids and sugar intake; inadequate calcium, Vitamin D, and iron; lack of a consistent meal and snack pattern |



therapy provided by state and federal resources. Nutrition services can be provided to young children within special educational programs and services both as preschoolers (3–5 years old) and toddlers up to 3 years old.[4,5] Services have to be culturally appropriate for various ethnic groups, reflecting food preferences, religious beliefs, and sensitivity to dress and language; otherwise, they are likely to be rejected.

What is confusing about nutrition services for chronically ill and at-risk toddlers and preschoolers is that the two systems, medical and educational, vary with regulations from state to state and country to country. Educational services categorize health problems differently than by medical diagnoses. This chapter (and Chapter 13) present both educational and medical systems to identify how nutrition services fit in (Table 11.1).

Educational categories of disabilities are not well aligned with nutrition diagnoses. More than half of the children eligible for special education services have specific learning disabilities or speech and language impairments, but these educational categories are unlikely to incorporate nutrition services. For example, there is no category of learning problems for children with obesity or feeding problems. An infant boy who had an early genetic test for ***Prader-Willi syndrome*** may need nutrition services as soon as the medical diagnosis is confirmed.[10] In contrast, educational categories for a toddler with Prader-Willi syndrome are developmental delay, speech or language impairment, or rare disorders. This is why a young boy with Prader-Willi syndrome may receive special education, but not be identified for nutrition services until obesity is evident.

One of the best resources for providers and families to find services is the National Dissemination Center for Children with Disabilities, funded by the U.S. Department of Education.[9] It identifies disabilities for toddlers and preschoolers and has outcome studies on the effectiveness of educational interventions. Families who learn to navigate the complexity of educational, medical, and nutrition resources for their young child deserve much respect for being good advocates for their children.

Many nutritionists work in community-based ***early intervention services*** funded by the Infants and Toddlers with Disabilities Program (Part C) of the Individuals with Disabilities Education Act (IDEA) (Table 11.2). A child's eligibility for services does not require a specific diagnosis. Early intervention programs are based on the following:[9]

- Developmental delay in one or more of the following areas: cognitive, physical, language and speech, psychosocial, or self-helping skills
- A physical or mental condition with a high probability of delay, such as Down syndrome
- At risk medically or environmentally for substantial developmental delay if services are not provided

A number of chronic conditions are suspected, but not obvious, in the first year of life. The diagnosis often becomes clear in the toddler and preschool years. Standardized developmental screening, evaluation, and testing for these ages show more reliability than they do for infants. Parents who were

**Prader-Willi syndrome** Condition in which partial deletion of chromosome 15 interferes with control of appetite, muscle development, and cognition.

**early intervention services** Federally mandated evaluation and therapy services for children in the age range from birth to 3 years under the Individuals with Disabilities Education Act.

TABLE 11.2 ▸ Early intervention nutrition services for children up to 36 months old

| | |
|---|---|
| Requirements | Align with Part C educational program state requirements<br>Align with the child's "Family Individualized Education Plan," which addresses:<br>• Where services are provided; the child's home, school, day care<br>• Who are team members, such as speech-language pathologist, case workers, medical providers, in addition to registered dietitian nutritionists<br>Document in local medical, educational, or other tracking systems to comply with funding sources |
| Service examples | Assess daily food and nutrient intake using a dietary analysis program<br>Assess safety of dietary supplements, over-the-counter products, and prescribed formulas<br>Evaluate nutrition care plan implementation at day care<br>Coordinate with the speech-language pathologist the plan for stimulating self-feeding<br>Track and interpret growth pattern<br>Observe developmental therapies in planning nutrition care<br>Communicate with specialty care providers about a specific nutrition problem |
| Supporting families | Respond to parent and grandparent questions about food choices<br>Attend care conference to plan a school transition<br>Arrange for menu adjustments at day care–provided meals<br>Educate caregivers in advocating for the child's access to a special formula<br>Educate about safe allergy-related food restrictions |
| Advocacy activities | Offer a continuing education session for colleagues about special formulas<br>Present nutrition recommendations to a parent advocacy group<br>Contribute nutrition educational resources for a school-based health fair |



told about possible disabilities during their child's infancy usually move beyond coping by denial or disbelief and are willing to seek out services. The tendency is to resist labeling a young child with a diagnosis, so some suspected conditions are not confirmed until school age if the delay in diagnosis will not harm the child.

# Nutrition Needs of Toddlers and Preschoolers with Chronic Conditions

**LO 11.2** Identify the more common nutrition problems in young children with special health care needs that result from chronic health conditions.

Toddlers or preschoolers with chronic health conditions are at risk for the same nutrition-related problems and concerns as are other children.[8] Consequently, every attempt should be made to meet their overall nutritional needs and to ensure normal growth and development. The DRIs for toddlers and preschoolers provide a good starting point for setting protein, vitamin, and mineral needs for children with chronic conditions.[11,12] The recommendations for typical children concerning dietary fiber, prevention of lead poisoning, and iron-deficiency anemia usually apply to children at risk or already diagnosed with special health care needs.[13]

Standard nutrition guidance does not apply for children with some specific conditions. Children with sickle-cell disease have specific blood iron and lead testing with interpretation that differs from the usual guidelines. Iron-rich foods to increase their iron stores may not be appropriate when iron also comes with blood transfusions. Consequently, nutrition assessments, diagnoses, and interventions must be customized to the child.[14]

Chronic conditions may result in poor appetite, although nutrition assessment may document increased energy needs (Table 11.3).[15] A child may have an interval of needing additional energy based on the course of the chronic condition. Changes in energy needs may explain why both underweight or overweight are more common in children with chronic conditions than in other children.[15] Overweight and obesity are commonly found with Down syndrome and spina bifida.[16] Nutrition assessment and diagnoses would include excessive energy intake as a consequence of low muscle mass, lower mobility, and short stature. Overall health status is worsened by excessive body weight, so matching energy intake to needs is important no matter how difficult.

TABLE 11.3 ▸ Chronic conditions generally associated with high and low energy needs

| HIGHER ENERGY NEEDS | LOWER ENERGY NEEDS |
|---|---|
| Cystic fibrosis | Down syndrome |
| Renal disease | Spina bifida |
| Ambulatory children with diplegia | Nonambulatory children with diplegia |
| Pediatric AIDS | Prader-Willi syndrome |
| Bronchopulmonary dysplasia (BPD) | Nonambulatory children with short stature |

Underweight results in part from the chronic illness and its medical treatment. Nutrition assessments for children with chronic illnesses often document weight loss with any illness. Nutrition interventions for underweight children with a chronic condition may or may not recommend food choices for weight gain. In underweight children, it is inappropriate to make some of the usual recommendations, such as reducing fat intake.

Nutrition interventions regarding food intake, vitamin and mineral supplementation, and mealtime behaviors also should be customized to the individual child. Children who are frequently sick or have low energy levels and appetites may dislike eating foods that are hard to chew or take a long time to eat. Some food-intake problems related to chronic illness may result from the child's behavior. It is age-appropriate for children to express their food likes and dislikes, insist on their independence, and go on food jags. It can be difficult but important to distinguish between food-intake problems related to the chronic condition and those related to normal growing up in the toddler and preschool years.

## Growth Assessment

**LO 11.3** Recognize approaches for completing a growth assessment in young children with special health care needs.

Most toddlers and preschoolers with chronic conditions are provided with an assessment of nutritional status as a first step in determining whether more intensive levels of nutrition services are needed. The need for nutrition services is identified by answers to these sorts of questions:

- Is the child's growth on track?
- Is his or her food and nutrient intake adequate?
- Are the child's feeding or eating skills appropriate for the child's age?
- Does the medical or nutrition diagnosis affect nutritional needs?

A variety of nutrition screening tools exist for assessing the nutritional status of young children.[17,18] Such tools are useful for children at risk as well as those with conditions such as asthma, HIV infection, allergies, and cerebral palsy. Screening tools identify those children who need in-depth nutrition services.[19] After assessment, nutrition intervention services provide methods to improve nutritional status. Several conditions that require nutrition intervention services include failure to thrive, celiac disease, breathing problems, and muscle coordination problems.

This example shows how in-depth nutrition services protect a child with special needs from inappropriate care. Imagine a thin and small-appearing child coming to a clinic for the first time. Within the nutrition assessment process, growth is assessed using growth charts, medical records reviewed, and body fat stores estimated. It is documented that this child has adequate fat stores, with a history of consistent low weight for age. As a part of a nutrition diagnosis, the nutritionist interprets the child's previous growth pattern and unusual body composition as being related to preterm birth medical records. The nutrition assessment process documents that this child has a healthy growth pattern. If the thin and small-appearing child was screened rather than given customized nutrition services, more energy for weight gain would likely be recommended. This would promote overweight from excess fat stores, and also frustrate the family to have increased food battles with the child Growth patterns in children with special health care needs are affected by feeding practices early in life, and nutrient adequacy, as well as prescribed medications, particularly those that change body composition, such as steroids.[10] Such factors are not assessed in healthy toddlers and preschoolers who only have screening nutrition services.

Children with special health care needs often have conditions that affect growth even when adequate nutrients are provided. Depending on age, either the 2006 WHO growth chart for children up to 24 months of age or the 2000 CDC growth charts is a good starting place to assess growth.[20,21] Specific growth charts developed for chronic conditions, when available, are recommended to be used.[18] Often both the CDC chart and the specialty chart give the best perspective of a growth pattern. For children up to age 3, who are born low birthweight (LBW) or very low birthweight (VLBW), various follow-up programs have clinical guidelines to adjust for preterm birth in interpreting growth over time. Correction for prematurity, as discussed in Chapter 9, and for catch-up growth are examples of such clinical guidelines.

Pediatric health care providers commonly use a special head growth chart. It provides head circumference percentiles from birth to age 18 years and is used to determine whether head growth falls within normal limits or indicates a neurological condition, such as ***Rett syndrome***.[22] Rett syndrome is a rare disorder which almost exclusively occurs in girls, characterized by a reduced rate of head growth beginning in the toddler years (see Illustration 11.1).[23] Later, over time, the rate of weight and height gain slows in girls with Rett syndrome.[23] Decreased rate of head growth in toddlers and preschoolers may be indicative of problems from infancy, such as prematurity, or consequences of infection such as ***meningitis***. Some clinics plot head circumference on the back of the standard growth chart as well as on the special head circumference growth chart.

**Rett syndrome** Condition in which a genetic change on the X chromosome results in severe neurological delays, causing children to be short, thin-appearing, and unable to talk.

**meningitis** Viral or bacterial infection in the central nervous system that is likely to cause a range of long-term consequences in infancy, such as intellectual disability, blindness, and hearing loss.

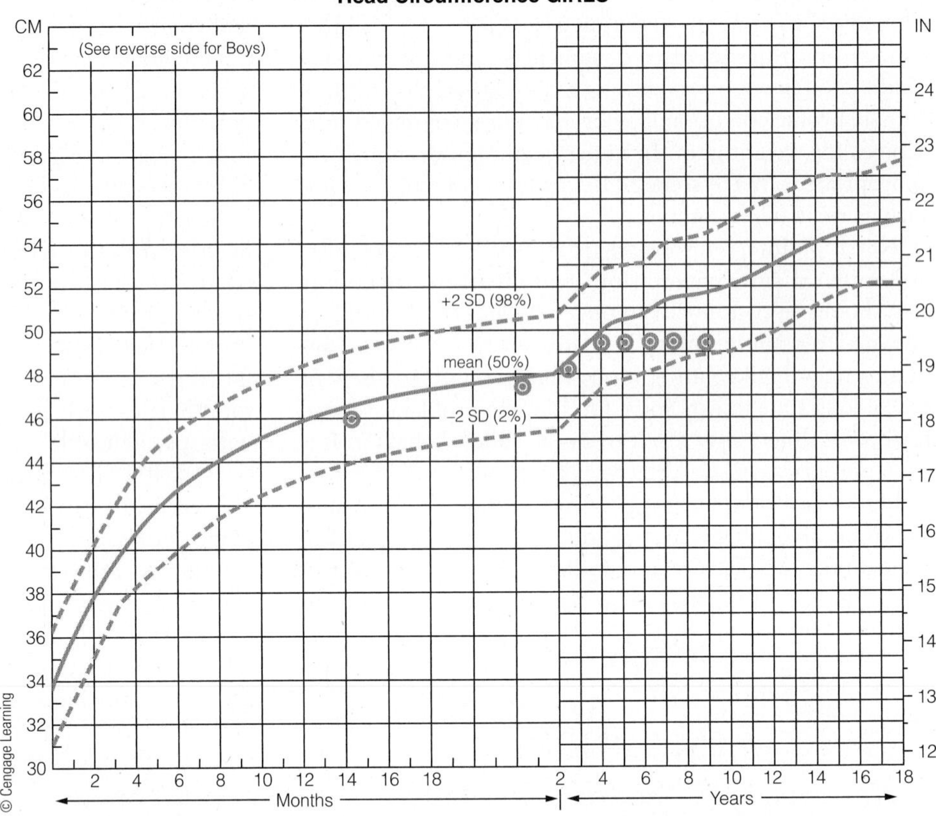


ILLUSTRATION 11.1 ▸ Nellhaus head circumference growth chart plotted for girl with Rett syndrome.

# Feeding Problems

**LO 11.4** Describe how feeding difficulties in preschoolers and toddlers are included in nutrition assessments and interventions.

Feeding problems are part of the continuum of health-related problems that require nutrition services. Children with special health care needs have many of the same developmental feeding issues as other children, such as using food to control their parents' behavior at mealtime and going on food jags. In hindsight, some feeding problems are signs of underlying health conditions that emerge in the toddler and preschool years on top of the usual feeding difficulties. These feeding problems turn out to be typical in children who are later diagnosed with a chronic condition. Children with complex health care needs have major feeding problems that may require them to be dependent on technology.[24] Examples of medical conditions that may present with signs of feeding problems include gastroesophageal reflux, asthma (and pulmonary problems in general), developmental delay, cerebral palsy, and ASD.[6,13] Nutrition assessments for such toddlers document signs of feeding problems, such as low interest in eating, long mealtimes (over 30 minutes), preferring liquids over solids, and food refusals. Children at risk for developmental delay often prove more difficult to feed as toddlers and preschoolers.[3] The child may drink liquids excessively, or eat foods usually preferred by younger children (see Case Study 11.1). Nutrition interventions for feeding problems often include recognizing that the child needs to be offered foods as if he or she is younger than his or her chronological age (Illustration 11.2). Offering food textures that he or she can eat successfully, even if a monotonous daily intake results, or continuing to offer liquids in a bottle, may be appropriate choices in these circumstances.

Table 11.4 shows an example of the likes and dislikes of a 2.5-year-old child. The child likes only a few foods, which are not especially nutritious. Usual recommendations are to add variety to the child's daily intake and to offer meats, milk, and vegetables. This recommendation is appropriate for a typical child, but this child's eating pattern suggests a feeding problem. The soft textures and mild tastes of preferred foods characterize a child closer to 1 year of age. The foods the child dislikes require higher oral skills. An evaluation of the child's overall level of functioning will likely indicate a developmental delay of the child's feeding skills.

## Behavioral Feeding Problems

> "Every mouth prefers its own soup."
>
> —Sephardic saying

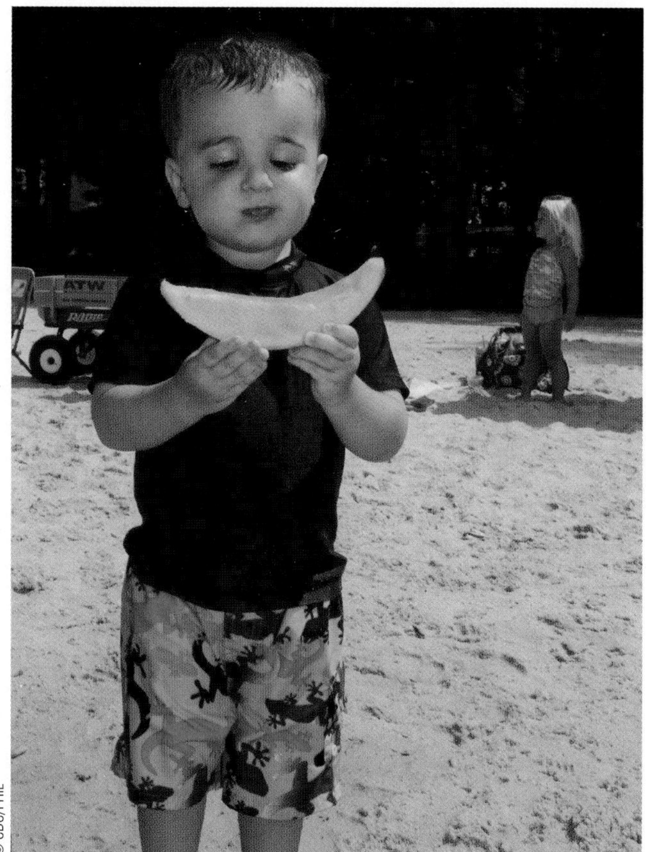


ILLUSTRATION 11.2 ▶ Toddlers with special health care needs may need foods that require fewer oral skills to consume.

Mealtime behavioral problems and food refusals are common in children with behavioral and attention disorders. These concerns often bring parents to nutrition experts for solutions. Behavioral disorders that affect nutritional status are ASDs and attention-focusing problems, such as *attention deficit hyperactivity disorder (ADHD)*. ADHD may be suspected during the preschool years, but it is primarily diagnosed during school years (Chapter 13).

TABLE 11.4 ▶ Food choices of a 2.5-year-old child with suspected developmental delay

| LIKES | DISLIKES |
|---|---|
| 3 packets instant Cream of Wheat with added sugar and margarine (refused offered apple slices) | Hamburger meats, or any other kind of meat |
| Macaroni and cheese (refused offered sandwich with lettuce and bologna) | Green beans or any kind of vegetables |
| Banana, with peel removed (refused other cut-up fruits offered) | Vegetable soup<br>Salads of all kinds |
| Pudding, only chocolate<br>Cheese puffs (refused corn chips) | Casseroles or any mixtures of foods |
| Juices of all kinds, in a sippy cup | Milk, and milk with any flavoring added |



Children with ASD may display feeding problems resulting in a self-restricted food selection (Table 11.5). A typical 2-year-old child with ASD may refuse to eat many foods and be rigid in what he will eat. He does not respond to feeling hungry, as other 2-year-old children do. When he is not given foods he likes, he refuses to eat at all and has temper tantrums during which he can injure himself. His self-restricted dietary intake is a part of the condition, which affects how he senses everything in his environment. He prefers to drink rather than eat foods, so a high proportion of his total energy comes from one type of drink. Interventions to improve the food and nutrient adequacy for this child may include a complete vitamin and mineral supplement, and adding one new food by offering it many times (15–20 times) over 1 or 2 months. Nutrition interventions should be incorporated into this child's overall treatment plan, provided within a special education program (see Case Study 11.1).

## Excessive Fluid Intake

The food intake noted in Table 11.5 highlights a common issue related to excessive fluids. Many young children prefer to drink rather than eat solid foods, especially when they are not feeling well. Families of chronically ill children tend to offer juices and lower-nutrient beverages in an effort to achieve growth when eating is difficult. The AAP recommendation to limit juice intake to 4–6 fluid ounces per day for ages 1–6 years applies to all children.[25] Calcium-fortified juices may be appropriate if other sources of calcium are limited, but these juices can also be overconsumed. In a child who already has gastrointestinal problems, it may not be clear if problems are caused by excessive juice intake.[25] In young children who may be less active due to chronic conditions, energy in excessive liquids is also a negative impact. Intake of high-sucrose beverages for young children raises concerns related to nutrient adequacy, as other more nutritious beverages are replaced.[26]

## Feeding Problems and Food Safety

Toddlers and preschoolers with chronic conditions are at greater risk for food-contamination problems. Some feeding problems result in prolonged needs for soft, easy-to-eat food textures well past the age when baby foods are eaten. Fork-mashing or blending foods may invite bacterial contamination or spoilage over time.[13] Liquid complete nutritional supplements and toddler formulas are subject to contamination once opened. Families with children dependent on feeding technology are aware of the high cost of such devices, and tend to use disposable items

**attention deficit hyperactivity disorder (ADHD)** Condition characterized by low impulse control and short attention span, with and without a high level of overall activity.

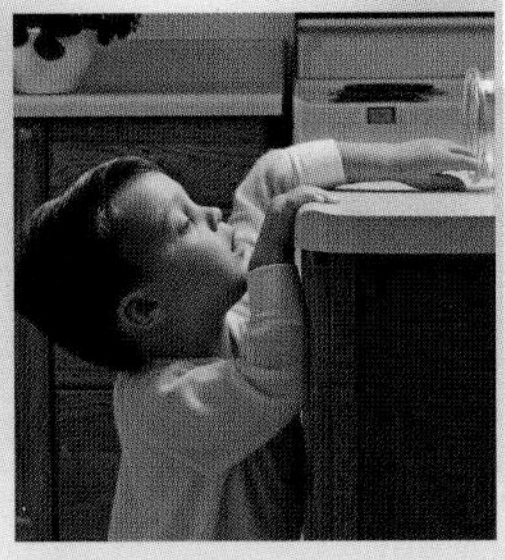
Photodisc

# CASE STUDY 11.1

## A Picky Eater

Nutrition assessment sources are the parent interview and physician records for Greg. Greg does not yet have a nutrition or medical diagnosis.

Greg is a well-groomed boy almost 3 years old. He has been growing as expected, but he does not talk. He can walk and move about well, but he prefers to play alone. Favorite foods are juices in his sippy cup, which he likes to carry around; macaroni and cheese; white bread without crusts; mashed potatoes; Honeycomb cereal; and crackers. Greg cries and throws food that he does not like, such as hamburgers, fruits, most vegetables, and any food combinations. He will periodically eat cheese pizza, scrambled eggs, and applesauce.

His mother tries talking to the pediatrician about his picky appetite, but the pediatrician reassures her that Greg will eat when he is hungry and she should not worry. Greg's mother is frustrated that he is so difficult to take out to eat because of the tantrums he throws in restaurants and friends' homes. He sometimes eats a large portion of a food he likes. Most of the time, he is satisfied just drinking juices all day from his sippy cup, and he is rarely interested in eating when others eat. He is able to eat with a spoon, but he does not like to touch foods with his hands. Greg has been referred for speech therapy, but his therapy does not address his eating. His medical history shows that he was born full-term and has had three ear infections but no major illnesses.

Nutrition assessment shows that Greg is consuming adequate energy at 1350 calories/day, or 85 cal/kg. His diet is excessive in vitamin C and B vitamins, with adequate protein at the RDA for his age. His sources of protein are mainly his starchy foods of bread, crackers, and dry cereal.

### Questions

1. What are the signs that Greg's feeding problem may be related to his speech?
2. Because Greg is growing well and meeting his energy needs, why not just wait for him to mature to accept other foods?
3. Why would there be concerns with the pediatrician's statement that Greg will eat when he is hungry?

longer than recommended. How often tubing and devices to deliver formulas are changed can be a food-safety issue.

## Feeding Problems from Disabilities Involving Neuromuscular Control

Children who have feeding problems related to muscle control of swallowing or control of the mouth or upper body may choke or cough while eating or refuse foods that require chewing.[15] These types of feeding problems result from conditions such as cerebral palsy or other ***neuromuscular disorders*** and genetic disorders such as Down syndrome. These signs of feeding and swallowing problems in toddlers or preschoolers generally appear more severe than the reactions of infants who are learning how to munch and chew foods.[13,15] The decrease in appetite expected in toddlers and preschoolers may be pronounced in children who find eating difficult and unpleasant. These feeding problems may require further study to make sure eating is safe for a child, and not related to frequent illness such as bronchitis or pneumonia.

A child with ***hypotonia*** or ***hypertonia*** in the upper body may experience difficulty sitting for a meal and self-feeding with a spoon.[8] If these feeding problems are not resolved by providing therapy in early-intervention programs or schools, children are likely to resist eating over time. When all nutrition cannot be provided orally, the child becomes technology dependent for feeding, requiring a form of nutrition support, such as placement of a ***gastrostomy***.[15]

Two concepts support services for families who have young children with complex health care needs:

1. *Every family deserves a plan for coordinated, interdisciplinary care that considers the child as a whole.* This is more likely to be accomplished with a *medical home*; this is a pediatrician or an experienced health care provider who oversees everything, such as keeping all medication records to protect the family from fragmented, bureaucratic, and duplicative services.[27]
2. *Young children thrive best when they live at home, even those*

**neuromuscular disorders** Conditions of the nervous system characterized by difficulty with voluntary or involuntary control of muscle movement.

**hypotonia** Condition characterized by low muscle tone, floppiness, or muscle weakness.

**hypertonia** Condition characterized by high muscle tone, stiffness, or spasticity.

**gastrostomy** Form of enteral nutrition support for delivering nutrition by tube directly into the stomach, bypassing the mouth through a surgical procedure that creates an opening through the abdominal wall and stomach.

*who are technology dependent and have complex health care needs.* They benefit when ongoing care is provided in the family home rather than in a hospital, or in a series of rehospitalizations.[27]

These concepts apply to nutrition services, too. Here is an example. A 20-month-old girl named Isabella has survived lengthy hospitalizations after birth and at 8 months of age. She now requires 12 daily medications, a mostly liquid diet modified in energy, both oral and non-oral feedings, physical therapy, speech and language therapy, and occupational therapy. When the family found out that such therapists come to a nearby day care center, they enrolled her since both parents needed to work. Isabella attends this day care center located in a school that participates in the USDA Child Nutrition Program. USDA regulations require a physician to sign an order for modifying the menu at school and child care sites. This paperwork cannot be signed by a nutrition expert who teaches the family how to implement the modified food and beverage choices at home. Additional paperwork is required for Isabella's expensive special formula for insurance coverage and for prescribed nutritional supplements. Isabella cannot chew well, so supplemental calcium and Vitamin D are prescribed in liquid form. Her mother is able to keep her job in part because the pediatrician coordinates all the required reports, prescriptions, and paperwork. Isabella progresses in her oral feeding skills now that her therapies are coordinated.

## Nutrition-Related Conditions

**LO 11.5** Identify conditions in young children with special needs in which nutrition services are a part of medical management.

### Failure to Thrive

Failure to thrive (FTT) is a condition in which an energy deficit is suspected.[13,28] FTT has a slightly different basis in toddlers and preschoolers, who may have grown adequately during the first year. Their decrease in growth rate occurs at the age when appetite typically decreases and control issues at mealtime are expected, making identifying the cause of FTT more difficult.[29] Generally FTT is suspected when a child's growth declines more than two growth percentiles, placing the child near or below the lowest percentile in weight-for-age, weight-for-length, and/or BMI. FTT may result from a complex interplay of medical and environmental factors, such as the following:[13,28]

- Digestive problems such as gastrointestinal reflux or celiac disease
- Asthma or breathing problems
- Neurological conditions such as seizures
- Pediatric AIDS

Children who have chronic illnesses or were born preterm have a higher risk of FTT as a result of abuse or ***medical neglect.***[29] They have greater needs than other children do, and they may be more irritable and demanding, which places them at risk. Often a specific nutrient or group of nutrients is suspected of being inadequate in children with FTT, when the more appropriate emphasis should be placed on energy and protein. As an example, copper and zinc in the blood of toddlers with FTT were reported to be the same as age-matched controls, although protein intake was lower.[30]

Recovery from FTT can include catch-up growth, which is acceleration in growth rate for age.[13] If energy is provided at a higher level than for a typical child of the same age, catch-up growth is likely (see Illustration 11.3). The length of time needed for catch-up growth varies, but some weight gain should be documented within a few weeks. For example, recovery from FTT for one 3-year-old was a gain of 6 pounds—more weight than is typical to gain in 1 year—within the first 3 months of living in a new home.

The opposite of FTT, obesity, is usually not a concern in the toddler and preschool age range when there is a medical history of a preterm birth. Increasingly, questions are being raised as to whether medical management of sick newborns does or does not increase the risk of diabetes and overweight later in childhood.[31] There is a growing group of overgrowth or obesity syndromes identified in the toddler and preschool age range that are quite different from typical childhood obesity. Prader-Willi syndrome is an example because the onset of obesity is typically after infancy.[10] Another example is Wiedemann-Beckwith syndrome, in which an usually high rate of weight gain is typical in toddlers.[15] Such conditions are not necessarily a result of excessive energy intake but rather from endocrine or metabolic abnormalities, body composition changes, or drug side effects. Many conditions have behavioral or developmental components that are found at older ages after the symptom of early obesity. Such conditions are good reminders of how nutrition services and recommendations have to be adjusted for children with special needs.

### Toddler Diarrhea and Celiac Disease

Toddlers are likely to develop diarrhea. The condition is called toddler diarrhea, in which otherwise healthy growing children have diarrhea so often that their parents bring them for a checkup.[13] Testing shows no intestinal damage and normal blood levels, without FTT or weight loss. The culprit is likely to be excessive intake of juices that contain sucrose or sorbitol. The diarrhea results from excess water being pulled into the intestine, so limiting juice intake may be recommended.[25,26]

**medical neglect** Failure of parent or caretaker to seek, obtain, and follow through with a complete diagnostic study or medical, dental, or mental health treatment for a health problem, symptom, or condition that, if untreated, could become severe enough to present a danger to the child.

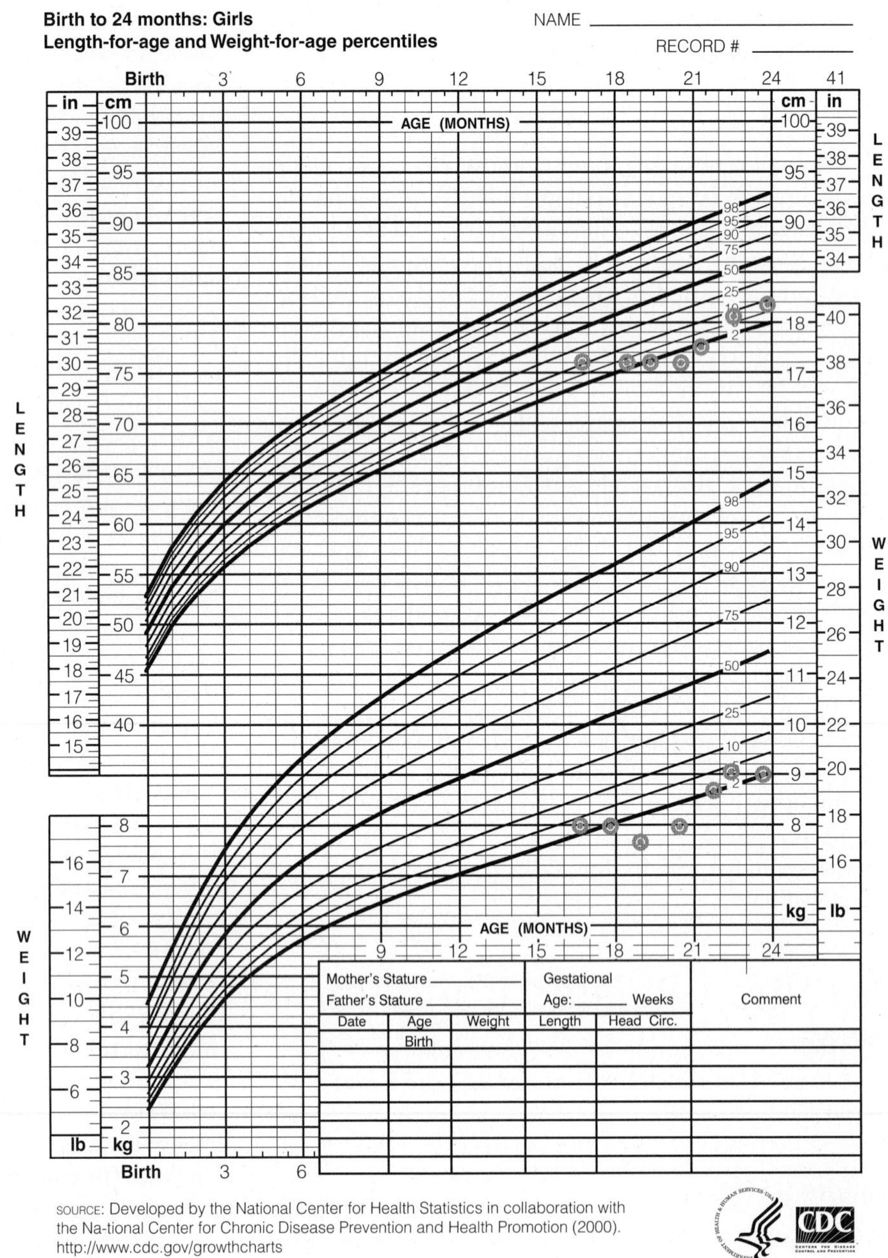


ILLUSTRATION 11.3 ▸ Growth chart for a girl with failure to thrive before and after intervention.

Toddlers and preschoolers with unexplained diarrhea need to have medical evaluations to rule out known conditions that cause diarrhea, such as lactose intolerance, prescribed medication side-effects, and celiac disease. Celiac disease occurs in people who are sensitive to gluten, a component of wheat, rye, and barley. Celiac disease is not the same as gluten intolerance, which is one symptom. It has a prevalence of 1 in 3,000 people within certain ethnic groups, such as those of Middle Eastern or Irish ancestry.[32] Celiac may be related to other chronic conditions, such as Down syndrome, and cancer treated by certain chemotherapy regimens. Symptoms of diarrhea and other digestive problems usually develop by 2 years of age. Confirmation of the condition is based on testing blood for the antibodies to gluten. Nutrition intervention is based on modifying food and nutrient intake with a complete restriction of any foods with gluten. This list includes everything made with flour, such as bread and pasta, as well as foods with wheat, barley, or rye as an additive.[32] The allowed foods include rice, soy, corn, and potato flours. Oats are gluten free but may be contaminated with gluten from wheat mixed in. Meats, fruits, and vegetables are not restricted, but many processed foods use wheat flour for thickening. After instituting food and nutrient intake restrictions, the intestinal damage heals, and the digestive symptoms disappear. The parents of preschoolers with celiac disease learn to be expert readers of food labels because intestinal damage recurs if gluten is eaten by mistake.

## Autism Spectrum Disorders

The term autism is more accurately described as ***autism spectrum disorders (ASD)*** since it is a group of developmental disabilities. These conditions were previously defined as autistic disorder, pervasive developmental disorder not otherwise specified (PDD-NOS), and Asperger syndrome.[33,34] ASD is presumably present at birth with symptoms apparent before age 3 years. (See also Chapter 13 for a discussion of ASDs in older children.) The toddler and preschool years are when behavioral signs of ASDs are noted by families. Early screening and diagnostic evaluations are recommended by the AAP for those with suspected speech delays, repetitive behaviors, and social skill deficits.[34] Preschoolers with ASDs are sensitive to all types of sensory information This sensitivity often results in a rigid, self-restricted range of food choices, which can lead to parent and caregivers concerns about the nutritional adequacy of the child's intake (Table 11.5). Nutritionists can offer families nutrition assessments of the child's food and nutrient intake and recommend nutrition interventions that assure the child's self-restricted food selections still meet their needs. Some families will restrict their child's intake of foods and beverages containing gluten and casein, in an attempt to improve behavior or gastrointestinal symptoms.[34] However, these dietary manipulations have not been endorsed by the AAP or other professional organizations due to lack to evidence of their efficacy. One recent systematic review evaluated the use of gluten and casein-free diets in children with ASD and found the evidence to be limited and weak. These authors recommended that these products should be eliminated in children with ASD's diets only when there is evidence of a true food intolerance or allergy.[35] Milk substitutes to avoid casein may or may not meet the child's need for calcium, vitamin D, protein, or other nutrients. Families of children with ASDs report a variety of gastrointestinal problems, but food and nutrient intake recommendations for ASDs are the same as for any other child of the same age who has feeding problems.[13] Nutritionists who work in early intervention programs and developmental evaluation centers become familiar with feeding problems in toddlers and preschoolers with ASDs because they are so prevalent. One recent study suggested that parent education along with experienced therapists could improve intake in dietary variety and decrease difficult mealtime behaviors in children ages 2–6 with ASD.[6]

**TABLE 11.5** Food and nutrient intake of 2-year-old child with a suspected autism spectrum disorder

| |
|---|
| Dry Fruit Loops cereal |
| 10 fl oz calcium-supplemented orange juice drink |
| Chicken fingers from a specific fast-food restaurant |
| French fries |
| 10 fl oz calcium-supplemented orange juice drink |
| Waverly crackers |
| Pringles potato chips |
| 10 fl oz calcium-supplemented orange juice drink |
| Oatmeal cake |
| 10 fl oz calcium-supplemented orange juice drink |



## Muscle Coordination Problems and Cerebral Palsy

Cerebral palsy (CP) is a shorthand name for a wide range of conditions in which medical diagnoses, educational categories, and nutrition diagnoses differ. Most children are diagnosed with CP by 1–2 years of age.[13] Some toddlers have muscle coordination problems combined with other developmental delays; others have a diagnosis of ***spastic quadriplegia***. The prevalence of cerebral palsy is 2.0–2.5 per 1000 children, with the highest risk found in children who were born prematurely. The more premature an infant is, the more likely he or she will develop CP.[37,5,24] Toddlers and preschoolers who were born preterm account for much of the increase in muscle coordination problems seen before cerebral palsy can be diagnosed.

Those at risk for or confirmed with cerebral palsy have a higher need for nutrition services than other toddlers and preschoolers, in part because the condition changes over the early childhood years. The lack of a clear diagnosis should not delay appropriate nutrition services, as growth and feeding problems worsen over time without intervention. Nutrition services start with nutrition assessments that include body composition indexes, such as fat stores.[24] Nutrition interventions are then based on these findings, and they may include encouraging weight gain if body fat stores are low. The child with muscle coordination problems may appear thin as a result of small muscle size and not low-fat stores; weight gain is not needed. Their growth tracking may not fit the WHO or CDC growth charts.[37,20,21] Part of the growth assessment for a preschooler with cerebral palsy may include an estimate of energy needs for activity, which may be higher or lower than expected. A girl may expend higher energy in her efforts to coordinate walking while receiving physical therapy 3 days per week at school. Her activity may be lower if she is in a wheelchair most of the time.

Feeding assessment for a child with severe cerebral palsy called *spastic quadriplegia* might be necessary as part of the overall nutritional assessment.[8,37]

**autism spectrum disorders (ASDs)** A group of developmental disorders characterized by deficits in communication, social interaction, and behaviors that meet diagnostic criteria in standardized testing, with onset generally before age 3.

**spastic quadriplegia** A form of cerebral palsy in which brain damage interferes with voluntary muscle control in both arms and legs.

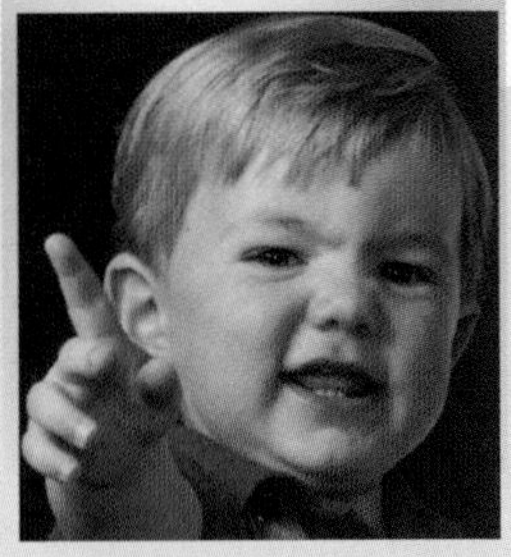
Photodisc

# CASE STUDY 11.2

## Early Intervention Services for a Boy at Risk for Nutrition Support

Roberto was born at 30 weeks gestation and is now 25 months old years old. His parents and extended families main concern is that "he is difficult to feed. He cries and refuses to eat when offered meals, even those with his favorite foods."

The registered dietitian nutritionist (RDN) who consults at the early intervention program meets with the family, assesses Roberto, and reviews his medical records. The first step by the RDN is to observe Roberto's feeding by his mother and to evaluate his growth pattern and nutritional intake. The nutritionist and occupational therapist are concerned that Roberto is choking so easily, and recommend he undergo a swallowing study. Roberto does not attend the early intervention program for the next 3 weeks. The swallowing study indicates he is aspirating some of his liquids into his lungs and so oral feeding is not safe for the moment. He requires a gastrostomy for tube feedings. His parents learn how to feed him a specialized formula through the gastrostomy tube.

Nutrition services provided in the early intervention program are now documenting his growth as adjustments are made in his gastrostomy feeding schedule. Roberto gains weight over the next 6 months and becomes more interactive with the staff at the early intervention center. He begins to progress in his walking and speaking skills. The occupational and speech therapist work with his oral motor skills. A repeat swallowing study will be conducted in the near future. The goal is for Roberto to consume all of his nutrition by mouth once his swallowing is normalized and he is no longer at risk of aspirating his feedings.

### Questions

1. What are the indications that Roberto needed to have a swallowing study?
2. Could the gastrostomy placement have been prevented if Roberto had gained weight?
3. Why is it important to have more than one health care discipline involved in Roberto's care?

The assessment may include an observation of eating to determine any restrictions in the type of foods that the child can eat, and whether coordinating muscles for chewing, swallowing, and/or using a spoon or fork are working well. Table 11.6 provides a food-intake record for a 4-year-old girl with spastic quadriplegia who does not walk and is receiving nutritional interventions for weight gain. Her meal pattern was adjusted because she tires easily while eating. She does not like to eat too much at a time, and she refuses to be fed by another person (which is appropriate for her age). She can chew foods such as fresh apple, but then is too tired to eat something else. She eats a larger portion if the food is soft and does not require her to work so hard. She has gained weight at a slow rate, and her fat stores are low. The first plan is to use regular foods that are easy for her to eat to meet her nutritional needs, including cooked rather than fresh vegetables and fruits, and to avoid hard-to-chew foods, such as roast beef or corn on the cob. If she does not gain weight by eating foods such as those suggested in Table 11.6, she may need nutritional supplementation to assure her nutritional needs are met within her feeding limitations (see Case Study 11.2).

## Pulmonary Problems

Breathing conditions are examples of common problems in children with special health care needs, and have major nutritional consequences. Breathing problems may carry a medical diagnosis such as ***asthma***, or reoccur without any diagnosis, such as respiratory symptoms related to suspected allergies or infections.[38] Asthma is self-reported in 58 of every 1000 children under 5 years of age.[38,36] Asthma results in more emergency-room visits for children under 5 years—at 121 visits per 10,000 people—than it does in older children with asthma.[38] Asthma per se does not require nutrition services, but some children with asthma may also have food allergies. Families may restrict specific food groups such as dairy with the unsubstantiated belief that "milk increases mucus."[39] There is also an in increased incidence of overweight and obesity in children with asthma.[40]

Nutrition diagnoses for a child with breathing problems are based on their impact on food and nutrient intake, such as excessive fluid intake, due to the difficulty with eating compared to drinking or involuntary weight loss as a result of frequent illness.[13]

Nutrition services are needed because recurrent breathing problems increase nutritional needs, lower interest in eating, and can slow growth rate (see Case Study 11.2).[13]

Infants who are born prematurely are more likely

**asthma** Condition in which the lungs are unable to exchange air due to lack of expansion of air sacs. It can result in a chronic illness and sometimes unconsciousness and death if not treated.

to have breathing difficulties carry into toddlerhood. Up to 80 percent of 1000-gram infants can develop what is known as chronic lung disease of infancy or ***bronchopulmonary dysplasia (BPD)***. BPD is thought to be the consequence of unresolved or unrepaired lung damage that occurs to a premature infant who receives supplemental oxygen and ventilator support in a neonatal intensive care unit.[37] Toddlers and preschoolers with BPD need extra energy due to the extra calories expended in breathing. Increased ***work of breathing (WOB)*** occurs with different pulmonary conditions and generally leads to low interest in feeding, partially as a result of tiredness.[41,42] Feeding difficulties have several causes in a toddler treated for BPD:[37]

- The normal progression of feeding skills is interrupted.
- Medications and their side effects contribute to high nutrition needs.
- Interrupted sleep and fatigue make hunger and fullness cues harder to interpret.

By the preschool years, the impact of BPD on slowing the rate of weight gain is usually clear. Exposure to common respiratory illnesses, which are minor in typical children, can require a trip back to the hospital for some children with BPD. Increased frequency of infections adds another limitation to proper weight gain and growth. Neither the CDC growth chart nor the WHO growth chart may be helpful in predicting a child with BPD's growth pattern, but periods of health are usually accompanied by an increase in weight and appetite.

Food and nutrient intake recommendations for toddlers with BPD are similar to those for children with weakness (Table 11.6). Small, frequent meals with foods that are concentrated energy sources are needed. Easy-to-eat foods may still be recommended so that fatigue from meals is low. If the toddler with breathing problems does not gain weight as a result of nutrition interventions (Table 11.6), the next step would be to add homemade or commercially prepared nutritional supplements to meet the higher energy and protein needs. These supplements, such as Pediasure® or KinderCal®, are designed to meet the needs of children ages 1–10. They are also a source of vitamins and minerals. Proper nutrition and growth is essential for toddlers and preschoolers with BPD as new lung tissue can grow until about 8 years of age. This lung growth allows for the resolution of BPD.[41]

### Developmental Delay and Evaluations

Developmental delay may be suspected when specific nutrients are consumed in inadequate or excessive amounts. Iron deficiency and lead toxicity are risk factors for developmental problems.[5] Developmental delay is a specific diagnosis that may be replaced by ***intellectual disability*** when the child is 6 or 7 years old.[44] Changes in growth rate are typical in children with developmental delay.[5,27] Short stature is common and part of the unusual growth pattern that often prompts referrals for genetic testing.[7] The evaluation of growth from a genetic expert may include more in-depth analyses, such as measurements of hand and foot size and bone age.[18] Genetic syndromes also can be associated with unusually fast growth. Soto's syndrome is a rare disorder in which the child is tall and large, but has delayed development.[18]

TABLE 11.6 ▸ Meal pattern and recommended foods for an underweight girl with feeding problems as a result of weakness

| MEAL PATTERN: SMALL, FREQUENT MEALS AND SNACKS TO PREVENT TIREDNESS AT MEALS | RECOMMENDED FOODS THAT ARE EASY TO CHEW, WITH SMALL PORTIONS |
|---|---|
| Breakfast at home | **Breakfast:** ½ cup oatmeal with added soft fruit, margarine, and brown sugar |
| Mid-morning snack<br>Lunch (at preschool)<br>Afternoon snack (at preschool)<br>After-school snack | **Snacks:** 1 slice deli meat with 6 fl oz whole milk with Carnation Instant Breakfast added ½ cup soft-cooked sliced apples with added margarine<br>Cake-type cookie (frosting allowed) |
| Dinner | **Dinner:** ½ cup mashed potato with added margarine<br>3 Tbsp meat loaf<br>3 Tbsp soft-cooked carrots with added margarine |
| Bedtime snack | **Bedtime snack:** Chocolate cake with frosting and 4 fl oz whole milk |



## Food Allergies and Intolerance

LO 11.6 Review food allergy and intolerance consequences for young children.

A true food allergy is a response by the body's immune system to a food or food additive. True food allergies are estimated to be present in 2–8 percent of children.[45] Food allergies are usually identified in toddlers and preschoolers because allergy testing in infancy is not useful due to the incomplete development of the immune system.[13,45] True food allergies can result in life-threatening

**bronchopulmonary dysplasia (BPD)** Condition in which the underdeveloped lungs in a preterm infant are damaged so that breathing requires extra effort.

**work of breathing (WOB)** A common term used to express extra respiratory effort in a variety of pulmonary conditions.

**intellectual disability** Substantially below-average intelligence and problems in adapting to the environment, which emerge before age 18 years.

episodes of ***anaphylaxis***.[13,45] Examples of food allergies that may result in anaphylaxis for some children include the following:[45]

- Cow's milk
- Eggs
- Wheat
- Peanuts
- Tree nuts
- Soy
- Crustacean shellfish

Cow's milk protein allergy rarely persists into the toddler and preschool years. However, when cow's milk protein allergy does persist, symptoms in the toddler and preschool years may appear as more general allergy symptoms, such as asthma or skin rashes.[45] Other food allergies are often present in a child with confirmed cow's milk protein allergy, with, for example, 35 percent reacting also to oranges or 47 percent reacting also to soy milk.[13,45]

True food allergies can greatly affect the family. Strict and complete avoidance of the food that causes the allergy is required. This abstinence includes all settings, such as eating nothing prepared at bake sales when the food ingredients are unknown. An extensively restricted therapeutic intervention for a preschooler includes how nutrient and energy adequacy is assured. Whatever is planned, restrictions are likely to result in mealtime behavioral problems. The parents may become overprotective, or the child may quickly learn to use restricted foods to get a parent's concern and attention. There are many resources available for caregivers who have children with food allergies such as The Food Allergy Research and Education Network (www.foodallergy.org). For children at risk for anaphylaxis, parents and caregivers should be given instruction in emergency lifesaving procedures and use of an injected form of epinephrine.[13,45]

# Dietary Supplements and Herbal Remedies

**LO 11.7** Compare use of dietary and herbal remedies in young children with and without special health care needs.

> "It is better to take food into the mouth than to take worries into the heart."
>
> —Yiddish saying

Families who are concerned that something may be wrong with their young children may be attracted to health and nutritional claims targeted and packaged for adults. The family that is having difficulty finding effective treatment for a child is most at risk for inappropriate or ineffective alternative products. Foods and supplements claiming probiotic benefits for adults are expanding into use for children, even though they not intended for chronically ill young children. Physicians recommend that their appropriate use in young children be safely limited, in spite of their expansion into the marketplace.[46] Use of dietary supplements in children with chronic conditions is more common than in healthy children, as most families take dietary supplements not prescribed or discussed with health care providers.[47] Examples of dietary supplements are vitamins, minerals, botanicals, amino acids, and fatty acids.[47] Parent coalitions and advocacy groups are excellent sources of networking for families, but they can also be sources of nutritional claims for products and food and nutrient intake regimens that have no scientific testing behind them.[48] Down syndrome, for example, is a disorder for which nutritional supplementation has been marketed to parents. No specific nutrients, combinations of nutrients, or herbal remedies have been shown to improve the intellectual functioning of individuals with Down syndrome.[16] The National Down Syndrome Society (www.ndss.org) cautions parents about the ineffectiveness of nutrient and herbal supplements to discourage their use, but interest continues.[49] It is important for care providers to be encouraged to discuss with a trusted health professional whatever supplements or over-the-counter products are of interest before giving them to young children.

# Sources of Nutrition Services

**LO 11.8** Explain how families access community and regional resources that provide nutrition services for toddlers and preschoolers with chronic health problems.

Most young children are healthy and do not see nutritionists as a part of routine care. Low-income families with young children are more likely to see a nutritionist than higher-income families, because of their participation in WIC. Registered dietitian nutritionists with training in pediatrics are best qualified to provide nutrition therapy to toddlers and preschool children with chronic conditions. Leadership Education in Neurodevelopmental and Related Disabilities (LEND) training programs are funded in part by the Maternal and Child Health Bureau and administered by the Health Resources and Service's Administration to improve the health of infants, children, and adolescents with disabilities. These programs train nutritionists and other health professionals to provide interdisciplinary, family-centered care to children with neurodevelopmental disabilities.[50] These programs also receive funding from legislation titled "Combating Autism Act of 2006" (Public Law 109–416),[51] designed to enable all infants, children, and adolescents who have, or are at risk for developing, ASD, and other

**anaphylaxis** Sudden onset of a reaction with mild to severe symptoms, including a decrease in ability to breathe, which may be severe enough to cause a coma.

developmental disabilities to reach their full potential by early screening, identification, and access to services.

Programs in which nutrition care may be accessed include the following:[9,50,51]

- State programs for children with special health care needs
- Early intervention programs (age 0 up to 36 months)
- Early childhood education programs (IDEA, ages 3–5 years)
- Head Start; regular program or special-needs category (ages 3–5 years)
- Early Head Start; regular program or special-needs category (0 up to 36 months)
- WIC
- Low-birthweight follow-up programs
- Child care feeding programs (USDA)

These programs are described in Chapters 8 and 10. Efforts to increase program accessibility come from state and federal governmental offices, toll-free outreach services, and websites. Specific outreach programs to locate toddlers and preschoolers at risk are funded in each state, under names such as "Child Find."[46] Because every child at risk is eligible for a screening, contacting a neighborhood public school is a good starting place to locate services, even if the child is not old enough to attend the school.

## KEY POINTS

1. Toddlers and preschoolers with special health care needs may have alterations in their nutritional needs, growth, and feeding skills. Early intervention programs and early childhood education programs are essential to help these children meet their intellectual, developmental, and growth potentials.
2. Toddlers and preschoolers with special health care needs are quite varied in their nutrition needs, but the basic concepts of supporting growth, typical feeding skill development, and meeting nutrition needs for age and activity still apply.
3. Families of children with special health care needs may use unsubstantiated over-the-counter products, such as herbal supplements, vitamins, or probiotic-containing foods for adults, which can be dangerous for young children.
4. Failure to thrive is often the reason children with special health care needs enter medical, educational, and developmental services. Such cases of failure to thrive cannot be corrected with additional energy, as it can be in children without special health care needs. Unusual growth patterns can be signs of conditions that are not directly related to nutrition.
5. Medical conditions with nutritional implications found in toddlers and preschoolers with special health needs are: autism spectrum disorder, ADHD, cerebral palsy, BPD, developmental delay, and food allergies.

## REVIEW QUESTIONS

1. What is an accurate statement about services for a boy with Down syndrome who has difficulty chewing when he turns 3 years old?
   a. He is now eligible to start receiving supplementary social security if his family meets the income requirements.
   b. He needs speech therapy to address his difficulty chewing.
   c. He is no longer eligible for early childhood programs under IDEA.
   d. His chewing difficulty cannot be included in his nutrition services, as it is a typical component of his underlying syndrome.
2. What is an accurate statement about a preschool girl who has a diagnosed milk-protein allergy?
   a. If she attends a public day care that participates in the USDA Child Nutrition Program, her family has to provide her lunch for her safety.
   b. Only if this allergy is a feature of an underlying condition is she considered a child eligible for educational modifications under IDEA.
   c. Her allergy would still let her have ice cream as a special treat on her birthdays.
   d. She may grow out of this allergy as she gets older.
3. A 4-year-old with asthma does not have food allergies. Her asthma routine requires a home breathing machine and two prescribed medications. Which statement is accurate about her nutrition needs?
   a. Her diagnosis is one of the more common types of special needs and is best managed by a reduced-calorie diet to compensate for restricted activity.
   b. Compliance with her nutrition recommendations can prevent emergency-room visits for flare-ups.
   c. Her prescribed medications could impact her appetite and growth and so require nutrition services.

d. Asthma is likely to interrupt the normal progression of eating skills in a young child.

4. Feeding and eating problems do not require nutrition services under which of these conditions?
   a. When a 3-year-old boy has a food jag and refuses to eat foods he usually likes.
   b. When the parents or caregivers are concerned that a toddler wants to drink milk or juice but refuses solid foods such as fruit.
   c. When a 3-year-old child has been diagnosed with ASD and is entering a behavioral management program.
   d. When a 3-year-old child is diagnosed with gastroesophageal reflux and prescribed medications again.

Questions 5, 6, and 7 concern growth assessment. Determine whether each is true or false.

5. Any child with a chronic condition should have a growth assessment as part of determining nutrition status.

   _____ True _____ False

6. A 4-year-old boy with cerebral palsy would have normal growth on the CDC growth charts.

   _____ True _____ False

7. A 21-month-old boy has a growth pattern that plots lower on the standard CDC growth chart than on the WHO growth charts; his growth is plotted incorrectly.

   _____ True _____ False

8. Briefly describe why measuring head size is a part of a nutritional assessment for a toddler or preschooler with a suspected special health care need.

9. Identify two examples of when standard nutrition guidance for healthy toddlers and preschoolers must be modified for a preschool-age child with special health care needs.

10. Identify two examples of when a vitamin or mineral supplement has to be a part of a nutrition services plan.

Visit www.cengagebrain.com to access MindTap, a complete digital course that includes additional resources.

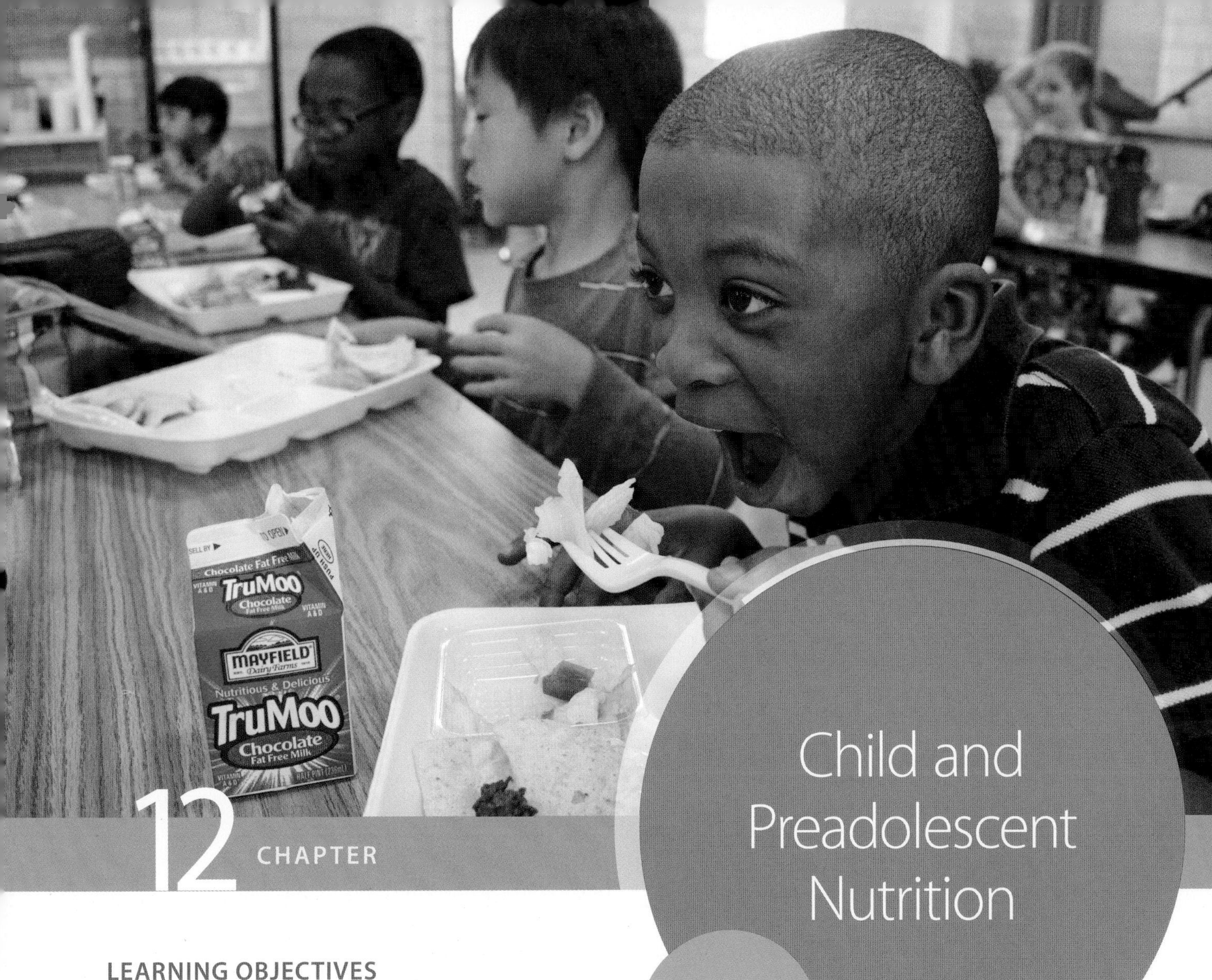


12 CHAPTER

# Child and Preadolescent Nutrition

*Prepared by*
**Beth L. Leonberg**

## LEARNING OBJECTIVES

After studying the materials in this chapter you should be able to:

**12.1** List two Healthy People 2020 objectives that specifically relate to middle childhood and preadolescence.

**12.2** Describe the expected pattern of growth of a healthy child during middle childhood and preadolescence.

**12.3** Define BMI rebound and describe the consequences of early BMI rebound.

**12.4** Explain what influences energy needs of school-age children.

**12.5** List two strategies for preventing dental caries in school-age children.

**12.6** Describe prevention strategies for overweight/obesity in school-age children.

**12.7** Describe the components of a healthy diet during middle childhood and preadolescence as recommended by health and professional organizations and agencies.

**12.8** List two strategies that parents/caretakers can employ to encourage school-age children to be more physically active.

**12.9** List three strategies that school health programs can use to promote healthy eating.

**12.10** Describe one component of the USDA's Child Nutrition Program and explain how this specific program addresses the health of school-age children.

# Introduction

This chapter focuses on the growth and development of school-age and preadolescent children and their relationships to nutritional status. Children continue to grow physically at a steady rate during this period, but development from a cognitive, emotional, and social standpoint is tremendous. This period in a child's life is preparation for the physical and emotional demands of the adolescent growth spurt. Having family members, teachers, and others in their lives who model healthy eating and physical activity behaviors will better equip children for making good choices during adolescence and later in life.

## Definitions of the Life-Cycle Stage

***Middle childhood*** is a term that generally describes children between the ages of 5 and 10 years. ***Preadolescence*** is generally defined as ages 9–11 years for girls and ages 10–12 years for boys. Both these stages of growth and development are also referred to as *school-age*.

## Importance of Nutrition

Adequate nutrition continues to play an important role during the school-age years in ensuring that children reach their full potential for growth, development, and health. Nutrition problems can still occur during this age, such as iron-deficiency anemia, undernutrition, and dental caries. Regarding weight, both ends of the spectrum are seen during this age. The prevalence of obesity is increasing, but the beginnings of eating disorders can also be detected in some school-age and preadolescent children. Therefore, adequate nutrition and the establishment of healthy eating behaviors can help to prevent immediate health problems as well as promote a healthy lifestyle. This may reduce the risk of the child developing a chronic condition, such as obesity, type 2 diabetes, and/or cardiovascular disease later in life.[1] Adequate nutrition, especially eating breakfast, has been associated with improved academic performance in school and reduced tardiness and absences.[2] Meeting energy and nutrient needs, addressing common nutrition problems, and preventing nutrition-related disorders while establishing healthy eating and physical activity habits will be discussed later in this chapter.

# Tracking Child and Preadolescent Health

**LO 12.1** List two Healthy People 2020 objectives that specifically relate to middle childhood and preadolescence.

In 2010, children under 18 years of age comprised nearly 25 percent of the U.S. population.[3] On the whole, Non-Hispanic White and Asian and Pacific Islander children have better child well-being outcomes compared with the other large racial and Hispanic origin groups.[3,4] For example, in 2010, more than one-third of American Indian, African American, and Hispanic children lived in households with incomes below the poverty level ($22,314 for a family of four in 2010), compared to less than one-eighth of Non-Hispanic White and Asian children.[3]

The environment in which a child lives affects the child's health status, including nutrition. In 2010, 7.3 million U.S. children younger than 18 years of age (representing 9.8 percent of the population) did not have health insurance.[3] A similar percentage of children, 9.3 percent, did not see a physician or other health care professional in the previous year for sick or well care. However, almost one-third of children living below the poverty level had visited an emergency room for care in the previous year, as compared to less than one-sixth of children living at twice the poverty level.[3] Lack of transportation is a significant limitation for many families. Disparities in nutrition status indicators exist among races and ethnicities. For instance, the odds of being obese are significantly higher for Non-Hispanic Black children and Mexican American children compared with Non-Hispanic White children.[5] In the discussions that follow regarding nutrition during childhood, the recommendations must always be considered in the context of the individual child's environment.

## Healthy People 2020

A number of objectives in the Healthy People 2020 document are specific to children's health and well-being. Table 10.1 lists Nutrition and Weight Status (NWS) objectives related to food and nutrient composition that pertain to the population aged 2 years and older. Table 12.1 lists additional Healthy People 2020 objectives that are pertinent to a discussion of middle childhood and preadolescence.

# Normal Growth and Development

**LO 12.2** Describe the expected pattern of growth of a healthy child during middle childhood and preadolescence.

During the school-age years, the child's growth is steady, but the growth velocity is not as great as it was during infancy or as great as it will be during adolescence. The average annual growth during the school years is 7 pounds

**middle childhood** Children between the ages of 5 and 10 years; also referred to as "school-age."

**preadolescence** The stage of development immediately preceding adolescence; 9–11 years of age for girls and 10–12 years of age for boys.

TABLE 12.1 ▸ Healthy People 2020 Objectives related to school-age children[6]

| HEALTHY PEOPLE 2020 OBJECTIVE | | BASELINE | TARGET |
|---|---|---|---|
| NWS-2.1: | Increase the proportion of schools that do not sell or offer calorically sweetened beverages to students. | 9.3% | 21.3% |
| NWS-2.2: | Increase the proportion of school districts that require schools to make fruits or vegetables available whenever other food is offered or sold. | 6.6% | 18.6% |
| NWS-10.2: | Reduce the proportion of children (aged 6–11 years) who are considered obese. | 17.4% | 15.7% |
| NWS-11.2: | Prevent inappropriate weight gain in children aged 6–11 years (developmental). | | |
| PA-4: | Increase the proportion of the nation's public and private schools that require daily physical education for all students. | | |
| | Elementary schools | 3.8% | 4.2% |
| | Middle and junior high schools | 7.9% | 8.6% |
| PA-6.2: | Increase the proportion of school districts that require regularly scheduled elementary school recess. | 57.1% | 62.8% |
| PA-8.2.2: | Increase the proportion of children and adolescents aged 6–14 years who view television, videos, or play video games for no more than 2 hours a day. | 78.9% | 86.8% |
| PA-8.3.2: | Increase the proportion of children and adolescents aged 6 to 14 years who use a computer or play computer games outside of school (for nonschool work) for no more than 2 hours a day. | 93.3% | 100% |
| PA-13.2: | Increase the proportion of trips to school of 1 mile or less made by walking by children and adolescents aged 5–15 years (developmental). | | |
| PA-14.2: | Increase the proportion of trips to school of 2 miles or less made by bicycling children and adolescents aged 5–15 years (developmental). | | |

SOURCE: U.S. Department of Health and Human Services

(3–3.5 kg) in weight and 2.5 inches (6 cm) in height.[7] Children of this age continue to have spurts of growth that usually coincide with periods of increased appetite and intake. During periods of slower growth, the child's appetite and intake will decrease. Parents should not be overly concerned with this variability in appetite and intake in their school-age children.

Periodic monitoring of growth continues to be important in order to identify any deviations in the child's growth pattern. Children should continue to be weighed on calibrated scales without shoes and in lightweight clothing. The child's stature or standing height should be measured without shoes and utilizing a wall-mounted stadiometer (see Illustration 10.3). A stadiometer consists of a non-stretchable tape on a flat surface like a wall, with a movable right-angle head board. The child's heels, buttocks, shoulders, and back of the head should be touching the wall or flat surface, and the child should be instructed to stand tall, looking straight ahead with arms by the sides, during the measurement. Both weight and height should be plotted on the appropriate 2000 CDC growth charts.

## The 2000 CDC Growth Charts

The "CDC Growth Charts: United States" are the recommended tool for monitoring the growth of a child.[8] The appropriate growth charts are gender-specific for children 2–20 years of age, and allow the user to plot weight-for-age, stature-for-age, and body mass index (BMI)-for-age. They can be downloaded from the CDC website www.cdc.gov/growthcharts /cdc_charts.htm. As described in Chapter 10, the growth charts are based on data from the second and third cycles of the National Health and Examination Survey (NHES) and the National Health and Nutrition Examination Surveys (NHANES) I, II, and III. However, weight data for children greater than 6 years of age who participated in NHANES III were not included because there was a known higher prevalence of overweight for these ages. Incorporating this information into the growth charts would reflect an unhealthy standard.[9] Children whose BMI-for-age is greater than or equal to the 85th percentile but less than or equal to the 94th percentile are classified as overweight, while children whose BMI-for-age is greater than or equal to the 95th percentile are classified as obese.[10,11]

A chart for weight-for-stature up to a height of 48 inches (122 cm) for the younger school-age child is available on the CDC website. As with the toddler and preschooler, it is the child's pattern of growth over time that is important rather than any single measurement (Illustration 12.1). The tracking of BMI-for-age percentile is an important screening tool for overweight and obesity as well as undernutrition (Illustration 12.2). Using the correct age of the child when plotting on the

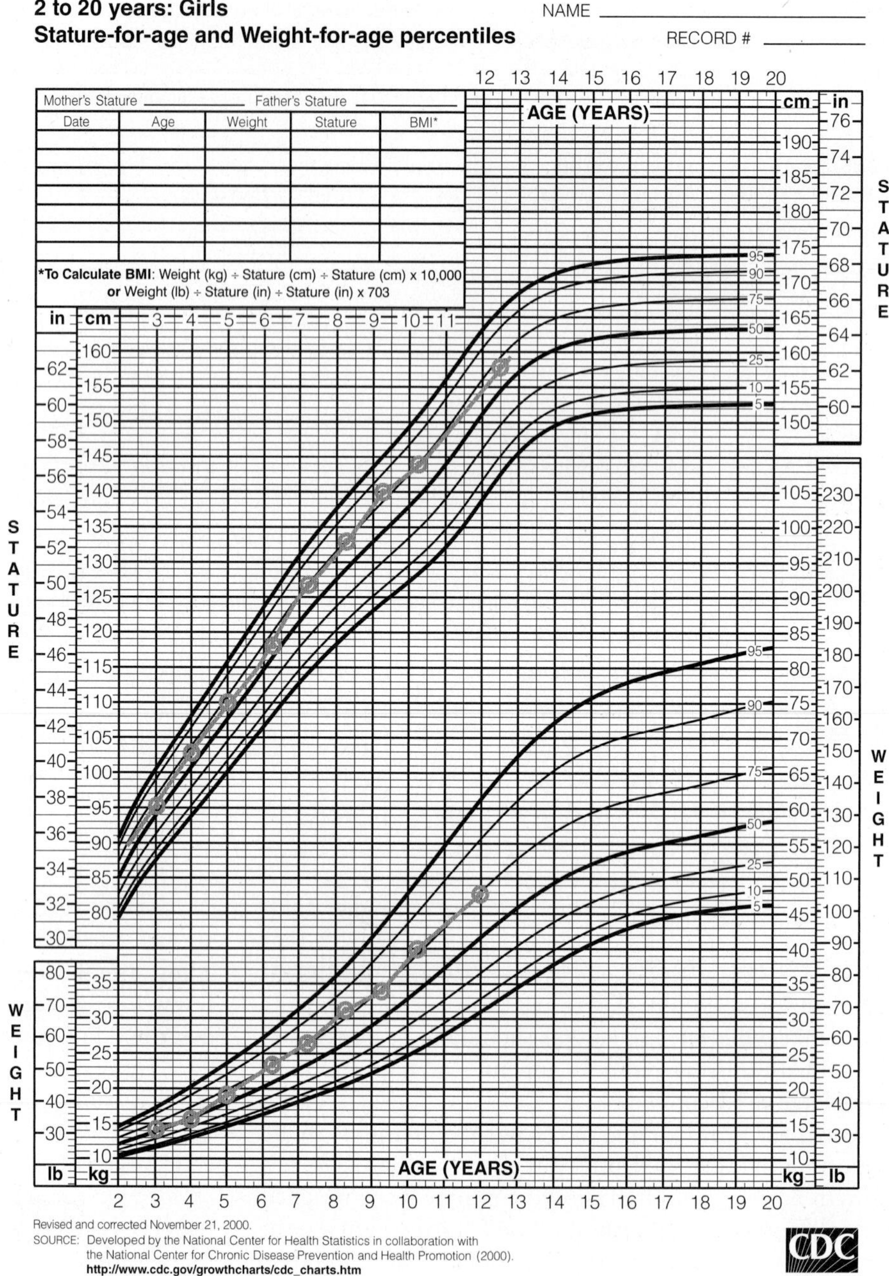


ILLUSTRATION 12.1 ▸ 2 to 20 years: Girls' stature-for-age and weight-for-age percentiles.[8]

growth charts will help to avoid plotting errors and possible misinterpretations of growth trends.

### WHO Growth References

In 2007, the World Health Organization (WHO) released growth references for older school-age children and adolescents, including height-for-age, weight-for-age, and BMI-for-age.[12] Unlike the WHO Child Growth Standards for 0–5 years, which were based on prospective growth data, and the growth reference for school-age children and adolescents was constructed using existing historical data. In most clinical settings in the United States, the CDC Growth Charts are used to monitor the growth of children.

## Physiological and Cognitive Development of School-Age Children

LO 12.3 Define BMI rebound and describe the consequences of early BMI rebound.

### Physiological Development

During middle childhood, muscular strength, motor coordination, and stamina increase progressively.[7] Children are able to perform more complex pattern movements,

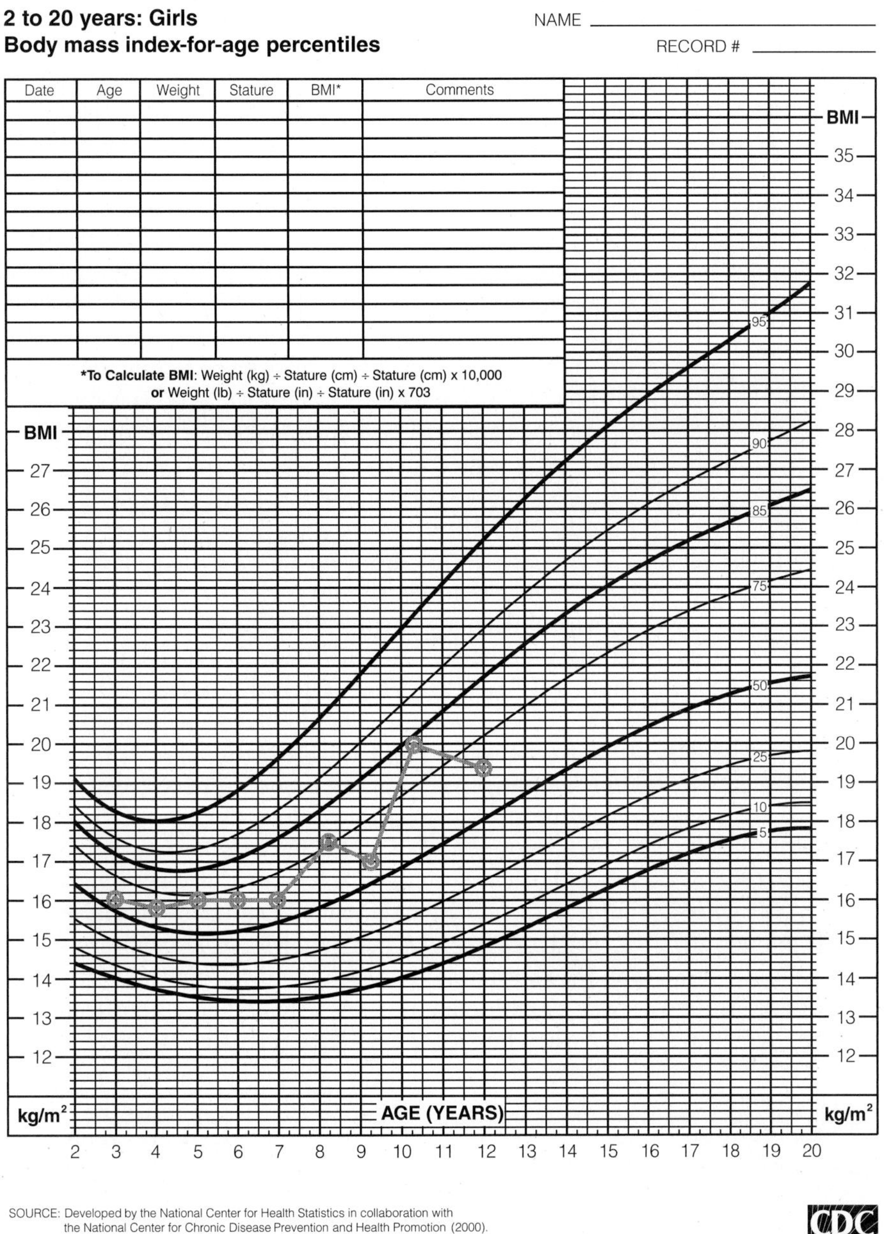


ILLUSTRATION 12.2 ▸ 2 to 20 years: Girls' body mass index-for-age percentiles.[8]

affording them opportunities to participate in activities such as dance, sports, gymnastics, and other physical activities.

During the early childhood years, body fat reaches a minimum of 16 percent in females and 13 percent in males. Percent body fat then increases in preparation for the adolescent growth spurt. This increase in percent body fat, which usually occurs on average at 6 years of age, is called BMI rebound, or adiposity rebound, and is reflected in the BMI-for-age growth charts.[13] An early BMI rebound has been associated with an increase risk of overweight and obesity.[14] The increase in percent body fat with puberty is earlier and greater in females than in males (19 percent for females versus 14 percent for males).[1] During middle childhood, boys have more lean body mass per centimeter of height than girls do. These differences in body composition become more pronounced during adolescence.[1] It is important to understand that BMI is not constant throughout childhood. This is because height is a component of the formula for BMI (weight in kg divided by height in meters squared), and a child's height is constantly increasing as he grows. Plotting BMI-for-age percentile on the growth charts is the only way to know if a child's BMI is outside the normal range for his age. The goal for children is not to strive for a certain range of BMI values, as it is in adults, but rather, to have a BMI-for-age percentile within the normal range.

With the increase in body fat, preadolescents, especially girls, may be concerned that they are becoming overweight. Parents need to be aware that an increase in body fat during this stage is part of normal growth and development. Parents need to be able to reassure their child that these changes are most likely not permanent; parents also need to be careful not to reinforce a preoccupation with weight and size. Boys may become concerned about developing muscle mass and need to understand that they will not be able to increase their muscle mass until middle adolescence (see Chapter 14).[1]

## Cognitive Development

The major developmental achievement during middle childhood is self-efficacy, the knowledge of what to do and the ability to do it. During the school-age years, children move from a developmental stage characterized by magical thinking and egocentrism to one of concrete operations.[7] This stage is characterized by being able to focus on several aspects of a situation at the same time; being able to have more rational cause/effect reasoning; being able to classify, reclassify, and generalize; and a decrease in egocentrism, which allows the child to see another's point of view. Schoolwork becomes increasingly complex as the child gets older. School-age children also enjoy playing strategy games, displaying growing cognitive and language development.

During this stage, the child is developing a sense of self. Children become increasingly independent and are learning their roles in the family, at school, and in the community.[1] Peer relationships become increasingly important, and children begin to separate from their own families by spending the night at a friend's or relative's house. More and more time is spent watching television, playing video games, and being on the computer and Internet. Older children may be able to walk or ride a bicycle to a neighborhood store and purchase snack items. Thus, influences outside the home environment play an increasing role in all aspects of the child's life.

## Development of Feeding Skills and Eating Behaviors

With increased motor coordination, school-age children develop increased feeding skills. During this period, the child masters the use of eating utensils, can be involved in simple food preparation, and can be assigned chores related to mealtime such as setting the table. By performing these tasks, the child learns to contribute to the family, which boosts developing self-esteem. The complexity of the tasks can be increased as the child grows older; for example, a six-year-old may be responsible only for putting napkins and silverware on the table, while a 10-year-old may also put on plates, pour beverages, and get out margarine or salad dressing. At the same time, the child is learning about different foods, simple food preparation, and some basic nutrition facts.

**Eating Behaviors** Parents and older siblings continue to have the most influence on a child's attitudes toward food and food choices during middle childhood and preadolescence. The eating behaviors and cultural food practices and preferences of parents will influence the child's food likes and dislikes. The feeding relationship between parent and child, as described in Chapter 10, still applies to the school-age child. Parents are responsible for the food environment in the home, what foods are available, and when they are served. The child is responsible for how much she eats.[15] Parents need to continue to be positive role models for their children in terms of healthy eating behaviors. They also need to provide the necessary guidance so that the child will be able to make healthy food choices when away from home.

**Family Mealtime** Although the trend over the last 15–20 years is for more meals to be consumed away from home, families should try to eat meals together. When children are involved in school-related activities, eating together is often difficult to achieve because of the family members' hectic schedules. Regardless, eating together as a family should be encouraged, allowing time for conversation (see Illustration 12.3). Excessive reprimanding and arguments should be avoided during mealtime.

Family mealtimes allow parents and caregivers to model healthy eating behaviors and have been shown to improve the nutritional quality of children's meals, as well as weight status.[16-17] A meta-analysis of 17 studies examining the relationship between family meals and nutritional status of children and adolescents found a significant impact when families ate at least three meals together each week.[16] The children in families who regularly ate three or more meals together weekly were 12 percent less likely to be overweight, 20 percent less likely to eat unhealthy foods, 35 percent less likely to have disordered eating, and 24 percent more likely to eat healthy foods.[16]

One study of 9- to 14-year-old children, who were participants of the Nurses' Health Study II, found a positive relationship between families eating dinner together and the overall quality of the children's diets.[15] Children who ate dinner with their families had higher energy intakes as well as higher intakes of nutrients such as fiber, calcium, folate, iron, and vitamins $B_6$, $B_{12}$, C, and E. These children also reported eating more fruits and vegetables, eating fewer fried foods when away from home, and drinking fewer soft drinks. The percentage of children who reported eating family dinner decreased with the age of the child, indicating that family dinner becomes more of a challenge as children get older.[18]

**Outside Influences** School-age children spend more and more time away from home, which is an important part of normal growth and development. Peer influence becomes greater as the child's world expands beyond the family.

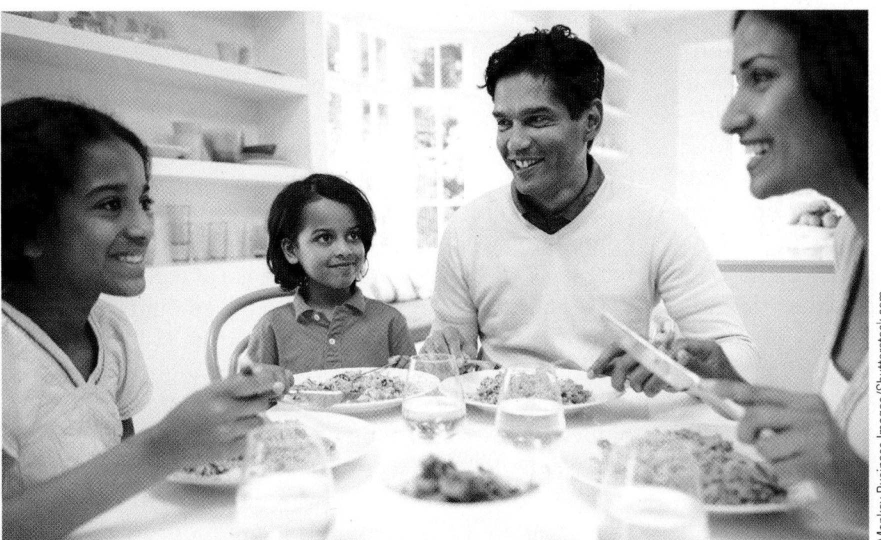

Monkey Business Images/Shutterstock.com

ILLUSTRATION 12.3 ▸ A family enjoying mealtime together.

The increased peer influence extends to attitudes toward foods and food choices. Children may suddenly request a new food or refuse a previous favorite food, based on recommendations from a peer.

Teachers and coaches have an increasing influence on the child's attitudes toward food and eating behaviors. Nutrition should be part of the health curriculum, and what is learned in the classroom should be reinforced by foods available in the school cafeteria. Vending machines present in school as a source of extra funding can also reinforce good nutrition with appropriate choices, or they can be a source of high-fat, high-sugar foods and beverages.

**Media Influence** In their expanding world, children come under the influence of the media. Children want to try foods they see advertised on television. One study analyzed the commercials aired during Saturday morning television programming and found that 49 percent of all advertisements were for food (Illustration 12.4).[19] Of these food advertisements, 91 percent were for foods or beverages high in fat, sodium, or added sugars or were low in nutrients, which is not in line with the recommendations of the U.S. Department of Agriculture's MyPlate (see Chapter 1).[19,20] The impact of advertising on nutrition choices has been evaluated by the Academy of Nutrition and Dietetics (AND) and is summarized in the Academy's Evidence Analysis Library (EAL).[19] The analysts reviewed seven published research studies and concluded that there is strong evidence that advertising can impact the amount of food consumed by children and that they have a preference for branded foods. The research also indicates that children are more likely to choose foods they have seen advertised, whether they are healthy or not. This finding suggests that there may be an opportunity to increase children's intake of healthier foods if they are advertised similarly to unhealthy foods.[21]

Fast-food establishments, with their playgrounds and giveaways, are also attractive to children. With more and more children having access to the Internet, food companies are finding new ways to market their products to children. The new forms of marketing include *advergames,* online games that feature the company's product or brand character; viral marketing that

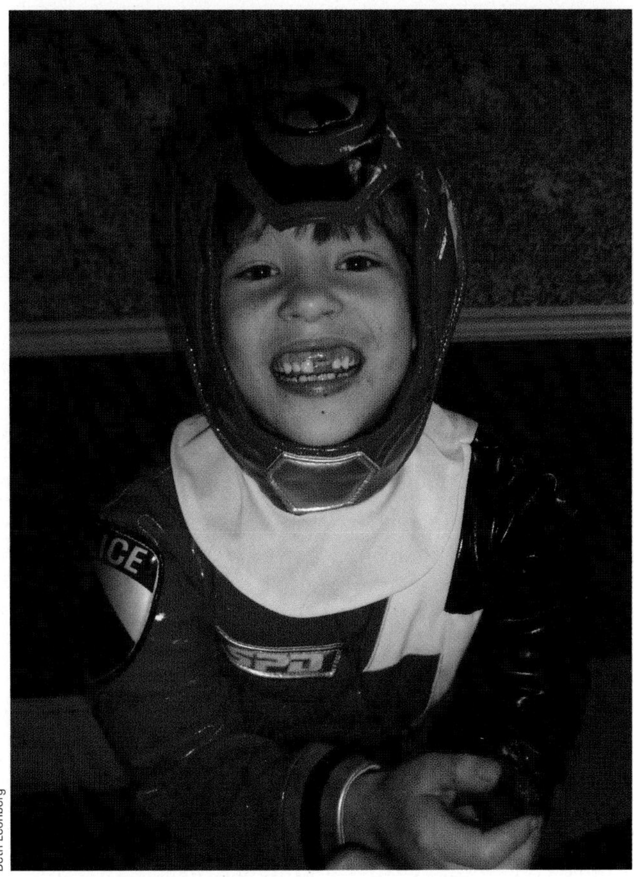

Beth Leonberg

ILLUSTRATION 12.4 ▸ Media have a large influence on children's food choices.

encourages children to send e-mails to their friends about a product; television advertising online, which blurs the lines between advertising and entertainment; and *advercation,* a combination of advertising and education. The impact of online marketing on children's food choices needs further study.[22]

There is some evidence that the food and beverage industry is making positive changes in its marketing targeted toward children;[23] however, critics claim they are unlikely to make substantial changes unless they are required to by law.[24]

**Snacking** Snacks continue to contribute significantly to a child's daily intake. During middle childhood, children cannot consume large amounts of food at one time and therefore need snacks to meet their nutrient needs. However, research shows that snacking has increased significantly in the last 30 years, with the greatest increase in salty snacks and candy, and the greatest overall snack calories coming from desserts and sweetened beverages.[25,26] Many children prepare their own breakfasts or after-school snacks. These children need to have a variety of foods available to them, be equipped with nutrition education for making their own food choices, and have some age-appropriate knowledge and skill in food preparation—assuming, of course, that the family has adequate access to food.

**Food Preference Development, Appetite, and Satiety** Food preference development, appetite, and satiety in young children were thoroughly discussed in Chapter 10. Researchers have described the innate ability of young children to internally control their energy intake and their responsiveness to energy density. The internal controls can be altered by external factors, such as child-feeding practices. Studies in 9- to 10-year-old children found that these older children were not as responsive to energy density as young preschool-age children were.[27] External factors such as the time of day, the presence of other people, and the availability of good food begin to override the internal controls of hunger and satiety as children get older.

Recent research has emphasized the importance of parents assuming responsibility for providing a healthy food environment, but not being overly controlling or restrictive of their child's intake.[28,29,30] When parents try to control their children's intake, especially by restricting their access to food, children become less able to regulate their intake to meet their needs and are more likely to become overweight.[28,29,30] Parents are encouraged to adopt a responsive feeding style, allowing the child to eat in response to their internal hunger and satiety cues.

**Body Image/Excessive Dieting** Parents who had difficulty controlling their own intakes seemed to impose more restrictions on their children. The more the mother is concerned with her own weight and with the risk of her daughter becoming overweight, the more likely she is to employ restrictive child-feeding practices. A study of mothers and their 5-year-old daughters found that this transfer of "restrictive" eating practices may begin as early as the preschool age.[31] These researchers hypothesize that chronic dieting and dietary restraints, which are commonly seen in adolescent girls and young women, may have their beginnings in the early regulation of energy intake and may be related to the amount of parental control exerted over the child's eating.[32] By imposing controls and restrictions over their daughters' intakes, mothers may actually be promoting the intake of the forbidden or restricted foods.[33] Similar results were found in 5-year-old girls whose parents restricted palatable snack foods.[34] Not only did parental restriction promote the consumption of these forbidden foods by the young girls, but also these children reported feeling badly about eating these foods.

Young girls seem to have a preoccupation with weight and size at an early age. With the normal increase in body mass index or body fatness in preadolescence, many girls and their mothers may interpret this phenomenon of normal growth and development as a sign that the child is developing a weight problem. Early "dieting" may actually be a risk factor for the development of obesity.[35] Dieting, which imposes restrictions, is similar to controlling child-feeding practices, which restrict children's intake. Both methods ignore internal cues of hunger and satiety. These types of child-feeding practices not only contribute to the onset of obesity and possibly a nutritionally inferior diet but may also be contributing to the beginnings of eating disorders. Eating disorders are discussed in more detail in Chapter 15.

Many studies of ethnic differences in body image and body-size preferences have been conducted hypothesizing that there are ethnic and gender differences in these parameters. The research conducted to date is not conclusive. One study of men and women of four ethnicities/races—Black, Hispanic, Asian, and White—found that ethnicity alone did not influence the preference for body shapes or tolerance for obesity.[36] In working with individual families, however, it is important to try to assess their health beliefs and their preference for body size, which may impact their readiness for nutrition counseling.

# Energy and Nutrient Needs of School-Age Children

LO 12.4 Explain what influences energy needs of school-age children.

Dietary Reference Intakes (DRIs) tables are provided on the inside front cover of this book. Children need a variety of foods that provide enough energy, protein, carbohydrate, fat, vitamins, and minerals for optimal growth and development.[1]

## Energy Needs

Energy needs of school-age children reflect the slow but steady growth rate during this stage of development. Energy needs of an individual child are dependent on the child's activity level and body size. Equations for estimating energy requirements have been developed as part of the Dietary Reference Intakes, based on a child's gender, age, height, weight, and physical activity level (PAL).[37] Estimated energy expenditure (EER) has been defined as total energy expenditure plus kilocalories for energy deposition. Categories of activity are defined in terms of walking equivalence. For example, an 8-year-old girl who weighs 56.4 pounds (25.6 kg) and is 50.4 inches (128 cm) tall will require 1360 kilocalories per day if sedentary, 1593 kcal/day if she is low-active, 1810 kcal/day if active, and 2173 kcal/day if very active. Energy allowances based on body weight are lower for school-age children than for toddlers and preschoolers. The decrease in the energy requirement per kilogram of body weight is a reflection of slowing growth rate. In addition to the DRI equations for estimating calorie requirements for children, online tools are available on websites such as MyPlate.gov and the website of the USDA/Agriculture Research Service's Children's Nutrition Research Center (see the "Resources" section).

## Protein

Based on the DRIs, the recommended protein intake for school-age children is 0.95 gram of protein per kg body weight per day for 4- to 13-year-old girls and boys.[37] School-age children can meet this recommendation by consuming diets that follow the MyPlate recommendations and the Dietary Guidelines for Americans, 2020.[20,38] Vegetarian diets are also appropriate for school-age children if they provide sufficient energy, complementary protein foods, a variety of foods, and adequate levels of intake of vitamins and minerals.[1] By meeting an individual child's energy needs, protein is spared for tissue repair and growth.

## Vitamins and Minerals

Dietary Reference Intakes (DRIs) for vitamins and minerals have been established for the school-age and preadolescent child (Table 12.2).[39,40] According to food-consumption surveys, children's mean intakes of most nutrients meet or exceed the recommendations. Still, certain subsets of children do not meet their needs for key nutrients such as iron and zinc, which are important for growth, and calcium, needed to achieve peak bone mass.

TABLE 12.2 ▸ Dietary Reference Intakes for key nutrients for school-age children[39,40]

| | RECOMMENDED DAILY ALLOWANCES | | |
|---|---|---|---|
| AGE | IRON (MG/D) | ZINC (MG/D) | CALCIUM (MG/D) |
| 4–8 years | 10 | 5 | 1000 |
| 9–13 years | 8 | 8 | 1300 |



# Common Nutrition Problems

LO 12.5 List two strategies for preventing dental caries in school-age children.

During the last century, common nutrition problems have shifted from problems of nutrient deficiencies to problems of excess nutrition, such as energy, fat, and salt. During middle childhood, some children still experience problems such as iron-deficiency anemia and dental caries, especially with easy accessibility to high-sugar foods. These nutrition problems are addressed here, followed by a thorough discussion of prevention of nutrition-related disorders.

## Iron Deficiency

Iron deficiency is not as common a problem in middle childhood as it is in the toddler age group. According to the NHANES 1999–2000 survey data, 4 percent of 6- to 11-year-old children were found to be iron deficient, compared to 7 percent of toddlers.[41] The American Academy of Pediatrics (AAP) and CDC both recommend screening for iron-deficiency anemia for children in whom anemia or an iron-deficient diet are suspected, such as those who consume a strict vegetarian diet without taking an iron supplement.[42, 43]

Age- and gender-specific cutoff values for anemia are based on the 5th percentile of hemoglobin and hematocrit for age from NHANES III. For children 5 to less than 8 years of age, the diagnosis of anemia is made if the hemoglobin concentration is <11.5 g/dL and hematocrit <34.5 percent. For children from 8 to less than 12 years of age, a hemoglobin value <11.9 g/dL or hematocrit <35.4 percent is diagnostic of iron-deficiency anemia.[41,43] Just as in early childhood, the treatment of iron-deficiency anemia in the school-age child consists of an oral iron trial for 4 weeks.[42] In addition, children and their caregivers should be educated on general dietary recommendations for preventing iron-deficiency anemia. These include eating plenty of iron-rich foods, such as meat, fish, poultry, and fortified breakfast cereals, and vitamin C-rich foods, such as citrus juice or fruit, which enhance iron absorption.

## Dental Caries

Approximately one in two children age 6–9 years has decay in primary or permanent teeth.[6] Children with poor oral health may also develop periodontal disease. The amount of time that children's teeth are exposed to carbohydrates influences the risk of dental caries or tooth decay. Complex carbohydrates such as fruits, vegetables, and grains are better choices than simple sugars, such as soft drinks or sports drinks and candy, in relation to oral health and nutrition. Sticky carbohydrate-containing foods, such as raisins and gummy candy, are strong caries promoters. Fats and proteins may have a protective effect on enamel. Choosing snacks that are combinations of carbohydrates, proteins, and fats may decrease the risk of developing dental caries. Having regular meal and snack times versus continually snacking throughout the day is also beneficial. Rinsing the mouth after eating—or, better yet, brushing teeth regularly—also decreases the development of caries.[44] It is important that the school-age child continue to have a source of fluoride, either from the water supply or through supplementation. Details about fluoride supplementation were reported in Chapter 10.

During middle childhood, children lose their primary or baby teeth and begin to get their permanent teeth. If several teeth are missing, children may experience difficulty in chewing some foods, such as meat. Also, the orthodontic appliances commonly worn by school-age children may interfere with their ability to eat certain foods. Modifying food, such as by chopping meat or slicing fresh fruit, can help.[1]

# Prevention of Nutrition-Related Disorders in School-Age Children

LO 12.6 Describe prevention strategies for overweight/obesity in school-age children.

The prevalence of overweight and obesity among children is at an alarming rate. Recent analysis of dietary data from NHANES indicates significant changes in dietary intake of school-age children over the 20 years from 1989 to 2010.[45] At the same time, decreases in physical inactivity may be a significant contributing factor to the increased prevalence of overweight.[46] The problem of increasing overweight in the United States needs to be addressed from a public health perspective.[47] Furthermore, children who are overweight are at increased risk for developing risk factors for chronic conditions, such as cardiovascular disease and type 2 diabetes mellitus.[46]

## Overweight and Obesity in School-Age Children

**Prevalence** According to the NHANES 2011–2012 data, approximately 17.7 percent of children ages 6 through 11 years are obese, with BMIs-for-age greater than or equal to the 95th percentile, with significant differences found by race/ethnicity.[48] In 2011–2012, 26.1 percent of Hispanic and 23.8 percent of Non-Hispanic Black children were obese (BMI for age percentiles > 95th percentile) as compared with 1 percent of Non-Hispanic White children.[48] Gender differences are also evident; 17.9 percent of Non-Hispanic white girls are obese, as compared to only 8.8 percent of Non-Hispanic white boys.[48] This gender difference is reversed in both Hispanic and Non-Hispanic Black children, where the incidence of obesity is higher among boys than girls (28.6 percent versus 23.4 percent among Hispanic children; 25.9 percent versus 21.7 percent among Non-Hispanic Black children).[48]

The prevalence of overweight among children has increased over the last 25 years; however, the most recent survey data indicate that the prevalence of high BMI appears to have reached a plateau.[5] BMI data for children older than 6 years of age were not included in the revised growth charts because of the known increased prevalence of overweight for these ages in NHANES III. Inclusion of this information in the revised growth charts would reflect a heavier population and would not be a healthy standard. Further analysis shows that the heaviest children are getting heavier. Extreme obesity is increasing in prevalence and has been associated with high risk for cardiovascular disease risk factors.[49]

**Characteristics of Overweight Children** Overweight children are usually taller, have advanced ***bone ages***, and experience sexual maturity at an earlier age than their non-overweight peers. From a psychosocial standpoint, overweight children look older than they are, and often adults expect them to behave as if they were older. Health consequences of obesity, such as hyperlipidemia, higher concentrations of liver enzymes, hypertension, and abnormal glucose tolerance, occur with increased frequency in obese children than in children of normal weight.[50] Analysis of data from the Bogalusa Heart Study, a community-based study of adverse risk factors in early life in a biracial population, confirms an increase in chronic disease risk factors with increasing BMI-for-age.[46] Increasing insulin levels, an indication of insulin resistance, show the strongest association with increasing BMI-for-age. Additionally, overweight children are more likely to have more than one chronic disease risk factor, especially those with BMI-for-age percentiles > 99th percentile.[49]

Type 2 diabetes mellitus, previously considered to be a disease of adults, is increasing in children and adolescents in the United States today. Between 2001 and 2009, there was a 30.5 percent increase in type 2 diabetes among children and adolescents aged 0 through 19 years of age,[51] with up to 85 percent of affected children being either overweight or obese at diagnosis.[52] According to the recommendations of a panel of experts in diabetes

**bone age** Bone maturation; correlates well with stage of pubertal development.

in children, any child who is overweight and who has other risk factors should be monitored for type 2 diabetes beginning at age 10 or at puberty. Other risk factors include a family history of type 2 diabetes, belonging to certain race and ethnic groups, including African American, Hispanic American, Asian and South Pacific Islander, and Native American, and having signs of insulin resistance.[52]

It is still unclear what effect an early onset of obesity in childhood has on the risk of adult morbidity and mortality.[50] Consequences of obesity and the precursors of adult disease do occur in obese children. More studies have been performed on the relationship between obesity during adolescence and the risks of obesity in adulthood than have been performed on the relationship between childhood obesity and obesity and type 2 diabetes in adulthood (see Chapter 15).[53]

**Predictors of Childhood Obesity** Dietz[13] describes critical periods in childhood for the development of obesity: gestation and early infancy, the period of BMI rebound, and adolescence. BMI rebound is the normal increase in body mass index that occurs after BMI declines and reaches its lowest point, between 5 and 7 years of age, and is reflected in the BMI-for-age growth chart.[14] Studies suggest that the age at which BMI rebound occurs may have a significant effect on the amount of body fat that the child will have during adolescence and into adulthood. Early BMI rebound is defined as beginning before 5.5 years of age, while the average age of BMI rebound is 6.0–6.3 years. BMI rebound after age 7 is considered late. Studies have shown that adolescents and adults who had an early BMI rebound as children have higher BMI than those subjects who had an average or late BMI rebound.[54] Several possible mechanisms may explain the relationship between BMI rebound and subsequent obesity.[14] The period of BMI rebound may be when children are beginning to express learned behaviors related to food intake and activity. Early BMI rebound may be related to infants who were exposed to gestational diabetes during fetal development and consequently have high birthweights. Although more study is needed, the conclusion is that preventive efforts need to focus on these developmental stages.[13]

Another predictor of childhood obesity is the child's home environment. Children from birth to 8 years of age were followed over a 6-year period as part of the National Longitudinal Survey of Youth.[55] Associations between the home environment and socioeconomic factors and the development of childhood obesity were examined. Maternal obesity was found to be the most significant predictor of childhood obesity, followed by low family income and lower cognitive stimulation.

Parental obesity is associated with an increased risk of obesity in children.[56] In one study, parental obesity doubled the risk of adult obesity for both obese and nonobese children less than 10 years of age. An analysis of data from NHANES III indicated a higher percentage of overweight youth among children who had one obese parent as compared to those children who had no obese parents. The percentage of overweight youth increased further if both parents were obese.[57] The connection between parental obesity and obesity in children is likely due to genetic as well as environmental factors.[56]

**Effects of Television Viewing and Screen Time on the Incidence of Overweight** One of the Healthy People 2020 objectives is to increase the proportion of children and adolescents who view television, videos, or play video games for no more than 2 hours per day from 78.9 percent to 86.8 percent. Related data analyzed by race and ethnicity, gender, and family income level are depicted in Table 12.3.[6,58] Young children commonly have ready access to computers, video games, and DVDs in addition to television. *Screen time* is the term now used to describe the time spent in these sedentary activities, which directly competes with time spent in physical activity. The AAP recommends that children have no more than 2 hours each day of screen time and that televisions and other screens be removed from the child's primary sleeping area.[59]

Many studies have demonstrated the strong relationship between TV viewing and childhood obesity, including studies that have followed subjects longitudinally from childhood to adulthood.[59] The proposed mechanisms by which television viewing contributes to obesity include reduced energy expenditure by displacing physical activity, increased dietary intake by eating during viewing or as a result of food advertising, and disruption of healthy sleep patterns.[59] Although some studies have demonstrated that increased screen time is associated with decreased physical activity, others have not.[59] One study found that energy expenditure during television viewing was actually

TABLE 12.3 ▸ Percentage of children and adolescents viewing television 2 or fewer hours per day by race/ethnicity, gender, and family income level[6,58]

| CHILDREN AND ADOLESCENTS AGED 6 TO 14 YEARS | TELEVISION 2 OR FEWER HOURS PER DAY 2007 |
|---|---|
| **Race and Ethnicity** | |
| Hispanic or Latino | 74.0% |
| Black or African American | 62.9 |
| White | 83.2 |
| **Gender** | |
| Female | 80.7 |
| Male | 77.3 |
| **Family Income Level (% Federal Poverty Level)** | |
| <100% | 70.1% |
| 100–199% | 73.2 |
| 200–399% | 80.5 |
| 400+% | 86.6 |

significantly lower than ***resting energy expenditure*** in 15 obese children and 16 normal-weight children who ranged in age from 8 to 12 years.[60] Other studies have found a direct relationship between screen time in children aged 9 to 16 years and their intake of junk foods, including sweet and salty snacks and sugar-sweetened drinks, as well as total calories.[61] At the same time, intakes of fruits and vegetables were inversely related to screen time, meaning there were fewer of these healthier choices consumed as screen time increased. The Academy of Nutrition and Dietetics (AND) conducted an analysis of the evidence of the impact of advertising on children's nutrition choices. They found good evidence that TV advertising affects children's intake, influences food and brand preferences, and may have a greater impact on obese children than their healthy-weight peers.[21] Based on these findings, it is hypothesized that screen time, and especially television viewing, does contribute to the prevalence of obesity, and that treatment for childhood obesity should include a reduction in the number of hours spent watching television and videos and playing video and computer games.

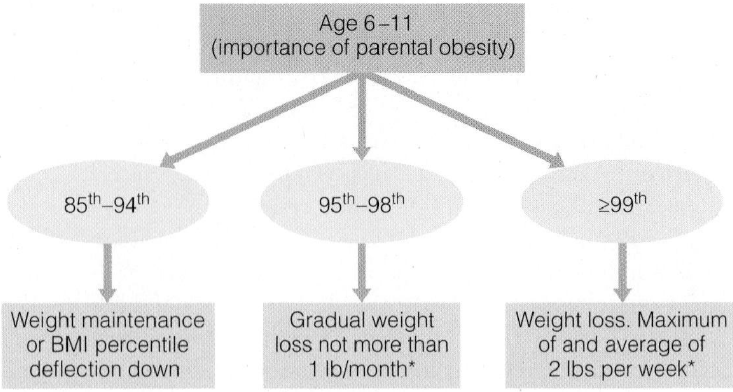


ILLUSTRATION 12.5 ▸ Suggested weight changes in staged treatment of pediatric obesity.

SOURCE: Based on data from B. A. Spear et al. Recommendations for treatment of child and adolescent overweight and obesity. *Pediatrics* 120 (2007): S254–S288.

## Addressing the Problem of Pediatric Overweight and Obesity

> "An ounce of prevention is worth a pound of cure."
>
> —Proverb

Recognizing the increase in the prevalence of childhood overweight and its associated chronic health problems, the AAP, AND, and eight other professional organizations joined together to develop a series of recommendations.[10,11,62] The expert committee's evidence-based recommendations address the topics of assessment, prevention, and treatment of pediatric obesity.

**Assessment of Overweight and Obesity** Body mass index-for-age percentile is recommended as the screening tool for assessment of pediatric overweight and obesity. A BMI-for-age percentile of greater than or equal to the 85th but less than or equal to the 94th is defined as overweight, and a BMI-for-age percentile greater than or equal to the 95th is defined as obesity.[10,11] Other components of assessment include evaluation of the child's medical risk, including parental obesity, and behavior risk, including dietary and physical activity behaviors. It is also essential to evaluate the child's and/or family's attitude toward and willingness to make behavior changes.[10,11]

**Prevention of Overweight and Obesity** All children should be targeted for prevention of overweight and obesity throughout their lives. The expert committee's recommendations for targeted behaviors in overweight and obesity prevention are described in detail in Chapter 10. The targeted behaviors address healthy eating and increased physical activity.[10,63]

**Treatment of Overweight and Obesity** The expert committee's recommendations for a four-stage approach to treatment of overweight and obesity in pediatrics are described in detail in Chapter 10.[10,62] Illustration 12.5 depicts suggested weight changes for 6- to 11-year-old children during treatment of overweight and obesity.[10,62] The four stages include:

- Stage 1: Prevention Plus
- Stage 2: Structured Weight Management (SWM)
- Stage 3: Comprehensive Multidisciplinary Intervention (CMI)
- Stage 4: Tertiary Care Intervention (reserved for severely obese adolescents)

The overall goal of treatment is for the child and family to develop healthy eating and physical activity behaviors for a lifetime. For children who fall into the overweight category based on a BMI-for-age between the 85th and 94th percentiles, the goal of treatment should be weight maintenance or a slowing of the rate of weight gain until a BMI-for-age < 85th percentile is achieved. For children with BMI-for-age of 95th to 98th percentiles, weight maintenance or gradual weight loss of no more than 1 pound per week is the goal until the BMI-for-age drops to < 85th percentile. Weight loss not to exceed 2 pounds per week is the goal of treatment for those children with BMI-for-age ≥ 99th percentiles until a BMI-for-age < 85th percentile is achieved.[10,62] See Case Study 12.1.

An evidence-based analysis of intervention literature showed positive effects of multicomponent,

**resting energy expenditure** The amount of energy needed by the body in a state of rest.

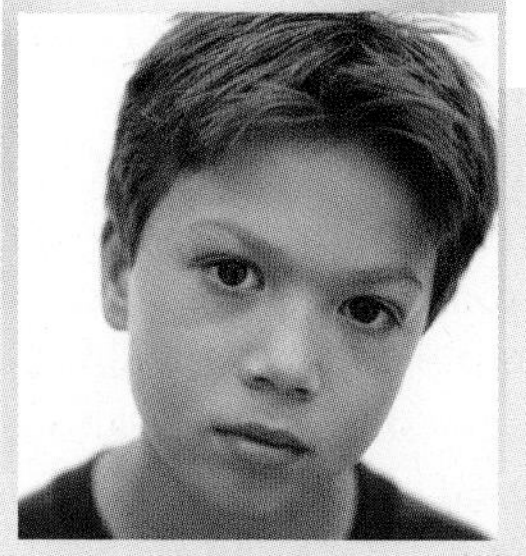
Photodisc

# CASE STUDY 12.1

## Pediatric Overweight

Seven-year-old Timothy's mother takes him to his pediatrician for his annual checkup. His weight is 68 pounds (31 kg), plotted at the 95th percentile, and his height is 50 inches (127 cm), between the 75th and 90th percentiles for his age. His body mass index of 19.25 kg/m² plots at the 95th percentile for his age. His growth percentiles have been increasing over the last several years.

Timothy's mother expresses concern to the pediatrician about her son's weight. His older and younger brothers are both thinner than Timothy. Timothy's mother is obese, but his father is a normal weight for height. Timothy is in the second grade. He rides the school bus to and from school. He participates in the School Lunch Program at his school, but his parents gave him extra money in case he wants to buy some additional à la carte food items from the cafeteria or items from the vending machines. After school, Timothy and his brothers stay in their home with a babysitter until one of their parents returns home from work. Timothy usually watches TV or plays video games after school. His parents leave snack foods—chips, cookies, and sodas—in the house for their sons to have after school. His mother usually prepares their evening meal, which consists of a meat, starch, vegetables, and a dessert item. After dinner, Timothy does his homework and then usually watches more TV with his parents. He usually has a dish of ice cream before going to bed.

### *Questions*

1. What is your assessment of Timothy's body size based on his weight-for-age, height-for-age, and BMI-for-age percentiles?
2. What suggestions do you have for Timothy's parents about improving his eating habits?
3. What suggestions do you have for Timothy's parents for increasing his physical activity level?
4. Is it significant that Timothy's mother also has a weight problem?

family-based programs for children between the ages of 5 and 12 years. Recommended components include parent training, dietary counseling/nutrition education, physical activity and addressing sedentary behaviors, and behavioral counseling.[64]

Some potential consequences of a weight-loss program in childhood are a slowing of linear growth and the beginnings of eating disorders. To reduce the risks associated with weight loss in childhood, the program must ensure nutritional adequacy of the diet, a nonjudgmental approach, and attention to the child's emotional state.[10,62]

## Nutrition and Prevention of Cardiovascular Disease in School-Age Children

In the new DRIs, no recommendations for total grams of fat per day in the diet of children have been made.[37] Studies have shown that as long as enough energy is provided for growth, no effect of fat intake on growth has been found. In addition, the evidence is still insufficient to be able to define the optimal fat intake for promoting growth while also preventing obesity and other chronic diseases. According to the DRIs, the Acceptable Macronutrient Distribution Range (AMDR) for fat is 25–35 percent of energy for children 4–18 years of age.[37]

The DRIs do stress the importance of including sources of linoleic acid (omega-6 fatty acid) and alpha-linolenic acid (omega-3 fatty acid) (Table 12.4). Sources of linoleic acid include vegetable oils, seeds, nuts, and whole-grain breads and cereals. Fish, as well as flaxseed, soy, and canola oils, are good sources of alpha-linolenic acid. (See Chapter 1.) A diet that emphasizes fruits, vegetables, low-fat dairy products, whole-grain breads and cereals, nuts, seeds, fish, and lean meats is recommended for promoting nutrition and preventing cardiovascular disease in school-age children.[37]

The American Heart Association and the American Academy of Pediatrics have jointly issued guidelines for cardiovascular health promotion in all children and adolescents and dietary recommendations.[65-67] The recommended diet is consistent with the Dietary Guidelines for Americans, MyPlate, and the DRIs, including a recommended total fat intake of 25–35 percent of total calories.[20,37,38] Emphasis is placed on adequate intakes of omega-3 fatty acids, with a recommendation of at least two servings of fish each week.

TABLE 12.4 ▸ Adequate intake of linoleic acid and alpha-linolenic acid[37*]

| GENDER AND AGE | LINOLEIC ACID G/DAY | ALPHA-LINOLENIC ACID G/DAY |
|---|---|---|
| Children 4–8 years | 10 | 0.9 |
| Boys 9–13 years | 12 | 1.2 |
| Girls 9–13 years | 10 | 1.0 |

* See Chapter 1 for a list of food sources.

SOURCE: Based on data from The Institute of Medicine, Food & Nutrition Board. Dietary Reference Intakes for energy, carbohydrate, fiber, fat, protein, and amino acids. Washington, D.C.: National Academy Press, 2002/2005.

Limiting the intake of fruit juice, sugar-sweetened beverages and foods, and salt is also recommended. For children over 2 years of age, these guidelines recommend limiting foods high in saturated fats (<7 percent of total calories per day), cholesterol (<300 mg per day), and *trans* fatty acids (<1 percent of total calories per day).[65–68]

As discussed in Chapter 10, the National Heart, Lung, and Blood Institute (NHLBI) convened a panel of experts to develop evidence-based cardiovascular health guidelines for pediatric care providers.[69] This panel recommends universal lipid screening between the ages of 9 and 11 years, as this age has been determined to be a stable time for lipid assessment. The panel recommends a Cardiovascular Health Integrated Lifestyle Diet (CHILD-1) for children with risk factors such as overweight and obesity as well as for children with a positive family history of early cardiovascular disease or risk factors such as obesity or primary hypertension. Children with hyperlipidemias require further dietary restrictions to help control LDL cholesterol, (CHILD-2-LDL diet) and/or triglycerides (CHILD-2-TG). Further restriction of dietary cholesterol to 200 mg per day and avoiding *trans* fatty acids as much as possible are recommended.[69] See Table 10.8 for more information about the CHILD-1, CHILD-2-LDL, and CHILD-2-TG evidenced-based recommendations. Increasing soluble fiber intake, emphasizing weight management and physical activity, and follow-up by a registered dietitian are also treatment recommendations.[69] Employing behavior change theory and motivational interviewing may be useful strategies when counseling children and families on these dietary recommendations.[68]

### Dietary Supplements

Children who are healthy and consume a diet of a variety of foods do not require a vitamin and mineral supplement to meet their nutrient needs. The AAP recommends vitamin and mineral supplementation for children who are at high risk of developing nutrient deficiencies or have one or more documented nutrition deficiency.[42] These deficiencies include:

1. With anorexia or an inadequate appetite or who follow fad diets
2. With chronic disease
3. From deprived families or who suffer from parental neglect or abuse
4. Who participate in a dietary program for managing obesity
5. Who consume a vegetarian diet without adequate intake of dairy products
6. With failure to thrive

If vitamin and mineral supplements are given to school-age children, the supplement should not exceed the DRI for age. Parents should be warned against giving amounts of vitamins and minerals that exceed the Tolerable Upper Intake levels designated in the DRI tables.[39,40]

It is not clear to what extent herbal supplements are given to school-age children. Herbal supplements are used in some cultures as home remedies. A recent report of complementary and alternative medicine (CAM) use in U.S. children aged 4–11 years showed that about 9.5 percent of the population had used some form of CAM in the 12 months prior to the survey.[70] The most commonly used type of CAM was nonvitamin, nonmineral dietary supplements, including fish oil, melatonin, probiotics or prebiotics, and echinacea. It is important to obtain this information from parents and caretakers as part of the child's health history. The use of herbal supplements, botanicals, and vitamin/mineral supplements may be a more prevalent practice by parents of children with special health care needs.

## Dietary Recommendations

**LO 12.7** Describe the components of a healthy diet during middle childhood and preadolescence as recommended by health and professional organizations and agencies.

The basic dietary recommendation for school-age and preadolescent children is to eat a diet of a variety of foods, which is why it remains so important throughout these school years for children to have a variety of foods available to them. The available food environment will affect children's food choices. Parents and other adult role models need to continue to model appropriate eating behaviors for children.

Dietary recommendations, as outlined by the USDA in the Dietary Guidelines for Americans and MyPlate, apply to school-age children as well as to other segments of the population.[20,38] Professional organizations, such as the American Heart Association, the AAP, and the AND, have also published positions on dietary guidance for healthy children, supporting the federal guidelines.[21,65–69]

**Recommendations for Intake of Iron, Fiber, Fat, Calcium, Vitamin D, and Fluids** Adequate iron nutrition is still important during middle childhood and preadolescence to prevent iron-deficiency anemia and its consequences. According to food-consumption surveys, children are not eating the recommended amounts of fiber in their diets, but they are exceeding the recommendations of total calories from fat and saturated fat. Calcium requirements increase during the preadolescent years, but calcium intake decreases with age.

**Iron** Although iron deficiency is not as prevalent during the school-age years as it was during the toddler and preschool-age years, adequate intake of iron is still important. The inclusion of iron-rich foods—such as meats,

TABLE 12.5 ▸ Adequate intake of total fiber[37]

| GENDER AND AGE | TOTAL FIBER, G/DAY |
|---|---|
| Children 4–8 years | 25 |
| Boys 9–13 years | 31 |
| Girls 9–13 years | 26 |

SOURCE: From the Institute of Medicine, Food & Nutrition Board.

fortified breakfast cereals, and dry beans and peas—in children's diets is important. A good vitamin C source, such as orange juice, will enhance the absorption of iron.

**Fiber** Many health effects of fiber intake have been identified—including prevention of chronic disease in adulthood, such as heart disease, certain cancers, diabetes, and hypertension. The recommendations for ***total fiber*** intake based on the DRIs can be found in Table 12.5. Total fiber is the sum of ***dietary fiber*** and ***functional fiber.*** Earlier recommendations were based on dietary fiber.[37] Although there is little research on the effect of fiber intake during childhood on health as an adult, there is agreement that the fiber intake of children is generally too low.[71]

To increase the dietary fiber in children's diets, parents and caretakers can begin by increasing the amount of fresh fruits and vegetables and whole-grain breads and cereals being offered. High-fiber fruits, such as apples with peels, have about 3 grams per serving, while fruit juices are low in fiber. High-fiber vegetables, such as broccoli, have about 2.5 grams per serving. Whole-grain breads, cereals, and brown rice have about 2.5 grams per serving. High-fiber cereals, such as bran flakes and raisin bran, have about 8–10 grams per serving. Served alone, these high-fiber cereals may not be well accepted by young children, but they can be mixed with other cereals or used in recipes for food items such as muffins. Dried beans and peas are also excellent sources of fiber, providing 4–7 grams of fiber per ½-cup serving.[72]

**Fat** Food intakes that follow the recommendations of the Dietary Guidelines for Americans and MyPlate provide an appropriate amount of fat for school-age and preadolescent children.[20,38] Healthy diets include whole-grain breads and cereals, beans and peas, fruits and vegetables, low-fat dairy products, and lean meats, fish, and poultry. Foods high in fat, especially those high in saturated fat and *trans* fatty acids, should be kept to a minimum. However, an appropriate amount of dietary fat is necessary to meet children's needs for calories, essential fatty acids, and fat-soluble vitamins.

**Calcium and Vitamin D** The recommendations for adequate daily intakes of calcium are 1000 milligrams for children aged 4–8 years and 1300 milligrams for children 9 through 13 years.[39] The higher recommendation for older children reflects the fact that most bone formation occurs during puberty. Adequate calcium intake during this time is necessary to achieve peak bone mass, which may prevent osteoporosis later in life.[73]

Good sources of calcium are listed in Chapter 1. It is difficult to meet the higher recommendations of calcium without the inclusion of dairy products, preferably low-fat dairy products. One cup of skim or low-fat milk contains about 300 mg calcium. Calcium-fortified foods such as fruit juice and soy milk are also available for children such as those on a vegan diet.

Adequate vitamin D is needed for calcium absorption. The revised DRIs for calcium and vitamin D set the Recommended Dietary Allowance (RDA), a value that meets the needs of most people, at 600 IUs per day for children 4–18 years of age.[39] Main sources of vitamin D include exposure to sunlight, vitamin D–fortified foods such as fortified cereals, and vitamin D–fortified milk (100 IU per 8 ounces).[73] Children who are at risk for vitamin D deficiency include those with increased skin pigmentation, including African Americans and Hispanics, and those with limited sunlight exposure. For children whose calcium and vitamin D intakes are inadequate or who are at increased risk for vitamin D deficiency, supplements need to be given under the guidance of a physician or registered dietitian.

***Lactose Intolerance*** Lactose intolerance, more commonly seen in older children than in younger children, is a common cause of abdominal pain. Lactose intolerance is a clinical syndrome of one or more gastrointestinal symptoms (e.g., abdominal pain, diarrhea, nausea, flatulence, or bloating) after consumption of lactose or lactose-containing foods or beverages. Lactose malabsorption, the disorder that manifests itself as lactose intolerance, is caused by reduced digestion of lactose because of the low availability of the enzyme lactase. Lactase breaks down lactose, the disaccharide in milk and milk products.[74]

Lactose intolerance can be caused by a primary lactase deficiency, which is the relative or absolute absence of the enzyme. Primary lactase deficiency is especially common in certain racial and ethnic groups, including Hispanics (50–80 percent), Black and Ashkenazi Jewish people (60–80 percent), and Asians and Native Americans (nearly 100 percent).[74] Affected individuals have varying degrees of lactose intolerance, and dairy products should be included in their diets as individually tolerated. Having lactose-containing foods in small amounts, spaced throughout the day, and eaten with other foods may be tolerated by many people with lactose intolerance. Additionally, yogurts, cheeses, and

**total fiber** Sum of dietary fiber and functional fiber.

**dietary fiber** Complex carbohydrates and lignins naturally occurring and found mainly in the plant cell wall. Dietary fiber cannot be broken down by human digestive enzymes.

**functional fiber** Nondigestible carbohydrates including plant, animal, or commercially produced sources that have beneficial effects in humans.

lactose-reduced dairy products have lower lactose content and may be well tolerated.

Secondary lactase deficiency can be caused by injury to the small bowel, such as from an acute infection. The underlying condition should be treated, and often the elimination of lactose from the diet is not necessary at all, but milk products should definitely be resumed once the underlying condition has resolved. The concern with both primary and secondary lactase deficiency is to avoid the total elimination of dairy products from the diet when it may not be necessary, as these foods are important sources of calcium, vitamin D, and other nutrients.[74]

**Fluids** School-age children need to drink enough fluids to maintain adequate hydration especially during periods of physical activity. Adults who are supervising children's physical activities need to make sure that children drink fluids before, during, and after exercise. The thirst mechanism may not work as well during exercise, and children may not realize that they need fluids. Cold water is the best fluid for children, and they should have free access to water, particularly during school hours.[75] Sports drinks, which contain 4–8 percent carbohydrate and diluted fruit juice, are most appropriate for children who are participating in prolonged vigorous physical activity, especially in hot and humid climates.[75] Some sports, such as football and hockey, require special protective gear that may prevent the body from being able to cool off. Children should never deprive themselves of food or water in order to meet a certain weight category, such as in wrestling. Children should not be given soft drinks or undiluted juice, because the carbohydrate load is too high to be hydrating and could cause stomach cramps, nausea, and diarrhea.[76] Energy drinks should not be consumed by children because they contain high amounts of caffeine and other stimulant substances, such as guarana, a plant extract that contains caffeine. Inappropriate use of sports drinks and energy drinks can contribute a significant amount of calories from carbohydrate to a child's diet and possibly contribute to excessive energy intake.[75]

***Soft Drinks*** School-age children consume more soft drinks than preschool-age children do, but not as much as adolescents—indicating an increase in consumption with age. Children's consumption of all sugar-sweetened beverages (SSB) increased by 20 percent among children age 6–11 years from 1988 to 2004. In 2004, SSBs add 229 calories per day to the school-age child's overall energy intake, with most of the SSB calories being consumed at home.[77] However, a more recent analysis of the top-10 food and beverage sources of energy for children aged 2–18 years shows that the peak intake of SSB may have been in 2003–2004, with a steady decline in intake since then.[45]

Children with high consumption of regular soft drinks (more than 9 ounces per day) consume less milk and fruit juice than do those with lower consumptions of regular soft drinks. A study of 548 ethnically diverse school-age children, with an average age 11.7 years, showed that BMI and the frequency of high BMI greater than 95th percentile increased along with increased consumption of SSB.[78]

Soft drinks can contribute significantly to children's overall calorie and caffeine intake while contributing little to the overall nutritional value of their diets and displacing more nutritious foods. A study of 30 children 6–13 years of age found that SSB consumption displaced milk from children's diets and resulted in intakes that were lower in protein, calcium, magnesium, phosphorus, and vitamin A but higher in calories.[79]

According to USDA food-consumption data, children's soft-drink consumption increases with age while milk consumption decreases at a time when calcium requirements are increasing.[39,80] Children who ate fast food consumed more carbonated nondiet beverages and less milk than children who did not eat fast food.[81] Diet soft drinks do not provide sugar, and the aspartame content of diet sodas does not appear to pose a risk to healthy children.[82] Soft drinks in excess are not recommended for school-age children because they provide empty calories, promote tooth decay, and are not a good fluid choice for hydration.

## Recommended Versus Actual Food Intake

The composition of children's diets, based on data from the report "What We Eat in America" (WWEIA), a joint project of the U.S. Department of Agriculture (USDA) and the U.S. Department of Health and Human Services (DHHS), can be found in Table 12.6.[83] According to the

TABLE 12.6 ▸ Mean percentages of food energy from carbohydrate, protein, total fat, saturated fatty acids, monounsaturated fat, and polyunsaturated fat intake of 6- to 11-year-old children[83]

| GENDER AND AGE | CARBOHYDRATE (%) | PROTEIN (%) | TOTAL FAT (%) | SATURATED FAT(%) | MONONUSATURATED FAT (MG/D) | POLYUNSATURATED FAT (MG/D) |
|---|---|---|---|---|---|---|
| Males: | | | | | | |
| 6–11 years | 55 | 14 | 32 | 11 | 11 | 7 |
| Females: | | | | | | |
| 6–11 years | 54 | 14 | 33 | 11 | 11 | 7 |

SOURCE: U.S. Department of Agriculture, Agricultural Research Service, www.ars.usda.gov

TABLE 12.7 ▶ Mean dietary fiber, sodium, and caffeine intake of 6- to 11-year-old children[83]

| GENDER AND AGE | DIETARY FIBER (G) | SODIUM (MG) | CAFFEINE (MG) |
|---|---|---|---|
| Males: | | | |
| 6–11 years | 15.4 | 3196 | 21.8 |
| Females: | | | |
| 6–11 years | 13.9 | 2954 | 17.2 |

SOURCE: U.S. Department of Agriculture, Agricultural Research Service, www.ars.usda.gov

data, both boys' and girls' percentage of total calories from fat is within the recommended range of 25–35 percent. However, both boys and girls are exceeding the recommendation for total calories from saturated fat of less than 7 percent.[66,68,83] The data further indicate that there are ethnic differences, with Non-Hispanic Asian boys and girls consuming more carbohydrate (58 percent) and less fat (29 percent).

Mean calcium intake for school-age children of 1137 mg for 6- to 11-year-old males and 1004 mg for 6- to 11-year-old girls falls short of the Recommended Dietary Allowance (RDA) of 1300 mg for 9- to 13-year-olds.[39,83] Table 12.7 depicts a further analysis of children's diets in relation to dietary fiber, sodium, and caffeine intake. School-age children's caffeine intake has risen dramatically for both males and females from the preschool years, indicating an increased consumption of caffeine with age. This coincides with an increase in soft-drink consumption. Thirty-three percent of U.S. children report consuming fast food on a typical day. Children who eat fast food consume more total energy, more total fat, more total carbohydrates, more added sugars, more sugar-sweetened beverages, less fiber, less milk, and fewer fruits and nonstarchy vegetables than children who do not eat fast food.[81] Analysis of food consumption data indicates that snacking among children has increased over the years. Approximately 50 percent of children aged 6–11 years report consuming two or three snacks a day, providing approximately 25 percent of the child's total energy intake and 35 percent of their total sugar intake.[83]

A measure of diet quality is provided by the Healthy Eating Index (HEI; available at www.usda.gov/cnpp), which utilizes data from the ongoing NHANESs.[84] The HEI measures the degree to which an individual's diet conforms to the Dietary Guidelines for Americans and uses the food-group standards found in MyPlate.[20,38] The index also measures total and saturated fat intake, cholesterol intake, sodium intake, and variety. According to data from 2007–2008, the average HEI score for children age 2–17 years was 49.8 out of 100, indicating that their diets needed improvement.[85] Data indicate that children had the best scores for dairy and protein foods, but especially need to increase their intake of whole grains, beans, and dark-green vegetables. One encouraging finding was that whole fruit intake was significantly higher, and empty calorie intake was significantly lower, in 2007–2008 when compared to 2003–2004.

## Cross-Cultural Considerations

One of the overarching goals of Healthy People 2020 is to "achieve health equity, eliminate disparities, and improve the health of all groups."[6] The reasons for the health disparities are complex but may include genetic variations, environmental factors, and health behaviors, including diet. Access to community-based, culturally competent, linguistically appropriate preventive health care is needed to eliminate these disparities.

A unique characteristic of every ethnic group in America is its culturally based foods and food habits.[86] As discussed earlier, children learn food habits within the context of their family's culture. It is important for a health care professional to try to learn as much as possible about the foods and diets of the ethnic groups served, including where food is purchased and how it is prepared.[1]

The next step is to evaluate the diet within the context of the culture. Which foods or food habits have positive health benefits and should be encouraged? Which food behaviors have harmful effects on health and should be limited or modified? For example, in working with the Latino population, it is important to first of all establish the country of origin. Latino immigrants may be from Mexico, Central America, South America, or the Caribbean. Food habits are unique for each of these ethnic groups. For example, Central Americans eat a lot of legumes, rice, and corn. Fruits and vegetables are also included in the diet. These dietary practices form the basis of a healthy diet. However, lard is the most commonly used fat. Encouraging Central Americans to use a vegetable oil instead of lard is an example of a modification of a food practice to make it healthier.

## Vegetarian Diets

Young children who are consuming vegetarian diets are usually following their parents' eating practices. Preadolescents, on the other hand, may choose to follow a vegetarian diet independently of the family, motivated by concerns about animal welfare, ecology, and the environment.[1] On the one hand, children following vegetarian and vegan diets can achieve growth comparable to the total population, but may be at higher risk for some nutrient deficiencies.[87] On the other hand, these children have a lower risk of becoming obese and better chance of meeting the dietary guidelines. Health care providers working with children following a vegetarian diet should pay special intake to their intakes of protein, essential fatty acids, calcium, iron, zinc, vitamin $B_{12}$ and vitamin C.[87,88]

# Physical Activity Recommendations

LO 12.8 List two strategies that parents/caretakers can employ to encourage school-age children to be more physically active.

Physical activity has many proven health benefits, including prevention of chronic diseases such as coronary heart disease, building muscle strength, and controlling energy balance. Physical activity is one of the health behaviors that are important to establish in childhood as part of a healthy lifestyle that will continue into adolescence and adulthood. With the increased prevalence of childhood obesity, increasing physical activity and decreasing sedentary behaviors become important factors in controlling childhood overweight.[64]

## Recommendations Versus Actual Activity

It is recommended that children engage in at least 60 minutes of physical activity every day (Illustration 12.6).[10,38]

Strategies for parents include the following:

- Set a good example by being physically active themselves and joining their children in physical activity.
- Encourage children to be physically active at home, at school, and with friends.
- Limit television and video/DVD watching, computer and video game playing, time at the computer, texting, and other inactive forms of play by alternating with periods of physical activity.

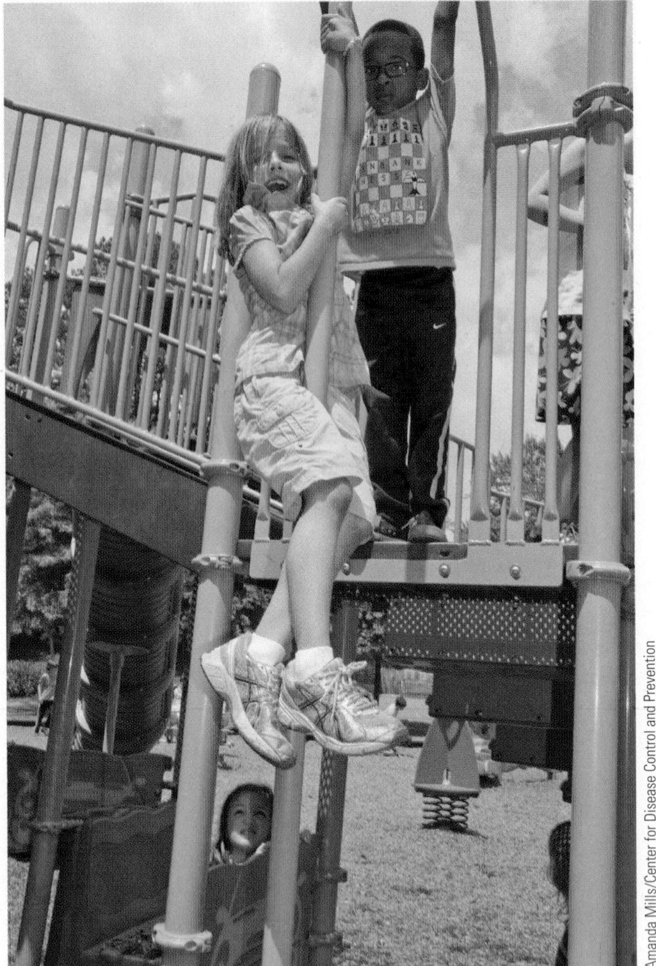

Amanda Mills/Center for Disease Control and Prevention

ILLUSTRATION 12.6 ▸ Children should engage in at least 60 minutes of physical activity daily.

As has already been mentioned, it is recommended that screen time for children be limited to not more than 2 hours per day, which is a Healthy People 2020 objective.[6] Televisions and other screens, such as computers, should be removed from children's bedrooms.[59] Additionally, physical activity and daily physical education should be encouraged at schools and during after-school care programs. Community-based sports and recreational activities for children are also encouraged, as well as using school-based facilities outside of school hours to give community access to appropriate locations for safe physical activity.

The American Academy of Pediatrics has recommended that schools reinstate daily physical education (PE) classes for all grade levels, to promote development of knowledge, skills, and attitudes to support a physically active lifestyle.[89] As of 2006, only 7.9 percent of middle and junior high schools required daily physical education for all students.[6] Healthy People 2020 objectives include increasing regularly scheduled elementary school recess in the United States and the proportion of trips that school-age children make to school by walking (one mile or less) and by bicycling (two miles or less).[6] In order to meet these goals, communities need to ensure that there are safe places for children to walk and ride their bicycles. The "built environment" is the term used to describe the overall structure of the physical environment of a child's community.[90]

The physical environment can be conducive to a healthy lifestyle by providing safe places such as parks for children to play in, sidewalks for walking to school, or bike paths (Illustration 12.7). Or the physical environment can be a barrier to a healthy lifestyle. In addition to the distances children must walk to school, parents are also concerned about traffic danger, followed by concerns about crime and weather.[90] Programs such as the "walking school bus" and the national Safe Routes to School Program help concerned parents, health professionals such as pediatricians, and other community leaders establish safe built environments in their communities. Safety measures, such as wearing a helmet when biking, need to be employed.

Communities can also offer youth sports and recreation programs that are developmentally appropriate and fun for all young people. To achieve such a community environment, partnerships need to be established among federal, state, and local governments, nongovernment organizations, and private entities. The U.S. Department of Health and Human Services has proposed strategies for

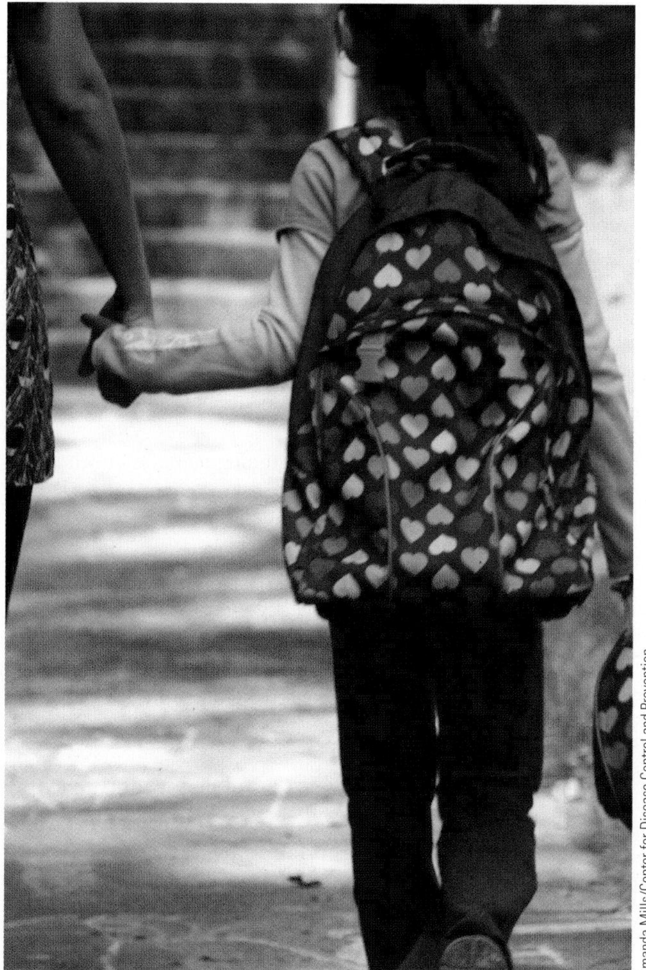

Amanda Mills/Center for Disease Control and Prevention

ILLUSTRATION 12.7 ▸ The physical environment can promote a healthy lifestyle by providing safe places for children to play and sidewalks for walking to school.

promoting physical activity for children in family, school, and community settings.[91]

## Determinants of Physical Activity

It is important to understand children's physical activity patterns and determinants of physical activity, so that vulnerable groups can be identified and appropriate intervention programs designed. Potential determinants of physical activity behaviors among children include physiological, environmental, psychological, social, and demographic factors.[92] Childhood physical activity has been difficult to assess and to track into adulthood. Many of the studies have identified correlates of physical activity behavior rather than predictors. The determinants of childhood physical activity are probably multidimensional and interrelated. More work needs to be done in this area, but some generalities resulting from existing studies are:

- Girls are less active than boys.
- Physical activity decreases with age.
- Seasonal and climate differences are seen in children's activity levels.
- Physical education in schools has decreased.

School and neighborhood safety is an important issue in promoting physical activity. In addition, parents have direct and indirect effects on children's physical activity levels.

## Organized Sports

Many school-age and preadolescent children participate in organized sport activities, through schools or other community organizations. An analysis of NHANES III data indicates that children who participate in team sports and exercise programs are less likely to be overweight as compared to nonparticipants (Illustration 12.8).[57] The AAP recognizes the fact that organized sports for children have become widely accepted in our society and do provide opportunities for physical activity for children. The AAP recommends that children be involved in sports that are appropriate for their physical and cognitive development.[93]

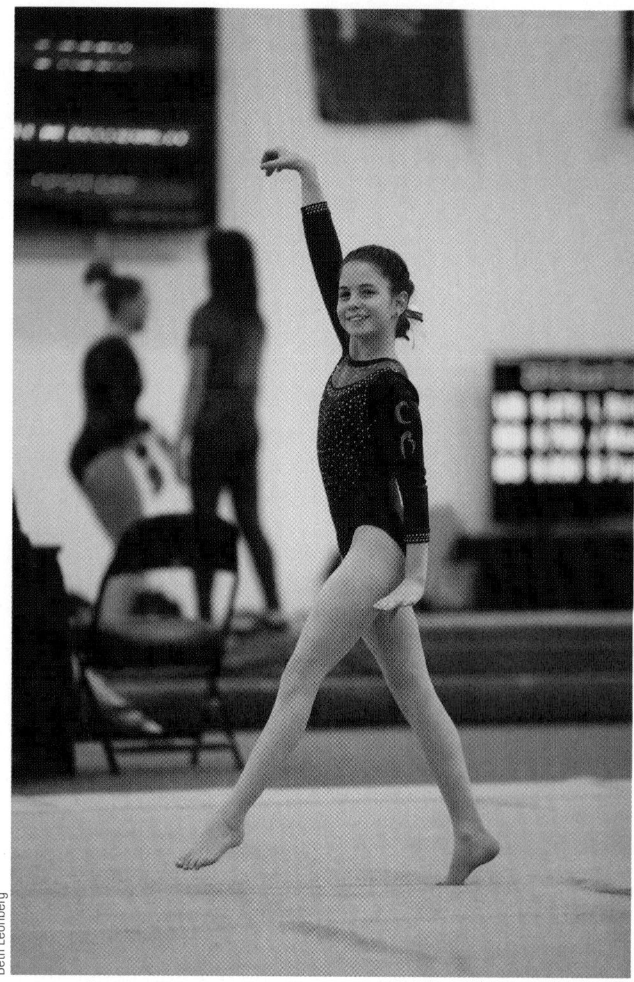

Beth Leonberg

ILLUSTRATION 12.8 ▸ Children who participate in organized sports are less likely to be overweight.

Emphasis should be placed on having fun and on family participation rather than on being competitive. Organized sports should not take the place of regular physical activity, such as physical education in school and free play.[93] The proper use of safety equipment, such as helmets, pads, mouth guards, and goggles, should be encouraged. The AAP warns against intensive, specialized training for children. Coaches should be educated about developmental and safety issues.[93] Recommendations for sports participation by children stress the importance of proper hydration. The AAP encourages the use of water for hydration in most instances, with carbohydrate and electrolyte-containing sports drinks being used only when a child is involved in vigorous or prolonged physical activity.[94] In spite of being heavily marketed at children and especially adolescents, the AAP has warned against the use of energy drinks in children because many of their ingredients, including added sugars, caffeine, and substances such as guarana, have known or potential harmful effects on children.[94]

# Nutrition Intervention for Risk Reduction

LO 12.9 List three strategies that school health programs can use to promote healthy eating.

> "It is the position of the Academy of Nutrition and Dietetics (AND), School Nutrition Association (SNA), and Society for Nutrition Education (SNE), that comprehensive, integrated nutrition services in schools, kindergarten through grade 12, are an essential component of coordinated school health programs and will improve the nutritional status, health, and academic performance of our nation's children."[95]
>
> —The Academy of Nutrition and Dietetics

## Nutrition Education

Eating a healthy diet and participating in physical activity are important components of a healthy lifestyle that may prevent chronic disease in childhood and into adolescence and adulthood. School age is a prime time for learning about healthy lifestyles and incorporating them into daily behaviors. Schools can provide an appropriate environment for nutrition education and learning healthy lifestyle behaviors. It has been reported that an average of 13 hours per year is spent in elementary school classrooms teaching lessons about nutrition; however, research demonstrates that 50 hours are required to facilitate behavior change.[96] One important driver for increasing nutrition education in schools was legislation that required that all school districts that participate in the National School Lunch Program (NSLP) develop a wellness policy by the 2006–2007 school year.[97] The Healthy, Hunger-Free Kids Act of 2010 further strengthened the requirements (see Table 12.8).

**TABLE 12.8** Local school wellness policy requirements[97]

At a minimum, a local school wellness policy must:

- Include goals for nutrition promotion and education, physical activity, and other school-based activities that promote student wellness.
- Include nutrition guidelines to promote student health and reduce childhood obesity for all foods available in each school district.
- Permit parents, students, representatives of the school food authority, teachers of physical education, school health professionals, the school board, school administrators, and the general public to participate in the development, implementation, and review and update of the local wellness policy.
- Inform and update the public (including parents, students, and others in the community) about the content and implementation of local wellness policies.
- Be measured periodically on the extent to which schools are in compliance with the local wellness policy, the extent to which the local education agency's local wellness policy compares to model local school wellness policies, and the progress made in attaining the goals of the local wellness policy, and make this assessment available to the public.

## Nutrition Integrity in Schools

> "It is the position of the American Dietetic Association (ADA, now the Academy of Nutrition and Dietetics) that schools and the community have a shared responsibility to provide students with access to high-quality, affordable, nutritious foods and beverages. School-based nutrition services, including the provision of meals through the National School Lunch Program and the School Breakfast Program, are an integral part of the total education program."[98]
>
> —The Academy of Nutrition and Dietetics

Health Education
Physical Education
Health Services
Nutrition Services
Counseling, Psychological, & Social Services
Healthy School Environment
Health Promotion for Staff
Family/ Community Involvement
Center for Disease Control

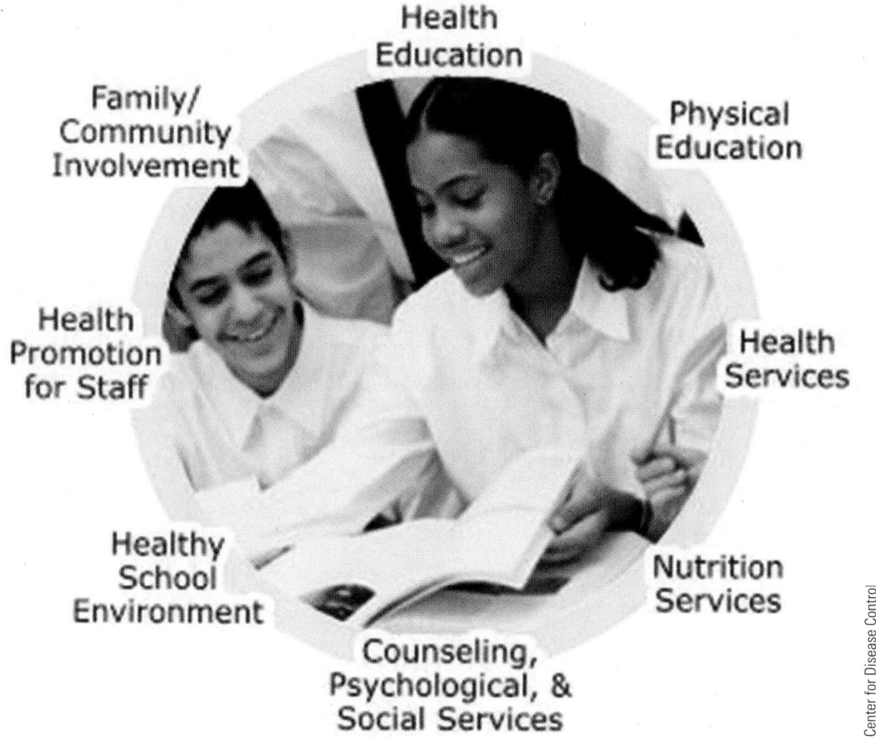

ILLUSTRATION 12.9 ▸ The School Health Index includes eight key areas for maintaining the well-being of young people.[103]
SOURCE: CDC

Nutrition integrity in schools is defined as ensuring that all foods available to children in schools are consistent with the U.S. Dietary Guidelines for Americans and the Dietary Reference Intakes.[38-40] School nutrition programs are vital to reinforcing healthy eating habits in school-age children. Sound nutrition policies need the support of the community and school environments, and these must involve students in order to be successful. Preparing community leaders for involvement in policy development is one of the nutrition integrity core concepts.[98] Training food-service personnel, teachers, administrators, and parents is an integral part of this process. Adequate time allotted for meals is another important component of a sound nutrition program. Students can be involved in a nutrition advisory council, providing feedback about menu preferences and meal environment and serving as a communication link with other students.

There are many challenges to nutrition integrity in schools. Foods sold from vending machines and snack bars often do not support healthy eating and may undermine sound nutrition programs. However, in some underfunded schools, vending machine proceeds are important sources of revenue. Many schools have ***pouring rights*** contracts with soft-drink companies and receive a percentage of the profits.[95] Many schools also sell à la carte items in addition to standard school lunches to increase revenue. One study of children in first through twelfth grade showed that 40 percent of children consumed at least one ***competitive food*** on a usual school day.[99] The competitive foods chosen were energy-dense and had few nutrients. Interestingly, children who ate a school lunch were significantly less likely to eat competitive foods. Data from the third School Nutrition and Dietary Assessment study in 2005 of 395 U.S. public schools in 38 states indicated that while there were vending machines in only 17 percent of elementary schools, there were vending machines in 82 percent of middle schools; à la carte items were sold in 71 percent of elementary schools and 92 percent of middle schools. The majority of the time, vending machines and à la carte items were sources of low-nutrient, energy-dense foods and beverages such as sugar-sweetened beverages and candy.[100] It is against USDA regulations to sell competitive foods of minimal nutritional value. However, it is not against USDA regulations to sell these foods to students at times other than mealtimes or in other areas of the school, outside of food-service areas.

In 2004, the AAP Committee on School Health has issued a policy statement about nutrition concerns regarding soft-drink consumption in schools.[101] It advocated for the elimination of sweetened beverages in schools and their replacement with beverages such as real fruit and vegetable juices, water,

**pouring rights** Contracts between schools and soft-drink companies, whereby the schools receive a percentage of the profits of soft-drink sales in exchange for the school offering only that soft-drink company's products on the school campus.

**competitive foods** Foods sold to children in food service areas during meal times that compete with the federal meal programs.

**N.5 All foods and beverages served and offered during the school day meet the USDA's Smart Snacks in School nutrition standards.**

Do all foods and beverages **served and offered** to students during the school day meet or exceed the USDA's **Smart Snacks in School** nutrition standards? This includes snacks that are not part of a federally reimbursed child nutrition program, birthday parties, holiday parties and school-wide celebrations.

### Smart Snacks in School – Nutrition Standards for Foods

**Any food sold in schools must:**

1. Be a grain product that contains 50% or more whole grains by weight or have whole grains as the first ingredient; or
2. Have as the first ingredient a fruit, a vegetable, a dairy product, or a protein food; or
3. Be a combination food that contains at least ¼ cup of fruit and/or vegetable; or
4. Contain 10% of the Daily Value (DV) of one of the nutrients of public health concern in the 2010 Dietary Guidelines for Americans (calcium, potassium, vitamin D, or dietary fiber).*

**Foods must also meet several nutrient requirements:**

1. Calorie limits:
   Snack items: ≤200 calories
   Entrée items: ≤350 calories
2. Sodium limits:
   Snack items: ≤230 mg**
   Entrée items: ≤480 mg
3. Fat limits:
   Total fat: ≤35% of calories
   Saturated fat: <10% of calories
   Trans fat: zero grams
4. Sugar limit:
   ≤35% of weight from total sugars in foods

*Beginning July 1, 2016, foods may not qualify using the 10% DV criteria.
**Beginning July 1, 2016, snack items must contain ≤200 mg sodium per item.

### Smart Snacks in School – Nutrition Standards for Beverages

**All schools may sell:**

1. Plain water (with or without carbonation)
2. Unflavored low fat milk
3. Unflavored or flavored fat free milk and milk alternatives permitted by NSLP/SBP
4. 100% fruit or vegetable juice
5. 100% fruit or vegetable juice diluted with water (with or without carbonation), and no added sweeteners

*There is no portion size limit for* ***plain*** *water.*
*Elementary schools may sell up to 8-ounce portions of milk and juice.*

### School Health Index – Elementary School

3 = Yes, **all** foods and beverages served and offered meet or exceed the USDA's Smart Snacks in School nutrition standards, **or** we do not serve or offer additional foods or beverages at our school.
2 = **Most** foods and beverages served and offered meet or exceed the USDA's Smart Snacks in School nutrition standards.
1 = **Some** foods and beverages served and offered meet or exceed the USDA's Smart Snacks in School nutrition standards.
0 = No, **no** foods and beverages served and offered meet or exceed the USDA's Smart Snacks in School nutrition standards.

ILLUSTRATION 12.10 ▸ School Health Index score card for foods and beverages served and offered in elementary schools.[103]

and low-fat white or flavored milk. It discouraged vended food or drink contracts, and stated that the health and nutritional interests of students should form the foundation of nutritional policies in schools. Because of the ongoing concern for the availability of competitive foods in the school environment, the AAP Council on School Health and Committee on Nutrition jointly issued a policy statement in 2015, urging continued efforts for improvement.[102]

While acknowledging that schools have made progress in making the school environment healthier in terms of food and beverage choices in the cafeteria, school faculty and parents are still struggling with achieving a reasonable balance when it comes to foods allowed for birthday parties, fundraisers, and holiday events. The AAP recommends that school wellness policies should avoid both prohibiting and allowing excessive consumption of added sugars; rather they encourage allowing minimal added sugars in foods that are not highly processed but are nutrient-rich.

The School Health Index (SHI) Self Assessment and Planning Guide: 2014 is an online tool for schools that is offered by the National Center for Chronic Disease Prevention and Health Promotion, Centers for Disease Control and Prevention.[103] The SHI helps schools:

- Identify strengths and weaknesses of health and safety policies and programs.
- Develop an action plan for improving student health, which can be incorporated into the school improvement plan.
- Engage teachers, parents, students, and the community in promoting health-enhancing behaviors and better health.[103]

The SHI has eight different modules for elementary schools and middle and high schools in the self-assessment, which correspond to the eight components of a coordinated school health program, as depicted in Illustration 12.9. Each module consists of a scorecard, a questionnaire with guidance for arriving at a score, planning questions, and recommendations for implementation. Recent versions of the SHI include an increased focus on the types of foods in the school environment, including:

- Food must not be used as a reward or punishment.
- Schools provide access to safe, free, unflavored drinking water throughout the school day.
- All foods and beverages sold or offered during the school day, including those for parties, events, and fundraisers, meet the USDA Smart Snacks in Schools standards (Illustration 12.10).
- Food and beverage advertising to students is limited.[103]

Schools are encouraged to assess their progress toward meeting these nutrition standards and to implement plans to promote continuous improvement.

## Nutrition Assessment

A nutrition assessment of a school-age child can identify nutrition-related concerns that pertain to the child's overall health status. Components of a nutrition assessment include a food/nutrition-related history, pertinent biochemical measurements, anthropometric measurements such as weight, height, body mass index percentile, and medical history. According to *Bright Futures: Guidelines for Health Supervision of Infants, Children, and Adolescents,* school-age children should be routinely screened for anemia and dyslipidemia by measuring pertinent biochemical indices (Table 12.9).[104] Based on this information, the nutrition professional can identify any nutrition diagnoses, design a nutrition intervention plan with family input, and make a plan for monitoring and evaluation (see Table 2.10 for the four steps of the Nutrition Care Process).

## Model Programs

The Fresh Fruit and Vegetable Program, is a public–private partnership of the CDC, Produce for Better Health, and other health organizations. Its public health initiative is called Fruits & Veggies—More Matters, which reflects the U.S. Dietary Guidelines in terms of recommendations for fruit and vegetable consumption. The Healthy Kids section of its website, www.fruitsandveggiesmorematters.org, includes coloring and activity pages for kids, online games, tips for parents to help them involve their children in choosing and preparing healthy meals, and links to educational resources to teach children about fruits and vegetables.[105] Kids can play a variety of games, and download coloring sheets, recipes, and activity pages on the Fruit and Veggie Color Champions website at www.foodchamps.org.

**TABLE 12.9** Normal values of biochemical nutritional parameters[42,104]

| TEST | NORMAL VALUES |
|---|---|
| **Iron Status** | |
| Hematocrit, % | 39 |
| Hemoglobin, g/dL | 14 |
| Serum ferritin, ng/mL | >15 |
| Serum iron, mcg/dL | >60 |
| Serum total iron binding capacity, mcg/dL | 350–400 |
| Serum transferrin saturation, % | >16 |
| Serum transferrin, mg/dL | 170–250 |
| Erythrocyte protoporphyrin, mcg/dl red blood cells | >70 |
| **Dyslipidemia Screen** | |
| Total cholesterol | >170 mg/dL |
| LDL cholesterol | >110 mg/dL |

SOURCE: From the Institute of Medicine, Food & Nutrition Board.

# Public Food and Nutrition Programs

LO 12.10 Describe one component of the USDA's Child Nutrition Program and explain how this specific program addresses the health of school-age children.

> "It is the position of the American Dietetic Association (now the Academy of Nutrition and Dietetics) that children and adolescents should have access to an adequate supply of healthful and safe foods that promote optimal physical, cognitive, and social growth and development. Nutrition assistance programs . . . play a vital role in meeting this critical need . . . ."[106]
>
> —The Academy of Nutrition and Dietetics

National child nutrition programs, which have had a federal legislative basis since 1946, contribute significantly to the food intake of school-age children. The purpose of the child nutrition programs is to provide nutritious meals to all children. These programs can also reinforce nutrition education, which takes place in the classroom. Since the school year 2006–2007, schools are required to develop a wellness plan that includes specific nutrition guidelines for all foods in the school, including competitive foods.[107] Child nutrition programs include the National School Lunch Program, School Breakfast Program, Child and Adult Care Food Program, Summer Food Service Program, and the USDA Fruit and Vegetable Program.[107]

## The National School Lunch Program

The federal government provides financial assistance to schools participating in the National School Lunch Program (NSLP) through cash reimbursements for all lunches served, with additional cash for lunches served to needy children, and through commodities.[107,108] Schools must meet five major requirements in order to participate in the NSLP:

1. Lunches must be based on nutritional standards.
2. Children who are unable to pay for lunches must receive lunches for free or at a reduced price, with no discrimination between paying and nonpaying children.
3. The programs operate on a nonprofit basis.
4. The programs must be accountable.
5. Schools must participate in the ***commodity program***.

In January 2012, the U.S. Department of Agriculture released revised nutrition standards in the National School Lunch and School Breakfast Programs, which marked the first major changes in school meals in 15 years.[108] The final standards included:

- Offering both fruits and vegetables every day of the week; substantially increasing offerings of whole grain-rich foods
- Offering only fat-free or low-fat milk varieties
- Limiting calories based on the age of children being served to ensure proper portion size
- Increasing the focus on reducing the amounts of saturated fat, *trans* fats, and sodium

The National School Lunch Program Meal Pattern (NSLP) is required to provide one-third of the DRIs based on the child's age or grade group (Table 12.10). In addition, school food-service personnel must make food safety a priority. These programs must also meet the needs of children with disabilities and special health care needs (see Chapter 13). Although not federally mandated, schools are encouraged to allow adequate time for children to eat their lunches. Schools receive payments from the federal government based on the number of meals served by category (paid, free, or reduced-price).

## School Breakfast Program

First authorized as a pilot program in 1966, the School Breakfast Program is a voluntary federal program. Many state legislatures have mandated breakfast programs for their districts, especially in schools serving needy populations. In general, the NSLP rules also apply to the School Breakfast Program. School breakfasts must provide one-fourth of the Dietary Reference Intakes for the children being served, based on age or grade groups, and comply with the U.S. Dietary Guidelines for Americans when analyzed over a week's time (Table 12.11). It is a special challenge for schools to allow enough time for school breakfasts before school when most of the participating children arrive at about the same time.

## Summer Food Service Program

The Summer Food Service Program provides meals to children from needy areas when school is not in session. Schools, local government agencies, or other public and private nonprofit agencies operate these programs. The federal government gives financial assistance to these programs for providing meals in areas where 50 percent or more of the participating children are from families whose incomes are lower than 185 percent of the poverty level. The Summer Food Service Program is an important source of food for many children from food-insecure families.

**commodity program** A USDA program in which food products are sent to schools for use in the child nutrition programs. Commodities are usually acquired for farm price support and surplus-removal reasons.[98]

TABLE 12.10 ▸ National School Lunch Program Meal Pattern[108]

| FOOD GROUP | NEW REQUIREMENTS K–12 |
|---|---|
| Fruit and Vegetables | ¾–1 cup of vegetables plus<br>½–1 cup of fruit per day |
| Vegetables | Weekly requirement for:<br>• Dark green<br>• Red orange<br>• Beans/peas (legumes)<br>• Starchy<br>• Other (as defined in 2010 Dietary Guidelines) |
| Meat/Meat Alternate | Daily minimum and weekly ranges:<br>Grades K–5: 1 oz equivalent minimum daily (8–10 oz weekly)<br>Grades 6–8: 1 oz equivalent minimum daily (9–10 oz weekly)<br>Grades 9–12: 2 oz Equivalent minimum daily (10–12 oz weekly) |
| Grains | Daily minimum and weekly ranges:<br>Grades K–5: 1 oz equivalent minimum daily (8–9 oz weekly)<br>Grades 6–8: 1 oz equivalent minimum daily (8–10 oz weekly)<br>Grades 9–12: 2 oz equivalent minimum daily (10–12 oz weekly) |
| Whole Grains | At least half of the grains must be whole grain–rich beginning July 1, 2012. Beginning July 1, 2014, all grains must be whole grain rich. |
| Milk | 1 cup<br>Must be fat-free (unflavored/flavored) or 1% low-fat (unflavored) |

SOURCE: U.S. Department of Agriculture, Food and Nutrition Service, www.usda.gov

## Team Nutrition

Team Nutrition is a program of the USDA's Food and Nutrition Service. The program is aimed at improving children's lifelong eating and physical activity habits through application of information in the Dietary Guidelines for Americans and MyPlate.[20,38,109] Team Nutrition is a partnership of public and private organizations, including private sector companies, nonprofit organizations, and advocacy groups that are interested in improving the health of the nation's children. Team Nutrition is an excellent example of a program that addresses the establishment of healthy eating and physical activity patterns for children on multiple fronts.

TABLE 12.11 ▸ School Breakfast Program meal pattern[108]

| FOOD GROUP | NEW REQUIREMENTS K–12 |
|---|---|
| Fruit | 1 cup per day (vegetable substitution allowed) |
| Grains and Meat/Meat Alternate (M/MA) | Daily minimum and weekly ranges for grains:<br>Grades K–5: 1 oz equivalent minimum daily (7–10 oz weekly)<br>Grades 6–8: 1 oz equivalent minimum daily (8–10 oz weekly)<br>Grades 9–12: 1 oz equivalent minimum daily 9–10 oz weekly)<br>Note: Quantity required School Year 2013–2014. Schools may substitute M/MA for grains after the minimum daily grains requirement is met. |
| Whole Grains | At least half of the grains must be whole grain rich beginning July 1, 2013. Beginning July 1, 2014, all grains must be whole grain rich. |
| Milk | 1 cup<br>Must be fat-free (unflavored/flavored or 1% low-fat (unflavored) |

SOURCE: U.S. Department of Agriculture, Food and Nutrition Service, www.usda.gov

Team Nutrition operates through three behavior-oriented strategies:

1. Provide training and technical assistance for child-nutrition food-service professionals to help them serve meals that meet nutrition standards while tasting and looking good.
2. Provide integrated nutrition education for children and their parents with the goal of establishing healthy food and physical-activity choices as part of a healthy lifestyle.
3. Provide support for healthy eating and physical activity by involving community partners, including school administrators and other school and community partners.

Communication channels utilized include: (1) food-service initiatives, (2) classroom activities, (3) school-wide events, (4) home activities, (5) community programs and events, and (6) media events and coverage.[109] Schools are recruited to become Team Nutrition schools with the benefit of receiving a resource kit of materials. Additional information is available on the Team Nutrition website at http://www.fns.usda.gov/tn/team-nutrition. The site includes activities for educators, parents, and students.[109]

## KEY POINTS

1. School-age and preadolescent children continue to grow at a slow, steady rate until the adolescent growth spurt.
2. Monitoring BMI-for-age percentiles is important for screening for overweight or underweight.
3. Family mealtimes should be encouraged, as there is a positive relationship between families eating together and the overall quality of the child's diet.
4. A child's food choices are being influenced by peers, teachers, coaches, the media, and the Internet.
5. The prevalence of overweight and obesity continue to increase in the school-age and preadolescent groups, but may be leveling out.
6. Complications of overweight and obesity in children and adolescents, such as type 2 diabetes mellitus, are increasing.
7. Sedentary lifestyles and limited physical activity are contributing factors to the increase in childhood overweight.
8. School-age and preadolescent children are encouraged to eat a variety of foods and increase physical activity as outlined by the U.S. Dietary Guidelines for Americans and MyPlate.
9. Consumption of sweetened soft drinks, which increases as children get older, is associated with increased calorie consumption and poorer diet quality.
10. Schools play an important community role in promoting healthy nutrition and physical activity patterns for children and adolescents.

## REVIEW QUESTIONS

Timothy in Case Study 12.1 returns to his pediatrician 6 months later at 7½ years of age for a weight check. He has gained 10 kg in 6 months and now weighs 90 pounds (41 kg). His height has increased to 51 inches (130 cm).

1. Calculate Timothy's BMI.
2. What is Timothy's BMI-for-age percentile? Use CDC growth curves to determine percentile.
3. Which of the following classifies Timothy's BMI-for-age percentile?
   a. Underweight
   b. Normal weight
   c. Overweight
   d. Obese
4. Based on the staged treatment plan for pediatric obesity, describe the recommended approach to treatment for Timothy.
5. Regarding fluid intake in school-age children, which of the following statements is most correct?
   a. Soft drinks are good choices for hydration during exercise because the high carbohydrate content provides quick energy.
   b. Children's caffeine consumption decreases as they get older.
   c. Diluted fruit juice is a good choice for hydration during exercise, as children are more likely to drink it than water.
   d. Adults who are supervising children during exercise can rely on the children to let them know when they are thirsty.
6. Name two strategies for increasing a school-age child's physical activity.
7. Name two strategies for decreasing a school-age child's sedentary behaviors.
8. Regarding child nutrition programs, which of the following statements is most correct?
   a. The nutritional analysis of the School Lunch Program includes à la carte items.
   b. Meals served as part of the School Lunch Program must provide one-third of the Dietary Reference Intakes of key nutrients for the age of the children being served.
   c. Meals served as part of the School Breakfast Program must provide one-third of the Dietary Reference Intakes of key nutrients for the age of the children being served.
   d. Team Nutrition refers to the component of the national child nutrition program that provides meals for student athletes.

Visit www.cengagebrain.com to access MindTap, a complete digital course that includes additional resources.

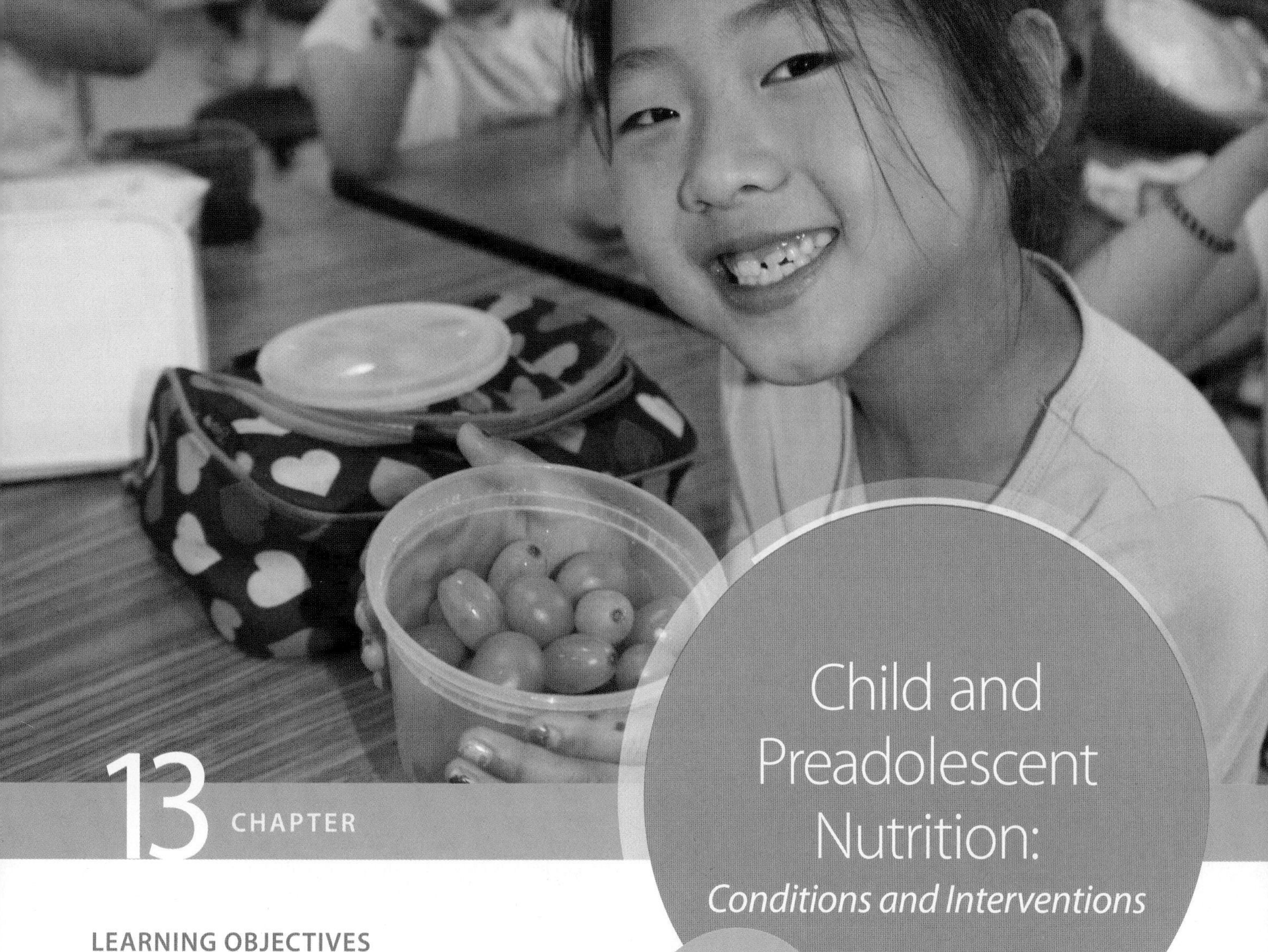

13 CHAPTER

# Child and Preadolescent Nutrition: *Conditions and Interventions*

*Prepared by*
Beth L. Leonberg

## LEARNING OBJECTIVES

After studying the materials in this chapter you should be able to:

**13.1** Explain why thinking that children are children first, even if they have conditions that affect their growth and nutritional requirements, suits child developmental milestones.

**13.2** Identify the common nutrition problems in children with special health care needs and chronic conditions.

**13.3** Describe how a growth assessment is modified in children with special health care needs.

**13.4** Characterize nutrition recommendations for children who are underweight and overweight, or have difficulties meeting known nutrient requirements.

**13.5** Describe the eating and feeding problems of children with special health care needs and chronic conditions.

**13.6** Compare use of dietary and herbal remedies in children with and without special health care needs.

**13.7** Explain why children who have special health conditions receive more intensive nutrition services in schools and health care settings than other children do.

Amanda Mills/Center for Disease Control and Prevention

# Introduction

Nutrition services need to be part of the goal to help a child reach his or her full potential. This chapter discusses the nutrition needs of children with chronic conditions, such as cystic fibrosis (CF), diabetes mellitus, cerebral palsy (CP), phenylketonuria (PKU), and behavioral disorders. Nutrition recommendations are based on those for children generally, but they may be modified by the condition and its consequences on growth, nutrient requirements, and/or eating abilities. Other factors such as activity that increase or decrease energy needs are also discussed. School and community resources include nutrition services for children with special health care needs, chronic conditions or those with developmental disabilities. Advocates for those with disabilities prefer "people-first language," which this chapter models. This convention names the person first and then the condition. An example is "a girl with Down syndrome" rather than "the Down's girl." Advocates for those with disabilities also prefer the word *disabilities* to the word *handicapped*. (Use of the term *handicap* comes from the practice of using a cap to beg.)

# "Children Are Children First"—What Does That Mean?

LO 13.1 Explain why thinking that children are children first, even if they have conditions that affect their growth and nutritional requirements, suits child developmental milestones.

Children with special health care needs are children first, even if their conditions change their nutrition, medical, and social needs. Children are expected to become more independent in making food choices, assisting with meal preparation, and participating at mealtime with other family members. These same expectations are appropriate for children with special health care needs. For example, the child with spina bifida should be encouraged to make a salad or set the table. Modifications may be needed to help the child be successful, such as storing plates and utensils on low shelves, or lowering counter heights to accommodate a wheelchair at a kitchen sink.

This concept has been acknowledged in schools through federal legislation in the Individuals with Disabilities Education Act (IDEA) (see also Chapter 11 for further discussion).[1,2] This law requires the least restrictive environment and is resulting in inclusive settings for more children with disabilities.[1] This concept of inclusion has major ramifications for how children receive all types of services, such as schools providing alternative foods as required in the main cafeteria. As a result of inclusion, children in wheelchairs or with Down syndrome spend time in regular classrooms with others of the same age. Nutritional problems related to food refusals, mealtime behavior, or special nutrition interventions are addressed in the neighborhood school, in the regular classroom, as often as possible.

This same concept of treating the child as a child first is recommended at home, too. Whatever special foods or dietary supplements required are in forms suitable for the child's developmental level, such as liquid supplemental calcium instead of chewable tablets. Children with diabetes or PKU do not benefit from being treated in a special manner at mealtime. As soon as possible, children are taught to take responsibility for making food choices consistent with their dietary plans. Consistency and structure in the home support a child's normal development. This structure includes regular meal and snack times, and the child accepting increasing levels of responsibility in preparing foods. These approaches lower the chance of the child being overprotected or manipulating adults because of her illness or its treatment.

## Counting Children with Special Health Care Needs

School-aged children with special health care needs are categorized differently than children under 5 years of age. A specific medical diagnosis is not required for providing educational services for younger children; they are eligible when considered at risk. Follow-up services after preterm birth are major reasons young children access educational and health services, but less a reason for older children. Educational terminology reflects a difference in young and older children. In young children, the name of the planning document is the family education services plan (IFSP). For those older than 3 years of age, the planning document is called the individualized education plan (IEP). U.S. education laws specify that by 8 years of age, stricter classifications of disability become the basis for eligibility.[2] Special educational services for those 8 years and older are not based on general terms such as *developmental delay* or *at risk*. Educational funding requires categories similar to a medical diagnosis for insurance coverage, and is subject to state-by-state guidelines. Because of this distinction, the Centers for Disease Control (CDC) is conducting ongoing research on the prevalence of autism spectrum disorder (ASD) among 8-year-old children.[3] ASD is a lifelong developmental disability, characterized by limited patterns of behavior, activity, or interests, and difficulty in social interaction and communication. The prevalence of ASD has been rising rapidly; the CDC reports that the prevalence in 2010 was about 1 in 68 8-year-old children, as compared to 1 in 150 children in 2000.

Estimates range widely about the number of children with chronic conditions and those with special health care needs. According to the U.S. Department of Education, approximately 6.5 million children between the ages of 3 and 21 received special education services in 2011–2012, or about 13 percent of all public school students.[4] Some factors that affect the different estimates of number of children with special health care needs include:

- *Duration*. Most agree a chronic condition in a child is one expected to last 12 months or more. However, state programs serving children with special health care needs differ in including or excluding pediatric cancers, genetic conditions, and recurrent infections, such as repeated ear infections.
- *Reporters*. Prevalence of chronic conditions in children differ if families are surveyed, or if educators or medical providers are reporting epidemiological research.[4,5,6,7]
- *Who makes the diagnosis*. Medical diagnoses, educational categories, and nutrition diagnoses result in different prevalence rates of children with chronic conditions. For example, obesity and overweight are rarely included in diagnoses of children with special health care needs.
- *Progress in health care*. What defines a diagnosis changes with medical knowledge, advocacy, and funding. Some conditions such as childhood mental health problems, consequences of concussions, obesity, and ASD are increasing over time.[3,7] Prevalence rates of lead poisoning, simple iron deficiency anemia, and infants with HIV born from HIV-affected mothers are decreasing over time in the United States.

U.S. educators consider asthma, learning disabilities, attention deficit hyperactivity disorder (ADHD), and speech problems the most prevalent chronic conditions in children.[4] Within each category, some children do require nutrition services, but most do not. The chronic conditions in children that require the most nutrition services, even though they are less prevalent—such as diabetes—are discussed in this chapter.

As most children are healthy, general nutrition guidelines for children, school nutrition educational materials, and nutrition prevention strategies may or may not be applicable to children with specific conditions. Many nutrition education curricula appropriately target the goals of preventing overweight, lowering fat intake, and increasing fruit and vegetable intake. These curricula provide appropriate education, for the most part, to children with conditions such as diabetes and Down syndrome. Conditions in which slow weight gain and underweight are common, such as CP and CF, may not fit such curricula.[8,9] Nutrition education may not address such children's need for high-fat foods as part of high energy needs. A child with PKU, for example, cannot ever have protein-rich meats or dairy products.[10] When the usual nutrition guidelines are discussed and encouraged, the child with PKU may feel isolated and confused about whether his restricted dietary selections are healthy. When possible, children with special health care needs are encouraged to participate in school nutrition education programs, with modifications as needed.

> "Train a child in the way he should go, and when he is old, he will not depart from it."
>
> —Proverb

# Nutritional Requirements of Children with Special Health Care Needs

**LO 13.2** Identify the common nutrition problems in children with special health care needs and chronic conditions.

Energy and protein needs are lower on a body-weight basis in childhood than during the preadolescence, toddler years, and preschool years.[11] Children with special health care needs have a wide range of nutrition requirements and more variability than other children do, based on these factors:[12,13]

- Low energy intake may be appropriate with small muscle size.
- High protein is needed with high protein losses, such as skin breakdown.
- High fluid volume is needed with frequent losses from vomiting or diarrhea.
- High fiber may be needed for chronic-constipation management.
- Long-term use of prescribed medications may increase or decrease vitamin or mineral requirements, or change the balance of vitamins and minerals needed as a result of medication side effects.
- Routine illness is more likely to result in hospitalization or resurgence of symptoms of the underlying disorder.

U.S. Dietary Guidelines and the Healthy People 2020 objectives may not fit some children with special health care needs.[14,15] In these cases, what replaces these tools is the individualized nutrition assessment that results in nutrition diagnoses and interventions.[13] Nutrition diagnoses augment and align with medical diagnoses within the child's medical and educational records.

## Energy Needs

Children with special health care needs may need more, less, or the same energy intake as other children of the same age. Energy needs are amazingly complex in children, let alone those with special needs. Under ideal conditions, the energy needs are measured by indirect calorimetry, but they are usually estimated using standard calculations that cannot take into account the specific conditions involved.[13] Professional guidelines recommend use of indirect calorimetry especially for very sick children, but they still can give only estimates of energy needs at rest, without considerations of energy needed for activity and growth.[16] Conditions that slow growth or decrease muscle size generally result in lower energy needs.[12,13] Energy needs in a child with Prader-Willi syndrome may be only 80 percent of the energy needs of a child of the same age and gender without the syndrome.[17]

Energy requirements are related to activity level and frequency of illnesses.[12] Children with a chronic condition are encouraged to participate in age-appropriate sports activities. Conditions in which activity may be especially beneficial include diabetes and mild CP. The level of activity of children with chronic conditions may be higher or lower than activity levels in other children. Children who are very active may appear thin as a result of low energy intake. Children with ASD and ADHD are generally more active and/or they may sleep less.[18] Such a range in level of activity is addressed as a part of a thorough nutrition assessment. Questions such as, "Is the child receiving physical therapy one to three times per week?" and, "How much time does the child use a walker compared to a wheelchair?" are examples of how activity can be assessed in determining energy needs.

### Protein Needs

Protein needs also can be higher than, lower than, or the same as those for other children, based on the condition. Healing burns and CF are examples of disorders with high protein needs—at 150 percent of the DRI.[19,20] Conditions such as PKU and other protein-based inborn errors of metabolism require greatly reduced amounts of natural protein consumed.[10] In contrast to these conditions that alter protein needs, children with many other chronic conditions, such as diabetes mellitus, do not have modified protein needs.[21] Protein is crucial for wound healing and for maintaining a healthy immune system; it is also a key requirement for various conditions with frequent illnesses or surgeries. For example, a child with CP who is scheduled to have hip surgery would have protein needs evaluated in a complete nutritional assessment.[22] Higher protein may be recommended for wound healing and the prevention of skin breakdown while in a cast after surgery.

Healthy children eat foods providing intact protein, but some conditions require hydrolyzed amino acids or specific amino acid mixtures rather than intact protein. Appropriate nutrition interventions for children with severe egg, soy, or milk allergies, chronic gastrointestinal conditions, or with inborn errors of metabolism include prescribed complete nutritional supplements because they fit altered protein requirements.[23]

### Other Nutrients

DRIs are good starting places to assess the need for vitamins and minerals in chronic conditions.[13] As in all children, if the allowed food selections provide sufficient choices to meet the needs for protein, fats, and carbohydrates, it is likely the vitamin and mineral needs are also met. However, children with chronic conditions may have more difficulty meeting the DRI for vitamins and minerals as a result of the following considerations:[13]

- Eating or feeding problems may restrict intake of foods requiring chewing, such as meats, so that certain minerals usually contributed in meats may be low.
- Prescribed medications and their side effects can increase turnover for specific nutrients, raising the recommended amount needed.
- Food refusals are common with recurrent illness, so total intake may be more variable day to day than in other children of the same age.
- Treatment of the condition necessitates specific food and nutrient restrictions, so that vitamins and minerals usually provided in restricted foods have to be supplemented.

Nutrients such as calcium that are low in the general population of children are also problem nutrients for children with chronic conditions. The 2010 Institute of Medicine Food and Nutrition Board statement that increased calcium RDA for children and also Vitamin D RDA applies to children with chronic conditions (see Chapter 12 for further discussion of these recommendations).[24] Children with neurologic impairment and developmental disabilities, such as CP, are at higher risk for osteopenia due to low mineral intakes, lack of weight-bearing activity, and use of anticonvulsant medications.[12] Vitamin D intake should be monitored and supplemented as needed in these children.

## Growth Assessment

LO 13.3 Describe how a growth assessment is modified in children with special health care needs.

The CDC 2000 growth charts are a good starting place for assessing the growth of any child.[25] Public health goals, such as identifying children at risk for overweight and preventing long-term cardiovascular risks, are important purposes underlying growth assessments of children. Such concerns may or may not apply to children with chronic conditions. Within the nutrition assessment process, a child's specific condition should be used to create individualized nutrition goals for weight gain and growth.

Children with special needs require in-depth growth assessments because interpretation of weight and height in the manner used for healthy children can be misleading. For example, body mass index (BMI) is a good indicator of growth for healthy children. However BMI has underlying assumptions that do not fit children with CP, so better indices based on weight and long-term mortality are recommended for children with CP.[8,9] For now, no BMI tables cover specific conditions or adiposity rebound in children with special health care needs.

If the nutritionist is especially skilled in interviewing families, parents may be willing to express their apprehension about growth in their child. They may have long-term concerns about caring for the child at home, when activities such as lifting him or her from the bathtub or out of a wheelchair may become more difficult. Also, children with degenerative conditions such as ***spinal muscular atrophy (SMA)*** have such major decreases in muscle size that growth may not occur. SMA is rare, but is the second most common autosomal genetic disease after CF.[26]

Most children with chronic conditions do grow, and assessing growth is an important component of nutrition services. If the child's condition is known to change the rate of weight or height gain—either slowing or accelerating it—the following signs need attention regardless of what growth chart is used:

- A plateau in weight
- A pattern of gain and then weight loss
- Not regaining weight lost during an illness
- A pattern of unexplained and unintentional weight gain

## Growth Interpretation in Children with Chronic Conditions

What a child eats usually does impact their growth. In children with chronic conditions, however, this may or may not be the case. Factors that affect growth assessment and interpretation in childhood are the age of onset of the condition, ***secondary conditions***, and activity. These factors might not have been detectable earlier in younger children.

The child's age when the condition started should influence growth interpretation. The fetal origins hypothesis (discussed in Chapter 9) supports this idea; early onset of a condition is more likely than later onset to affect growth in children with short stature, seizures, and asthma.[27,28,29] Such conditions are now understood to reflect fetal programming that overrides the impact of current food and nutrient intake on growth. Global maternal and health data on growth stunting has shown that the process begins *in utero*, even though the diagnosis is made years later.[27]

Children who were born with severe prematurity may have experienced undernutrition that results in unusual growth patterns, in spite of adequate food and nutrition in childhood. Even though infants and young children are not diagnosed with asthma until childhood, the developmental origins of asthma are seen in low birthweight infants who require respiratory support.[29] Nutritionists use such information to interpret growth and help avoid frustration for families who are told to increase energy for a child to promote growth, which does not end up showing any benefit.

Another example of the impact of the age of onset of a chronic condition on growth interpretation is in children with seizures. If the child's seizures started in middle childhood, the standard growth chart may be appropriate because the child's growth pattern is already established. Onset of seizures in younger years requires careful interpretation of growth, as uncontrolled seizure or medication side effects on food and nutrient intake may slow growth rate. This is another example of when the child's own growth record over time would be the best indicator of future growth.

Children, but not toddlers and preschoolers, with CP are assessed for developing secondary conditions.[22] ***Scoliosis*** is a secondary condition that interferes with accurate measurement of stature.[13,19] It may develop as a result of muscle incoordination and asymmetrical weakness in one group of muscles. If a child with CP has stature measurements that plateau or decline, it may be a result of CP, scoliosis, lack of adequate nutritional intake, or a combination of these three factors. Nutritional interventions cannot prevent scoliosis, although nutritional consequences of its treatment may arise. Children may be provided with custom-fitted back braces, so weight gain means the brace needs to be replaced. Children with scoliosis braces also may become less active because the brace restricts some types of movement. If scoliosis surgery is performed, the child may become slightly taller immediately, again showing that stature measurements have to be interpreted with care.

## Body Composition and Growth

Nutritionists use body composition as another factor in interpreting growth in an in-depth assessment. Children with special health care needs may or may not be typically proportioned in muscle size, bone structure, and fat stores. Some children with good nutritional status may plot at or below the lowest percentile on a standard growth chart for height. In fact, low-percentile heights are usual for a child with Down syndrome if growth is plotted on the CDC chart.[30] Short stature, low muscle tone, and low weight compared to age-matched peers should not be attributed to low energy intake. They characterize the natural consequences of the ***neuromuscular*** changes within Down syndrome.

Similarly, a child with low muscle size could have a low weight and short stature (muscle contractions cause resistance, which promotes skeletal growth) compared to children with regular-sized muscles.[19] It would be unfair to assume

**spinal muscular atrophy** Condition in which muscle control declines over time as a result of nerve loss, causing death in childhood.

**secondary condition** Common consequence of a condition, which may or may not be preventable over time.

**scoliosis** Condition in which the vertebral bones in the back show a side-to-side curve, resulting in a shorter stature than expected if the back were straight.

**neuromuscular** Term pertaining to the central nervous system's control of muscle coordination and movement.

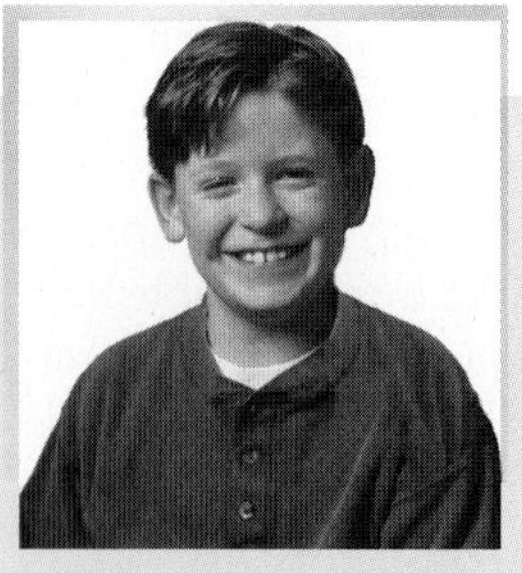
Photodisc

# CASE STUDY 13.1

## Adjusting Energy Intake for a Child with Spina Bifida

This case study is about appropriate nutrition interventions, monitoring, and evaluation within the Nutrition Care Process. The nutrition diagnosis is excess energy intake related to spina bifida as evidenced by weight gain over the last year.

Sam is a third-grader in regular classes at his public school. He uses a wheelchair all the time and can transfer from his wheelchair to a chair by himself. He is on a toileting schedule at school with the assistance of a nurse. He participates in modified physical education as part of his physical therapy treatment. He likes to eat with his friends at school. His mother tries to make him cut back at the evening meal and has stopped buying some of his favorite snacks. He is mad at his mother because he likes his snacks after school when he is bored.

Nutrition assessment from Sam's last visit at the spina bifida clinic at the local hospital showed that he was overweight by measuring his fat stores. Because he cannot stand, his stature was estimated by measuring his length lying down and comparing it with his last length measurement. Standard methods could not be used to measure him, which limits the interpretation of his growth using the CDC growth chart. The chart showed Sam at the 75th percentile in weight for his age, which is not overweight for his age. His rate of weight gain of 8 pounds per year, typical for a boy his age, is too fast for his low level of activity. His estimated energy need is 1,100 calories per day due to low activity and short stature, or about two-thirds of the energy needs of others his age. Sam says he does not care about his size or being overweight. His mother is quite concerned that she would not be able to assist him if he fell or needed to be lifted.

**Interventions:** The nutritionist at the clinic completes a school lunch prescription to reduce Sam's energy intake from 650 calories to 350 calories per lunch. His meal pattern is adjusted to two meals (breakfast and lunch) and two snacks per day at home, which better fits his low energy needs. Sam is allowed to choose his favorite snack foods to replace his evening meal. Giving him choices about his snacks increases Sam's sense of being in control and lowers the instances of expressing anger at his mother about snack foods. The clinic nutritionist calls the school to review Sam's level of activity and confirm that the lunch changes are being implemented. His physical therapist has found after-school swimming lessons and recommends them to Sam's mother as a way to increase his activity and socialization.

To motivate Sam to pay attention to his eating and weight gain, his teacher and his mother set up a monthly nonfood reward for him if he does not gain any weight. The effectiveness of the plan to cut Sam's energy intake and increase his activity will be assessed at his next clinic visit, when he will be weighed and have his fat stores measured.

### *Questions*

1. Since Sam does not care about his size or being overweight, why is a diet plan necessary?
2. What are the risks from Sam's weight, since he is only at the 75th percentile for his age on the standard growth chart?
3. Will Sam grow taller when he goes through puberty and be able to eat more each day?

that the child's food choices result in a low weight in this example. Conditions with altered muscle size may be described using terms such as *hypotonia* or *hypertonia*. Examples include CP, Down syndrome, and spina bifida.[22,30] Not all muscles are affected. For example, some children with spina bifida have larger muscle size in the upper body and smaller muscle size in the lower body. Variation in size of muscles may make growth interpretation more difficult. Standard interpretation may suggest a risk of overweight, but it may not accurately reflect that short stature is part of the child's condition (see Case Study 13.1).

A thorough assessment that includes body composition is necessary, such as measuring fat stores in a standard manner.[31] A thin-appearing child needs to have body fat stores measured before nutrition recommendations are made; if body fat stores are fine, adding food as extra energy just contributes to overweight. Measuring fat stores in children is not like measuring fat stores in adults, because of the changes in body composition that come with age and growth. Calculated methods for evaluating body composition in children are not the same as those for adults.[19,32] Estimates of body composition for children with chronic conditions may be based on smaller sample sizes than for other children, but such information is still helpful. Identified low fat stores trigger recommendations to boost food energy.

Prescribed growth hormone is another major factor in interpreting growth.[33] It is now prescribed for more conditions than decades before, including children with CF, Down syndrome, Prader Willi syndrome, and other chromosomal disorders. If a child is prescribed growth hormone, the time of initiation and discontinuation should be noted during the growth assessment, so that growth patterns may be interpreted correctly.

In-depth growth assessment may include head circumference measurement for all ages, with plotting and interpretation based on the Nellhaus head circumference growth chart, as discussed in Chapter 9.[34] Head circumference is important because children with unusually small heads have smaller brains, a characteristic associated with short stature. Even with good food choices and no eating problems, children with some genetic disorders tend to be shorter than their age-matched peers.[35]

### Special Growth Charts

Special growth charts have been published for a variety of genetic conditions (Table 13.1).[36] The number of children reported in such growth charts is not as large, nor as representative as the CDC 2000 growth charts.[25] Special growth charts are revised often, based on new information emerging about the natural course of rare conditions. For example, the American Academy of Pediatrics does not recommend Down syndrome growth charts that have been used for decades continue to be used since the population reported in the old growth charts does not reflect current practice guidelines.[30] New growth charts for those with Down syndrome are being developed. Some special growth charts are based on only the most severe forms of the condition, such as for children living in residential care. Many chronic conditions have such a wide range of severity that special growth charts cannot be developed. Conditions without a specialty growth chart in which growth patterns can be variable include the following:

- ***Juvenile rheumatoid arthritis***
- Cystic fibrosis
- Rett syndrome
- Spina bifida
- Seizures
- Diabetes type 1 and type 2

**TABLE 13.1** Examples of specialty growth charts[2,19]

| CONDITIONS WITH SPECIAL GROWTH CHARTS | COMMENT |
|---|---|
| Achrondroplasia | Form of dwarfism |
| Down syndrome | Short stature, variable weight |
| Trisomy 13 | |
| Trisomy 18 | |
| Fragile X syndrome | Short stature, primary in males |
| Prader-Willi syndrome | Short stature, overweight |
| Rubinstein-Tabyi syndrome | Short stature |
| Sickle-cell disease | Short stature |
| Turner syndrome | Short stature |
| Spastic quadriplegia | Short stature, low weight |
| Marfan syndrome | Tall stature |



## Nutrition Recommendations

**LO 13.4** Characterize nutrition recommendations for children who are underweight and overweight, or have difficulties meeting known nutrient requirements.

Children with chronic conditions require nutrition assessments to determine whether they are meeting their nutrient and energy needs. Then nutrition diagnoses and interventions are provided based on the assessment. The more frequent nutrition diagnoses are derived from assessments showing underweight and overweight, or having difficulties meeting known nutrient requirements. The goal is for the child to maintain good nutritional status, and to prevent nutrition-related problems from being superimposed on the primary condition. (See Case Study 13.1.)

Children with special health care needs benefit from the same nutritional recommendations that other children do, particularly in general areas such as dietary fiber or appropriate intake of soft drinks (Illustration 13.1). Often children with special health care needs have

**juvenile rheumatoid arthritis** Condition in which joints become enlarged and painful as a result of the dysfunction of the immune system; generally occurs in children or teens.

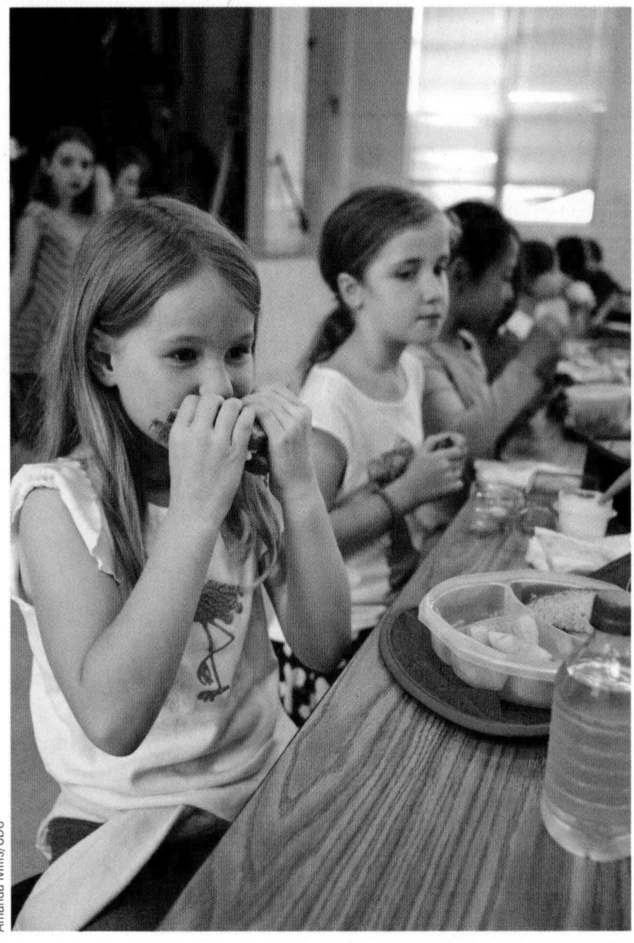



**ILLUSTRATION 13.1** Children with special needs still need to follow general dietary guidelines.

nutritional diagnoses and interventions that require particular supplements and methods of delivering energy and nutrients not needed for healthy children.

The starting place for nutrition interventions is to view the child in the context of her family. The goal is for the child to live at home and be educated in spite of her health care needs. This requires close attention to meeting all known food and nutrient requirements. Most children with and without special health care needs eat and drink to obtain their needed nutrients and energy, like everyone else. Nutrition experts are involved mainly with those children unable to meet their needs in the usual manner. They range from children who need just a little help to those who are technology dependent for both eating and breathing.[37]

The quality of the child's life, his or her ability to live at home and avoid frequent hospital visits, and the ability of the parents to work and take care of other family members are examples of factors that nutritionists consider in planning nutrition interventions.[37,38] Nutrition interventions may include prescribing nutrition products that are digested in the usual manner, termed enteral supplements, to maintain health and to assure growth is not being limited (Table 13.2).[19] Children less than 10 years of age are generally prescribed a pediatric form, but adult complete nutritional supplements may be safely consumed by children. (Energy and nutrients that do not go into the gastrointestinal tract but, rather, directly into the blood stream is called parenteral nutrition; see Chapter 9.)

## Methods of Meeting Nutritional Requirements

Since feeding a child is such an important part of caring for him, nutritionists give parents and caregivers a large role in deciding about the type and form of nutrition support provided. Part of the decision-making process often hinges on trying various interventions to improve nutrition status. A common nutrition intervention is supplementing or partially replacing meals or snacks with complete nutritional supplements consumed orally. Most complete nutritional supplements can be consumed as beverages. Nutritionists try to avoid the word *formula* when talking about the complete nutritional supplements, to highlight that these are for children, not infants.

If this does not improve nutrition status over time, complete nutritional supplements can be administered through a feeding *gastrostomy, which is a tube placed semi-permanently through the abdominal wall.*[38] Most families experience difficulty accepting a gastrostomy for meeting nutritional requirements because eating is such an important aspect of parenting.[38] Medical providers conduct the tests and surgical procedures to create a gastrostomy and monitor it over time. Nutrition experts recommend what goes into the gastrostomy to meet nutrition requirements. Children who have a gastrostomy may or may not also require other types of technology, such as mechanical pumps. Sometimes the term *technology dependent* is used when technology is required for feeding and breathing. Gastrostomy feeding may be required in children with kidney diseases, some forms of cancer, and severe forms of CP and CF.[37-39] Insurance coverage and financial questions of paying for complete nutritional supplements are major concerns for some families.

Children fed by gastrostomy can have many different schedules, such as eating orally during school and supplemented by gastrostomy feeding overnight (Table 13.3). If medications are required, they can also be given through the gastrostomy. For example, for children with pediatric AIDS who require many medications during the day, compliance with taking the drugs improved after gastrostomies were placed.[40,41] The parents spent less time trying to administer the medications to their children, and some children's health improved as a result of taking all of the required medications. Another example is a child who cannot safely drink liquids as a result of CP. The child could have fluids given by gastrostomy but eat solid foods. Children with gastrostomies can swim, bathe, and do any activities they could do before the gastrostomy was placed.

When possible, gastrostomy feeding is planned as a temporary measure, with a return to oral eating later. For example, a child who has a gastrostomy because of a kidney condition may have a kidney transplant that allows

TABLE 13.2 ▸ Examples of nutritional supplements and formula for children[13]

| FORMULA | COMMENTS |
|---|---|
| Pediatric versions of complete nutritional supplements, such as Pediasure | Generally recommended for children under 10 years of age; can be used for gastrostomy or oral nutrition support |
| Adult complete nutritional supplements, such as Ensure | Generally 1 calorie per milliliter strength is recommended for children |
| Enrichment of beverages, such as Carnation Instant Breakfast added to milk | Requires that milk is tolerated |
| Predigested formula with amino acids and medium-chain fatty acids, such as Peptamen Junior | For conditions in which intestinal absorption may be impaired |
| Special formulas for inborn errors of metabolism (PKU), such as Phenex-2 | Usually a powder that is mixed as a beverage, but other forms such as bars and capsules are available |
| High-energy booster for cystic fibrosis, such as Scandishake | Generally 2.5 calories per milliliter to concentrate energy in a small volume |

TABLE 13.3 ▸ Example of a feeding and eating schedule for an 8-year-old who eats by mouth and by gastrostomy

| DAILY SCHEDULE | COMMENTS |
| --- | --- |
| 6:30 a.m. Night feeding pump turned off<br>7:15 a.m. Breakfast: refused<br>8:00 a.m. Bus to school | Overnight feeding by gastrostomy runs from 9:30 p.m. until 6:30 a.m., providing about 3 fl oz per hour, so no hunger in the morning is common |
| 11:30 a.m. School lunch offered and about half is eaten: ½ chicken sandwich, all of french fries, with ⅓ pint of whole milk | Child has slow eating pace and is easily distracted by school lunchroom sounds |
| 3:30 p.m. After-school snack at home of 4 oz pudding cup, two plain cookies, and 4 fl oz orange drink | Mealtime behavior at home includes many attempts to leave the table, with prompting to eat from parents |
| 6:30 p.m. Evening meal at home: ½ cup mashed potato, 6 fl oz whole milk, refused vegetable and meat<br>8:30 p.m. Bedtime | Parents hook up night feeding pump while the child is sleeping |



removal of the gastrostomy after recovery. Other nutrition supplements fed by gastrostomy have specific components that cannot be in beverages because they have such a strange taste. For example, those containing individual amino acids generally are accepted only by those used to this taste from infancy, such as the metabolic foods prescribed for those with PKU. If a child required a new product with amino acids in place of intact protein, he or she will probably reject drinking it. Administering the product through a gastrostomy would be more successful in improving nutritional status over time.

**Vitamin and Mineral Supplements for Chronic Conditions** Children's complete vitamin and mineral supplements are recommended for a variety of chronic conditions to assure that the DRIs for essential nutrients are provided. However, most over-the-counter supplements are in the form of chewable tablets, so children who cannot chew well may require a liquid form of vitamins and minerals. The composition of vitamin and mineral supplements may be important because some have ingredients that are not allowed. Examples are vitamin and mineral brands with added carbohydrates, which are not allowed on a ***ketogenic diet***, or those made with an artificial sweetener containing phenylalanine not recommended for children with PKU. (The ketogenic diet and PKU are discussed later in this chapter.)

The underlying diagnosis can make specific nutrients so important that they may be prescribed as pharmaceuticals. CF treatment (discussed later in this chapter) requires fat-soluble vitamin supplements due to poor intestinal absorption of these nutrients.[20] Vitamins A, D, E, and K are all supplemented in those with CF.[20] Vitamin $B_{12}$ injections are needed for some protein-based inborn errors of metabolism.[10] Vitamin C may be prescribed above the DRI for some children with spina bifida who have frequent bladder infections.[19] The high dose of vitamin C functions as a medication rather than as a nutrient in this instance.

All medications, prescribed and over-the-counter, should be identified in a nutrition assessment. Inadvertently, excessive levels of vitamins and minerals can be consumed through a combination of diet and supplements, and are risky, especially for underweight children. One family may be told to give the child an adult nutrition supplement such as Carnation Instant Breakfast daily, while another provider adds a complete nutritional supplement and is unaware that the child also takes a chewable children's vitamin/mineral tablet, too. This is why determination of the total intake of supplemented nutrients is part of a nutrition assessment.

Children with chronic conditions that limit activity or require medications that affect bone growth need special attention to their calcium and vitamin D intake.[42] ***Galactosemia***, in which all food choices with lactose are eliminated, and CP are two examples of conditions affecting calcium. Some children with these conditions are like older women with ***osteoporosis*** in that their calcium may move out of bones faster than it goes in. Providing additional calcium, phosphorus, and vitamin D may be recommended, raising concerns about supplements needed for years or decades.[42]

## Fluids

Guidelines for fluids for all children are appropriate. Particular considerations for children with special health care needs are high fluid losses—for example, from uncontrollable drooling—or problem behaviors that result in low fluid intakes.[19] Children with limited ability to talk may have more difficulty indicating thirst. Because constipation is common in children with neuromuscular disorders, adequate fluids are often stressed as part of a bowel management program. Many chronic health conditions carry higher risks for dehydration due to side effects of prescribed medications. A chronic condition generally does not change the fluid requirement when the child is well.

**ketogenic diet** High-fat, low-carbohydrate meal plan in which ketones are made from metabolic pathways used in converting fat as a source of energy.

**galactosemia** A rare genetic condition of carbohydrate metabolism in which a blocked or inactive enzyme does not allow breakdown of galactose. It can cause serious illness if not identified and treated soon after birth.

**osteoporosis** Condition in which low bone density or weak bone structure leads to an increased risk of bone fracture.

# Eating and Feeding Problems in Children with Special Health Care Needs

LO 13.5 Describe the eating and feeding problems of children with special health care needs and chronic conditions.

By the middle childhood years, abilities and/or disabilities that limit eating independently and using utensils are clear, as feeding and eating skills develop during toddler and preschool years. Eating or feeding-related problems are diagnosed when children have difficulty accepting foods, chewing them safely, or ingesting sufficient foods and beverages to meet their nutritional requirements. A variety of health care providers are involved in the process of assessment, diagnosis, and interventions of eating or feeding-related problems, and in radiological studies of swallowing, including occupational therapists, speech therapists, registered dietitians, pediatricians, and psychologists. When drinking and eating is unsafe, raising the risk of respiratory failure, nutrition interventions to avoid eating by mouth are lifesaving. Parents and caregivers recognize over time that children who cannot eat independently nor enjoy mealtimes need help with eating and its stressful impact on both the family and the child. About 70 percent of children with developmental delays have feeding difficulties, independent of whether neuromuscular problems have been identified.[19]

## Feeding Challenges for Children with Health Care Needs

Examples of these feeding problems for children with special health care needs and chronic conditions include the following situations:

- Self-feeding skills are lower than the child's chronological age, requiring assistance and supervision to ensure adequate intake.
- Meals take so long or so much food is lost in the process of eating that the actual food intake is too low.
- The condition requires adjustment in the timing of meals and snacks at home and at school.

In children without intellectual disabilities, eating problems may include behavioral problems at mealtimes, conflicts about control over food choices, and variability in appetite. Families of children with chronic conditions may focus on mealtimes and foods as methods of coping with their own concerns about the child. For example, families may be overprotective and restrict a child from eating at friends' homes, when such activities may be appropriate for social development.

## Specific Disorders

**Cystic Fibrosis** CF is one of the most common lethal genetic disorders, with an incidence of 1 in 1,500–2,000 live births.[13] It has a higher incidence among Caucasians, and is less common in African Americans. The CF gene is located on the long arm of chromosome 7, and it has hundreds of gene versions. The most common genetic mutation characterizes 67 percent of the cases. CF affects all the exocrine functions in the body, with lung complications often causing death during the adult years. Its major nutrition-related consequence is malabsorption of various nutrients due to the lack of pancreatic enzymes. This can result in a slower rate of weight and height gain, and higher energy needs due to chronic lung infections. Children with CF require close monitoring to avoid malnutrition as the condition progresses. Intensive nutrition interventions may be required to meet higher energy needs.[12,43]

Nutrition interventions for CF include monitoring growth, assessing food and nutrient intake, and increasing energy and protein by two to four times the usual recommendations to compensate for malabsorption.[20] Every time a child with CF eats a meal or snack, he must take pills containing enzymes. Frequent eating and large, calorie-dense meals are encouraged. Gastrostomy feeding at night to boost energy is sometimes required. Vitamin and mineral supplementation, particularly fat-soluble vitamins, is a part of daily management. Children with CF are at risk for developing diabetes because the pancreas is a target organ of CF damage.[43] Nutrition experts struggle to balance the children's high nutrient needs with their frequent illnesses that throw off their appetite to eat. Many children with CF have slow growth and are lower in weight and shorter than expected. Even with nutrition support, decline in pulmonary function over time continues. Some children with CF have lung transplants if they meet strict eligibility requirements. CF is on the leading edge of gene therapy research and has new medications in development, giving hope to families with young children.

**Diabetes Mellitus** Diabetes mellitus is a disorder of glucose metabolism and ***insulin*** regulation in which nutrition intervention is crucial.[12,44] Early signs of abnormal glucose regulation, such as insulin resistance, have been found in the childhood years in those born preterm and in those with unusual patterns of catch-up growth.[45] Type 1 diabetes is related to immune function and results in virtually no insulin production. Children with type 1 diabetes have both high and low blood sugars, not just high blood sugars, as in type 2 diabetes.[44] Increasingly, children with type 1 diabetes mellitus are managed with insulin pumps set to inject small amounts of insulin continuously and in response to meals. Continuous insulin pumps change food timing and nutrition guidelines from those older guidelines

**insulin** Hormone usually produced in the pancreas to regulate movement of glucose from the bloodstream into cells within organs and muscles.

based on using less frequent injections of different types of insulin and also from those for managing type 2 diabetes.

The prevalence of both type 1 and type 2 diabetes among US youth (up to 20 years of age) increased between 2001 and 2009; prevalence of type 1 increased by 21 percent, and of type 2 increased by 30.5 percent.[46] This increase in prevalence has occurred in both sexes and across all racial groups. Overall, type 1 diabetes is about four times more prevalent than type 2 diabetes in youth; however, the larger increase in type 2 diabetes makes its prevention and treatment a high priority. Currently, type 2 diabetes is most prevalent in American Indian youth (at approximately 10 times the prevalence in White youth), followed by Black, Hispanic, Asian Pacific Islander, and White.[46]

Treatment for both types of diabetes includes regulation of the timing and composition of meals and exercise, along with insulin injections or medications.[44] Type 1 diabetes requires families and children to master a carbohydrate counting system for all consumed foods, as that is what is used to adjust insulin doses accompanying meals. A third-grader with type 1 diabetes requires a school diabetes management plan describing oversight and modification of school breakfast, school lunch, and snack time based on physical activity in school and during after-school activities. If the child is invited to a birthday party, the timing of meals and snacks can be adjusted to allow the child to attend the party and eat most of the foods there. Common colds, or foods a child refuses to eat, can cause wide variation in blood sugar, contributing to irritability, sleepiness, or difficulty with schoolwork. Many localities organize summer camps for children with diabetes; food and nutrition education and controlled access to food choices are provided, along with the usual camp activities. Such disease-specific camps are good for breaking the social isolation that children experience when they feel they are the only ones required to limit food choices.

**Seizures** Seizures are uncontrolled electrical disturbances in the brain. Epilepsy and seizures are the same disorder. Seizures in children are a relatively common condition, with an incidence of 3.5 per 1,000 children.[12] Seizure activity has a range of outward signs, from uncontrollable jerking of the whole body to mild blinking. Currently, no known nutrients bring on seizures. Children who have seizures are usually treated by medications that prevent them. After some types of seizures, the child may have a period of semiconsciousness called a ***postictal state*** and appear to be sleeping, but he or she is difficult to wake.[12] Feeding or eating during the postictal state is not recommended, because the child may choke. Some children have long enough postictal states to miss meals. In this case, adding other eating times is needed to make up for the lost energy and nutrients.

When seizures are controlled by medications, growth usually continues at the rate typical for that child. Food and nutrient consequences of controlled seizures are primarily related to drug–nutrient side effects, such as changes in hunger or sleepiness. Some drugs should be taken without food, and others may be offered with snacks or meals. Most drugs have to be taken on a strict schedule and are not stopped without medical supervision.

Some children have uncontrolled seizures that may cause further brain damage over time. For reasons that remain unknown, seizures decrease when brain metabolism is switched from the usual fuel, glucose, to *ketones* from fat metabolism.[47] Specialty neurology clinics administer the *ketogenic diet* for uncontrolled seizures. The diet severely limits food sources of carbohydrates and increases fat content, but is adequate in energy and protein. Vitamins and minerals have to be added as supplements because the allowed food sources of carbohydrates are not sufficient to meet vitamin and mineral requirements. The ketogenic diet may allow seizure medications to be reduced or eliminated over time.[51] However, many difficulties, such as measuring growth, blood glucose, and ketones in urine, lie in monitoring the body's reaction to such a severe carbohydrate restriction. Growth during the time on a ketogenic diet may be different from that seen in the child's previous pattern. Some children improve in both weight and height when seizure activity declines. The ketogenic diet is so high in fat that some children gain weight faster than expected. This diet is generally recommended for two years, if it is effective in reducing seizures, to optimize its effectiveness. After that time, some children are able to resume a typical diet and remain seizure free, while others may be able to control their seizures with medications.

**Cerebral Palsy** CP is one of the most common conditions in children with severe disabilities (Illustration 13.2).

**postictal state** Time of altered consciousness after a seizure; appears to be like a deep sleep.

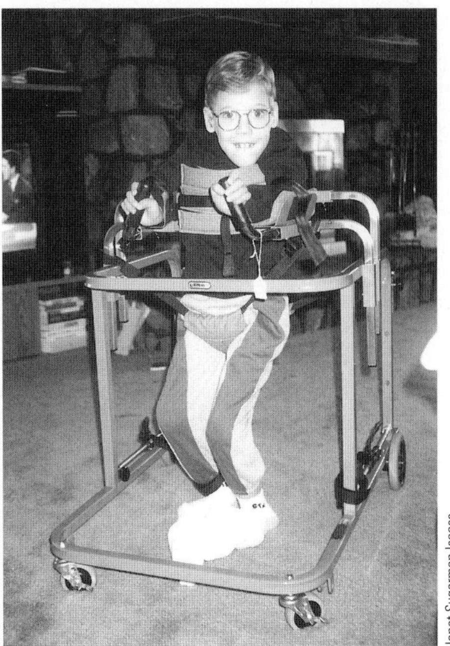
Janet Sugarman Isaacs

ILLUSTRATION 13.2 ▸ Boy with CP in a walker.

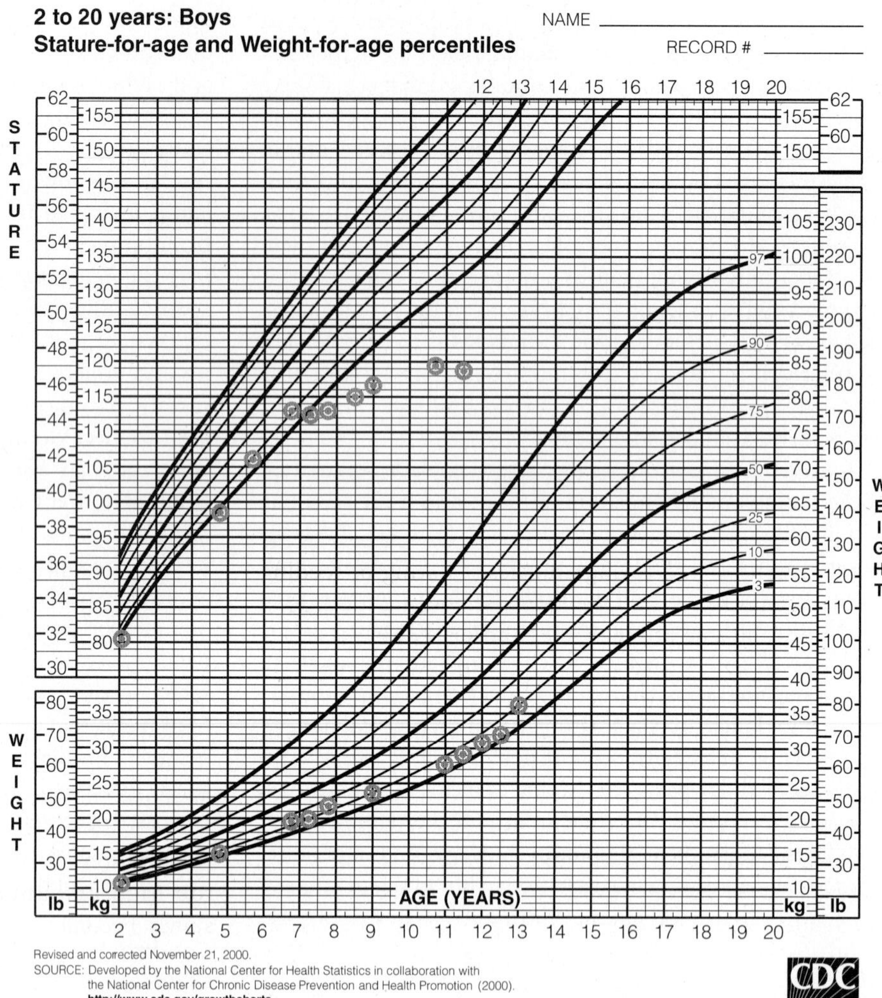


ILLUSTRATION 13.3 ▸ Growth chart of a child with spastic quadriplegia and scoliosis, who is fed by gastrostomy tube.

Revised and corrected November 21, 2000.

Overall incidence of CP is about 1.4–2.4 per 1,000 children.[48] CP is a general term well understood by the public; it covers a broad range of conditions resulting from brain damage. Causes of CP all involve damage to the brain early in life, either before or after birth. The initial site of brain damage does not progress, but progression of secondary effects occurs over time. Secondary effects may include contractures, scoliosis, gastroesophageal reflux, and constipation.[22] Many children with CP have constipation because coordinated muscle movements are part of bowel emptying, including the muscles in and over the intestines. Muscle coordination problems most easily seen in movements of the arms and legs may occur in muscles all over the body, including the abdominal muscles that assist in bowel evacuation.[48]

The form of CP that presents the most nutrition problems is spastic quadriplegia, involving all limbs.[8,9] Most children with spastic quadriplegia appear thin, but this appearance may be a result of smaller muscle size. Children with CP often have other forms of brain damage as well: 39–44 percent have intellectual disability, 26–36 percent have seizures, and 14–18 percent have severe visual impairment.[48] Causes of CP are unknown for more than one-third of affected children, and the condition may or may not be related to preterm birth. About half the time after a preterm birth, a basis for CP can be identified from the perinatal period.[48] The prevalence of CP in children born with very low birthweight has been increasing, but this trend may be a consequence of the overall increase in survivors of severe prematurity. Children with CP can enjoy many activities, attend school, and later contribute to society. Persons with CP display a wide range of abilities. Children with spastic quadriplegia grow, but their growth is slower than that in others, with or without gastrostomy feeding (Illustration 13.3).[8,9]

Nutritional consequences of spastic quadriplegia are slow weight gain and other growth concerns, difficulty with feeding and eating, and changes in body composition. No specific vitamins or minerals are known to correct CP. Problem nutrients are likely to be those related to bone density, calcium, and vitamin D, or nutrients needed in higher amounts as a result of medication side effects. Recommendations for energy needs are difficult to determine, even with an in-depth growth assessment. Children with small or weak muscles have lower energy needs because they are less active as a result of little voluntary muscle control. In contrast, types of CP characterized by increased uncontrolled movement require extra energy as a result of a higher activity level. ***Athetosis*** is an example of this less common form of CP, in which increased energy needs have been documented.[9]

Altered body composition affects many aspects of the child's nutrition and eating abilities.[37] Eating or feeding problems may appear in the forms of spilling food, long mealtimes, fatigue at mealtime, and/or requiring assistance to eat. Difficulty in controlling muscles such as those in the neck and back, those used in head position and sitting, and those in the jaw, tongue, and lips and used in swallowing may contribute to feeding and eating problems.[13,22]

Nutrition experts who provide services for children with CP assess their growth and then make recommendations for food choices that fit the children's abilities for eating, for nutritional supplements if food and beverages are not providing sufficient nutrients, and for nutrition support if needed. Nutrition interventions may include the following:

- Stimulating oral feeding
- Promoting healthy eating at school
- Adjusting menus and timing of meals and snacks at home or school for meeting nutrient needs from foods that minimize fatigue during meals
- Assessing and adjusting the child's dietary plan over time
- Using adapted self-feeding utensils or other types of feeding equipment

**Inborn Errors of Metabolism** PKU is a well-known example of a group of genetic disorders called inborn errors of metabolism.[10,49] More children are found to have inborn errors of metabolism in recent years as a result of more genetic disorders being identified with better survival after newborn screening. (Newborn screening and genetic screening is discussed in Chapter 9.) These disorders require interventions to manage breakdown products from foods and beverages that contain protein, fats, and carbohydrates being metabolized incompletely or inadequately. Inborn errors of metabolism involve molecular- or cellular-level blocks and have little or nothing to do with the gastrointestinal level of digestion and absorption of nutrients. Examples of inborn errors of metabolism diagnosed during childhood are glycogen-storage diseases (inborn errors of carbohydrate metabolism) and medium-chain fatty acid disorders (inborn errors of fat metabolism) diagnosed in older siblings or family members after the birth of an infant identified with the same disorder by newborn screening.

PKU best demonstrates the importance of nutrition interventions in an inborn error of metabolism. PKU has a prevalence of 1 in 12,000 live births.[10] The main treatment is lifelong nutrition intervention in which more than 80 percent of protein intake from foods and beverages is replaced by a mixture of amino acids from which phenylalanine has been removed. The enzyme that uses phenylalanine as a substrate is either not working at all or only partially active in the liver of a person with PKU. For children with specific types of blood phenylalanine elevations, a prescribed medication can adjust the degree of nutrition intervention required.[49] Both medication and nutrition intervention reduce intake of this amino acid to the minimum amount needed as an essential amino acid. This strategy limits toxic breakdown products of accumulated phenylalanine, which the body has difficulty clearing. How excess phenylalanine causes intellectual disability is not known, but is a side effect of PKU. The PKU diet is required throughout life (Illustration 13.4). If foods with protein are consumed in too-high amounts, PKU slowly becomes a degenerative disease affecting the brain at whatever age the treatment is stopped.

**athetosis** Uncontrolled movements of the large muscle groups as a result of damage to the central nervous system.

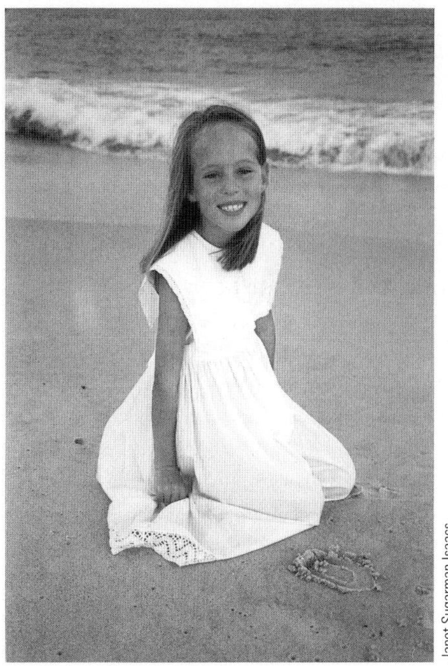
Janet Sugarman Isaacs

ILLUSTRATION 13.4 ▶ This girl does not appear to have a chronic illness, but she has PKU.

When their dietary prescription is set correctly, children with PKU appear to be eating meals providing less food than the meals of other children. The diet is adequate in all vitamins, minerals, protein, fats, and energy, but more nutrients are in liquid rather than solid forms. Foods to be avoided completely are protein-rich foods such as meats, eggs, regular dairy products, peanuts, and soybeans in all forms. Allowed natural sources of protein are limited amounts of regular crackers, potato chips, rice, and potatoes. Many fruits and vegetables are encouraged, if offered without added sources of protein. Some foods that are high in fats and/or sugars and generally low in natural protein, such as fried vegetables or candy canes, are safe for children with PKU.

The phenylalanine-deficient protein is generally served as a liquid, called a medical food or formula. The vitamins and minerals required to meet the RDA are in the phenylalanine-deficient protein powder. If the child does not drink enough of the PKU formula, foods that the child eats to meet her vitamin, mineral, and energy needs will elevate the blood phenylalanine. The phenylalanine-deficient protein is also available as bars and pills (Table 13.4). It can be expensive to buy substitute low-protein alternative foods, such as low-protein pizza crusts, low-protein cheese, and low-protein baking mixes. Successful compliance requires use of low-protein foods to allow variety, such as low-protein pasta.

**Attention Deficit Hyperactivity Disorder** Attention deficit disorder and ADHD are the most common ***neurobehavioral*** conditions in children. The number of 4- to 17-year old children whose parent's report that their child has been diagnosed with ADHD is increasing by approximately 5 percent per year (Illustration 13.5).[50] In 2011, this number was 11 percent, as compared to only 7.8 percent in 2003. While not all parents of children with ADHD choose to treat it with medication, approximately 6.1 percent of US children were being treated for ADHD with medication in 2011.[50] The most common type of medications used to treat children with ADHD are stimulants, which have a number of well-recognized side effects.

Nutritional concerns in ADHD include ***psychostimulant*** medication side effects that decrease appetite, resulting in weight loss or slow weight gain and growth. The effect of ADHD medications on appetite is variable; it depends on the type of medication, timing of the medications compared to meals, dosage and medication schedule, and on how long the child has had to adjust to the

TABLE 13.4 ▸ Food and nutrient recall for a 5-year-old child with well-controlled PKU

| |
|---|
| **Breakfast** |
| 2 slices low-protein bread with jelly and margarine |
| 6 cut-up orange pieces |
| 8 fl oz PKU metabolic food |
| **Lunch** |
| ½ cup fruit cocktail in heavy syrup |
| 1 cup tossed salad (lettuce, tomato, celery, cucumber only) with 2 Tbsp ranch dressing |
| 17 french fries with ketchup |
| 6 fl oz apple juice |
| **After-school snack** |
| ½ cup microwave popcorn |
| 8 fl oz PKU metabolic food |
| **Dinner** |
| Pickle spears (dill, 3 wedges) |
| 1 cup low-protein imitation rice containing 1.5 Tbsp margarine |
| ½ cup grilled onions, green peppers, and mushrooms (on rice) |
| 1 cup canned peaches in heavy syrup |
| 8 fl oz PKU metabolic food |
| **Snack** |
| Skittles candy (small snack-size) |
| 4 fl oz apple juice |



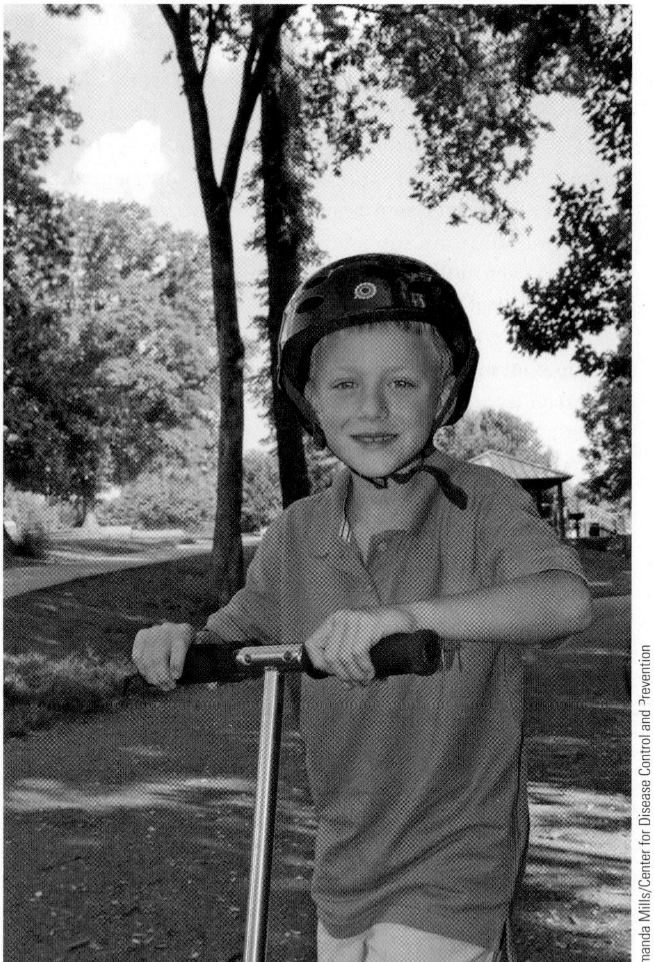


ILLUSTRATION 13.5 ▸ The number of children reported to have ADHD is increasing.

**neurobehavioral** Pertains to control of behavior by the nervous system.

**psychostimulant** Classification of medication that acts on the brain to improve mental or emotional behavior.

medication. Less interference with appetite and growth is likely if the child does not take the medication during school holidays. Long-term or continuous treatment with stimulants has been associated with delays in weight and height, although it's not clear whether these delays will persist into adulthood.[51]

Regardless of the child's dosage schedule, the peak activity for ADHD medication is aimed for school hours, which includes school lunch. Nutrition interventions for children on psychostimulant medications call for timing meals and snacks around the medication's action peaks. For example, adding a large bedtime snack when the medication's effects are low is a typical recommendation. Monitoring weight and height carefully over time helps identify growth plateaus. Education for the school's lunchroom supervisors and teachers may be helpful to deal with food refusals and mealtime behavior for the child with ADHD.

Children with ADHD who are not on medication may have a chaotic meal and snack pattern and the inability to stay seated for a meal. They may be given fewer opportunities to use kitchen appliances and get their own snacks due to impulsiveness. Theories about specific foods or nutrients causing ADHD have not been proven scientifically, but high interest in nutrition as a cause and treatment continues. The sale of herbal medicines and nutritional supplements to families with children with ADHD is common. One large survey found that 64 percent of children with ADHD had tried at least one type of alternative therapy and that 13 percent of children took some sort of multivitamin supplement.[52] Megavitamins and herbal supplements were found ineffective in treating ADHD, but such information has not stopped claims made for them or marketing and sales.[52-54]

**Pediatric HIV** Most children with HIV were infected at around the time of birth. HIV in children under age 13 is classified differently than it is in adults, by age-based categories as well as level of immunosuppression from the virus. Only in the last few years have affected children lived long enough to benefit from the combination highly active antiretroviral therapy that became available in the mid-1990s.[40,41] As experience has accumulated with these potent medications, growth of children with low viral loads has improved, and opportunistic infections have occurred at a lower rate.

Nutrition is an important component of HIV management. For children too young to be in charge of their own medication and eating schedules, educating the family, referring them for financial and support services may be part of the nutrition intervention. Other nutrition concerns include food-related infection-control measures, assuring access to complete nutritional supplements, and referrals to food banks. If weight-gain and medication compliance problems are unresolved, gastrostomy placement for medications and supplemental feedings may be needed.[40]

Working with children with HIV is complicated in part because the mother is likely to have HIV, and/or there has already been family disruption from this condition. Nutrition interventions have to be customized to the behavioral and developmental realities of each child. For example, an 11-year-old girl is being treated for HIV and its related illnesses. Her diet prescription includes a high-protein/high-energy plan, with one complete vitamin/mineral supplement daily and three meals and three snacks. Her family members are to check her weight at home weekly and call in if they observe weight loss and low appetite. The girl takes four kinds of HIV-related medications, totaling 17 capsules per day. Two medications have no food-related restrictions, one is best taken with food at two different times per day, and one is best taken on an empty stomach (30 minutes before a meal or 2 hours after a meal). She also gets an injection every other week to strengthen her blood counts.

**Childhood Celiac Disease** Celiac disease is a chronic condition that seems to be increasing in prevalence, without explanation. A recent study of the prevalence of celiac disease in the United States found 1 in 141 individuals, aged 6 years or older, tested positive for the disease or reported having been diagnosed by a doctor.[55] Among those diagnosed in this study, 83 percent were unaware of their condition. Celiac disease in children presents differently than in adults, and is also underdiagnosed.[56] It may interfere with growth and learning and be confused with various laboratory markers of malnutrition.[57] Diagnostic criteria are based on intestinal biopsy results showing specific pathology. Understandably, a trial avoiding gluten-containing foods is often what families want to try first. When celiac disease has been diagnosed, nutrition intervention by avoiding gluten, a component of wheat, rye, oats and barley, for life is the most effective treatment. Increasing interest in avoiding gluten for a variety of possible conditions has resulted in many more gluten-free foods in the food supply.

# Dietary Supplements and Herbal Remedies

**LO 13.6** Compare use of dietary and herbal remedies in children with and without special health care needs.

Children with special health care needs are found to use complementary and alternative medicine at a higher rate, 30–70 percent, than healthy children.[52] This includes various types of nutritional supplements and vitamins and minerals.[53] Families with children in a lengthy process of diagnosis—where the diagnosis does not lead to a definite treatment and when expense, insurance-coverage, and administrative problems tax their ability to cope—are more likely to seek alternative therapies. Some of these alternatives have questionable effectiveness and are perhaps even harmful. No herbal remedies or nutritional supplements have been found effective to prevent or treat the conditions covered in this chapter; however, nutritional claims abound for various chronic conditions. Families hear from one another about micronutrients—such as magnesium, zinc, and $B_6$—sold with various combinations of amino acids for Down syndrome and ASDs.[58] Restrictive food choices, such as avoiding dairy products or gluten, have been researched for one condition and then extrapolated for another. Sports drinks and high-protein products marketed for athletes may attract families with children who have difficulty gaining weight.

Strategies to counter unscientific nutritional claims for various products include the following:

- Recognize the benefits of support for families, such as advocacy groups.
- Improve communication with health care providers, so that families ask more questions about nutrition claims of alternative treatments.
- To give them some control over decision making for their children, give families reliable information, such as scientific literature or fact sheets, without endorsing any claim.

## Sources of Nutrition Services

LO 13.7 Explain why children who have special health conditions receive more intensive nutrition services in schools and health care settings than other children do.

Children with special health care needs and chronic conditions need more intensive nutrition services than healthy children. More resources are available, but due to the complexity of chronic conditions and their low frequency, problems locating quality nutrition services persist. Public health nutrition services are more widely available than nutrition services for children with chronic conditions. Here are sources to help families find the appropriate level of nutrition services in their communities.

- Supplemental Social Insurance (SSI). This is insurance coverage and financial support for low-income families with eligible children. Conditions usually eligible for SSI are chromosomal disorders; intellectual disability; and severe forms of seizures, CP, and CF. A child with treated PKU is generally not eligible for SSI because treatments prevent decline in learning abilities.
- The Americans with Disabilities Act applies to all ages. It requires, for example, that school cafeteria lines accommodate wheelchairs. The Americans with Disabilities Act may protect children from having their special food and nutrient needs being the basis for discrimination against them.
- The U.S. Department of Agriculture Child Nutrition Program (described in Chapters 1 and 11) requires that school breakfast and lunch menus be modified for children with diagnosis-specific dietary interventions or changes in the texture of foods. Parents who want their children to participate in the Child Nutrition Program cannot be charged an additional fee for providing prescribed food choices. Physicians complete a prescription ordering special breakfasts or lunches. Examples of diet prescription orders are a reduced-energy school lunch and breakfast, a pureed diet, or a nutrient-modified diet, such as a PKU diet (see Case Study 13.2). Complete nutritional supplements administered by gastrostomy are not required to be supplied by the Child Nutrition Program.
- Department of Education public school regulations, called 504 Accommodation and IDEA, guide how schools can fund nutrition services in addition to those from the Child Nutrition Program. Children in regular education have different access to services than do children eligible for special education. They may have a 504 Accommodation that modifies the regular curriculum teaching methods to fit a child's educational needs. For example, a child with diabetes who needs a snack before physical education or a child who has refrigerated nutrition supplements may have this need described in the 504 accommodation plan. Under IDEA, special education services may have specific nutrition services written into a child's IEP [1,2] (Table 13.5). For this particular plan, the child's education includes learning to eat by mouth with prompting and assistance. Nutritional supplements may be purchased as part of an education intervention called for in the child's IEP. For a child with PKU, diabetes, or another chronic condition, the food intake restrictions apply to classroom birthday parties or when food is used in classroom projects. These regulations do not apply in private schools.
- U.S. Department of Health and Human Services (HHS) Maternal and Child Health block grants designate a portion of funding for services for children with special health care needs in every state.[59] Nutrition services may be funded in specialty clinics, in county health departments, or contracted from community nutrition providers. Thus, nutrition experts can work with children in various settings, including schools, early-intervention programs, homes, clinics, and facilities.

**TABLE 13.5** Example of nutrition objectives in an individualized education plan for an 8-year-old boy with limited oral feeding skills

1. In three of five trials, J. R. will hold food on the spoon as he moves it to his mouth without hand-over-hand assistance from his aides during three meals per week.
2. J. R. will point to what he wants to eat with his left hand in three trials after two prompts per meal, three days each week.
3. J. R. will cooperate in having his gastrostomy site checked at feedings by pulling up his shirt three days in a row each week.

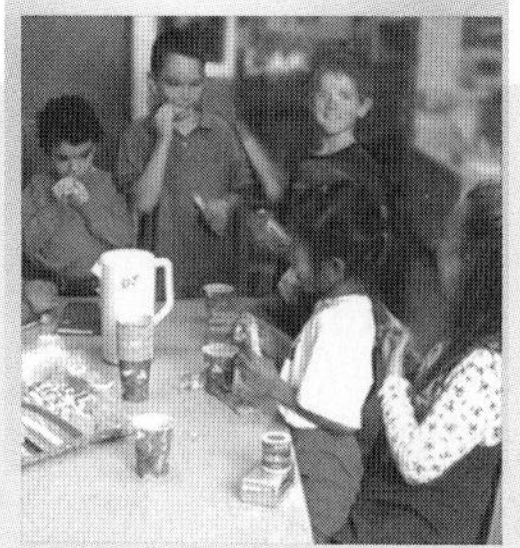
Photodisc

# CASE STUDY 13.2

## Dealing with Food Allergies in School Settings

Judy is to start regular kindergarten. When she was 2 years old, she was diagnosed with a peanut food allergy after many episodes of asthma and hives. Her health has improved as a preschooler with avoidance of peanuts in all forms. The family has carefully watched what she eats. However, at age 4, she had an episode of breathing difficulty that required an emergency-room visit. This incident makes the family quite concerned about Judy's eating at school. She is generally not allowed to go to friends' homes to play; friends come to her house so the family can watch out for her. She has been instructed not to take any food from anyone. She has not been in day care or preschool, so starting school is a big step for the family.

**Interventions:** A meeting was held at the school after receiving the physician's statement and diagnosis. Judy's mother met with the school staff to discuss plans for Judy at school to avoid exposure to peanuts in any form. The family did not want to participate in the school lunch program. Her mother proposed to pack Judy a lunch from home, although most children eat food provided at school. With the school staff, Judy's mother discussed snack time for Judy and her eating at the cafeteria, which periodically serves food cooked in peanut oil, or food containing peanuts. The snack at kindergarten was discussed, as it is provided by parents based on a rotation schedule. It is usually milk or juice with cookies or fruit.

**Monitoring Recommendations:** A plan was put in place for the teacher to check the snack foods and offer a replacement snack provided by Judy's mother if she is unsure whether that day's snack contains peanuts. The school working group had written out a 504 accommodation plan for Judy's peanut allergy. It included making sure that tables where children eat peanut-containing foods are washed well, with signs in the cafeteria with Judy's picture to make sure she does not inadvertently get peanut-containing food from another child or in a food activity.

After Judy has been in school for one month, the family meets with the school group. In that month, two episodes resulted in what may have been hives, and her family is worried that Judy is not adjusting well. At snack time Judy did not recognize some of the foods; she refused to eat a snack most days. She appeared hungry at home after school. Her mother says she would like to send to school a snack that she knows her daughter will eat, and she wants to attend school during snack time to make sure Judy is not being teased.

### *Questions*

1. Why is it the school's job to check for peanuts when other parents are sending snacks?
2. Do you think the mother's reaction to the situation is reasonable? Are there any alternative accommodations you could recommend?
3. What are the chances that Judy will outgrow the peanut allergy by next year?

- Every state identifies, advocates, and trains parents to be advocates for children with special needs. An example is the Developmental Disabilities Council in each state.

### Nutrition Intervention Model Program

The Maternal and Child Health Bureau (MCH), a part of HHS, funds nutrition services among other types of services.[59] MCH develops and promotes model programs by funding competitive grants that emphasize training health care providers, including nutrition experts. Training programs vary in length from short, intensive courses to year-long traineeships. Topics vary from nutrition for infants receiving intensive care services to nutrition problems of adolescence, such as warning signs of anorexia nervosa. Two MCH initiatives directly impacting children with special health care needs are the Family/Patient Centered Medical Home Program and Family/Professional Partnerships Program.

- The Family/Patient Centered Medical Home Program encourages parent–provider–community partnerships so that children with complex medical conditions, who are only a small minority in any community, have access to coordinated, well-planned services.[60] This approach lowers overall medical costs in communities as such families use medical services so often.[61] Medical homes support families so that children with complex medical conditions can live at home.[37]
- The Family/Professional Partnerships Program provides health information centers that are staffed by families who themselves have children with special health care needs.[62] These information centers help parents access resources to help support their child and make informed choices for their care.

## KEY POINTS

1. Children with chronic health conditions still want to fit in with everyone else and be treated like others their age. Paying too much attention to their special needs may not help them become independent over time.
2. Nutrition requirements have to be customized to the individual: guidelines for healthy children may not be appropriate.
3. Energy needs are based on the child's activity as affected by the underlying condition; calories each day may be higher or lower than others the same age.
4. Eating problems are likely to interfere with appetite and meal patterns for conditions that require medications that have side effects.
5. The goal for meeting nutritional needs is to eat by mouth, if this is enjoyable and safe. An alternative may be to drink complete nutritional supplements or add overnight feedings.
6. Vitamins and minerals are needed for some conditions at levels that are higher or lower than usually recommended.
7. Nutrition interventions for CF and diabetes mellitus are examples of lifelong approaches that align with medical treatment for children with special health care needs.
8. CP is one of the more severe conditions in which nutritionists assess how growth and eating are impacted, and offer interventions suited to the child rather than standard growth and eating guidelines.
9. Children with special health care needs attend school like everyone else, but they may need to have a modified school lunch or eat different foods than others based on their underlying condition.
10. Nutrition and medical providers help families find in their communities the educational, medical, and specialty services suitable for their children.

## REVIEW QUESTIONS

1. Which child requires an interpretation of growth modified from the usual CDC growth chart interpretation?
   a. A child with ADHD
   b. A child with type 1 diabetes
   c. A child with mild cerebral palsy with scoliosis
   d. A child with PKU
2. Which child requires in-depth nutrition assessment due to changes in body composition?
   a. A child with drug–nutrient interactions that increase sleepiness
   b. A child who appears thin and uses a wheelchair most of the time
   c. A child with seizures with a BMI at the 50th percentile
   d. A child with ASD who looks thin and refuses a variety of foods
3. When a child has a chronic condition that limits activity, such as spina bifida, what is the greatest long-term nutrition concern?
   a. Protein limiting growth
   b. Modified food textures to avoid eating difficulties
   c. Excessive calorie intake further limiting mobility
   d. Intake of calcium and vitamin D to prevent bone fractures
4. An 8-year-old child with diabetes is eating birthday cake at school. What is a likely explanation?
   a. The child has type 2 diabetes and is obese.
   b. The child has type 1 diabetes and he has adjusted his insulin pump to cover the cake.
   c. The child's chronic condition is not managed well, as cake is not allowed.
   d. The child had eaten a high-protein food with little carbohydrate at lunch.

Sue has a chronic condition with a pattern of weight gain and then loss, without growth over the last year. Identify as true or false statements 5, 6, and 7.

5. Sue's condition can modify her energy needs compared to a healthy child.
   _____ True _____ False
6. The family may be worried about handling Sue if she grows as expected for her age.
   _____ True _____ False
7. Sue's nutritional intake must not be sufficient, since her growth is not as expected.
   _____ True _____ False
8. What are two examples of family support that would assist a child with a chronic condition?
9. When a child with ADHD refuses to eat, what are two possible explanations?
10. Explain why a child could need an IEP that includes nutrition services.

Visit www.cengagebrain.com to access MindTap, a complete digital course that includes additional resources.

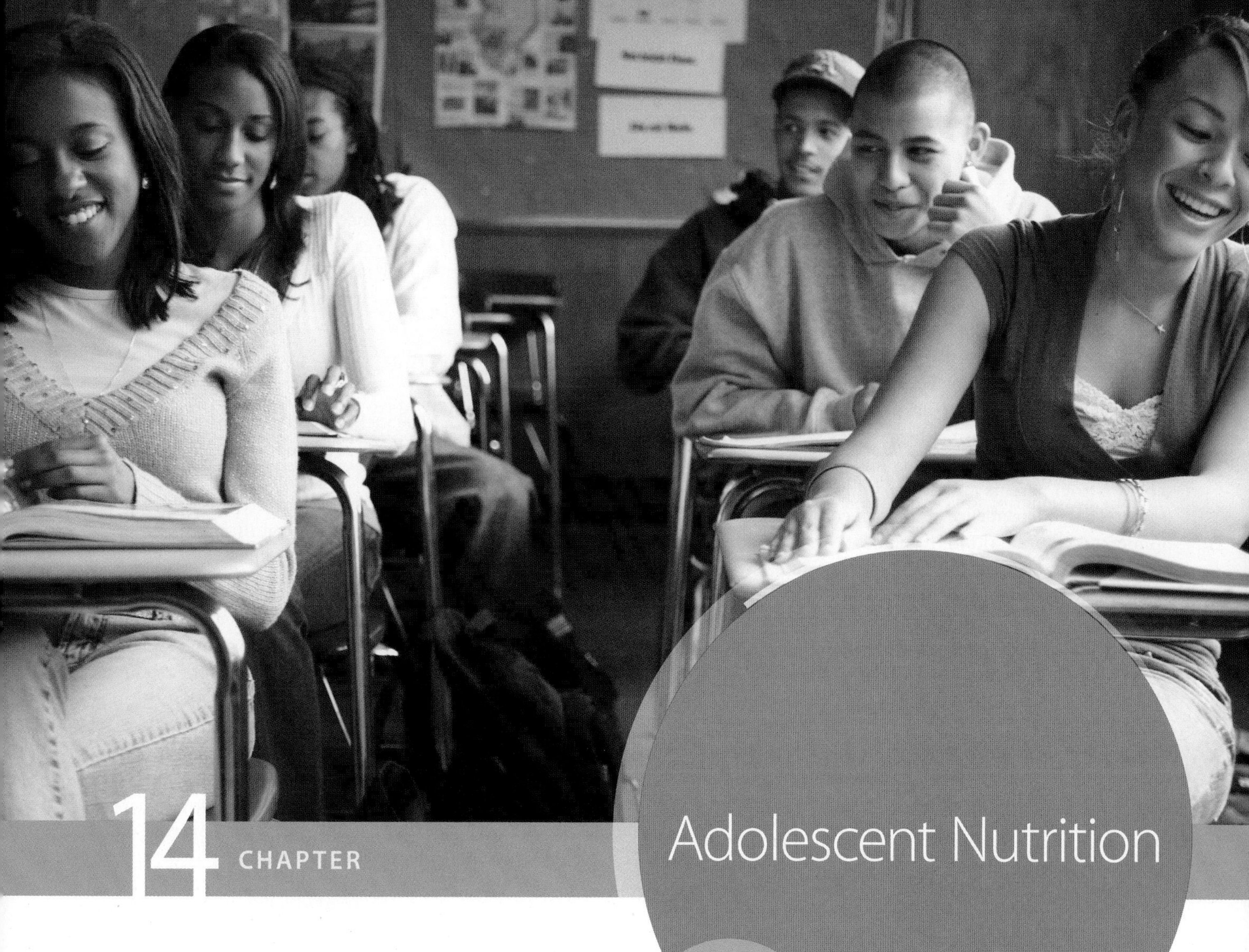

# 14 CHAPTER Adolescent Nutrition

*Prepared by*
Jamie Stang

## LEARNING OBJECTIVES

After reading this chapter you should be able to:

**14.1** Explain why sexual maturity and biological maturity (biological age) are better determinants of nutritional needs than chronological age.

**14.2** Explain how the psychosocial developmental stages of adolescence, including levels of abstract reasoning and critical thinking abilities, affect the types of health education messages and intervention components that are effective with teens.

**14.3** Describe at least three eating behaviors commonly seen among adolescents and the potential consequences of these behaviors on nutritional status.

**14.4** Compare which nutrients adolescents consume in lower than recommended amounts and which nutrients they consume in higher than recommended amounts, and how these behaviors may impact overall health status.

**14.5** Identify the key components of nutrition assessment and screening of adolescents and how resulting data can be used during nutrition education and counseling.

**14.6** Describe the roles that peers, families, schools, and communities play in determining the dietary behaviors and nutritional status of adolescents.

Blend Images/Shutterstock.com

# Introduction

Adolescence is usually defined as the period of life between 11 and 21 years of age. It is a time of profound physical, emotional, and cognitive changes during which a child develops into an adult. Physical, psychosocial, and cognitive maturity are largely accomplished during this life stage (Illustration 14.1). In the United States, adolescence is often viewed as a tumultuous, irrational phase that children must go through. However, this view does disservice to its developmental importance. The tasks of adolescence, comparable to those experienced during the toddler years, include the development of a personal identity and a unique value system separate from parents and other family members, a struggle for personal independence accompanied by the need for economic and emotional family support, and adjustment to a new body that has changed in shape, size, and physiological capacity. When adolescence is viewed in light of these dramatic developmental tasks, it can be appreciated as a unique, positive, and integral part of human development.

## Nutritional Needs in a Time of Change

The physical, psychosocial, and cognitive changes associated with adolescence have direct effects on nutritional status. The dramatic physical growth and development experienced by adolescents, which matches and can even exceed the rate of growth experienced during infancy, significantly increases their needs for energy, protein, vitamins, and minerals. However, the simultaneous search for personal autonomy and peer acceptance that characterizes adolescent psychosocial development often leads to the development of health-compromising eating behaviors, such as meal skipping and the adoption of unhealthy weight control behaviors. These behaviors may create a challenge for health care professionals, but can also become opportunities for teens to change at a time during when adult health behaviors are being formed.

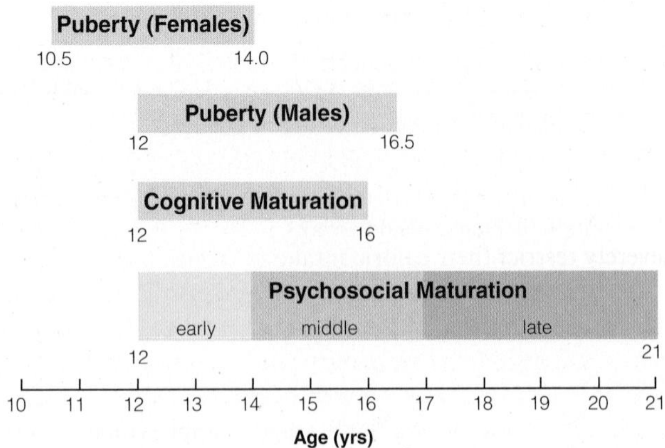


ILLUSTRATION 14.1 ▸ Average ages of pubertal, cognitive, and psychosocial maturation.

SOURCE: "Adolescent Growth and Development" by R. L. Johnson, in Adolescent Medicine 2/e by A. Hofmann and D. Greynaus, Fig. 2.1, p. 9. Copyright © 1988 McGraw-Hill Companies. Reprinted with permission.

This chapter provides an overview of normal biological and psychosocial growth and development among adolescents and how these experiences affect the nutrient needs and eating behaviors of teens. Common concerns related to adolescent nutrition and effective methods for educating and counseling teens are also discussed. Health conditions that require specific nutrition interventions such as obesity and eating disorders are discussed in Chapter 15.

# Normal Physical Growth and Development

LO 14.1 Explain why sexual maturity and biological maturity (biological age) are better determinants of nutritional needs than chronological age.

Early adolescence encompasses the occurrence of puberty, the physical transformation of a child into a young adult. The biological changes that occur during puberty include sexual maturation, increases in height and weight, accumulation of skeletal mass, and changes in body composition. Even though the sequence of these events during puberty is consistent among adolescents, the age of onset, duration, and tempo of these events may vary a great deal between and within individuals. Thus, the physical appearance of adolescents of the same chronological age covers a wide range. These variations in development directly affect the nutrition requirements of adolescents. A 14-year-old male who has already experienced rapid linear growth and muscular development will have noticeably different energy and nutrient needs than a 14-year-old male peer who has not yet entered puberty. For this reason, sexual maturation should be used to assess biological growth and development (or biological age), and the individual nutritional needs of adolescents rather than chronological age.

Sexual Maturation Rating (SMR), also known as *Tanner Stages*, is a scale of ***secondary sexual characteristics*** that allows health professionals to assess the degree of pubertal maturation among adolescents, regardless of chronological age (Table 14.1). SMR is based on breast development and the appearance of pubic hair among females, and on testicular and penile development and the appearance of pubic hair among males.[1] SMR stage 1 corresponds with prepubertal growth and development, while stages 2 through 5 denote the occurrence of puberty. At SMR stage 5, sexual maturation has concluded. Sexual maturation correlates highly with linear growth, changes in weight and body composition, and hormonal changes.[1]

***Puberty*** usually occurs earlier among females than males, with a 2.5 year gender difference on average.[2] There

**secondary sexual characteristics** Physiological changes that signal puberty, including enlargement of the testes, penis, and breasts and the development of pubic and facial hair.

**puberty** The time frame during which the body matures from that of a child to that of a young adult.

TABLE 14.1 ▸ Sexual maturity rating for girls and boys

| STAGE GIRLS | BREAST DEVELOPMENT | PUBIC HAIR GROWTH |
|---|---|---|
| 1 | Prepubertal; nipple elevation only | Prepubertal; no pubic hair |
| 2 | Small, raised breast bud | Sparse growth of hair along labia |
| 3 | General enlargement of raising of breast and areola | Pigmentation, coarsening, and curling, with an increase in amount |
| 4 | Further enlargement with projection of areola and nipple as secondary mound | Hair resembles adult type, but not spread to medial thighs |
| 5 | Mature, adult contour, with areola in same contour as breast, and only nipple projecting | Adult type and quantity, spread to medial thighs |
| **STAGE BOYS** | **GENITAL DEVELOPMENT** | **PUBIC HAIR GROWTH** |
| 1 | Prepubertal; no change in size or proportion of testes, scrotum, and penis from early childhood | Prepubertal; no pubic hair |
| 2 | Enlargement of scrotum and testes; reddening and change in texture in skin of scrotum; little or no penis enlargement | Sparse growth of hair at base of penis |
| 3 | Increase first in length, then width of penis; growth of testes and scrotum | Darkening, coarsening, and curling; increase in amount |
| 4 | Enlargement of penis with growth in breadth and development of glands; further growth of testes and scrotum, darkening of scrotal skin | Hair resembles adult type, but not spread to medial thighs |
| 5 | Adult size and shape genitalia | Adult type and quantity, spread to medial thighs |

SOURCE: Growth at Adolescence, J. M. Tanner, Copyright © 1962 Blackwell Publishers. Reprinted with permission of John Wiley & Sons, Inc.

is a great deal of variation in the timing of puberty based on racial and ethnic background, however. The National Health and Nutrition Examination Study III (NHANES III) found that Non-Hispanic Black and Mexican American females experienced thelarche (breast development, SMR stage 2) at 9.6 years old, which was about 8 months earlier than White females.[2] Early thelarche (by age 9.6 months) was twice as common among overweight and obese girls, suggesting that variations in body weight and composition may play a role in ethnic and racial differences in the onset of puberty. Pubarche (the presence of pubic hair, SMR stage 3) was found to occur approximately one year earlier among Black girls compared to White or Mexican American girls as well.[2] Among males, pubarche occurred approximately 6 months earlier among White and Black males compared to Mexican American males; however, no significant relationship between pubarche and body weight or composition was noted among adolescent males.

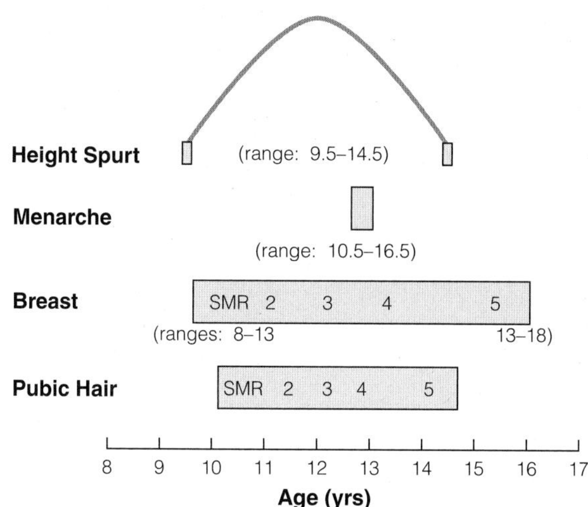


ILLUSTRATION 14.2 ▸ Sequence of physiological changes during puberty in females.

SOURCE: Growth at Adolescence, J. M. Tanner, Copyright © 1962 Blackwell Publishers. Reprinted with permission of John Wiley & Sons, Inc.

The onset of ***menses*** and changes in height relative to the development of secondary sexual characteristics that occur in females during puberty is shown in Illustration 14.2. ***Menarche*** occurs 2–4 years after the initial development of breast buds and pubic hair, most commonly during SMR stage 4. The average age of menarche is 12.5 years, but menarche can occur as early as 8 years or as late as 17 years of age.[2] Early onset of menarche (by age 10.6 years) is four times more likely among overweight and obese females than those who are at a lower body weight. Menarche may be delayed in highly competitive athletes or in girls who severely restrict their caloric intake to reduce body weight.

The onset of the linear growth spurt occurs most commonly during SMR stage 2 in females, beginning between the ages of 9.5 and 14.5 years in most females (Illustration 14.2). Peak velocity in linear growth occurs during the end of SMR stage 2 and during SMR stage 3, approximately 6 to 12 months prior to menarche. As much as 15 percent to 25 percent of final adult height will be gained during puberty, with an average

**menses** The process of menstruation.

**menarche** The occurrence of the first menstrual cycle.

increase in height of 9.8 inches (25 cm).[3] During the peak of the adolescent growth spurt, females gain approximately 3.5 inches (8–9 cm) a year. The linear growth spurt lasts 24–26 months, ceasing by age 16 in most females. Some adolescent females experience small increments of growth past age 19 years, however. Linear growth may be delayed or slowed among females who excessively restrict their caloric intake.

Enlargement of the ***testes*** and change in scrotal coloring are most often the first signs of puberty among males (Illustration 14.3), occurring between the ages of 10.5 and 14.5 years, with 11.6 years being the average age. The development of pubic hair is also common during SMR stage 2. Testicular enlargement begins between the ages of 9.5 and 13.5 years in males (SMR 2 to 3) and concludes between the ages of 12.7 and 17 years. The average age of spermarche (the age at which via sperm is produced by the tests) is approximately 14 years among males.

On average, peak velocity of linear growth among males occurs during SMR stage 4, coinciding with or just following testicular development and the appearance of faint facial hair. The peak velocity of linear growth occurs at 14.4 years of age, on average. At the peak of the growth spurt, adolescent males will increase their height by 2.8–4.8 inches (7–12 cm) a year. Linear growth will continue throughout adolescence, at a progressively slower rate, ceasing at about 21 years of age. The use of stimulant medications for conditions such as attention deficit hyperactivity disorder has been suggested to reduce or delay linear growth velocity among adolescent males, with effects most pronounced among 14–16 year olds.[4] Higher doses of stimulant medication appear to be associated with more pronounced variations in linear growth velocity. Due to the smaller number of females using these medications, it is not clear if this phenomenon also occurs among girls.

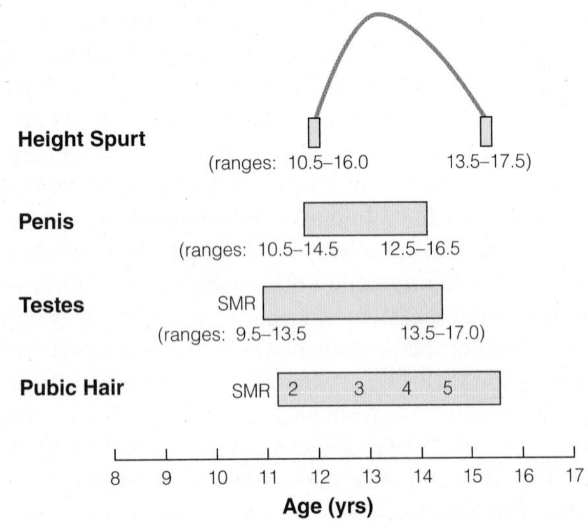


ILLUSTRATION 14.3 ▸ Sequence of physiological changes during puberty in males.

SOURCE: Growth at Adolescence, J. M. Tanner, Copyright © 1962 Blackwell Publishers. Reprinted with permission of John Wiley & Sons, Inc.

## Changes in Weight, Body Composition, and Skeletal Mass

As much as 50 percent of ideal adult body weight is gained during adolescence. Among females, peak weight gain follows the linear growth spurt by 3–6 months. During the peak velocity of weight change, which occurs at an average age of 12.5 years, girls will gain approximately 18.3 lb (8.3 kg) per year.[3] Weight gain slows around the time of menarche, but will continue into late adolescence. Adolescent females may gain as much as 14 lb (6.3 kg) during the latter half of adolescence. Peak accumulation of muscle mass occurs around or just after the onset of menses.

Body composition changes dramatically among females during puberty, with average lean body mass falling from 80 to 74 percent of body weight while average body fat increases from 16 to 26 percent at full maturity. Females experience a 44 percent increase in lean body mass and a 120 percent increase in body fat during puberty.[5] Adolescent females gain approximately 2.5 lb (1.14 kg) of body fat mass each year during puberty. Body fat levels peak among females between the ages of 15 and 16 years. Research by Frisch suggests that a level of 17 percent body fat is required for menarche to occur and that 25 percent body fat is required for the development and maintenance of regular ovulatory cycles.[6] Normal changes in body fat mass can be mediated by excessive physical activity and/or caloric restriction.

Even though the accumulation of body fat by females is obviously a normal and physiologically necessary process, adolescent females often view it negatively. Weight dissatisfaction is common among adolescent females during and immediately following puberty, leading to potentially health-compromising behaviors such as excessive caloric restriction, ***fasting***, use of diet pills or laxatives, and, in some cases, the development of body image distortions and eating disorders (see Chapter 15).

Among males, peak weight gain coincides with the timing of peak linear growth and peak muscle mass accumulation.[3] During peak weight gain, adolescent males gain an average of 20 lb (9 kg) per year. Body fat decreases in males during adolescence, resulting in an average of approximately 12 percent by the end of puberty.

Almost half of adult peak bone mass is accrued during adolescence. By age 18, more than 90 percent of adult skeletal mass has been formed, thus adolescence is a critical time for osteoporosis prevention.[7] A variety of factors contribute to the accretion of bone mass, including genetics, hormonal changes, weight-bearing exercise, cigarette smoking, consumption of alcohol, and dietary intake of calcium, vitamin D, vitamin K, phosphorus, boron, strontium, magnesium, and iron.[7] Bone is composed largely of calcium, phosphorus, and protein. A great deal of bone mass is accrued during adolescence, making adequate intakes of these nutrients critical to support optimal bone growth and development.

**testes** One of the two male reproductive glands located in the scrotum.

**fasting** Going 24 hours or more without eating.

# Psychosocial and Cognitive Development

LO 14.2 Explain how the psychosocial developmental stages of adolescence, including levels of abstract reasoning and critical thinking abilities, affect the types of health education messages and intervention components that are effective with teens.

During adolescence, individuals develop a sense of personal identity, a moral and ethical value system, feelings of self-esteem or self-worth, and a vision of occupational aspirations.[8,9] While each individual experiences psychosocial development at their own rate, it is most readily understood when it is divided into three periods: early adolescence (11–14 years), middle adolescence (15–17 years), and late adolescence (18–21 years). Each period of psychosocial development is marked by the mastery of new emotional, cognitive, and social skills.

During this stage of biological changes, young adolescents experience the development of body image and an increased awareness of sexuality are central psychosocial tasks during this period of life.[9] The dramatic changes in body shape, size, and composition can cause a great deal of ambivalence among adolescents, often leading to the development of poor body image and sometimes leading to disordered eating if not addressed by family or health care professionals (see Chapter 15).

The wide chronological age range during which pubertal growth and development begins and proceeds can become a major source of personal dissatisfaction for some adolescents. Males who enter puberty late often feel physically inferior to their peers who mature earlier and may resort to the use of anabolic steroids and other supplements in an effort to increase linear growth and muscle development. Females who mature early have been found to have more eating problems and poorer body image than their later-developing peers.[10] They are also more likely to initiate risky behaviors such as smoking, drinking alcohol, and engaging in sexual intercourse at an earlier age.[10,11] Education of young adolescents on normal variations in tempo and timing of growth and development can help to facilitate a positive self-image, which may reduce the likelihood of engaging in health-compromising behaviors.

Peer influence is very strong during early adolescence.[8,9] Young teens, conscious of their physical appearance and social behaviors, strive to fit in with their peer group. The need to fit in can affect nutritional intake among adolescents. Qualitative research has revealed that situational factors, such as who students ate with and where they ate, were important factors in the food choices they made.[12,13] Consequently, teens express their ability and willingness to fit in with a group of peers by adopting food preferences and making food choices based on peer influences and by refuting family preferences and choices. In some cases, choices based on peer pressure can lead to improved dietary intake, such as reduced intake of animal protein due to moral (animal welfare) concerns or choosing foods that are sustainably produced. In other cases, the choices based on peer pressure may lead to poor dietary intake, such as frequent consumption of fast foods, convenience foods, sweetened beverages, and other highly processed foods that are high in added fats and sugars.

Cognitively, early adolescence is a time dominated by concrete thinking, egocentrism, and impulsive behavior.[8,9] Abstract reasoning abilities are not yet developed to a great extent in most adolescents, limiting their ability to understand complex health and nutrition issues. Young adolescents also lack the ability to see how their current behavior can affect their future health status or health-related behaviors. This can make nutrition education efforts difficult unless the messages provided focus on how nutritional status and eating behaviors can impact daily concerns, such as physical attractiveness, academic ability or physical performance.

Middle adolescence marks the development of emotional and social independence from family, especially parents. Conflicts over personal issues, including eating and physical activity behaviors, are heightened during mid adolescence. Physical growth and development are mostly completed during this stage.[9] Body image issues are still of concern, especially among males who are late to mature and females.[10,11] Peer groups become more influential, and their influence on food choices peaks, which can lead to the initiation of health-compromising behaviors such as fasting, use of diet pills and laxatives, and alcohol use. Adolescents lack the ability to connect current behaviors with future health outcomes and often believe they are invincible during this stage of development.

The emergence of abstract reasoning skills occurs rapidly during middle adolescence; however, these skills may not be applied to all areas of life.[9] Adolescents will revert to concrete thinking skills if they feel overwhelmed or experience psychosocial stress; thus, health information should be presented in very concrete, understandable examples. Toward the end of this phase, some teens begin to understand the relationship between current health-related behaviors and future health, even though their need for peer acceptance may supplant this understanding.

Late adolescence is characterized by the development of a personal identity and individual moral beliefs.[8,9] Physical growth and development is largely concluded, and body image issues are less prevalent. Older teens become more confident in their ability to handle increasingly sophisticated social situations, which is accompanied by reductions in impulsive behaviors and peer pressure. Adolescents become less economically and emotionally dependent on parents. Relationships with one individual become more influential than the need to fit in with a large group of peers. Personal choice emerges and can affect eating behaviors in both positive and negative ways. For instance, some individuals become more health conscious as they approach young adulthood, and may improve eating habits. Other older adolescents become less influenced by parental advice regarding eating, thus may rely more on convenience and fast foods. The use of motivational counseling methods is recommended during this phase to engage older adolescents in making health and nutrition choices.

Abstract thinking capabilities are realized during late adolescence, which assists teens in developing a sense of future goals and interests. Adolescents are now able to understand the perspectives of others and can fully perceive future consequences associated with current behaviors. This capability is helpful in nutrition counseling to reduce chronic disease risk factors and is especially important among adolescent females who become pregnant.

## Health and Nutrition-Related Behaviors During Adolescence

LO 14.3 Describe at least three eating behaviors commonly seen among adolescents and the potential consequences of these behaviors on nutritional status.

Eating patterns and behaviors of adolescents are influenced by many factors in addition to peer attitudes and behaviors, including parental modeling, food availability, food preferences, cost, convenience, personal and cultural beliefs, mass media, and body image. Teens report that food preferences, accessibility of foods, cost, busy schedules, and social support from family and friends are key factors in their food choices.[12,13]

Illustration 14.4 presents a conceptual model of the many factors that influence eating behaviors of adolescents. The model depicts three interacting levels of influence that impact adolescent eating behaviors: personal or interpersonal, environmental/community, and macrosystem. Personal and interpersonal factors that influence eating behaviors include family and peer attitudes and beliefs, food preferences, role modeling, self-efficacy, and biological/physical changes; these are daily influences that may have a profound effect on food choices. Environmental/community factors include food availability in schools and communities, accessibility of fast-food outlets and convenience stores, and social and cultural norms. These factors can either prohibit or promote access to healthy food choices. Macrosystem factors, which include food production and distribution systems and mass media and advertising, play a more distal and indirect role in determining food patterns, yet can exert a powerful influence on specific food choices. To improve the eating patterns of youth, nutrition interventions should be aimed at each helping the youth understand the three levels of influence.

Eating habits of adolescents are not static; they fluctuate throughout adolescence in relation to physical, psychosocial, and cognitive development. Longitudinal data suggest

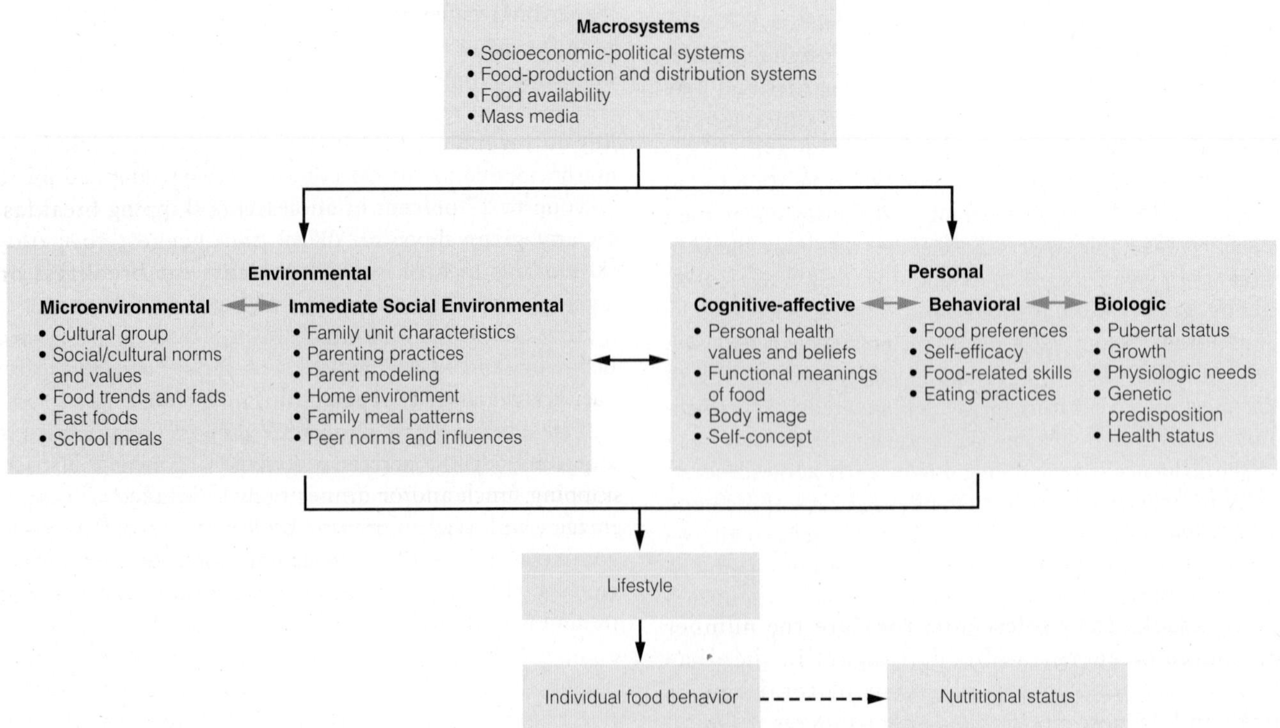


ILLUSTRATION 14.4 ▸ Conceptual model for factors influencing eating behavior of adolescents.

SOURCE: From M. Story and I. Alton, "Becoming a Woman: Nutrition in Adolescence," in D. A. Krummel and P. M. Kris-Etherton (Eds.), in Nutrition in Women's Health. Copyright © 1996 Aspen Publishers. Reprinted with permission.

that while body-weight percentiles track throughout adolescence for many individuals, there is more variability in the intake of energy, nutrients, vitamins, and minerals from early to late adolescence.[14] These changes often result from increasingly hectic schedules and greater perceived barriers to healthy eating as adolescents mature and take on additional responsibilities such as participation in extracurricular activities at school and employment outside of the home. Health professionals should take the time to assess the current dietary intake and habits and nutritional status of adolescents as both eating behaviors and nutritional status are likely to change over time.

## Snacking

Adolescents lead busy lives. Many are involved in extracurricular sports or academic activities, others are employed, and many must care for younger children in a family for part of the day. These activities, combined with the increased need for social contact and approval, and increasing academic demands as they proceed through school, leave little time for adolescents to sit down to eat a meal. Snacking, skipping meals, and eating foods that are cheap and quick, such as vending machine snacks and fast foods, are commonplace behaviors among adolescents who report a lack of time as a major barrier to healthy eating.

Eighty-three percent of adolescents report snacking, with a mean 1.7 snacks on any given day.[12] Nearly half of teens (47 percent of males, 45 percent of females) report eating three or more snacks per day.[15] Eating patterns that consist of frequent snacking result in a higher total energy intake and greater proportion of calories from added and total sugars.[16] Snacks account for approximately one-quarter of daily food energy among adolescents, with 27–35 percent of discretionary calories, 21–24 percent of total fats, and 37–39 percent of added sugars provided by snacks alone.[17-19] National data suggest that the proportion of energy and nutrients from foods consumed as snacks has risen during the past three decades. Foods and beverages consumed during snacks contribute significantly to daily nutrient intake, providing 17 percent of folate, 31–39 percent of vitamin C, 18–22 percent of vitamin D, 22–27 percent of calcium, and up to 20 percent of iron.[19]

Unfortunately, the food choices made by adolescents while snacking tend to favor foods high in sugar, sodium, and fat, and are relatively low in vitamins and minerals. Soft drinks are among the most commonly chosen snacks for adolescents; they are the number one source of energy and added sugars in the diets of teens, accounting for 9 percent of total energy intake and 45 percent of added sugar intakes.[20] On an average day, an adolescent consumes 286 calories from sugar-sweetened beverages; however, about 1 in 8 teens consumed 500 or more calories from these drinks.[21] The 2013 Youth Risk Behavior Surveillance (YRBS) reported that 27 percent of adolescents consume one soda per day, 19 percent consume two per day, and 11 percent consume three or more sodas per day.[22] Males are much more likely to report having two or more sodas per day than are females (22 percent compared to 17 percent). Black and Hispanic students report consuming the most soda, with 25 percent of Black students and 16 percent of Hispanic students reporting consumption of two or more sodas per day. Longitudinal examination of YRBS data suggest that twice daily or more frequent consumption of soda decreased between 2007 and 2013 (from 24 percent to 19 percent for two or more servings/day and 14 percent to 11 percent for three or more servings per day), with almost all of the decrease occurring between 2007 and 2011.[22]

Other snack foods that are significant sources of energy, fat, and sugars in the diets of teenagers include fruit drinks, dairy desserts, salty snacks, and pizza.[17,20] Health practitioners working with adolescents need to understand that snacking is a commonplace behavior among adolescents and should work with adolescents to improve food choices rather than discouraging snacking. Due to the frequency of snacking, an improvement in food choices during snacking toward more nutrient-dense foods has the potential to significantly impact the dietary intake and adequacy of adolescents. Although increased frequency of snacking among teens is associated with greater energy intakes, a greater frequency of snacking among adolescents does not seem to be associated with higher BMI values.[23]

## Meal Skipping

The occurrence of meal skipping increases as adolescents mature. Breakfast is the most commonly skipped meal, with up to 27 percent of adolescents skipping breakfast on any given day.[24,25] YRBS data suggest that only 38 percent of high school students eat breakfast on a daily basis.[22] Skipping breakfast can dramatically decrease intakes of energy, protein, fiber, calcium, and folate due to the absence of breakfast cereal or other nutrient-dense foods commonly consumed at breakfast.[24] Lunch is skipped by almost 25 percent, and dinner is skipped by up to 8 percent of teens.[25,26] As with breakfast, skipping lunch and/or dinner reduces intakes of energy, protein, and other nutrients. Adolescents who skip meals should be counseled on convenient, portable, and healthy food choices that can be taken with them and eaten as meals or snacks.

## Eating Away from Home and Family Meals

Eating away from home becomes prevalent during adolescence. More than one-third of daily energy, protein and carbohydrate intakes are consumed away from home each day, along with 39 percent of total fat and sugar intake.[27] Common sources of foods eaten away from home include school meals programs, vending machines, school canteens and stores, fast-food restaurants, and convenience or corner stores. Analysis of empty calories as a component of total energy intake among U.S. youth suggests that stores (33 percent), school food sources (32 percent), and fast-food restaurants (35 percent) contribute similarly to nutrient profiles of youth.[28] Food purchased in stores provided more energy from sugar (15 percent) than those from schools and fast-food outlets (10 percent for both) but fast food provided more energy from solid fats (24 percent) than food from schools (22 percent) or stores (18 percent).

In 2014, more than 30.4 million students ate school lunches; 72 percent of these meals were served as free or reduced price options.[29] During the same year, 13.6 million students ate school breakfasts, of which 86 percent were free or reduced price meals. A national study suggests that vending machines are accessible in 72 percent of middle schools and 87 percent of high schools, though hours of availability and contents can vary greatly between schools and districts.[30] School stores are available in about 20 percent of middle schools and one-quarter of high schools have school stores or canteens that sell food items. New federal regulations assuring that all foods sold in schools, including those sold outside of the hot lunch program, meet national nutrition guidelines help to assure that many adolescents eat well when eating away from home.[31] This is discussed in great detail at the end of this chapter (see "School-Based Education, School Meals, and Wellness Activities").

As adolescents spend more time with peers, participation in family meals tends to steadily decline.[32] Only about one-third of 15- to 17-year-olds report eating meals with their family at least 6 days per week, compared to half of 12- to 14-year-olds. This is an unfortunate occurrence, as more frequent family meals are associated with improved dietary intake among adolescents, including higher intakes of fruits, vegetables, and foods that are good sources of calcium, and decreased intake of soft drinks.[33] Family meals can promote long-term healthy eating habits as parents have the opportunity to model healthy eating attitudes and introduce teens to a wide variety of foods, behaviors that may track into adulthood.[34] Teens who participate in family meals at least 6 days per week are less likely to utilize substances such as alcohol and street drugs, are less likely to smoke and experience better academic outcomes.[35] Similar improvements in dietary intake are found among older adolescents living away from their parents who eat meals with others compared to those who eat alone.[26]

TABLE 14.2 ▸ Types of vegetarian diets and foods excluded

| TYPE OF VEGETARIAN DIET | FOODS EXCLUDED |
|---|---|
| Semi- or partial-vegetarian | Red meat |
| Lacto-ovo-vegetarian | Meat, poultry, fish, seafood |
| Lacto-vegetarian | Meat, poultry, fish, seafood, eggs |
| Vegan (total vegetarian) | Meat, poultry, fish, seafood, eggs, dairy products (may exclude honey) |
| Macrobiotic | Meat, poultry, eggs, dairy, seafood, fish (fish may be included in the diets of some macrobiotic vegetarians) |

SOURCE: Reprinted with permission. Haddad E., Johnston P. "Vegetarian Diets and Pregnant Teens." In: Stang J, Story M., eds. *Nutrition and the Pregnant Adolescent: A Practical Reference Guide*. Minneapolis. MN: Center for Leadership, Education, and Training in Maternal and Child Nutrition, University of Minnesota, 2010.

## Vegetarian Diets

The term *vegetarian* is used quite broadly and can consist of many different eating patterns. Table 14.2 lists the most common vegetarian diet patterns, along with the foods most commonly excluded. Among low-literacy populations or those who do not speak English as a first language, *vegetarian* may be thought to refer to a person who eats vegetables. Therefore, health professionals should ask adolescents to define what type of vegetarian diet they consume and elicit a complete list of foods that are avoided.

The prevalence of vegetarianism among adolescents is small—approximately 4 percent of adolescents report currently consume a vegetarian diet, but almost 11 percent report having identified themselves as vegetarian at some point in time.[36] Adolescents adopt vegetarian eating plans for a variety of reasons, including cultural or religious beliefs, moral (animal welfare) or environmental/sustainable food systems concerns, health beliefs, as a means to restrict calories and/or fat intake, and as a means of exerting independence by adopting eating behaviors that differ from those of their family. Regardless of the reason for consuming a vegetarian diet, the adolescent's diet should be thoroughly assessed for nutritional adequacy. As a rule, the more foods that are restricted in the diet, the more likely it is that nutritional deficiencies will result.

Adolescents who follow vegetarian diets have been found to be shorter and leaner and to enter puberty at a later age than omnivores. On average, menarche occurs 6 months later in vegetarians than among omnivores.[37,38] After puberty, teens who consume vegetarian diets are as tall as or taller than omnivores and are generally leaner, although final adult height may be reached at a later age.[37,38]

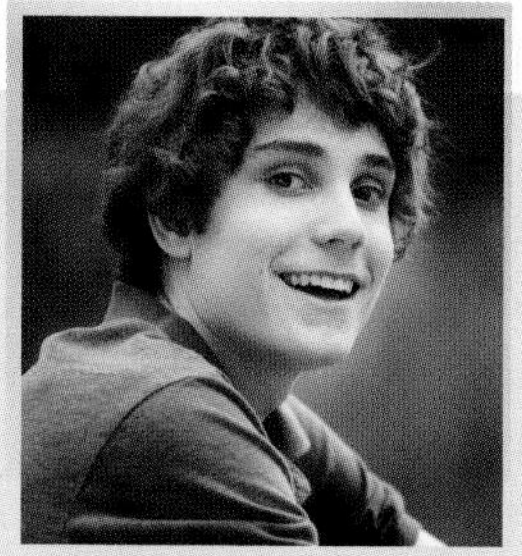
sianc/Shutterstock.com

## CASE STUDY 14.1

### Moral and Ethical Dietary Considerations Leading to Changes in Dietary Habits in Late Adolescence

Darden is an 18-year-old male who is in his first year of undergraduate education at the state university. He hasn't yet declared a major but is leaning toward a dual degree in economics and environmental studies. Darden lives in a residence hall on campus, where he has a 12-meal-per-week meal plan. He usually skips breakfast because he doesn't get up early enough to get to the cafeteria before his 8 a.m. class. He does stop at a coffee shop on his way to class several times per week, where he usually orders a macchiato or mocha coffee drink.

Darden eats lunch and dinner at the cafeteria most days of the week. He tends to focus on foods that are quick to eat, such as chicken sandwiches, pizza, french fries, chicken fingers, and burgers. Occasionally, he will focus on the salad bar or sandwich bar, but often doesn't feel he has the time to do this. On weekends, he usually eats brunch late in the morning, snacking the rest of the day. Darden does have a mini-fridge and microwave in his dorm room, which he shares with a roommate. He keeps nonperishable foods in his room such as chips, cookies, ramen noodles, and microwave popcorn; the mini-fridge is mostly used to store soft drinks and sports drinks. There are no grocery stores on campus so he buys his food and beverages at either the big-box pharmacy chain store or the convenience store close to his residence hall.

#### Questions

1. What food choices might you recommend to Darden to improve his weekend food intake? Specifically, what foods and beverages might be available at the pharmacy or convenience store that would provide more nutrient-dense diet?
2. What food groups seem to be lacking in Darden's diet, and what recommendations would you make to improve his intake on weekdays?

Darden has an interest in sustainable foods, so he joined an environmental justice group on campus. The group frequently discusses topics related to animal welfare and the impact of feedlots on climate change. Darden has decided to follow the lead of his fellow group members and become a vegetarian, eliminating red meat, poultry, and fish from his diet. Within 2 months of becoming a vegetarian, he decided to give up all animal protein, including eggs and milk. He also avoids foods with high fructose corn syrup and preservatives when possible.

#### Questions

1. What type of diet did Darden originally adopt? What type of diet is he currently consuming?
2. What are nutrients of concern for Darden, given his current diet?
3. What are potential benefits of Darden's dietary choices?
4. Is Darden's choice of diet developmentally normal? Is it likely to affect his growth?
5. What are food items that Darden can keep in his dorm room for weekend consumption, given his dietary beliefs?

Well-planned vegetarian diets can offer many health advantages to adolescents, such as a high intake of fiber, a lower intake of saturated fat, and relatively high intake of the vitamins and minerals found in plant-based foods. Data suggest that vegetarian adolescents consume more fruits and vegetables, fewer sweets, fewer salty snack foods, and less fat compared to omnivorous teens.[36] With planning, vegetarian diets can provide adequate protein to promote growth and development among pubescent adolescents, particularly if small amounts of animal-derived foods, such as milk or eggs, are consumed at least two times per week. If vegetarian diets restrict intake of all animal-derived food products such as in vegan diets, however, careful attention must be paid to ensure adequate intakes of protein, calcium, zinc, iron, long-chain n-3 fatty acids, and vitamins D, $B_6$, and $B_{12}$.[38] Supplements of vitamins $B_{12}$ and D, iron, zinc, and calcium are often required among vegans unless fortified foods are routinely consumed. Fortification can vary widely among brands of dairy products and milk substitutes, thus label reading should be encouraged and taught. A suggested dietary food guide for adolescent vegetarians is listed in Table 14.3.

TABLE 14.3 ▸ Suggested daily food guide for lacto-ovo and vegan vegetarians 11 years and older requiring 2200–2800 kcals per day

| FOOD GROUPS | LACTO-OVO VEGETARIANS | VEGAN VEGETARIANS |
|---|---|---|
| Breads, grains, cereal | 9–11 | 10–12 |
| Legumes | 2–3 | 3 or more |
| Vegetables | 4–5 | 5 or more |
| Fruits | 4 | 4 or more |
| Nuts, seeds | 1 | 4–6 |
| Milk, yogurt, cheese | 4 | — |
| Soy, almond, or rice milk (fortified with calcium and vitamin D) | — | 4 |
| Eggs | ½–1 | — |

SOURCE: Data used with permission from E. H. Haddad (1994), "Development of a Vegetarian Food Guide," in American Journal of Clinical Nutrition, 59: 307–316; and M. Story, et al. (eds.), Bright Futures in Practice: Nutrition. © 2000 National Center for Education in Maternal and Child Health.

## Physical Activity

Physical activity is defined as any bodily movement produced by skeletal muscles, which results in energy expenditure.[39] This definition is distinguished from exercise, which is a subset of physical activity that is planned, structured, and repetitive and is done to improve or maintain physical fitness. Physical fitness is a set of attributes that are either health- or skill-related. The Physical Activity Guidelines for Americans recommends that all adolescents be physically active daily, or nearly every day, as part of play, games, sports, work, transportation, recreation, physical education, or health promotion.[39] Further, they recommended that adolescents engage in muscle- and bone-strengthening activities at least three days per week.

Regular physical activity leads to many health benefits. It improves aerobic endurance and muscular strength, may reduce the risk of developing obesity, and builds bone mass density.[39,40] Physical activity among adolescents is consistently related to higher levels of self-esteem and self-concept and lower levels of anxiety and stress. Thus, physical activity is associated with both physiological and psychological benefits, which offers opportunities to positively influence the adoption of lifelong activity patterns. Increasing physical activity among adolescents is an important goal because regular physical activity declines during adolescence and many American teens are inactive.

Despite common knowledge about the importance and benefits of physical activity, only 27 percent of U.S. adolescents are active every day of the week, while 15 percent of adolescents report no moderate to vigorous physical activity on any day in a week.[22] More males than females meet daily physical activity guidelines during adolescence. Approximately 62 percent of adolescent males engage in muscle-building activities three or more times per week compared to only 42 percent of females.[22] Moreover, physical activity has been shown to decline steadily throughout adolescence, especially among females. Racial and ethnic differences are also noted in physical activity; White teens are more likely to meet physical activity targets, while Black students are more likely to report no physical activity.[22]

Individual, social, and environmental factors are associated with physical activity among adolescents.[41] Individual factors positively associated with physical activity among young people include male gender, confidence in one's ability to engage in exercise (i.e., self-efficacy), perceptions of physical or sports competence, having positive attitudes toward physical activity, enjoying physical activity, and perceiving positive benefits associated with physical activity (i.e., excitement, fun, adventure, staying in shape, improved appearance, weight control, improving skills).[41] Social factors associated with engaging in physical activity are family affluence and peer and family support. Environmental factors associated with physical activity are having easy access to safe and convenient venues, sports equipment, and transportation to sports or fitness programs.

# Dietary Requirements, Intake, and Adequacy Among Adolescents

LO 14.4 Compare which nutrients adolescents consume in lower than recommended amounts and which nutrients they consume in higher than recommended amounts, and how these behaviors may impact overall health status.

## Energy and Nutrient Requirements of Adolescents

Increases in lean body mass, skeletal mass, and body fat that occur during puberty result in energy and nutrient needs that exceed those at any other point in life. Energy and nutrient requirements of adolescence correspond with the degree of physical maturation that has taken place. Unfortunately, there is little available data that define optimal nutrient and energy intakes during adolescence. Most existing data are extrapolated from adult recommendations. Suggested intakes of energy, protein, and some other nutrients are often based on adequate growth as opposed to optimal physiological functioning. The Dietary Reference Intakes (DRIs) provide the best estimate of nutrient requirements for adolescents (Table 14.4).[42]

TABLE 14.4 ▸ Dietary Reference Intakes of selected nutrients for adolescents

| | CALCIUM (MG/D) | PHOSPHORUS (MG/D) | MAGNESIUM (MG/D) | VITAMIN D (IU/D)[a,b] | FLUORIDE (MG/D) | THIAMIN (MG/D) | RIBOFLAVIN (MG/D) | NIACIN (MG/D)[c] |
|---|---|---|---|---|---|---|---|---|
| **Males** | | | | | | | | |
| 9–13 years | 1300* | **1250** | **240** | 600* | 2* | **0.9** | **0.9** | **12** |
| 14–18 years | 1300* | **1250** | **410** | 600* | 3* | **1.2** | **1.3** | **16** |
| **Females** | | | | | | | | |
| 9–13 years | 1300* | **1250** | **240** | 600* | 2* | **0.9** | **0.9** | **12** |
| 14–18 years | 1300* | **1250** | **360** | 600* | 3* | **1.0** | **1.0** | **14** |
| **Pregnancy** | | | | | | | | |
| ≤18 years | 1300* | **1250** | **400** | 600* | 3* | **1.4** | **1.4** | **18** |
| **Lactation** | | | | | | | | |
| ≤18 years | 1300* | **1250** | **360** | 600* | 3* | **1.4** | **1.6** | **17** |

| LIFE-STAGE GROUP | VITAMIN $B_6$ (MG/D) | FOLATE, (MG/D) | VITAMIN $B_{12}$ (MG/D) | PANTOTHENIC ACID (MG/D) | BIOTIN (MG/D) | CHOLINE (MG/D)[d] | VITAMIN C (MG/D) | VITAMIN E (MG/D) | SELENIUM (MG/D) |
|---|---|---|---|---|---|---|---|---|---|
| **Males** | | | | | | | | | |
| 9–13 years | **1.0** | **300** | **1.8** | 4* | 20* | 375* | **45** | **11** | **40** |
| 14–18 years | **1.3** | **400** | **2.4** | 5* | 25* | 550* | **75** | **15** | **55** |
| **Females** | | | | | | | | | |
| 9–13 years | **1.0** | **300** | **1.8** | 4* | 20* | 375* | **45** | **11** | **40** |
| 14–18 years | **1.2** | **400** | **2.4** | 5* | 25* | 400* | **65** | **15** | **55** |
| **Pregnancy** | | | | | | | | | |
| ≤18 years | **1.9** | **600** | **2.6** | 6* | 30* | 450* | **80** | **15** | **60** |
| **Lactation** | | | | | | | | | |
| ≤18 years | **2.0** | **500** | **2.8** | 7* | 35* | 550* | **115** | **19** | **70** |

NOTE: This table presents Recommended Dietary Allowances (RDAs) in bold type and Adequate Intakes (AIs) in ordinary type followed by an asterisk (*). RDAs and AIs may both be used as goals for individual intake. RDAs are set to meet the needs of almost all (97–98 percent) individuals in a group. For healthy and breastfed infants, the AI is the mean intake. The AI for other life stage and gender groups is believed to cover needs of all individuals in the group, but lack of data or uncertainty in the data prevent being able to specify with confidence the percentage of individuals covered by this intake.

[a] As cholecalciferol. 1 mg cholecalciferol = 40 IU vitamin D.

[b] In the absence of adequate exposure to sunlight.

[c] As niacin equivalents (NE). 1 mg of niacin = 60 mg tryptophan; 0–6 months = pre-formed niacin (not NE).

[d] Although AIs have been set for choline, there are few data to assess whether a dietary supplement of choline is needed at all stages of the life cycle, and it may be that the choline requirement can be met by endogenous synthesis at some of these stages.

SOURCE: Reprinted with permission from Dietary Reference Intakes: Recommended Intakes for Individuals, © by the National Academy of Sciences. Courtesy of the National Academy Press, Washington, D.C.

It should be noted, however, that these nutrient recommendations are classified according to chronological age, as opposed to individual levels of biological development. Thus, health care professionals must use prudent professional judgment based on SMR status, and not solely on chronological age, when determining the nutrient needs of an adolescent. Nutrients of particular concern for teens are discussed in greater detail in the following sections.

## Energy

Energy needs of adolescents are influenced by activity level, basal metabolic rate, and increased requirements to support pubertal growth and development. Basal metabolic rate (BMR) is closely associated with the amount of lean body mass of individuals. Because adolescent males experience greater increases in height, weight, and lean body mass, they have significantly higher caloric requirements than do females. The estimated energy requirements for adolescents are listed in Table 14.5. Due to the great variability in the timing of growth and maturation among adolescents, the determination of energy needs based on velocity of growth will provide a better estimate than one based on chronological age.

The DRI for energy is based on the assumption of a light to moderate activity level. Therefore, adolescents who participate in sports, those who are in training to increase muscle mass, and those who are more active than average may require additional energy to meet their individual needs. Conversely, adolescents who are not physically active or those who have chronic or handicapping conditions that limit their mobility will require less energy to meet their needs. Physical activity has been found to decline throughout adolescence, therefore caloric needs of older adolescents who have completed puberty and are less active may be significantly lower than those of younger, active, still-growing adolescents.

Physical growth and development during puberty is sensitive to energy and nutrient intakes. When energy intakes fail to meet requirements, linear growth may be retarded and sexual maturation may be delayed. The standard way to gauge adequacy of energy intake is to assess height, weight, and body composition. If, over time, height as well as weight-for-height continuously fall within the same percentiles when plotted on gender-appropriate National Center for Health Statistics growth charts, it can be assumed that energy needs are being met. If percentile of weight-for-height measurements begin to fall or rise, a thorough assessment of energy intake should be done, and adjustments in energy intake should be made accordingly. The use of body-fat measurements, such as triceps and subscapular skinfold measurements, can provide useful information when weight-for-height does not remain consistent. Remember, however, that transient increases and decreases in body fat are commonly noted among adolescents during puberty due to the variation in timing of increases in height, weight, and accumulation of body fat and lean body mass. Repeated measurements of weight, height, and body composition over a several-month period are needed to accurately assess adequacy of growth and development.

## Protein

Protein needs of adolescents are influenced by the amount of protein required for maintenance of existing lean body mass, plus allowances for the amount required to accrue additional lean body mass during the adolescent growth spurt. The estimated protein need for adolescents is 0.85 g/kg body weight/day, slightly higher than that of adults.[42] Because protein needs vary with the degree of growth and development, requirements based on developmental age will be more accurate than absolute recommendations based on chronological age.

Recommended protein intakes are shown in Table 14.5. Protein requirements are highest for females at 11 to 14 years and for males at 15 to 18 years, when growth is at its peak. Similar to energy needs, estimation of protein needs based on timing of growth rather than chronological

TABLE 14.5 ▸ Recommended intakes of macronutrients based on IOM Daily Recommended Intakes

| | ESTIMATED ENERGY | CARBOHYDRATE (G) | % OF DAILY ENERGY FROM CARBOHYDRATE | FIBER (G) | % OF DAILY ENERGY FROM FAT | LINOLEIC ACID A (G) | ALPHA-LINOLENIC ACID (G) | PROTEIN (G) FROM PROTEIN | % ENERGY REQUIREMENTS |
|---|---|---|---|---|---|---|---|---|---|
| **Males** | | | | | | | | | |
| 9–13 | 2279 | 130 | 45–65 | 31 | 25–35 | 21 | 1.2 | 34 | 10–30 |
| 14–18 | 3152 | 130 | 45–65 | 38 | 25–35 | 16 | 1.6 | 52 | 10–30 |
| **Females** | | | | | | | | | |
| 9–13 | 2071 | 130 | 45–65 | 26 | 25–35 | 10 | 1.0 | 34 | 10–30 |
| 14–18 | 2368 | 130 | 45–65 | 26 | 25–35 | 11 | 1.1 | 46 | 10–30 |

age is most accurate. As with energy, growth is affected by protein intakes. Subgroups of adolescents may be at risk for marginal or low protein intakes, including those from food-insecure households, those who severely restrict calories, and those who consume vegetarian diets, most notably vegans.

## Carbohydrates

Carbohydrates provide the body's primary source of dietary energy. Carbohydrate-rich foods such as fruit, vegetables, whole grains, and legumes are also the main source of dietary fiber. The recommended intake of carbohydrate among teens is 130 g/day, or 45–65 percent of daily energy needs (Table 14.5).[42] Sweeteners and added sugars provide approximately 21 percent of energy intake by teens. Males consume 35 tsp and female teens consume 26 tsp of added sugar per day.[43] Soft drinks, candy, baked goods, and sweetened beverages are major sources of added sweeteners in the diets of adolescents.

## Dietary Fiber

Dietary fiber is important for normal bowel function and may play a role in the prevention of chronic diseases such as certain cancers, coronary artery disease, and type 2 diabetes mellitus. Adequate fiber intake is also thought to reduce serum cholesterol levels, moderate blood sugar levels, and reduce the risk of obesity. The DRIs set the recommended intake of dietary fiber for adolescent females at 26 g/day, for males $<$14 years of age at 31 g/day, and for older adolescent males at 38 g/day.[42]

National data indicate that adolescent males consume 16.4 grams of fiber per day, while adolescent females consume 12.6 g/day, well short of AAP and DRI recommendations.[27] During adolescence, fiber intake among males increases slightly with age, while it decreases with age among females. A low intake of fruits and vegetables, combined with an average intake of less than one serving of whole grains per day among adolescents, are contributing factors affecting fiber intake among adolescents.[43]

## Fat

The human body requires dietary fat and essential fatty acids for normal growth and development. Current recommendations suggest that children over the age of 2 years consume no more than 25–35 percent of calories from fat, with no more than 10 percent of calories derived from saturated fat.[42] Data on energy and macronutrient intakes among adolescents suggest that approximately 33 percent of total calories consumed are derived from fat.[44] Approximately two-thirds of teens meet the recommendations for fat intake. The DRIs recommend specific intake of linoleic and alpha-linolenic acid to support optimal growth and development (Table 14.5).[42]

## Calcium

Achieving an adequate intake of calcium during adolescence is crucial to physical growth and development. Calcium is the main constituent of bone mass. Because about half of peak bone mass is accrued during adolescence, calcium intake may be of great importance for the development of dense bone mass and the reduction of the lifetime risk of fractures and osteoporosis.[7] Additionally, calcium needs and absorption rates are higher during adolescence than any other time except infancy.[7,45] Female adolescents appear to have the greatest capability to absorb calcium at about the time of menarche, with calcium absorption rates decreasing from then on.[7,45] Calcium absorption rates in males also peak during early adolescence, a few years later than in females. Young adolescents have been found to retain up to four times as much calcium as young adults. Males accrue more bone mass than females at all ages during puberty, possibly due to lower intake of calcium, less weight-bearing stress on bone tissue, or hormonal influences among females.

The DRI for calcium for 9- to 18-year-olds is 1300 mg per day (Table 14.4).[42] National data suggest that many adolescents, most notably females, do not consume the DRI for calcium. Adolescent females consume 937 mg calcium per day, while adolescent males have been found to consume about 1311 mg calcium each day.[46] The level of dietary intake among females is not adequate to support the development of optimal bone mass. Supplements may be warranted for adolescents who do not consume adequate calcium from dietary sources.

Research suggests that adolescents are not able to meet daily calcium needs in diets that do not include dairy products without the use of calcium-fortified foods.[47] Adolescents increasingly consume their calcium in the form of fortified foods. A longitudinal study of individuals followed from childhood into young adulthood found that breads/grains, vegetables, nonalcoholic beverages, and cheese are common sources of calcium, with milk supplying less than 25 percent of daily intake.[48] Soy beverages are another source of calcium consumed by youth that can be served in school meal programs. The availability of calcium from soy beverages appears low, however, and the equivalency of soy versus dairy as a calcium source is highly debated.[49] Other food sources of calcium must be carefully chosen when dairy intake is not adequate to meet daily needs.

Calcium consumption drops as age increases among both male and female adolescents; however, males consume greater amounts of calcium at all ages than do females.[47,48] Calcium intakes among adolescents are highly correlated with energy intakes. When dietary calcium intake is adjusted for energy intake, no differences in calcium density of diets are found between males and females. This fact suggests that females who restrict calories in an effort to control their weight are at particularly high risk for inadequate calcium intakes. Some variation in calcium intake follows race categories among females: Cuban, Asian, and Black females consume less calcium on average than do Mexican American, Puerto Rican, and White, Non-Hispanic females.

## Iron

The rapid rate of linear growth, the increase in blood volume, and the onset of menarche during adolescence increase a teen's need for iron. The DRIs for iron for male and female adolescents are shown in Table 14.4.[42] These recommendations are based on the amount of dietary iron intake needed to maintain a suitable level of iron storage, with additional amounts of iron added to cover the rapid linear growth and onset of menstruation that occur in male and female adolescents, respectively. Note that even though DRIs are based on chronological age, the actual iron requirements of adolescents are based on sexual maturation level. Iron needs of an adolescent will be highest during the adolescent growth spurt in males, and after menarche in females.

The age-specific hemoglobin and hematocrit values used to determine iron-deficiency anemia are listed in Table 14.6. Hemoglobin and hematocrit levels, although commonly used to screen for the presence of iron-deficiency anemia, are actually the last serum indicators of depleted iron stores to drop. More sensitive indicators of iron stores include ***serum iron, plasma ferritin, and transferrin saturation***. These measures are expensive and not commonly used in the traditional medical setting, however. Dietary intakes of iron are estimated at 18.8 mg/day among 12- to 19-year-old males and 12.0 mg/day among 12- to 19-year-old females.[46]

Estimates of iron deficiency among adolescents are 9 percent of 12- to 15-year-old females, 5 percent of 12- to 16-year-old males, 11 percent of 15- to 19-year-old females, and 2 percent of 15- to 19-year-old males.[50] While iron deficiency occurs more frequently in all adolescents, iron-deficiency anemia occurs almost exclusively in females, with a prevalence of <1 percent of males and 2 percent among females.[50] Therefore, it is assumed that although the prevalence of iron-deficiency anemia may be relatively low among adolescents, a larger proportion may have inadequate iron stores. Rates of iron deficiency and anemia are twice as high among Black and Mexican American females compared to White females and among adolescents from low-income families.[50]

**TABLE 14.6** Common biochemical indices

| | IDEAL | BORDERLINE ACCEPTABLE | UNACCEPTABLE |
|---|---|---|---|
| Total cholesterol (mg/dL) | <170 | 170–199 | ≥200 |
| LDL cholesterol (mg/dL) | <110 | 110–129 | ≥130 |
| Non-HDL cholesterol (mg/dL) | <120 | 120–144 | ≥145 |
| HDL cholesterol (mg/dL) | >45 | 40–45 | <40 |
| Triglycerides (mg/dL) | <90 | 90–129 | ≥130 |
| Apolipoprotein A-1 | >120 | 115–120 | ≤115 |
| Apolipoprotein B | <90 | 90–109 | ≥110 |
| Hemoglobin (g/dL) | Males<br>≥12.5 (12–15 yr)<br>≥13.3 (16–18 yr)<br>≥13.5 (181 yr)<br>Females<br>≥11.8 (12–15 yr)<br>≥12.0 (16 + yr) | | |
| Hematocrit (%) | Males<br>≥37.3 (12–15 yr)<br>≥39.7 (16–18 yr)<br>≥39.9 (181 yr)<br>Females<br>≥35.7 (12–15, 18 + yr)<br>≥35.9 (16–18 yr) | | |



## Vitamin D

Vitamin D is a fat-soluble vitamin that plays an essential role in facilitating intestinal absorption of calcium and phosphorus that is required to maintain adequate serum levels of these minerals.[42] Vitamin D can be synthesized by the body through exposure of skin to ultraviolet B rays of sunlight. However, individuals who live in northern latitudes may not receive adequate exposure to sunlight in the winter months to facilitate synthesis of adequate amounts of vitamin D.[51] Individuals with dark skin pigmentation may also experience limited vitamin D production by the body.[51,52]

Vitamin D is essential for optimal bone formation. There appears to be an inverse relationship between serum parathyroid hormone (PTH) and vitamin D levels.[42,52] Even in the earliest states of vitamin D deficiency, when no overt symptoms of deficiency are seen, PTH is elevated in order to maintain serum calcium levels through demineralization of bone. As deficiency progresses, absorption of calcium from the gastrointestinal tract is reduced, resulting in even higher levels of PTH being released into circulation and further bone demineralization. Low levels of vitamin D

**serum iron, plasma ferritin, and transferrin saturation** Measures of iron status obtained from blood plasma or serum samples.

among adolescents have been found to be inversely related to systolic blood pressure, fasting plasma glucose levels, hypertriglyceridemia, and metabolic syndrome.[53] Low vitamin D status is also associated with low HDL cholesterol levels and higher BMI and abdominal obesity measurements.

Data from NHANES surveys have demonstrated that serum 25 (OH) vitamin D levels decreased among adolescents during the past few decades.[51] NHANES III (1988–1994) found average serum 25 (OH) vitamin D levels of 32 ng/mL among 12- to 19-year-olds, while average levels measured during NHANES 2001–2004 in the same age group were 24 ng/mL. Reductions in serum vitamin D status were seen among all groups, but were particularly pronounced among Black subjects. Greater decreases in serum vitamin D status were found among females than among males. This has long-term implications for teenage females, given their low calcium intake during the teen years and higher life-long risk for osteoporosis.

When the criteria of <10 ng/mL for deficiency and $30 ng/mL are used to determine sufficiency, it appears that <1 percent of White adolescents are vitamin D deficient; however, 39 percent of girls and 29 percent of boys do not have adequate vitamin D status.[51] Approximately 2 percent of Mexican American girls and <1 percent of boys in the United States are vitamin D deficient; however, 59 percent of male and 76 percent of female Mexican American adolescents had insufficient vitamin D status. The highest rates of vitamin D deficiency and insufficiency are noted among Black teens, with 4 percent of males and 10 percent of females experiencing deficiency and 75 percent of Black boys and 92 percent of Black girls found to be vitamin D insufficient. While deficiency may be uncommon, insufficiency in vitamin D status is a major public health nutrition concern.

The AAP has recommended that the criterion for deficiency be 20 ng/mL, which is lower than that used in the NHANES surveys.[52] A report by the Institute of Medicine concluded that a serum 25-OH-D level of 20 ng/mL would meet the requirement of 97.5 percent of the population.[54] However the Endocrine Society has recommended that individuals at risk for vitamin D deficiency maintain a higher level of 30 mg/mL.[55]

Both the Institute of Medicine and American Academy of Pediatrics have recommended that all adolescents who do not consume at least 400 IU (10 $\mu$g) of vitamin D per day through dietary sources receive a supplement of 400 IU per day Vitamin D intake to meet the RDA of 600 IU per day.[54,56] Average daily intakes are 6.9 $\mu$g per day among male and 4.3 $\mu$g per day among female adolescents.[46] Vitamin D adequacy should be assessed for all adolescents of high-risk groups, particularly those who live in northern climates, who have limited sun exposure, who have lactose intolerance or milk allergy, who have developmental disabilities that may limit outdoor activities, or who have darkly pigmented skin or frequently use sunscreen.

## Folate

Folate is an integral part of DNA, RNA, and protein synthesis. Thus, adolescents have increased requirements for folate during puberty. The DRI for folate is listed in Table 14.4.[42]

Severe folate deficiency results in the development of megaloblastic anemia, which is rare among adolescents. Evidence, however, indicates that a significant proportion of adolescents have inadequate folate status. Red blood cell and serum folate levels drop during adolescence as sexual maturation proceeds, suggesting that increased folate needs during growth and development are not being met. Serum levels were found to drop significantly between childhood and adolescence in data gathered through NHANES 2005–2006, with levels of 16.1 ng/mL measured in children 4–11 years of age and levels of 11.6 ng/mL measured in adolescents.[57] According to national data, adolescents have the lowest red blood cell folate levels of any age group in the United States, with levels of 229 ng/mL among both males and females.[57,58]

Poor folate status among adolescent females presents an issue related to reproduction. Studies show that adequate intakes of folate prior to pregnancy can reduce the incidence of spina bifida and selected other congenital anomalies, and may reduce the risk of Down syndrome among offspring.[57] The protective effects of folate occur early in pregnancy, often before a woman knows she is pregnant. Thus, it is imperative that all women of reproductive age (15–44 years old) consume adequate folic acid, preferably through dietary sources, or if needed, through supplements.

Despite the low serum and red blood cell levels of folate, national data suggest that many adolescents consume adequate amounts of folate. Mean intakes of folate among adolescent males average 687 $\mu$g/day, while females consume 453 $\mu$g/day.[46] The DRI for folate among adolescents is 400 $\mu$g/day.[42] Teens who skip breakfast or do not commonly consume orange juice, fortified breads and ready-to-eat cereals are at an increased risk for having a low consumption of folate.

## Dietary Intake and Nutritional Adequacy

Nutrient intakes of U.S. adolescents suggest that many consume inadequate amounts of vitamins and minerals; this trend is more pronounced in females than in males.[46] It is not surprising, given the fact that most adolescents do not consume diets that comply with MyPlate or the Dietary Guidelines for Americans. On average, adolescents consume diets inadequate in several vitamins and minerals, including folate; vitamins A, B6, C, and E; and iron, zinc, magnesium, phosphorus, and calcium.[46] Dietary fiber intake among adolescents is also low. Diets consumed by many teens exceed current recommendations for total and saturated fats, cholesterol, sodium, and added sugar.

Few adolescents meet recommendations for fruit or vegetable consumption. Nationally representative data suggest that 17 percent of adolescent males and 14 percent of adolescent females met recommendations for vegetable intake (excluding fried potatoes), while 24 percent of males and 20 percent of females met recommendations for fruit intake.[22] Six percent of male and 4 percent of female teens consume no fruit and 8 percent of males and 6 percent of females consume no vegetables on a given day.[22] Inadequate fruit intake is higher among Black students than White or Hispanic students while inadequate vegetable intake is almost twice as high among Black and Hispanic students compared to their White peers. Fruit and vegetable intake by teens does not appear to be adequate to promote optimal health and reduce risk of chronic diseases.

Adequate intake of servings of grains are reported by 64 percent of teenage males and 48 percent of teen females; however, intake of whole grains are below recommended levels.[59] Intake of meat/meat alternatives was low among adolescents surveyed; 10 percent of males and 18 percent of females reported less than one serving per day, with only 50 percent of males and 17 percent of females meeting recommended intakes.[59] Intake of dairy products is especially low among adolescents. The YRBS found reported that 19 percent of adolescents report drinking no milk on a given day.[22] Lack of dairy consumption is reported twice as often by female adolescents compared to male adolescents (25 percent vs. 13 percent) and almost twice as often by Black students compared to Hispanic and White students (34 percent, 18 percent and 16 percent, respectively). Seventeen percent of adolescent males and 8 percent of teen females report consuming the recommended three or more glasses of milk per day, according to YRBS data.[22]

# Nutrition Screening, Assessment, and Intervention

**LO 14.5** Identify the key components of nutrition assessment and screening of adolescents and how resulting data can be used during nutrition education and counseling.

## Dietary Assessment and Screening

Annual screening of all adolescents for indicators of nutritional risk is recommended. Common concerns that should be investigated during nutrition screening include overweight, underweight, eating disorders, hyperlipidemia, hypertension, iron deficiency and/or anemia, food insecurity, and excessive intake of high-fat or high-sugar foods and beverages (Table 14.7). Pregnant adolescents should also be assessed for adequacy of weight gain and compliance with prenatal vitamin/mineral supplement recommendations.

Nutrition screening should include an accurate measurement of height and weight, and calculation of BMI (body mass index). These data, plotted on age- and gender-appropriate National Center for Health Statistics 2000 growth charts, indicate the presence of any weight or other growth problems. Table 14.8 shows the percentile range for each weight status category, as well as an example of BMI-for-age percentiles for an adolescent boy. Teens below the 5th percentile of weight-for-height or BMI-for-age are considered to be underweight and should be referred for evaluation of metabolic disorders, chronic health conditions, or eating disorders.[60]

Adolescents with a BMI above the 85th percentile but below the 95th percentile are considered to be overweight.[60] They should be evaluated to determine the presence or absence of obesity-related co-morbid complications and referred for treatment as necessary. Teenagers with a BMI greater than the 95th percentile are considered to be obese and should be referred for a full medical evaluation.[60] Referral to a weight-management program specially designed to meet the needs of adolescents may also be warranted for overweight adolescents who have completed physical growth (see Chapter 15 for additional information).

Nutrition screening should include at least a brief dietary assessment. Food frequency questionnaires, 24-hour recalls, and food diaries or food records are all appropriate for use with adolescents. Table 14.9 lists the advantages and disadvantages of each dietary assessment method. Less formal dietary assessment questionnaires that target specific behaviors, such as consumption of savory snacks and high-sugar beverages, can also be used for initial nutrition screening. These rapid-assessment questionnaires and screening tools can be completed quickly and may be used to identify those adolescents in need of additional dietary assessment and nutrition counseling. Online dietary assessments tools such as the ASA24 may be used with teens during nutrition assessment and counseling sessions or by teens on their own for self-assessment of dietary intake.[61]

Nutrition risk indicators that may warrant further nutrition assessment and counseling are listed in Table 14.10. Adolescents who have a poor-quality diet characterized by an excessive intake of high-fat or high-sugar foods and beverages or meal skipping should be provided with nutrition counseling that provides concrete examples of ways to improve dietary intake. Adolescents who have been found to have a nutrition-related health risk, such as hyperlipidemia, hypertension, iron-deficiency anemia, overweight, or an eating disorder, should be referred for in-depth medical assessment and nutrition counseling. Pregnant adolescents may also benefit from in-depth nutrition assessment and counseling.

Adolescents who consume vegan diets must be assessed for adequacy of vitamin and mineral intake (particularly vitamins D and $B_{12}$, iron and zinc) and total fat and essential fatty acid intakes. Docosahexaenoic acid (DHA) is derived from alpha-linolenic acid. Although it is found in

TABLE 14.7 ▸ Recommended health assessment and screening for prevention of chronic disease and promotion of optimal health

| HEALTH ISSUE | YOUNG ADOLESCENT (12–17 Y.O.) | OLDER ADOLESCENT (18–21 Y.O.) |
|---|---|---|
| Dietary behaviors | - Assess usual food intake using age-appropriate method.<br>- Provide appropriate nutrition intervention and/or medical nutrition therapy as needed. | - Assess usual food intake using age-appropriate method.<br>- Provide appropriate nutrition intervention and/or medical nutrition therapy as needed. |
| Physical activity and sedentary activity | - Review usual daily physical and sedentary behavior patterns.<br>- Discuss recommendation for 60 minutes or more of moderate-to-vigorous physical activity per day.<br>- Emphasize importance of limiting sedentary activity, with no more than 2 hours of screen time per day. | - Review usual physical and sedentary behavior patterns with client.<br>- Discuss recommendation for 60 minutes or more of moderate-to-vigorous physical activity each day.<br>- Emphasize importance of limiting sedentary activity and recommend no more than 2 hours of screen time per day. |
| Anthropometric measurements | - Assess and plot height, weight and BMI using appropriate methods.<br>- Review weight status with adolescent and parent(s).<br>- Refer overweight adolescents to weight management program for Step 1 counseling (see Chapter 15) and schedule follow-up appointment.<br>- Refer obese adolescents to a comprehensive weight management program for Step 2 counseling. | - Assess and plot height, weight and BMI using appropriate methods.<br>- Review weight status with client.<br>- Thoroughly assess dietary intake and physical activity and sedentary activity behaviors and provide appropriate counseling for overweight and/or obese clients.<br>- Refer overweight and obese clients to primary health provider for full medical assessment and treatment. |
| Family history of premature cardiovascular disease, diabetes and obesity | - Update family history at each visit.<br>- Provide primary care referral and preventive dietary counseling based on family history as necessary. | - Update family history annually.<br>- Provide primary care referral and preventive dietary counseling based on family history as necessary. |
| Blood pressure | - Interpret and review blood pressure readings with adolescent.<br>- Counseling adolescents and caregivers on the DASH diet.<br>- Request follow-up visit.<br>- Assess changes in blood pressure at follow-up visit. Refer to primary care provider for blood pressure management with medication as needed, if dietary changes have not successfully reduced blood pressure.<br>- Refer to adolescent weight management program if overweight and/or obese. | - Interpret and review blood pressure readings with client.<br>- Counseling client on the DASH diet.<br>- Request follow-up visit.<br>- Assess changes in blood pressure at follow-up visit. Refer to primary care provider for blood pressure management with medication as needed, if dietary changes have not successfully reduced blood pressure.<br>- Refer overweight or obese clients to weight management program or provide appropriate dietary counseling. |
| Blood lipids | - Interpret and review blood lipid levels with adolescent and caregiver.<br>- Refer adolescent to primary care provider and request a blood lipid panel for overweight or obese adolescents if laboratory data are not available.<br>- Provide medical nutrition therapy as appropriate, based on blood lipid levels.<br>- Refer overweight teens to a weight management program for Step 1 weight management or provide appropriate counseling (see Chapter 15).<br>- Refer obese teens to a comprehensive weight management program.<br>- Up to 2 g/day of plant sterols or stanols can be recommended for use by adolescents.<br>- Refer to primary care provider for management of dyslipidemia including medication if dietary changes are not effective. | - Interpret and review blood lipid levels with client.<br>- Refer client to primary care provider and request a blood lipid panel for overweight or obese adolescents if laboratory data are not available.<br>- Provide medical nutrition therapy as appropriate, based on blood lipid levels.<br>- Refer to a weight management program or provide appropriate counseling to promote weight loss if client is overweight or obese.<br>- Up to 2 g/day of plant sterols or stanols can be recommended for use by adolescents.<br>- Refer to primary care provider for management of dyslipidemia including medication if dietary changes are not effective. |

(Continued)

TABLE 14.7 ▸ Recommended health assessment and screening for prevention of chronic disease and promotion of optimal health (*Continued*)

| HEALTH ISSUE | YOUNG ADOLESCENT (12–17 Y.O.) | OLDER ADOLESCENT (18–21 Y.O.) |
| --- | --- | --- |
| Diabetes | - Assess for family history of diabetes, presence of acanthosis nigricans, and symptoms consistent with diabetes among overweight or obese adolescents.<br>- Review fasting blood glucose levels with teens and caregivers or refer to primary care provider for treatment and drawing of a fasting blood glucose level if laboratory data are not available.<br>- Provide medical nutrition therapy and nutrition counseling as appropriate.<br>- Refer overweight and obese teens to a comprehensive weight management program. | - Assess for family history of diabetes, presence of acanthosis nigricans, and symptoms consistent with diabetes among overweight or obese clients.<br>- Review fasting blood glucose levels with clients or refer to primary care provider for treatment and drawing of a fasting blood glucose level if laboratory data are not available.<br>- Provide medical nutrition therapy and nutrition counseling as appropriate.<br>- Provide weight management counseling to overweight and obese clients. |

Adapted from: U.S. Department of Health and Human Services, National Institutes of Health, National Heart, Lung and Blood Institute: Expert panel on integrated guidelines for cardiovascular health and risk reduction in children and adolescents. Summary report. NIH Publication No 12-7486A, October 2012.

soy products, flaxseed, nuts, eggs, and canola oil, intake is very low in the diets of vegans. Diets that are low in fat may not supply an adequate ratio of linoleic acid to alpha-linolenic acid (5:1 to 10:1) to facilitate the metabolism of alpha-linolenic acid to DHA.[38] Therefore, particular attention should be paid to sources of fat in the diets of vegans and other dietary regimens with low fat contents.

Teens who consume a vegetarian diet, particularly if they report doing so for health- or weight-related reasons, should be carefully assessed for the presence of eating disorders, chronic dieting, and body-image disturbances. Surveys of adolescents have shown that those who consume vegetarian diets are somewhat more likely to report binge eating, almost twice as likely to report frequent or chronic dieting, four times more likely to report purging, and up to eight times more likely to report laxative use than nonvegetarian peers.[36] These results seem to reflect the fact that many individuals who are chronic dieters or who have disorder eating patterns adopt a vegetarian diet as a means of restricting fat intake or practicing self-denial rather than the vegetarian diet causing the restrictive behaviors. Adolescent vegetarians, especially adolescent males, have been found to be at high risk for engaging in unhealthy and often extreme weight-loss behaviors.[36] Therefore, it is imperative that practitioners working with adolescents who consume a vegetarian diet explore reasons for adopting this eating style and encourage adolescents to follow a nutritionally balanced and healthy diet.

TABLE 14.8 ▸ Example of height and weight status for adolescents

| WEIGHT STATUS CATEGORY | PERCENTILE RANGE |
| --- | --- |
| Underweight | Less than the 5th percentile |
| Healthy weight | 5th percentile to less than the 85th percentile |
| Overweight | 85th to less than the 95th percentile |
| Obese | Equal to or greater than the 95th percentile |

In-depth nutrition assessment should include a review of the full medical history, a review of psychosocial and physical development, and evaluation of all laboratory data available. A complete and thorough dietary assessment should be performed, preferably using two dietary assessment methods. Most commonly, a food frequency questionnaire or a 3- to 7-day food record is combined with a 24-hour recall to provide accurate dietary intake data. Specific areas of nutrition concern can be identified during a complete nutrition assessment, and recommendations for nutrition education and counseling can be made accordingly.

## Nutrition Education and Counseling

Providing nutrition education and counseling to teenagers requires a great deal of skill and a good understanding of normal adolescent physical and psychosocial development. Health professionals need to remember that developmentally, adolescents may look like young adults, but they are not. Their psychosocial development can vary tremendously, and they may not respond favorably to traditional adult counseling methods. It is also important to not provide nutrition education messages or materials that are too childish in nature. Adolescence is a unique developmental stage between young adulthood and childhood and requires its own approach to education and counseling. When working with teens, it is important to treat them as individuals with unique needs and concerns. This capitalizes on their developmental process of becoming autonomous and helps to foster a sense of respect and self-reliance. Messages containing concrete recommendations (such as choose foods with 5 grams or less of fat per serving) and that incorporate activities or concerns from their daily lives will be most effective with teens. Such daily life activities and concerns might include improvements in academic achievement, clearer skin, shinier hair, improved athletic performance, or increased energy levels.

The initial component of the counseling session should involve getting to know the adolescent, including personal health or nutrition-related concerns. After establishing a rapport with the teen, the counselor should provide an

TABLE 14.9 ▸ Strengths and limitations of various dietary assessment methods used in clinical settings

| | STRENGTHS | LIMITATIONS | APPLICATIONS |
|---|---|---|---|
| 24-hr recall | • Does not require literacy<br>• Relatively low respondent burden<br>• Data may be directly entered into a dietary analysis program<br>• May be conducted in person or over the telephone | • Dependent on respondent's memory<br>• Relies on self-reported information<br>• Requires skilled staff<br>• Time consuming<br>• Single recall does not represent usual intake | • Appropriate for most people as it does not require literacy<br>• Useful for the assessment of intake of a variety of nutrients and assessment of meal patterning and food group intake<br>• Useful counseling tool |
| Food frequency | • Quick, easy, and affordable<br>• May assess current as well as past diet<br>• In a clinical setting, may be useful as a screening tool | • Does not provide valid estimates of absolute intake of individuals<br>• Can't assess meal patterning<br>• May not be appropriate for some population groups | • Does not provide valid estimates of absolute intake for individuals, thus of limited usefulness in clinical settings<br>• May be useful as a screening tool; however, further development research is needed |
| Food record | • Does not rely on memory<br>• Food portions may be measured at the time of consumption<br>• Multiple days of records provide valid measure of intake for most nutrients | • Recording foods eaten may influence what is eaten<br>• Requires literacy<br>• Relies on self-reported information<br>• Requires skilled staff<br>• Time consuming | • Appropriate for literate and motivated population groups<br>• Useful for the assessment of intake of a variety of nutrients and assessment of meal patterning and food group intake<br>• Useful counseling tool |
| Diet History | • Able to assess usual intake in a single interview<br>• Appropriate for most people | • Relies on memory<br>• Time consuming (60 to 90 minutes)<br>• Requires skilled interviewer | • Appropriate for most people, as it does not require literacy<br>• Useful for assessing intake of nutrients, meal patterning, and food group intake<br>• Useful counseling tool |

SOURCE: Used with permission. Story M, Stang I, eds. Nutrition and the Pregnant Adolescent: A Practical Reference Guide. Minneapolis, MN: Center for Leadership, Education, and Training in Maternal and Child Nutrition, University of Minnesota; 2000.

TABLE 14.10 ▸ Key indicators of nutrition risk for adolescents

| INDICATORS OF NUTRITION RISK | RELEVANCE | CRITERIA FOR FURTHER SCREENING & ASSESSMENT |
|---|---|---|
| | **Food Choices** | |
| Consumes fewer than 2 servings fruit or fruit juice per day | Fruits and vegetables provide dietary fiber and several vitamins (such as A and C) and minerals. Low intake of fruits and vegetables is associated with an increased risk of many types of cancer. In females of childbearing age, low intake of folic acid is associated with an increase risk of giving birth to an infant with neural tube defects. | Assess the adolescent who is consuming less than 1 serving of fruit or fruit juice per day. |
| Consumes fewer than 3 servings of vegetables per day | | Assess the adolescent who is consuming fewer than 2 servings of vegetables per day. |
| Consumes fewer than 6 servings of bread, cereal, pasta, rice, or other grains per day | Grain products provide complex carbohydrates. | Assess the adolescent who is consuming fewer than 3 servings of bread, cereal, pasta, rice, or other grains per day. |
| Consumes fewer than 3 servings of dairy products per day | Dairy products are a good source of protein, vitamins, and calcium and other minerals. Low intake of dairy products may reduce peak bone mass and contribute to later risk of osteoporosis. | Assess the adolescent who is consuming fewer than 2 servings of dairy products per day. Assess the adolescent who is consuming more than 20 ounces of soft drinks per day. |

(Continued)

TABLE 14.10 ▸ Key indicators of nutrition risk for adolescents (*Continued*)

| INDICATORS OF NUTRITION RISK | RELEVANCE | CRITERIA FOR FURTHER SCREENING & ASSESSMENT |
|---|---|---|
| Consumes fewer than 2 servings of meat or meat alternatives (e.g., beans, eggs, nuts, seeds) per day | Protein-rich foods (e.g., meats, beans, dairy products) are good sources of B vitamins, iron, and zinc. Low intake of protein-rich foods may impair growth and increase the risk of iron-deficiency anemia and of delayed growth and sexual maturation. Low intake of meat or meat alternatives may indicate inadequate availability of these foods at home. Special attention should be paid to children and adolescents who follow a vegetarian diet. | Assess the adolescent who is consuming fewer than 2 servings of meat or meat alternatives per day or who consumes a vegan diet. |
| Has excessive intake of dietary fat | Excessive intake of total fat contributes to the risk of cardiovascular diseases and obesity and is associated with some cancers. | Assess the adolescent who has a family history of premature cardiovascular disease.<br>Assess the adolescent who has a body mass index (BMI) greater than or equal to the 85th percentile. |
| | **Eating Behaviors** | |
| Exhibits poor appetite | A poor appetite may indicate depression, emotional stress, chronic disease, or an eating disorder. | Assess the adolescent if BMI is less than the 15th percentile or if weight loss has occurred.<br>Assess if irregular menses or amenorrhea have occurred for 3 months or more.<br>Assess for organic and psychiatric disease. |
| Consumes food from fast-food restaurants three or more times per week | Excessive consumption of convenience foods and foods from fast-food restaurants is associated with high fat, calorie, and sodium intakes, as well as low intake of certain vitamins and minerals. | Assess the adolescent who is at risk for overweight/obesity, or who has diabetes mellitus, hyperlipidemia, or other conditions requiring reduction in dietary fat. |
| Skips breakfast, lunch, or dinner/supper 3 or more times per week<br>Consumes a vegetarian diet | Meal skipping is associated with a low intake of energy and essential nutrients and, if it is a regular practice, could compromise growth and sexual development. Repeatedly skipping meals decreases the nutritional adequacy of the diet.<br>Vegetarian diets can provide adequate nutrients and energy to support growth and development if well planned. Vegan diets may lack calcium, iron, and vitamins D and $B_{12}$. Low-fat vegetarian diets may be adopted by adolescents who have eating disorders. | Assess the adolescent to ensure that meal skipping is not due to inadequate food resources or unhealthy weight-loss practices.<br>Assess the adolescent who consumes fewer than 2 servings of meat alternatives per day.<br>Assess the adolescent who consumes fewer than 3 servings of dairy products per day.<br>Assess the adolescent who follows a low-fat vegetarian diet and experiences weight loss for eating disorder and adequacy of energy intake. |
| Skips breakfast, lunch, or dinner/supper 3 or more times per week | Meal skipping is associated with a low intake of energy and essential nutrients and, if it is a regular practice, could compromise growth and sexual development. Repeatedly skipping meals decreases the nutritional adequacy of the diet. | Assess the adolescent to ensure that meal skipping is not due to inadequate food resources or unhealthy weight-loss practices. |
| Consumes a vegetarian diet | Vegetarian diets can provide adequate nutrients and energy to support growth and development if well planned. Vegan diets may lack calcium, iron, and vitamins D and $B_{12}$. Low-fat vegetarian diets may be adopted by adolescents who have eating disorders. | Assess the adolescent who consumes fewer than 2 servings of meat alternatives per day.<br>Assess the adolescent who consumes fewer than 3 servings of dairy products per day.<br>Assess the adolescent who follows a low-fat vegetarian diet and experiences weight loss for eating disorder and adequacy of energy intake. |
| | **Food Resources** | |
| Has inadequate financial resources to buy food, insufficient access to food, or lack of access to cooking facilities | Poverty can result in hunger and compromised food quality and nutrition status. Inadequate dietary intake interferes with learning. | Assess the adolescent who is from a family with low income, is homeless, or is a runaway. |

| INDICATORS OF NUTRITION RISK | RELEVANCE | CRITERIA FOR FURTHER SCREENING & ASSESSMENT |
|---|---|---|
| | **Weight and Body Image** | |
| Practices unhealthy eating behaviors (e.g., chronic dieting, vomiting, and using laxatives, diuretics, or diet pills to lose weight) | Chronic dieting is associated with many health concerns (fatigue, impaired growth and sexual maturation, irritability, poor concentration, impulse to binge) and can lead to eating disorders. Frequent dieting in combination with purging is often associated with other health-compromising behaviors (substance use, suicidal behaviors). Purging is associated with serious medical complications. | Assess the adolescent for eating disorders.<br>Assess for organic and psychiatric disease.<br>Screen for distortion in body image and dysfunctional eating behavior, especially if adolescent desires weight loss, but BMI is <85th percentile. |
| Is excessively concerned about body size or shape | Eating disorders are associated with significant health and psychological morbidity; 85% of all cases of eating disorders begin during adolescence. The earlier adolescents are treated, the better their long-term prognosis. | Assess the adolescent for distorted body image and dysfunctional eating behaviors, especially if adolescent wants to lose weight, but BMI is <85th percentile. |
| Has exhibited significant weight change in past 6 months | Significant weight change during the past 6 months may indicate stress, depression, organic disease, or an eating disorder. | Assess the adolescent to determine the cause of weight loss or weight gain (limited to too much access to food, poor appetite, meal skipping, eating disorder). |
| | **Physical Activity** | |
| Is physically inactive: engages in physical activity fewer than 5 days per week | Lack of regular physical activity is associated with overweight, fatigue, and poor muscle tone in the short term and a greater risk of heart disease in the long term. Regular physical activity reduces the risk of cardiovascular disease, hypertension, colon cancer, and type 2 diabetes mellitus. Weight-bearing physical activity is essential for normal skeletal development during adolescence. Regular physical activity is necessary for maintaining normal muscle strength, joint structure, and joint function; contributes to psychological health and well-being; and facilitates weight reduction and weight maintenance throughout life. | Assess how much time the adolescent spends watching television/videotapes and playing computer games.<br>Assess the adolescent's definition of physical activity. |
| Engages in excessive physical activity | Excessive physical activity (nearly every day or more than once a day) can be unhealthy and associated with menstrual irregularity, excessive weight loss, and malnutrition. | Assess the adolescent for eating disorders. |
| | **Medical Conditions** | |
| Has chronic diseases or conditions | Medical conditions (diabetes mellitus, spina bifida, renal disease, hypertension, pregnancy, HIV infection/AIDS) have significant nutritional implications. | Assess adolescent's compliance with therapeutic dietary recommendations. Refer to dietitian if appropriate. |
| Has hyperlipidemia | Hyperlipidemia is a major cause of atherosclerosis and cardiovascular disease in adults. | Refer adolescent to a dietitian for cardiovascular nutrition assessment. |
| Has iron-deficiency anemia | Iron deficiency causes developmental delays and behavioral disturbances.<br>Another consequence is increased lead absorption. | Screen adolescents if they have low iron intake, a history of iron-deficiency anemia, limited access to food because of poverty or neglect, special health care needs, or extensive menstrual or other blood losses. Screen annually. |
| Has dental caries | Eating habits have a direct impact on oral health. Calcium and vitamin D are vital for strong bones and teeth, and vitamin C is necessary for healthy gums. Frequent consumption of carbohydrate-rich foods (e.g., lollipops, soda) that stay in the mouth a long time may cause dental caries. Fluoride in water used for drinking and cooking as well as in toothpaste reduces the prevalence of dental caries. | Assess the adolescent's consumption of snacks and beverages that contain sugar, and assess snacking patterns.<br>Assess the adolescent's access to fluoride (e.g., fluoridated water, fluoride tablets). |

(Continued)

TABLE 14.10 ▸ Key indicators of nutrition risk for adolescents (*Continued*)

| INDICATORS OF NUTRITION RISK | RELEVANCE | CRITERIA FOR FURTHER SCREENING & ASSESSMENT |
|---|---|---|
| Is pregnant | Pregnancy increases the need for most nutrients. | Refer the adolescent to a dietitian for further assessment, education, and counselling as appropriate. |
| Is taking prescribed medication | Many medications interact with nutrients and can compromise nutrition status. | Assess potential interactions of prescription drugs (e.g., asthma medications, antibiotics) with nutrients. |
| | **Lifestyle** | |
| Engages in heavy alcohol, tobacco, and other drug use | Alcohol, tobacco, and other drug use can adversely affect nutrient intake and nutrition status. | Assess the adolescent further for inadequate dietary intake of energy and nutrients. |
| Uses dietary supplements | Dietary supplements (e.g., vitamin and mineral preparations) can be healthy additions to a diet, especially for pregnant and lactating women and for people with a history of iron-deficiency anemia; however, frequent use or high doses can have serious side effects. Adolescents who use supplements to "bulk up" may be tempted to experiment with anabolic steroids. Herbal supplements for weight loss can cause tachycardia and other side effects. They may also interact with over-the-counter prescription medications. | Assess the adolescent for the type of supplements used and dosages.<br>Assess the adolescent for use of anabolic steroids and megadoses of other supplements. |

SOURCE: Adapted from Tool D, from K. Holt, N. Wooldridge, M. Story, and D. Sofka, eds. *Bright Futures: Nutrition*, 3rd ed. 2011.

overview of the events of the counseling session, including which specific nutrition topics will be discussed. Once again, the adolescent should be encouraged to add his or her own nutrition concerns to the list of topics to be discussed during the education session. After agreeing on a list of topic areas to be covered during the nutrition education session, a complete nutrition assessment should be performed. Upon completion of the assessment, the counselor and teen should work together to establish goals for improving dietary in-take and reducing nutrition risk.

It is important to involve the adolescent in decision-making processes during nutrition counseling. Allowing teens to provide input as to what aspects of their eating habits they think need to be changed and what changes they are willing to make accomplishes several important tasks during the counseling session. First, the importance of the adolescent in the decision-making process is stressed, and she or he is encouraged to become engaged in personal decisions about health. Second, a good rapport established between the health professional and the adolescent may lead to greater interaction between both parties. Finally, behavior change is more likely when the adolescent has suggested ways to change, thus becoming engaged in the education process and owning a willingness to change.

One or two goals during a counseling session are a reasonable number to work toward. Setting too many goals reduces the probability that the adolescent can meet all of the goals and may seem overwhelming. For each goal set, several potential behavior-change strategies should be mutually agreed upon for meeting that goal. These strategies should be concrete in nature and instigated by the teen. The adolescent and the counselor should also work together to decide how to determine when a goal is met. The MyPlate website can be utilized by teens as a means of assessing how changes in food choices affect changes in nutrient intake across time. Frequent follow-up sessions also help to provide feedback and monitor progress toward individual goals.

The use of technology to facilitate nutrition education and counseling for adolescents should be implemented whenever possible to engage adolescents and to provide nutrition information between client visits. Electronic communications methods such as text messaging, podcasts, YouTube, and social media (e.g., Instagram, Twitter, and Tumbler) are commonly accessed by adolescents and can serve as a means to convey nutrition information in a highly engaging way. In a study of health screening prior to a well visit delivered through the use of personal digital assistants, a significantly greater number of discussions related to fruit and vegetable intake occurred compared to well visits for teens without the use of technology.[62]

# Promoting Healthy Eating and Physical Activity Behaviors

LO 14.6 Describe the roles that peers, families, schools, and communities play in determining the dietary behaviors and nutritional status of adolescents.

Meeting the challenge of improving the nutritional health of teenagers requires the integrated efforts of teenagers, parents, educators, health care providers, schools, communities, the food industry, and policy makers all working together to create more opportunities for healthful eating.

Health professionals need to rethink how they frame messages to youth. Decades ago, Leverton pointed out that too often, teenagers have been given the message that good nutrition means "eating what you don't like because it's good for you." Rather, they should be told to "eat well, because it will help you in what you want to do and become."[63] This still applies to adolescents today. Teenagers are present-oriented and tend not to be concerned about how their eating will affect them in later years. However, they are concerned about immediate, socially relevant issues such as their physical appearance, achieving and maintaining a healthy weight, and having lots of energy. Many are also interested in optimizing sports performance. Others are concerned with environmental or moral aspects of food. Even though adolescents need to be aware of the long-term risks of an unhealthy diet and benefits of a more healthful one, focusing on the short-term or tangible benefits will have more appeal to them and is more likely to result in behavior change.

## The Home Environment and Parental Involvement

Parents should be targets for nutrition education as well as teenagers, because they fill the role of gatekeepers of foods and serve as role models for eating behavior. Even though parents may have little control over what their teenagers are eating outside the home, they have more control in the home environment. Teenagers tend to eat what is available and convenient. Parents can capitalize on this by stocking the kitchen with a variety of nutritious ready-to-eat foods and limiting the availability of high-sugar, high-fat foods within the home. Research has shown that availability of healthy foods including fruits and vegetables in the home is associated with higher intake of these foods and lower BMI, while availability of unhealthy foods in the home is associated with higher intakes of snack foods and fast foods and lower intakes of fruits and vegetables.[64–66]

Focus groups of parents of teenagers suggest that parents have concerns over whether or not they should involve teens in choosing foods served at meals, prepare alternative foods for teens when they don't like what is served, or restrict intake of specific foods.[67] In general, adolescents should be involved in food purchasing and preparation as often as possible to provide them with food-preparation and decision-making skills. Parents should refrain from offering specially prepared foods for adolescents who do not like what is served, and should instead be encouraged to provide a balanced meal. Research has found that serving adolescents fruits, vegetables, and dairy at dinner time is related to higher intakes of these foods both during adolescence and five years later, during young adulthood.[66] While parental modeling of fruit, vegetable, and dairy intake has not been found to predict adolescent intake of these foods, it has been found to have a longer-term impact, improving intakes of these foods during young adulthood.

## School-Based Education, School Meals, and Wellness Activities

School-based programs can play important roles in promoting lifelong healthy eating and physical activity. Efforts to promote physical activity and healthful eating should be part of a comprehensive, Coordinated School Health (CSH) program and should include school health instruction (curriculum), school physical education, school food service, health services (screening and preventive counseling), school-site health promotion programs for faculty and staff, and integrated community efforts. The Centers for Disease Control and Prevention (CDC) championed this approach in 1987 and have created a developmental framework for comprehensive school nutrition and physical activity programs to be used by school administrators, educators, health professionals, and policy makers (Table 14.11).[68] The guidelines include recommendations to promote healthy eating and lifelong physical activity, including school policies and physical and social environments that encourage and enable physical activity and healthy eating; developmentally appropriate nutrition and physical education curricula and instruction; personnel training; family and community

**TABLE 14.11** School health guidelines to promote healthy eating and physical activity

| | |
|---|---|
| **Guideline 1.** | Use a coordinate approach to develop, implement, and evaluate health eating and physical activity policies and practices. |
| **Guideline 2.** | Establish school environments that support healthy eating and physical activity. |
| **Guideline 3.** | Provide a quality school meal program and ensure that students have only appealing, healthy food and beverage choices offered outside of the school meal program. |
| **Guideline 4.** | Implement a comprehensive physical activity program with quality physical education as the cornerstone. |
| **Guideline 5.** | Implement health education that provides students with the knowledge, skills, and experiences needed for healthy eating and physical activity. |
| **Guideline 6.** | Provide students with health, mental health, and social services to address healthy eating, physical activity, and related chronic disease prevention. |
| **Guideline 7.** | Partner with families and community members in the development and implementation of healthy eating and physical activity policies, practices, and programs. |
| **Guideline 8.** | Provide a school employee wellness program that includes healthy eating and physical activity services for all school staff members. |
| **Guideline 9.** | Employ qualified persons, and provide professional development opportunities for physical education, health education, nutrition services, and health, mental health, and social services staff members, as well as staff member who supervise recess, cafeteria time, and out-of-school-time programs. |

SOURCE: Centers for Disease Control and Prevention, School Health Guidelines to Promote Healthy Eating and Physical Activity. *Morb Mortal Wkly Rep.* (September 16, 2011) / 60(RR05), 1–71.

involvement; and program evaluation. The CDC has also published the School Health Index for Middle School/High School, which can be used when planning and evaluating school health and nutrition programs.[69] This tool will help schools identify strengths and weakness of their specific policies and programs, can help them determine areas for improvement, provides examples for action items that can be incorporated into future plans, and gives guidance on how to engage parents, teachers, students and the broader community in developing comprehensive school health and nutrition services.

The CDC has developed the Whole School, Whole Community, Whole Child (WSCC) model to expand the CSH approach (Illustration 14.5). The WSCC focuses on 10 components of child health, many of which nutrition play key roles in overall adolescent health and wellbeing. For instance, the CDC specifically recommends nutrition and healthy eating as components of a comprehensive school health education curriculum. The WSCC advises that all schools meet Smart Snacks in Schools Nutrition Standards (discussed later in this section) and stresses the need to market healthy foods and beverages and the importance of assuring that school staff role model healthy eating behaviors. The recommendations included for employee wellness focus on healthy eating as a risk reduction strategy for chronic diseases. There are many additional ways in which nutrition can be incorporated into the WSCC model to assure that schools provide healthy eating and nutrition education options for youth, school staff, and families.

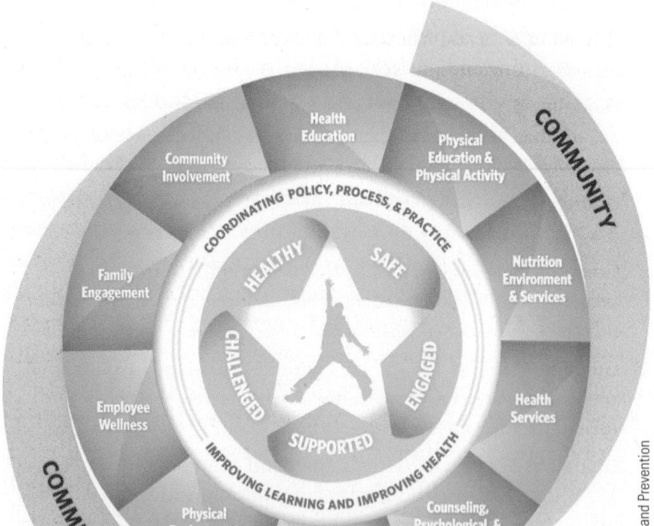

**ILLUSTRATION 14.5** ▸ Whole School, Whole Community, Whole Child Model.

SOURCE: Centers for Disease Control and Prevention, Adolescent and School Health. Available at http://www.cdc.gov/healthyyouth/images/schoolhealth/wsccmodel.png

Centers for Disease Control and Prevention

Schools offer an ideal setting for promoting physical activity through physical education classes. Under half (48 percent) of U.S. adolescents attend a physical education class at least once a week, and only 29 percent attend physical education classes daily.[22] Physical education classes may not offer significant health benefits to some students, as many students spend less than 50 percent of class time being active.[70] Community programs that offer noncompetitive activities where all teens get an opportunity to participate for at least 30 minutes or more are essential to meeting physical activity goals for youth, because most physical activity among adolescents, particularly among females, occurs outside of schools. Activities that allow students to participate fully for most or all of the time include walking, stationary or nonstationary bicycling, hiking, noncompetitive swimming, yoga, zumba and other dance classes, pilates, golf, and tennis. These are also activities that can be done throughout the lifespan, on an individual or group basis.

Nationally, the inclusion of content specific to nutrition and dietary behavior is mentioned in health education policies in 83 percent of middle school and 86 percent of high school district policies.[71] Only violence, alcohol, and drug use prevention were more commonly required, with physical activity being required in similar numbers of high school district health education policies. The mean percentages of school districts that taught specific content related to nutrition and dietary behaviors are listed in Table 14.12.[72]

The 2012 School Health Policies and Practice Survey found that 84 percent of states provided technical assistance to schools in the area of nutrition and dietary behavior education, but only 63 percent of school districts and 74 percent of states provided funding for training related to this topic.[71] This suggests a need for free or low-cost training opportunities for secondary-education health education teachers related to nutrition and eating behaviors. Training may be most effective if teachers have the opportunity to examine their own nutrition and health beliefs, identify their personal body image, and assess their personal eating behaviors. Teacher training typically increases the time spent on teaching nutrition in the classroom.

By high school, students are in the process of cognitive and social development changes that permit more advanced nutrition education concepts and activities. The ability for more abstract thinking, coupled with the changing psychosocial terrain of young adolescents, provides both a challenge and a unique opportunity for educators to offer new learning and teaching strategies to encourage them to make healthful food choices. Early adolescence is an ideal time to teach students how to assess their own behavior and set goals for change. As adolescents begin the social process of individuation, they become ready and eager to make their own decisions and show their individuality. Nutrition education often fails to take advantage of the social

TABLE 14.12 ▸ The mean percentages of school districts that taught specific content related to nutrition and dietary behaviors[72]

| TOPIC | % DISTRICTS |
|---|---|
| Benefits of health eating | 95% |
| Current Dietary Guidelines for Americans | 90% |
| Use of food labels | 90% |
| Balancing food intake and physical activity | 93% |
| Eating more fruits, vegetables, and whole grains | 94% |
| Choosing foods low in total fat, saturated fat, and cholesterol | 92% |
| Using sugars in moderation | 92% |
| Using salt and sodium in moderation | 90% |
| Eating more calcium-rich foods | 86% |
| Food safety | 80% |
| Preparing healthy meals and snacks | 86% |
| Risks of unhealthy weight-control practices | 91% |
| Accepting body size differences | 87% |
| Signs and symptoms for eating disorders | 84% |
| All of the above nutrition and dietary behavior topics | 68% |

SOURCE: Z. Demissie, N. D. Brener, T. McManus, S. L. Shanklin, J. Hawkins, and L. Kann. Results from the School Health Profiles, 2012: Characteristics of Health Programs Among Secondary Schools. Atlanta: Centers for Disease Control and Prevention, 2013. Available at http://www.cdc.gov/healthyyouth/profiles/index.htm.

and cognitive transitions of adolescence to promote the adoption of more healthful behaviors.

Because knowledge alone is inadequate when students must decide which foods to eat and how to deal with peer and social influences, as well as with a widely available supply of high-fat, high-sugar foods, the focus of nutrition education and teaching methods should be on behavior-change strategies and skill acquisitions to make healthful food decisions. Teaching methods found to be most effective in school health education curricula include the following:

- Use of discovery learning
- Use of student learning stations, small work groups, and cooperative learning techniques
- Cross-age and peer teaching
- Positive approaches that emphasize the intrinsic value of good health
- Use of personal commitment to change
- Goal setting
- Provision of opportunities to increase self-efficacy in modifying health behaviors

Most important, adolescents need to be given repeated opportunities to develop, demonstrate, practice, and master the skills needed to make informed decisions and cope with social

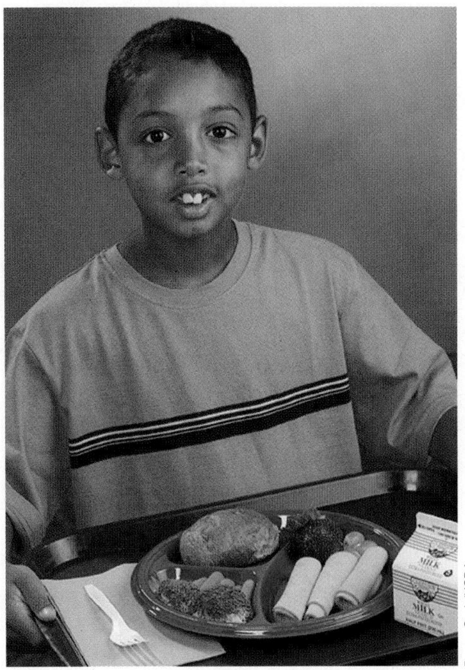


Peggy Greb/USDA

ILLUSTRATION 14.6 ▸ School meals are a significant source of energy and nutrients for adolescents.

influences (Illustration 14.6). To be effective, programs also must take into account cultural factors as well as the developmental processes of adolescents. The integration of technology as a means of assessing and monitoring eating behaviors needs to be encouraged within schools and school districts.

As previously mentioned, teens eat a significant amount of food at school, whether through a la carte choices, vending, school stores, or school meal program offerings. Thus, assuring healthy school food options at schools can have a big impact on the health and nutritional status of adolescents. The National School Lunch Program (NSLP) and School Breakfast Program (SBP) are federally sponsored nutrition programs administered by the U.S. Department of Agriculture (USDA) in conjunction with state and local education agencies. Youth from households with incomes between 130 percent and 185 percent of the poverty level receive meals at reduced rates; youth from households with incomes 130 percent of poverty and below receive meals free of charge.[73] Over 31 million students receive lunch and more than 13 million students receive breakfast through school meals programs each day, in more than 100,000 educational institutions, at an annual cost of about $16 billion.[73] The Healthy, Hunger Free Kids Act of 2010 updated the nutrition standards required for school meals, and for the first time required that all foods and beverages sold to students during regular school hours meet these standards.[74] These nutrition standards are listed in Table 14.13.

In addition to the Smart Snacks requirements, there are food-based requirements for the NSB and NSLP. In accordance with the final rule for nutrition standards published in January 2012, reimbursable meals must provide a minimum amount of specific types of vegetables served

TABLE 14.13 ▸ Nutrition standards for foods sold in schools: "Smart Snacks in Schools"

**Nutrition Standards for Schools**[74]

Any food sold in schools must:

- Be a whole grain-rich product, or
- Have the first ingredient a fruit, a vegetable, a dairy product, or a protein food, or
- Be a combination food that contains at least ¼ cup of fruit and/or vegetable, or
- Contain 10% of the Daily Value of at least one nutrient of public health concern (calcium, potassium, vitamin D, or dietary fiber).

Foods must also meet several nutrient requirements:

- Calorie limits
  - Snack items: ≤200 kcals
  - Entree items: ≤350 kcals
- Sodium limits
  - Snack items: ≤230 mg
  - Entree items: ≤480 mg
- Fat limits
  - Total fat: ≤35% of kcals
  - Saturated fat: <10% of kcals
  - Trans fat: 0 g
- Sugar limit
  - ≤35% by weight of total sugars

**Nutrition Standards for Beverages**

All schools may sell:

- Plain carbonated or uncarbonated water
- Unflavored low-fat milk
- Flavored or unflavored fat-free milk and milk alternatives
- 100% fruit or vegetable juice
- 100% fruit or vegetables juice diluted with water, no added sweeteners

Elementary schools may sell up to 8-oz portions of milk and juice
Middle schools and high schools may sell up to 12-oz portions of milk and juice.
Additional "no calorie" and "lower calorie" beverage option for high school students:

- No more than 20-oz portions of
  - Calorie-free, flavored carbonated or uncarbonated water
  - Flavored and/or carbonated beverages that contain <5 kcals/8 oz or <10 kcals/20 oz
- No more than 12-oz portions of
  - Beverages with ≤40 kcals/8 oz
  - Beverages with ≤60 kcals/12 oz

**Other Requirements**

**Fundraisers**

- The sale of foods and beverages that meet nutrition requirements are not limited.
- The standards do not apply outside of school hours, at off-campus events or on weekends.
- Infrequent fundraising activities may be exempted by state agencies to allow the sale of items that do not meet nutrition standards.

**Accompaniments**

- Items such as salad dressing, butter, cream cheese, and other condiments must be included in the nutrient profile of the food items as sold.

SOURCE: U.S. Department of Agriculture, Food and Nutrition Service. Smart Snacks in School: USDA's "All Foods Sold in Schools" Standards. USDA 2014. Available at http://www.fns.usda.gov/sites/default/files/allfoods_flyer.pdf.

each week (see Table 14.14).[75] Limits on trans fats and sodium were also revised.

Originally enacted in 2006 as part of the Child Nutrition Reauthorization Act, the United States Congress included a provision requiring that all school districts with a federally funded school meals program develop and implement wellness policies that address nutrition and physical activity by the beginning of the 2006–2007 school year (P.L. 108–265). At a minimum, each local policy was to include these benchmarks:

- Goals for nutrition education, physical activity, and other school-based activities that are designed to promote student wellness in a manner that the local educational agency determines is appropriate
- Nutrition guidelines selected by the local educational agency for all foods available on each school campus under the local educational agency during the school day, with the objectives of promoting student health and reducing childhood obesity
- Guidelines for reimbursable school meals
- A plan for measuring implementation of the local wellness policy, including designation of one or more persons within the local educational agency or at each school, as appropriate, charged with operational responsibility for ensuring that each school fulfills the district's local wellness policy
- Community involvement—including parents, students, and representatives of the school food authority, the school board, school administrators, and the public—in the development of the school wellness policy

The Healthy, Hunger-Free Kids Act of 2010 expanded the scope of the school wellness policy requirements, with additional requirements:

- Public updates will be provided on the content and implementation strategies of local policies.
- Physical education teachers and school health professionals will be allowed to become involved with the development of school wellness policies and related activities.

TABLE 14.14 ▸ Nutrition standards and meal patterns in the National School Lunch and School Breakfast Programs, Final Rule, 2012

| | BREAKFAST | | LUNCH | |
|---|---|---|---|---|
| | GRADES 6–8 | GRADES 9–12 | GRADES 6–8 | GRADES 9–12 |
| MEAL PATTERN | AMOUNT PER WEEK (MINIMUM PER DAY) | | | |
| Fruits (cups) | 5 (1) | 5 (1) | 2½ (½) | 5 (1) |
| Vegetables (cups) | 0 | 0 | 3¾ (¾) | 5 (1) |
| Dark Green | 0 | 0 | ½ | ½ |
| Red/Orange | 0 | 0 | ¾ | 1¼ |
| Beans/Peas/Legumes | 0 | 0 | ½ | ½ |
| Starchy | 0 | 0 | ½ | ½ |
| Other | 0 | 0 | ½ | ¾ |
| Additional Vegetables to Reach Total | 0 | 0 | 1 | 1½ |
| Grains (oz/equivalent) | 8–10 (1) | 9–10 (1) | 8–10 (1) | 10–12 (2) |
| Meats/Alternatives (oz/equivalent) | 0 | 0 | 9–10 (1) | 10–12 (2) |
| Fluid Milk (cups) | 5 (1) | 5 (1) | 5 (1) | 5 (1) |
| **Other Requirements: Daily Amount Based on the Average for a 5-Day Week** | | | | |
| Minimum-maximum kcals | 400–500 | 450–600 | 600–700 | 750–850 |
| Saturated fat (% total energy) | <10 | <10 | <10 | <10 |
| Sodium (mg) | ≤470 | ≤500 | ≤710 | ≤740 |
| Trans fat (g/serving) | 0 | 0 | 0 | 0 |

SOURCE: Federal Register. Volume 77, No. 17, Part II. 7 CFR Parts 210 and 220. Nutrition Standards in the National School Lunch and School Breakfast Programs; Final Rule. January 26, 2012.

- All stakeholders will be allowed to participate in the implementation of school wellness policies as well as periodic review and updates of policies.
- School wellness committees periodically (at least once every 3 years) measure progress of the wellness policy:
  - Extent of compliance with USDA regulations
  - How well the local policy compares to model school wellness policies
  - Achievement of goals of local policies
- Committees must designate at least one school official or education agency responsible for assuring compliance with USDA school wellness policy regulations.
- Resources will be made available to local districts and state agencies from the USDA and CDC to assist with the development, implementation and evaluation of school wellness policies.[75]

A promising practice to assist youth in making healthy choices in the lunchroom, which can be implemented as part of a comprehensive school wellness policy, is that of behavioral economics.[76] Sometimes referred to as *nudging*, behavior economics strategies utilize the principle that most people make food choices based on perceptions rather than knowledge. Behavioral economics strategies to improve eating behaviors usually focus on the four "Ps" of marketing: price, placement, promotion and product. Such strategies focus on "making the healthy choice the easy choice." Schools can utilize these "Smart Lunchroom" strategies that are based on behavioral economics principles:

- Place healthy foods at the beginning of food lines and in front of less healthy foods.
- Place less healthy foods just out of reach, making it inconvenient to access them.
- Price healthier food products more competitively and less healthy food items at a higher level.
- Provide healthier food products through a "preorder" or "quick service line" to encourage their selection.
- Promote fruit and salads by serving them in attractive bowls and containers.
- Promote fruits and salads by placing them just before the cash register where students will be waiting and where last-minute "grabs" are made.

Another behavioral economics strategy that has been shown to improve food choices is that of providing foods with interesting and appealing names. Research suggests that students eat twice the amount of carrots given an appealing name compared to those just labeled as carrots or vegetable of the day, with even more robust results for other vegetables such as broccoli and green beans.[77]

The concept of *libertarian paternalism,* which is defined as influencing but not restricting choices in an effort to change behavioral cues, is a key concept of behavioral economics.[76] In this case, students are given a variety of healthy choices, as opposed to only one healthy choice, and are reminded of their ability to still make a choice. Asking students in the lunch line if they'd rather have the baby carrots or roasted beets still provides the student the ability to make a healthy choice, while also assuring that the school meal pattern requirement of a red or orange vegetable is met. Prompting students to make a choice with phrases such as, "Looks like you forgot to take a vegetable. How about trying . . .?" or, "That meals comes with another side. You can grab a piece of fruit or a salad just before you get to the cash register." Such strategies and prompts can be made at home and in food venues outside of schools as well, to encourage healthy food choices in all settings.

## Community Engagement to Create Nutritionally Supportive Environments

Promoting lifelong healthy eating and physical activity behaviors among adolescents requires attention to the multiple behavioral and environmental influences in a community. Adolescents are most likely to adopt healthy behaviors when they receive consistent messages through multiple channels (e.g., community, home, school, and the media) and from multiple sources (e.g., parents, peers, teachers, health professionals, and the media). Because most physical activity occurs outside the school setting, community parks and recreation programs are essential for promoting physical activity among young people. Healthy eating can be integrated into these efforts by providing nutritious snacks, food-preparation activities, and other skill-based learning activities. Community coalitions or task forces can be established to assess community needs and to develop, implement, and evaluate physical activity and nutrition programs for young people. The use of different creative settings and outlets to deliver innovative nutrition education programs to parents to encourage recommended behaviors—including such settings as work sites, places of worship, community centers, libraries, supermarkets, hair and nail salons, shopping centers, housing complexes, and restaurants—should be explored.

One example of a model community-based nutrition intervention program is Urban Roots, located in St Paul, Minnesota. The goal of Urban Roots is to build vibrant, healthy communities through food, conservation and youth development (Illustration 14.7).[78] The program offers three main youth development programs that strive to improve eating behaviors and engage and educate youth:

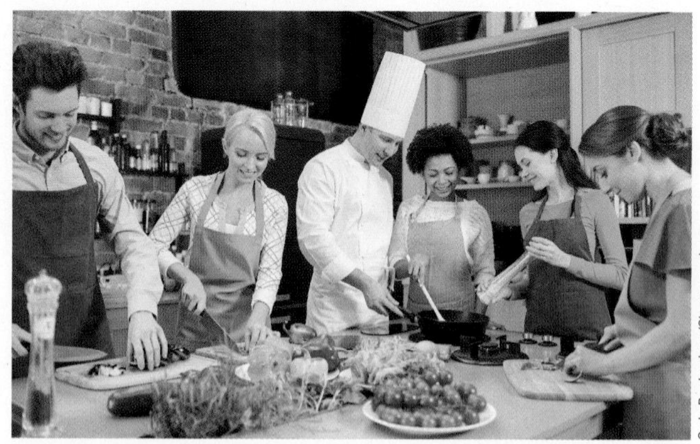

Syda Productions/Shutterstock.com

ILLUSTRATION 14.7 ▸ Reinforcing healthy eating habits through active learning and cooking.

- *The Market Garden Program.* This program offers paid internships to youth who plant, maintain and harvest urban garden plots. The produce is offered for sale to the community through a community supported agriculture (CSA) program and a farmers market stand, is sold to local restaurants, is used in the cooking program, and is donated to local food shelves, in addition to providing produce for the families of the youth involved. Youth learn entrepreneurial and business skills in addition to gardening and growing skills.
- *The Conservation Program.* This program offers paid internships to youth who install and maintain rain gardens, renovate local parks and nature sanctuaries, create attractive streetscapes and work to remove invasive species from native planting areas. Interns and staff also provide classes and activities for elementary- and middle-school aged youth.
- *The Cooking and Wellness Program.* Paid interns and staff teach hands-on cooking classes, provide nutrition education, develop recipes, and provide affordable meals to local residents. Weekly after-school classes are offered for youth and families along with fourth-grade nutrition lessons.

Evaluation data from Urban Roots suggests that the organization provided 45 paid internships to teens and reached over 1420 people in the community in 2011–2012 through education programs and CSA participation.[78] All of the participants reported an increase in knowledge of a healthy lifestyle and could identify at least one action they took as a result of the knowledge they gained through participation in Urban Roots programs. The program offers a blog of their activities, including their Youth Intern Cooking Competition at http://urbanrootsmn.org/blog/. Programs such as Urban Roots show how adolescents can be engaged in activities that promote healthy, sustainable eating habits as well as empower teens to become agents for change in their communities.

## KEY POINTS

1. Rapid rates of physical growth and development experienced by adolescents significantly increase their needs for energy, protein, vitamins, and minerals.
2. Body composition changes dramatically during puberty, with the percentage of body fat increasing among females but decreasing among males.
3. Adolescents will not fully develop abstract reasoning and critical thinking skills until late in adolescence or early adulthood; therefore, nutrition education messages should be simple and concrete, and should relate to activities common in their current everyday lives.
4. Snacking among adolescents is extremely common, and provides a significant proportion of daily energy and nutrient intakes.
5. Meal skipping is common during adolescence, with breakfast the most commonly skipped meal.
6. Family meals provide many benefits, including improved dietary intake, better academic performance, and reduced risk for substance use.
7. Only 27 percent of teens meet the current physical activity guidelines and 15 percent report no physical activity on an average day.
8. Soft drinks and sweetened beverages provide approximately 9 percent of the daily energy intake and 45 percent of added sugars in the diets of adolescents.
9. School environments play a major role in shaping the dietary habits of teens. Strong school food standards and comprehensive school health guidelines help assure that school eating and physical activity environments mirror national recommendations. The use of behavioral economics principles can help assure students frequently make healthy choices.

## REVIEW QUESTIONS

1. Which of the following is considered a risk factor for low vitamin D status?
   a. Dark skin pigmentation
   b. Light skin pigmentation
   c. Low calcium intake
   d. High calcium intake
2. Sexual maturation rating is a method of determining when adolescents have completed menarche or spermarche.
   _____ True _____ False
3. Which of the following factors contributes to increased iron needs among adolescents?
   a. Increased growth velocity during puberty
   b. Low dietary intake of iron
   c. Onset of menarche
   d. All of the above
4. School wellness policies are only required for schools that offer à la carte foods for sale.
   _____ True _____ False
5. The nutrients most likely to be missing from the diets of vegan adolescents are:
   a. Vitamins A, D, E, iron, and zinc
   b. Vitamins B6, D, B12, iron, and calcium
   c. Vitamins B6, B12, E, zinc and choline
   d. Vitamins A, D, E, folate, and iron
6. Which of the following is NOT a behavioral economics strategy to improve food choices?
   a. Competitive pricing of healthy foods
   b. Hanging MyPlate posters in the cafeteria
   c. Placing fruit in attractive bowls
   d. Creating quick food lines that offer salads and vegetarian entrees
7. What is biological age (SMR) and why should it be used instead of chronological age to determine adolescent nutrient needs?

   Biological age is based on sexual maturation rating. It assesses the degree of physical development, which can vary greatly among individuals of the same gender and age, thus is a better indicator of the nutrient needs of individuals as it provides a physiological estimate of needs based on growth velocity, body composition, and reproductive capacity.
8. Which of the following is a result of eating family meals most days of the week?
   a. Higher intake of fruits and vegetables
   b. Less risk of drug and alcohol use
   c. Better academic performance
   d. All of the above
9. Which of the following pieces of legislation determines components of school wellness policy guidelines?
   a. Child Nutrition and WIC Reauthorization Act
   b. School Health Programs and Policies
   c. Whole School Whole Community Whole Child
   d. Healthy, Hunger-Free Kids Act

Visit www.cengagebrain.com to access MindTap, a complete digital course that includes additional resources.

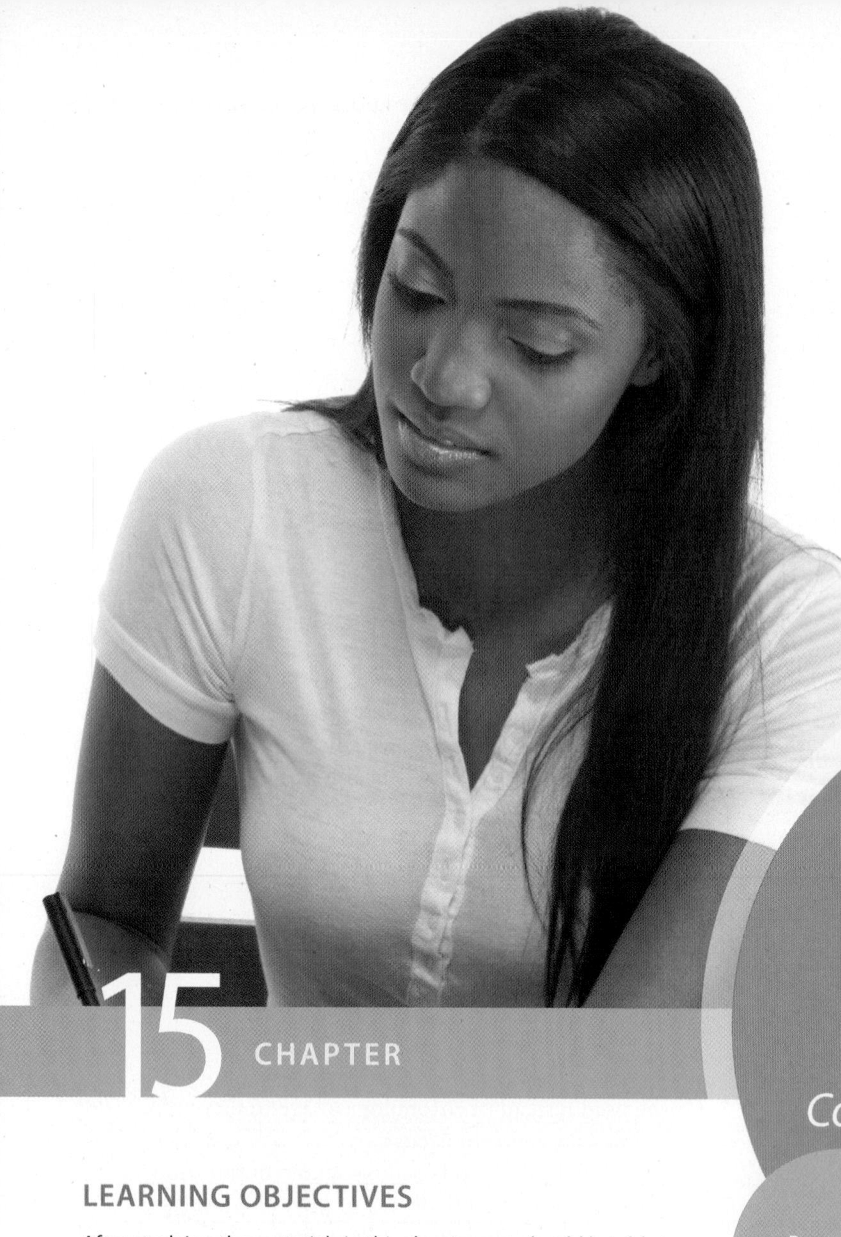

15 CHAPTER

# Adolescent Nutrition: *Conditions and Interventions*

*Prepared by*
Jamie Stang

OLJ Studio/Shutterstock.com

## LEARNING OBJECTIVES

After studying the materials in this chapter, you should be able to:

**15.1** Describe at least five chronic health issues that are considered comorbid conditions of adolescent obesity, including the proposed mechanisms by which obesity raises the risk for these conditions.

**15.2** Determine the unique energy, protein, and micronutrient needs of competitive adolescent athletes who have not yet completed growth and development.

**15.3** Compare and contrast national dietary recommendations to prevent and treat hypertension and hyperlipidemia in adolescents.

**15.4** Differentiate between disordered eating behaviors and eating disorders based on frequency and severity of symptoms and anticipated outcomes.

# Introduction

Multiple factors influence the nutritional needs and behaviors of adolescents. This chapter presents specific nutrition concerns that affect significant numbers of adolescents, including overweight, participation in competitive sports, substance abuse, eating disorders, hypertension and hyperlipidemia. Because overweight, sports participation, and eating disorders affect a larger group of adolescents than other conditions, they are presented in greater detail.

# Overweight and Obesity

**LO 15.1** Describe at least five chronic health issues that are considered comorbid conditions of adolescent obesity, including the proposed mechanisms by which obesity raises the risk for these conditions.

The increase in the prevalence of overweight and obesity among adolescents has nearly doubled during the past two decades. Exact reasons for this increase have not been identified. Environmental factors, or interactions between genetic and environmental factors, are the most likely causes of the dramatic rise in overweight and obesity. Risk factors for the development of overweight and obesity among children and adolescents include having at least one overweight or obese parent; low socioeconomic status; being of African American, Hispanic, or American Indian/Native Alaskan race/ethnicity; and being diagnosed with a chronic or disabling condition that limits mobility.[1] Inadequate levels of physical activity and consuming diets high in total calories and added sugars and fats are behavioral risk factors common among a significant proportion of adolescents.[2] These environmental factors increase the risk of developing obesity if an adolescent is genetically predisposed to obesity.

Weight status among adolescents should be assessed by calculating body mass index (BMI). BMI is calculated by dividing a person's weight (kg) by his or her height$^2$ (m$^2$). The Centers for Disease Control and Prevention has an online BMI calculator (available at http://nccd.cdc.gov/dnpabmi/Calculator.aspx) that can be used to quickly and accurately calculate BMI values for youth. BMI values are compared to age- and gender-appropriate percentiles to determine the appropriateness of the individual's weight for height. Youth with BMI values greater than the 85th but lower than the 95th percentile are considered overweight; those with BMI values above the 95th percentile are considered obese.[2] Growth curves based on BMI values for children and adolescents are available from the National Center for Health Statistics. An example of a BMI growth curve is shown in Illustration 15.1.

Data from the 2009–2010 National Health and Nutrition Examination Survey (NHANES) suggest that 34 percent of U.S. adolescents are overweight and 18 percent are obese.[3] Table 15.1 provides prevalence estimates of overweight among adolescents in the United States, by gender and race/ethnicity. In general, the prevalence of being overweight or obese among females is highest among Black teens, while among males the prevalence is highest among Mexican American teens. Data on American Indian youth are not available through NHANES or the Youth Risk Behavioral Surveillance (YRBS) survey, but regional surveillance data suggest that 20% of urban American Indian children are obese and 48 percent of American Indian male and 46 percent of American Indian females between 5 and 17 years olds are overweight or obese.[3,4]

The persistence of overweight from childhood throughout adulthood has not been well quantified. Research suggests that the persistence of obesity from infancy to adulthood increases with age. As many as 90 percent of

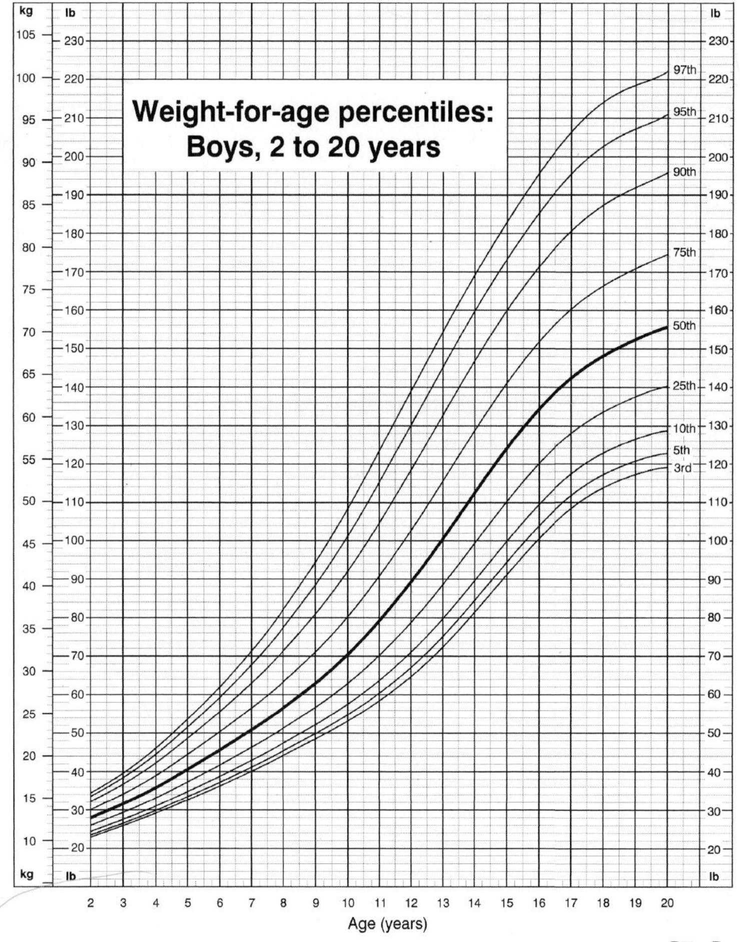


ILLUSTRATION 15.1 ▸ CDC Growth Charts: United States.

Developed by the National Center for Health Statistics in collaboration with the National Center for Chronic Disease Prevention and Health Promotion, 2000.

**TABLE 15.1** ▸ Prevalence of at-risk-for overweight and overweight by race and gender among 12- to 19-year-olds in NHANES 2009–2010

| | OVERWEIGHT | OBESE |
|---|---|---|
| **Males** | | |
| White | 32.2 | 17.5 |
| Black | 37.4 | 22.6 |
| Hispanic | 42.9 | 23.9 |
| Male Total | 34.6 | 19.6 |
| **Females** | | |
| White | 27.6 | 14.7 |
| Black | 45.1 | 24.8 |
| Hispanic | 41.9 | 19.8 |
| Female Total | 32.6 | 17.1 |

SOURCE: All data taken from Ogden, CL, Carroll MD, Kit, BK, Flegal, KM. Prevalence of Obesity and Trends in Body Mass Index in U.S. Children and Adolescents, 1999–2010. JAMA 2012; 307(5): 483–490.

overweight adolescents can be expected to remain overweight into adulthood.[5] Identification of overweight at an early age is important, as research data suggest that children with BMI above the 85th percentile are more than twice as likely as children with BMI below the 50th percentile to continue to gain weight and reach overweight status by adolescence.[1,5] The risk of persistence of obesity from childhood into adulthood increases if at least one parent is overweight.[5] The risk of persistence of overweight is also higher among the most overweight individuals, especially those whose weight is more than 180 percent of ideal weight.

## Health Implications of Adolescent Overweight and Obesity

A range of medical and psychosocial complications accompanies overweight among adolescents, including hypertension, dyslipidemia, insulin resistance, type 2 diabetes mellitus, sleep apnea and other hypoventilation disorders, orthopedic problems, hepatic diseases, body image disturbances, and lowered self-esteem.[6,7] Longitudinal studies of obesity and chronic disease risk among youth suggest an increased risk of morbidity and premature mortality from coronary heart disease, stroke, diabetes, asthma, and hypertension among adults who were overweight or obese during adolescence.[7]

## Assessment and Treatment of Adolescent Overweight and Obesity

All adolescents should be screened for appropriateness of weight-for-height on a yearly basis, or more frequently if concerns about excessive weight gain are present. Teens with multiple risk factors for obesity require an in-depth medical assessment to diagnose potential co-morbid complications.[2] Illustration 15.2 provides recommended screening and referral procedures for adolescents with a BMI ≥ 85th percentile for age and gender.

National guidelines for the treatment of child and adolescent overweight and obesity recommend a staged care process based on BMI, co-morbid conditions, age, and progress with previous stages of treatment.[8] Adolescents advance through the stages based on age, biological development, presence of co-morbid conditions, and success with previous stages of treatment (see Table 15.2). A brief overview of the stages is included below.

**Stage 1: Prevention Plus** Adolescents with BMI of ≥85th but <95th percentile may start out in Stage 1 if they do not exhibit significant co-morbid conditions and/or have not completed their adolescent growth spurt.[8] This level of treatment builds upon basic nutrition and physical activity guidance recommended to promote health and prevent disease for all youth. Specific topics that should be included as components of Stage 1 obesity treatment include consumption of at least 5 servings of fruits and vegetables per day, limiting sweetened-beverage consumption, achieving at least 60 minutes of physical activity per day, and limiting screen time (including DVDs, Internet, television, and computer or video games) to no more than 2 hours of non-academic time per day. Additional nutrition issues that may be addressed in

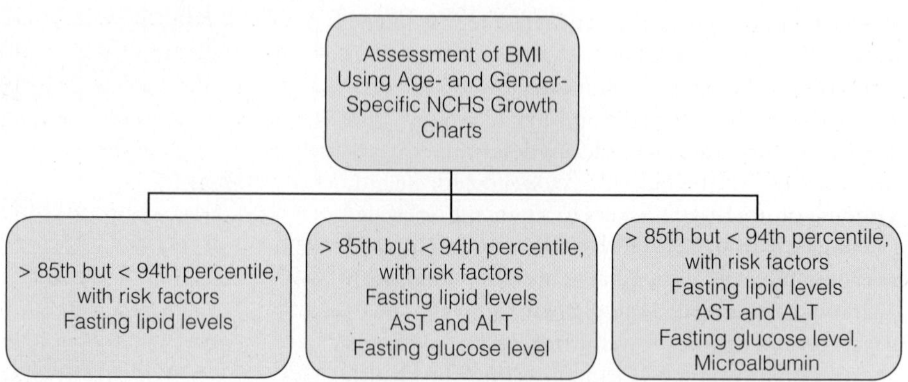


**ILLUSTRATION 15.2** ▸ Primary care assessments based on adolescent BMI.

TABLE 15.2 ▸ How BMI is calculated and interpreted for children and teens

Calculating and interpreting BMI using the BMI Percentile Calculator involves the following steps:

1. Before calculating BMI, obtain accurate height and weight measurements. See Measuring Children's Height and Weight Accurately At Home. (www.cdc.gov/healthyweight/assessing/bmi/childrens_bmi/about_childrens_bmi.html)
2. Calculate the BMI and percentile using the Child and Teen BMI Calculator (http://nccd.cdc.gov/dnpabmi/Calculator.aspx). The BMI number is calculated using standard formulas (www.cdc.gov/healthyweight/assessing/bmi/childrens_bmi/about_childrens_bmi.html).
3. Review the calculated BMI-for-age percentile and results. The BMI-for-age percentile is used to interpret the BMI number because BMI is both age-and sex-specific for children and teens. These criteria are different from those used to interpret BMI for adults—which do not take into account age or sex. Age and sex are considered for children and teens for two reasons:
   - The amount of body fat changes with age. (BMI for children and teens is often referred to as BMI-for-age.)
   - The amount of body fat differs between girls and boys.

   The CDC BMI-for-age growth charts for girls and boys (www.cdc.gov/growthcharts) take into account these differences and allow translation of a BMI number into a percentile for a child's or teen's sex and age.
4. Find the weight status category for the calculated BMI-for-age percentile as shown in the following chart. These categories are based on expert committee recommendations.

| Weight Status Category | Percentile Range |
|---|---|
| Underweight | Less than the 5th percentile |
| Healthy weight | 5th percentile to less than the 85th percentile |
| Overweight | 85th to less than the 95th percentile |
| Obese | Equal to or greater than the 95th percentile |

The CDC BMI-for-age growth charts are available at: CDC Growth Charts: United States (hht://www.cdc.gov.nchs/about/major/nhanes/growthcharts/charts.htm).

SOURCE: Centers for Disease Control and Prevention, from http://www.cdc.gov/healthyweight/assessing/bmi/childrens_bmi/about_childrens_bmi.html#How%20is%20BMI%20calculated.

Stage 1 include the importance of daily breakfast consumption, limiting take-out and restaurant meals (including fast food), participating in family meals at least 5 times per week, and encouraging youth to self-regulate their intake. Stage 1 treatment can be provided by a single healthcare provider, including physicians, nurses, physician assistants, nurse practitioners, dietitians, and other allied healthcare providers who have training in pediatric weight management.[8]

**Stage 2: Structured Weight Management** The second stage of pediatric weight management addresses the same behaviors as Stage 1, but does so in a more structured manner. Monitoring of food and nutrition behaviors by the adolescent and/or their parent(s) is a key component of this stage.[8] All of the goals of Stage 1 should be reinforced, but several are modified in Stage 2. Screen time is limited to < 1 hour per day in this stage, and a meal plan is introduced to emphasize nutrient-dense food choices while minimizing energy-dense foods. Journals or log books may be provided for monitoring target behaviors. Achievement of goals should be rewarded with nonfood items such as new clothing or jewelry or tickets to a concert or event.[8]

Stage 2 can be offered by a health care provider with training in behavioral pediatric weight management. Skills required to successfully implement this stage of treatment include motivational counseling, monitoring and reinforcement, and family conflict resolution.[8] Referrals for physical therapy, mental health counseling, and medical nutrition therapy may be necessary for some adolescents with significant co-morbidities. Monthly follow-up and assessment of progress is suggested.

**Stage 3: Comprehensive Multidisciplinary Intervention** Stage 3 targets the same behavioral goals as Stage 2, but does so in a more structured, multidisciplinary format with more frequent client contact. This treatment stage is provided by a team of healthcare professionals who specialize in pediatric obesity management. A detailed eating and physical activity plan that is designed to lead to negative caloric balance is implemented in this phase.[8] A structured behavior-modification program is recommended, with weekly visits for at least 8–12 weeks followed by bimonthly or more frequent contact with the adolescent and his or her family. The recommended membership of the multidisciplinary team includes a physician, physician assistant or pediatric nurse practitioner; a behavioral health specialist, social worker, or mental health counselor; a registered dietitian; an exercise physiologist or physical therapist; and a nurse.

**Stage 4: Tertiary Care Intervention** The use of Stage 4 treatment is appropriate with severely obese teens or those who have significant, chronic co-morbid conditions that necessitate intensive intervention.[8] Adolescents should be evaluated for their level of maturity to be sure they are able to understand the high level of commitment required as well as the potential risks associated with Stage 4 treatment. This level of treatment is provided through a tertiary weight management center that specializes in adolescent obesity; access to these programs may be limited outside of large metropolitan areas. In addition to diet and activity counseling and behavior modification, more intensive treatments such as meal replacement, a very-low-energy diet, medication, and surgery may be implemented. These treatments are particularly warranted when multiple co-morbid conditions or potentially life-threatening conditions such as pseudotumor cerebri occur.

Few data on the effectiveness of very-low-energy diets or meal replacements are available; however, these measures appear to be safely used for short periods of time.[8] The use of very-low-calorie diets or protein-sparing modified fasts should only be done under continuous medical supervision, as these diets have been associated with many health risks, including orthostatic hypotension, diarrhea, hyperuricemia, cholelithiasis, electrolyte imbalance, and reduced serum protein levels.[9] The use of these diets should not exceed 12 weeks in duration.

**Weight Loss Medication** There is currently only one medication that have been FDA-approved for use by adolescents: orlistat, an pancreatic lipase inhibitor that causes fat malabsorption.[10] Approved for use by youth 12 years and older, side effects include steatorrhea, flatulence, fecal incontinence, and fat-soluble vitamin deficiencies.[10] The gastrointestinal side effects may be reduced among adolescents who successfully follow a low-fat diet. The use of a multivitamin supplement is recommended due to reductions in fat soluble vitamin absorption. Results of trials with orlistat on improvements in weight status, insulin sensitivity and lipid profiles are mixed.[10] While some trials have shown significant differences in weight loss among teens who took orlistat while implementing lifestyle (diet and physical activity) changes, others have shown no differences and have attributed weight loss primarily to the lifestyle changes.[10] Long-term follow-up data on the effectiveness of orlistat on weight status is lacking.

Metformin, a drug commonly used to address insulin resistance and diabetes, is often used as an off-label (non-FDA approved) treatment for obesity in youth over 10 years of age.[10] Metformin reduces hepatic glucose production, reduces glucose absorption by the intestines, increases insulin sensitivity, inhibits fat cell formation and may reduce food intake.[10] Data from clinical trials suggests that metformin improves weight loss and glucose control over lifestyle changes alone, however results varied among studies based on initial degree of insulin sensitivity and racial/ethnic background.

**Surgical Weight Loss** Gastric bypass has been used for several decades to treat severely obese adolescents who were not successful with behavior modification and lifestyle changes. Guidelines for the use of bariatric surgery among adolescents have been published (Table 15.3).[11,12] In order to be considered as a candidate for bariatric surgery, adolescents must have a BMI of >35 with medical major complications or a BMI of >40 with minor

**TABLE 15.3** Recommendations for consideration of bariatric surgery in adolescents

- Failure to obtain adequate weight loss after minimum of 6 months of intensive weight loss program participation.
- SMR/Tanner is at stage IV or higher or 95% of adult physical maturity.
- BMI ≥35 with major medical co-morbidities or ≥40 with mild comorbidities.
- Strong indications for bariatric surgery in adolescents include major comorbidities, including:
    - type 2 diabetes
    - moderate to severe obstructive sleep apnea
    - Nonalcoholic fatty liver disease
    - Pseudotumor cerebri
- Mild comorbid conditions that may indicate a need for bariatric surgery include:
    - mild obstructive sleep apnea
    - mild nonalcoholic fatty liver disease
    - hypertension
    - dyslipidemia
    - significantly impaired quality of life
- Candidate participates in psychological and medical counseling before surgery with agreement to continue counseling after surgery.
- Candidate must have adequate support of family and a home environment conducive to long-term dietary change.
- Candidate has the capability to follow medical nutrition therapy protocol after surgery.
- Candidate agrees to prevent pregnancy for at least 1 year after surgery.
- Roux-en-Y gastric bypass should be considered safe and effective.
- Adjustable gastric banding and laparoscopic sleeve gastrectomy should be considered investigative and are not currently approved for use among adolescents in the United States by the FDA.
- Biliopancreatic diversion and duodenal switch surgical procedures are not recommended in adolescents due to the risk of malnutrition and potential effects on growth, development, and reproductive outcomes.

SOURCES: Based on American Pediatric Surgical Association Clinical Task Force on Bariatric Surgery 2004; Pratt, J. S. A., Lenders, C. M., Dionne, E. A., et al. 2009. Best practice updates for pediatric/adolescent weight loss surgery. *Obesity* 17: 901–910; Ibele, A. R., Mattar, S. G. 2011. Adolescent bariatric surgery. *Surg Clin N Am* 91: 1339–1351.

co-morbidities. In addition, teens should have completed the majority of their adolescent growth spurt before undergoing bariatric surgery in order to minimize potential side effects such as stunting of growth. Once the adolescent growth spurt is completed, nutrient needs are reduced, so it is less likely that nutrient deficiencies will occur among adolescents who have limited food intakes following bariatric surgery. The two most commonly performed procedures for adolescents in the United States are the adjustable gastric band and the Roux-en-Y gastric bypass procedures, though the adjustable gastric band has not been approved by the FDA for use in individuals under 18 years of age.[12] Sleeve gastrectomy is a surgical option that some bariatric surgery centers are offering to extremely obese adolescents.

The long-term success rate of bariatric surgery among teens is not well established. Research suggests that adolescents had an mean estimated weight loss of 15 percent to 87 percent following bariatric surgery.[11] Complications occur in up to 27 percent or more of patients; however, mortality is rare.[11] A meta-analysis of adjustable gastric banding outcomes among adolescents suggests that 8 percent of teens experience complications requiring further surgery, with the most common issue being band slippage.[13] Iron deficiency was noted in 2 percent of adolescents following gastric banding.[13] A study of one-year outcomes following bariatric surgery among adolescents found that two of the 30 patients began regaining weight within the first year following surgery, with one adolescent regaining more than 50 percent of lost body weight.[14]

Detailed recommendations for pre- and post-operative nutrition recommendations specific to adolescents have been published.[15] The post-operative diet is high in protein and modest in fat content to preserve lean body mass. Sugars and simple carbohydrates should be avoided or severely limited to reduce the risk of diarrhea secondary to high osmolarity.[15] Supplementation with multivitamin/mineral preparations following bariatric surgery is imperative for adolescents. While all nutrients may require supplementation when food intake is severely limited following surgery, nutrients that are particularly important to assess and monitor include: protein; iron; calcium; vitamins D, $B_6$, $B_{12}$; thiamin; and folic acid.[13–15] The risk of dehydration is elevated following bariatric surgery due to the restricted stomach capacity as well as nausea and vomiting, thus fluid intake should be closely monitored.

# Supplement Use Among Adolescents

## Vitamin/Mineral Supplements

Supplements may be used by adolescents for a variety of reasons, including improving health, treating iron deficiency, increasing energy, building muscle, and losing weight. National data suggest that more than 28% of adolescents consume vitamin/mineral supplements, while studies in Canada show a prevalence of vitamin/mineral use of 43 percent.[16,17] More than half of adolescents who report using vitamin/mineral supplements take them occasionally, with slightly less than half using them daily. Approximately half of vitamin/mineral supplements consumed by adolescents are multivitamins without minerals, 34 percent are individual vitamins or minerals, 18 percent are multivitamins with minerals, and 17 percent are iron with vitamin C tablets.[17–19] Among the individual nutrient supplements used, vitamin C is the most common, followed by calcium, iron, vitamin E, and B-vitamin complex.[18,19]

Data on demographic differences in adolescent supplement use are apparent; supplement use is directly correlated with household income, high food-security status, having some form of health insurance, and parental education.[16–19] Adolescents who take vitamin/mineral supplements tend to consume a more nutritionally adequate diet than those who don't.[16,18-19] Supplement use is also directly correlated with health behaviors such as meeting physical activity goals, consuming more fruits and vegetables, and spending less than 2 hours per day watching television, playing video games, or using a computer. BMI status and intakes of total and saturated fat and cholesterol are negatively correlated with supplement use.

Few data are available to quantify the use of nonnutritional supplements such as herbs (including herbal weight-loss products) among adolescents. Data suggest that as many as 29 percent of U.S. teens may use herbal products.[19,20] A study of 353 teens from Canada found that 4 percent of adolescents used herbal weight-control products, 6 percent used energizers (e.g., bee pollen), 2 percent used L-carnitine, and 5 percent used creatine.[17] Adolescents who use herbal supplements have been found to be more likely to engage in health-compromising behaviors, such as the use of cigarettes, marijuana, alcohol, and other street drugs.[20]

The use of herbs and supplements by youth is highly controversial. Adolescents may take herbal supplements for several reasons, including weight loss, treatment of attention deficit disorder, and to increase energy and stamina. Youth with special health care needs, such as autism spectrum disorders, attention deficit disorder, and cystic fibrosis, may use supplements more frequently than other adolescents. Teens may also use herbal supplements to help them lose weight, build muscle, or improve athletic performance. Studies are needed to determine exactly what types of herbal products are used by adolescents, because many herbs are known to have potentially dangerous side effects, and few recommendations are available to guide the use of herbs by children or adolescents.

## Ergogenic Supplements Used by Teens

Youth Risk Behavior Surveillance (YRBS) system data suggest that 3 percent of adolescents report having used steroids without medical supervision.[21] Steroid use is reported more frequently among male (4 percent) than female (2 percent) adolescents, and appears to decrease with age, peaking during ninth grade.[21] Other U.S. data suggest that the use of muscle-enhancing supplements may be higher, with 6 percent of males and 5 percent of females using them.[22-24] International data suggest that up to 91 percent of elite adolescent athletes use dietary supplements to enhance athletic performance.[23,24] Steroids and other ergogenic supplements are taken orally, injected, or absorbed through transdermal patches.[21,22] The most common sources of ergogenic aids are parents and coaches.[23] Supplements used by adolescent athletes include creatine; individual amino acids or protein powders; dextrose; caffeine; carnitine; anabolic-androgenic steroids; anabolic steroid precursors, including dehydroepiandrosterone (DHEA) and androstenedione; beta-hydroxy-beta-methylbutyrate; growth hormone; Xenadrine; and ephedra.[21-23] They are most often used outside of the direct sport season to avoid detection of use in situations where urine testing may be used.

Anabolic-androgenic steroids are controlled substances used to increase lean body mass and improve strength.[24] Steroids and ergogenic supplements are often taken in 1- to 3-month periods and are "stacked" so that the peak dose of one substance may overlap the introduction of another substance.[24] While the use of steroids and ergogenic aids is forbidden by national and NCAA regulations, few high school athletic programs test athletes for their use. The use of these steroids has been linked to infertility, hypertension, physeal closure, depression, aggression, and increased risk of atherosclerosis.[24]

DHEA and androstenedione are precursors of testosterone and estrogen. Androstenedione is also a controlled substance, while DHEA is widely available as a supplement.[24] Naturally produced in the human body by the adrenal glands, DHEA levels fall in humans as age increases. Its reputed effects include reducing body fat, decreasing insulin resistance, increasing immune system function, increasing lean body mass, and decreasing risk of osteoporosis; however, no scientific evidence backs such claims.[24] As steroid precursors, androstenedione and DHEA may induce many of the same side effects as steroids, such as irreversible gynecomastia (breast enlargement) and prostate enlargement among males and hirsutism (facial hair) among females.[24,25] As many as 4 percent of adolescents take androstenedione.[25]

Growth hormone (GH) has been shown to decrease subcutaneous body fat and may strengthen ligaments and tendons, resulting in fewer injuires.[24] Side effects of its use include physeal closure, hyperlipidemia, glucose intolerance, and myopathy.[24] Few data are available on the use of GH by adolescents, as it is a substance available only by prescription for the treatment of growth disorders in youth. The extent of illegal use of GH among adolescents is unknown. Given the possibility of significant side effects in pubescent adolescents undergoing hormonal changes, steroids or their precursors and GH should not be used by adolescents.

Creatine is sold as a nutritional supplement to increase lean body mass. Creatine, formed in the liver and kidney of the human body, can be obtained in more than adequate amounts from the consumption of meat. Eleven percent or more of adolescent athletes report the use of creatine; however, the prevalence among male athletes has been found to be as high as 51 percent.[25] Creatine use has been found to be most prevalent in athletes who are involved with football, gymnastics, hockey, wrestling, and baseball. Studies of creatine use in adults show mixed results; data on adolescent performance are sparse.[26] It appears to be of minimal benefit to endurance athletes, and marginal benefit to those involved in short-duration, anaerobic, strength-related sports.[26] Side effects of creatine use, which seem to be dose-related, include abdominal pain and cramping, nausea, diarrhea, headache, dehydration, reduced renal function, increased tendency toward muscle strains, and muscle soreness.[24,25] No available data document the long-term health effects related to creatine use; however, chronic use may be associated with renal damage.[24-26]

Ephedrine was sold as an over-the-counter supplement until 2004, when the FDA banned its sale. While it has been proven to increase metabolic rate, no known benefits on athletic performance have been documented.[24] Ephedrine was removed from the market due to side effects including cardiac arrhythmia, hypertension, increased risk of myocardial infarction and cerebral vascular accidents, and, in extreme cases, death. Ephedrine use has been reported to be at high as 26 percent among female and 12 percent among male adolescents.[25]

# Nutrition for Adolescent Athletes

LO 15.2 Determine the unique energy, protein, and micronutrient needs of competitive adolescent athletes who have not yet completed growth and development.

More than half (54 percent) of U.S. adolescents report playing on one or more organized sports teams through their school or a community organization.[21] Participation is higher among male adolescents than female adolescents (60 percent versus 49 percent) and reduces with age. White and Black adolescents report participation in organized sports more often than do Hispanic students.

High levels of physical activity, combined with growth and development, increase adolescents' needs for energy, protein, and select vitamins and minerals. Participation in competitive sports often means an adolescent will participate in intense training and competition during an athletic season. If the athlete competes in several sports, energy and nutrient needs will remain relatively stable throughout the year. If an athlete participates in only one sport and does not maintain a training routine off-season, energy and nutrient needs may fluctuate based on the timing of the sports season. Therefore, adolescents must be assessed for seasonal and yearly physical activity when energy and nutrient needs are determined.

The energy and nutrient needs of adolescent athletes vary widely. Many of the recommendations available are based on needs of young adult athletes or are extrapolated from usual nutrient needs of adolescents. The best method of assessing the nutrient needs of athletes is to begin with general dietary needs based on Sexual Maturation Rating (SMR, see Chapter 14), adding additional allowances based on the unique needs of the individual and the intensity of physical activity he or she engages in. In order to assess individual nutrient needs, health care professionals must gather information such as the following:

- What sport(s) does the adolescent engage in, and what is the duration of the competition season?
- What is the level of competition of the adolescent? Is participation recreational, competitive, or elite?
- What kind of training does the adolescent engage in? The method(s), intensity, and duration of training activities should be noted.
- Does the athlete typically sweat profusely or lose body weight during competition? Weighing before and after practice and competition is a good idea, especially during outdoor activities in hot and humid weather or in cases where gear may cause sweating (e.g., hockey goalies).
- Does the athlete follow a special diet or take supplements to improve athletic performance? The type, amount, and frequency of supplement use should be noted and counseling provided as necessary.

General energy and protein needs are discussed in Chapter 14. These guidelines should provide the foundation for calculating protein and energy needs for athletes. Competitive athletes may require 500–1500 additional calories per day to meet their energy needs. Athletes and their parents should be encouraged to monitor weight stability throughout the sports season. During the season, particularly during intense training phases or at the beginning of a season, athletes should weigh themselves before and after practice and sporting events. Any change in body weight during the activity signals a loss of body water, which could lead to dehydration. Any weight loss that is not transient (transient losses are often due to dehydration) signifies that the caloric intake is inadequate to support growth and development. A thorough assessment of energy and protein intakes, accompanied by measurements of body composition, should be taken when unexpected weight loss occurs. Protein should supply no more than 30 percent of calories in the diet. Groups at risk for inadequate intake would include athletes who follow vegan diets or restrict caloric intake to maintain a particular weight. When the main sources of protein are plant-based, additional protein intake may be needed because plant-based sources of protein may be less bioavailable.

Dietary intakes of athletes should follow the MyPlate recommendations, with the realization that the increased energy needs of athletes may require them to consume the upper limit of food-group recommendations. Athletes should be encouraged to eat a pre-event meal at least two to three hours prior to exercise; eating too close to exercise may lead to indigestion and physical discomfort.[27,28] Table 15.4 provides an overview of meal and snack recommendations for adolescent athletes. Foods that are high in fat, protein, and/or dietary fiber should be avoided for at least four hours prior to exercise, because they take longer to digest and may cause physical discomfort during exercise. Protein and fat also displace complex carbohydrates, which are the most readily available source of energy during athletic events. Post-event meals should contain approximately 400–600 calories and should comprise high-carbohydrate foods and adequate amounts of noncaffeinated fluids.[27]

**Calcium** Calcium intakes have been shown to be below the DRIs in a significant proportion of adolescents, especially females. Athletes' increased risk for bone fractures makes adequate calcium intake extremely important.[27] Although

**TABLE 15.4** Recommendations for food and beverage prior to sports events

| MEAL/SNACK COMPOSITION | TIMING | EXAMPLES OF RECOMMENDED FOODS AND BEVERAGES |
|---|---|---|
| Snack with 15–20 g CHO and <5% of energy from fat | 30–60 mins prior to event | Cereal bar, water, and ½ cup juice |
| Light meal with 30–40 g CHO and 5% to 15% of energy from fat | 2–4 hours before event | Turkey and cheese sandwich, ½ C grapes, water, 1 cup lemonade |
| Full meal with 50–60 g CHO and 15% to 25% of energy from fat | 4–5 hours prior to event | Roasted chicken, mashed potatoes, ½ cup carrots, small banana, and water OR peanut butter and jelly sandwich, 1 cup low-fat milk, 1 orange, water |

Based on: Holt, K., Wooldridge, N., Story, M., and Sofka, D., eds. (2011). *Bright Futures Nutrition*. 3rd ed. Elk River, IL: American Academy of Pediatrics, pp. 186.

the mechanism responsible for this tendency has not been identified, female adolescent athletes with low calcium consumption appear to be the highest-risk group of all adolescents for bone fractures, and they therefore should make every effort to consume adequate calcium in their diets. Teen athletes who cannot or will not consume calcium from dietary sources should be counseled to take a daily calcium supplement that meets their daily requirements.

**Fluid Level and Dehydration** Fluid intake is an important issue in sports nutrition for adolescents. Young adolescents and those who are prepubertal present a particular vulnerability to heat illnesses because their bodies do not regulate body temperature as well as those of older adolescents.[27,28] Adolescents can become so mentally and physically involved in physical activities that they do not pay attention to physiological signals of fluid loss, such as excessive sweating and thirst. Some athletes commonly assume they do not need additional fluids if they are not actively moving all of the time during exercise. Other factors, such as ambient temperature and humidity levels and weight of equipment (helmets, padding, etc.) worn or utilized during exercise also play a role. For instance, hockey goalies may not skate for great distances during a match, yet they may lose five or more pounds of body weight due to the weight of the padding and equipment they wear. Therefore, all athletes should be counseled to regularly consume fluids, even if they do not feel thirsty.

Table 15.5 provides recommendations for fluid intake before, during, and after strenuous physical activity. Athletes should consume 6–8 oz of fluid prior to exercise, 4–6 oz every 15–20 minutes during physical activity, and at least 8 oz of fluid following exercise.[27] Recommendations encourage athletes to weigh themselves periodically before and after exercise or competition to determine whether they have lost body weight. Each pound of body weight lost during an activity requires ingestion of 16 oz of fluid following the activity to maintain proper hydration.

**TABLE 15.5** Recommendation for fluid intake during strenuous physical activity

| TIME | AMOUNT OF FLUIDS |
|---|---|
| 1–2 hours prior to event | 12–22 oz cool water* |
| 10–15 minutes before event | 10–20 oz cool water |
| During event | 4–6 oz cool water every 15–20 minutes |
| After event | 2–3 cups of cool fluid for every pound of body weight loss |

*Cool water and fluids should be 50°F–60°F and lower than ambient temperature.

Based on: Holt, K., Wooldridge, N., Story, M., and Sofka, D., eds. (2011). *Bright Futures Nutrition*. 3rd ed. Elk River, IL: American Academy of Pediatrics. pp. 187.

Athletes should drink no more than 16 oz of fluid each 30 minutes, however, to avoid potential side effects, such as nausea.

The type of fluid an athlete drinks is affected more by peer pressure and mass media than by actual physiological need. Sports drinks and energy drinks are very popular among teens, even those who do not participate in sports. Data on children suggest that even though water is an economical, easily available fluid, it may not provide optimal benefits for athletes who participate in physically intense events or those of great duration.[27,28] In such events, juice diluted at a ratio of 1:2 with water, or sports drinks that contain no more than 6 to 8 percent carbohydrate, may allow for better hydration and physical performance. Undiluted juices, fruit drinks, carbonated beverages, energy drinks, and sports drinks that contain more than 6 to 8 percent carbohydrate are not recommended during exercise because they may cause gastric discomfort. Their high carbohydrate content may also delay gastric emptying. Some carbonated soft drinks and many energy drinks contain significant amounts of caffeine, which promotes diuresis.

**Training Diets** Adolescent athletes may follow special diets or consume nutritional and non-nutritional supplements in an effort to improve physical performance and increase lean body mass. Special diets that are noted among adolescent athletes include carbohydrate-loading regimens and high-protein diets. Distance runners and other endurance athletes traditionally used carbohydrate loading to improve the glycogen content of muscle.[27] It involves the manipulation of training intensity and duration, along with the carbohydrate content of meals to improve glycogen formation in muscle tissue. Carbohydrate loading is traditionally a week-long process that begins with intense training one week prior to competition. For the first three days of a carbohydrate-loading week, athletes choose low-carbohydrate foods, but continue to exercise in an attempt to deplete muscle glycogen stores. During the three days prior to competition, athletes rest, or exercise minimally, while consuming a high-carbohydrate diet to promote glycogen formation and storage. Many athletes follow a modified version of this regimen rather than the full traditional method.

High-protein diets may take many forms for teen athletes. In general, athletes who follow high-protein diets may consume three to four times the recommended protein intake, accompanied by a relatively low intake of carbohydrate. High-protein diets should be discouraged as pre-performance dietary regimens among athletes for several reasons.[27] First, many dietary protein sources are also sources of total and saturated fats, which may increase lifetime risk of coronary artery disease. Second, high protein and fat intakes result in reduced carbohydrate intake and may delay digestion and absorption, limiting the amount of energy available for use during physical activity. Finally, more water is required for the breakdown of protein than for either fat or carbohydrate due to the increased water loss that accompanies the excretion of nitrogen. This factor places an athlete at increased risk for dehydration, often accompanied by a decrease in physical performance. High protein intake appears to be more effective in recovering from intense physical activity than in preparing for an event.

# Special Dietary Concerns Among Adolescents

LO 15.3 Compare and contrast national dietary recommendations to prevent and treat hypertension and hyperlipidemia in adolescents.

## Substance Use

The use of substances such as tobacco, alcohol, and recreational drugs can affect the nutritional status of adolescents. YRBS data suggest that 9 percent of adolescents self-report cigarette smoking, with 4 percent smoking at least one cigarette each day.[21] Smoking is slightly more prevalent among male vs. female adolescents and White students are the most likely to smoke cigarettes (11 percent), followed by Hispanic students (6 percent) and Black students (4 percent).[21] Tobacco exposure through chewing tobacco is as prevalent as smoking cigarettes, with about 9 percent of students reporting using smokeless tobacco.[21] Males are more likely to use smokeless tobacco products, with 15 percent of male and 3 percent of female adolescents using these products. Smokeless tobacco use is highest among White males (21 percent), followed by Hispanic males (8 percent), Black males (4 percent) and Hispanic females (4 percent).[21] Other forms of smokeless tobacco and ecigarettes may be used by teens; however, national data on the prevalence of use is not available. Adolescents who use tobacco have been shown to have higher vitamin C requirements compared to peers who do not use tobacco.

Data from the YRBS suggest that 35 percent of teens report current alcohol use; 21 percent reported binge drinking (drinking five or more alcoholic drinks during one occasion) on at least one day during the past month.[21] Alcohol use is higher among White (36 percent) and Hispanic (38 percent) youth compared to Black youth (30 percent). Binge drinking is more common among White and Hispanic teens than among Black students (23 percent, 23 percent and 12 percent, respectively) and increases with age.[21] The consumption of alcohol may replace nutritious foods and beverages in the diet, compromising nutritional status. Thiamin and other B-vitamin requirements may be higher among adolescents who frequently consume large quantities of alcohol.

According to YRBS data, illicit drug use is reported by a significant number of adolescents.[21] Twenty-three percent report current marijuana use, 6 percent report cocaine use, 9 percent have used inhalants, 7 percent have used Ecstasy (MDMA), 3 percent have used methamphetamine, 7 percent had used hallucinogens, 2 percent have used heroin, and 2 percent have used other injectable drugs.[21] Illicit drug use may alter dietary intake patterns through influences on appetite and metabolism as well as dietary choices made while under the influence of these substances. In addition, for older adolescents who are financially independent, money used to purchase alcohol and illicit substances may reduce the amount of money available to purchase food and pay for other daily living expenses, thus increasing the risk of food insecurity and/or homelessness.

Recent data on the effects of substance use on eating behaviors have focused exclusively on the risk for disordered eating behaviors, particularly on bulimia nervosa and binge-eating disorder. Disordered eating is seen more frequently among females who report smoking cigarettes, drinking alcohol, and using inhalants.[29] Among males, the use of marijuana, steroids, and inhalants was related to higher risk for disordered eating. It is believed that substance use may result in depleted stores of vitamins and minerals, including thiamin, vitamin C, and iron. Chronic ingestion of alcohol and drug use can result in a reduced appetite, leading to low dietary intakes of protein, energy, vitamins A and C, thiamin, calcium, iron, and fiber (see Table 15.6).

## Iron-Deficiency Anemia

Iron-deficiency anemia is the most common nutritional deficiency noted among children and adolescents. Several risk factors are associated with its development among adolescents, including rapid growth, inadequate dietary intake of iron-rich foods or foods high in vitamin C,

TABLE 15.6 ▸ Potential effects of substance use on nutrition status

- Appetite suppression
- Reduced nutrient intake
- Decreased nutrient bioavailability
- Increased nutrient losses/malabsorption
- Altered nutrient synthesis, activation, and utilization
- Impaired nutrient metabolism and absorption
- Increased nutrient destruction
- Higher metabolic requirements of nutrients
- Inadequate weight gain/weight loss
- Iron deficiency anemia
- Decreased financial resources for food

SOURCE: Reprinted with permission. Alton I. Substance Abuse During Pregnancy. In: Story M, Stang J, eds. 2010. Nutrition and the Pregnant Adolescent: A Practical Reference Guide. Minneapolis, MN: Center for Leadership, Education, and Training in Maternal and Child Nutrition, University of Minnesota.

TABLE 15.7 ▸ Maximum hemoglobin concentration and hematocrit values for iron-deficiency anemia

| SEX/AGE[a] | HEMOGLOBIN (<G/DL) LESS THAN: | HEMATOCRIT (<%) LESS THAN: |
|---|---|---|
| **Males and Females** | | |
| 8–12 years | 11.9 | 35.4 |
| **Males** | | |
| 12–15 years | 12.5 | 37.3 |
| 15–18 years | 13.3 | 39.7 |
| 18+ years | 13.5 | 39.9 |
| **Females[b]** | | |
| 12–15 years | 11.8 | 35.7 |
| 15–18 years | 12.0 | 35.9 |
| 18+ years | 12.0 | 35.7 |

SOURCE: Abridged from Centers for Disease Control and Prevention. Recommendations to Prevent and Control Iron Deficiency Anemia in the United States. 2002. *Morb Mortal Wkly Rep*. 51(40): 897–899.

[a]Age and sex-specific cutoff values for anemia are based on the 5th percentile from the third National Health and Nutrition Examination Survey.

[b]Nonpregnant and lactating adolescents.

vegan diets, calorie-restricted diets, meal skipping, participation in strenuous or endurance sports, and heavy menstrual bleeding.[28,30] The effects of iron-deficiency anemia include delayed or impaired growth and development, fatigue, increased susceptibility to infection secondary to depressed immune system function, reductions in physical performance and endurance, and increased susceptibility to lead poisoning. Pregnant teens that are iron deficient in the early stages of gestation are at increased risk of preterm delivery and delivery of a low-birthweight infant.

Assessment of iron-deficiency anemia compares individual hemoglobin and hematocrit levels to standard reference values. Table 15.7 lists the Centers for Disease Control and Prevention criteria for determining anemia, based on age and gender. Adjustments to these values must be made for individuals who live at altitudes greater than 3,000 feet and for smokers. An adjustment of 10.3 g/dL is required for adolescents who smoke.[30] Because adolescent males are not at high risk for iron-deficiency anemia, they do not need to be screened unless they exhibit one or more of the risk criteria listed. All adolescent females should be screened every five years for anemia; those with one or more risk factors for anemia should be screened annually.

Treatment that follows a diagnosis of iron-deficiency anemia needs to include increased dietary intake of foods rich in iron and vitamin C as well as iron supplementation. Adolescents under the age of 12 should be supplemented with 60 mg of elemental iron per day, and teenagers over the age of 12 should receive 60 mg (for males) to 120 mg (for females) of elemental iron per day.[28,30] These recommendations spark some controversy, however, given the high doses of elemental iron.

Adolescents often report gastrointestinal side effects from iron supplementation, such as constipation, nausea, and cramping. These side effects can be lessened by giving smaller doses of iron more frequently throughout the day and counseling the adolescent to take the iron supplement at mealtimes or with food sources of vitamin C. Calcium supplements, dairy products, coffee, tea, and high-fiber foods may decrease absorption of iron supplements; these foods should be avoided within one hour of taking an iron supplement.

## Hypertension

Criteria for the detection and diagnosis of hypertension are shown in Table 15.8. Adolescents are considered to have pre-hypertension if blood pressure readings are ≥ the 90th percentile but < the 95th percentile for age and gender, or > 120/80.[31] Hypertension is diagnosed if the average of three systolic and/or diastolic blood pressure readings exceeds the 95th percentile, based on age, sex, and height.[31] Blood pressure levels for the 95th percentiles for males and females are shown in Table 15.9.

TABLE 15.8 ▸ Consensus statement guidelines for detection and diagnosis of hypertension and hyperlipidemia

| | GUIDELINES |
|---|---|
| **Hypertension** | |
| Normal Blood Pressure | Systolic and diastolic blood pressure <90th percentile for age and gender |
| Pre-hypertension | Systolic or diastolic blood pressure >90th but <95th percentile for age and gender or 120/80 mm Hg |
| Stage 1 Hypertension | Systolic or diastolic blood pressure >95th but <99th percentile +5 mm Hg for age and gender on 3 consecutive visits |
| Stage 2 Hypertension | Systolic or diastolic blood pressure >99th percentile +5 mm Hg for age and gender |
| **Hyperlipidemia** | |
| Total cholesterol, mg/dL | |
| acceptable | <170 |
| borderline | 170–199 |
| abnormal | ≥200 |
| LDL cholesterol, mg/dL | |
| acceptable | <110 |
| borderline | 110–129 |
| abnormal | ≥130 |
| Triglycerides, mg/dL | |
| abnormal | >150 |

Based on: Holt, K., Wooldridge, N., Story, M., and Sofka, D., eds. (2011). *Bright Futures Nutrition*. 3rd ed. Elk River, IL: American Academy of Pediatrics.

TABLE 15.9 ▸ Blood pressure levels for the 90th and 95th percentiles of blood pressure for boys and girls, aged 10 to 17 years

| AGE | BP PERCENTILE* | SYSTOLIC BP (MM HG), BY HEIGHT PERCENTILE FROM STANDARD GROWTH CURVES | | | | | | | | | | | | | |
|---|---|---|---|---|---|---|---|---|---|---|---|---|---|---|---|
| | | BOYS | | | | | | | GIRLS | | | | | | |
| | | 5% | 10% | 25% | 50% | 75% | 90% | 95% | 5% | 10% | 25% | 50% | 75% | 90% | 95% |
| 10 | 90th | 110 | 112 | 113 | 115 | 117 | 118 | 119 | 112 | 112 | 114 | 115 | 116 | 117 | 118 |
| | 95th | 114 | 115 | 117 | 119 | 121 | 122 | 123 | 116 | 116 | 117 | 119 | 120 | 121 | 122 |
| 11 | 90th | 112 | 113 | 115 | 117 | 119 | 120 | 121 | 114 | 114 | 116 | 117 | 118 | 119 | 120 |
| | 95th | 116 | 117 | 119 | 121 | 123 | 124 | 125 | 118 | 118 | 119 | 121 | 122 | 123 | 124 |
| 12 | 90th | 115 | 116 | 117 | 119 | 121 | 123 | 123 | 116 | 116 | 118 | 119 | 120 | 121 | 122 |
| | 95th | 119 | 120 | 121 | 123 | 125 | 126 | 127 | 120 | 120 | 121 | 123 | 124 | 125 | 126 |
| 13 | 90th | 117 | 118 | 120 | 122 | 124 | 125 | 126 | 118 | 118 | 119 | 121 | 122 | 123 | 124 |
| | 95th | 121 | 122 | 124 | 126 | 128 | 129 | 130 | 121 | 122 | 123 | 125 | 126 | 127 | 128 |
| 14 | 90th | 120 | 121 | 123 | 125 | 126 | 128 | 128 | 119 | 120 | 121 | 122 | 124 | 125 | 126 |
| | 95th | 124 | 125 | 127 | 128 | 130 | 132 | 132 | 123 | 124 | 125 | 126 | 128 | 129 | 130 |
| 15 | 90th | 123 | 124 | 125 | 127 | 129 | 131 | 131 | 121 | 121 | 122 | 124 | 125 | 126 | 127 |
| | 95th | 127 | 128 | 129 | 131 | 133 | 134 | 135 | 124 | 125 | 126 | 128 | 129 | 130 | 131 |
| 16 | 90th | 125 | 126 | 128 | 130 | 132 | 133 | 134 | 122 | 122 | 123 | 125 | 126 | 127 | 128 |
| | 95th | 129 | 130 | 132 | 134 | 136 | 137 | 138 | 125 | 126 | 127 | 128 | 130 | 131 | 132 |
| 17 | 90th | 128 | 129 | 131 | 133 | 134 | 136 | 136 | 122 | 123 | 124 | 125 | 126 | 128 | 128 |
| | 95th | 132 | 133 | 135 | 136 | 138 | 140 | 140 | 126 | 126 | 127 | 129 | 130 | 131 | 132 |

| AGE | BP PERCENTILE* | DIASTOLIC BP (MM HG), BY HEIGHT PERCENTILE FROM STANDARD GROWTH CURVES | | | | | | | | | | | | | |
|---|---|---|---|---|---|---|---|---|---|---|---|---|---|---|---|
| | | BOYS | | | | | | | GIRLS | | | | | | |
| | | 5% | 10% | 25% | 50% | 75% | 90% | 95% | 5% | 10% | 25% | 50% | 75% | 90% | 95% |
| 10 | 90th | 73 | 74 | 74 | 75 | 76 | 77 | 78 | 73 | 73 | 73 | 74 | 75 | 76 | 76 |
| | 95th | 77 | 78 | 79 | 80 | 80 | 81 | 82 | 74 | 74 | 75 | 75 | 76 | 77 | 78 |
| 11 | 90th | 74 | 74 | 75 | 76 | 77 | 78 | 78 | 74 | 74 | 75 | 75 | 76 | 77 | 77 |
| | 95th | 78 | 79 | 79 | 80 | 81 | 82 | 83 | 78 | 78 | 79 | 79 | 80 | 81 | 81 |
| 12 | 90th | 75 | 75 | 76 | 77 | 78 | 78 | 79 | 75 | 75 | 76 | 76 | 77 | 78 | 78 |
| | 95th | 79 | 79 | 80 | 81 | 82 | 83 | 83 | 79 | 79 | 80 | 80 | 81 | 82 | 82 |
| 13 | 90th | 75 | 76 | 76 | 77 | 78 | 79 | 80 | 76 | 76 | 77 | 78 | 78 | 79 | 80 |
| | 95th | 79 | 80 | 81 | 82 | 83 | 83 | 84 | 80 | 80 | 81 | 82 | 82 | 83 | 84 |
| 14 | 90th | 76 | 76 | 77 | 78 | 79 | 80 | 80 | 77 | 77 | 78 | 79 | 79 | 80 | 81 |
| | 95th | 80 | 81 | 81 | 82 | 83 | 84 | 85 | 81 | 81 | 82 | 83 | 83 | 84 | 85 |
| 15 | 90th | 77 | 77 | 78 | 79 | 80 | 81 | 81 | 78 | 78 | 79 | 79 | 80 | 81 | 82 |
| | 95th | 81 | 82 | 83 | 83 | 84 | 85 | 86 | 82 | 82 | 83 | 83 | 84 | 85 | 86 |
| 16 | 90th | 79 | 79 | 80 | 81 | 82 | 82 | 83 | 79 | 79 | 79 | 80 | 81 | 82 | 82 |
| | 95th | 83 | 83 | 84 | 85 | 86 | 87 | 87 | 83 | 83 | 83 | 84 | 85 | 86 | 86 |
| 17 | 90th | 81 | 81 | 82 | 83 | 84 | 85 | 85 | 79 | 79 | 79 | 80 | 81 | 82 | 82 |
| | 95th | 85 | 85 | 86 | 87 | 88 | 89 | 89 | 83 | 83 | 83 | 84 | 85 | 86 | 86 |

SOURCE: Adapted from the National Heart, Lung, and Blood Institute, National High Blood Pressure Education Working Group on Hypertension Control in Children and Adolescents. Fourth Report on the Diagnosis, Evaluation, and Treatment of High Blood Pressure in Children and Adolescents. Bethesda, MN: National Institutes of Health; 2005.

*Blood pressure percentile determined by a single movement.

Classifications of blood pressure are based on the average of three readings:

- Normal blood pressure: <90th percentile
- Prehypertensive: >90th and <95th percentiles
- Stage 1 hypertension: >95th and <99th percentile + 5 mm Hg
- Stage 2 hypertension: >99th percentile + 5 mm Hg

Risk factors for hypertension among adolescents include a family history of hypertension, high dietary intake of sodium, overweight or obesity, hyperlipidemia, inactive lifestyle, and tobacco use.[31] Adolescents who display one or more of these risk factors should be routinely screened for hypertension. Nutrition counseling to decrease sodium intake, to limit fat intake to 30 percent or less of calories, and to consume adequate amounts of fruits, vegetables, whole grains, and low-fat dairy products should be provided when hypertension is diagnosed.[31] Table 15.10 outlines the dietary recommendations suggested for adolescents to promote health and reduce cardiovascular risk factors. Weight loss is recommended for adolescents who are hypertensive in the presence of overweight or obesity. If medications are prescribed, teens still must adhere to general dietary recommendations and should still be encouraged to reach and maintain a healthy weight for their height.

## Hyperlipidemia

Approximately one in four adolescents in the United States has an elevated cholesterol level.[28] Table 15.8 provides the classification criteria for elevated blood lipid and cardiovascular disease markers in children and adolescents. It should be noted that total and LDL cholesterol levels drop by 10–20 percent during puberty; thus, the best time to screen for hyperlipidemia is around age 10 (before the onset of puberty) or after age 17, when growth is largely completed.[31] Youth who have family risk factors for hyperlipidemia or who are overweight or obese should undergo blood lipid and cardiovascular disease risk marker screening, but routine screening for all adolescents is not warranted.[31] Risk factors for hypercholesterolemia include a family history of cardiovascular disease or high blood cholesterol levels, cigarette smoking, overweight, hypertension, diabetes mellitus, and

**TABLE 15.10** ▸ DASH eating plan to reduce hypertension and other chronic diseases: servings per day by food group and total energy intake

| FOOD GROUP | SERVING SIZE | 1,400 KCALS | 1,600 KCALS | 1,800 KCALS | 2,000 KCALS |
|---|---|---|---|---|---|
| Grains (with whole grains the majority of choices) | 1 slice bread<br>1 oz dry cereal<br>½ cup cooked rice, pasta or cereal | 6 | 6 | 6 | 6–8 |
| Vegetables | 1 cup raw leafy greens<br>½ cup raw or cooked vegetable<br>½ cup vegetable juice | 3–4 | 3–4 | 4–5 | 4–5 |
| Fruits | 1 medium fruit ¼ cup dried fruit<br>½ cup fresh, frozen or canned fruit<br>½ cup fruit juice | 4 | 4 | 4–5 | 4–5 |
| Milk and milk products (fat free or low-fat choices) or substitutes | 1 cup milk or yogurt<br>1 cup soy, almond, rice, or other milk substitute<br>1.5 oz cheese | 2–3 | 2–3 | 2–3 | 2–3 |
| Lean meats, poultry or fish | 1 oz cooked meats, poultry or fish<br>1 egg | 3–4 | 3–4 | ≤6 | <6 |
| Nuts, seed and legumes | ⅓ cup or 1.5 oz nuts<br>2 Tbsp peanut or other nut butter<br>2 Tbsp or 0.5 oz seed<br>½ cup cooked legumes | 3/week | 3–4/week | 4/week | 4–5/week |
| Fats and Oils | 1 tsp margarine<br>1 tsp vegetable oil<br>1 Tbsp mayonnaise<br>2 Tbsp salad dressing | 1 | 2 | 2–3 | 2–3 |
| Sweets and added sugars | 1 Tb sugar<br>1 Tb jelly or jam<br>½ cup sorbet or gelatin<br>1 cup lemonade | ≤3 oz/week | <3 oz/week | <5 oz/week | <5 oz/week |

SOURCE: Based on the U.S. Department of Health and Human Services, National Institutes of Health, National Heart, Lung and Blood Institute: Expert panel on integrated guidelines for cardiovascular health and risk reduction in children and adolescents. Summary report. NIH Publication No 12-7486A, October 2012.

low level of physical activity. Early intervention among adolescents who have high cholesterol levels may reduce their risk of coronary artery diseases later in life.

The NHLBI has developed the CHILD 1 (Cardiovascular Health Integrated Lifestyle Diet) diet and nutrition guidelines, which integrate dietary approaches to prevention hypertension, hyperlipidemia, and obesity. These guidelines include the DASH dietary guidelines (Table 15.10) as well as recommendations to consume 14 g of dietary fiber per day/1,000 Kcals, limiting intake of juice to 4–6 oz per day, limiting sodium intake and choosing low-sodium foods when available, limiting fast food meals, and encouraging daily breakfast consumption and family meals.[31]

## Diabetes and Metabolic Syndrome

The prevalence of diabetes among adolescents is not available based on national data. The CDC suggests that approximately 215,000 people 20 years or young have diabetes with the majority of the cases being type 1 diabetes.[32] National data show that type 1 diabetes and youth less than 19 years old occurs in 1.7 per 1,000 youth in the United States. Type 2 diabetes typically has few symptoms; thus, is harder to detect in adolescents. Differentiating between type 1 and type 2 can be very difficult among youth. Teens with type 2 diabetes often are obese and may have a strong family history for the disease. The risk of type 2 diabetes among teens appears to be highest among 15–19-year-old American Indian youth (4.5/1,000 among all tribal groups and 50.9/1,000 among Pima Indian teens). Type 2 diabetes prevention includes reaching and maintaining a healthy body weight, engaging in regular physical activity, and following the DASH diet listed in Table 15.10.

Risk for metabolic syndrome is often not assessed among teens, though this clustering of risk factors for cardiovascular disease can have a significant impact on adolescent health. National estimates suggest that between 2 and 9 percent of all U.S. teens have metabolic syndrome; however, rates among obese teens are considerably higher, estimated at 12 to 44 percent.[31] Older adolescents with a family history of cardiovascular disease and/or diabetes and those who are overweight or obese should be considered as candidates for screening for metabolic syndrome. Females who are diagnosed with polycystic ovary syndrome also benefit from screening for metabolic syndrome.

## Children and Adolescents with Chronic Health Conditions

Approximately 18 percent of children and adolescents have a chronic condition or disability.[28] These children and adolescents are at increased risk for nutrition-related health problems because of (1) physical disorders or disabilities that may affect their ability to consume, digest, or absorb nutrients; (2) biochemical imbalances caused by medications or internal metabolic disturbances; (3) psychological stress from a chronic condition or physical disorder that may affect a child's appetite and food intake; and/or (4) environmental factors, often controlled by parents who may influence the child's access to and acceptance of food.[28]

Reports of children and adolescents with special health care needs estimate that as many as 40 percent have nutrition risk factors that warrant a referral to a dietitian.[28] Common nutrition problems in adolescents with special health care needs include the following:

- Altered energy and nutrient needs (e.g., inborn errors of metabolism, spasticity of movement, enzyme deficiencies)
- Delayed growth
- Oral-motor dysfunction (e.g., neurological disorders, swallowing disorders)
- Elimination problems
- Drug/nutrient interactions
- Appetite disturbances
- Unusual food habits (e.g., rumination)
- Dental caries, gum disease

Malnutrition has been implicated as a major factor contributing to poor growth and short stature in adolescents with a variety of diseases (e.g., chronic inflammatory bowel disease, cystic fibrosis). Factors such as inadequate nutrient and energy intakes, excessive nutrient losses, malabsorption, and increased nutrient requirements all lead to the chronic malnourished state. Studies have shown that the energy requirements for adolescents with cystic fibrosis or inflammatory bowel disease may be 30–50 percent higher than the RDA for adequate growth.[28] In addition to the increased energy needs caused by malabsorption (or in the case of adolescents with cystic fibrosis, the increased work of breathing), fever, infection, and inflammation also increase energy requirements. Whereas undernourishment is frequently seen in adolescents with chronic illnesses, obesity is common among youth with gross motor limitations or immobility.[28] Because of limited activity, caloric requirements are lower, and the balance between intake and expenditure is often difficult to achieve, resulting in obesity.

Consideration of nutrition needs of children with chronic disabling conditions or illnesses is complex and requires specialized, individualized care by an interdisciplinary team. Assessment of nutrition status followed by nutrition intervention, when necessary, and monitoring will help ensure the health and well-being of adolescents with chronic and disabling conditions. Also, during adolescence, issues of personal responsibility and independent-living skills related to food purchasing and preparation may need to be addressed.

# Dieting, Disordered Eating, and Eating Disorders

LO 15.4 Differentiate between disordered eating behaviors and eating disorders based on frequency and severity of symptoms and anticipated outcomes.

Eating concerns and disorders lie on a continuum ranging from mild dissatisfaction with one's body shape to serious eating disorders such as anorexia nervosa, bulimia nervosa, and binge-eating disorder. Along the continuum, between these endpoints, lie normative dieting behaviors and more severe disordered eating behaviors such as self-induced vomiting and binge eating (Illustration 15.3). Although engagement in anorexic behaviors and unhealthy dieting may not be frequent or intense enough to meet the formal criteria for being defined as an eating disorder, these behaviors may negatively impact health and may lead to the development of more severe eating disorders. All eating disorders present a serious public health concern in light of their prevalence and their potentially adverse effects on growth, psychosocial development, and physical health outcome.

Dieting behaviors among adolescents, and in particular among adolescent girls, tend to be alarmingly high. National data suggest that 63 percent of female and 33 percent of male adolescents have dieted in the past month to lose weight.[21] Dieting was once considered to be a phenomenon of White, middle-class females, however current data suggests that dieting is more prevalent among Hispanic females (67 percent) than White females (63 percent), with Black females dieting at a lower, although still elevated, rate (55 percent).[21] Nearly half of Hispanic males (42 percent) report dieting, compared to 31 percent of White and 26 percent of Black males. The prevalence of dieting drops slightly with age among males but increases with age among females. Dieting remains a significant issue for adolescents of all ages, races, and ethnicities, which persists into adulthood.

Dieting and the use of unhealthy weight-control behaviors may also place adolescents at increased likelihood of being overweight in the future. Neumark-Sztainer and colleagues found that over a 10-year period, adolescents who initially reported dieting or using unhealthy weight-control behaviors were more likely to be overweight a decade later than were peers who did not report using weight-control behaviors.[33] Effective nutrition messages aimed at teens should focus on making healthy lifestyle changes, rather than focusing on short-term dieting behaviors that are often difficult to sustain. Shifting focus toward long-term behavior changes is needed for prevention of both eating disorders and overweight.

Dieting behaviors among youth are of concern in that they are often used by youth who are not overweight. Furthermore, unhealthful dieting behaviors in which meals are skipped, energy intake is severely restricted, or food groups are lacking are common. Dieting behaviors have been found to be associated with inadequate intakes of essential nutrients, particularly when an entire food group or category is avoided. Restricting behaviors (e.g., avoiding all sweet-tasting foods) can lead adolescents to experience hunger or cravings for specific foods, which may place them at risk for binge-eating episodes. Finally, dieting behaviors may be indicative of increased risk for the later development of eating disorders; research has found that during a 3-year period, restrained eating was a significant predictor of eating-disorder risk among female adolescents.[34] Therefore, dieting should not be viewed as a normative and acceptable behavior, in particular among teenagers.

During adolescence, body image and self-esteem tend to be closely intertwined; therefore, body-image concerns should not be viewed as acceptable and normative components of adolescence. Furthermore, body dissatisfaction is a main contributing factor to dieting behaviors, disordered eating behaviors, and clinical eating disorders.[35-37] Body dissatisfaction appears to increase dramatically following the body-weight increase that normally occurs in females around the time of menarche and remains a significant concern for females for the next 1–2 years. Binge eating and/or purging has been found to occur within 6–12 months of menarchial weight changes.[35-37] Adolescents with low levels of body satisfaction are also at greater risk for using other unhealthy weight-control behaviors, and are less likely to participate in physical activity.[35-37] Although actual weight status is directly associated with perceived weight status, a considerable number of teens who are not overweight perceived of themselves as overweight, particularly around the time of puberty.

In working with overweight or obese youth who express body dissatisfaction, health professionals are challenged to help them improve their body image while simultaneously working toward weight control. All adolescents, including overweight or obese youth, should be encouraged to appreciate the positive aspects of their bodies. Overweight adolescents may need help in accepting the fact that they

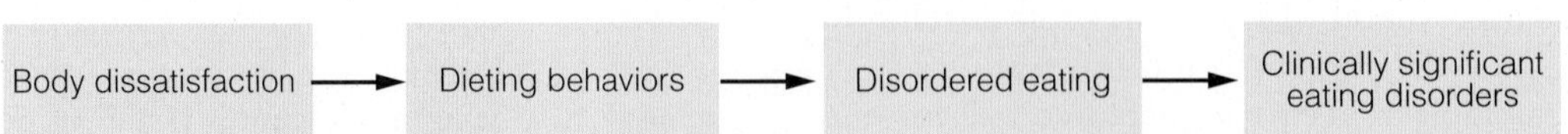


ILLUSTRATION 15.3 ▸ The continuum of weight-related concerns and disorders.

may never achieve the thin ideal portrayed in the media, but they may strive toward a leaner and healthier body that is realistic for them.

## Disordered Eating Behaviors and Eating Disorders

Some adolescents engage in restricting or binge/purge eating behaviors, but with less frequency or intensity than required for a formal diagnosis of an eating disorder. Behaviors typically considered in this category include self-induced vomiting, fasting or extremely restrictive dieting, binge eating, compensatory physical activity, and the use of laxatives, diuretics, or diet pills. The heterogeneity of these behaviors makes it more difficult to estimate their prevalence. Data from the YRBS show that 13 percent of adolescents had gone for 24 hours or longer without eating (fasting) as a means of losing weight.[21] Fasting was more commonly reported among females (19 percent) than among males (7 percent). Eighteen percent of White females reported fasting to lose weight, compared to 17 percent of Black and 23 percent of Hispanic females; rates are lower among males with 6 percent of White, and 10 percent of Hispanic and Black males reporting fasting.

Five percent of students surveyed in YRBS reported using diet pills or other diet formulae to lose weight.[21] The use of diet pills was reported by 6 percent of White females, 10 percent of Hispanic females and 5 percent of Black females, compared to 3 percent of Hispanic and 3 percent of Black and White males. The use of vomiting and/or laxatives to lose weight was reported by 4 percent of students (7 percent among female teens, 2 percent among male teens). Hispanic females reported the highest rates of vomiting or using laxatives, with a prevalence of 10 percent, followed by White females (6 percent), Black females (4 percent), Black and Hispanic males (3 percent), and White males (1 percent).[21] Data on compensatory exercise, or exercise for the purpose of purging calories eaten rather than for health benefits, is difficult to find. Adolescents who report more than 60 minutes of physical activity per day should be carefully assessed for the purpose of excessive exercise. Teens who work out until they have "burned off" all of the calories eaten that day should be considered at high risk for disordered eating.

The types of questions used to assess disordered eating behaviors may influence prevalence estimates and may account for the disagreement on how common this issue is among teens. Based on research findings, it can be reasonably estimated that between 10 and 20 percent of adolescents have engaged in disordered eating behaviors. These behaviors are often overlooked in overweight adolescents, but overweight adolescents have reported the use of unhealthy and extreme weight-control behaviors, which can include purging, laxative use, self-restriction, and excessive exercise.[37] Disordered eating behaviors such as self-induced vomiting and binge eating have serious implications for health and may be precursors to a diagnosed eating disorder. Therefore, interventions aimed at their prevention are essential.

**TABLE 15.11** Estimated prevalence and brief description of weight-related concerns/disorders among adolescents

| DISORDER | ESTIMATED PREVALENCE |
|---|---|
| Anorexia nervosa | Approximately 0.2% to 1.0% of adolescent females and young women. |
| Bulimia nervosa | Approximately 1% to 3% of adolescent females and young women. |
| Binge-eating | Estimated 30% of population currently dieting; 2% of general population. |
| Disordered eating behaviors | Estimated 10% to 20% of adolescents, although estimates vary. |
| Dieting behaviors | Estimates vary; they range from about 44% of adolescent females, 15% adolescent males, to 50% to 65% of all adolescent females attempting to lose weight. |
| Body dissatisfaction | Estimates vary in accordance with type of measurement used and age, gender, and ethnicity of population; approximately 60% of girls and 35% of boys are not satisfied with their weight. |



An awareness of the prevalence of eating disorders is critical in effective planning for interventions aimed at their treatment and prevention. Conditions prevalent among youth, such as disordered eating behaviors and obesity, warrant interventions such as community-based and school-based programs that have the potential to reach large numbers of youth. The small percentage of the adolescent population affected by eating disorders requires more intensive individual or small-group interventions. Estimates as to the prevalence of each of the eating disorders on the continuum are presented in Table 15.11.

**Anorexia** *Anorexia nervosa* and its impact on morbidity and mortality make it the most severe condition on the continuum of eating disorders. Among adolescent girls and young women, prevalence estimates of anorexia nervosa range from 0.2 percent to 1.0 percent.[38,39] Anorexia nervosa presents more frequently among females than among males; about 9 out of 10 individuals with anorexia nervosa are female. Only in recent years has attention been directed toward males with this condition; they may not be suspected of having anorexia nervosa and therefore may be diagnosed at later stages of the disease, when treatment is more difficult.

Characteristics of anorexia nervosa include preoccupation with food,

**anorexia nervosa** An eating disorder characterized by extreme weight loss, poor body image, and irrational fears of weight gain and obesity.

**TABLE 15.12** ▸ Diagnostic criteria for anorexia nervosa

- Refusal to maintain body weight at or above a minimally normal weight for age and height (e.g., weight loss leading to maintenance of body weight less than minimally normal weight in adults; or failure to make expected weight gain during period of growth, leading to body weight less than minimally normal weight)
- Intense fear of gaining weight or becoming fat, even though underweight
- Disturbance in the way in which one's body weight or shape is experienced, undue influence of body weight or shape on self-evaluation, or denial of the seriousness of the current low body weight
- Amenorrhea in postmenarchial women; that is, the absence of at least three consecutive menstrual cycles (a woman is considered to have amenorrhea if her menstrual periods occur only following hormone/estrogen administration)

**Restricting Type**

- During the episode of anorexia nervosa, the person has not regularly engaged in binge eating or purging behavior (i.e., self-induced vomiting or the misuse of laxatives, diuretics, or enemas).

**Binge-Eating/Purging Type**

- During the episode of anorexia nervosa, the person has regularly engaged in binge-eating or purging behavior (i.e., self-induced vomiting or the misuse of laxatives, diuretics, or enemas).

SOURCE: Adapted from the American Psychiatric Association: Diagnostic and Statistical Manual of Mental Disorders, Fifth Edition. Arlington, VA, 2013, American Psychiatric Association.

self-starvation, and strong fears of being fat.[39] An adolescent may begin with dieting behaviors due to social pressures to be thin, comments by others about weight, or as a result of their discomfort with the normal pubescent weight gain. Weight loss may result in adolescents feeling more in control of their body or other aspects of their life, which further reinforces the restricting behavior. If the weight loss and accompanying body-image and self-esteem issues are not addressed early on, anorexia nervosa develops. Diagnostic criteria for anorexia nervosa are shown in Table 15.12. Key features of anorexia nervosa are refusal to maintain body weight over a minimal normal weight for age and height; intense fear of gaining weight or becoming fat, even though underweight; a distorted body image; and amenorrhea (in females).

The two subtypes of anorexia nervosa are restricting and non-restricting. In the restricting subtype, the individual does not regularly engage in binge-eating or purging behaviors. The nonrestricting subtype exhibits regular episodes of binge-eating and purging behaviors. However, both subtypes present with a refusal to maintain a minimally normal body weight, which differentiates them from other types of eating disorders.

An estimated 10–15 percent of patients with anorexia nervosa die from their disease, although difficulties arise in assessing mortality rates from anorexia nervosa.[38,39] Reasons for fatality from anorexia include a weakened immune system due to undernutrition, gastric ruptures, cardiac arrhythmias, heart failure, and suicide. The adolescent or the family commonly denies the condition, which delays the diagnosis and treatment, resulting in a poorer prognosis for recovery. Early recognition of possible signs of anorexia nervosa and seeking out professional help significantly affect the time and intensity of treatment and improve chances for a successful recovery. Full recovery rates are estimated at less than 50 percent of individuals with anorexia nervosa; 33 percent show improvements; and 20 percent are chronically affected by this mental illness.[38–40]

**Bulimia** *Bulimia nervosa* is an eating disorder characterized by the consumption of large amounts of food with subsequent purging by self-induced vomiting, laxative or diuretic abuse, enemas, and/or obsessive exercising.[38,39] Whereas anorexia nervosa is characterized by severe weight loss, bulimia nervosa may show weight maintenance or extreme weight fluctuations due to alternating binges and fasts. In some individuals, anorexia and bulimia nervosa overlap. Reliable estimates of bulimia nervosa range from 1.0 percent to 3.0 percent.[38–40] As with anorexia nervosa, the vast majority of individuals with bulimia nervosa are female.

Diagnostic criteria for bulimia nervosa are shown in Table 15.13. Key features of bulimia nervosa include

**bulimia nervosa** A disorder characterized by repeated bouts of uncontrolled, rapid ingestion of large quantities of food (binge eating) followed by self-induced vomiting, laxatives or diuretic use, fasting, or vigorous exercise in order to prevent weight gain.

**TABLE 15.13** ▸ Diagnostic criteria for bulimia nervosa

A. Recurrent episodes of binge eating. An episode of binge eating is characterized by both of the following:
   - Eating, in a discrete period of time (e.g., within any 2-hour period), an amount of food that is definitely larger than most people would eat during a similar period of time and under similar circumstances.
   - A sense of lack of control over eating during the episode (e.g., a feeling that one cannot stop eating or control what or how much one is eating).

B. Recurrent inappropriate compensatory behavior in order to prevent weight gain, such as self-induced vomiting; misuse of laxatives, diuretics, enemas, or other medications; fasting; or excessive exercise.

C. The binge eating and inappropriate compensatory behaviors both occur, on average, at least once a week for 3 months.

D. Self-evaluation is unduly influenced by body shape and weight.

E. The disturbance does not occur exclusively during episodes of anorexia nervosa.

SOURCE: Adapted from the American Psychiatric Association: Diagnostic and Statistical Manual of Mental Disorders, Fifth Edition. Arlington, VA, 2013, American Psychiatric Association.

recurrent episodes of binge eating (rapid consumption of a large amount of food in a discrete period of time), a feeling of lack of control over eating during the binge, some form of purging food and calories from the body, and a persistent overconcern with body shape and weight.[38-40] There are two categories of bulimia nervosa: purging and nonpurging. Individuals with the purging subtype of bulimia nervosa regularly engage in self-induced vomiting and/or the use of laxatives, diuretics, or enemas to purge calories from the body. Individuals with the nonpurging subtype may fast in between binge episodes and utilize compensatory exercise as a means of compensating for caloric intake. People with bulimia nervosa can be overweight, underweight, or of average weight for their height and body frame. Bulimia nervosa may be preceded by a history of dieting or restrictive eating, which are thought to contribute to the binge–purge cycle.

Mortality for bulimia nervosa appears to be lower than for anorexia nervosa. Based on a review of the existing literature in this area, it has been estimated that approximately 2 to 3 percent of patients die of their disease.[38-40] Recovery rates for bulimia nervosa are estimated at 48 percent for full recovery, 26 percent for improvement, and 26 percent for chronicity.[40] Early diagnosis and treatment and less severe behaviors are associated with better outcomes for bulimia nervosa, while having a comorbid psychological condition such as borderline personality disorder, anxiety, or alcohol abuse is associated with poorer outcomes.

**Binge-eating disorder (BED)** ***Binge-eating disorder*** is a condition in which an individual engages in eating large amounts of food and feels that these eating episodes are not within one's control.[39] BED is defined by recurrent episodes of binge eating at least 1 day a week for at least 3 months (Table 15.14). In addition, the person feels a subjective sense of a loss of control over binge eating, which is indicated by the presence of three of the following five criteria: eating rapidly, eating when not physically hungry, eating when alone, eating until uncomfortably full, and feeling self-disgust about bingeing. BED differs from bulimia nervosa in that binge eating is not followed by compensatory behaviors such as self-induced vomiting, as occurs in bulimia nervosa.

Dieting may be a risk factor for BED; however, 35 percent to 55 percent of women may experience binging before dieting.[41] Females who report dieting before bingeing are more likely to have experienced sexual or physical abuse, which may lead to feelings of loss of control and the desire to participate in restricting behaviors to regain a sense of control. Females who experienced stressful situations, such as the death of someone close to them, were more likely to report bingeing prior to dieting, consistent with an emotional eating response. Age of onset of BED is somewhat lower for women who report bingeing first (20 years) versus those who report dieting first (25 years).

BED appears to be more prevalent among overweight clinical populations (30 percent) than among community samples (5 percent of females and 3 percent of males).[38,39] Studies on adolescents that assess the prevalence of binge eating include few that document prevalence rates of BED. In a college-student sample, the rate of BED was 2.6 percent. In contrast to other weight-related conditions, significant differences were not found between male and female students. Further study of the prevalence and etiology of BED among adolescents seems critical in light of the high rates of obesity among youth.

**TABLE 15.14** ▸ Diagnostic criteria for binge-eating disorder

A. Recurrent episodes of binge eating. An episode of binge eating is characterized by both of the following:
- Eating, in a discrete period of time (e.g., within any 2-hour period), an amount of food that is definitely larger than most people would eat in a similar period of time and under similar circumstances.
- A sense of lack of control over eating during the episode (e.g., a feeling that one cannot stop eating or control what or how much one is eating).

B. The binge-eating episodes are associated with three (or more) of the following:
- Eating much more rapidly than normal
- Eating until feeling uncomfortably full
- Eating large amounts of food when not feeling physically hungry
- Eating alone because of being embarrassed by how much one is eating
- Feeling disgusted with oneself, depressed, or guilty after overeating
- Experiencing marked distress regarding binge eating
- Occurring, on average, at least 1 day a week for 3 months

C. The method of determining frequency differs from that used for bulimia nervosa; future research should address whether the preferred method of setting a frequency threshold is counting the number of days on which binges occur or counting the number of episodes of binge eating.

D. The binge eating is not associated with the regular use of inappropriate compensatory behaviors (e.g., purging, fasting, excessive exercise) and does not occur exclusively during the course of anorexia nervosa or bulimia nervosa.

SOURCE: Adapted from the American Psychiatric Association: Diagnostic and Statistical Manual of Mental Disorders, Fifth Edition. Arlington, VA, 2013, American Psychiatric Association.

## Causes of Disordered Eating and Eating Disorders

The causes of eating disorders are multifactorial including social norms emphasizing thinness, being teased about one's weight, familial relations (e.g., chaotic lifestyles, lack of boundaries between family members, poor patterns of communication), physical and sexual abuse experiences, personal body shape and size, body

**binge-eating disorder** An eating disorder characterized by periodic binge eating, which normally is not followed by vomiting or the use of laxatives. People must experience eating binges twice a week on average for over six months to qualify for this diagnosis.

image, and self-esteem (Table 15.15). A genetic component to eating disorders has been proposed in response to studies that have shown a higher prevalence of these disorders within families and/or twins. These factors do not operate in isolation, but rather, an interaction between genetics and environmental risk factors may be necessary to increase an adolescent's risk for engaging in potentially harmful eating and dieting behaviors.[41]

In considering the causes of eating issues, it is essential to realize that different pathways may lead to weight-related disorders in different adolescents. For some adolescents, family issues may be major factors, while for others social norms may be the key factors leading to the onset of a condition. Furthermore, different conditions tend to be influenced by different factors. Potential contributory factors for eating disorders can be categorized into environmental, familial, interpersonal, and personal domains.

An understanding of the causes of eating disorders is essential to the development of effective interventions aimed at their treatment and prevention. An individual clinical setting needs to allow time to assess the factors leading to the onset of the condition for that particular adolescent. In developing prevention programs to reach larger groups of adolescents, it is more feasible to identify and address factors that may be contributing to the onset of weight-related behaviors and conditions for a broad sector of the targeted population. Although not all factors may be addressed within one intervention, it is important to be aware of the broad range of factors coming into play and the interactions among them.

The complex causes of eating disorders and their potentially life-threatening psychosocial, physical, and behavioral consequences highlight the need for a multidisciplinary treatment approach. The health-care team caring for an adolescent with an eating disorder will often include a physician, dietitian, nurse, psychologist, and/or psychiatrist.[28,42,43] The role of the dietitian is paramount to the treatment of eating disorders at the stages of assessment, treatment, and maintenance. Initially, an adolescent may be more willing to discuss his or her concerns with a dietitian than with a psychologist.

**Treatments for Eating Disorders** The treatment of eating disorders may take many forms.[42,43] Individuals with eating disorders who are medically and psychologically stable are generally treated through outpatient programs. The frequency of contact with the health care team is usually weekly, but it may be more frequent if required. Day treatment programs, often referred to as partial-inpatient programs, may be recommended for individuals who require daily contact with the health care team and whose body weight is sufficient to remain treated as an outpatient. Day treatment programs may vary in the number of weekly visits from 3–7 days per week, depending on the facility and

TABLE 15.15 ▸ Screening elements and warning signs for individuals with eating disorders

| SCREENING | WARNING SIGNS |
|---|---|
| Body image and weight history | Distorted body image<br>Extreme dissatisfaction with body shape or size<br>Profound fear of gaining weight or becoming fat<br>Unexplained weight change or fluctuations greater than 10 lbs |
| Eating and related behaviors | Very low caloric intake; avoidance of fatty foods<br>Poor appetite; frequent bloating<br>Difficulty eating in front of others<br>Chronic dieting despite not being overweight<br>Binge-eating episodes<br>Self-induced vomiting; laxative or diuretic use |
| Meal patterns | Fasting or frequent meal skipping to lose weight<br>Erratic meal pattern with wide variations in caloric intake |
| Physical activity | Participation in physical activity with weight or size requirement (e.g., gymnastics, wrestling, ballet)<br>Overtraining or "compulsive" attitude about physical activity |
| Psychosocial assessment | Depression<br>Constant thoughts about food or weight<br>Pressure from others to be a certain shape or size<br>History of physical or sexual abuse or other traumatizing life event |
| Health history | Secondary amenorrhea or irregular menses<br>Fainting episodes or frequent light-headedness<br>Constipation or diarrhea unexplained by other causes |
| Physical examination | BMI <5th percentile<br>Varying heart rate, decreased blood pressure after arising suddenly<br>Hypothermia; cold intolerance<br>Loss of muscle mass<br>Tooth enamel demineralization |

SOURCE: Based on Herpetz-Dahlmann, B. Adolescent eating disorders: Definitions, symptomatology, epidemiology and co-morbidity. 2009. *Child Adolesc Psychiatr Clin N Am* 18(1): 31–47; American Psychiatric Association: Diagnostic and Statistical Manual of Mental Disorders, 5th ed. Arlington, VA, 2013, American Psychiatric Association; Mazzeo, S. E., and Bulik, C. M. Environmental and genetic risk factors for eating disorders: What the clinician needs to know. 2008. *Child Adolesc Psychiatr Clin N Am* 18: 67–82; Shaw, H., Stice, E., and Becker, C. B. Preventing eating disorders. 2008. *Child Adolesc Psychiatr Clin N Am* 18: 199–207.

TABLE 15.16 ▸ Suggested criteria for inpatient treatment of eating disorders

| MEDICAL CRITERIA | PSYCHOSOCIAL CRITERIA |
|---|---|
| Failure to thrive (BMI <3rd percentile) | Social isolation |
| Rapid and dramatic weight loss | Depression |
| Very low caloric intake | Obsessive-compulsive disorder |
| Refusal to eat or drink | Suicidal thoughts or tendencies |
| Hypokalemia | Lack of parental support |
| Alkalosis | Poor family communication and dynamics |
| Bradycardia | Poor response to outpatient or day treatment |
| Pancreatic dysfunction | |
| Liver dysfunction | |

SOURCE: Based on Herpetz-Dahlmann, B., and Slaback-Andrae, H. 2008. Overview of treatment modalities in adolescent anorexia nervosa. *Child Adolesc Psychiatr Clin N Am* 18: 131–145.

the client. Inpatient programs are required for individuals with life-threatening comorbidities, unstable medical or psychological status, or severely low body weight. The criteria for inpatient care of adolescents are listed in Table 15.16.

The goal of eating disorder treatment programs is to restore body weight, to improve social and emotional well-being, and to normalize eating behaviors. While programs vary, the core components of any eating-disorder treatment program include: [42,43]

- Treatment of medical comorbidities
- Restoration of body weight to a normal level
- Nutrition education and counseling to normalize food-related thoughts and beliefs
- Individualized psychotherapy to improve social well-being and emotional health
- Family therapy to improve communication and family function
- Group therapy

During treatment, a major role of the dietitian is to help the adolescent normalize eating patterns and to feel comfortable with these changes. Some of the key goals of the nutritional care include the following:

- Thoroughly assess dietary intake and adequacy.
- Recommend nutrition-related therapeutic interventions based on nutrition-assessment data.
- Provide counseling to client to establish a regular pattern of nutritionally balanced meals and snacks.
- Monitor dietary intake and physical activity levels to determine adequate but not excessive levels of energy intake or physical activity, with the goal of reaching and maintaining a healthy body weight.
- Counsel clients to consume adequate dietary fat and fiber intake to promote satiety.
- Provide counseling in conjunction with the psychologist or other mental health care provider on strategies to help clients avoid dieting behaviors and excessive exercise.
- Assist clients with strategies to gradually include formerly forbidden foods into the diet, which may include role-modeling appropriate food intake at mealtimes, arranging for groups of clients to practice eating out at restaurants, and assisting clients in preparing meals.
- Periodically evaluate effectiveness of interventions.
- Monitor client nutritional status.

For some adolescents, denial of the condition or a lack of motivation for change makes nutrition counseling quite challenging. It is important for the nutritionist to work in close conjunction with other members of the health team to ensure that roles of different members of the team are clearly defined.

The high prevalence of eating disorders and their potentially harmful consequences point to a need for interventions aimed at their prevention. One of the most pressing current public health issues that needs to be addressed concerns the prevention of eating disorders described in previous sections and the prevention of obesity. Even the prevention of a small percentage of these conditions, at a population level, returns huge benefits in terms of reducing physical, emotional, and financial burdens.

**Prevention of Eating Disorders** In the development of interventions aimed at the prevention of eating disorders, it is essential to address factors that contribute to the onset of these conditions for a large proportion of the targeted population, factors that are potentially modifiable, and factors suitable for addressing within the designated setting. For example, media awareness and advocacy has been suggested as a suitable approach toward preventing eating concerns and disorders. Participants may learn about how the media influence one's body image and about techniques used within the media to improve the appearance of models, and then take action toward making changes in the media. This approach is suitable in that media influences, and the internalization of media messages, may contribute to weight concerns among a large sector of the adolescent population. These adolescent perceptions are potentially modifiable and suitable for addressing within clinical, community, and school-based settings where interventions may be implemented.

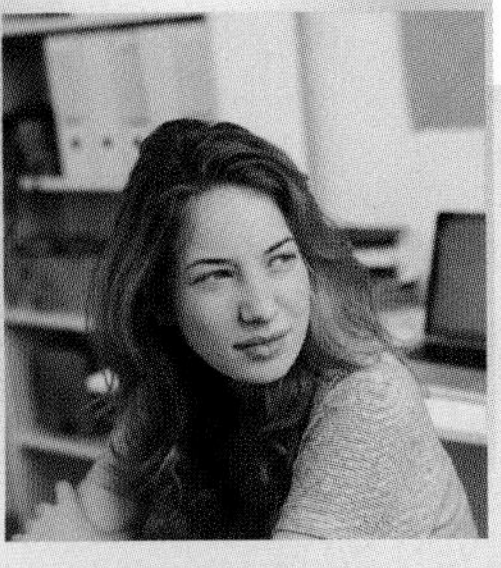
racorn/Shutterstock.com

# CASE STUDY 15.1

## Following Ana's Medical History

Ana is a 15-year-old high school student who is active in school activities, loves to run and bike, and has a 3.95 grade point average. She has a close group of friends that she spends her free time with; her parents are very proud of her for her outstanding academic performance.

**School Nurse Visit** Ana being seen at the school clinic for a sore throat and fever. The nurse takes her height (5'3") and weight (107 lb). Ana is diagnosed with strep throat infection and is given antibiotics.

**Sports Physical Visit** Ana is seen 4 months later (in early fall) by her pediatrician for a sports physical, since she is planning to join the cross-country running team. Weight at this time is 96 pounds. The physician notes that Ana seems to be tired and has lost weight since her most recent visit to the clinic. Ana replies that she has had a lot of sinus and other infections, which causes her to lose her appetite. She also notes that she has been training hard to make the cross-country team but that her training should become less intense now that she has made the team. Ana assures the physicians that she will try to eat more in the future. They physician encourages her to eat a lot of carbohydrates and protein to improve her sports performance.

**Pre-employment Physical Visit** Ana is seen by her family physician for a preemployment physical in early June. At this time her weight is 91 pounds.

The physician is concerned about her weight, but Ana assures her that she looks and feels fine. The MD refers her to the outpatient clinical dietitian. During the interview with the dietitian, it is noted that Ana eats only twice a day, with many diet beverages in between these meals. The dietitian suggests that Ana increase her weight to at least 95 pounds, but she refuses, stating that at this weight she would "have too much fat in her thighs" for running. When asked about the use of diet pills, laxatives, and other diet aids, Ana states that she doesn't need these because she has enough willpower to reduce her food intake on her own. She also denies vomiting after eating. When asked about her willingness to reduce her running so that she could reach a more healthy weight, Ana get agitated. The dietitian asks Ana how she determines how much or how long she needs to run. Ana states that she runs as long as she needs to so that she can use up all of the calories she has eaten. When the dietitian suggests that this is compensatory exercise and is a form of purging, Ana becomes upset and leaves. The dietitian looks for her parents in the waiting room, and lets Ana's mother know that she thinks there may be an eating issue that the family should deal with. The mother thanks the dietitian for letting her know and leaves, as Ana has already gone to the parking lot.

The dietitian confers with the physician and her parents are send information about eating disorders, including possibly outcomes and treatment options. Three months later, the clinic is notified that Ana has fainted at gym class in school and that the hospital where she was taken has referred her for an in-patient eating disorder evaluation.

### Questions

1. For the school nurse visit, what is Ana's BMI?
2. What percentile does Ana's weight fall at during the school nurse visit?
3. How would you classify Ana's weight status at the school nurse visit?
4. Calculate BMI and percentile from the sports physical visit.
5. How would you classify her weight status at the sports physical visit?
6. What advice would you give to Ana in terms of pre-event sports nutrition?
7. What advice would you give her about post-event eating?
8. Calculate BMI and percentile from the preemployment physical visit.
9. How would you classify her weight during the preemployment physical visit?
10. What eating issue would you suspect Ana has? Why?
11. What are the long-term outcomes and prognosis of this issue?

Any efforts toward prevention first must consider the target audience. An important question is whether to direct interventions to all adolescents or to adolescents at increased risk for eating disorders. Reasons for providing interventions for all adolescents include the high prevalence of eating concerns among adolescents, difficulties inherent in identifying and targeting high-risk individuals, and the advantages of developing positive social norms regarding eating issues within the peer group. Taking a more targeted approach offers the advantages of better use of limited resources, more intensive interventions, and interventions developed for specific high-risk groups (e.g., ballet dancers, youth with diabetes, or overweight girls). In order to be most effective at preventing eating disorders, both types of interventions seem necessary; more general approaches address the issues of the general adolescent population, while more refined approaches can better meet the needs of specific high-risk groups.

Prevention interventions may be implemented within clinical, community, and school-based settings that serve adolescents. A meta-analysis of eating-disorder prevention programs suggests that more than half of published eating-disorder prevention programs reduced at least one risk factor for disordered eating, and 29 percent reduced the severity of disordered eating among youth.[44] Programs that focused on changing weight-related attitudes of youth and promoted healthy weight-control strategies were found to be the most effective, with effects lasting up to two years. Other characteristics of successful eating-disorder prevention programs included:

- Selective targeting of high-risk groups rather than all youth
- Programs targeting adolescents >15 years of age
- Programs with information provided by trained interventionists rather than counselors, teachers, or health care providers
- Programs that included multiple sessions rather than a single encounter
- Integrated interactive learning (role-playing, computer technology, etc.) rather than providing only didactic learning experiences

Most eating-disorder prevention programs have focused on females. There is a need to develop prevention programs for males as well, especially those who exhibit a high concern about muscularity or thinness.[45]

## KEY POINTS

1. More than one-third of adolescents are overweight and 18 percent are obese.
2. National guidelines specify a four-stage approach to weight management for adolescents, which may include bariatric surgery in the presence of extreme obesity or life-threatening comorbid conditions.
3. Teen athletes should consume 6–8 oz of fluid prior to exercise, 4–6 oz every 15–20 minutes during physical activity, and at least 8 oz of fluid following exercise to maintain proper hydration.
4. Dieting is common among adolescents, with 33 percent of males and 63 percent of females reporting dieting during the past month.
5. Thirteen percent of teens report going for more than 24 hours without food (fasting) in an attempt to lose weight.
6. Risk factors for iron deficiency anemia, the most common nutrition deficiency among adolescents, include rapid growth, low dietary iron intake, meal skipping, dieting, athletic participation, and heavy menstrual bleeding.
7. Cholesterol levels drop during puberty, thus routine screening for hyperlipidemia should be done before age 10 and again after age 17.
8. Disordered eating behaviors occur in 10 to 20 percent of adolescents, while eating disorders occur at much lower rates.

## REVIEW QUESTIONS

1. Stage 2 treatment for adolescent obesity can be offered by a single provider.

   _____ True _____False

2. At which state of obesity treatment is a structured eating plan designed to create a caloric deficit?
   a. Stage 1
   b. Stage 2
   c. Stage 3
   d. Stage 4

3. Which of the following nutrients may be required in greater amounts by adolescents who use alcohol and tobacco?
   a. Thiamin
   b. Iron
   c. Vitamin C
   d. All of the above

4. Which is not a criterion for inpatient treatment of eating disorders?
   a. Social isolation or depression
   b. Excessive parental expectations
   c. Weight loss of more than 10 lb in 3 months
   d. Unwillingness to eat or drink
5. All of the following criteria are required for adolescent bariatric surgery, except:
   a. Failure to lose weight during intensive lifestyle program
   b. BMI $>$ 40 with medical complications
   c. Family history of obesity-related deaths
   d. Supportive home environment
6. How does binge-eating disorder differ from bulimia nervosa?
7. How does the use of substances such as alcohol, tobacco, and recreational drugs affect the nutritional status of adolescents?
8. Why don't adolescent BMI charts use a single cutoff point for determining obesity in the same way adult BMI charts do?
9. Which of the following is NOT part of national guidelines for physical activity for adolescents?
   a. Engage in at least 60 minutes of strenuous aerobic physical activity at least 5 days a week.
   b. Engage in bone-strengthening activities at least 3 days a week.
   c. Engage in muscle-strengthening activities at least 3 days a week.
   d. Engage in at least 60 minutes of physical activity almost every day.

Visit www.cengagebrain.com to access MindTap, a complete digital course that includes additional resources.

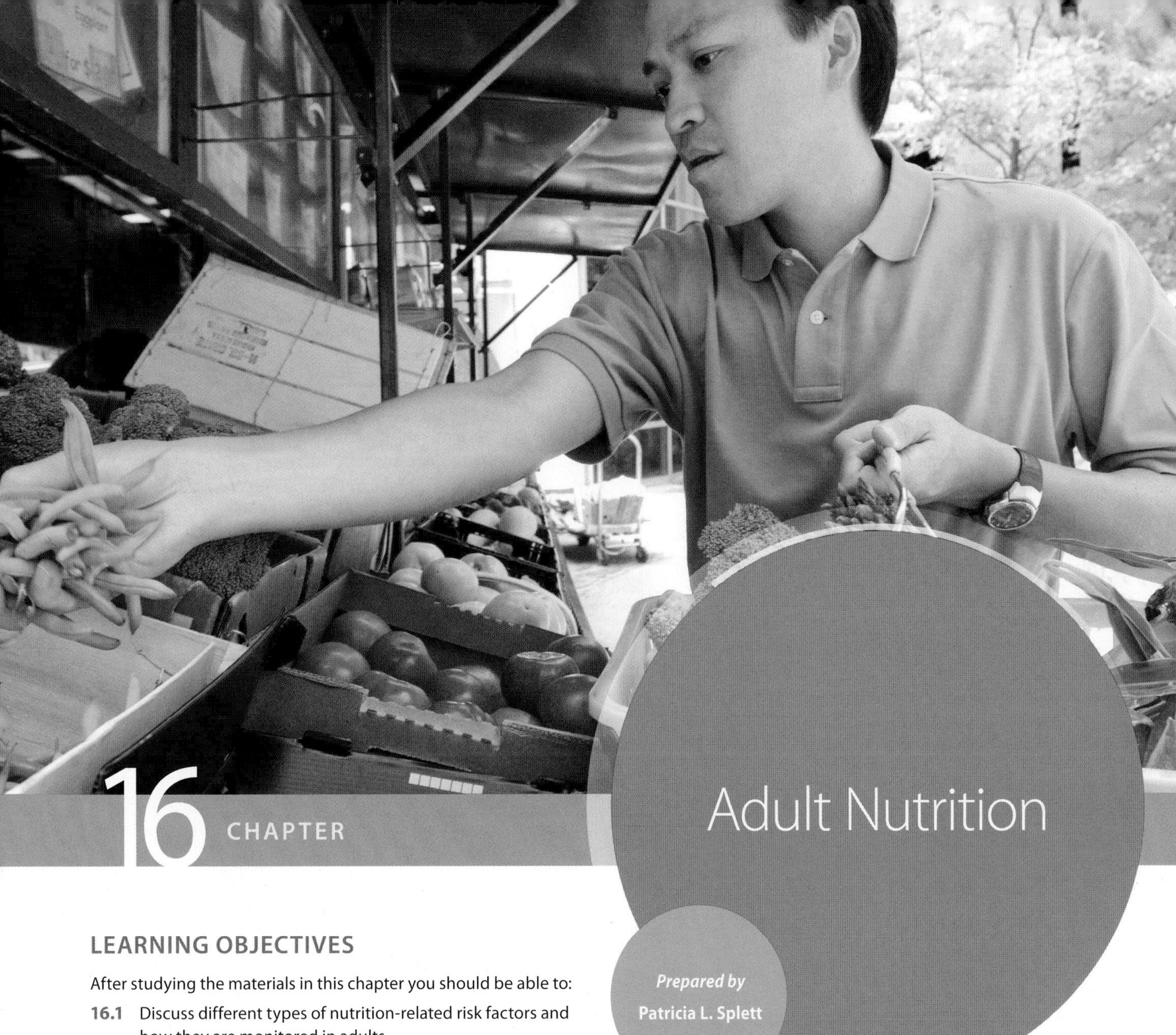

# 16 CHAPTER Adult Nutrition

*Prepared by*
Patricia L. Splett

## LEARNING OBJECTIVES

After studying the materials in this chapter you should be able to:

**16.1** Discuss different types of nutrition-related risk factors and how they are monitored in adults.

**16.2** Describe normal physiological changes in adulthood and how they are associated with the development and progression of chronic diseases.

**16.3** Estimate your daily energy needs using three methods and discuss factors that affect energy expenditure of adults.

**16.4** Identify nutrients that are consumed in excessive and inadequate levels and the consequences for adult health.

**16.5** Explain the purpose of dietary guidance and how it translates science into healthful food and beverage choices and pleasurable eating experiences for adults.

**16.6** Describe national recommendations for physical activity and the benefits of regular physical activity.

**16.7** Contrast strategies for promoting and supporting good nutrition of adults.

Amanda Mills/CDC

# Introduction

> "Healthy living is the best revenge."
>
> —Earl S. Ford[1]

Adulthood marks a long period between the active growth and development phases of infancy, childhood, and adolescence and the older adult phases where a concern is sustaining physical and mental capacity. Adulthood is subdivided into the following segments.

**Early Adulthood:** The twenties generally involve becoming independent, leaving the parental home, finishing formal schooling, entering regular employment and starting a career, developing relationships, and choosing a partner. Planning, buying, and preparing food are newly developing skills for many. The thirties could be characterized by increasing responsibilities to and for others, including having children, providing for and caring for family, building a career, and involvement in community and civic affairs. There may be renewed interest in nutrition at this time "for the kids' sake."

**Midlife:** The forties are a period of active family responsibilities (that may include nurturing children and teenagers and, for some, building new relationships and blending families), as well as expanding work and professional roles. Managing schedules and meals becomes a challenge. Sociologists say that this is a time of reviewing life's accomplishments and beginning to recognize one's mortality.

The phase around the fifties is referred to as the ***sandwich generation***. Many, especially women, are multigenerational caregivers who juggle the roles of caring for children and aging parents while maintaining a career. Work and career continue to be priorities for most adults. In the fifties, health concerns frequently are added to the picture. Dealing with a ***chronic disease*** or managing identified risk factors to prevent diseases is an added responsibility.

**Later Adulthood:** By their early sixties, many adults are making the transition to retirement, have more leisure time, and are able to give greater attention to physical activity and nutrition. While many are "empty-nesters," significant numbers have children living at home and/or have responsibilities as guardians and caretakers of grandchildren, parents, or others. Food choices and lifestyle factors may take on added significance for those who are dealing with a chronic disease.

This chapter explores the nutritional needs of adults and nutrition guidance and interventions aimed at helping meet those needs. During the adult years the focus is on preserving health, maintaining a ***healthy weight***, and delaying or preventing the onset of chronic diseases.

## Importance of Nutrition

The span of years between ages 20 and 64 is a time when diet, physical activity, smoking, and body weight strongly influence the future course of health and wellness. During these 44 years, lifestyle choices interact with genetic endowment, social forces, and environmental factors to determine years of life and quality of life.[2] Today, about half of all American adults are living with one or more preventable chronic diseases.

The onset and severity of heart disease, stroke, diabetes, some cancers, and liver disease (5 of the 10 leading causes of death in adults) have risk factors that can be modified through changes in nutrition and physical activity. Overweight and obesity, experienced by two-thirds of American adults, is a factor in all of the major chronic diseases.[3] Dietary practices that are common in American diets can be labeled as carcinogenic, atherogenic, and obesogenic; and, if changed, could reduce the occurrence of these widespread chronic diseases (Table 16.1).

# Tracking Adult Nutritional Health and Its Determinants

LO 16.1 Discuss different types of nutrition-related risk factors and how they are monitored in adults.

Nutrition status and factors that promote or interfere with achieving optimum nutrition status of the adult population are tracked using standard indicators. Data at the local, state, and national level are used to identify problem areas, shape interventions, and measure progress. The monitoring process starts with assessing food intake, nutrient adequacy, and weight status at the individual level. Then data are summarized across population groups. At the national level, data on many cross-cutting indicators of chronic disease risk are collected and reported (Table 16.2). The table includes values for the United States.[4] Using the website below the table, go to Prevalence and Trends Data and fill in the values for your state, race/ethnic group, age group, and income group.

What adults eat is not strictly a matter of individual choice; what they eat and the resulting nutrition status are shaped by many external factors. Where people learn, work, and play, the community they live in, as well as policies and politics all affect their ability to access a variety of affordable, healthful food and live a healthful lifestyle.[5] The complexity of external factors is depicted in Illustration 16.1. Understanding the external factors that contribute to individual and population health is important for identifying the

**sandwich generation** Refers to middle-aged adults, usually women, who are multigenerational caregivers dealing with the complex roles of wife, mother, daughter, caregiver, and employee.

**chronic diseases** Slow-developing, long-lasting diseases that are not contagious (e.g., heart disease, cancer, diabetes).

**healthy weight** A weight range compatible with normal function and long, healthy life.

TABLE 16.1 ▸ Modifiable nutritional risk factors for chronic diseases*

| | |
|---|---|
| Cancer | *Carcinogenic diet*<br>• Low fruit and vegetable intake<br>• Low level of antioxidants (especially vitamins A, C)<br>• Low intake of whole grains and fiber<br>• High dietary fat intake<br>• Nitrosamines, burnt and charred food<br>• High intakes of pickled and fermented food<br>• Alcohol consumption<br>• High animal-food, low plant-food intake |
| Heart Disease | *Atherogenic diet*<br>• High saturated fat (>10% calories)<br>• *Trans*-fatty acid intake<br>• Dietary cholesterol intake >300 mg<br>• Low fruit and vegetable intake<br>• Low antioxidants<br>• Low intake of whole grains<br>• No or excess alcohol intake**<br>• High sodium intake<br>• Low potassium intake<br>• Low intake of milk and dairy foods<br>• High waist circumference (men >40 inches, women >35 inches) |
| Obesity | *Obesogenic diet*<br>• Caloric intake exceeding needs<br>• Unstructured eating<br>• Frequent fast-food consumption<br>• High fat intake<br>• Sugar-sweetened beverage consumption<br>• Energy-dense, low-nutrient food choices |
| Diabetes | Atherogenic diet<br>Obesogenic diet |

*Obesity (BMI >.30) and physical inactivity are also independent risk factors for all of the chronic conditions.

**In middle-aged adults, moderate alcohol intake reduces risk of heart disease (for men, after age 45; and for women, after age 55).



problem, planning interventions, and monitoring progress. The ***social determinants of health*** model goes beyond the biological and genetic makeup and behaviors at the individual level. It organizes the complex and interacting factors that determine health and nutritional well-being of the population and provides a framework so these factors can be monitored (Illustration 16.2).[7]

## Health Objectives for the Nation

Healthy People 2020 objectives address multiple health improvement goals for adults.[8] Each objective has a defined data source for monitoring progress. Data from the last decade show that heart disease, cancer, and stroke deaths have declined, and fat intake (as percentage of total calories) has declined. However, rates of obesity and diabetes have continued to increase, sugar intake has risen, and health care disparities still exist.[9] The current objectives for the Nutrition and Overweight topics are listed in Table 16.3. As you read them, think about how the objectives address risk factors for the major chronic diseases, and also signal a shift away from nutrition as something for which the individual is solely responsible toward its being a focus for community planners, retailers, employers, and health care providers.

## Health Disparities Among Groups of Adults

Some population groups have a higher prevalence of chronic diseases than others. This is illustrated by comparisons of disease prevalence in adults of different racial/ethnic backgrounds and income levels:[8,10]

- Obesity patterns vary by race/ethnicity and income. Among women, non-Hispanic Black women have the highest obesity rates, followed by women of Mexican origin
- An inverse association exists between family income and obesity prevalence among White females of all ages

TABLE 16.2 ▸ Chronic disease indicators: physical activity and nutrition

| INDICATOR | U.S. PREVALENCE RATE | YOUR STATE* | RACE/ETHNIC GROUP | AGE GROUP | INCOME GROUP |
|---|---|---|---|---|---|
| Consume fruit (one or more times/day) | 60.8% (2013) | | | | |
| Consume vegetables (one or more times/day) | 77.1 (2013) | | | | |
| Obesity (BMI ≥30) | 29.4% (2013) | | | | |
| Overweight and Obese (BMI ≥25) | 64.8% (2013) | | | | |
| 150 minutes or more aerobic physical activity/week | 50.8% (2013) | | | | |

*Check the chronic disease indicators for your state and for your race/ethnic, age and income groups. Go to CDC, Behavioral Risk Factor Surveillance System at www.cdc.gov/brfss.



**carcinogenic diet** A pattern of eating and food choices that increases the risk of some cancers.

**atherogenic diet** A pattern of eating and food choices that promotes deposits of plaque in arterial walls and contributes to the development of cardiovascular disease.

**obesogenic diet** A pattern of eating and food choices that leads to excessive energy intake and accumulation of body fat.

**social determinants of health** Socioeconomic and environmental factors that are powerful determinants of health and are largely outside of the control of individuals and groups.

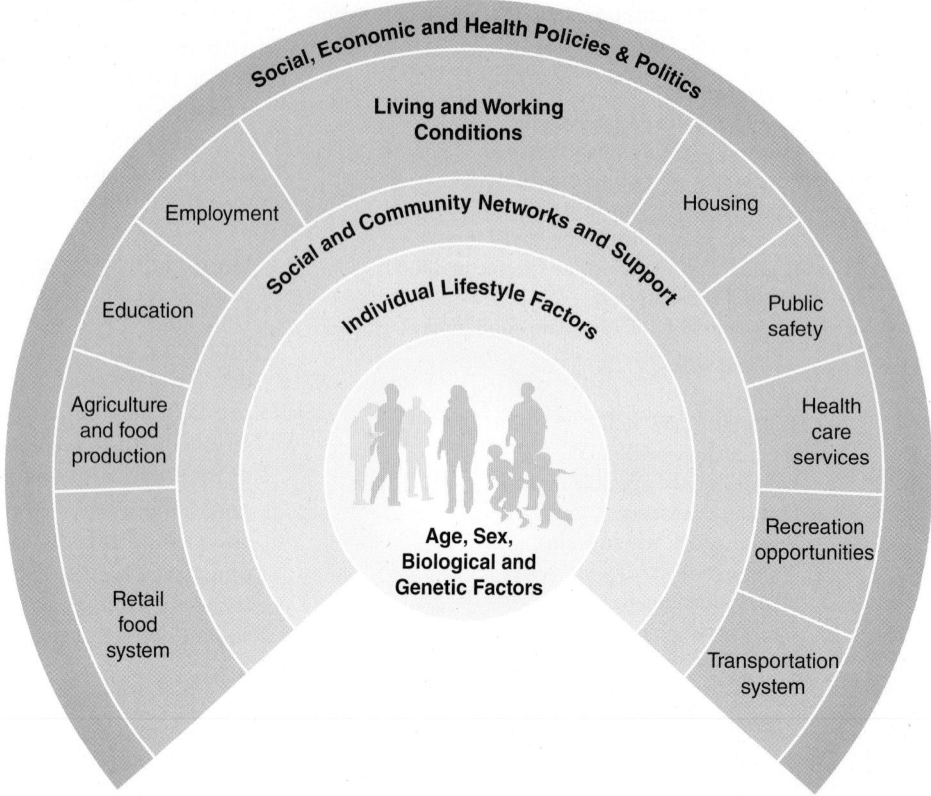


ILLUSTRATION 16.1 ▸ External factors affecting nutrition and health.

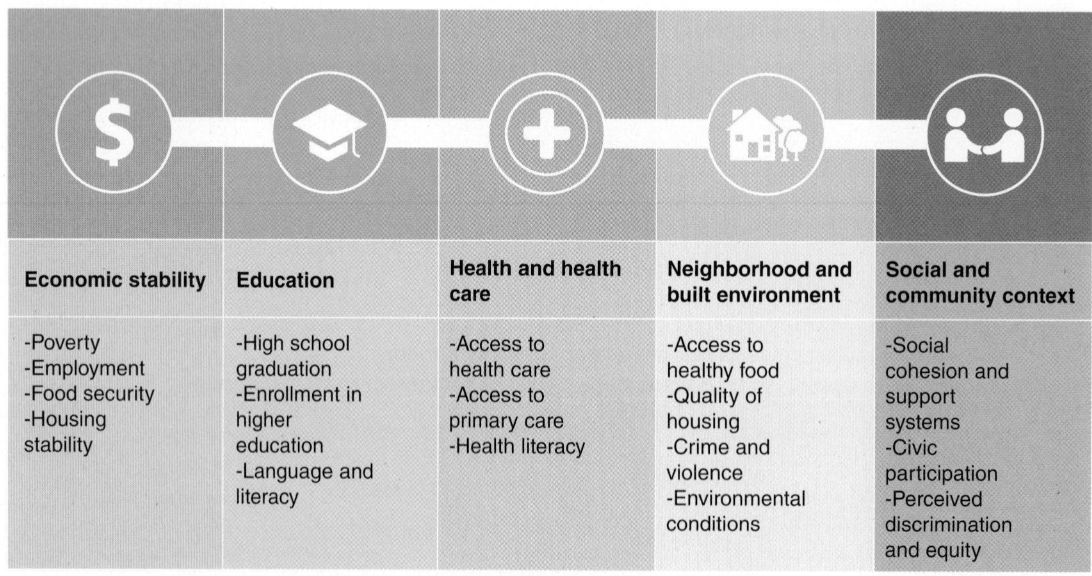

| Economic stability | Education | Health and health care | Neighborhood and built environment | Social and community context |
|---|---|---|---|---|
| -Poverty<br>-Employment<br>-Food security<br>-Housing stability | -High school graduation<br>-Enrollment in higher education<br>-Language and literacy | -Access to health care<br>-Access to primary care<br>-Health literacy | -Access to healthy food<br>-Quality of housing<br>-Crime and violence<br>-Environmental conditions | -Social cohesion and support systems<br>-Civic participation<br>-Perceived discrimination and equity |

ILLUSTRATION 16.2 ▸ Healthy People 2020 Social determinants of health.

- While new cases of cancer have been going down for most groups, the number of new cases has increased for American Indian women.
- Blacks and Hispanics are 77 percent and 66 percent, respectively, more likely to be diagnosed with diabetes than Whites.

Some groups have a genetic predisposition for certain diseases. American Indians have a predisposition for diabetes; Asians develop cardiovascular disease at lower BMI and smaller waist circumference; and African-Americans have greater salt sensitivity and earlier onset of hypertension.[11] However, genetics, environment, and lifestyle

TABLE 16.3 ▸ Healthy People 2020 objectives: Nutrition and overweight

| | | | Progress |
|---|---|---|---|
| **Weight** | | | |
| Increase the proportion of adults who are at a healthy weight | Baseline: 30.8% | Target: 33.9% | |
| Reduce the proportion of adults who are obese | Baseline: 34.0% | Target: 30.6% | ✓ |
| Prevent inappropriate weight gain in youth and adults | Developmental* | | |
| **Food and Nutrient Consumption (for population aged 2 years and older)** | | | |
| **Increase contribution to the diet** | | | |
| Fruit | Baseline: 0.5 cup** | Target: 0.9 cup | |
| Total vegetables | Baseline: 0.8 cup | Target: 1.1 cup | |
| Dark green and orange vegetables, & legumes | Baseline: 0.1 cup | Target: 0.3 cup | |
| Whole grains | Baseline: 0.3 oz** | Target: 0.6 oz | |
| Calcium | Baseline: 1118 mg | Target: 1300 mg | ✓ |
| **Reduce percent of total calories consumed from** | | | |
| Solid fats | Baseline: 18.9% | Target: 16.7% | |
| Added sugars | Baseline: 15.7% | Target: 10.8% | |
| Saturated fats | Baseline: 13.3% | Target: 9.5% | ✓ |
| Sodium | Baseline: 3641 mg | Target: 2300 mg | |
| **Community Actions** | | | |
| Increase the number of states that have state-level policies that incentivize food retail outlets to provide foods that are encouraged by the Dietary Guidelines. | Baseline 8 | Target 18 | ✓ |
| Increase the proportion of worksites that offer education related to weight reduction, nutrition, or physical activity. | Developmental* | | |
| **Primary Health Care Settings** | | | |
| Increase the proportion of primary care physicians who regularly assess body mass index (BMI) in their adult patients. | Baseline 48.7% | Target 53.6% | |
| Increase the proportion of physician office visits that include counseling or education. | | | |
| • Related to diet and nutrition for patients with a diagnosis of cardiovascular disease, diabetes, or hyperlipidemia | Baseline: 20.8% | Target: 22.9% | |
| • Related to physical activity for patients with a diagnosis of cardiovascular disease, diabetes, or hyperlipidemia | Baseline: 12% | Target: 14.3% | |
| • Related to weight reduction, nutrition, or physical activity for adult patients who are obese | Baseline: 28.9% | Target: 31.8% | |

*Baselines and targets have not been set for new, developmental objectives.

**equivalents per 1,000 calories.

SOURCE: U.S. Department of Health and Human Services. Office of Disease Prevention and Health Promotion. Healthy People 2020. Washington, DC. Available at healthypeople.gov/2020.

behaviors interact to determine the actual development of the disease. Groups experiencing ***health disparity*** not only have higher prevalence of certain conditions and experience worse health but also tend to have less access to environmental conditions that support health, such as healthy food, good housing, quality education, and safe neighborhoods. The impact of racism and other forms of discrimination is also recognized as a significant contributor to health disparity.[11] For these reasons, strategies directed to the social determinants of health are necessary to get at the fundamental causes behind health disparity. Eliminating health disparity is a priority within Healthy People. Goals for 2020, and objectives under many topic areas, including nutrition, aim to create social and physical environments that promote good health for all. Social and environmental risk factors can be gradually changed; however, to speed progress, more data about the determinants of health are being monitored and policy and environmental change strategies are receiving greater emphasis.[5,7,8,11]

# Physiological Changes During the Adult Years

LO 16.2 Describe normal physiological changes in adulthood and how they are associated with the development and progression of chronic diseases.

For the most part, individuals have stopped growing by the time they reach

**health disparity** Significant differences in the incidence, prevalence, mortality, and burden of disease and other adverse conditions that exist among specific population groups. Health disparity is closely linked to social and economic disadvantage.

their twenties. Men and women continue to develop bone density until roughly age 30. Peak bone mass is related to the amount of dietary calcium and weight-bearing exercise in prior years. Muscular strength peaks around 25–30 years of age and later dexterity and flexibility begin to decline, although regular use of muscles and weight training affects strength as well as muscle size and retention. The type and amount of physical activity has a significant impact on body composition, including ***lean body mass***, fat accumulation and relocation, and bone density.[12] Sensory and perceptual abilities change. Hearing loss begins as early as age 25 (or earlier with exposure to loud music), and vision changes often become noticeable by age 40. Blood flow to muscle, skin, and all tissues of the body are impacted by gradual changes in cardiovascular function include decrease in maximal heart rate and increase in rigidity (stiffness) of blood vessels.[13] Other body composition changes slowly occur in tandem with hormonal shifts.

## Hormonal and Climacteric Changes

Changes associated with the end of reproduction are referred to as ***climacteric changes.*** The decline of estrogen production, which begins in women during their early fifties, begins ***perimenopause*** and continues through ***menopause***, the end of reproductive capacity. Women with greater body mass tend to have a later menopause. Menopause is associated with an increase in abdominal fat and significant increase in risk of cardiovascular disease and accelerated loss of bone mass.[14] In addition to effects on the female reproductive system, estrogen, in both men and women, is involved in the supply of calcium to bones, health of blood vessel walls, blood cholesterol and triglyceride levels, and elasticity of the skin. Obesity is associated with higher estrogen levels in men and women due to the production of estrogen by fat cells. After age 30, men experience a gradual decline in testosterone level and muscle mass. Physical activity and weight training to increase muscle mass also result in small and transient increases in testosterone level.

## Body Composition Changes in Adults

**Bone** Bone shape is modified in response to physiological influences and mechanical forces. The ongoing process of bone remodeling preserves bone strength and mineral (calcium and phosphorus) homeostasis. Around age 40, men and women begin to gradually lose bone mass. The risk of developing osteopenia (low bone mineral density) and osteoporosis (weak, porous bones with high risk for fracture) depends on the peak bone mass achieved in the late twenties.[15]

**Adiposity** Positive ***energy balance*** typical between ages 20 and 64 results in weight gain and storage of excess energy in adipose tissues. Storage begins with hypertrophy of subcutaneous fat cells, then shifts to deposits in the central and intra-abdominal space (visceral fat) and other tissues such as heart, blood vessels, liver, and muscle (ectopic fat). Obesity and visceral fat are strongly related to development of inflammation and metabolic disturbances, which are connected to insulin resistance, diabetes, gallbladder disease, hypertension, stroke, and coronary artery disease. Furthermore, risks for these diseases increase as weight and adiposity increase.[16]

**Gut Microbiome** The constellation of bacteria and other microbes that inhabit the gut is determined early in life. This complex microbial community shifts and adapts with age, diet, geographic location, stress, supplements, and medications; but each individual has a gut microbiota "fingerprint" that is relatively stable. The composition of gut microbiota (formerly called gut flora) determines the balance between beneficial and harmful actions in the gut lumen. Healthy gut microbiota functions to activate and support the immune system, protect against opportunistic pathogens, digest food to release nutrients and energy from diet, ferment nondigestible carbohydrates, synthesize vitamins (K, $B_{12}$, biotin, carnitine), stimulate renewal of cells of intestinal lining, control colonic motility and transit time, and provide regulatory signals through the gut–brain axis.[17] A breakdown in the balance between protective and harmful intestinal bacterial, ***gut dysbiosis***, produces in an inflammatory state that may present with acute symptoms, or result in insidious changes in body weight, insulin sensitivity, glucose metabolism, dyslipidemia, and other cardio-metabolic and carcinogenetic factors. Interventions (including probiotics, prebiotics, and fecal transplant) can improve or prevent some pathological conditions.[18]

## Continuum of Nutritional Health

With good genes, good habits, good environment, and good luck, the effects of aging can be minimized and nutritional and physical health can be maintained throughout adulthood. More likely, the interaction of those factors over the years results in "nutritional injury," which leads to alteration or loss of function at the cellular level. Nutritional injury

**lean body mass** Sum of fat-free body tissue: muscle, mineral (as in bone), and water.

**climacteric change** Point in life where crucial changes occur; refers to the loss of reproductive activity, marked by menopause in women and reduction in testosterone production in men.

**perimenopause and menopause** An approximately 4-year period of decreasing estrogen production followed by the end of menstruation; a marking point for increased risk of cardiovascular disease and other chronic conditions for women.

**energy balance** An equilibrium state in which the number of calories consumed equals the number of calories expended.

**gut dysbiosis** Breakdown in the balance of protective and harmful bacterial in the intestines.

| *Nutritional state* | Resilient and healthy | Altered substrate availability | Nonspecific signs and symptoms | Clinical condition | Chronic condition | Terminal illness and death |
|---|---|---|---|---|---|---|
| *Metabolic, physiological, functional status* | Metabolic homeostasis Able to defend against injury | Reduction of nutrient stores or accumulation of excess Subclinical changes | Metabolic and physiologic alterations are observable | Evident illness and medical diagnosis | Altered metabolism and structural changes in tissues become permanent | Complications advance, body systems shut down |
| *Focus of nutrition guidance, education, or therapy* | Dietary guidance to support adequate intake and anticipate risks | Dietary guidance and education to inform about risks and encourage healthy eating and lifestyle choices | Nutrition education and counseling to reduce or reverse specific risk factors | Intensive medical nutrition therapy or therapeutic lifestyle change programs to delay progression | Medical nutrition therapy and patient education to enable self-management of the condition and prevent complications | Comfort care |

← *Continuum of nutritional health and intervention* →

ILLUSTRATION 16.3 ▸ Continuum of nutritional health.



may be minor, of short duration, and reversible, or, if it continues, permanent changes in cells and tissues can develop.[18] Several principles of human nutrition, presented in Chapter 1, bear repeating here to emphasize their relevance to nutritional health during the adult years:

- Health problems related to nutrition originate within cells.
- Poor nutrition can result from both inadequate and excessive levels of nutrient intake.
- Humans have adaptive mechanisms for managing fluctuation in food intake.
- Malnutrition can result from poor diets and from disease states, genetic factors, or combinations of these causes.
- Poor nutrition can influence the development of certain chronic diseases.
- Adequacy, variety, and balance are key characteristics of healthy diets.

Nutritional health can be viewed as a continuum (Illustration 16.3), ranging from "healthy" and resilient to the terminal state in which the body systems shut down and life ceases. According to the ***Continuum of Nutritional Health***, adapted from nutritional-injury models put forth by Arroyave and Leyse-Wallace,[20,21] changes occurring at the cellular level are initially insidious and unnoticed. Alterations progress over a long period and are reversible up to a point. But in the face of continued poor nutrition, permanent damage occurs. Altered nutrient intakes produce early changes in metabolic process that are preclinical stages of illness. This "injury" may not manifest itself until permanent damage has occurred. In the absence of signs and symptoms and awareness of a "problem," adults might not be especially concerned about food choices or motivated to adjust lifestyle behaviors.

## States of Nutritional Health

The continuum of nutritional health can be represented in six states or stages.

**Resilient and "Healthy"** In this state, metabolic systems are in homeostasis, and organs are functioning at optimum level. The body's defenses and immune system can counter assaults from toxins, pathogens, and stress. In this stage, nutritional guidance and education are used to encourage adequate intake—not too much, not too little—of a variety of healthful foods. The mantra is "moderation, variety, and balance." Anticipatory guidance is used to enable

**Continuum of Nutritional Health** Stages of nutritional status that range from optimal to unable to sustain life. The stages are resilient and healthy, altered substrate availability, nonspecific signs and symptoms, clinical conditions, chronic conditions, and terminal illness and death.

healthy individuals to anticipate and plan for possible risks so they are able to make informed choices that sustain resilience and prevent nutritional injury.

**Altered Substrate Availability** This early, subclinical state of nutritional harm occurs when intake does not meet needs. There is a loss of reserves and/or accumulation of excesses. Nutrients are drawn out of other body compartments, such as protein out of muscle or lung tissue and calcium from bones. There may be a buildup of byproducts resulting from inefficient or altered metabolism. When substrates are not available in appropriate amounts, adaptive mechanisms kick in, but they reach limits. If measured, blood and other biochemical markers could show subclinical changes, but without physical signs or risk indicators, such laboratory testing normally is not done. Nutrition education and ***dietary guidance*** directed at the public attempts to inform people about common risks and encourages healthful diets and lifestyle choices to minimize or reverse subclinical changes.

**Nonspecific Signs and Symptoms** Eventually, insufficient or excessive intake of nutrients or energy leads to observable changes. Examples include the accumulation of subcutaneous fat and central adiposity, elevated blood pressure, and insulin resistance. These changes are well-recognized risk factors for the development of chronic diseases. By this stage, immune function is affected and there is reduced resistance to pathogens, chemical exposures, radiation, and stress, including the continued stress of nutrient imbalance. Screening should identify these changes and signal the need for intervention. Dietary guidance, nutrition counseling, and medical nutrition therapy, delivered individually or in groups, are potential interventions to assist individuals in making changes at this stage. Goals of intervention target specific risk factors and observable signs and symptoms. These can be measured and monitored over time to assess progress in halting or reversing nutritional injury and risk factors for disease.

**Clinical Condition** Genetic predisposition, interacting with dietary components and other environmental factors, influence whether and when the clinical condition develops. If changes aren't made and the nutritional injury persists, frank signs and symptoms of illness are now present and a medical diagnosis such as atherosclerosis, osteoporosis, cancer, type 2 diabetes, or depression is made. A clear medical diagnosis is the turning point for serious lifestyle change for some adults. Change is difficult, and intensive intervention such as medical nutrition therapy or therapeutic behavior change programs (presented in detail in Chapter 17) may be necessary to manage the disease and prevent or delay its progression and the development of side effects and complications.

**Chronic Condition** At this stage, altered metabolism and structural changes in tissues become permanent and irreversible. Examples are structural damage to coronary arteries, invasive and metastatic cancer, loss of kidney function, or blindness. Major adjustments of life are necessary to manage the chronic disease and accommodate conditions that have significant impact on quality of life. Intervention at this stage is aimed at managing the condition, preventing further complications, reducing the degree of disability, and optimizing quality of life.

**Terminal Illness and Death** At the final stage in the continuum, complications advance, body systems shut down, and life ceases.

# Energy Recommendations

**LO 16.3** Estimate your daily energy needs using three methods and discuss factors that affect energy needs of adults.

Energy requirements are defined as the amount of dietary energy intake needed to be consumed by individuals to sustain stable body weight consistent with long-term good health that would allow for adequate levels of physical activity to maintain social, cultural, and economic activity.[22] A healthy weight for most individuals is a BMI of 18.5 up to 25 $Kg/m^2$.

## Age-Related Changes in Energy Expenditure

Metabolic rate and energy expenditure begin to decline in early adulthood at a rate of about 2.9 percent for men and 2.0 percent for women per decade.[23] These reductions generally correspond to declines in physical activity and lean muscle mass. Between ages 25 and 65, physical working capacity (measured by $VO_2$ max) declines by 5–10 percent per decade. The presence of musculoskeletal disease, obesity, and other conditions can accelerate declines in energy expenditure and physical capacity.

In young, healthy adults, there is compensatory adjustment between physical activity and calorie intake. Early studies indicate this is also true for older adults.[24] In the mid-1960s, researchers at the Baltimore Longitudinal Study on Aging (BLSA) reported that caloric intake in men decreased 22 percent, from 2,700 to 2,100 calories, between age 30 and age 80.[25] They suggested that the decrease was due to lowered metabolic rates as well as decreased activity levels. However, the current trend of higher body weight and the increasing rate of overweight and obesity through the adult decades indicates that behavioral, social, and environmental factors supersede the innate physiological ability to adjust caloric intake with energy expenditure.[26]

**dietary guidance** Providing concise recommendations and consumer information to guide daily food choices.

TABLE 16.4 ▸ Estimated caloric needs per day by age, gender, and physical activity level

| GENDER | AGE | SEDENTARY | MODERATELY ACTIVE | ACTIVE |
|---|---|---|---|---|
| Female | 19–30 | 1800–2000 | 2000–2200 | 2400 |
| | 31–50 | 1800 | 2000 | 2200 |
| | 51–65 | 1600 | 1800 | 2000–2200 |
| Male | 19–30 | 2400–2600 | 2600–2800 | 3000 |
| | 31–50 | 2200–2400 | 2400–2600 | 2800–3000 |
| | 51–65 | 2000–2200 | 2400 | 2600–2800 |

Adapted from Dietary Guidelines for Americans 2010 Report. Based on Estimated Energy Requirements (EER) using reference heights and weights from the Institute of Medicine, Dietary Reference Intakes for Energy, Carbohydrate, Fiber, Fat, Fatty Acids, Cholesterol, Protein, and Amino Acids. Washington (DC): The National Academies Press; 2002.

## Estimating Energy Needs in Adults

Energy needs are based on an individual's ***basal metabolic rate (BMR)***, the ***thermic effect of food (TEF)***, and ***activity thermogenesis***. The largest component of daily energy expenditure, 60–75 percent for most adults, is the involuntary process of internal chemical activities that maintain the body.[27] While the brain, liver, gastrointestinal tract, heart, and kidney make up less than 5 percent of body weight, the active metabolic processes and functions of these organs account for about 60 percent of BMR. Additional energy is required for the digestion, absorption, and metabolism of food—referred to as the thermic effect of food (TEF). This amounts to approximately 10 percent of energy needs but varies with diet composition and across individuals. TEF is lower in some obese individuals, suggesting that more efficient digestion and absorption of food may be a factor in obesity.[28] The most variable component of energy expenditure is activity thermogenesis (which includes energy expended through exercise and nonexercise activity such as fidgeting), accounting for 20–40 percent of total energy expenditure.

Energy needs of an individual can be estimated in several ways. The Food and Nutrition Board determined ***estimated energy requirements (EER)*** from studies that measured total daily energy expenditure by the doubly labeled water technique (DLW).[22] The DLW technique is a very precise method of measuring energy utilization in real living conditions (i.e., not the laboratory). Subjects are given a dose of "tagged" water containing "heavy" isotopes of hydrogen and oxygen. Excretion of isotopes in saliva and urine is used to calculate average energy utilization over several days. For the EER in Table 16.4, the reference man is 5 feet 10 inches tall and weighs 154 pounds, and the reference woman is 5 feet 4 inches tall and weighs 126 pounds. For each 2 inches of extra height, add 90 calories if female and 125 if male. For overweight and obese individuals (BMI 25–40 Kg/m$^2$), energy requirements are higher (by 120–400 calories/day) due to the increased energy cost of carrying extra weight.

Indirect calorimetry is used to determine ***resting energy expenditure (REE)***, a measure closely related to basal metabolic rate. Indirect calorimetry is done by measuring the exchange of gases during respiration, for a specific period of time, using a metabolic cart in hospitals or newer portable technology and handheld devices in clinics and gyms. The respiratory quotient ($VCO_2/VO_2$) is used to estimate 24-hour energy expenditure.

REE can also be calculated using a validated estimation formula. The Mifflin–St. Jeor formula was developed for healthy, normal-weight, and moderately overweight men and women. It requires accurate measures of height (cm) and weight (kg).[29]

**Mifflin–St. Jeor Energy Estimation Formula**
**Males:** REE $= (10 \times 3\text{ wt}) + (6.25 \times \text{ht}) - (5 \times \text{age}) + 5$
**Females:** REE $= (10 \times \text{wt}) + (6.25 \times \text{ht}) - (5 \times \text{age}) - 161$

After the REE has been determined, the value is multiplied by an activity factor (1.2 sedentary, 1.55 moderately active, or 1.725 very active) to arrive at the estimated daily calorie expenditure.[22]

Numerous energy calculators based on height and weight are available online. Many are based on the older Harris-Benedict equation, which is less accurate.[30] For more athletic individuals, a formula based on lean body mass is recommended, which produces a higher and more accurate EER reflecting the effect of greater lean muscle mass on BMR.[31] A simple calculation can also be used to "ballpark" caloric levels for weight maintenance, weight loss, or weight gain. Approximately 15 calories per pound of body weight per day are needed to maintain weight. Cutting to 13 calories/lb per day can result in weight loss, and increasing to 17 calories/lb per day can produce weight gain.[32]

## Energy Adjustments for Weight Change

A pound of body weight is the equivalent of approximately 3,500 calories. To lose 1 pound a week, an adult would need to create a negative calorie balance of 500 calories daily. These

**basal metabolic rate (BMR)** Amount of energy required for cellular metabolic processes and function of organs. It is measured in an individual who has been awake less than 30 minutes and is still at absolute rest, has fasted for 10 hours or more, and is in a quiet room with normal, comfortable temperature.

**thermic effect of food (TEF)** Energy required for the digestion, absorption, and metabolism of food; approximately 10 percent of energy needs.

**activity thermogenesis** Energy expended through physical activity and nonexercise activity such as fidgeting.

**estimated energy requirement (EER)** The average dietary energy intake for adults in good health, by age, gender, weight, height, and level of physical activity, that is predicted to maintain energy balance and is consistent with good health.

**resting energy expenditure (REE)** Measured or estimated energy expenditure in an individual at rest.

500 calories can be generated from a combination of decreased calorie intake and increased physical activity. For instance, briskly walking two extra miles uses roughly 200 calories, and eliminating 12 ounces of regular cola and a single-serving bag of potato chips (1 ounce) allows subtraction of 300 calories, summed to total 500 calories. Seven days of burning 200 extra calories through physical activity and eating 300 fewer calories leads to a weight loss of approximately 1 pound. On the other hand, a positive balance of just 100 extra calories per day will result in a gain of 10 pounds in a year!

### Energy Balance

Adults need to pay attention to the delicate balance between energy in and energy out. A myriad of lifestyle, social, and environmental factors make consumption of extra calories easy and burning those calories up thorough physical activity more difficult. Studies have linked the obesity epidemic to small, reoccurring excesses in energy intake over energy enpenditure.[33]

Reduction of total energy intake enhances weight loss regardless of the macro composition of the diet.[34] It doesn't matter if the diet is low fat, high protein, low carb, or a balanced combination (as long as micronutrient needs are met); the point is to consume fewer calories and to incorporate more physical activity.

## Nutrient Recommendations

> "Poison is in everything, and no thing is without poison. The dosage makes it either a poison or a remedy."
>
> —Paracelsus, Swiss alchemist, 1493–1541

**LO 16.4** Identify nutrients that are consumed in excessive and inadequate levels and the consequences for adult health.

### Macro and Micro Nutrient Recommendations

The Institute of Medicine's recommendations for macronutrient (carbohydrate, fat, and protein), intake are expressed in ranges of percentage of total calorie intake. The wide ranges account for the fact that various eating patterns can be healthful.[22]

Acceptable Macronutrient Distribution Ranges for adults are:

- Fat — 20–35 percent of calories
- Carbohydrate — 45–65 percent of calories
- Protein — 10–35 percent of calories

For comparison, the 2000–2012 NHANES found that the average macronutrient distribution for adults was about one-third fat and one-half carbohydrate.

Table 16.5 lists recommended nutrient intakes for adults using the DRIs or the Daily Values (DV) used in food labeling,[35] shows average intakes based on NHANES survey data[36] and highlights (in yellow and green, respectively) risk nutrients where intake falls below or exceeds recommendations. Physiological and metabolic mechanisms can be compromised with excessive, inadequate or imbalanced intake of these risk nutrients.

### Risk Nutrients

**Fiber** Dietary fiber decreases the energy density of the diet and a high-fiber diet is linked with lower body weight and less weight gain overtime. Fiber slows gastric emptying time and produces a longer sensation of fullness. Fiber has many benefits beyond its effect on bowel mobility. The action of dietary fiber depends on its form. ***Viscous fiber*** such as that in oatmeal decreases the absorption of cholesterol, increases fecal excretion of cholesterol-rich bile, and results in lower blood levels of total and LDL cholesterol. ***Fermentable fiber***, such as the skin of fruit and wheat or corn bran, enters the colon undigested and is fermented by gut bacteria. Higher intake of fermentable fiber promotes the development of a beneficial mix of microbiota in the gut, which stimulates the immune system that is formed in the lining of the gut. As microbes ferment fiber, short-chain fatty acids and other metabolites are produced.[37] Through these mechanisms, fiber is associated with beneficial impacts on obesity, diabetes, inflammatory bowel disease, and cardiovascular disease. ***Functional fiber***, such as resistant starch, has been approved as a food ingredient by FDA and is being added to many food products. Because of these beneficial physiological effects, health claims attributed to dietary fiber are allowed on the food labels.[38]

**Calcium and Vitamin D** Low vitamin D intake is associated with decreased calcium bioavailability. Combined with low dietary calcium intake by adults, especially women, this leads to loss of calcium from bones, which, in turn, leads to osteopenia—and progression to osteoporosis.[39] The mechanism behind this is that Vitamin D assists calcium absorption from the gut, calcium resorption from bones by osteoclasts, and calcium resorption from the distal renal tubules. Both vitamin D intake and dermal synthesis from sun exposure contribute to serum levels. The substitution of other

**viscous fiber** Types of fiber characterized by their ability to form a gel solution when combined with liquid. Formerly called soluble fiber.

**fermentable fiber** Type of fiber that enters the large colon undigested, where it is acted on by the bacteria of the gut. Formerly called insoluble fiber.

**functional fiber** Isolated or purified undigestible carbohydrates that have beneficial physiological effects in humans.

TABLE 16.5 ▸ Selected nutrient intakes of adults, NHANES 2009–2010, compared to recommendations

| | INTAKE | | | | |
|---|---|---|---|---|---|
| | ACTUAL | | | | RECOMMENDED[a] |
| | 20–29 YEARS | | 40–49 YEARS | | 31–50 YEARS |
| NUTRIENT | MALES | FEMALES | MALES | FEMALES | MALES/FEMALES |
| Energy, kcal | 2764 | 2019 | 2734 | 1841 | — |
| Protein, g | 103 | 72 | 105 | 66 | 56/46 |
| Total fat, g | 102 | 76 | 105 | 66 | 65 (DV)[b] |
| Saturated fat, g | 33 | 25 | 35 | 22 | 20 (DV)[b] |
| Alpha-linolenic acid (omega 3), g | 2.2 | 1.7 | 2.2 | 1.5 | 1.6/1.1 |
| Cholesterol, mg | 341 | 227 | 371 | 232 | ≤300 (DV)[b] |
| Total carbohydrate, g | 332 | 255 | 317 | 231 | 300 (DV)[b] |
| Fiber, g | 20 | 16 | 20 | 15 | 38/25 |
| Total sugar, g | 146 | 114 | 137 | 108 | 125 (DV)[b] |
| Sodium, mg | 4477 | 3294 | 4646 | 3089 | <2400 |
| Vitamin A, mcg RE | 612 | 593 | 764 | 574 | 900/700 |
| Vitamin $B_{12}$, $\mu$g | 6.6 | 4.6 | 6.3 | 3.9 | 2.4 |
| Folate, $\mu$g | 661 | 543 | 684 | 460 | 400 |
| Vitamin C, mg | 95 | 83 | 72 | 78 | 90/70 |
| Vitamin D IU ($\mu$g) | 4.9 | 3.7 | 6.2 | 3.8 | 15[f] |
| Vitamin E, mg TE | 10.2 | 6.4 | 8.0 | 7.6 | 15 |
| Vitamin K, $\mu$g | 117 | 121 | 129 | 130 | 120/90 |
| Choline, mg | 391 | 272 | 430 | 273 | 550/425 |
| Calcium, mg | 1194 | 908 | 1238 | 856 | 1000 |
| Iron, mg | 18.0 | 14.4 | 18.5 | 12.8 | 8/18 |
| Magnesium, mg | 346 | 266 | 375 | 275 | 420/320 |
| Potassium, mg | 2983 | 2334 | 3329 | 2397 | 3500 |
| Zinc, mg | 14.0 | 10.0 | 14.6 | 9.3 | 11/8 |
| Caffeine, mg | 114 | 94 | 229 | 185 | Up to 250[c] |
| Alcohol, g[e] | 16.6 | 7.8 | 16.6 | 7.8 | 20/8[d] |

SOURCE: *What We Eat in America*, NHANES, 2011–2012. U.S. Department of Agriculture, Agriculture Research Service, 2014. Available from www.ars.usda.gov

[a]Recommended intake according to DRI 2002 or to DV nutrient reference amount used on food labels, relevant to a 2000 kcal diet.[47]

[b]Based on a 2000 kcal diet; for other caloric levels, the 2010 Dietary Guidelines recommendation is no more than 30% of calories from fat, 10% from saturated fat, and 25% of calories from sugar.

[c]250 mg is an average moderate intake; safety > 400 is unclear, 800 mg is considered excessive.

[d]Based on Dietary Guidelines for Americans.

[e]Alcohol intake is reported for ages 20 and over because of wide variability within groups.

[f]Assumes inadequate exposure to sunlight.

beverages for milk, which is high in calcium and enriched with vitamin $D_3$ (the most available form of vitamin D), contributes to the fact that 50 percent of the population has low serum 25 hydroxy (OH) vitamin D.[40] Studies of nonskeletal effects of calcium and vitamin D intake have produced mixed findings, including mortality risk, prostate, breast and colon cancers, and diabetes.[41]

**Vitamin A and Vitamin E** Vitamin A and vitamin E are fat-soluble vitamins with strong antioxidant functions. Oxidation reactions produce free radicals, which start chain reactions that damage cells. Antioxidants terminate these chain reactions. The roles of vitamin E and vitamin A in DNA transcription has led to investigation of their potential protective effects in various cancers.[42] Both are also involved in the functioning of the immune system. Vitamin A is essential in maintaining the integrity of the skin and mucosal cells, which function as a mechanical barrier and defend the body against infection. Vitamin A also plays a central role in the development and differentiation of white blood cells that defend the body against pathogens.[43] Vitamin E has anti-inflammatory properties and is involved in maintenance and repair of cellular membranes.

**Choline** Choline comes from the diet and is also synthesized within the body. Dietary deficiency has been shown to cause fatty liver and muscle deterioration. Choline and its derivatives serve as components of cell membranes and as a precursor of the neurotransmitter acetylcholine, which signals between neurons and is involved in brain function.[44] Along with folate and vitamin B12, choline is involved in the conversion of homocysteine to methionine, suggesting a role in cardiovascular disease; and it is a methyl donor during RNA replication and gene expression.[45]

**Potassium and Sodium** Sodium and potassium have opposing effects on blood vessels. High sodium decreases vasodilation and raises blood pressure, and potassium increases vasodilation.[46] High dietary potassium intake is associated with low blood pressure and is recommended for primary prevention of hypertension, but potassium supplementation does not appear to have added benefit. Research using a diet high in fruits and vegetables and low-fat dairy products (all good sources of potassium) and low in sodium (the DASH diet) was found to reduce blood pressure. Studies show that sodium intake limited to 2400mg/d can prevent and reduce high blood pressure.[47]

**Magnesium** A cellular magnesium deficit elicits a calcium-activated inflammatory cascade independent of injury or pathogens. Elevated C-reactive protein (CRP), an indictor of low grade or chronic inflammation, is more frequently found in adults with magnesium intakes below 50 percent of the RDA.[48] This chronic inflammation may contribute to the occurrence of atherosclerosis, hypertension, osteoporosis, diabetes, cancer, and heart failure. Eating a small handful of peanuts (¼ cup) daily is an easy way to increase magnesium intake.

**Iron** Sustained low dietary intake of iron leads to depletion of iron stores, reduced synthesis of hemoglobin, and iron-deficiency anemia with decreased oxygen transport to tissues. Iron depletion, with or without anemia, is associated with lower work performance, athletic performance, cognitive function, reproductive function (see Chapter 2), and reduced immune function. Adiposity has an inhibiting role in iron absorption from the small intestine.[49] Premenopausal women may have low iron status due to losses in menstrual blood.

# Dietary Recommendations for Adults

LO 16.5 Explain the purpose of dietary guidance and how it translates science into healthful food and beverage choices and pleasurable eating experiences for adults.

Knowing about nutrients and their roles in health and disease is one thing; but how is that translated into foods adults should eat? This is where dietary guidance systems come in. ***Dietary guidance systems*** are sets of dietary and lifestyle recommendations, based on the latest scientific evidence related to nutrition and health that are developed to promote health and prevent disease. They include technical reports of the scientific evidence, recommendations on types and amounts of food to eat, and tools and resources to help the public and professionals put recommendations into action. Another component of dietary guidance systems is recommendations for community action and policy changes to help create an environment where achievement of the dietary and lifestyle recommendations is possible.

Guidelines are updated periodically in response to priority health issues, new research, current nutrient intakes, and eating patterns of the population. They also take into account changes in the food system and the hospitality industry, food product development, and, more recently, environmental impacts. The ***Dietary Guidelines*** for Americans and MyPlate are major components of the U.S. dietary guidance system.[26,50,51] (See Chapter 1 for background information.) They are the foundation for U.S. nutrition policy and for federal nutrition program regulations and education activities.

Voluntary (i.e., nonprofit) health organizations also make science-based dietary recommendations for healthy adults related to the organization's mission. For example, the American Cancer Society has Nutrition and Physical Activity Guidelines[52] and the American Heart Association has Diet and Lifestyle Recommendations.[53] Along with the Dietary Guidelines for Americans, these guidelines identify an urgent need to address obesity and are generally consistent in their dietary advice to adults. They encourage adults to do the following:

- Consume greater amounts of fruits and vegetables, whole grains and fiber and low-fat dairy; and reduce refined carbohydrates.
- Avoid *trans* fats, limit saturated fat intake, and select healthy fats and oils to replace saturated fat.
- Select fish, poultry, and meat alternatives (nuts, seeds, beans, tofu), lean meats and avoid processed meats.
- Select more nutrient-rich food and less nutrient-poor food.
- Limit sugar, especially beverages with added sugar and grain-based desserts.
- Keep sodium low.
- Get regular physical activity.
- Balance energy intake with energy expenditure to maintain or achieve a healthy weight.

**dietary guidance system** A comprehensive set of dietary and lifestyle recommendations, based on the latest scientific information, that are developed to promote heath and prevent disease or its complications, ensure adequate intake of nutrients of concern, and offer guidance on what and how much to eat.

**Dietary Guidelines** A report, including scientific information and rationale, on dietary information and guidelines for the general public or a defined subpopulation. The guidelines provide a cohesive set of recommendations that are adopted by the government or organization. They represent policy and are integrated into food, nutrition, and health programs.

Which of these women is making food choices consistent with the dietary recommendations?

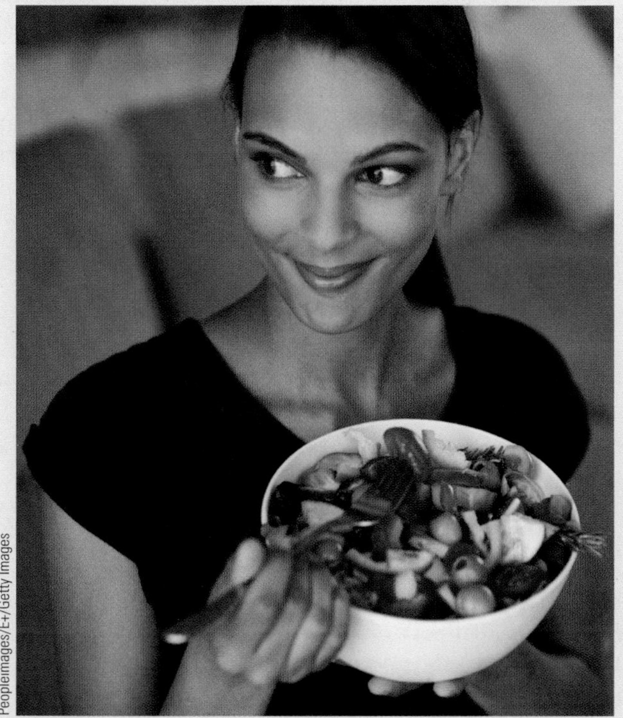

Peopleimages/E+/Getty Images

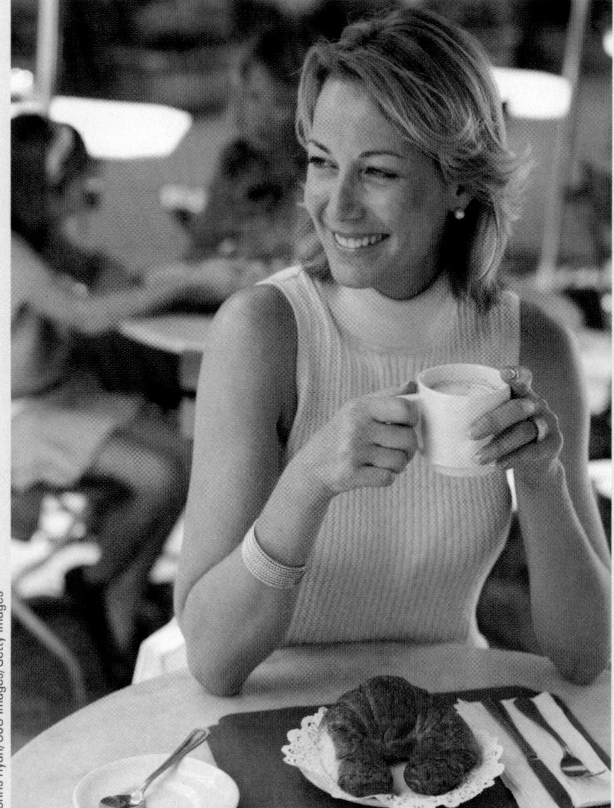

Chris Ryan/OJO Images/Getty Images

ILLUSTRATION 16.4 ▸ Contrast of eating choices.

## Total Diet Approach

Beginning with the 2010 Dietary Guidelines for Americans and USDA Food Patterns, a ***total diet approach*** was adopted.[50,51] This approach recognizes that food choices vary from day to day and across seasons. The aim is the selection of a combination of foods and beverages that provide energy and nutrients and meet an individual's nutritional requirements, on average, over time.[54] There is no assumption that every day is the same; rather, selecting a variety of foods within each food group and from day to day helps assure all nutrient needs are met.

Using resources available at ChooseMyPlate.gov, adults can determine calorie needs and access a corresponding food plan that specifies the amount of each food group necessary to achieve nutrient adequacy for their calorie level. MyPlate resources help consumers translate amounts into food choices and personalized menus. The goal is a nutrient-rich total diet—a balanced grouping of a variety of foods among all the food groups, consumed in moderation—that is culturally appealing, offers pleasurable eating experiences, and promotes health among Americans.[5] Which woman in the photos comes closer to meeting these goals? (Illustration 16.4)

There are two important cautions when applying the USDA food patterns to yourself and other adults.

1. *Choose **nutrient-dense foods**.* The recommended amounts in the USDA food patterns assume that all choices are nutrient-dense forms without added sugar and keep oil within the recommended amount. The dilemma is that nutrient-dense food choices are available in the marketplace, but they often are not the form typically consumed. When "typical" rather than "ideal" nutrient-dense food choices are made, energy, total fat, saturated fat, cholesterol, and sodium exceed limits in all USDA patterns, often by substantial margins, even when the recommended quantity is selected. Consider for example: a fried breaded chicken patty on a white bun, fries, and soda versus a grilled skinless chicken breast on a whole grain bun, green salad, and low-fat milk. A study found that with typical choices, calories were 15 to 30 percent (350 to 450 kcal) above the target calorie level for each pattern. However, goals for adequacy of nutrients were not substantially affected by the use of typical food choices.[56]

**total diet approach** Guidance based on overall eating patterns that meet needs with a variety of foods over time.

**nutrient-dense food** A food that provides substantial amounts of vitamins, minerals, and other biologically active food components with relatively few calories. Also called nutrient-rich.

2. *Don't eat too much.* Portion sizes specified by MyPlate are smaller than the amounts in conventional food packaging and as commonly served in restaurants. Foods must be chosen keeping in mind recommended serving sizes and amount per day or week rather than the amount in a package or the amount served. Large serving sizes increase calorie intake and also contribute more fat and added sugar.[57] Calorie, fat, and sugar intake can be minimized by selecting fewer and smaller portions of energy-dense foods and replacing with foods of lower energy density.[58]

A nutrient-rich, calorie-balanced diet can be implemented in many ways to meet cultural and taste preferences. Systemic reviews of research point to three eating "styles" associated with the positive impacts on heart disease, cancer, and diabetes—the DASH diet (featuring fruits and vegetables, low-fat dairy, and low sodium), the Mediterranean style of eating (featuring vegetables, fish and seafood, and olive oil), and vegetarian diets (featuring fruits and vegetables and meat alternatives).[26,50] What these eating styles have in common is a shift toward a more plant-based, lower-sodium diet that includes a moderate amount of healthy fat. The USDA food plans include a typical U.S. pattern containing meat as well as a vegetarian plan to provide guidance to current vegetarians or those interested in shifting to a plant-based diet.

## Water Intake Recommendations

The Food and Nutrition Board defines the adult adequate intake (AI) level for water based on median total water intake (from fluids and food) from NHANES III data for young adults aged 19 to 30 years.[59] The panel did not set an upper level for water; however, water toxicity can occur.

Total Water AI for Adults

| | | |
|---|---|---|
| Men | 3.7 liters | (125 oz) |
| Women | 2.7 liters | (91 oz) |

According to the NHANES survey, drinking water and other beverages supplied 81 percent of total water needs of adults, and the moisture in food provided the remaining 19 percent.[60] Following a review of the science, the 2010 Dietary Guidelines Task Force concluded that the combination of thirst and typical behaviors, such as drinking beverages with meals, provides sufficient total water intake.[26]

## Beverage Intake Recommendations

Adults (19 years and older) consume an average of 400 calories per day as beverages. By order of calorie contribution they include regular soda, energy and sport drinks, alcoholic beverages, milk, 100 percent fruit juices, and fruit drinks.[26] Coffee drinks, flavored with syrup and topped with whipped cream, account for more calories and take a big bite out of the allowance for solid fats and added sugars (SoFAS). Sugar-sweetened beverages are associated with metabolic syndrome and fatty liver disease. "Diet" soda is not the answer, as the safety of noncaloric sweeteners is under question.[50] Another issue is that calories consumed in liquid form may have less satiety value and may not be compensated for with adjustments in food intake.[61] Except for milk and fruit juices, beverages contribute little to essential nutrient needs. To meet fluid needs while managing calories and contributing to nutrient needs, a plan for daily beverage selections could be:

- Choose water as the preferred beverage, 3–5 12-ounce containers.
- Limit unsweetened coffee or tea to 3–4 cups.
- Drink two 8-ounce glasses of low-fat milk.
- Drink a small (4-ounce) glass of 100 percent fruit juice, or choose fresh fruit.
- Avoid sugar-sweetened soda; if using diet soda, limit to one 12-ounce can.

Resources such as the CDC's "Rethink Your Drink" help consumers make smarter fluid selections.[63]

## Caffeine and Coffee Intake

What about fluids containing caffeine? Occasionally, someone suggests that coffee, tea, or other caffeine-containing beverages not be counted as fluid intake because they have a diuretic effect on the body. Caffeine temporarily increases urine production at high doses, but no evidence connects these beverages with dehydration.[63] The Food and Nutrition Board concluded that caffeine-containing beverages contribute to daily total water intake.[59]

Caffeine is known for its stimulating effects on the central nervous system, but other biologically active compounds in regular and decaffeinated coffee exert anticarcinogenic, antimicrobial, neuroprotective, and hypoglycemic effects that may protect against cancer, dental caries, Parkinson's disease, diabetes, and weight gain. How coffee is roasted and brewed affects its taste and aroma, as well as its content of caffeine and other compounds. Naturally occurring caffeine routinely consumed by healthy adults in the range of 400–800 mg/dL has not been found to be harmful and is associated with the above positive effects.[64] However, products supplemented with caffeine are proliferating in the marketplace, raising concern about its safety at high levels of intake. Adverse effects of high doses include increased heart rate and blood pressure and headaches, and depend on individual sensitivity.

## Alcoholic Beverages

Alcohol is a popular beverage with significant social and cultural significance, but it is also a psychoactive drug with potential for abuse. While moderate alcohol intake is a recognized contributor to heart health, alcohol also increases the risk of oral, esophageal, liver, and colorectal cancers, and breast cancer in women and it adds calories.[51]

Approximately 61 percent of adults in the United States drink alcohol, with the highest rates among persons aged 25 to 44 years (76 percent of males, 63 percent of females).[65] Rates of alcohol consumption decline with age. The U.S. guideline is: "If alcohol is consumed, it should be consumed in moderation," defined as no more than 2 drinks per day for males, and no more than 1 drink per day for females.[51]

What is a drink? A drink contains roughly 13–15 grams of alcohol or 0.5 ounce of ethanol (Table 16.6). Additional calories needed to be added if mixers are used.

## Dietary Supplements and Functional Foods

Dietary supplements include vitamins, minerals, amino acids, herbal and botanical supplements, enzymes, prebiotics, and probiotics. There are circumstances in which vitamin and mineral supplements are indicated to assure nutritional adequacy, such as during pregnancy, with certain illness, or when low-calorie or nutrient-restricted diets are consumed. Estimates from national survey data indicate that 44 percent of males and 53 percent females take a vitamin and/or mineral; most of these do so daily.[66] Supplemental vitamin and mineral use gradually increases with age. For example, at perimenopause, many women begin to take calcium or calcium with vitamin D supplements to prevent bone loss.

Botanical and herbal supplements are used by many adults to "treat" or "prevent" a particular health-related concern. Research supporting the purported benefits is often lacking, but this is an area of active research. For example, there is some evidence supporting Echinacea for upper respiratory infections and ginger for nausea; mixed results on the use of St. John's wort for depression and concern about its interaction with other medications; and no conclusive evidence on the effects of cinnamon for diabetes or heart disease.[67] Research on health effects and safety is challenging because of variations in, the growing, extraction, manufacturing, and marketing of these products.

TABLE 16.6 ▸ Alcoholic beverages: alcohol and calorie content

| AMOUNT | BEVERAGE | ALCOHOL GRAMS | CALORIES |
|---|---|---|---|
| 12 oz | Regular beer | 13 | 153 |
| 12 oz | Light beer | 12 | 100 |
| 1.5 oz | Distilled spirits: gin, whiskey, rum, vodka | 15 | 90 |
| 5 oz | Red wine | 15 | 125 |
| 5 oz | Dry white wine | 14 | 107 |
| 2 oz | Sherry | 9 | 80 |



**Functional Foods** Numerous products are available that blur the lines among conventional food, supplement, and therapeutic agent. These cover many categories, as defined in Table 16.7.[68] ***Functional foods*** is the term used for food products or ingredients that have a physiological benefit beyond the nutritional value provided. There is a growing body of evidence linking diet and biologically active components of food to immune function, antioxidant and anti-inflammatory effects, and to chronic-disease risk reduction. Consumer interest in managing health and performance is increasing demand such as use of ergogenic products to enhance physical performance and prebiotics and probiotics for gut health.

## The Eating Competence Model

Eating behaviors begin within the individual and his or her beliefs and attitudes about food and eating. The *Eating Competence Model* offers a paradigm for nutrition education and dietary guidance that is different from but complementary to dietary guidelines that are focused on risk reduction. This model recognizes the special value of the social and sensory aspects of food and eating. The goal is to encourage "competent eaters who are positive, comfortable, and flexible with eating and are matter-of-fact and reliable about getting enough to eat of enjoyable, nourishing food."[69]

The model has four components:

1. **Eating attitudes:** Includes positive interest in foods and eating; self-trust about managing food and eating; and finding harmony among food desires, food choices, and amounts eaten.
2. **Food acceptance:** Recognizes that enjoyment and pleasure are primary motivators for food selection, and that nutritional excellence is supported by enjoyment of a variety of food, including nutritious food. Food acceptance means being comfortable eating a preferred food, even if it isn't the most nutritious, but it also means being able to settle for less-preferred food when necessary to satisfy caloric or other nutritional needs.
3. **Regulation of food intake:** Emphasizes internally regulated eating and attention to sensations of hunger and fullness. See Table 16.8 for hunger-related cues.[70] One who has learned self-regulation has the ability to tolerate hunger when there is

**functional foods** A food product that has a physiological benefit or reduces the risk of chronic disease beyond basic nutritional functions

**Eating Competence Model** A new paradigm for nutrition education and dietary guidance that considers four components: eating attitudes, food acceptance, regulation of food intake, and eating context. A competent eater is positive, comfortable, and flexible with eating and is matter-of-fact and reliable about getting enough to eat of enjoyable, nourishing food.

TABLE 16.7 ▸ Definition and examples of supplements and functional food categories

| CATEGORY | DEFINITION | EXAMPLES |
|---|---|---|
| **Supplement** | Vitamin, mineral, amino acid, herbal or other botanical, or combination ingested in pill, capsule, or liquid form | Multiple vitamin<br>Calcium<br>Glucosamine and chondroitin<br>Amino acids |
| **Functional Food Category** | | |
| Conventional foods (whole foods) | Unmodified food rich in bioactive components that have health benefits | Nuts reduce risk of cardiac death<br>Cruciferous vegetables reduce risk of cancer<br>Flaxseed oil for omega-3 fatty acids |
| Modified foods<br>• Fortified<br>• Enriched<br>• Enhanced | • Bioactive component added<br>• Replacement or addition of component naturally in the food<br>• Food product formulated with bioactive components | • Calcium-fortified orange juice, iodized salt<br>• Flour enriched with vitamins and iron<br>• Margarine with plant stanols or sterol esters for cholesterol lowering<br>• Energy bars, yogurt, or bottled water formulated with amino acids, lutein, fish oil, probiotics, ginkgo biloba, caffeine |
| Medical foods (available only by prescription) | A food formulated to be used under the supervision of a physician, intended for the specific dietary management of a disease or condition | Phenylketonuria (PKU) formula free of phenylalanine |
| Foods for special dietary use (available at the retail level) | Food designed to meet a special dietary need due to physical, physiological, pathological, or other condition; supplement the diet; or replace a meal or daily food intake | Gluten-free foods<br>Sports drinks with electrolytes<br>Nutrient-dense beverage for protein and calorie supplementation<br>Meal replacements for weight-reducing diets |

SOURCE: Based on C. M. Hasler et al. Position of the American Dietetic Association: Functional foods. *J Am Diet Assoc* 109 (2009): 735–746.

TABLE 16.8 ▸ Cues for regulating food intake

| APPETITIVE CUES | PHYSICAL SENSATION | EMOTIONAL FEELING OR COGNITION |
|---|---|---|
| Famished | Extreme hunger, pronounced discomfort: shakiness, crankiness, headache | Urgency and desperation to eat<br>Often results from food insecurity (no assurance of being able to get enough to eat)<br>May result from extreme self-restraint |
| Hunger, increased appetite | Physical experience of emptiness; may include mild discomfort | Tolerable anticipation of eating<br>Awareness that adequate amounts of rewarding food will soon be available |
| Hunger goes away | Physical feeling of emptiness subsides, along with discomfort from energy deficit | Sense of relief increases; however, most people are reluctant to stop eating at this point because eating is still rewarding |
| Appetite goes away | Satiety: positive experience of readiness to stop eating<br>This is a more sustaining and rewarding endpoint to eating for most people than when hunger goes away | Food stops tasting good; a subjective experience of losing interest in eating |
| Feeling full | For most, this is a pleasant, if occasional, endpoint to eating; it is a positive state of feeling filled up | Eating past satiety is rewarding if it follows a deliberate decision to eat more than usual, perhaps on a ceremonial occasion, because food tastes exceptionally good or because energy needs have suddenly increased |
| Feeling Stuffed | Negative physical state, including extreme fullness, lethargy, physical discomfort, perhaps nausea; virtually universally experienced as being a negative endpoint to eating | Accompanied by a sense of chagrin at overeating and self-indulgence; often arrived at as an unthinking or impulsive suspension of self-restraint |

SOURCE: Based on Satter Eating Competency Model.

confidence that adequate, rewarding food will be available; the ability to stop when satisfied; and the ability to accept the body weight that evolves from internally regulated eating.

4. **Eating context:** Puts priority on structure and meal planning. Meals are a predictable time to eat adequate amounts of preferred food. Eating is intentional and deliberate, and it requires discipline. The model teaches that going to some trouble to procure rewarding food, scheduling eating times, and setting aside time to eat are important. Intentional, deliberate eaters are able to postpone snacking and grazing when they are confident that there will be satisfying food at the next meal.

Within the eating competence model, nutrition education, and dietary guidance are used to help people be more attuned to their needs and feelings; to encourage them to try and learn to like a wide variety of nutritious foods; and to remind them of the importance of taking time and having the self-discipline to plan and prepare satisfying meals.

# Physical Activity Recommendations

**LO 16.6** Describe national recommendations for physical activity and the benefits of regular physical activity.

Healthy eating and increased physical activity are the featured duo for combating obesity at the individual and population level and are primary and secondary prevention strategies for several chronic diseases, including cardiovascular disease, diabetes, hypertension, osteoporosis, and colon and breast cancer.[5,19,50,52,53] Physical activity increases muscle strength, balance, and endurance, and cardiorespiratory fitness; it supports physical and mental health and improves cognitive function; and it helps manage weight and reduces risk factors for disease including high blood cholesterol and blood pressure. Regular physical activity and resulting fitness enables adults to meet the physical demands of daily living, work, and leisure and enhances quality of life.[71]

## Guidelines for Physical Activity

Any physical activity is better than none; even short, 10-minute intervals of intentional physical activity above usual activity can have positive health benefits.[31] The degree of benefit increases as the duration and intensity increase.[71] Government agencies and health organizations around the world recommend that adults integrate moderate to vigorous intensity physical activity (that increases breathing or heart rate) into their routine lifestyle.[72] Based on the review and synthesis of research, the amount of physical activity needed to achieve positive effects is 2.5 hours per week (Table 16.9).[71]

**TABLE 16.9** Physical Activity Guidelines for Americans: Adults (aged 18–64)

- **Basic recommendation:** 2 hours and 30 minutes a week (150 minutes) of moderate-intensity, or 1 hour and 15 minutes a week (75 minutes) of vigorous-intensity aerobic physical activity, or an equivalent combination. Aerobic activity should be performed in episodes of at least 10 minutes, preferably spread throughout the week.
- **For additional health benefits:** Increase to 5 hours (300 minutes) a week of moderate-intensity aerobic physical activity or 2 hours and 30 minutes (150 minutes) of vigorous-intensity physical activity.
- **Muscle strengthening:** Adults should also do muscle-strengthening activities that involve all major muscle groups (legs, hips, back, abdomen, chest, shoulders, and arms) on 2 or more days per week.

Moderate or vigorous intensity?

**Take the talk test:**
If you can talk, but not sing, you are doing moderate-intensity activity. If you can't say more than a few words without pausing for a breath, you are doing vigorous-intensity activity.

**Moderate-intensity activity examples:**
Baseball, brisk walking, cycling, golf (carrying bag), raking leaves, vacuuming, water aerobics

**Vigorous-intensity activity examples:**
Aerobic exercise classes, basketball, fast dancing, hiking with backpack, jumping rope, running, swimming laps



The basic recommendation could be met with a brisk 30-minute walk five days a week, or an individualized plan using "Be Active Your Way."[73] It is easier said than done. According to recent surveys a quarter of adults reported no physical activity in the past month while about half were meeting the Physical Activity Guidelines. Some segments of the adult population get little or no physical activity. Younger adults, men, Non-Hispanic whites, and those with greater education have higher rates of physical activity.[74]

## Promotion of Physical Activity

Overcoming a sedentary lifestyle is a challenge. Habitual physical activity starts with intentional, repetitive actions that become enjoyable, rewarding and outweigh alternative uses of time. Personal (e.g., time, motivation, skill), social, and environmental factors influence the degree to which physical activity is a routine part of lifestyle. Socioeconomic constraints, cultural preferences, and baseline levels of sedentariness or obesity are barriers; while community-wide campaigns, social encouragement, and access to facilities help promote physical activity. Social

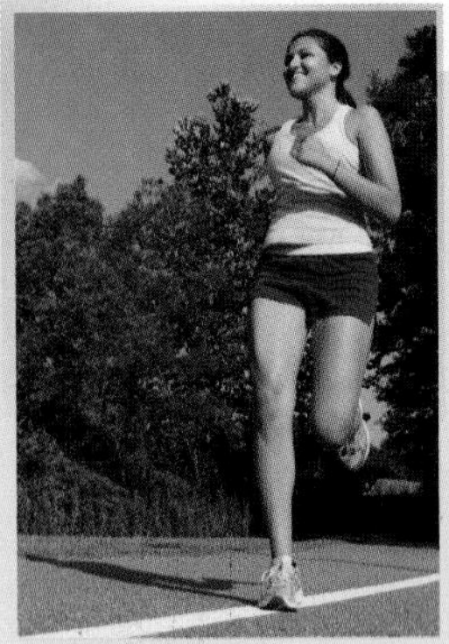
Amanda Mills/CDC

# CASE STUDY 16.1

## Run, Kristen, Run

Kristen, who was active in competitive sports throughout high school, has decided to run a marathon with some of her college friends. She is 25 years old, 5 foot, 8 inches tall, and weighs 135 pounds. She eats all sorts of foods, likes fruits and vegetables, but tries to avoid greasy foods. She says coffee is her downfall—she drinks 4–6 cups a day. She doesn't like sweets, although she keeps ice cream in her freezer. A family history notes that her mother needed angioplasty to treat occluded arteries shortly after menopause and that her father is not at risk for any chronic conditions. Although she would eventually like to have children, Kristen is not pregnant now.

An analysis of a 24-hour dietary recall shows the following:

2090 calories
352 g carbohydrate (67% of calories)
41 g total fiber
98 g protein (19% of calories)
33 g fat (14% of calories)
(7 g saturated fat, 1 g trans fat,
1.5 g omega-3 fatty acid,
99 mg cholesterol)
3343 mg sodium

34 mg iron
958 g calcium
117 mcg vitamin A
158 mg vitamin C
0.5 mcg vitamin D
7.4 IU vitamin E
1548 mcg folic acid
283 mg choline

### Questions

1. How many calories does Kristen need to maintain her weight?
2. Is she eating enough to support daily workouts?
3. Describe three health-promoting aspects of Kristen's diet.
4. Make three suggestions that could improve Kristen's diet.

support interventions such as buddy systems and walking groups, and structural changes in the environment such as accessible walking trails and the creation of exercise facilities, are strategies that have been feasible, sustainable, and effective in many communities and among different populations including racial/ethnic minority groups.[50] Widespread efforts to change the environment to foster a variety of opportunities for physical activity and accommodate a wide range of preferences and abilities have developed into the ***active living movement***. Private businesses, nonprofit organizations, and government sectors are collaborating to foster social, environmental, and policy changes to reduce sedentary lifestyles and enable greater physical activity in all aspects of life.[50]

Healthy People 2020 Objectives for physical activity are targeted to promote physical activity in all the ways just mentioned and to encourage health care providers to routinely assess physical activity levels and provide counseling and education about physical activity.[8]

## Physical Activity, Body Composition, and Metabolic Change

Individuals who are habitually sedentary should progressively increase the duration and intensity of regular physical activity to allow for adaptations in capacity and efficiency of the body's structures and functions (e.g., cardiorespiratory fitness and muscle strength).[71] Favorable body composition changes (reduced fat mass and increased lean muscle mass) occur with the adoption of regular physical activity.[71] Even in the absence of caloric restriction, aerobic physical activity equivalent to walking at 4 miles per hour for 150 minutes a week or jogging at 6 miles per hour for 75 minutes a week results in decreases in total and abdominal adiposity that are consistent with improved metabolic function. When more physical activity is done, intra-abdominal fat losses are greater. Moreover, research indicates that abdominal fat loss is greater during exercise-induced weight loss and among those with the greatest level of adiposity.[71] Recent studies indicate that exercise can result in beneficial changes in circulating insulin and inflammatory biomarkers, which may explain the positive effect of physical activity on cardiovascular disease, diabetes, and cancer.[75]

## Diet and Physical Activity

The concerns a person might have when starting an intensive training program are illustrated in Case Study 16.1. Healthy adults who exercise regularly and follow a healthful diet, as recommended by the Dietary Guidelines don't need dietary modifications to support physical activity. For some starting an exercise program provides an

**active living movement**
Building a culture where regular physical activity and healthy eating are the accepted norm for people of all ages, abilities and income levels. Involves partnerships of public and private entities and the local community to bring about changes.

**TABLE 16.10** ▸ Nutrient and fluid consideration for intensive exercise program

| |
|---|
| Macronutrients:<br>• Carbohydrate: 6–10 g/kg (2.7–4.5 g/lb) to maintain blood glucose and replace muscle glycogen<br>• Protein: 1.2–1.7 g/kg (0.5–0.8 g/lb) along with sufficient calories for protein sparing<br>• Fat: 20–35% of total calories for energy and source of antioxidents |
| Vitamins and Minerals: Supplements generally not needed if consuming a healthful diet with adequate calories. Numerous recommendations exist on performance-enhancing effect of various supplements. |
| Fluid: Sufficient water and other liquids for hydration and to replace sweat losses:<br>• Weigh before and after exercise to determine sweat loss.<br>• Drink 16–24 oz fluid for every lb (0.5 kg) of body weight lost.<br>• Observe urine; A dark color indicates dehydration.<br>• Adjust fluid intake before, during, and after exercise to minimize or prevent dehydration. |
| Exercise: Impact of type of training or intensive physical activity on nutrient needs:<br>• Endurance sport—Carbohydrate and energy needs higher to sustain blood glucose and replace muscle glycogen.<br>• Bodybuilder training—Protein and calorie needs higher for muscle growth and repair.<br>• Exercise or training program to improve fitness and drop body fat—Carbohydrate intake lower, moderate caloric reduction. |

SOURCE: Adapted from Position Paper of the American Dietetic Association and the Canadian Dietetic Association: Nutrition and Athletic Performance.[76]

incentive to examine and improve eating practices. Adults who engage in a strenuous exercise program or competitive sports have increased nutrient and hydration needs to meet demands of training, competition, and recovery (Table 16.10).[76] Nutritional ***ergogenic aids***—nutritional products that are purported to enhance performance—range from caffeine beverages and protein powders to sport drinks and energy gels and bars. Few improve performance, and some may be harmful. In spite of the popularity of energy and sports drinks, water is sufficient for hydration for routine physical activity.[76] The bottom line for all adults is making healthful eating and regular physical activity a routine and enjoyable part of everyday life.

# Nutrition Intervention for Risk Reduction

LO 16.7 Contrast strategies for promoting and supporting good nutrition of adults.

Many strategies are used to promote nutritional health and reduce the risk for obesity and chronic disease among adults. These range from individual, client-centered interventions such as education and counseling, to multicomponent programs that take advantage of social and environmental supports, to policy and system changes that affect the quality, availability, and affordability of food.

Nutrition intervention for adults takes place at many levels and in many settings. Education and counseling can be directed to the individual to increase knowledge and encourage behavior change. Discussions about BMI and eating habits are becoming a more common part of primary health care. Environmental changes, such as point-of-purchase signage about calorie or fat content of foods, or healthier food options in vending and convenience outlets, are being implemented to enable healthier food choices.[77] Other interventions affect availability and access to healthful foods, such as menu guidelines for worksite cafeterias and food policies for organization-sponsored events, more community gardens and farmers markets, and limits on the number of fast-food outlets in low-income neighborhoods.[50] Health-promotion programs that include healthy eating and physical activity are sponsored by churches, community organizations, and employers.[50,72] Community campaigns promote healthy eating messages to the general public or specific messages tailored to identified needs and risk factors within subgroups. Enrichment of commonly eaten foods with nutrients lacking in the diet is a policy intervention that changes nutrient intake without requiring nutrition education or behavior change. Reducing risk and improving the nutritional and health status of adults requires multiple strategies that combine individual, social, organizational, and policy-level changes such as those mentioned.

## A Model Health-Promotion Program

"Sisters Together: Move More, Eat Better" illustrates the components of a comprehensive, effective program for adults. Sisters Together, a national initiative of the Weight-control Information Network (WIN), is a health awareness program that encourages African-American women 18 years and older to maintain a healthy weight by becoming more physically active and by eating nutritious foods (Illustration 16.5). It is a culturally relevant, community-based program that is flexible and can be tailored to African-American women of all ages, communities, and demographics. The program design combines social marketing with community-building strategies.

Dedicated individuals and organizations can start a program at the local level using the Sisters Together Program Guide and materials. The manual outlines the steps to creating a successful program:[78]

- Assess needs and select the audience.
- Identify community resources and partners.

**ergogenic aids** Nutritional products that are purported to enhance performance. Examples range from caffeine and protein powders to sports drinks and energy gels and bars.

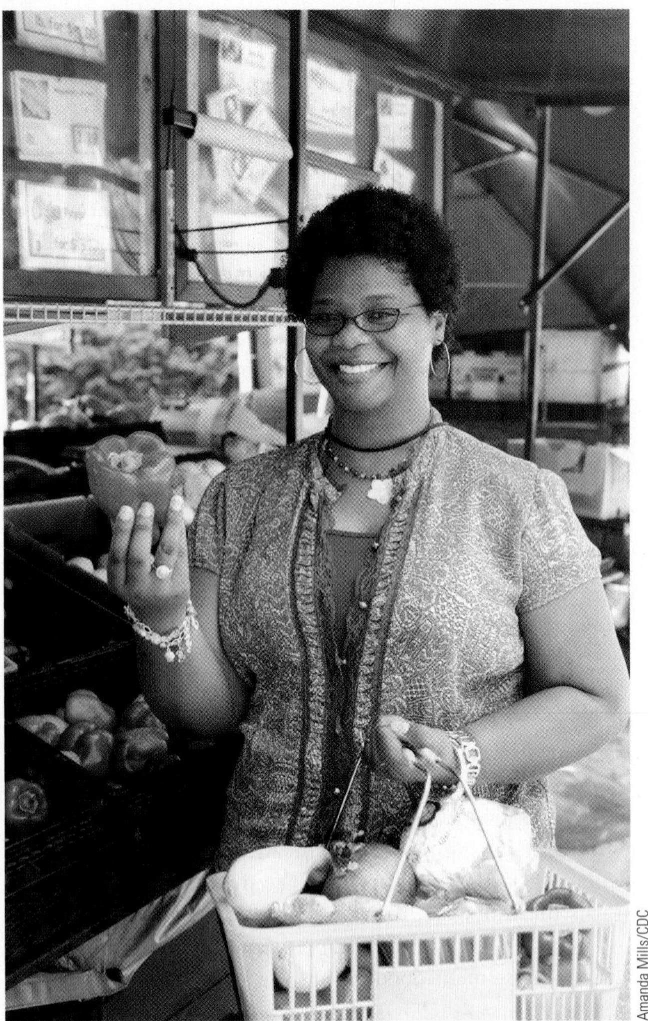

ILLUSTRATION 16.5 ▸ Multicomponent programs like Sisters Together foster healthy eating.

Amanda Mills/CDC

- Set realistic goals and objectives.
- Work with media to raise awareness.
- Decide on core activities and events.
- Measure success.

Sisters Together initiatives bring together respected leaders and organizations in the community that have goals similar to those of Sisters Together, address women's issues and concerns, and have credibility with African American women in the community. Programs are based in settings that range from churches to beauty salons. They partner with community centers and YWCAs for space for group meetings or exercise classes, and link up with public programs such as WIC and SNAP. Media, including radio, newspapers and newsletters, and social media, are used to increase the visibility of the Sisters Together program, cover special events, and raise awareness about relevant issues.

Core activities are determined at the local level and are designed to fill knowledge gaps, reduce barriers, increase opportunity, provide social support, and complement other community resources. Activities are selected to match the expressed needs of women in the community such as desires to have more energy, relieve stress, look good, and feel better about themselves. Program content emphasizes how physical activity and nutrition help achieve these needs. Examples of successful activities include classes where food is prepared and tasted, featuring easy-to-prepare recipes that are low in calories, fat, and salt; and organized groups and buddy systems to support physical activity such as walking clubs and classes.

Approaches encourage physical activity versus exercise and feature traditional ethnic foods and flavors but with more health-conscious ingredients and preparation methods. Positive changes in fruit and vegetable intake and physical activity have been documented through pre- and post-evaluations. Ongoing and periodic "booster" programs are strategies to maintain changes over time.

The model of raising awareness and improving health through the establishment of community-based groups and campaigns is applicable in a wide range of adult nutrition and health issues. Multicomponent programs such as this help create a "culture of health" that supports positive diet, physical activity, and lifestyle behaviors.

## Public Food and Nutrition Programs

Having a low income makes it difficult to consistently provide enough food for family members and to access a variety of healthful foods. People living in poverty tend to have poorer diets and increased rates of obesity, and adverse health outcomes.[8-11,19,50] Improving the food security of the population is part of the national health goal of eliminating heath disparity. Food insecurity—difficulty providing enough food for all family members at some time during the year due to a lack of resources—is a fact of life for nearly 15 percent of U.S. households, but impacts some segments of the population at much higher rates (see Table 16.11).[79]

TABLE 16.11 ▸ Healthy People 2020 food-security target compared to 2008 levels

| OBJECTIVE | TARGET | 2013 LEVEL |
|---|---|---|
| Reduce household food insecurity and in doing so, decrease hunger | | |
| All households | 6% | 14.3% |
| Households at or <130% of poverty | | 38.9% |
| African-American, not Hispanic | | 26.1% |
| Mexican American | | 23.7% |
| White, not Hispanic | | 10.6% |
| Other | | 11.7% |
| Single women with children | | 34.4% |

SOURCE: U.S. Department of Health and Human Services. Office of Disease Prevention and Health Promotion. Healthy People 2020. Washington, DC. Available at healthypeople.gov. Household Food Security in the United States in 2013/ERR-173, Economic Research Service, USDA.

According to Census Bureau estimates for 2013, the poverty rate for the United States is 14.5 percent; however, there is great disparity. The rate is 9.7 percent for Whites, compared to 27.2 percent for Blacks, 23.5 percent for Hispanics, and 10.5 percent for Asians, and the highest rate is for American Indians and Alaskan Natives (27.6 percent). For adults aged 18–64 years, the rate is 13.6 percent.[80] The poverty threshold is derived by calculating the cost of foods needed for basic dietary requirements (according to the Thrifty Food Plan) and multiplying that cost by 3. This poverty index was developed in the early 1960s by the Social Security Administration; at that time, food costs made up about one-third of the average household budget. Currently, households spend 7–40 percent of after-tax income on food, depending on household income. Poor households spend disproportionately higher levels of their income on food.

For 2015, a person was considered to live in poverty if his or her annual income was $11,770 or less.[81] Poverty guidelines are calculated according to household size and adjusted for higher living costs in Alaska and Hawaii. For a four-person household, the poverty guideline is $24,250 in the contiguous states and Washington, D.C. The federal poverty guideline is published annually in the Federal Register. Multiples of the poverty guideline (125 percent, 150 percent, and 185 percent) are used to determine eligibility for food and nutrition assistance programs that are administered by the USDA.

By far, the largest of all nutrition assistance programs is the Supplemental Nutrition Assistance Program (SNAP). It provides economic support for food purchases to low-income households, and also nutrition education. Participation in SNAP, which rises and falls with changes in the economy and poverty rate, has been shown to result in greater expenditures on vegetables, fruit, grain products, meat, and meat alternatives.[82]

Many other programs work to help hungry individuals and families gain food security. For example:

- Government extension programs teach budgeting, shopping, meal planning, and food-safety skills.
- The Second Harvest food bank network keeps wholesome food items out of the waste stream, coordinates charitable giving programs, and supplies food shelves and community kitchens.
- Soup kitchens and shelters provide hot meals and snacks for hungry and homeless people.
- Meals-on-Wheels programs serve homebound adults. Some are funded through the Agency on Aging, but many operate as voluntary community efforts.

Together, governmental and private organizations help individuals and families gain consistent access to safe, wholesome foods that are culturally acceptable. Such access is the basis of food security.

### Putting It All Together

Adults need access to a variety of healthful foods, knowledge to guide food choices, and positive attitudes about food and eating, balanced with discipline. Food choices that result in nutrient adequacy and energy balance matter throughout the adult years. Good choices, a variety of nutritious foods, and not too much food intake in early adulthood years affect health and nutritional status in future years. Food and nutrient intakes, along with physical activity and other lifestyle factors, genetics, and environment, determine one's ability to maintain or restore health and minimize the development and advancement of chronic disease. The overarching message is to follow the principles of variety, moderation, and balance in choosing a diet that will be satisfying and that will achieve a healthy body weight and maintain health.

## KEY POINTS

1. Individual choices as well as external factors strongly influence the course of health and wellness for adults.
2. There are significant disparities in the incidence and prevalence of disease across population groups. Social and economic disadvantage, along with other factors, are important determinants of nutritional and health outcomes.
3. Beginning early in the adult years, bone mass begins to decline, and there is an increase in body fat that is associated with increased risk of chronic diseases.
4. Subclinical nutritional injury begins long before observable signs and symptoms emerge. Early alterations in nutritional state can be reversed with changes in nutrition and physical activity.
5. Metabolic rate and energy expenditure decline through the adult years. Balancing energy intake and physical activity is necessary to maintain a healthy body weight. Several methods can be used to estimate energy needs.
6. Risk nutrients for adults include excessive saturated fat and sodium intake and inadequate intake of several vitamins, minerals, and fiber with important metabolic consequences.
7. Various eating patterns can be healthful, provided energy intake is not excessive, recommended amounts of nutrients are consumed over time, and nutrients are balanced to support their interdependent functions.

8. Dietary guidance systems are designed to reduce risks of specific diseases, ensure that the population consumes adequate levels of required nutrients from food and beverages, and help the public understand what, and how much, to eat.
9. Current dietary recommendations emphasize nutrient-dense foods but not too much, allow for flexibility, and recognize the social and sensory aspects of food and the importance of pleasurable eating experiences.
10. Regular physical activity has crucial effects on weight, body composition, and development of chronic diseases.
11. Reducing risk and improving the nutritional and health status of adults requires multiple strategies that combine individual, organizational and policy level changes.

## REVIEW QUESTIONS

1. What are the differences between individual and external or environmental factors that determine nutrition status and health? Give examples for how each type is monitored.
2. Describe the physiological changes that occur during the adult years. How do those changes relate to the continuum of health? Which changes have implications for development of chronic diseases?
3. How many calories do you need? Use three methods discussed in the chapter to estimate daily energy requirement. What factors would increase or decrease the number of calories you need to eat in a day?
4. If you are a typical male or female as represented in Table 16.5, what nutrient shortfalls and excesses should you be worried about and why?
5. You have been appointed to the Campus Dietary Guidelines Committee. What things do you need to consider when developing dietary guidelines for the campus community?
6. What do you need to do to meet the Physical Activity Guidelines for Americans? What are the benefits if you do? What are the consequences if you don't?
7. Make a table of different types of strategies for helping adults achieve good nutritional health.

Visit www.cengagebrain.com to access MindTap, a complete digital course that includes additional resources.

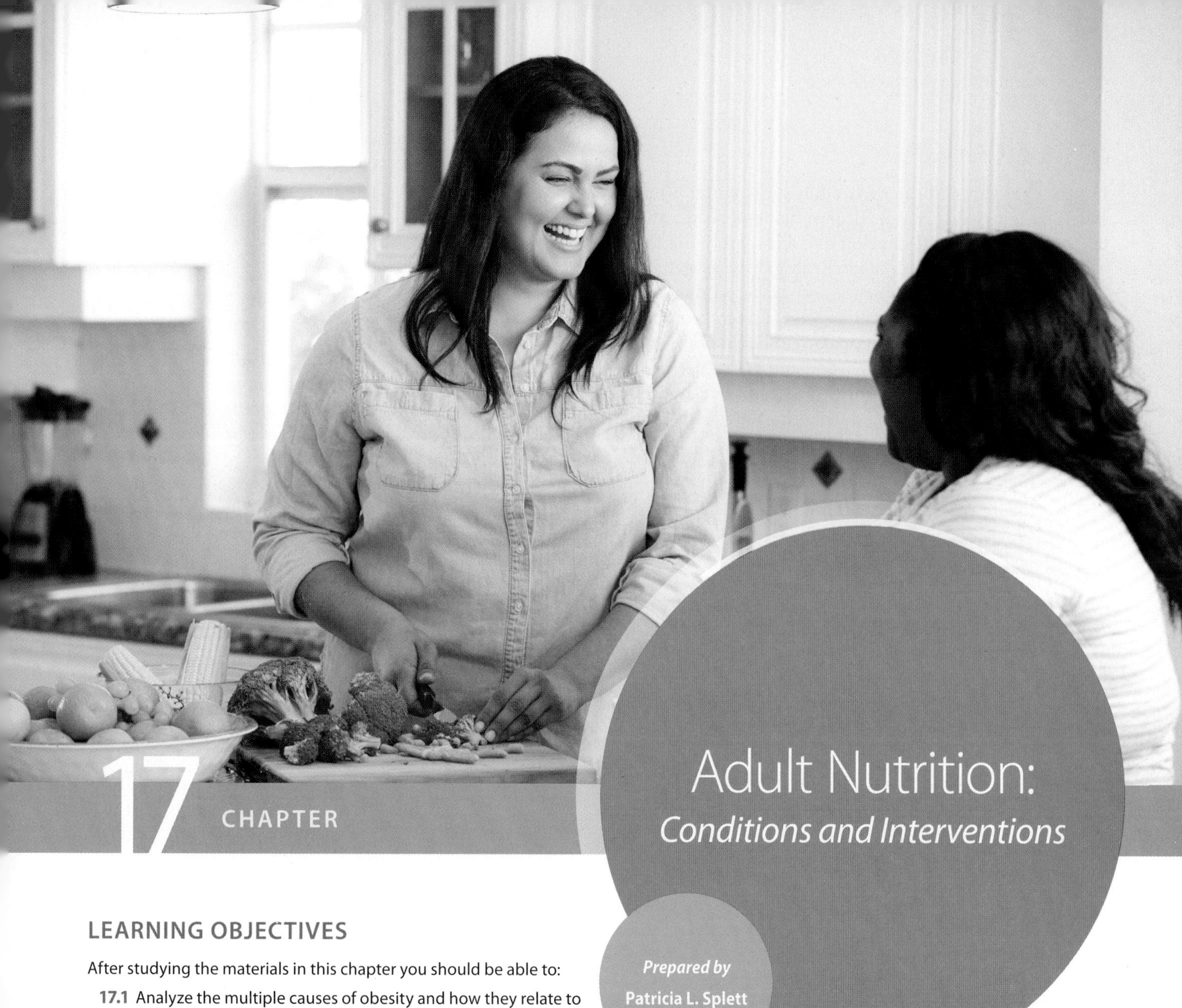

# 17 CHAPTER

# Adult Nutrition: *Conditions and Interventions*

*Prepared by*
Patricia L. Splett

## LEARNING OBJECTIVES

After studying the materials in this chapter you should be able to:

**17.1** Analyze the multiple causes of obesity and how they relate to nutrition assessment and intervention for adults.

**17.2** Explain how atherosclerosis is the basis for cardiovascular diseases and how assessment and intervention are used for prevention and treatment of CVD.

**17.3** Describe metabolic syndrome and its assessment and effects.

**17.4** Differentiate the types of diabetes and how they are diagnosed and managed.

**17.5** Describe the development of cancer and contrast nutrition assessment and intervention priorities at each of the four stages of cancer care.

**17.6** Describe HIV and its physiological changes and how key components of nutrition assessment and intervention are tailored to the stage of disease.

# Introduction

If adults get through the early adult years without being killed by injury or drug or alcohol induced death, about half (47 percent) will develop and ultimately die from one or more nutrition-related chronic disease including obesity, heart disease, diabetes, and cancer (Table 17.1).[1] Medically, obesity and cancer are considered chronic diseases, although they are not popularly thought of that way. Lifestyle, interacting with environment, and genetics, determines risks and opportunities and adults' response to them. Diseases that develop during the adult years result from the cumulative effects of:

- Diets high in calories, saturated fats, and sodium
- Diets low in vegetables, fruits, and fiber
- Tobacco, drug, and alcohol use
- Physical inactivity

The development and progression of chronic diseases, which are commonly diagnosed at midlife (45–65 years), significantly impact the quality and length of life of adults. Nutrition plays an important role in primary prevention (maintaining a healthy state) and secondary prevention (reducing risk factors and delaying advancement to overt disease), as well as treatment of the major chronic diseases.

This chapter starts with obesity and then addresses the three nutrition-related diseases that are the highest contributors to premature death among adults—cancer, cardiovascular diseases, and diabetes—and concludes with HIV/AIDS. The reader should recognize the interrelatedness of the chronic diseases and be alert to the risk factors that these diseases have in common, and note a core set of intervention strategies used to prevent and manage all of the nutrition-related chronic diseases.

**TABLE 17.1** Leading causes of death by age group

| | 24–44 YEARS | 45–54 YEARS | 55–65 YEARS |
|---|---|---|---|
| 1 | Injury* | Cancer | Cancer |
| 2 | Drug/alcohol induced | Heart disease | Heart disease |
| 3 | Cancer | Injury* | Injury* |
| 4 | Heart disease | Drug/alcohol induced | Respiratory disease |
| 5 | Liver disease | Liver disease | Diabetes |
| 6 | Diabetes | Diabetes | Drug/alcohol induced |
| 7 | Stroke | Stroke | Liver |
| 8 | HIV/AIDS | Respiratory disease | Stroke |
| 9 | Influenza, pneumonia | Septicemia | Septicemia |
| 10 | Respiratory disease | HIV/AIDS | Kidney disease |

*Injury includes deaths from accidents, homicide and suicide

SOURCE: National Center for Health Statistics. Deaths: Final Data for 2013.

# Overweight and Obesity

**LO 17.1** Analyze the multiple causes of obesity and how they relate to nutrition assessment and intervention for adults.

Obesity is an unhealthy accumulation of body fat. In technical terms, obesity is a chronic disease involving pathophysiological processes that result in an excess accumulation of adipose tissue, which increases morbidity and mortality.[2] Adipocytes (fat cells) are not passive deposits of excess fat. They comprise an active endocrine organ that secretes hormone-like factors associated with chronic low-grade inflammation and ***insulin resistance***.[3]

## Prevalence of Obesity and Overweight

About one-third of U.S. adults are obese, and another third are overweight. Since the 1980s, obesity has developed as an epidemic throughout the United States and the world.[4] In 1990, the obesity rate across states ranged from less than 10 percent to 15 percent. By 2013, all states had obesity rates above 20 percent, and 19 exceeded 30 percent.[5]

Obesity and overweight have increased in all segments of the population, but vary across age, gender, race-ethnicity, and income categories and geographic region.[5] Although some data suggest that the overall rate of overweight and obesity may be leveling off, the rates of severe obesity (BMI $> 40$) are expected to double by 2030 to 10 percent of the population, indicating a shift to higher weight and greater adiposity.[6]

## Etiology of Obesity

Overweight and obesity are not simply a matter of intake exceeding output. They are complex and chronic conditions, stemming from numerous interacting physiological, individual, environmental, and genetic factors. These factors affect the type, frequency, and quantity of food and beverages consumed and the body's metabolic processes. Physiological and psychological mechanisms are involved in weight gain leading to obesity, which can be characterized as metabolic or hedonic obesity Illustration 17.1 contrasts these mechanisms with the normal state.[7]

Normally body weight is determined by a neuroendocrine regulatory system that tends to maintain weight at a relatively stable "set point" through homeostatic feedback processes. Leptin, insulin, gut hormones, and levels of other metabolic products signal anabolic or catabolic responses, adjustment of resting energy expenditure, appetite, and food intake.

**insulin resistance** A condition in which cells "resist" the action of insulin in facilitating the passage of glucose into cells.

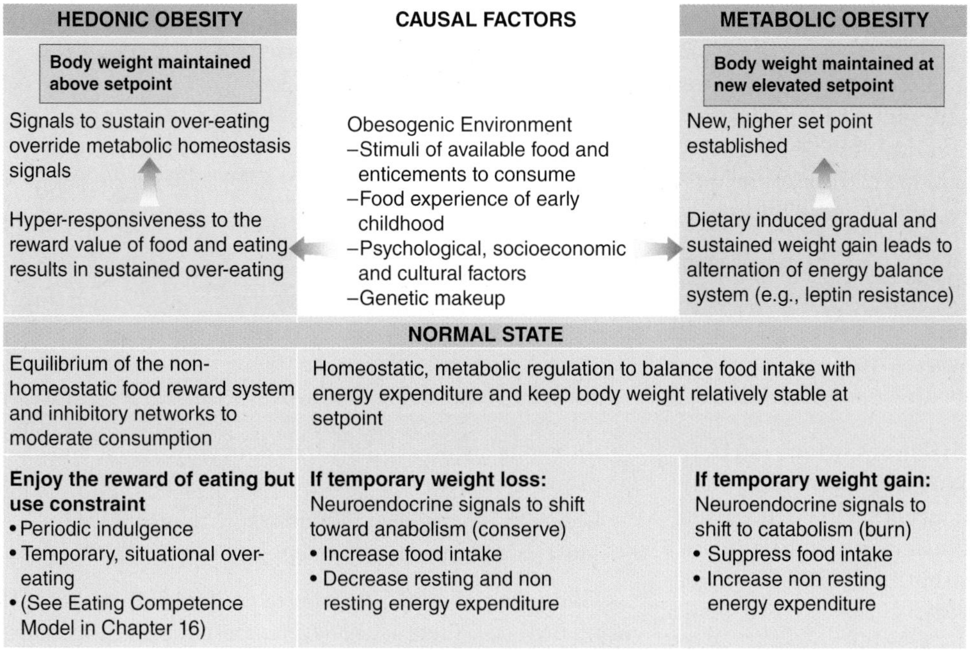

<table>
<tr><th>HEDONIC OBESITY</th><th>CAUSAL FACTORS</th><th>METABOLIC OBESITY</th></tr>
<tr><td>Body weight maintained above setpoint<br>Signals to sustain over-eating override metabolic homeostasis signals<br>↑<br>Hyper-responsiveness to the reward value of food and eating results in sustained over-eating ←</td><td>Obesogenic Environment<br>–Stimuli of available food and enticements to consume<br>–Food experience of early childhood<br>–Psychological, socioeconomic and cultural factors<br>–Genetic makeup</td><td>Body weight maintained at new elevated setpoint<br>New, higher set point established<br>↑<br>→ Dietary induced gradual and sustained weight gain leads to alternation of energy balance system (e.g., leptin resistance)</td></tr>
<tr><th colspan="3">NORMAL STATE</th></tr>
<tr><td>Equilibrium of the non-homeostatic food reward system and inhibitory networks to moderate consumption</td><td colspan="2">Homeostatic, metabolic regulation to balance food intake with energy expenditure and keep body weight relatively stable at setpoint</td></tr>
<tr><td>Enjoy the reward of eating but use constraint<br>• Periodic indulgence<br>• Temporary, situational over-eating<br>• (See Eating Competence Model in Chapter 16)</td><td>If temporary weight loss:<br>Neuroendocrine signals to shift toward anabolism (conserve)<br>• Increase food intake<br>• Decrease resting and non resting energy expenditure</td><td>If temporary weight gain:<br>Neuroendocrine signals to shift to catabolism (burn)<br>• Suppress food intake<br>• Increase non resting energy expenditure</td></tr>
</table>

ILLUSTRATION 17.1 ▸ Mechanism of weight gain leading to metabolic and hedonic obesity.

Figure 1 (Metabolic and hedonic obesity) from Yu, Y-H., et al. Metabolic vs. hedonic obesity: a conceptual distinction and its clinical implications. *Obesity Reviews* 2015; 16: 234–247 (p. 236).

***Metabolic obesity*** occurs when an individual's set point shifts and stabilizes at a higher weight level. Genetic and environmental influences, including food experiences in infancy and childhood, are causes. ***Hedonic obesity*** occurs when the energy homeostatic signals are overridden by hyper-responsiveness to the reward value of food. These mechanisms behind weight gain and obesity distinguish between the metabolic brain responsible for homeostatic regulation, and the cognitive and emotional brain, which responds to perceived pleasantness, liking, wanting, and reward.[7]

Backing up a step, what is the cause behind these altered obesity pathways? Research has led to the identification of genetic traits and epigenetic factors that determine an individual's susceptibility to metabolic alternations, weight gain, and potential responsiveness to weight management strategies.[8,9] Phenotypes (i.e., observable traits the results from interactions between genetics and the environment) help explain why some people are obese yet "metabolically healthy" and some people are normal weight, but laboratory tests indicate they are "metabolically obese."[9]

At the individual level, genetic factors interact with other factors involved in the development of obesity. Psychological, socioeconomic, and cultural factors play a role in shaping attitudes, behaviors, and lifestyle patterns. Stress, anxiety and depression, and life-changing events such a transition to college life[10] and pregnancy are associated with weight gain.

The prevailing ***obesogenic environment*** seems to stack the deck against controlled eating. Food advertising, the easy availability of highly palatable and highly processed, energy-dense snack foods and beverages, larger retail package sizes, larger portions served in fast-food and sit-down restaurants, the relatively low cost of fast food, and the added fat and sugar in many foods work against healthy eating and contribute to the obesity epidemic.[11] Technological advances in every dimension of life—work, leisure time, transportation—have replaced physical activity with sedentary activity and further contributed to the obesity epidemic.[11,12]

Egger and Dixon describe layers of influence from lifestyle and environmental "inducers" that incite low-level, persistent, systemic inflammation in susceptible individuals.[12] Obesity has been linked to other diseases through adipose-related inflammation. Egger and Dixon postulate that inflammation can arise in direct response to nutrition, inactivity, stress, technology, inadequate sleep, the built environment, occupation, drugs, smoking and alcohol, sunlight exposure, relationships and social factors. This low-grade inflammation is an independent, determinant of many chronic diseases, including obesity.[12]

## Effects of Obesity

Being overweight or obese increases the risk of pathological conditions in most organs of the body, and is related to development of a long list of conditions (Table 17.2). The risks rise as the degree of excess weight rises. Persons who

**metabolic obesity** Body weight set point shifts to a higher level due to alterations of the energy balance system.

**hedonic obesity** Body weight maintained above set point due to sustained overeating.

**obesogenic environment** The sum of influences that promote overeating and minimize physical activity and lead to weight gain and hinder weight loss.

TABLE 17.2 ▸ Conditions associated with overweight and obesity

| CARDIOMETABOLIC CONDITIONS | BIOMECHANICAL CONDITIONS | OTHER CONDITIONS |
|---|---|---|
| Cardiovascular disease | Disability and immobility | Some cancers (endometrial, breast, prostate, colon) |
| Dyslipidemia | Gastrointestinal reflux disease | Depression and other psychological disorders |
| Hypertension | Musculoskeletal disorders | Gall bladder disease |
| Metabolic syndrome | Osteoarthritis | Infertility |
| Nonalcoholic liver disease | Sleep apnea | Respiratory problems |
| Prediabetes | Urinary stress incontinence | Social stigmatization |
| Type 2 diabetes mellitus | | |
| Polycystic ovary syndrome | | |

Adapted from: AACE/ACE Consensus Conference on Obesity 2014

are obese might have physical disabilities, which interfere with the routine activities of daily living, and they may face psychosocial complications, including low self-esteem and depression, social and job discrimination, and social stigma.[13] Life expectancy is shortened by 6–19 years, depending on the severity of obesity.[14]

## Screening and Assessment

### BMI for Classification of Obesity and Associated Risks

Body mass index (BMI) is significantly correlated with total body fat. BMI, calculated from height and weight, is used internationally for classifying overweight and obesity.[4] Overweight in adults is defined by BMI of 25.0–29.9 and obesity by BMI of 30 or greater. A BMI of 30 is roughly equivalent to being 30 or more pounds overweight for a 5-foot, 4-inch person. Although BMI approximates body fat for most healthy individuals, there are exceptions:

- Athletes or others with greater-than-average percentages of muscle mass
- Individuals with dense, large bones
- Individuals who are dehydrated, overhydrated, and prone to edema
- Sedentary or disabled individuals with atrophied muscles and increased fat deposits (sarcopenic obesity)

Clinically, obesity is further classified as I, II, and III using BMI (see Table 17.3). Severe obesity (also called morbid obesity because of its high correlation with premature death), defined as a BMI of 40 or more, is a dangerous condition that places the person at extremely high risk for cardiovascular and other diseases as well as physical disability and severely impaired quality of life.

**Waist Circumference for Central Adiposity** The distribution of body fat is a more important indicator of health risk than weight or BMI.[15] Body fat, or adipose tissue, is stored in three compartments: subcutaneous fat layered underneath the skin, visceral or intra-abdominal fat packed between internal organs, and ectopic fat stored in liver, pancreas, heart, and skeletal muscles. Visceral fat, recognized as a potbelly or apple shape, and known clinically as *central adiposity,* is highly correlated with metabolic abnormalities

TABLE 17.3 ▸ Classification of overweight and obesity by BMI and waist circumference values associated with high risk

| | | | WAIST CIRCUMFERENCE | | |
|---|---|---|---|---|---|
| | BMI (KG/M²) | WHO OBESITY CLASS | COUNTY/ETHNIC GROUP | MALE | FEMALE |
| Underweight | <18.5 | | North American | ≥102 | ≥88 |
| Normal | 18.5–24.9 | | European | ≥94 | ≥80 |
| Overweight | 25.0–29.9 | | Sub-Saharan Africans | ≥94 | ≥80 |
| Obesity | 30.0–34.9 | I | Eastern Mediterranean & Middle East (Arab) populations | ≥94 | ≥80 |
| | 35.0–39.9 | II | Ethnic South and Central American | ≥90 | ≥80 |
| Severe Obesity | ≥40 | III | South Asian/Chinese | ≥90 | ≥80 |
| | | | Japanese | ≥85 | ≥90 |

SOURCE: Adapted from Clinical Assessment and Management of Adult Obesity[17]

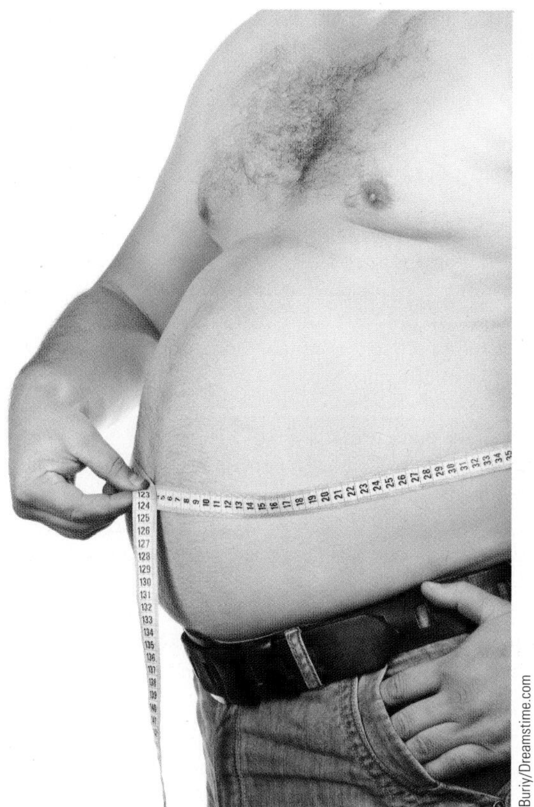

Buriy/Dreamstime.com

ILLUSTRATION 17.2 ▸ Central adiposity assessed by waist circumference.

and chronic diseases (Illustration 17.2). Waist circumference (WC) is used to assess central adiposity and it allows further stratification of risk beyond BMI. To assess WC, place a tape measure around the abdomen just above the hip bone, level with the navel and parallel to the floor. The tape should be snug but not compressing the skin. Measure after exhaling.[16] The measurement is compared to ethnic-specific values, shown in Table 16.2, for males and females. WC is important in the assessment of obesity because increased central adiposity is associated with higher risk even in person with normal BMI, and the threshold for risk varies across racial and ethnic groups.[17]

**Weight Change** A third metric for assessment of obesity is weight change since young adulthood. A modest amount of gain (<5 kg) is significantly associated with increased risk and earlier onset of chronic disease and 11–19 kg gain is associated with a twofold increase in risk.[15]

## Nutrition Assessment

After the need for weight management is identified, a comprehensive assessment is used to understand the individual's experience with overweight, current eating and physical-activity patterns, psychosocial and medical factors, and his/her motivation and readiness to change and goals. Table 17.4 outlines possible factors to consider during an assessment for weight management. A patient-centered interview approach allows the client's priorities and perceptions to be expressed and provides information for jointly planning appropriate goals and treatment strategies.[18]

**Motivation** Several factors contribute to understanding the client's motivation to engage in a weight-loss program: reasons and motivation for weight reduction, previous weight-loss attempts, the patient's understanding of causes of obesity and how obesity contributes to several diseases, existing comorbidities, attitude toward physical activity, capacity to engage in physical activity, time available for weight-loss intervention, and financial considerations.[19,20] Patient's nutrition knowledge, food access, food selection, and functional capacity to prepare food and engage in physical activity are all important for individualized treatment planning.

## Intervention in Obesity and Overweight

The good news is that relatively small amounts of weight loss (3–5 to 10 percent of body weight) can reduce or prevent the health risks associated with obesity.[2,17,26] Because of this, the U.S. Preventive Services Task Force recommends that all patients with a BMI ≥30 should be referred for comprehensive weight management.[21] Weight reduction is recommended even for those who are mildly overweight (BMI 25–29) when an obesity-related complication is present.[3] The national guidelines for treatment of overweight and obesity use BMI, waist circumference, and presence of obesity-related risks and complications and patient motivation to prioritize individuals for treatment.[2,17]

## Comprehensive Weight Management Program

A comprehensive, multicomponent weight management program is needed for successful weight loss, including diet, physical activity and behavior therapy.[2,17,20,22,23] Many options exist for delivery of weight management programs, ranging from online programs to community-based programs at the YMCA, to clinic-based medical nutrition therapy provided by registered dietitians.[11]

Men and women have different preferences for type of program, delivery options, and outcome goals.[24,25] A successful weight-loss plan is tailored to the individual and includes an eating plan that reduces caloric intake relative to calories burned, provides for nutrient needs at a safe level, incorporates physical activity, and is compatible with the individual's lifestyle. In addition to behavioral modification to alter eating and physical-activity patterns, pharmacotherapy can be used to support weight loss. Bariatric surgery is reserved for patients with high-risk comorbid conditions.

## Weight Loss Goals

Goals of weight management are to (1) prevent further weight gain, (2) reduce body weight, (3) maintain a lower

TABLE 17.4 ▸ Nutrition assessment of adults with overweight or obesity and obesity-related diseases and conditions

**Anthropometrics**
- Height, weight, BMI, waist circumference, waist–hip ratio

**Food and Nutrition History**
- Weight history: age of onset of overweight, highest/lowest adult weights, patterns of weight gain and loss, environmental triggers to weight gain, triggers to excessive or disordered eating
- Dieting experience: number and types of diets, weight-loss medications, success of previous efforts
- Current eating patterns: meal and snack patterns (skipped meals, largest meal, snacks/grazing)
- Eating location and environment: meals eaten out (cafeteria, fast food, restaurant, carry lunch), family meals, television on at mealtime
- Types and amounts of food typically eaten: 24-hour recall or food frequency, food preferences, ethnic foods, cultural practices
- Nutritional intake: assessment of reported intake for energy and adequacy of key nutrients
  - Total caloric intake
  - Type and amount of fat (saturated, mono saturated, polyunsaturated, *trans* fats, omega-3 fatty acid)
  - Sources of key nutrients: fruits and vegetables (vitamins A, C, antioxidants and phytochemicals, potassium, fiber), bread and grains (fiber, B-vitamins, iron, folic acid), milk and dairy (calcium, vitamin D), fish, meat, beans, nuts (protein, iron, omega-3 fatty acid)
  - Energy-dense foods (bakery goods, such as cookies, cake, sweet rolls), chips and crackers, candy, salad dressings and toppings, specialty coffee drinks, alcoholic beverages, fried foods)
  - Salty foods: salt-shaker use, processed meats, chips and crackers, nuts, convenience foods, restaurant foods
  - Supplement use: nutrient-enhanced food or beverage products, vitamin/mineral supplements, herbal supplements

**Physical Activity**
- Level of activity at work, school, home; and leisure-time activities
- Frequency, intensity, and duration of planned exercise beyond routine work and leisure time activities

**Laboratory**
- Lipid profile: total serum cholesterol, HDL, LDL, triglycerides
- Glucose: random or fasting glucose, hemoglobin A1C, glucose tolerance test

**Medical and Health History**
- Obesity severity, extent of physical limitations, impact on activities of daily living
- Potential contributing causes: endocrine, neurological, physical disability, genetics/family history, medications
- Obesity-associated conditions: diabetes, hypertension, cardiovascular diseases, cancer, fatty liver disease, GERD, sleep apnea, osteoarthritis
- Mental health: daily stress level, recent life-changing events (birth, death, marriage, job change or loss, new medical diagnosis), depression, post-traumatic stress disorder, eating disorder (binge eating, bulimia)
- Active medical diagnoses and medication use

**Social History**
- Occupation, family composition, caretaking responsibilities
- Economic constraints, food insecurity, food/nutrition program participation, access to health care, coverage for nutrition intervention

**Nutrition Knowledge and Attitudes**
- Basic understanding about foods and nutrition, guidelines for healthy eating, and recommended serving sizes
- Role of nutrition in patient's diseases or conditions; previous diet instruction or lifestyle-management program
- Level of self-care regarding nutrition: experience in meal planning, food purchasing and preparation
- Confidence in ability

**Readiness to Change**
- Reasons to lose weight at this time, weight-loss goals
- Stage of change: precontemplation, contemplation, preparation, action, maintenance, relapse
- Support system



body weight for the long term, and prevent or reduce complications. Accomplishing this requires sustainable lifestyle changes.

A moderate rate of weight loss of ½ to 1 pound per week is recommended, but accelerated weight loss of up to 2 pounds per week can also be used and may provide positive reinforcement to continue.[26] A deficit of 3500 kcal is necessary to lose one pound of weight; thus a weight loss of ½, 1, or 2 pound per week requires a calorie deficit of 300, 500, or 1,000 kcal/day, respectively.

**Medical Nutrition Therapy for Weight Management** The nutrition prescription for weight loss is an eating plan that is deficient in calories but otherwise meets guidelines for healthy eating. A balanced vitamin/mineral supplement may be recommended. Strategies for reducing caloric intake include following a menu plan and tracking calories, fat grams, or carbohydrate grams; portion control; and eating four to five meals/snacks, including breakfast. Replacing one or two meals a day with ***meal replacements*** (liquid meals, meal bars, or packaged meals) is helpful for individuals who have difficulty with portion control. Very-low-energy diets (800 kcal/day) can produce rapid weight loss but should only be used under close medical supervision.[26] Research comparing low-fat and low-carbohydrate diets has shown that either approach can produce weight loss and have positive effects on disease biomarkers, but following a low-carbohydrate plans had some advantage in terms of longer-term weight maintenance.[27] The prescribed diet approach should be determined with the patient, considering his or her preferences, cooking style, and culture.[17,26]

## Cognitive Behavioral Therapy for Weight Management

Successful programs developed for weight management, diabetes education, and other lifestyle changes utilize ***cognitive behavioral therapy.*** Programs are 12–16 weeks long to build knowledge, modify beliefs and attitudes, and integrate new behaviors through a combination of skills training and analysis of behavior and thought processes. Key features are helping the client recognize and replace automatic and irrational thoughts and beliefs (cognitive restructuring) and increasing awareness and control of cues associated with eating (stimulus control).[28,29]

There are 12 components of weight-management programs based on cognitive behavioral therapy:

1. *Realistic goals:* Identify a healthy weight goal and a feasible rate of loss (0.5–1.0 lb/week), and provide the ability to self-monitor progress.
2. *Caloric deficit:* Develop an individualized meal plan with intake adjusted to lose weight gradually.
3. *Meal plan:* Build meal plans around a variety of foods that fit with the patient's lifestyle and budget, can be readily obtained, and can be enjoyed by the entire household.
4. *Skill development:* Provide tools and skills training, including teaching, practicing within sessions, homework, review, and feedback.
5. *Problem-solving techniques:* Assist with development of strategies to anticipate and solve potential weight-management problems.
6. *Self-monitoring and self-management:* Provide tools for keeping food and activity records and build confidence in ability to monitor and adjust.
7. *Cognitive restructuring:* Help client examine thought processes and recognize dysfunctional thinking.
8. *Stress management:* Teach strategies other than eating to deal with stressful situations.
9. *Support system:* Encourage having someone to check in with and receive support.
10. *Regular exercise:* Advise initiation and gradual increase of physical activity, tailored to the patient's ability, aiming for 30–60 minutes most days of the week and including aerobic and muscle-strengthening activities.
11. *Maintenance:* Make available support for weight loss and for maintenance of the loss.
12. *Long-term effectiveness:* The weight-management plan is built around learning and practicing behaviors that can be maintained for a lifetime.

## Physical Activity for Weight Management

Added physical activity contributes to the energy deficit required for weight loss. Cardiorespiratory fitness and screening for musculoskeletal problems may need to be reviewed before making physical activity recommendations. For obese individuals, exercise should be initiated slowly and the intensity increased gradually. Even 10-minute sessions of moderate to vigorous intensity physical activity have been shown to have beneficial effects.[11,30,31] Depending on body size, fitness level, and exercise intensity, 30 minutes of moderate physical activity five days a week would burn approximately 1000 calories. Increasing physical activity has the additional benefit of reducing diabetes and cardiovascular risk beyond that produced by weight loss alone, through its effect on blood cholesterol, blood pressure, and blood glucose.[30]

Physical activity is crucial to the prevention of weight regain. Studies indicate that a high level of daily energy expenditures in the range of 380 to 600 kcal per day may be necessary to sustain energy balance without overly restricting food intake.[32]

## The Challenge of Weight Maintenance

After six months, the rate of weight loss usually declines and weight plateaus, due in part to a decline in metabolic rate—the body's physiological response to protect against starvation.[7] This metabolic compensation, termed an *energy gap,* is about 8 kcal/lb lost/day.[32] Long-term maintenance of weight loss requires lifelong personal adherence to behaviors that balance

**meal replacement** A nutritionally balanced beverage, meal bar, or packaged meal used to replace a meal in weight management.

**cognitive behavioral therapy** Programs designed to build knowledge, modify beliefs and attitudes, and integrate new behaviors through a combination of skills training and analysis of behavior and thought processes over a period of several weeks. Key features are cognitive restructuring and stimulus control.

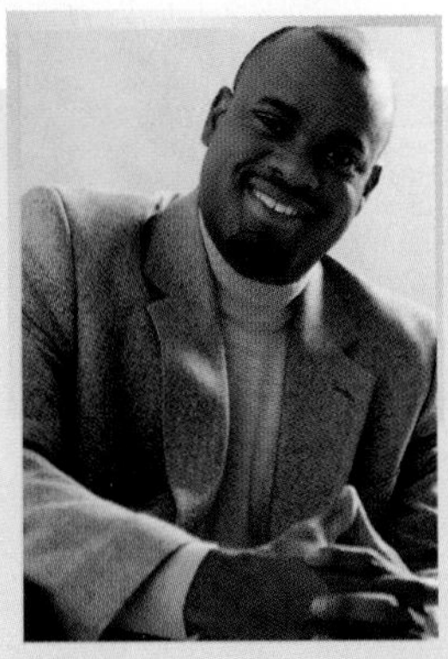
Photodisc

## CASE STUDY 17.1

### Maintaining a Healthy Weight

Adam is 5′11″ tall and weighs 190 pounds. He is a single father with two teenage sons. The commute to and from his software development job takes about 90 minutes. He likes his coworkers and the work environment and is happy that his workplace provides a cafeteria so he doesn't have to bring a lunch. He believes it is important for the family to have a "hot meal" every night, but he mostly relies on frozen entrees or take-out to accomplish this. Frequently, the evening meal is from the drive-through window of a fast-food restaurant on the way to his sons' sport events. Adam is an avid football and basketball fan and spends many hours watching televised games. In his spare time, he is restoring an old car with his sons.

#### Questions

**Assessment**

1. Calculate Adam's current BMI. How would you classify his weight status based on the clinical classifications in Table 17.3?
2. What would you consider a healthy BMI and "healthy weight" for Adam?
3. What lifestyle and dietary factors are related to Adams weight status?

**Diagnosis**

4. What is Adam's nutrition diagnosis? What modifiable factors cause or contribute to this problem? What evidence do you have for the problem?

**Intervention**

5. What dietary prescription would you have for Adam? What goal would you recommend? *Hint:* Calculate a calorie intake level and estimate the number of weeks it would take for Adam to reach a healthy weight.
6. What interventions would you use to help Adam reach the goal? What topics and suggestions would you discuss with Adam?

**Monitoring and Evaluation**

7. What would you measure later to determine if Adam was making progress?

calories consumed with energy burned in an environment that pushes food and fosters sedentary lifestyles.[27,33]

A widely held misconception is that most people regain all lost weight and more. Follow-up studies have found that while most regain some weight, up to 50 percent are below their baseline weight 1–5 years after completing therapy, and over 20 percent are successful at maintaining a 10 percent weight loss for at least one year.[33,34]

Individuals who use more behavioral strategies to support weight loss and maintenance. These behaviors include consistently controlling caloric intake (through restricted intake of certain types or classes of food, limiting fast food, eating all foods but in limited quantities, counting calories, or limiting percentage of daily energy from fat), exercising more often and more strenuously, tracking weight, and eating breakfast.[11,35]

Follow-up weight maintenance programs are strongly recommended.[2,21] National guidelines acknowledge that weight maintenance for many individuals requires ongoing therapy, yet this service is not covered by most health plans unless the patient has a ***comorbidity***. Some health plans employ lifestyle coaches who use telephone and electronic media to assist patients in sustaining behavioral changes and maintaining the health benefits of reduced risk for diseases. Research backs up the effectiveness of this strategy.[11] Apps and wearable devices for monitoring and managing weight are proliferating. Older-generation technology-based programs were found to be effective in weight loss and maintenance, but less successful than in-person individual or group interventions.[36] The effectiveness of new technology is unknown at this time. See Case Study 17.1 for a realistic example of weight challenges faced by adults.

## Pharmacotherapy for Weight Loss

For some, comorbidities and risk factors warrant addition of weight-loss drugs to the comprehensive intervention plan. Research has found that medications combined with lifestyle modification produces slightly greater weight loss than lifestyle modification and placebo.[37] Mechanisms for drug action include appetite suppression and inhibiting fat absorption from the gut. Numerous over-the-counter and herbal weight-loss preparations offer hope for those seeking help, but most have not been tested for efficacy and safety and are not recommended.[38,39]

**comorbidity** The presence of one or more diseases or conditions in addition to the primary disease or disorder.

### Bariatric Surgery

Bariatric surgery is reserved for patients with clinically severe obesity who meet criteria (BMI ≥40 or ≥35 with high risk for obesity-related morbidity or mortality, and generally after other therapy has been tried for six or more months without success). In such patients, surgery is the most effective therapy for weight management. Bariatric surgery impacts the mechanisms of metabolic and hedonistic obesity and has been shown to result in improvement or resolution of obesity-related comorbidities (e.g., lower blood glucose, better lipid profile, lower blood pressure, reduced cardiovascular disease risks, and increased mobility).[40] Surgical procedures reduce stomach size and restrict intake (by stapling, banding, or insertion of balloon) or produce malabsorption by bypassing a section of the small intestine (Roux-en-Y procedure). Patients considered for gastric surgery must be highly motivated to adhere to aftercare guidelines to prevent the onset of post-operative complications (nausea, vomiting, dehydration, and dumping syndrome) and prevent long-term nutritional deficiencies.[19] Patients treated with bariatric surgery are at risk for micronutrient deficiencies and should have ongoing monitoring of serum nutrient levels.[41]

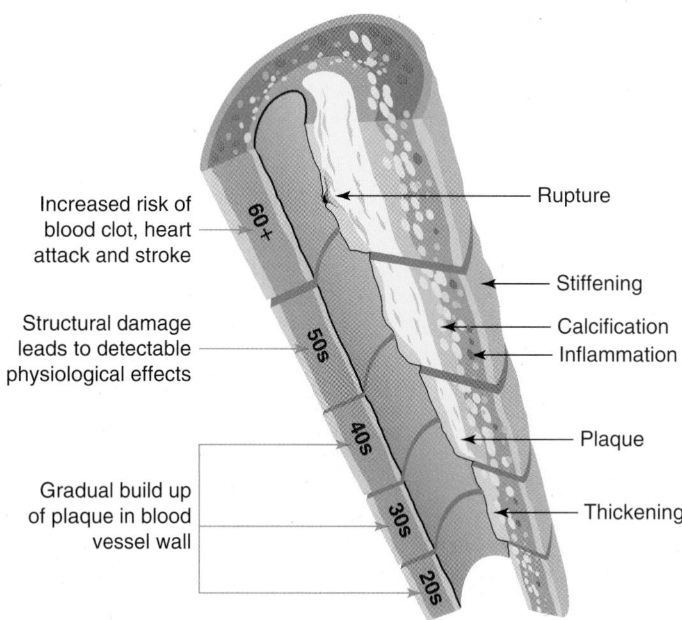


ILLUSTRATION 17.3 ▸ Atherosclerotic blood vessel changed during the adult years.

## Cardiovascular Disease

LO 17.2 Explain how atherosclerosis is the basis for cardiovascular disease and how assessment and intervention are used for prevention and treatment of CVD.

Cardiovascular diseases (CVD) are diseases related to the heart and blood vessels and are usually associated with atherosclerosis (hardening of the arteries), which is a buildup of plaque in the blood vessel wall. The areas affected include the heart (coronary heart disease or CHD), the brain (cerebral vascular disease leading to stroke), and blood vessels in the legs (peripheral arterial disease, or PAD). Atherosclerotic lesions begin to form in childhood and adolescence and gradually develop through the decades (Illustration 17.3). Lesions remain asymptomatic until the thickening wall reduces blood flow leading to ***ischemia***, or a lesion ruptures and a blood clot forms resulting in a heart attack (myocardial infarction) or stroke.

Hyperlipidemia and hypertension are important factors in the progression of CVD. Tracking for Healthy People 2020 objectives indicates that progress is being made in reducing the numbers of adults with these conditions (Table 17.5). Other objectives track the proportion of adults with elevated LDL cholesterol (1) who are advised by health care professionals regarding lifestyle changes to manage cholesterol, and (2) who adhere to the prescribed LDL-lowering lifestyle changes, including a cholesterol-lowering diet, physical activity, weight control, and, if indicated, medication.[42]

### Prevalence of CVD

Over 83.6 million adults have one or more CVD diagnoses. Men develop CVD at a younger age, but women catch up after menopause. Many people think of CVD as an "old person's" disease, but sclerotic blood vessel changes begin by the thirties and hyperlipidemia and hypertension are early biomarkers

**ischemia** Inadequate blood supply to a local area due to partial or complete blockage of a blood vessel.

TABLE 17.5 ▸ Healthy People 2020 nutrition-related health objectives to reduce heart disease and stroke among adults

| | PERCENTAGE OF ALL ADULTS | | |
|---|---|---|---|
| OBJECTIVE | TARGET | 2008 | 2009–2012 |
| Increase the proportion of adults with hypertension whose blood pressure is under control | 61.2% | 43.7% | 48.9% |
| Reduce the proportion of adults with high total blood cholesterol (240 mg/dL or greater) | 13.5% | 15% | 12.9% |

SOURCE: *Healthy People* 2020. Washington, D.C.: U.S. Department of Health and Human Services.

TABLE 17.6 ▸ Deaths from heart disease and stroke compared to national goals to reduce mortality

| | PER 100,000 POPULATION | | | |
|---|---|---|---|---|
| | | | 2011 | |
| OBJECTIVE | TARGET | BASELINE (2007) | FEMALES | MALES |
| **Reduce stroke deaths** | 34.8 | 43.5 | 60.1 | 39.1 |
| **Reduce coronary heart disease deaths** | 103.4 | 129.2 | 81.6 | 145.6 |
| BY RACE/ETHNICITY | | | STROKE | CHD |
| American Indian or Alaska Native | | | 27.1 | 81.4 |
| Asian or Pacific Islander | | | 31.6 | 62.7 |
| Black or African American | | | 50.9 | 125.3 |
| Hispanic or Latino | | | 36.5 | 84.2 |
| White | | | 36.7 | 109.3 |

SOURCE: *Healthy People 2020*. Washington, D.C.: U.S. Department of Health and Human Services.

for CVD. (See Chapter 19 for greater detail regarding hypertension and stroke.) Racial/ethnic differences in risk factors for CVD are linked with earlier disease onset and higher death rates. Compared to Whites, Blacks develop hypertension at an earlier age and have higher blood pressure levels, and Mexican American men have the highest cholesterol levels.[43]

CHD is the number two cause of death for adults aged 34–64. Table 17.6 shows death rates for males and females and for racial/ethnic groups. Blacks and females have the highest rates of stroke, and Blacks, Whites and males have highest rates of CHD. Overall death rates from CHD and stroke have declined significantly in the recent decade for all racial/ethnic groups; however, CVD death rates for women 35–54 years appear to be increasing, likely due to the obesity epidemic.[44]

## Etiology of Atherosclerosis

***Atherosclerosis*** begins when fatty deposits become part of tissues that form over injured arterial wall cells. Fibrous plaques (containing fats, cholesterol, triglycerides, collagen, muscle, white blood cells, and other cells and metabolites) form. These lesions gradually become calcified and blood vessels stiffen, increasing the extent of atherosclerosis.[45] Chronic vascular inflammation makes arteries susceptible to plaque development.[46] High blood levels of homocysteine, abnormal blood clotting factors, central adiposity, elevated blood glucose and insulin levels, and other conditions also influence the development of atherosclerosis.[47] The progression of atherosclerosis can be slowed, neutralized, or partially reversed by dietary and lifestyle modifications.[48]

## Physiological Effects of Atherosclerosis

The buildup of lesions and plaque inside the blood vessels (atherosclerosis) reduces blood flow and vessels lose flexibility. To compensate for this, the heart has to work harder to pump blood through this narrower space to reach all parts of the body, leading to higher blood pressure levels. Atherosclerosis decreases blood circulation to the heart, resulting in decline in organ function. CHD can present as decreased energy and shortness of breath after exertion or chest pain (angina) and death from a heart attack. Plaque in carotid and cranial arteries, complicated by hypertension, leads to stroke, with transient or permanent changes in mental and physical functioning. Poor circulation to the extremities due to PAD causes pain and limits physical activity. The progression of these cardiovascular diseases significantly interferes with activities of daily living, reduces quality of life, and can result in early death.

## Risk Factors for CVD

The risk factors for the various CVDs have been known and targeted for intervention for many years, and they include ***dyslipidemia*** (elevated low-density lipoprotein (LDL), low level of high-density lipoprotein (HDL), and high total cholesterol, and high triglycerides), high blood pressure, and the lifestyle factors of diet, physical inactivity, and smoking. Genetics, evidenced through a family history of CVD and inherited types of dyslipidemias, and older age are also risk factors. LDH and HDL have been referred to as "bad" cholesterol and "good" cholesterol, respectively; however, recent research is uncovering different metabolic impacts attributed to subtypes of LDL ("large-fluffy" vs. "small-dense") and malfunctioning HDL.[49] Risk for development and progression of CVD is interconnected with obesity, diabetes, infection, and inflammation.

## Screening and Assessment of CVD

Screening should occur about every five years beginning at age 20. Conventional risk factors noted above have been incorporated into screening tools to determine lifetime and ten-year risk for having a major adverse cardiac event (e.g., heart attack).[50] (Go to www.cvriskcalculator.com to calculate risk using the 2013 guidelines) Race/ethnicity is also considered because of known differences in susceptibility to risk factors by some populations. Levels of the factors listed in Table 17.7 are used to target interventions and determine the aggressiveness of therapy. The table includes well-established indicators, as well as screening criteria for metabolic syndrome, and additional

**atherosclerosis** A disease of the arterial blood vessels (arteries) in which the walls of the blood vessels become thickened and hardened by cholesterol and calcium-containing plaque.

**dyslipidemia** Abnormal blood levels of cholesterol and/or triglycerides resulting from altered lipid metabolism.

TABLE 17.7 ▸ Risk factors and criteria for CVD and CHD

| RISK FACTOR | CRITERIA FOR RISK |
|---|---|
| **Major Risk Factors for CHD** | |
| Hyperlipidemia | ATP III classification (lipid profile following 9- to 12-hour fast) |
| Low-density lipoprotein (LDL) mg/dL | Optimal: <100<br>Borderline high: 130–159<br>High: 160–189<br>Very high: ≥190 |
| Total cholesterol levels mg/dL | Desirable: <200<br>Borderline high: 200–240<br>High: >240 |
| High-density lipoprotein (HDL) mg/dL | Low: <40<br>High: ≥60 (good, high HDL compensates for other risk factor) |
| Clinical atherosclerotic disease | CHD, PAD, carotid artery disease, abdominal aortic aneurysm |
| Diabetes | Diagnosis of diabetes or prediabetes |
| Hypertension | Blood pressure ≥140/90 mmHg or on antihypertensive medication |
| Cigarette smoking | Current smoker |
| Family history of premature CHD | Parent or sibling with CHD<br>If male <55 years<br>If female <65 years |
| Age and gender | Men ≥45 years<br>Women ≥55 years |
| **Risk Factors for Metabolic Syndrome** | |
| Abdominal obesity | Waist circumference<br>Men: ≥40 inches (102 cm)<br>Women: ≥35 inches (88 cm) |
| Elevated blood triglyceride (TG) mg/dL | Normal: <150<br>Borderline high: 150–199<br>High: 200–499<br>Very high: ≥500 |
| High-density lipoprotein (HDL) cholesterol mg/dL | Men: <40<br>Women: <50 |
| Blood pressure | Blood pressure ≥130 (systolic) or >85 (diastolic) mmHg |
| Fasting blood glucose mg/dL | ≥110 |
| Hemoglobin A1C | ≥6.4 |
| Overweight/Obesity | BMI >25 (overweight) or >30 (obese) |
| Comorbidities | HIV/AIDS<br>Diabetes, especially if uncontrolled<br>Elevated fasting plasma insulin levels |
| **Lifestyle Factors** | |
| Food intake patterns | Consumption of few vegetables, fruits, and whole grains<br>High saturated fats and *trans*-fatty acid intake<br>Infrequent intake of fish (low omega-3 fatty acid intake)<br>Inadequate folate intake |
| Sedentary lifestyle<br>Lack of physical activity | Less than 30 minutes of moderate physical activity on most days of the week (<150 minutes a week) |
| Emotional stress | Unresolved emotional stress<br>Hostility, angry personality |
| **Emerging Risk Factors** | |
| Elevated levels of high-sensitivity C-reactive protein (indicator of inflammation) mg/L | Average risk: 1.0 to 3.0<br>High risk: >3.0 |
| Elevated plasma apolipoprotein B (apo B) (the protein constituent of LDL cholesterol) mg/L | ≥1.20 (75th percentile) increased risk for CHD |
| High plasma homocysteine levels μmol/L (related to folic acid and B-vitamin intake) | ≥15 |

biomarkers that are associated with CVD but not routinely used as screening factors.[51,52]

## Nutrition Assessment

People identified at high risk should be referred to a registered dietitian for an nutrition assessment (Table 17.4) and individualized intervention.[49,53] Key assessment components include:

- Food and nutrition history to determine usual intake, especially amount and type of fat, fruits and vegetables, bread and grains, meat, fish, and dairy foods; meal and snack patterns; and supplement use
- Nutrition knowledge of healthy-eating recommendations and relationship of food choices to CVD risk, and attitudes about food choices and change
- Physical activity
- Anthropometric measurements of weight, height, BMI, and waist circumference and weight gain history
- Laboratory values for lipid profile and blood glucose
- Medical and social history to clarify other health and lifestyle factors that impact nutritional status, food choice and access, and motivation and ability to initiate and maintain lifestyle changes

## Nutrition Interventions for CVD

Nutrition intervention for CVD should begin early in life to prevent or delay the development of atherosclerosis. Population-oriented messages and dietary guidance are primary prevention strategies. Intervention shifts to the individual level with medical nutrition therapy and ***therapeutic lifestyle change*** programs when risk factors develop or CVD is diagnosed.

**Primary Prevention** Eating for cardiometabolic health is not on the top of the agenda for many young adults, but eating habits during those years influence the development of atherosclerosis and risk for CHD and stroke. All young and middle-aged adults, with risk factors or not, should follow the principles of a ***cardio-protective diet*** that emphasizes plant foods (vegetables, fruits, and whole grains), appropriate fats (polyunsaturated), fish, poultry, legumes and nuts, and low-fat dairy.

The American Heart Association (AHA) has prevention guidelines to reduce risk for CVD across the population and to modify diet (see Table 17.8), physical activity, and smoking to reduce risk factors.[49,54] The aim is to prevent subclinical signs and symptoms from developing into overt acute and chronic CVD. AHA also provides recommendations for systems that influence the foods people eat and the physical activities they are able to include in their daily routine.[55] Table 17.9 lists AHA evidence-based recommendations for changes that can be made by big industries such as the media and the food industry, and for changes at worksites that impact what adults choose to eat.

**TABLE 17.8** Diet recommendations to reduce LDL-C, blood pressure and obesity

1. **Dietary Pattern** Consume a dietary pattern that emphasizes intake of vegetables, fruits, and whole grains; includes low fat dairy products, poultry, fish, legumes, nontropical vegetable oils and nuts; and limits intake of sweets, sugar-sweetened beverages and red meats.
   a. Adapt this dietary pattern to appropriate calorie requirements, personal and cultural food preferences, and nutrition therapy for other medical conditions (including diabetes mellitus).
   b. Achieve this pattern by following plans such as the DASH dietary pattern, the USDA Food Pattern, or the AHA Diet
2. **Type of Fat** Reduce percent of calories from sat fat; aim for 5–6% of calories from sat fat. Reduce *trans* fat (by avoiding hydrogenated oil and reducing meat intake).
3. **Sodium** For those who could benefit from blood pressure reduction (two-thirds of adult population) Lower sodium intake to 2400 mg or preferably 1500 mg per day; or reduce by at least 1000 mg/day.
4. **Calorie Restriction** For those who need to lose weight based on BMI or WC (2/3 of population) 1200–1500 kcal/day women, 1500–1800 kcal/day men (adjusted for current body weight), or 500–750 kcal/day energy deficit
   a. Prescribe evidence-based diet that restricts certain food types; chose based on patient preference and health status
   b. Aim for 3–5% weight loss for clinical outcomes, but aim for greater loss to get greater clinical changes and avoid need for medications
   c. Refer to nutrition professional for counseling and/or recommend comprehensive lifestyle program of at least 6 months to assist in adhering to diet and increasing physical activity.

SOURCE: Adapted from 2013 AHA/ACC Guideline on Lifestyle Management to Reduce Cardiovascular Risk: A Report of the American College of Cardiology /American Heart Association Task Force on Practice Guidelines

**Therapeutic Lifestyle Changes** A more intensive intervention called Therapeutic Lifestyle Changes (TLC), with behavioral counseling and follow-up by health care providers, is recommended for individuals identified at high-risk.[49,53] Diet and lifestyle change is the cornerstone of therapy and is recommended even when ***pharmacotherapy*** (lipid-lowering medication) is implemented. Medical nutrition therapy provided by a registered dietitian tailors behavioral change and outcome goals to each individual's situation. Higher-intensity

**therapeutic lifestyle change (TLC)** A higher-intensity dietary approach for reducing risk of cardiovascular disease with defined targets for type and amount of fat and dietary fiber, physical activity, and weight reduction. This is considered the first line of treatment.

**cardio-protective diet** A diet that emphasizes plant foods (vegetables, fruits, grains, especially whole grains, and legumes), appropriate fats, and fish, along with smaller amounts of lean meat and dairy.

**pharmacotherapy** Treatment of disease through the use of drugs.

TABLE 17.9 ▸ Evidence-based population approaches for improving diet

| | |
|---|---|
| Media and education | Sustained, focused media and education campaigns for increasing consumption of specific healthful foods and decreasing consumption of specific less healthful foods or beverages |
| Labeling and information | Mandate nutrition information panels or front-of-package labels or icons as a means to influence industry behaviors and product formulations |
| Economic incentives | Subsidy strategies to lower prices of more healthful food and beverages<br>Tax strategies to increase prices of less healthful food and beverages<br>Changes in both agriculture subsidies and related policies to create an infrastructure that facilitates production, transportation, and marketing of healthier foods, sustained over several decades |
| Workplaces | Comprehensive worksite wellness programs with nutrition, physical activity, and tobacco cessation/prevention components<br>Increased availability of healthier food/beverage options and/or strong standards for foods and beverages served, in combination with vending machine prompts, labels, or icons to make healthier choices |
| Local environment | Increase availability of supermarkets near homes |

SOURCE: Adapted from Population Approaches to Improve Diet, Physical Activity, and Smoking Habits: A Scientific Statement of the American Heart Association.



intervention is important to support the individual in making lifestyle changes to reduce risk factors and halt or reverse atherosclerotic processes and prevent a coronary event (heart attack) or death. This intensive approach, developed by the National Cholesterol Education Program, has stood the test of time. (See: www.nhlbi.nih.gov/health/resources/heart/cholesterol-tlc.) Making therapeutic lifestyle changes requires ongoing intervention using many strategies as discussed in the cognitive behavior change section.

After years of recommending low-fat diets, focus has been redirected to the type of fat with emphasis on keeping saturated to less than 5–6 percent of calories, consuming polyunsaturated fat (from fish and vegetable oils) and avoiding *trans* fats.[56,57] Stanols/sterols and additional viscous fiber (5–15 grams) intake are also being encouraged.[58]

**Stanols/Sterols** Plant stanol and sterol esters are an essential component of plant cell membranes that resembles the chemical structure of animal cholesterol. When eaten, they block particles responsible for cholesterol transport, which results in less cholesterol absorption. Regular consumption of 2–3 grams per day (divided into two servings) with meals is associated with a 7–15 percent reduction in LDL.[59] Stanol and sterol esters have been added to food products such as margarines, salad dressings, beverages and bars and are available as softgel capsules, making them readily available. The safety of more than 3 grams per day has not been studied and high plant sterol serum levels can be detrimental for persons with genetic differences in sterol metabolism.[60]

**Viscous Fiber** Viscous fiber is the "sticky" type of soluble fiber found in oats, barley, and flax, psyllium-enriched cereals, legumes (beans and lentils), some fruits (apples, mangoes, plums, kiwi, pears, berries, peaches, citrus fruits, and dried apricots, prunes, and figs) and certain vegetables (such as okra and eggplant). Viscous fiber is responsible for the fiber-related physiological effects of decreased LDL. Viscous fiber holds water in the gut, forming a thick gel that reduces absorption of cholesterol-rich bile acids and carries them out of the body. When this happens, the liver shifts from producing cholesterol that ends up in the blood to producing bile acids that are necessary for digestion. In addition, fermentation by colonic bacteria inhibits fat absorption and cholesterol transport and synthesis. Eating 5–10 grams of viscous fiber (1½ cups of cooked oatmeal provides 3 grams) a day has been shown to reduce LDL by 10–15 percent.[61]

## Pharmacotherapy of CVD

Lipid-lowering medications are prescribed when LDL is >190 mg/dL, or 70–189 mg/dL if the individual has an increased 10 year risk score or diabetes.[62] Two types of drugs are used to lower blood cholesterol levels. Ezetimibe inhibits intestinal absorption of cholesterol. Statins work by blocking the enzyme (HMG-CoA) responsible for making cholesterol in the liver. They also stabilize plaques, making them less prone to rupturing and forming clots that can block arteries. Statins also reduce arterial inflammation, which contributes to atherosclerosis. Lowered blood cholesterol results in reduced formation of new plaques and reduced size of existing plaques lining arterial walls.

# Metabolic Syndrome

LO 17.3 Describe metabolic syndrome and its assessment and effects.

***Metabolic syndrome*** (also known as syndrome X or the dysmetabolic syndrome) designates a cluster of altered metabolic conditions that come together in a single individual, and place that person at high risk for coronary artery disease, stroke, and type 2 diabetes. The metabolic conditions include abdominal obesity indicated by large waist circumference, elevated blood pressure, insulin resistance indicated by elevated fasting glucose, and dyslipidemia indicated by elevated triglycerides and low HDL cholesterol.[63] The diagnosis of metabolic syndrome is made when an individual has any three of these five indicators. Cutpoints used in diagnosing metabolic syndrome and diabetes are included in Table 17.10.

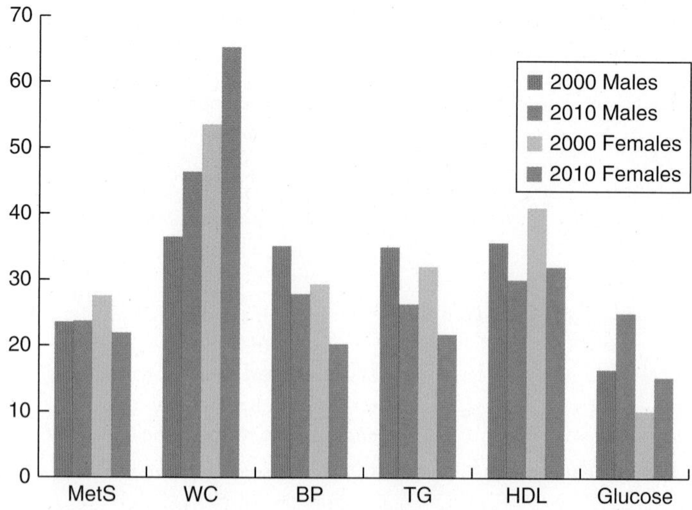


ILLUSTRATION 17.4 ▸ Ten-year shift in metabolic syndrome prevalence and diagnostic components for adult males and females.

TABLE 17.10 ▸ Laboratory values used for prediabetes and diabetes screening and management in adults

| | NORMAL RANGE | SCREENING & ASSESSMENT | TREATMENT GOAL |
|---|---|---|---|
| Screening | | | |
| Random capillary glucose, mg/dL[a] | 70–150 | ≥200 | |
| Clinical Assessment | | | |
| Fasting plasma glucose, mg/dL | 70–100 | | |
| Prediabetes | | 100–125 | |
| Diabetes | | ≥126 | <126 |
| 2-hr, 75-gram OGTT[b], mg/dL | <140 | | |
| Prediabetes | | 140–199 | |
| Diabetes | | ≥200 | |
| A1C, % | 4.0–5.9 | | |
| Prediabetes | | 5.7–6.4 | |
| Diabetes | | ≥6.5 | <7.0 |
| Individualized A1C, % | | | 7.5–8.5 |
| Self-monitored Blood Glucose | | | |
| Preprandial capillary glucose, mg/dL | | | 80–130 |
| 1–2 hr Postprandial capillary glucose, mg/dL | | | <180 |

[a] To convert these Conventional Units to SI Units see Appendix B: Conventional Units to SI Units table.
[b] OGTT–Oral glucose tolerance test.

SOURCE: Based on American Diabetes Association (2015). Standards of Medical Care in Diabetes—2015. *Diabetes Care* 38 (Suppl 1): S11–S63.

## Prevalence of Metabolic Syndrome

Metabolic syndrome affects over a fifth of U.S. adults.[64] Prevalence has declined slightly in 10 years, but the metabolic conditions leading to diagnosis have changed substantially (see Illustration 17.4). Waist circumference, especially among women had increased; and elevated glucose has increased, especially among men. Declines in rates of suboptimum blood pressure, triglycerides, and HDL cholesterol are attributed to increased awareness and medication management.[64] Metabolic syndrome is present in nearly 10 percent of people with normal body weight, one-third of those who are overweight, and two-thirds of those who are obese. The prevalence increases from 20 percent for ages 20–39 to 41 percent for ages 40–59.[65]

The prevalence of metabolic syndrome varies substantially by gender and ethnicity even after accounting for a person's BMI, age, socioeconomic status, and other factors. American Indian and Alaskan Native subpopulations have a wide range of metabolic syndrome rates that parallel the subgroups' rates of diabetes.[66] Mexican American males have the highest prevalence and Black males have the lowest. Among females, Mexican American and Black females have 1.5 times the rate of White females.[64] African Americans with very high BMIs and very high levels of insulin resistance can have very low levels of triglycerides, even though they have a significantly higher prevalence of cardiovascular disease and diabetes compared to Whites.[67] The diagnosis criteria that

**metabolic syndrome**
A constellation of metabolic abnormalities that increases the risk of type 2 diabetes and cardiovascular diseases. It is characterized by insulin resistance, abdominal obesity, high blood pressure and triglyceride levels, low HDL cholesterol, and elevated fasting glucose or impaired glucose tolerance. Also called Syndrome X, insulin-resistance syndrome, and the dysmetabolic syndrome.

relies on triglyceride levels as a marker for metabolic syndrome may result in underdiagnosis in African Americans. Asians, especially South Asians, can develop metabolic syndrome with only moderate excess in abdominal fat.[18] Thus, African Americans and Asians could be at risk for metabolic syndrome with only two metabolic risk factors.

### Etiology of Metabolic Syndrome

The underlying cause of metabolic syndrome is not entirely clear, but it is thought to result from central adiposity and insulin resistance. Insulin resistance refers to the diminished ability of cells to respond to the action of insulin in promoting the transport of glucose from blood into muscles and other tissues. To compensate, the pancreas produces more insulin, resulting in ***hyperinsulinemia***. A sedentary lifestyle and a pro-inflammatory, atherogenic diet (high calories, total fat and saturated fat, and low in whole grains, vegetables, and fruits) contribute to insulin resistance. Progressive weight gain and high body fat (especially central obesity), inflammation, existing cancer, and HIV also increase risk.[63]

As is true with many medical conditions, genetics and the environment both play important roles in the development of the metabolic syndrome. Genetic factors influence each individual component of the syndrome, and the syndrome itself. A family history that includes type 2 diabetes, hypertension, and early heart disease greatly increases the chance that an individual will develop the metabolic syndrome.[63]

### Effects of Metabolic Syndrome

The hyperinsulinemic state related to insulin insensitivity is considered a prediabetic condition, but it is also recognized as a major risk factor for the development of early atherosclerotic cardiovascular disease.[49,63] The presence of metabolic syndrome increases the risk of developing type 2 diabetes fivefold, heart disease by 2–4 times, and nearly doubles the risk of stroke.[43] Metabolic syndrome is also associated with fat accumulation in the liver (fatty liver disease or steatahepatitis), chronic kidney disease, obstructive sleep apnea, polycystic ovary syndrome, and cognitive decline and dementia in the elderly, as well as a general proinflammatory and prothrombotic state.[68]

### Screening and Assessment

Waist circumference is a simple, low-cost method that can be used to screen for metabolic syndrome in community or clinic settings and identify those who should be referred for laboratory tests.[63] A fasting lipid profile providing LDL cholesterol, HDL cholesterol, and triglyceride levels, and fasting blood glucose, along with blood pressure, are necessary for diagnosis and provide baseline measures to track changes over time.[63,64,68] Screening for metabolic syndrome is recommended beginning at age 45 for asymptomatic adults or earlier for individuals who are overweight and have one additional risk factor, such as smoking or physical inactivity. With identification, earlier treatment can be initiated to minimize the effects noted above.

Insulin resistance, a hallmark of metabolic syndrome and type 2 diabetes, can present with phenotypic manifestations (physical signs). These are hyperpigmentation of the skin at the back of the neck (acanthosis nigricans),[69] "buffalo hump" (fat accumulation at the base of the neck), and double chin.[70] These signs suggest high risk and should signal further assessment. Case Study 17.2 presents a somewhat typical picture of metabolic syndrome.

### Nutrition Interventions for Metabolic Syndrome

The goal of clinical management of metabolic syndrome is to reduce the risk of atherosclerotic diseases and progression to diabetes. Intervention is directed to the problem identified: for central adiposity, reduce weight and fat mass; for dyslipidemia, achieve an optimal lipid profile; for hypertension, normalize blood pressure; and for elevated glucose, reduce fasting blood glucose and increase insulin sensitivity.[63,68] The first-line therapy, guided by the dietitian or other healthcare provider, is diet and lifestyle modification to adopt healthy eating, increase physical activity, and reduce weight. Medical nutrition therapy sections for CVD and diabetes provide details. Adherence to a Mediterranean-style dietary pattern reduces risk factors.[71] Exercise has beneficial effects on blood pressure, cholesterol levels, and insulin sensitivity, even if weight loss is not achieved.[72] If a period of lifestyle intervention does not reduce risk factors, or the individual is in a high-risk category, medications to treat the dyslipidemia, hypertension, elevated blood glucose, and/or insulin resistance are added.[68]

## Diabetes Mellitus

LO 17.4 Differentiate the types of diabetes and how they are diagnosed and managed.

Diabetes is a chronic disease associated with abnormally high levels of glucose in the blood (***hyperglycemia***). The hyperglycemia is due to one of two mechanisms: minimal or no production of the hormone insulin by the pancreas (type 1 diabetes), or defective production of insulin and insulin resistance (type 2 diabetes). In type 2 diabetes, circulating insulin is high, and cholesterol, triglycerides, and blood pressure are commonly elevated. Overweight is also characteristic of type 2 diabetes. Another type of diabetes,

**hyperinsulinemia** A state of excess levels of insulin circulating in the blood. It is common among persons with metabolic syndrome and type 2 diabetes and is caused by the pancreas trying to compensate for insulin resistance of cells.

**hyperglycemia** Abnormally high levels of glucose in the blood.

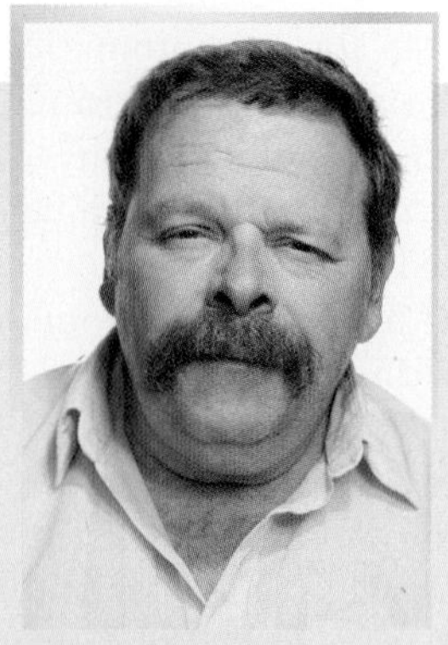

Image Source/Getty Images

## CASE STUDY 17.2

## Managing Metabolic Syndrome in Adults: Dan Goes Dancing

Dan Beek is 59 years old, semiretired, and lives with his wife in a midtown apartment complex. Dan was diagnosed with metabolic syndrome 10 years ago, and he has since gained 15 pounds. He attributes his weight gain to lazy afternoons in front of the television and frequent suppers at a local buffet restaurant. Though he plans to take his wife ballroom dancing on the evening of their wedding anniversary, Dan fears he will be out of shape and uncomfortable in the tight confines of his old suit. His wife suggests that the couple speak with a health professional regarding the management of his metabolic syndrome before attempting to lose weight. The following information is obtained at a recent medical follow-up.

Height: 5′9″
BMI: 32 kg/m²
Waist circumference: 42″

TCHOL: 218 mg/dL
HDL: 33 mg/dL
LDL: 154 mg/dL

Weight history (lb):
Current: 225
Highest: 225
At age 20: 175
Healthy body weight: 155 to 165

TRIG: 155 mg/dL
FBS: 125 mg/dL
TSH: Normal
HgbA1C: 7.1%
Blood pressure: 130/90

### Questions

1. From the information gathered at his medical visit, how well do you think Dan is managing his metabolic syndrome? Why?
2. What are the desired goals for metabolic syndrome factors (i.e., anthropometric and laboratory indicators)?
3. List the primary sequelae of poorly managed metabolic syndrome.
4. What sort of lifestyle modifications would you discuss with Dan in order to improve the management of his condition?

gestational diabetes, is discussed in Chapter 5. Of primary concern for adults is type 2 diabetes.

### Prediabetes

There is a long presymptomatic phase called ***prediabetes*** in which blood glucose levels are marginally elevated and vascular changes occur.[73] If untreated, prediabetes converts to type 2 diabetes in 5–10 years. The landmark Diabetes Prevention Program (DPP) study found that an intensive program of weight loss (7 percent of body weight) and physical activity (150 minutes/week) reduced the conversion from prediabetes to diabetes by 58 percent and reduced cardiovascular risk factors.[74] The DPP and similar studies have led to a greater emphasis on screening for prediabetes and intervention before typical diabetes symptoms occur.

### Prevalence of Diabetes

In the United States, over 28.9 million adults over age 20 years (12.3 percent) have diabetes and of these 8.1 million are undiagnosed. It is estimated that over a third of adults have prediabetes.[75] The rising prevalence of diabetes correlates with the rise in overweight and obesity. Although most often diagnosed in people over the age of 40, type 2 diabetes is becoming increasingly common in children, adolescents, and younger adults who are overweight. Type 1 diabetes accounts for 5–10 percent of diabetes cases.

Racial and ethnic minorities bear a disproportionate burden of the diabetes and its complications. They have higher prevalence rates, worse diabetes control, and two to four times the rate of complications such as renal disease requiring dialysis, blindness, amputations, and cardiovascular mortality of Whites.[76] Many customized, culturally specific diabetes outreach, care, and education programs have been developed to address these disparities.

### Etiology of Diabetes

***Type 1 diabetes*** is a progressive autoimmune disease in which the beta cells of the pancreas that produce insulin are destroyed by the body's own immune system. It has a relatively quick onset. A genetic predisposition, along with environmental factors, such as a childhood viral infection, are involved.

**prediabetes** A condition in which blood glucose levels are higher than normal but not high enough for the diagnosis of diabetes. It is characterized by impaired glucose tolerance, or fasting blood glucose levels between 100 and 125 mg/dL.

**type 1 diabetes** A disease characterized by high blood glucose levels resulting from destruction of the insulin-producing cells of the pancreas. This type of diabetes was called juvenile-onset diabetes and insulin-dependent diabetes in the past.

*Type 2 diabetes* develops over time. Insulin is present but it cannot do its job of facilitating transport of glucose into cells. This insulin resistance is strongly associated with visceral adiposity.[77] It affects muscle, fat, and liver cells in different ways. Insulin resistance in fat cells leads to the mobilization of stored lipids in these cells and elevates free fatty acids in the blood plasma. Insulin resistance in muscle cells reduces glucose uptake and interferes with muscle storage of glucose as glycogen. Insulin resistance in liver cells results in impaired glycogen synthesis and a failure to suppress glucose production. These metabolic alterations contribute to hyperglycemia. High plasma levels of insulin and glucose due to insulin resistance are believed to be the origin of metabolic syndrome and type 2 diabetes, including its complications.[68] High insulin also affects the arterial walls throughout the body and leads to hypertension.

## Physiological Effects of Diabetes

Diabetes is a progressive disease. In the short run, untreated or poorly controlled diabetes with sustained hyperglycemia produces frequent urination as the body tries to excrete extra glucose, increased thirst, increased hunger, fatigue, weight loss, blurred vision, increased susceptibility to infection, and delayed wound healing. In the long run, diabetes contributes to heart disease, hypertension, blindness, kidney failure, stroke, and the loss of limbs due to circulatory and neurological changes.

Micro- and macro-vascular complications typically develop in people with diabetes. Oxidative stress (see Chapter 3) related to hyperglycemia is believed to be a mechanism underlying vascular changes. Microvascular damage to capillaries in the back of the eye results in retinopathy and eventual blindness; in the kidneys, it causes nephropathy leading to reduced kidney function and renal failure requiring renal dialysis; and in nerves, it causes neuropathy and loss of feeling in hands and feet. Macrovascular changes (atherosclerosis in large vessels) are accelerated by diabetes, resulting in earlier onset of cardiovascular diseases. As a result, heart disease, not diabetes, is the number one cause of death among people with diabetes.[78]

## Screening and Assessment

**Diabetes Status** The American Diabetes Association recommends that adults should be screened for type 2 diabetes or prediabetes if they are 45 years old, or earlier, if they are overweight and have one or more additional risk factors.[79] The risk factors for diabetes and prediabetes include:

- Parent or sibling with diabetes
- History of gestational diabetes or delivery of an infant weighing more than 9 pounds
- Elevated A1C, IFG, or IGT on a previous test
- Racial or ethnic background associated with an increased risk (African American, Native American, Asian American, Pacific Islander, or Hispanic American/Latino)
- Sedentary lifestyle and physical inactivity
- Hypertension
- Low HDL cholesterol, high triglycerides, or CVD
- Woman with polycystic ovary disease[79]

Go to the American Diabetes Association website and look at the "Are You At Risk" tab, determine your risk for type 2 diabetes. The diagnosis of diabetes requires confirmed glucose intolerance verified by either a A1C test, fasting plasma glucose tests or an oral glucose tolerance test.[79] Criteria for screening and for assessment of glycemic control during treatment are shown on Table 17.10.

After diabetes is diagnosed, fasting plasma glucose and A1C are tested and compared to treatment goals to assess glycemic control. The A1C indicates the average blood glucose concentration over the previous 120 days. A1C levels can range from below 6 percent (normal range) to as high as 25 percent in uncontrolled diabetes.

## Nutrition Assessment

Nutrition assessment of the person with diabetes includes many of the same areas as listed in Table 17.4. In diabetes, the following are important for determining the individual's needs, tailoring a diabetes management plan and patient education and counseling, and monitoring progress over time.[79,80,81]

- Weight status
- Current eating pattern; types and amounts of food typically eaten throughout the day, especially types and amounts of carbohydrate
- Knowledge about diabetes and how food intake and physical activity relate to blood glucose changes
- Usual physical activity and opportunities and interests for increasing physical activity
- Laboratory values for glycemic control (see Table 17.10), self-monitored blood glucose records, and hypoglycemia or hyperglycemia events
- Medical history relevant to management of diabetes and comorbidities, CVD risk factors and disease, lipid profile, and blood pressure
- Medications for glycemic management and others, and supplement use
- Social, financial, and environmental factors impacting diabetes self-management
- Past education and experience with meal planning, carbohydrate counting, or exchange lists; and attitudes about diabetes and expectations for medical management and outcomes

**type 2 diabetes** A disease characterized by high blood glucose levels due to the body's inability to use insulin normally, or to produce enough insulin. This type of diabetes was called adult-onset diabetes and non-insulin-dependent diabetes in the past.

## Interventions for Diabetes

**Management of Diabetes** Diabetes studies in the 1990s with people newly diagnosed with type 1 and type 2 diabetes demonstrated that intensive lifestyle change interventions with target A1C levels at near normal levels (<7 percent) could prevent or delay the development of microvascular complications of diabetes (retinopathy and nephropathy) by several years.[74,82] These intervention programs were intensive in terms of the amount of time dedicated to diabetes self-management education, coaching, and support, and in terms of the targeted level of glucose control. A significant contribution of these studies was verifying the effectiveness of interventions that incorporate cognitive behavioral change strategies (as described earlier in this chapter). Subsequent studies among people with longer duration of diabetes found significant, but smaller, benefits in cardiovascular outcomes and an added risk associated with hypoglycemia.

The clinical goals for management of prediabetes and diabetes are to normalize blood glucose and glucose metabolism, and prevent or slow the development of diabetes complications, as well as to normalize lipid levels and blood pressure. This is accomplished utilizing medical nutrition therapy, physical activity, and medications.[79,80] Principles at the foundation of diabetes care are: *patient-centered diabetes care* and *self-management education and support*.[79]

***Patient-centered care*** is provided by a collaborative, interdisciplinary team that includes a physician, nurse, dietitian, and the patient. Additional team members might be a pharmacist, health educator, exercise physiologist, or psychologist. The person with diabetes is the central member of the team because the treatment focus is on empowering him/her to self-manage diabetes and maintain good control of blood glucose levels and other metabolic indicators throughout life. ***Diabetes self-management education and support*** is an ongoing process of facilitating the knowledge, skill, and ability necessary for prediabetes and diabetes self-care and quality of life. Education is based on a curriculum, tailored to each person's treatment goals and individualized plan for behavior change. Support is provided to encourage behavior change and maintenance of healthy diabetes-related behaviors and to address psychosocial concerns.[83]

The goal for diabetes management is an A1C of 7 percent or below. Less stringent A1C goals may be set depending on the duration of diabetes, age/life expectancy, awareness of hypoglycemia and other individual patient considerations.[79,84] Weight loss, with a target of 5–10 percent of body weight, is frequently a goal for those with prediabetes and type 2 diabetes because of its positive effect on insulin resistance, lipid profile, and longer term complications.[79]

**Medical Nutrition Therapy for Diabetes** There is no "diabetes diet." The current philosophy of dietary management of diabetes is diet flexibility within an individualized plan that is consistent with Dietary Guidelines.[79,80] For most newly diagnosed, and many with longstanding diabetes, this means modifying their usual eating practices and shifting to regular eating times and a healthful meal pattern that incorporates nutrient-rich food choices and appropriate portion sizes (balanced with physical activity and glucose-managing medications). To achieve this, individualized medical nutrition therapy from a registered dietitian familiar with comprehensive diabetes management should be an ongoing part of care. The dietitian determines a caloric level matched to weight goals (maintain or reduce) and a plan that balances dietary intake with physical activity and prescribed medications to keep blood glucose within normal ranges throughout the day. In addition, comorbidities and risk factors are taken into consideration. The plan and nutrition intervention should:

a. Enable the individual to achieve glycemic and weight goals as well as lipid and blood pressure goals.
b. Be responsive to personal and cultural preferences, and maintain the pleasure of eating.
c. Provide practical guidance and tools for day-to-day meal planning, taking into account health literacy and numeracy, access to healthful choices, willingness and ability to make behavioral changes, and barrier to change.
d. Promote and support healthful eating patterns, with a variety of food choices to meet basic nutrient needs (RDA and DRI), rather than focus on macro- or micronutrients or single foods.
e. Include ongoing counseling and education and follow up, and make adjustments as needed based on life circumstances, preferences and disease course.

The types, amounts, and timing of foods and beverages consumed determines blood glucose, as well as the response of insulin secretion, if available. Digestion converts dietary carbohydrate (both naturally occurring in food and added sugar and starch) to glucose. A consistent eating pattern or ***eating plan*** (regular timing of meals and snacks and amount eaten, especially carbohydrates) helps moderate blood glucose levels, and minimize spikes and valleys throughout the day. Strategies for managing carbohydrate intake include the plate method based on MyPlate to counting grams of carbohydrate at each meal and snack. The more complicated method of exchange lists for all food groups is being phased out. Selecting foods based on glycemic index and glycemic load

**patient-centered care** An approach to care that is respectful of and responsive to the patient's preferences, needs, and values and ensures that the patient's values guide all clinical decisions.

**diabetes self-management education and support** An ongoing process of individualized education and support to facilitate the knowledge, skill, and ability necessary for prediabetes and diabetes self-care and quality of life.

**eating plan** A plan for timing of meals and snacks and types and amount of foods eaten to achieve nutrition goals.

is controversial.[80] Some studies found a modest benefit (reduction of A1c by 0.2–0.5 percent).[79] Ongoing counseling and education is important for managing the nutrition component of diabetes managment.[79,80,84]

## Carbohydrate Management

**Carb Counting** Foods are classified in groups that have similar carbohydrate, protein, and fat profiles and thus have approximately the same effect on blood glucose as other foods in the group. This makes carbohydrate counting ("carb counting") easier as the focus is on the carbohydrate content of foods. See Table 17.11. The amount of carbohydrate allowed per meal is based on body size and activity level and typically ranges from 45 grams (women) to 60 grams (men) or 2–3 carb servings per meal. Planned snacks are typically 10–30 grams. Using reference lists, servings of food are selected to reach a specific number of grams of carbohydrate at a meal. Or based on a meal being served or choosing from a menu, what and how much to eat can be determined by knowing that each serving from the grain, starchy vegetable, fruit, legume, and dairy groups is counted as having 15 grams/servings. Nutrition Facts on food labels can also be used to determine grams and serving size. Using an eating plan and carb counting helps achieve consistent intake at meals and snacks throughout the day, and from day to day. Those using insulin strive for consistency, but can adjust units of insulin to the amount of carbohydrate in a meal. Measuring food and using carb counting food lists and Nutrition Facts on food labels is recommended at the beginning.

After becoming well versed in carbohydrate counting and understanding their blood glucose response, some adults can routinely use experience-based estimates instead of counting carbohydrate grams at each meal.

**Plate Method** The plate method is not as accurate as carb counting, but is easier to learn and is a good starting point for persons newly diagnosed with prediabetes and type 2 diabetes. A small dinner plate is divided in half. The first half is filled with about 1 cup of nonstarchy vegetables (e.g., mixed green salad, green beans). The other half is divided again. One quarter is used for a serving of a lean protein source (e.g., 3 oz. skinless chicken). On the other quarter, place a serving of starchy food (brown rice, potato, whole grain bread, pasta). Dairy is included as a small glass of low-fat milk or a serving of yogurt. After becoming familiar with serving sizes and types of food, many advance to carb counting, which allows greater flexibility of food choices and combination dishes.

## Self-Monitored Blood Glucose

Self-monitoring of blood glucose (SMBG) levels through the use of a glucometer is a part of everyday life for persons with diabetes. Recording the values helps the individual see his or her pattern of blood glucose and how it responds to physical activity and eating various amounts and combinations of food. Information about current blood glucose levels can be used to adjust diet and exercise (and to adjust insulin, if used) to minimize blood glucose swings. The record is also reviewed at

TABLE 17.11 Food lists for carbohydrate counting 1 serving = about 15 grams of carbohydrate

| BREADS & CEREALS | STARCHY VEGETABLES |
|---|---|
| • 1 slice bread (1 oz)<br>• 1 tortilla (6-in. size)<br>• ¼ large bagel (1 oz)<br>• ½ hamburger or hot dog bun (1 oz)<br>• ¾ cup ready-to-eat cereal<br>• ½ cup cooked cereal<br>• This should be 1/3 cup<br>• ⅛ of 12-in. pizza crust | • ½ cup peas, corn, or winter squash (cooked)<br>• This should be 1/3 cup<br>• ½ cup lentils, pinto beans (cooked)<br>• ½ cup mashed or boiled potatoes (cooked)<br>• ½ med baked potato (regular or sweet)<br>• 10–15 french fries<br>• 1 cup vegetable soup |
| **FRUIT** | **SWEETS & SNACKS** |
| • 1 small fresh fruit (4 oz)<br>• ½ cup canned fruit<br>• ¼ cup dried fruit (2 Tbsp)<br>• 17 small grapes (3 oz)<br>• 1 cup melon or berries<br>• ½ cup fruit juice | • 2-inch square cake (unfrosted)<br>• 2 small cookies (This should be 2/3 oz)<br>• ½ cup pudding<br>• ½ cup ice cream or frozen yogurt<br>• ¾ oz pretzels, potato or tortilla chips<br>• 3 cups popcorn (popped) |
| **MILK & DAIRY** | **CASSEROLES & MIXED DISHES** |
| • 1 cup fat-free or reduced-fat milk<br>• 1 cup soy milk<br>• 6 oz yogurt (light or sugar-free) | • Count 1 cup of casserole or other mixed foods as two carbohydrate servings |

each clinic visit to assess control and make adjustments in individual's diabetes management plan.

### Physical Activity in Diabetes Management

Physical activity is an integral part of lifestyle interventions to prevent progression of prediabetes, and it is important in the management of type 1 and type 2 diabetes. The benefits of regular physical activity include aiding weight loss and maintenance and improvement of the insulin/glucose profile, as well as reducing lipids and blood pressure.[32,79,85] National physical activity recommendations, as described in Chapter 16, also apply to persons with diabetes.[79,85] Exercise facilitates the uptake of glucose by muscle cells, therefore individuals with type 1 diabetes must learn to reduce their insulin dose and increase carbohydrate intake to minimize blood glucose swings during and after exercise. Frequent SMBG is recommended to learn how the body responds to various types, duration, and intensities of physical activity. Consistent daily physical activity that includes aerobic exercise supplemented with resistance exercise is recommended over sporadic, intensive bouts of physical activity.[85] Further, duration of sedentary time (sitting) should be reduced by breaking up session of 90 minutes or more by standing, stretching and moving.[86]

### Pharmacotherapy for Type 2 Diabetes

Lifestyle change (diet and exercise) is successful for about 30 percent of patients with type 2 diabetes. However, metformin, which reduces blood glucose by decreasing the amount of glucose released by the liver and increases glucose uptake by the muscles, is typically prescribed along with lifestyle changes for newly diagnosed type 2 diabetes.[79,84] Oral antihyperglycemic drugs are used in type 2 diabetes if glycemic goals are not reached in six weeks of lifestyle interventions.[79] They have four primary mechanisms of action: (1) stimulate the pancreas to produce more insulin; (2) increase the response to insulin at cell receptor sites; (3) decrease amount of glucose released by the liver; and (4) reduce digestion of polysaccharides to delay absorption of glucose from the gut into the blood. Insulin, injected intramuscularly, is required in type 1 diabetes and is sometimes used in type 2 diabetes.

### Herbal Remedies and Other Dietary Supplements

Numerous dietary supplements are promoted as being effective for blood glucose control and the prevention of diabetes complications. Many botanicals have been tested in studies, and a few are supported to some extent by scientific evidence of safety and effectiveness. For example, bitter melon, cinnamon, and funugreek have hypoglycemic action, ginseng may decrease carbohydrate absorption and increase glucose transport, and gymnema may stimulate beta cells and increase insulin release.

Chromium supplementation along with biotin may reduce insulin resistance. Dietary supplements are pharmacologically active substances that have side effects as well as potential drug interactions. If used to complement diabetes treatment, caution is necessary.[87]

## Cancer

**LO 17.5** Describe the development of cancer and contrast nutrition assessment and intervention priorities at each of the four stages of cancer care.

Cancer is a group of diseases in which genes malfunction, resulting in unregulated cell growth and tumor formation. ***Carcinogenesis***, the process by which normal cells are transformed into cancer cells, is complex and moves through several stages. The stages are activation (from inactive or quiescent state), initiation (injury or insult to DNA by a carcinogen such as free radicals, toxin, virus, or radiation), promotion (damaged DNA divides during a lag period, potentially over 10–30 years), progression (uncontrolled growth of cancer cells), invasion and metastasis (spread to other tissues and organs), and possible remission (successful treatment or reversal). Dietary elements can modify carcinogenesis at several points along the continuum—some by promoting (e.g., aflatoxins, red meat, alcohol) others by inhibiting (e.g., cruciferous vegetables, phytoestrogens in soybeans).[88] Cancers can originate in any cell, but the majority develop in epithelial tissue, where cells replicate at a high rate. Examples of epithelial cancers include the skin, lungs, prostate, breast, colon and rectum, uterus, pancreas, oral cavity, esophagus, stomach, and urinary tract. Since most cancers take many years to develop, the chance of a cancer diagnosis increases with age.

Cancer is considered a preventable disease because modifiable environmental exposures and lifestyle factors are a factor in most cancers. Cancer is also considered a chronic disease, because the majority of those diagnosed have an extended post-treatment survival period where the disease is in remission or "cured." Cancer survivorship is a growing practice area dedicated to improving the length and quality of life of those diagnosed with cancer.[89]

### Prevalence of Cancer

Each year, over 1.6 million people are diagnosed with cancer; and deaths from cancer total nearly 600,000. Cancer is the first leading cause of death for adults aged 45–65 and the third leading cause of death for adults 24–44.[90] Cancer deaths have declined in all groups except American Indians/Alaska Natives

**carcinogenesis** The process by which normal cells are transformed into cancer cells. It includes activation, initiation, promotion, progression, and invasion and metastasis. Dietary constituents can modify the process at several points along the continuum.

since the 1990s.[91] The American Cancer Society (ACS) estimates that there are 12 million cancer survivors.[92] Cancer types and rates very across populations, with African American males and White females having the highest incidence rates (new cases) of cancer. Five-year survival rates are lowest for African Americans. Economic and social barriers to cancer prevention programs, screening for early detection, and access to high-quality, ongoing treatment services are factors behind the disparity in cancer morbidity and mortality.[91]

## Etiology of Cancer

Cancer development is age associated but not age dependent. As people age, it becomes more likely that some insult or error will damage RNA or adversely affect the DNA replication process, and ultimately cause cancer. In healthy, resilient individuals, initiation may be repaired and subsequent cancer avoided or delayed. In a person with impaired immunity or suffering from major physiological stress, initiation may proceed through promotion and progression.[93]

Cancer is caused by exogenous (environmental) and endogenous factors. Environmental factors include tobacco, infectious agents, radiation, chemicals (some of which become concentrated in the food supply), and carcinogenic agents in food or resulting from food preservation or cooking methods.[88] Epithelial tissue, where a majority of cancers originate, has the greatest exposure to these environmental carcinogens. Endogenous factors include inherited genes, genetic mutations, accumulated genetic defects as people age, oxidative stress, inflammation response, and hormonal activity. Obesity is a factor in the development of some cancers.[93] In addition to promoting chronic low-grade inflammation, nutrient excess establishes a state of cellular and systematic anabolism characterized by increased expression of growth factors, including insulin. This produces a cellular environment conducive to survival and growth of cancer cells.[93]

Lifestyle behaviors such as smoking, food choices, alcohol use, sleep patterns, and physical activity, ultimately affect inflammatory, endocrine, and metabolic pathways that intensify or diminish cellular exposure and response to cancer promoting agents.[94] A European study of cancer and nutrition confirmed that the risk of developing most types of cancer was significantly related to the number of lifestyle recommendations followed (see modifiable risk factors, below).[95]

## Physiological and Psychological Effects of Cancer

A cancer lesion damages the cells, and eventually the function of the organ and system where it is located. The impact could be localized as in skin cancer, or have widespread effects such as the impact of pancreatic cancer on digestion, absorption and metabolism. Pain, fatigue, and emotional stress are also common. Psychological stress is compounded by the loss of income and health care costs.

## Screening and Assessment

### Modifiable Risk Factors and Primary Prevention

Although smoking is the most recognized contributor to cancer occurrence and death, there are other factors including obesity and insulin resistance; excess alcohol consumption; and poor dietary habits are important nutrition-related risk factors for developing cancer.[88,95] The list of foods, nutrients and biologically active components of food that have been implicated in cancer promotion or cancer protection grows continually. Table 17.12 lists many of them. Different dietary components have been implicated in different types of cancer. Obesity is associated with cancer occurrence, recurrence, and mortality; and high BMI and insulin resistance are predictive of poor cancer prognosis.[96] Excess weight and low physical activity adversely affect the quality of life for cancer survivors and may worsen prognosis.[92]

**Primary Prevention** Early screening of lifestyle behaviors, conducted through worksite wellness and community programs, fitness centers, clinics, online assessments, and smartphone apps, identifies behaviors that, if changed, can

TABLE 17.12 ▸ Nutrition-related factors associated with cancer risk

| INCREASE CANCER RISK* | DECREASE CANCER RISK** |
|---|---|
| Aflatoxins | Allium vegetables |
| Alcoholic drinks | Coffee, green tea |
| Arsenic in drinking water | Dietary fiber |
| Cantonese-style salted fish | Fruits |
| Diets high in calcium | Garlic |
| Maté | Milk |
| Red meat, processed meat | Nonstarchy vegetables |
| Salt | Foods containing folate, carotenoids, beta-carotene, lycopene, vitamin C, selenium |
| Salted and salty foods | Calcium supplements |
| Beta-carotene supplements | Selenium supplements |
| Greater birthweight | Lactation |
| Body fatness, abdominal fatness, adult weight gain | Physical activity |
| Overweight and obesity: increase risk through energy-dense foods, fast foods, sugary drinks, sedentary living, television viewing | Normal bodyweight: decrease risk through low energy-dense foods, being breastfed |

*Probable or convincing evidence for increased risk.

**Probable or convincing evidence for decreased risk.

SOURCE: Based on World Cancer Research Fund/American Institute for Cancer Research. Food, Nutrition, Physical Activity and the Prevention of Cancer: A Global Perspective. Washington, D.C.: AICR, 2007.

reduce individuals' risks for development of cancer. Cancer screening during medical checkups and tests such as the Pap test, mammogram, and colorectal cancer screening seek to identify cancer at an early treatable stage.

## Nutrition Assessment Following Diagnosis and During Treatment

Nutrition assessment determines the complete nutritional status of the patient and identifies if and what nutrition therapy is needed. Nutrition assessment areas are outlined in Table 17.4. Areas of focus for cancer include:

- Anthropometrics: usual weight and recent weight loss or gain
- Food and nutrition history: appetite, food tolerance, energy intake, nutrient adequacy or shortfalls, supplement use, knowledge of appropriate strategies to optimize nutritional intake in the context of the specific type of cancer and treatment
- Medical and social history: cancer type and treatment, side effects, support system, and resources to meet nutritional needs

Finding and treating nutrition problems early may help the individual with cancer gain or maintain weight, improve the patient's response to therapy and reduce complications of treatment, and improve the patient's prognosis. Assessment is done before beginning anticancer therapy, and assessment and monitoring continues throughout treatment.

## Nutrition Interventions for Cancer

Nutrition intervention for cancer differs significantly, depending on the stage of care, as follows.

**Prevention** Healthy diet and physical activity (see Table 17.13) with caloric intake adjusted to achieve and maintain weight within normal ranges to reduce risk of cancer development.[97]

**Treatment** Medical nutrition therapy is a part of care during treatment with chemotherapy, radiation, and surgery and recovery to restore nutrient shortages, maintain nutritional health, and prevent or manage complications. Anticancer medications and radiation treatments are associated with nausea, vomiting, diarrhea or constipation, fatigue, and weight loss. Nutrition modifications help the people with cancer cope with the effects of cancer and its treatment. In addition to those mentioned above, side effects that interfere with eating include taste aversions, anorexia (loss of appetite for food), mouth sores, trouble swallowing, pain, depression, and anxiety. Loss of weight, fat, and muscle is common in cancer and is due to a combination of eating fewer calories, altered absorption, and increased nutrient and energy demands of the tumor and/or response to treatment.[98] Dietitians individualize nutrition recommendations according to each patient's symptoms, treatment, nutritional status, and tastes for food. Foods and beverages that are high in calories, protein, vitamins, and minerals are usually advised. Some cancer treatments are more effective and better tolerated if the patient is well nourished. Enteral or parenteral nutrition supports (nutrition formulas delivered by tube to the gastrointestinal tract or directly into the circulatory system) are sometimes used. Getting enough calories and protein is important for healing, fighting infection, and providing energy and maintaining stamina and being well nourished are linked to better prognosis.[99]

TABLE 17.13 Nutrition and physical activity guidelines for cancer prevention

**Achieve and maintain a healthy weight.**

- Be as lean as possible throughout life without being underweight.
- Avoid excess weight gain at all ages, avoid increasing waist circumference.
- If overweight, losing even a small amount of weight can be beneficial.

**Make physical activity a part of daily routines.**

- Any intentional physical activity above usual activity provides some benefit.
- As a general goal, get 30 minutes or more of physical activity in daily routines.
- Strive to meet national recommendations for physical activity of moderate to vigorous intensity.
- Minimize sedentary behaviors such as sitting, lying down, watching TV, and other types of screen time.

**Eat a healthy diet, with emphasis on plant foods.**

- Choose foods and drinks in amounts that maintain a healthy weight.
- Base diet on vegetables and fruits of different colors (red, purple, green, yellow, and orange) and other food from plant sources such as whole grains and beans.
- Choose whole, relatively unprocessed grains rather than refined grain products.
- Minimize intake of energy-dense foods (>225–275 kcal/100 gm).
- Use fruits and vegetables to replace snacks and empty calories.
- Avoid sugary drinks.
- Avoid salt-preserved, salted, and salty foods.
- Avoid processed meat and meats cooked at high temperatures.
- Limit consumption of red meat to <18 oz/week, and minimize saturated fat intake.

**If you drink alcohol, do so in moderation.**

- Limit to no more than 1 drink per day for women and 2 per day for men.
- Cancer risk increases with the amount of alcohol and the years of regular drinking.

SOURCE: Adapted from American Cancer Society, Mayo Foundation for Medical Education and Research, National Cancer Institute, World Cancer Research Fund/American Institute for Cancer Research, and World Health Organization.

**Periods of Remission** Healthy eating is encouraged in the same way as for the general population. Lifestyle interventions can optimize health and nutritional status and help achieve or maintain normal weight. Intervention may include an individualized plan for weight management and physical activity.

**Nutrition Care During Advanced Stages of the Disease** Food and fluid intake are adjusted in accordance with the patient's wishes, to manage symptoms and improve quality of life.

### Alternative Medicine and Cancer Treatment

The hope for remission and cure is a powerful motivator to consider alternative medicine therapies. Many cancer patients or their families seek complementary or alternative treatments, including special regimens and nutritional and herbal supplements. Some herbal products have potentially useful roles in cancer treatment to ameliorate nausea and common symptoms. Examples include ginger capsules before and after chemotherapy treatment to prevent nausea,[100] chamomile or ginger tea for gastrointestinal discomfort, and peppermint tea as a digestive aid. The National Cancer Institute and the National Center for Complementary and Alternative Medicine are sources of information regarding complementary and alternative treatments for cancer.

## HIV Disease

LO 17.6 Describe HIV and its physiological changes and how key components of nutrition assessment and intervention are tailored to the stage of disease.

The multiple aspects of disease initiated by or surrounding infection with the human immune deficiency virus are referred to as HIV disease. In the early latency stage, the body is able to contain the virus. Without diagnosis or treatment, the virus destroys immune cells and chronic symptoms occur, including weight loss, diarrhea, and cough.

The latency stage can last from several weeks to 20 years. AIDS, acquired immunodeficiency syndrome, is the advanced stage that develops when the body's immune system is severely damaged and unable to contain the virus or defend against opportunistic infections or tumor development. Not all individuals with HIV go on to develop AIDS. Advances in drug therapy have changed HIV/AIDS from a terminal disease characterized by malnutrition and severe wasting to HIV as a chronic condition that can be managed over many years. As the years of life are extended, HIV-infected persons are more likely to develop cancer and cardiovascular disease, which are now becoming the primary cause of death for this population.[101]

### Prevalence of HIV

Over 1.2 million people (13 years and older) in the United States are living with HIV/AIDS. Annually, approximately 50,000 new cases are diagnosed and nearly 27,000 existing HIV cases convert to AIDS. New cases are highest among males. Black, White, and Latino racial/ethnic groups and the 45- to 54-year age group have the highest number of persons living with HIV.[102]

### Etiology of HIV

The human immune deficiency virus is able to make its own DNA and replicate itself by using genetic material from the host's cells. It penetrates the body's immune cells and eventually destroys the cells. Oxidative stress related to continued activation of the inflammatory process plays a role in disease progression. Decreased function of the immune system increases the risk that people with HIV will develop infections and cancer.

### Physiological Effects of HIV

HIV infection raises energy requirements by 10 percent.[103] Macro- and micronutrient needs increase with high viral load, decline of immune function, secondary infections, and altered absorption and metabolism.[104] Nutrient malabsorption due to changes in the gut and gastrointestinal pathogens can further compromise nutrient stores.[105] Unmet nutrient needs lead to antioxidant depletion, anemia, and protein-energy malnutrition. Vitamin and mineral supplementation has been found to slow progress on HIV for those not yet on antiretroviral (ARV) therapy.[104] There is a loss of lean tissue (e.g., muscle mass) throughout the HIV disease process regardless of weight maintenance. Weight maintenance and adequate protein stores improve a person's ability to survive HIV disease.[106]

The introduction of ARV drugs was associated with lipodystrophy—a redistribution of body fat stores.[101] HIV-associated lipodystrophy is characterized by loss of body fat from the arms, legs, face, and buttocks and with abnormal buildup of fat in the breasts, on the back of the neck and upper shoulders ("buffalo hump"), deep within the abdomen ("protease paunch"), or in fatty growths known as *lipomas*. Some of these changes are reversed or avoided with newer classes of ARV drugs; however, newer ARV drugs induce other metabolic abnormalities, including glucose impairment and bone disorders.[101,107,108]

Like other adults, the accumulation of central fat in persons with HIV is associated with insulin resistance, dyslipidemia, and metabolic syndrome. Adults with HIV have high rates of bone alterations, and have earlier onset of cardiovascular disease and type 2 diabetes.[101,106,107]

The medication regimen and drug side effects of ARV often require adjustment of meal spacing to minimize gastrointestinal disturbances and food–drug interactions.

In later stages of AIDS, oral lesions, nausea, and diarrhea make eating difficult.[106]

HIV disease imposes significant psychosocial burdens. Many people with HIV disease face social isolation and stigmatization, and some experience economic insecurity and have food access and housing issues. Substance abuse or comorbidities including mental illness and physical disability complicate the disease and its treatment.[106] Alcohol use significantly reduces compliance with HIV meds, dietary recommendations, and clinic appointments.[109]

Nutrition status is strongly predictive of survival and functional status of people living with HIV. Nutritional problems can occur at any stage of disease and can contribute to impaired immune response, accelerated disease progression, increased frequency and severity of infections, and impede the effectiveness of medications.

## Nutrition Assessment in HIV

Nutrition concerns during HIV include macro- and micronutrient inadequacies, altered metabolism, and body composition changes that include muscle wasting, lipodystrophy and obesity.[110] Assessment is important for identifying nutritional problems, tailoring nutrition intervention plans to the individual's needs and preferences, and monitoring ongoing care. Areas of focus vary with the stage of HIV disease and the presence of comorbidities, but include the following:

- Anthropometric: weight change (percent of usual body weight) and body composition—muscle wasting and fat distribution (electrical impedance, waist/thigh and waist/calf ratios[111])
- Food and nutrition history: eating pattern and nutrient adequacy (current food and beverage intake, usual meal pattern, medication and food timing, use of supplements, food intolerances)
- Physical activity: regular exercise to prevent muscle wasting, barriers to physical activity (fatigue, neuropathy), physical performance (strength/weakness, stamina)
- Laboratory: viral load, glucose tolerance, inflammatory and lipid profiles, measures of protein and vitamin and mineral stores
- Nutrition-focused physical assessment: muscle wasting, subcutaneous fat, oral health, gastrointestinal symptoms (nausea, diarrhea), appetite, pain, weakness
- Medical history: intercurrent health events (including infections and hospitalizations), comorbidity diagnoses (metabolic syndrome, atherosclerosis, diabetes) body-image concerns, mental health
- Social history: psychosocial issues, economic constraints, food security, lifestyle, support system
- Knowledge: knowledge of nutritional needs and strategies for managing disease and medication side effects, adherence to past recommendations, personal goals

TABLE 17.14 Energy and macronutrient recommendations for HIV management

| **Energy** |
|---|
| • To maintaining weight: 17 kcal per lb body weight<br>• To gain weight: 20 kcal per lb body weight<br>• To reverse weight loss: 25 kcal per lb body weight |
| **Protein** |
| • Men: 100–150 grams per day<br>• Women: 80–100 grams per day |
| **Fat** |
| • Healthy fat at every meal and snack |
| **Carbohydrate** |
| • Limit simple sugars, use whole-wheat grain products |

## Nutrition Interventions in HIV

Maintaining good nutritional status is important for overall health and immune system function. Nutrition care, provided by a registered dietitian with HIV experience, supports optimum nutrition, as well as medication therapy, symptom management, resistance against infections and complications, and increased quality of life.[106]

Individualized nutrition plans are an essential feature of medical nutrition therapy for persons with HIV infection and AIDS.[112] See Table 17.14 for energy and macronutrient recommendations. Nutrition goals in the early phase of disease include:

- Consume sufficient calories to maintain a healthy weight and prevent rapid weight loss.
- Consume adequate protein and other nutrients and engage in regular physical activity (Table 17.12), including weight-bearing resistance exercise to maintain lean muscle mass.[112]
- Follow a nutrient-rich, heart-healthy diet to maintain nutrient stores and reduce risk of cardiovascular disease and diabetes.
- Choose calcium-rich and vitamin D–fortified food and calcium supplements to prevent progressive bone loss.
- Consider vitamin/mineral supplement to support body stores of micronutrients.

As a result of greater longevity, managing elevated lipids, insulin resistance, and other metabolic changes become part of the nutrition intervention plan.[101] Medical nutrition therapy guidelines for CVD and diabetes, as described earlier, are added to those for HIV.

Nutrition goals and intervention strategies are adjusted for patients who transition into the symptomatic stages of AIDS, including:

- Encourage energy and nutrient-rich foods and supplements to maintain weight and body nutrient stores as long as possible.

- Use dietary strategies to manage symptoms—nausea, vomiting, diarrhea, anorexia, pain, chewing/swallowing difficulties, and taste changes.
- Adjust timing of eating occasions to accommodate medication regimens and potential side effects.

Currently, even the best nutritional advice and self-care cannot restore immune function and prevent the eventual progression of HIV. However, nutritionally adequate diets can help people with the disease maintain weight and avoid depletion of nutrient stores, and increase their level of control and sense of well-being.

## KEY POINTS

1. Overweight, obesity, and central adiposity are associated with the major chronic diseases—cardiovascular disease, diabetes, metabolic syndrome, and cancer—and many other conditions in a dose-response manner.
2. Relatively small amounts of weight loss (5–10% of body weight) can reduce risk for insulin resistance, diabetes, hypertension, and cardiovascular disease.
3. Within the categories of nutrition assessment (anthropometrics, food and nutrition history, physical activity, laboratory tests, medical and health history, social history, nutrition knowledge and attitudes, and readiness to change), different things are emphasized relating to the etiology, physiological effects, and risk factors for each of the chronic diseases presented in this chapter.
4. Modifiable risk factors for cardiovascular disease are blood lipid levels, high blood pressure, and the lifestyle factors of diet, physical activity, and smoking.
5. Therapeutic lifestyle changes, alone or with pharmacotherapy, can halt or reverse the atherosclerotic process and prevent coronary events.
6. Metabolic syndrome is very common among overweight and obese adults. Therapy is directed to normalizing blood lipids, blood pressure, and blood glucose through diet and physical activity.
7. Among overweight people with prediabetes, progression to type 2 diabetes can be halted or delayed with a weight loss of 7 percent and 150 minutes of physical activity per week; and among persons with diabetes, complications can be delayed when blood glucose levels are maintained at near-normal levels.
8. Intensive and ongoing education and counseling are necessary to make lifestyle changes to manage chronic disease and prevent complications.
9. Nutrition intervention in cancer depends on the stage of care: prevention, treatment, remission, or advanced stage.
10. HIV infection raises nutrient requirements; and nutrition intervention is directed toward maintaining weight, lean body mass, and nutrient stores, improving resistance against infections, and increasing quality of life.

## REVIEW QUESTIONS

1. How would you design a lifestyle-change program based on cognitive behavioral therapy?
2. What three things differentiate population recommendations to minimize cardiovascular disease risk from therapeutic lifestyle changes for individuals at high risk?
3. List the metabolic changes that characterize metabolic syndrome. How many are required for a diagnosis of metabolic syndrome? What is the easiest way to screen for metabolic syndrome?
4. Why is it better to start intervention in the prediabetic state rather than waiting for the diagnosis of diabetes?
5. List the main considerations in developing a diet plan (nutrition prescription) for an individual with diabetes.
6. What are a dietitian's priorities for nutrition intervention in each of the four stages of cancer care?
7. What nutrition-related concerns develop as a result of having HIV?

   The following six questions concern Rebecca, who is 36 years old, weighs 182 pounds, and is 5 feet 4 inches tall. She just found out her LDL cholesterol is 170 and her HDL is 37.
8. Rebecca is obese.

   _____ True _____ False
9. Rebecca should be assessed for metabolic syndrome.

   _____ True _____ False
10. Rebecca needs to lose over 20 pounds to reduce her risk of developing type 2 diabetes.

    _____ True _____ False

11. Eating high-fiber foods a few times a week will help lower her LDL cholesterol.

    _____ True _____ False

12. What other information do you need to determine Rebecca's 10-year risk of having a heart attack?
13. Rebecca quit smoking a few years ago. What else can she do to reduce the development of cardiovascular disease?
14. Identify and discuss at least three themes that are common across all the conditions—overweight and obesity, cardiovascular disease, metabolic syndrome, diabetes, cancer, and HIV disease—presented in this chapter.

Visit www.cengagebrain.com to access MindTap, a complete digital course that includes additional resources.

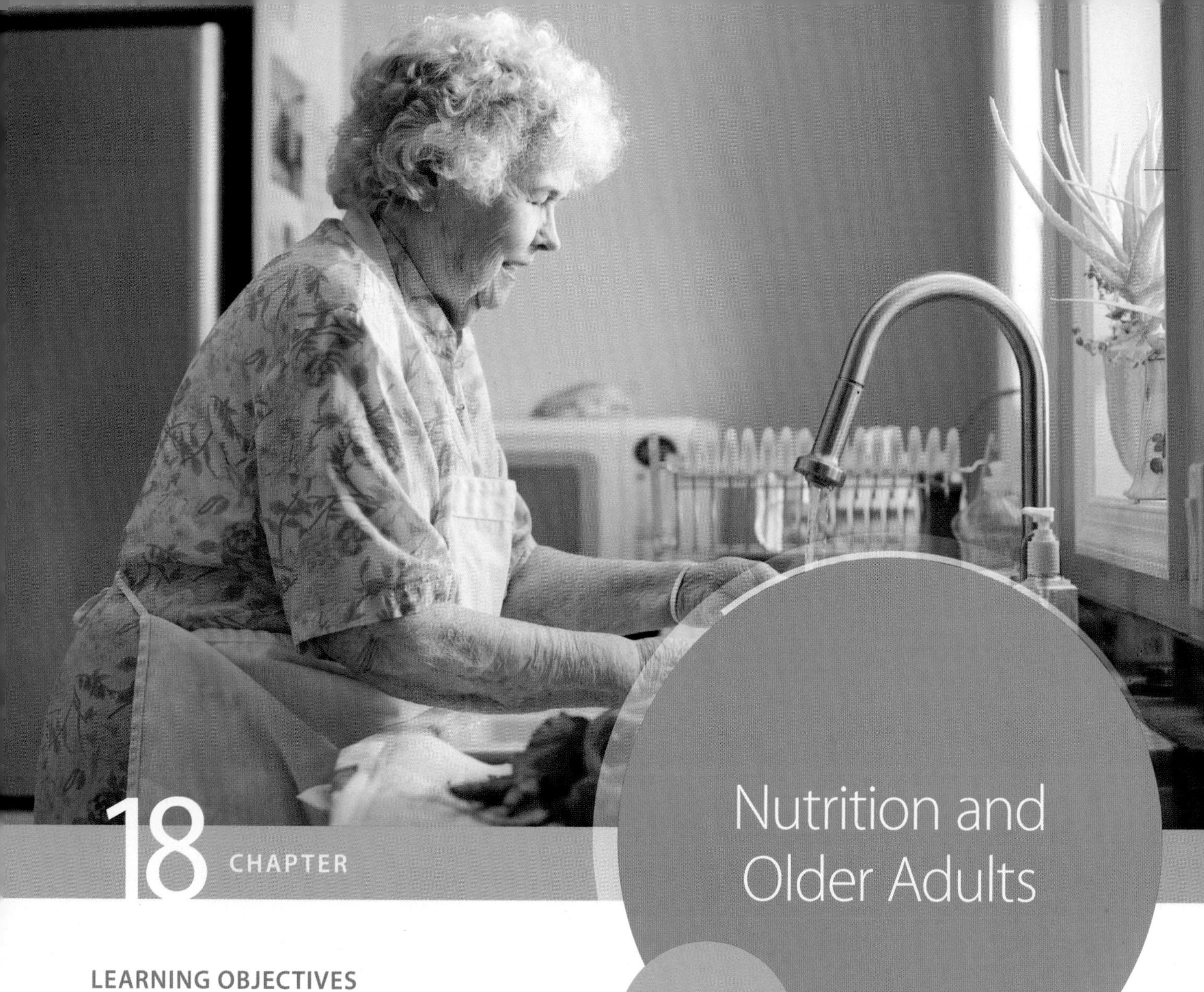

# 18 CHAPTER

# Nutrition and Older Adults

Prepared by
Nadine R. Sahyoun

## LEARNING OBJECTIVES

After studying the materials in this chapter, you should be able to:

**18.1** Distinguish three or more reasons why functional status is a better indicator of health in older adults than chronological age.

**18.2** Discuss the distinctions between life expectancy and life span, and address implications for society of increases in both.

**18.3** Defend the statement: "Diseases and disabilities are *not* inevitable consequences of aging."

**18.4** List five physiological changes occurring at ages 70+ and describe nutritional implications for each.

**18.5** Describe the relative effectiveness of two nutrition screening and assessment tools.

**18.6** Relate how enjoying a varied diet contributes to mental and physical well-being.

**18.7** Compare nutrient recommendations of old and young adults, citing five or more nutrients of concern for older populations.

**18.8** Explain how good food safety practices contribute to the health of older adults, and how increasing functional decline can be accommodated.

**18.9** Summarize the heterogeneity of older adult populations and suggest two or more reasons to tailor health promotion.

**18.10** Describe one or more nutrition programs serving older adults.

CDC/PHIL

# Introduction

LO 18.1 Distinguish three or more reasons why functional status is a better indicator of health in older adults than chronological age.

Aging is a natural phenomenon. It reflects the physiological changes that the body undergoes over the course of a lifetime. Many of the changes may lead to a decline in resilience, however, aging is not all loss or decline. Rather, healthy aging is associated with continuing psychosocial, personal, moral, cognitive, and spiritual development.

Aging is a heterogeneous process. Everyone ages differently. Genetics, lifestyle, and disease processes all affect the way people age. Although older adults are more vulnerable to disease because of biological changes that occur over time, aging is not synonymous with disease. Aging is an ongoing process; however, there is no single way of defining old age. *Old* has been defined chronologically, biologically, psychologically, and socially. Definition of old age is important for political, economic, and medical reasons. Chronological age is being used most frequently, but one 80-year-old individual may be playing tennis while another may be in a wheelchair.

Despite the prevalence of chronic diseases that accompanies older age, 72.4 percent of adults aged 75 and older consider themselves to be in good, very good, or even excellent health.[1] More than anything, older adults want to remain independent and living in their own home.[2] Older adults believe that good nutrition and exercise will help them maintain autonomy and independence.

What constitutes good nutrition in later life? Older adults need fewer calories but their nutrient needs remain the same or even increase for some of them. This means that older adults must consume more nutrient-dense foods. Diet quality is linked to the ***longevity*** of older men and women.[3,4] Eating adequate amounts of vegetables, fruits, and whole grains, choosing unsaturated fats, drinking enough water to stay hydrated, and drinking alcohol only in moderation will reduce risks of developing a disease. Good health habits help to delay mortality and achieve ***compression of morbidity*** in older populations.[5–7] In fact, 4 of the 10 leading causes of death for people aged 65 and older[8] in the United States have nutritional risk factors—namely, heart disease, cancer, stroke, and diabetes. Of these, heart disease and cancer accounted for nearly half of all deaths in the United States in 2010.[9]

This chapter defines aging and provides information about the nutrient requirements, dietary recommendations, and food and nutrition programs designed to support healthy aging. Chronic conditions that affect older persons' health are discussed in Chapter 19.

## What Counts as Old Depends on Who Is Counting

Societal and governmental definitions use various chronological ages to designate who is *old*. Based on nutritional needs, the Dietary Reference Intakes (DRIs) created a category for persons aged 70 and older. Due to the increase in the older population, the U.S. Census Bureau expanded the classification of people aged 65 and older to *young old*, *old*, and *oldest old* categories. The World Health Organization uses age 60 when referring to aging populations. How does this match the perceptions of older adults? A survey by the Pew Research Center found that the average older adult does not feel old, and that what is considered as *old* depends on one's age.[10] Overall, adult survey respondents said that old age begins at 68. However, adults under 30 considered 60 to be old, while respondents over age 65 believe that old age begins at age 75.

Establishing an age cut-off to define old age is used for policy decisions such as, determining retirement age, disbursement of pensions and social security benefits, and eligibility for other programs and services. For example, the Older Americans Act Nutrition Program, first funded in 1972, uses eligibility criteria of 60 years and older. The Social Security Program identifies people 65 years old as being eligible for ***Medicare***. These different age limits for program eligibility reflect society at the time the laws were enacted, and they affect program funding; adjusting them to meet public health needs will happen as science and the public's perceptions evolve. The arbitrarily set retirement age of 65 years to denote an *older adult* is commonly used, and we will use it here. Chronological age is just one of many factors that affect the nutritional status of individuals.

Since there is no single biological benchmark that signals a person's becoming old, chronological age commonly serves as a proxy measure for predicting health status and functional abilities. However, functional status, a description of how well one can accomplish the desired tasks of daily living, is more indicative of health than chronological age. Rather than ask, "How old are you?" we should ask, "Can you independently do the things you want and need to do?" and "Can you shop for food?" and "Can you see or smell well enough to know if your food is moldy or spoiled?"

## Food Matters: Nutrition Contributes to a Long and Healthy Life

It is human nature to seek magic bullets and super foods, but a balanced, varied and healthy diet throughout life contributes to optimal growth, to appropriate weight, and to nutrient levels in blood and other tissues that boost immunity and provide disease resistance. In trying to assess the contribution that good nutrition can make to longer life, the Centers for Disease Control and Prevention (CDC) suggest that longevity depends 19 percent on

**longevity** Length of life, measured in years.

**compression of morbidity** Shortening the period of illness and decreased functional capabilities at the end of life.

**Medicare** Federal health insurance for all people age 65 and older, and for younger individuals with certain disabling conditions.

genetics, 10 percent on access to high-quality health care, 20 percent on environmental factors such as pollution, and 51 percent on lifestyle factors.

Besides not smoking, diet and exercise are estimated to be the lifestyle factors contributing most to decreased mortality, or longer life. From a prospective study of over 3000 older adults and 10 years of mortality follow-up, the results showed that individuals who consumed the "Healthy Foods" dietary pattern, characterized by relatively higher intake of fruit, vegetables, whole grains, poultry, fish, low-fat dairy products, and lower consumption of meat, fried foods, sweets, high-calorie drinks, and added fats, had reduced risk of mortality and more years of healthy life than individuals who consumed other dietary patterns.[4]

Diet contributes to reducing risk of disease and delaying death and also contributes to wellness. Wellness means having the energy and ability to do the things one wants to do and to feel in control of one's life. Being able to choose, purchase, or prepare, and eat a satisfying diet every day; enjoying traditional foods at holidays, birthdays, and other special occasions; and having the resources to purchase desired foods on a regular basis all contribute to independence and a higher quality of life. Good nutrition, as defined by dietary guidelines covered later in this chapter, can help "add life to years" as well as add years to life.

# A Picture of the Aging Population: Vital Statistics

LO 18.2 Discuss the distinctions between life expectancy and life span, and address implications for society of increases in both.

Life expectancy varies by state and county. In Florida, where Ponce de Leon was associated with the Fountain of Youth, the U.S. Census Bureau 2013 estimates put the number of residents aged 65 and older at 18.7 percent of the population, the highest density in all states and territories.[11] Alaska has the lowest older-adult population density at 9.0 percent, and Utah in the lower 48 comes closest, at 9.8 percent.

During Roman times, fewer than 1 percent of the population reached age 65, in 1900 it was 4 percent. The last census in 2010 estimated the number of adults aged 65 and older at 40.3 million, an increase of 15.3 percent since the 2000 census.[1] This rapid rise of aging adults turning 65 is driven by baby boomers, born between 1946 and 1964, starting after the end of World War II, when soldiers returned home. Today, 13 percent of the North American population is aged 65 and older, expected to increase to 19 percent by 2030.[12] Persons aged 85 years and older are the fastest-growing segment of the population, expected to increase from 2.5 percent of the population in 2030 to 4.5 percent in 2050. Their growth rate is twice that of those 65 and over and almost four times that for the total population. The 1995 White House conference on aging called this age wave "a demographic revolution" and predicted that it will change the twenty-first century much as information technologies revolutionized the twentieth century.[13] Housing, transportation, and medical systems will need to adapt their programs and services to meet the needs of ever-increasing numbers of older adults.

## Global Population Trends: Life Expectancy and Life Span

Today, ***life expectancy*** at birth in the United States is 78.8 years (see Table 18.1 and Illustration 18.1) compared to 47 years for someone born in 1900. At age 65, an individual can expect to live another 19.3 years, and someone reaching age 85 can expect to live another 6.6 years.[9]

Life expectancy varies by race, and gender (see Illustration 18.1). Between 2003 and 2013, life expectancy at birth increased 1.9 years for males and 1.5 years for females. The gap in life expectancy between males and females narrowed from 5.2 years in 2003 to 4.8 years in 2013. Also, between 2003 and 2013, life expectancy at birth increased more for the black than for the White population, thereby narrowing the gap in life expectancy between these two racial groups. In 2003, life expectancy at birth for the White population was 5.3 years longer than for the Black population; by 2013, the difference had narrowed to 3.6 years.

Since the early 1900s, immunizations and other risk-reduction measures, treatment of infectious

**life expectancy** Average number of years of life remaining for persons in a population cohort or group; most commonly reported as life expectancy from birth.

TABLE 18.1 ▸ Life expectancies in selected countries, using 2011 data

| RANK | COUNTRY | YEARS* |
|---|---|---|
| 1 | Monaco | 90 |
| 3 | Japan | 84 |
| 4 | Singapore | 84 |
| 9 | Australia | 82 |
| 10 | Italy | 82 |
| 12 | Canada | 81 |
| 14 | France | 81 |
| 15 | Spain | 81 |
| 16 | Sweden | 81 |
| 44 | Puerto Rico | 79 |
| 50 | United States | 78 |

The CIA ranks 224 countries. Some of the shortest life expectancies are found in Chad, at 49 years; Afghanistan, at 50 years; and Haiti; at 63 years.

*Years rounded to nearest whole number.

SOURCE: Central Intelligence Agency. *The World Factbook*. Available at https://www.cia.gov/library/publications/the-world-factbook/rankorder/rawdata_2102.txt, accessed 6/9/15.

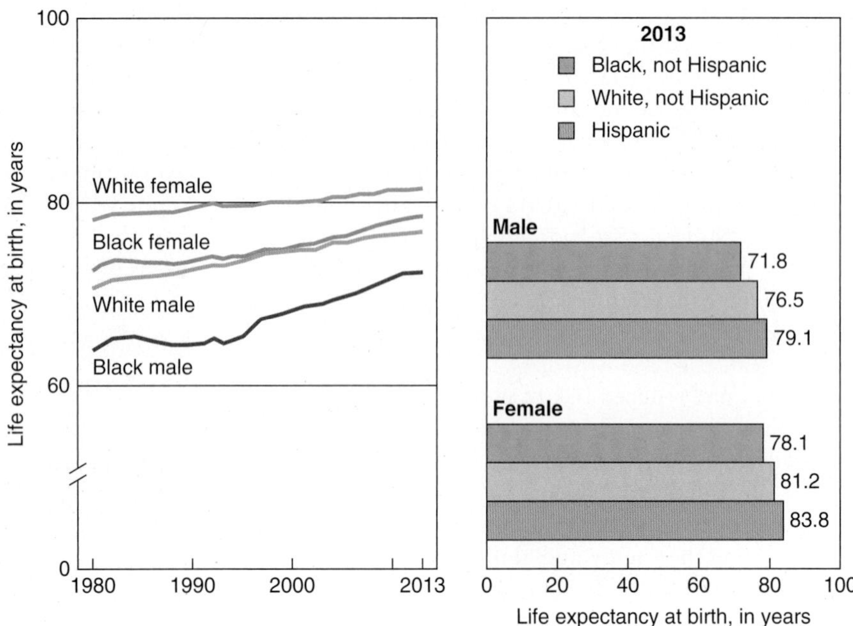


ILLUSTRATION 18.1 ▸ Life expectancy at birth, by race, sex.[9]

SOURCE: Centers for Disease Control and Prevention, from http://www.cdc.gov/nchs/hus/contents2014.htm#fig01, accessed 6/14/15.

diseases, decreased infant and childhood mortality rates, and clean water and safe food have increased average life expectancies. Additionally, by the mid-twentieth century, there was and continues to be a decline in mortality from chronic diseases. These factors contributed to the increase in life expectancy. The baby boomers, who are living longer than previous generations, started turning 65 in 2011, leading to a rapid increase in the older population. The increase in proportion of older adults is a worldwide phenomenon. This is known as the ***demographic transition***, which is the confluence of improved health and longevity, decline in fertility leading to growing numbers and proportions of older population in most parts of the world.

Although life expectancy is rising and populations are aging, human ***life span*** remains stable at around 110–120 years.[14] Jeanne Calment of France was the oldest known person, living to age 122. In the United States, Sarah Knauss lived to age 119 and Gertrude Weaver to age 116.[15] In May 2015, Jeralean Talley, the oldest person alive, turned 116 years old. Reaching age 100 has been rare enough that the president of the United States sends personal greetings to individuals for their 100th birthday. By 2050, when nearly 1 percent of the population is expected be a ***centenarian***, the president might have to reserve this special goodwill gesture for ***supercentenarians***.[15]

### Health Objectives for Older Adults

The most recent Healthy People 2020 national health goals emphasize overall fitness and the health consequences of obesity.[16] The objectives specified for older adults set a 10 percent improvement goal for behaviors related to disease prevention and management (see Table 18.2). Nutrition-specific goals are the same as those for individuals aged 2 and older. The greatest dietary improvement in the older-adult population would be to eat more vegetables and grains, especially whole-grain products.

## Theories of Aging

LO 18.3 Defend the statement: "Diseases and disabilities are *not* inevitable consequences of aging."

What triggers aging? Theories explaining aging grow from human desire to understand the biological processes that determine how long and how well we live. Aging theory tries to explain the mechanisms behind loss of physical resilience, decreased resistance to disease, and other physical and mental changes that accompany aging.

Biological systems are so complex that no single theory has been robust enough to explain the mechanisms of aging. Genetics are thought to account for up to one-third of longevity.[17] Environmental factors influence expression of the genetic code by aggravating or improving certain traits. Nutritional genomics is a

**demographic transition** Transition from high birth and death rates to low birth and death rates.

**life span** Maximum number of years someone might live; human life span is projected to range from 110 to 120 years.

**centenarian** Person who reaches age 100 or more.

**supercentenarian** Person who has reached age 110 or more, validated.

TABLE 18.2 ▸ Healthy People 2020, Objectives for older adults (target percentage, equals a 10% improvement from baseline)[16]

**Prevention:**

Reduce the proportion of older adults who have moderate to severe functional limitations (25.5%)

Increase the proportion of older adults:

- Who use the Welcome to Medicare benefit (7.0%)
- Who are up to date on a core set of clinical preventive services (males 44.6%, females 46.8%)
- Who receive Diabetes Self-Management Benefits (2.2%)
- Who have moderate to severe functional limitations (26.4%)
- With reduced physical or cognitive function who engage in light, moderate, or vigorous leisure-time physical activities (35.9%)
- With one or more chronic health conditions who report confidence in managing their condition (developmental)
- Increase the proportion of the health care workforce with geriatric certification (all types <5%)

**Long-Term Services and Supports** (2 of 5 directly related to nutritional status)

Reduce the rate of pressure ulcer-related hospitalizations among older adults (0.9%)

Reduce the rate of emergency department visits due to falls among older adults (4.7%)

SOURCE: Healthy People 2020: Improving the Health of Americans, U.S. Department of Health and Human Services.

field that examines the interplay between genetics and nutrition; it can help to promote healthy aging by tailoring interventions to specific risk factors, such as adding omega-3 fatty acid to one's diet in an attempt to enhance gene-controlled responses to inflammation. Body composition is another area that demonstrates reactions between genes and environment. While height and weight are strongly influenced by genetic factors, individuals have some ability to control diet, activity levels, and other environmental exposures (such as smoking) to determine what their body composition will be in later life.[6,18] Understanding how people age can help to separate the effects of age-associated disease from changes naturally caused by aging. Such an understanding can guide prevention efforts, leading to compression of morbidity and mortality.

Theories of aging can be examined from two perspectives: (1) programmed aging theories and (2) "wear-and-tear" theories. Caloric restriction is an intervention that incorporates aspects of several aging theories to manipulate life span and morbidity.

## Programmed Aging

**Hayflick's Theory of Limited Cell Replication** Hayflick proposed that all cells contain a genetic code that directs them to divide a certain number of times during their life span.[14] After cells divide according to their programmed limit, and barring disease or accident, cells begin to die (some call this replicative ***senescence***). For example, if individual cells of a fly have a 3-day life span and replicate 15 times, a fly can live 45 days. Using this theory, Hayflick calculated the potential human life span to be in the range of 110–120 years, estimating that human cells replicate from 40–60 times. Although most human cells can regenerate (e.g., blood, liver, kidney, and skin cells reproduce themselves), not all cells have that capacity (e.g., spinal cord nerves and brain cells). Hayflick's theory is difficult to prove in humans because we die from age-associated chronic disease more often than from old age itself.

**Molecular Clock Theory** Another theory of programmed aging is that of the molecular clock. ***Telomeres*** that cap the ends of chromosomes act to mark time, becoming a bit shorter with each cell division. Eventually loss of telomeres stops the ability of chromosomes to replicate. Loss of chromosomal replication may produce signs of aging because new cells cannot be formed, and the function of existing cells declines with time. A major thrust of aging research is to identify ways to limit loss of telomeres and thus prolong cell replication.[19]

## Wear-and-Tear Theories of Aging

Wear-and-tear theories are built on the premise that things wear out with use. Errors in the replication of cells and accumulation of damaging byproducts eventually destroy the organism. Cytotoxicity (poisoning of the cell) results when damaged cell components reach critical mass and become toxic to healthy cells. Glucose binding to proteins (glycosylation) leads to accumulation of AGEs (Advanced Glycosylation End-products); cross-linking between cells stiffens collagen fibers, including those in tendons, ligaments, blood vessels, and kidneys. According to wear-and-tear theories, the accumulation of damaged cells and waste byproducts leads to declining function and aging.

**Free-Radical or Oxidative Stress Theory** Oxygen is an integral and versatile part of metabolic processes; it can both accept and donate electrons during chemical reactions. One cause of aging is thought to be oxidative stress due to the buildup of reactive (unstable) oxygen

**senescence** The condition or process of deterioration with age.

**telomere** A caplike structure that protects the ends of chromosomes; it erodes during replication.

compounds. Unstable oxygen, formed normally during metabolism, can also initiate reactions that break down cell membranes and damage cells needed to keep the immune system intact. Exposure to oxidizing agents is increased by smoking, ozone, solar radiation, and environmental pollutants. Unstable oxygen compounds are neutralized, however, when they combine with an antioxidant. This prevents them from interfering with normal cell functions. The body produces antioxidant enzymes (such as catalases, glutathione, peroxidase reductases, and superoxide dismutase), but part of our need for antioxidants is met from the diet. Dietary antioxidants include selenium, vitamins E and C, and phytochemicals such as beta-carotene, lycopene, flavonoids, lutein, zeaxanthin, resveratrol, and isoflavones.

**Rate-of-Living Theory** The rate-of-living theory is similar to the oxidative stress theory in that it suggests that "faster" living results in faster aging. For example, higher metabolic rate and greater energy expenditure leads to greater turnover of all body tissues. Theoretically, fast-paced living shortens life span, whereas living more slowly leads to a longer life. Scientists have not adequately examined old people, including centenarians, to fully understand this theory.

## Calorie Restriction to Increase Longevity

If you search PubMed today, most of studies listed include non-primate organisms. Animal studies (e.g., of fruit flies, water fleas, spiders, guppies, mice, rats and other rodents, and primates) show that an energy-restricted diet that meets micronutrient needs can prolong healthy life.[20] For example, laboratory mice and rats fed calorie-restricted diets live longer and have fewer age-associated diseases than their counterparts whose diets are unrestricted. In the 1930s, McCay and colleagues suggested that delays in aging result after food restriction, due to slowed growth and development.[21] But since then, rodent studies have shown that instituting ***caloric restrictions*** in midlife, after growth and development were completed, results in longer life spans.[20]

Studies of caloric restriction (CR) in primates have shown conflicting results. Researchers at the Wisconsin National Primate Research Center found that adult rhesus monkeys fed calorie-restricted diets (at 70 percent of their previous energy maintenance level) had significantly fewer age-related deaths (the controls were three times more likely to die than the CR monkeys during the 20-year study period). They also found that CR led to delayed onset of age-related illnesses, maintenance of muscle mass at a higher level, and delayed gray matter atrophy. The authors suggest one mechanism driving these results might be that CR leads to changes in cell signaling pathways that induce metabolic reprogramming and subsequent life extension.[22] A similar study conducted by the National Institute on Aging (NIA) did not show a significant difference in survival between the CR- and control-fed monkeys.[23] Coleman and colleagues, who took a closer look at both sets of data, suggested that a possible reason for the difference in results may be that the control monkeys in the NIA study had lower body weight than the control monkeys in the Wisconsin study or even the weights of healthy, nonexperimental captive Rhesus monkey housed in research facilities across the United States. This seemed to imply that the NIA control animals were already fed a restricted diet and the difference in caloric intake between the NIA control and CR-fed animals was not large enough to show a significant difference in survival.[24] More research is needed to get a better understanding of the aging process.

Could calorie-restricted diets also extend human life? Experimental findings in small animals have led some individuals, such as Dr. Roy Walford of Biosphere 2, to personally adopt very-low-calorie diets. Walford coordinated the calorie-restricted diets of eight normal-weight people living in Biosphere 2.[25] However, such a small study lasting 2 years is too limited to determine human life-span extension results from caloric restriction, especially in the closed terrarium-like setting of the Biosphere. Luigi Fontana and colleagues tested the theory that caloric reduction also reduces a thyroid hormone (T3) that controls cell respiration and free-radical production.[26] They compared hormone levels of healthy, lean, weight-stable adults eating an 1800-kcal diet for 3–15 years with those of two matched groups eating typical Western diets of 2400 (sedentary group) or 2800 kcal (exercise group). Fontana's results suggest that reducing metabolic rate and oxidative stress may slow the rate of aging.

From an ecological view, people in France and Japan have lower caloric intake than do people in the United States, and people in both of those countries also live longer (see Table 18.1). Willcox and colleagues[27] studied a cohort of older Japanese residents of Okinawa whose nutrient-dense diets provided approximately 11 percent fewer calories than estimated to meet their energy needs. Population records show that this Okinawan cohort experienced caloric restriction at least until middle age, some longer. Lower caloric intake was coupled with reduced mortality from age-associated diseases. The authors concluded that, consistent with animal literature supporting caloric restriction, "an adaptive response to early and mid-life energy restriction in the older cohort of Okinawans may be implicated in their low morbidity and exceptionally long survival."

We know that nutrition affects human longevity by moderating risks of developing chronic diseases, ameliorating certain chronic conditions, and aiding in the healing of acute conditions. Many physiological relationships seem

**calorie restriction** Decreasing the energy level of one's diet by 25–30 percent while meeting protein, vitamin, and mineral needs.

TABLE 18.3 ▸ Age-associated physiological system changes that affect nutritional health*

**Cardiovascular System**
- Reduced blood vessel elasticity, blood volume, stroke volume output
- Increased arterial stiffening, blood pressure

**Endocrine System**
- Reduced levels of estrogen, testosterone
- Decreased secretion of growth hormone
- Increase in cortisol (stress hormone)
- Reduced glucose tolerance
- Reduced levels of thyroid gland secretions
- Decreased ability to convert provitamin D to previtamin D in skin

**Gastrointestinal System**
- Reduced secretion of saliva and of mucus
- Missing or poorly fitting teeth
- Dysphagia, or difficulty in swallowing
- Damaged, less-efficient mitochondria produce less ATP, less energy
- Reduced secretion of hydrochloric acid and digestive enzymes
- Slower peristalsis
- Reduced vitamin $B_{12}$ absorption

**Musculoskeletal System**
- Reduced lean body mass (bone mass, muscle, water)
- Increased fat mass
- Decreased resting metabolic rate
- Reduced work capacity (strength)

**Nervous System**
- Blunted appetite regulation
- Blunted thirst regulation
- Declining number of olfactory receptors, blood flow to nasal smell organ, and increased thickness of nasal mucus
- Reduced nerve conduction velocity, affecting sense of smell, taste, touch, cognition
- Changed sleep as the wake cycle becomes shorter

**Renal System**
- Reduced number of nephrons
- Slowed glomerular filtration rate

**Respiratory System**
- Reduced breathing capacity
- Reduced work capacity (endurance)

*Some of these age-associated changes, such as the increase in blood pressure, are usual but not normal.



to function well in a mid-range, between the dangerous zones of insufficiency and excess. Body weight is an example. Severe caloric restriction during famine leads to malnutrition and starvation, with poor outcomes in human reproduction, growth, development, immune status, and healing, while severe obesity leads to early death. Researchers are seeking the perfect balance of nutrient and energy intake to maintain a long, healthy life.

# Physiological Changes

**LO 18.4** List five physiological changes occurring at ages 70+ and describe nutritional implications for each.

Normal aging is associated with changes in most physiological systems, which may eventually lead to functional and structural deterioration (Table 18.3). As scientists come to understand the human aging process, they will learn to sort through age-associated physiological changes to be able to distinguish which changes are due to genetic factors and which are due to poor diets, inactivity, or other lifestyle-related factors.

## Body-Composition Changes

**Lean Body Mass (LBM) and Fat** Of all physiologic changes that occur during aging, the biggest effect on nutritional status and physical ***resilience*** is due to the shifts in the musculoskeletal system. On average, there is a decline in ***fat-free*** or ***lean body mass*** of 2–3 percent per decade from age 30–70, even when weight is stable.[7] This leads to the loss of up to 15 percent of muscle mass ***(sarcopenia)*** (Table 18.4).

During this time, body fat increases, especially in the visceral region. The increase is gradual so individuals might not notice, especially since weight stays relatively stable because muscle is replaced by fat. But maybe one day, the person puts on his or her favorite old swimsuit, and the shift is obvious. Of course, the extra fat does provide a reserve of energy for periods of low food intake or recovery from illness or surgery, acts as an insulator in cold weather, and cushions falls. Losses of fat-free mass leave older people with lower mineral, muscle, and water reserves to call on when needed. After age 70, weight, including fat at all sites, begins to decline.[7] Body-composition changes of aging are associated with lower levels of physical activity, food intake, and hormonal changes.[28]

**resilience** Ability to bounce back, to deal with stress, and recover from injury or illness.

**fat-free mass** Used interchangeably with lean body mass, comprising bone, muscle, water.

**lean body mass** Sum of fat-free body tissues: muscle, mineral as in bone, and water.

**sarcopenia** Age-associated loss of skeletal muscle mass and function.

TABLE 18.4 ▸ Comparison of body composition of a young and an old adult

| | 20 TO 25 YEARS | 70 TO 75 YEARS |
|---|---|---|
| Protein/cell solids | 19% | 12% |
| Water | 61% | 53% |
| Mineral mass | 6% | 5% |
| Fat | 14% | 30% |

SOURCE: Data from Chernoff, R., ed. *Geriatric Nutrition: The Health Professional's Handbook*. Sudbury, MA: Jones and Bartlett, 2014: p. 442. Based on Shock, N. W., *Biological Aspects of Aging*. New York, NY: Columbia University Press, 1962.

**Muscles: Use It or Lose It** Many older people expect decreases in physiologic function with increasing age. However, physical activity and regular exercise can mitigate the physiological effects of a sedentary lifestyle and delay onset or progression of chronic disease. For example, the HEalth, RIsk Factors, Training, And GEnetics (HERITAGE) Family Study compared the effects of a 20-week strength-training program on older and younger men and women, finding that the training response differed by gender and by race, but *not* by age.[29] Training exercises led to increases in fat-free mass; decreases in total, subcutaneous, and visceral fat mass; and to weight loss. Weight-bearing and resistance exercise increase lean muscle mass and bone density.[7,30] Building muscle also results in added water stores because muscle tissue contains more water than fat tissue does. Regular physical activity, including strengthening and flexibility exercise, contributes to maintenance of ***functional status.***

**Weight Gain** Weight gain tends to accompany aging. Large cross-sectional studies show that mean body weight increases gradually during adulthood. Weight and body mass index (BMI) peak between 50 and 59 years, then stabilize and start slowly dropping around age 70.[7,31] Reasons for age-associated gains are uncertain, but longitudinal studies are showing that decreased physical activity and lower metabolism could be factors.[32] For example, men in the Baltimore Longitudinal Study on Aging decreased their energy expenditure by 17–24 calories per day after age 55, and gained weight.[33] In the Fels Longitudinal Study, men gained 0.7 pounds per year, and women gained an average of 1.2 pounds as they aged.[28] Subjects were 40–66 years old when entering the study and were followed for up to 20 years. Weight gains were concurrent with decreases in lean body mass and increases in body fat. This overall weight and body-composition shift was moderated by physical activity. For example, the two groups with moderate or high physical activity levels (as opposed to the least active group) increased lean body mass and decreased total and percentage of body fat as age increased. Physical activity effects differed by gender. In women, higher levels of physical activity were associated with higher levels of lean body mass. However, lack of estrogen seems to promote fat accumulation, and total weight increased regardless of the group's activity level. Men in the highest physical activity groups in the Fels Longitudinal Study slowed their total body-weight and body-fat gains.

## Changing Sensual Awareness: Taste and Smell, Chewing and Swallowing, Appetite and Thirst

**Taste and Smell** Although there is some argument about the extent to which aging affects the sense of taste, there is general agreement that taste and smell senses are generally robust until age 60, when they start declining. Approximately 75 percent of individuals over age 80 have some olfactory impairment, compared to 6 percent of adults in their fifties.[34,35] Women retain their sense of smell better than men do. Other than aging (see Table 18.3), conditions leading to impaired olfaction include congestion, upper respiratory tract infections, stroke, epilepsy, medications, and current smoking.

Eating is a sensuous activity, involving not just taste buds but also the olfactory nerves and, many believe, the eyes. A blunted sense of smell can lead to blunted enjoyment of food, which anyone with a stuffy nose can easily affirm. Declining taste and smell also result in decreased ability to detect spoiled or burnt foods.

It is difficult to sort out whether aspects of sensory decline are due to illness or age. The number and structure of taste buds are not significantly altered during aging. In addition, taste perception for sucrose does not decline with age. Taste has been so important to biological survival that the body developed redundant systems. Several pathways of nerves and receptors control taste mechanisms. All of the pathways would have to be damaged before the ability to identify tastes is lost.

Disease, medications, and covering part of the palate with dentures may affect taste more than does age itself. Yet age matters. For example, during illness or with the use of medications, younger individuals maintained greater ability than older individuals to detect salty, bitter, sour, sweet, and savory tastes.[36]

**Oral Health: Chewing and Swallowing** Poor dietary habits are a modifiable risk factor that can contribute to caries and potential tooth loss. Approximately 1 in 4 (2 percent) of adults aged 65 and over have no natural teeth (edentulous), although this statistic varies greatly by income, education level, and state.[37] Tooth loss is associated with poor nutritional status,[38] disability, and mortality in old age.[39] What and when we eat affects oral health. Oral health affects what we eat and, in turn, nutritional status and health. Oral health depends on several organ systems working together: gastrointestinal secretions (saliva), the skeletal system (teeth and jaw), mucous membranes, muscles (tongue, jaw), taste buds, and olfactory nerves for smelling and tasting. Disturbances in oral health and tooth loss are associated with, but not necessarily caused by, aging.

Healthy teeth are protected by an enamel layer, but bacterial action on the breakdown products of food slowly erodes tooth enamel. For about 15 minutes after we ingest food or drink, oral bacteria feast on the food breakdown products, especially those of sucrose. Foods such as caramels or raisins stick around longer, especially when they lodge between teeth. Frequent eating and drinking of sugary beverages provides a continuous substrate for bacteria. The acid in carbonated beverages adds to the corrosive

**functional status** Ability to perform daily activities to meet basic needs and live independently, including telephoning, grocery shopping, food preparation, and eating.

potential of food. In addition, poor oral hygiene and a diet deficient in Vitamin C and in zinc contribute to periodontal disease.[40]

Saliva, which lubricates the mouth and begins the digestive process (amylase in "spit" begins starch breakdown), also helps to keep tooth enamel clean. However, saliva seems to become thicker and more viscous with age. Lack of saliva slows nutrient absorption. Lack of sufficient and effective saliva, especially in the presence of gingivitis and periodontal disease, also makes the oral cavity more sensitive to temperature extremes and coarse textures, resulting in pain while eating. Keeping the oral cavity moist through frequent sips of water and artificial saliva is beneficial.

Pain and discomfort with chewing foods can result in eating fewer fruits, vegetables, and whole grains. A loss of self-esteem associated with missing teeth and worry regarding how to pay for dental care can affect quality of life. Edentulous (no natural teeth) older people are less likely to visit the dentist for oral care (denture adjustment, periodontal disease management) than are those individuals having their natural teeth.

An oral health assessment is particularly important for older adults because they are more likely to have conditions that exacerbate periodontal disease. It includes review of soft tissues, teeth, and other factors that may affect dietary intake. One such factor is functional status, which can affect the ability to brush, floss, and obtain regular dental care, potentially resulting in periodontal disease, which can precipitate tooth loss and lead to a vicious cycle.

**Appetite and Thirst** Hunger and satiety cues are weaker in older than in younger adults. Roberts and colleagues examined the ability of 17 young men (mean age 24) and 18 older men (mean age 70) to adjust caloric intake after periods of overeating and of undereating.[41] All men were healthy and not taking medications. Food intake and weight were monitored for 10 days, and then men were overfed by roughly 1000 calories, or underfed by about 800 calories, for 21 days. Periods of over- or underfeeding were followed by 46 days of "ad lib" intake during which all men were free to eat as much or as little as desired. After the periods of over- and underfeeding, young men adjusted their caloric intake to get back to their initial calorie intake level and weight. Older men kept overeating if they had been in the overfed group, and undereating if they had been in the underfed group. The authors suggest that older adults may need to be more conscious of food intake levels because their appetite-regulating mechanism may be blunted. Whereas healthy young people adjust to cycles of more and less food intake, healthy older people's inability to adapt to these changes may lead to overweight or anorexia.

Elderly people don't seem to notice thirst as clearly as younger people do. A set of papers by Phillips and Rolls demonstrated that the thirst-regulating mechanism of older adults was less effective than that of younger individuals.[42–44] Researchers compared thirst response to fluid deprivation in a group of seven 20- to 31-year-old men, and seven 67- to 75-year-old men. Subjects lost 1.8–1.9 percent of body weight during 24 hours without fluids. Both groups were asked about feeling thirsty, mouth dryness, and how pleasant it would be to drink something. After fluid deprivation, the younger group reported being thirsty and having dry mouth. The older group, however, reported no change in thirst or mouth dryness. Both the older and younger groups thought that it would be pleasant to drink something after fluid deprivation. Blood measures showed that older men lost more blood volume than younger men did, indicated by their plasma concentrations of sodium. Researchers also measured how much water the men drank in the hour after their 24-hour period of fluid deprivation. Older men drank less water than their younger counterparts did. Younger people made up for fluid loss in 24 hours; older people did not drink enough to achieve their prior state of hydration. It appears that dehydration occurs more quickly after fluid deprivation and that rehydration is less effective because of lower thirst sensation and reduced renal water-conservation capacity. The prevalence of water-loss dehydration is estimated to be 20–30 percent in the older adult population.[45]

# Nutritional Risk Factors

**LO 18.5** Describe the relative effectiveness of two nutrition screening and assessment tools.

Identifying nutritional risk factors before chronic illness occurs is basic to health promotion. Risk-factor reduction forms the basis of dietary guidance. In adults of all ages, dietary risk factors that increase the likelihood of developing heart disease, cancer, diabetes, and stroke are consuming a diet that is high in saturated fat; low intake of vegetables, fruits, and whole-grain products; and poor nutritional habits leading to obesity. Healthy People 2020, the Dietary Guidelines for Americans, and MyPlate graphics all emphasize eating patterns designed to reduce the risk of the leading killer diseases.

Identifying risk-factors potentially leading to malnutrition can also be done by comparing dietary intake to nutrient intake recommendations such as the Dietary Reference Intakes. For example, sodium is a risk factor for hypertension, which is a problem for many older adults. How many of them limit sodium to amounts that would reduce their high blood pressure? More women aged 51 and over (31 percent) than men (9 percent) stay below 2300 mg per day, probably due to a lower caloric intake. But less than 3 percent of men and women aged 71 and older limit their daily sodium intake to the Adequate Intake (AI) of 1200 mg.[46] High sodium intake is a nutrition risk factor that is amenable to prevention efforts.

Another approach is to screen a population for risk factors that lend themselves to interventions to prevent or delay the onset of chronic conditions or prevent further deterioration of health. Several screening tools are available, such as the Nutrition Screening Initiative (NSI), the Mini Nutritional Assessment (MNA) and the Malnutrition Universal Screening Tool (MUST). Each of the tools has advantages and limitations, and the choice of which one to use is dependent on the objective of the screening and the resources available.

The NSI is the first nutrition screening tool developed and was based on the accumulating evidence that nutritional risk factors affect the health status of individuals. The American Academy of Family Physicians, the Academy of Nutrition and Dietetics, and the National Council on the Aging sponsored the development of this screening and assessment tools. A consortium of care providers, policy makers, and researchers used literature review, expert discussion, and a consensus process to generate a list of warning signs of poor nutritional health in older adults.[47,48] These warning signs were integrated into a screening tool, the NSI DETERMINE checklist (Table 18.5 and Illustration 18.2), and pilot-tested for use in community settings. Ten risk factors remained after testing a longer list.[49] This tool is freely available for use and many community agencies, educators, and care providers have integrated parts or all of NSI tools into their own materials to screen for nutrition risk factors.

The nutritional risk factors identified during the NSI process[48] are reflected in the list of risk factors identified in the Academy of Nutrition and Dietetics' position on nutrition and aging.[3] Any of the following conditions potentially place older adults at nutritional risk:

- Hunger
- Poverty
- Inadequate food and nutrient intake
- Functional disability
- Social isolation
- Living alone
- Urban and rural demographic areas
- Depression
- Dementia
- Dependency
- Poor dentition and oral health; chewing and swallowing problems
- Presence of diet-related acute or chronic diseases or conditions
- Polypharmacy (use of multiple medications)
- Minority status
- Advanced age

Why are factors such as poverty and minority status included in a list of nutritional risk factors? Although older people on average are less likely to live in poverty than are children, several subpopulations of older adults are at high risk of poverty (see Table 18.6).

**TABLE 18.5** DETERMINE: Warning signs of poor nutritional health

*Disease.* Any disease, illness, or chronic condition (i.e., confusion, feeling sad or depressed, acute infections) that causes changes in the way you eat, or makes it hard for you to eat, puts your nutritional health at risk.

*Eating poorly.* Eating too little, too much, or the same foods day after day, or not eating fruits, vegetables, and milk products daily, will cause poor nutritional health.

*Tooth loss/mouth pain.* It is hard to eat well with missing, loose, or rotten teeth, or dentures that do not fit well or cause mouth sores.

*Economic hardship.* Having less or choosing to spend less than $47.00 (female) to $52.50 (male) weekly for groceries makes it hard to get the foods needed to stay healthy. (These costs are calculated for individuals living in four-person households; 20 percent will be added to adjust for living alone. All meals and snacks are prepared at home.)

*Reduced social contact.* Being with people has a positive effect on morale, well-being, and eating.

*Multiple medicines.* The more medicines you take, the greater the chance for side effects such as change in taste, increased or decreased appetite and thirst, constipation, weakness, drowsiness, diarrhea, nausea, and others. Vitamins or minerals taken in large doses can act like drugs and can cause harm.

*Involuntary weight loss or gain.* Losing or gaining a lot of weight when you are not trying to do so is a warning sign to discuss with your health care provider.

*Needs assistance in self-care.* Older people who have trouble walking, shopping, and buying and cooking food are at risk for malnutrition.

*Elder years above 80.* As age increases, risk of frailty and health problems also rises.

SOURCE: Warning signs adapted from Nutrition Screening Initiative, a project of the American Academy of Family Physicians, the American Dietetic Association (Academy of Nutrition and Dietetics), and the National Council on the Aging, Inc., and funded by a grant from Ross Products Division, Abbott Laboratories, Inc.; dollar amounts under economic hardship inserted by author using the May 2015 USDA low-cost food plan.

Economic security contributes to food security. Lack of food security in older adults is associated with inadequate food intakes, especially for energy, protein and several micronutrients.[50,51] Minority status is related to economic status; older Blacks are nearly twice as likely as Non-Hispanic White older adults to live in low-income households and are also more likely to be food-insecure.[52] Black and Hispanic populations aged 65 and over are more likely to be poor or nearly poor (living at or below 199 percent of the poverty guideline). Furthermore, minority populations are more likely to be in fair or poor health, while Non-Hispanic Whites are most likely to be in excellent or good health. Similarly, women live longer than men, have more disabilities and a larger population live in poverty. Health care costs may contribute to food insecurity; for some, that means choosing between drugs and food.

*The Warning Signs of poor nutritional health are often overlooked. Use this checklist to find out if you or someone you know is at nutritional risk.*

# DETERMINE YOUR NUTRITIONAL HEALTH

Read the statements below. Circle the number in the yes column for those that apply to you or someone you know. For each yes answer, score the number in the box. Total your nutritional score.

| | Yes |
|---|---|
| I have an illness or condition that made me change the kind and/or amount of food I eat. | 2 |
| I eat fewer than 2 meals per day. | 3 |
| I eat few fruits or vegetables, or milk products. | 2 |
| I have 3 or more drinks of beer, liquor, or wine almost every day. | 2 |
| I have tooth or mouth problems that make it hard for me to eat. | 2 |
| I don't always have enough money to buy the food I need. | 4 |
| I eat alone most of the time. | 1 |
| I take 3 or more different prescribed or over-the-counter drugs a day. | 1 |
| Without wanting to, I have lost or gained 10 pounds in the last 6 months. | 2 |
| I am not always physically able to shop, cook, and/or feed myself. | 2 |
| TOTAL | |

**Total your nutrition score. It it's . . .**

**0–2** **Good!** Recheck your nutritional score in 6 months.

**3–5** **You are at moderate nutritional risk.** See what you can do to improve your eating habits and lifestyle. Your office on aging, senior nutrition program, senior citizens center, or health department can help. Recheck your nutritional score in 3 months.

**6 +** **You are at high nutritional risk.** Bring this checklist the next time you see your doctor, dietitian, or other qualified health care or social service professional. Talk with them about any problems you may have. Ask for help to improve your nutritional health.

***Remember: warning signs suggest risk, but do not represent diagnosis of any condition.***

*These materials developed and distributed by the Nutrition Screening Initiative, a project of: AMERICAN ACADEMY OF FAMILY PHYSICIANS, THE AMERICAN DIETETIC ASSOCIATION, and NATIONAL COUNCIL ON AGING, INC.*

ILLUSTRATION 18.2 ▸ Determine your nutritional health checklist.

SOURCE: The Nutrition Screening Initiative, originated as a project of the American Academy of Family Physicians, The American Dietetic Association and the National Council on the Aging, Inc., with funding by a grant from Ross Products Division, Abbott Laboratories, Inc.; screening questions have been adopted by state agencies and private health care companies. http://nutritionandaging.fiu.edu/downloads/NSI_checklist.pdf, accessed 6/14/15

Poverty is one risk factor for malnutrition; polypharmacy is another. Prescription drug use increases with age; three of four adults aged 60 and over used two or more prescription drugs in the previous month in 2007–2008 and 37 percent used five or more, compared to less than 10 percent children (under age 12), who used two or more prescription drugs in the past month and only 1 percent used five or more.[53] Between prescription drugs, vitamin and mineral supplements, and over-the-counter products, it is not uncommon for someone to take 10 pills a day. Such use of multiple medications invites adverse drug events from potentially inappropriate drugs and from drug–drug interactions. Healthcare expenditures related to the use of potentially inappropriate drugs are estimated to be over $7 billion annually.[54] The most commonly used medications of older adults include cholesterol-lowering agents, diuretics, and beta-blockers often used for heart disease and hypertension.

TABLE 18.6 ▸ By the numbers: Food budgets and poverty statistics

| FOOD BUDGET FOR 1 YEAR, BASED ON USDA'S LOW-COST FOOD PLAN (APRIL 2015 FIGURES) | |
|---|---|
| Female aged 71 and older: $2,907 ($46.60/week plus 20% for single household) | |
| Male, aged 71 and older: $3,251 ($52.10/week plus 20% for single household) | |
| Median Income for a person aged 65+ (2013): | $21,225 |
| **Defining Poverty:** | |
| 2015 Poverty Guidelines (Health and Human Services) for a one-person household (any age) | |
| For the 48 contiguous states and the District of Columbia | $11,770 |
| For Hawaii | $13, 550 |
| For Alaska | $14,720 |
| By race (U.S. Census Bureau, 2013), poverty statistics for adults aged 65 and older: | |
| Percent living below the poverty level | |
| All races | 9.5% |
| White | 7.4% |
| Asian | 13.6% |
| Hispanic | 19.8% |
| Black | 17.6% |
| Race disparities become more disparate at age 75. For reference, during this same time period, 19.9% of children under age 18 lived below the poverty level. | |
| By geography: the fewest poor elders live in the Northeast, the most in the South. | |
| Take away: A 71-year-old female, living alone in one of the 48 contiguous states, would spend 25% of her income on food to meet nutritional needs if all food is prepared at home. She has $55.92 per week to meet her nutritional needs; every bite counts when you are living in poverty and 25% of your income goes for food. The average American spends 13.1% of income on food. | |

SOURCE: http://www.cnpp.usda.gov/sites/default/files/CostofFoodApr2015.pdf, accessed 6/13/2015; http://www.pensionrights.org/publications/statistic/income-today%E2%80%99s-older-adults, accessed 6/13/15, http://aspe.hhs.gov/poverty/15poverty.cfm, accessed 6/13/15, https://www.census.gov/content/dam/Census/library/publications/2014/demo/p60-249.pdf, accessed 6/14/2015.

Taken individually, the risk factors identified in the DETERMINE acronym are not unique to older adults. But each is more likely to lead to nutritional problems in a frail, vulnerable population. For instance, functional disability can affect dietary intake at any age, but very old people are more likely to live alone and to have fewer resources to compensate for lost function. Consequently, diet quality may decline. Fewer 65-year-olds live alone than 75- and 85-year-olds, and more women than men live alone. Race and ethnicity affect living situations; Hispanic and Asian men and women aged 65 and over are least likely to live alone, whereas Non-Hispanic White and Black women are most likely to live alone.

A common perception is that older adults living alone eat poorly. Although living alone is a nutritional risk factor, it's not clear whether the issue is eating alone, living alone, or lack of social contact.[55] On average, meals eaten with other people last longer and supply more calories than do meals eaten alone.[56] The effect of living alone starts at a younger age for men and affects nutrition more extensively than for women.[57] Women aged 75 and older eat less protein and also less sodium than those living with others; men aged 65 and older eat less protein, beta-carotene, vitamin E, phosphorus, calcium, zinc, and fiber.

The purpose of a screening tool is primary prevention. Screening for nutritional risk should identify conditions that need further exploration, such as detecting significant weight loss. The NSI DETERMINE tool includes a cumulative score. The score was shown to weakly predict mortality in an aging population of mostly White, educated adults.[58] and did not consistently identify all those individuals who had poor health or low nutrient consumption.[49] Therefore, although the NSI scoring system is not necessarily useful in identifying existing malnutrition, its individual questions address common risk factors that could potentially lead to interventions to prevent malnutrition. The advantage of this screener is that it alerts older adults and caregivers of potential nutritional risk factors. This tool is a mandatory requirement for screening older adults who participate in the federally funded home-delivered meal program.

The MNA short form uses six screening items, including BMI, to identify individuals at risk of malnutrition (Illustration 18.3). It replaces a longer 18-item form available for screening and assessment, and does not require blood work or other biochemical tests, unlike hospital-based screening tools.[59] MNA has been used in clinical, home-care, and community settings. Note that the MNA uses a BMI of 23 or greater as presenting the least risk of malnutrition in older adults. The MNA is an easy to use, validated tool that identifies individuals at risk of malnutrition.

The Malnutrition Universal Screening Tool (MUST) is another brief tool that was developed for institutional and community use to identify adults who are malnourished

# Mini Nutritional Assessment MNA®

**Nestlé NutritionInstitute**

Last name: First name:

Sex: Age: Weight, kg: Height, cm: Date:

Complete the screen by filling in the boxes with the appropriate numbers. Total the numbers for the final screening score.

## Screening

**A Has food intake declined over the past 3 months due to loss of appetite, digestive problems, chewing or swallowing difficulties?**

0 = severe decrease in food intake
1 = moderate decrease in food intake
2 = no decrease in food intake ☐

**B Weight loss during the last 3 months**

0 = weight loss greater than 3 kg (6.6 lbs)
1 = does not know
2 = weight loss between 1 and 3 kg (2.2 and 6.6 lbs)
3 = no weight loss ☐

**C Mobility**

0 = bed or chair bound
1 = able to get out of bed / chair but does not go out
2 = goes out ☐

**D Has suffered psychological stress or acute disease in the past 3 months?**

0 = yes 2 = no ☐

**E Neuropsychological problems**

0 = severe dementia or depression
1 = mild dementia
2 = no psychological problems ☐

**F1 Body Mass Index (BMI) (weight in kg) / (height in $m^2$)**

0 = BMI less than 19
1 = BMI 19 to less than 21
2 = BMI 21 to less than 23
3 = BMI 23 or greater ☐

IF BMI IS NOT AVAILABLE, REPLACE QUESTION F1 WITH QUESTION F2.
DO NOT ANSWER QUESTION F2 IF QUESTION F1 IS ALREADY COMPLETED.

**F2 Calf circumference (CC) in cm**

0 = CC less than 31
3 = CC 31 or greater ☐

## Screening score (max. 14 points)

**12–14 points:** Normal nutritional status
**8–11 points:** At risk of malnutrition
**0–7 points:** Malnourished ☐☐

**References**

1. Vellas B, Villars H, Abellan G, *et al.* Overview of the MNA® - Its History and Challenges. *J Nutr Health Aging.* 2006;**10**:456-465.
2. Rubenstein LZ, Harker JO, Salva A, Guigoz Y, Vellas B. Screening for Undernutrition in Geriatric Practice: Developing the Short-Form Mini Nutritional Assessment (MNA-SF). *J. Geront.* 2001; **56A**: M366-377
3. Guigoz Y. The Mini-Nutritional Assessment (MNA®) Review of the Literature - What does it tell us? *J Nutr Health Aging.* 2006; **10**:466-487.
4. Kaiser MJ, Bauer JM, Ramsch C, et al. Validation of the Mini Nutritional Assessment Short-Form (MNA®-SF): A practical tool for identification of nutritional status. *J Nutr Health Aging.* 2009; **13**:782-788.



**For more information:** www.mna-elderly.com

ILLUSTRATION 18.3 ▸ MNA nutritional screening and assessment.

or at risk of malnutrition.[60] Assessment of nutritional status is a five-step process:

1. Use height and weight measurement to calculate BMI.
2. Score unplanned weight loss.
3. Assign an acute disease effect score (e.g., no nutritional intake due to illness for more than 5 days rates the maximum risk score of 2).
4. Sum scores to determine overall risk of malnutrition.
5. Use the score to plan management.

When height and weight cannot be measured, alternative calculations using the ulna, knee height, and mid–upper-arm circumference are suggested. The focus of scoring the MUST tool is to predict ability to combat disease; MUST uses a BMI of 20 or less to flag potential malnutrition. A BMI of 30 or more is scored as *obese*. MUST is the most commonly used screening tool in the United Kingdom and is validated. It is most applicable to frail older adults. Several other screening tools are available; however, the best tool to use is dependent on the purpose for the screening and the options available for follow-up.[61]

**TABLE 18.7** ▸ USDA Food Intake Patterns that meet nutritional needs for older adults at various activity levels (see Chapter 1 for food measure equivalents)

| | FEMALE, AGE 76, SEDENTARY | FEMALE, AGE 61 AND OLDER, ACTIVE | MALE, AGE 65, MODERATELY ACTIVE |
|---|---|---|---|
| Calorie level | 1600 | 2000 | 2400 |
| Fruits | 1.5 cups | 2 cups | 2 cups |
| Vegetables | 2 cups | 2.5 cups | 3 cups |
| Grains | 5 oz equivalent | 6 oz equivalent | 8 oz equivalent |
| Protein foods | 5 oz equivalent | 5.5 oz equivalent | 6.5 oz equivalent |
| Dairy | 3 cups | 3 cups | 3 cups |
| Oils | 22 gm | 27 gm | 31 gm |

SOURCE: www.fns.usda.gov/sites/default/files/Appendices.pdf, accessed 6/14/2015 (Reference[62] Appendix 7, USDA Food Patterns).

# Dietary Recommendations for Older Adults

**LO 18.6** Relate how enjoying a varied diet contributes to mental and physical well-being.

Sometimes, in all the discussions about nutritional effects on health and disease status of older adults, we forget that old age is not a disease. No matter what the health status of a person is, however, recommendations for specific nutrients change with age, and food consumption patterns need to adjust accordingly. USDA and HHS 2015 Dietary Guidelines for Americans (DGA)[62] do not single out older adults as a special group with unique dietary needs. Instead, age categories are combined with activity levels to generate energy needs, which are then used to determine a recommended food pattern (see Table 18.7). As age increases, the number of calories required decreases.

Part of the dietary guideline update was replacing the pyramid with a plate icon, which prompted educators to create new tools targeting subpopulations based on the MyPlate graphic. Two universities adapted MyPlate to the needs of older adults; Tufts University and the University of Florida. Both tools reflect the need for greater nutrient density and adequate fluid, for activities appropriate to functional ability, and for adapting communications to a diverse audience (Illustrations 18.4 and 18.5).

The Tufts MyPlate relies almost exclusively on icons. Food product illustrations emphasize whole grains and all forms of fruits and vegetables, not just fresh ones. Both tools offer vegetarian options in the protein group. Adequate fluid intake is emphasized by seven beverage containers and a soup plate in Illustration 18.4. In Illustration 18.5, a text paragraph suggests, "Drink water and other beverages that are low in added sugars." Older adults' potential need for supplemental nutrients is reflected in the graphics of the Tufts adaptation, while the Florida version adds a sentence about meeting vitamin D and $B_{12}$ requirements.

The Florida MyPlate is more detailed and uses text to describe food groups and corresponding serving sizes for adequate food intake. Food patterns constituting a range of calorie levels are needed to meet the needs of older adults

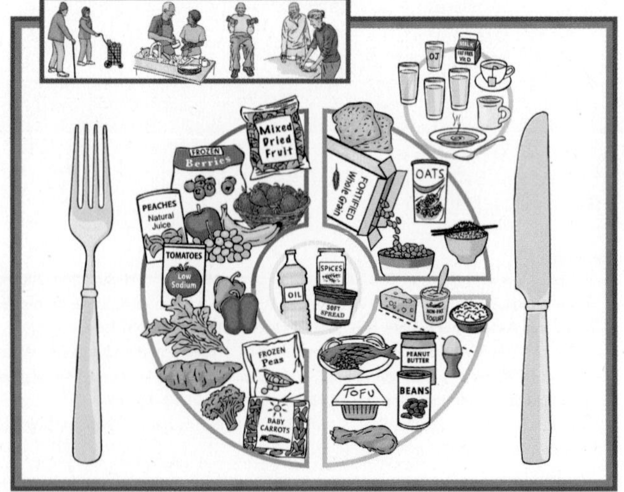


**ILLUSTRATION 18.4** ▸ Tufts University modified food guide for 70+ adults.

 For details about the MyPlate for Older Adults, http://nutrition.tufts.edu/research/myplate-older-adults, accessed 6/14/15.

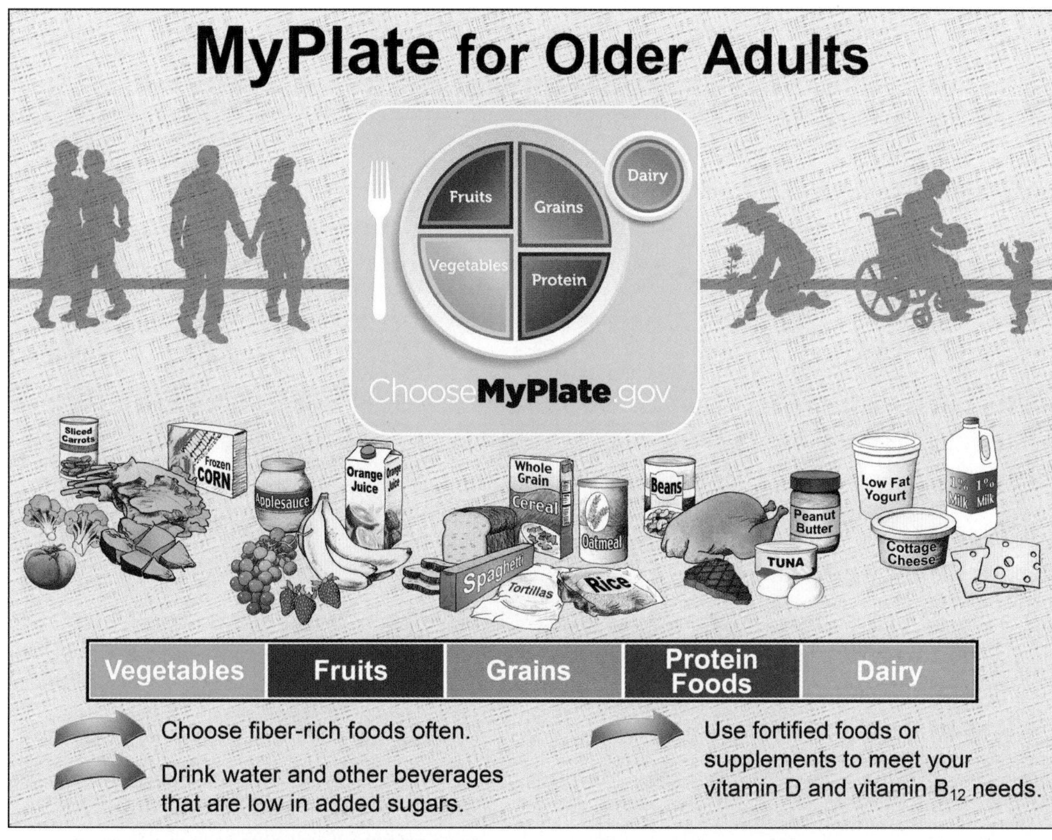


| VEGETABLES<br>Vary your veggies | FRUITS<br>Focus on fruits | GRAINS<br>Make half your grains whole | PROTEIN FOODS<br>Go lean with protein | DAIRY<br>Get your calcium-rich foods |
|---|---|---|---|---|
| Eat more dark-green veggies, like broccoli, salad greens, and cooked greens.<br><br>Eat more orange vegetables, such as carrots and sweet potatoes.<br><br>Eat more dried beans and peas, like pinto, black, or kidney beans, and lentils. | Eat a variety of fruits, like bananas, berries, grapes, and oranges.<br><br>Choose fresh, frozen, canned, or dried fruit.<br><br>Eat fruit rather than drinking juice for most of your fruit choices. | Eat at least 3 oz. of whole-grain cereals, breads, rice, crackers, or pasta every day.<br><br>1 oz. is about 1 slice of bread, 1 cup of cold breakfast cereal, or ½ cup of cooked cereal, rice, or pasta.<br><br>Eat cereals fortified with vitamin $B_{12}$. | Choose low-fat or lean meats and poultry.<br><br>Bake, broil, or grill.<br><br>Vary your protein sources. Include eggs, dried beans, tofu, fish, nuts, and seeds. | Choose low-fat or fat-free milk, yogurt, and other milk products.<br><br>If you don't or can't consume milk, choose lactose-free products or other calcium sources, such as fortified foods and beverages. |

**For an 1,800-calorie diet, you need the amounts below from each food group. To find the amounts that are right for you, go to ChooseMyPlate.gov.**

| Eat 2½ cups every day | Eat 1½ cups every day | Eat 6 oz. every day | Eat 5 oz. every day | Eat 3 cups every day |
|---|---|---|---|---|

## Eat Right

- **Choose foods rich in fiber to help keep you regular.**
- **Drink plenty of fluids to stay hydrated.**
- **Limit sweets to decrease empty calories.**
- **Get your oils from fish, nuts, and liquid oils such as canola, olive, corn or soybean oils.**
- **Choose and prepare foods with less salt or sodium.**
- **Talk to your doctor or pharmacist about supplements you are taking.**

## Be Active

- **Go for a walk.**
- **Play with your grandchildren and/or a pet.**
- **Work in your yard or garden.**
- **Take an exercise or dance class at a community center or gym.**
- **Share a fun activity with a friend or family member.**
- **Remember: all activity adds up! You don't have to do it all at once.**

Enjoy Life: **Spend time with caring people doing things you enjoy.**

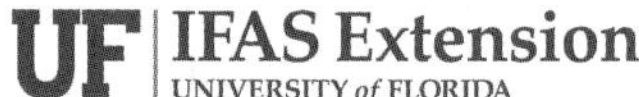


**MyPlate for Older Adults** was adapted from USDA's MyPlate by nutrition faculty in the Department of Family, Youth and Community Sciences, IFAS, University of Florida, Gainesville, Florida 32611. 2011

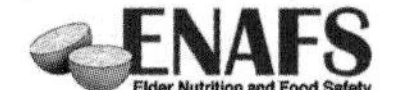


Elder Nutrition and Food Safety Program, University of Florida

ILLUSTRATION 18.5 ▸ UF/IFAS Extension: MyPlate for Older Adults.

Aging Health & Well-being, University of Florida http://fycs.ifas.ufl.edu/extension/hnfs/myplate/MyPlate/MyPlate_for_Older_Adults_Front.pdf and http://fycs.ifas.ufl.edu/extension/hnfs/myplate/MyPlate/MyPlate_for_Older_Adults_Back.pdf, accessed 6/14/15

(Table 18.7). Calorie levels can be modified by choosing more or less nutrient-dense foods from each group. For instance, citrus and berries are among the most nutrient-dense fruits. A baked potato has more vitamins and minerals per calorie than french fries do. Among grain-based products, whole-grain breads and cereals provide fiber as well as the usual nutrients found in grain. Consistently choosing nutrient-dense foods minimizes caloric intake. With the increase in food fortification, it is sometimes hard to know whether to count an item as food or supplement. For instance, adequate folic acid intake was problematic before 1998, when folic acid fortification of grain products became mandatory. Now, older adults consume more than enough folic acid and could easily exceed the 1000 mcg Tolerable Upper Intake Level (UL) if they take supplements.[63]

**The "Discretionary Calories"** Food group patterns in the DGAs suggest that SoFAS (solid fats and added sugars) can make up 8–19 percent of total calories of a health-promoting meal plan, depending on total energy levels (see Table 18.7). Often, these SoFAS are snacks. While many older adults grew up during an era when people did not snack, let alone graze all day, NHANES data showed that snacks provide nearly one-fourth of their daily energy intake.[64] But snacks contribute more than fat and sugar. In the diets of older adults, snacks make up 14 percent of protein and 12 percent of the alcohol consumed.

In contrast to nutrient recommendations, dietary guidance tends to be addressed to the general public. For older adults, that guidance is focused on disease risk reduction and quality of life enhancements. What are some of the specific nutrients that will enhance the nutritional status of older adults? Read on.

# Nutrient Recommendations

**LO 18.7** Compare nutrient recommendations of old and young adults, citing five or more nutrients of concern for older populations.

Nutrient recommendations change as scientists learn more about the effect of foods on human lives. Before 1997, nutrient recommendations for older adults were for the combined age group of 51 and over; however, nutrient levels specific for population groups ages 51–70 and 71+ were first established in 1997 as the DRIs.[63] The complete tables, including UL, are found on the inside covers of this text. This section addresses current intakes and energy recommendations (see Tables 18.8 to 18.10), followed by vitamin and mineral recommendations (Table 18.11).

## Estimating Energy Needs

The main goal for energy calculations is to maintain a healthy body weight. The DRI energy calculations are based on age and physical activity (see Table 18.8). NHANES data (Table 18.9) shows caloric intake as adults age.[65] Women aged 70 and older report the lowest intake and may be especially vulnerable to malnutrition, even though the prevalence of obesity is high (BMI = 30 or more).[66] What matters is the nutrient density of the calories consumed.

From early to late adulthood, a decrease of physical activity and basal metabolic rate leads to an estimated decrease of 7–10 calories in energy needs per year. Over a decade, daily energy needs would decline by 70–100 calories. Energy expenditure is primarily determined from basal metabolic rate (BMR), which slows with age, diet-induced thermogenesis, and physical-activity energy needs. However, genetics, hormones, and body composition also influence metabolic rates, resulting in broad ranges of energy needs for older populations. Doubly labeled water measurement, which uses stable isotopes to measure energy expenditure and is a form of indirect calorimetry, is used

**TABLE 18.8** Dietary reference intake values for energy by active individuals with sample calculations

| LIFE STAGE GROUP[A] | EER (KCAL/D)[B] (REPRESENTING ACTIVE PAL[C]) | |
|---|---|---|
| ALL ADULTS | MALE | FEMALE |
| >18 y[E] | 3067[D] | 2403[D] |

SOURCE: Institute of Medicine. *Dietary Reference Intakes for Energy, Carbohydrate, Fiber, Fat, Fatty Acids, Cholesterol, Protein, and Amino Acids*, 2002.
[A] For healthy, moderately active Americans and Canadians.
[B] EER = estimated energy requirement.
[C] PAL = Physical Activity Level Factor.
[D] TEE = Total Energy Expenditure, which is the intake that meets the average energy expenditure of individuals at reference height, weight, and age.
[E] Subtract 10 kcals/d for males and 7 kcals/d for females *for each* year above 19 years old (y).

| MALE EXAMPLE | FEMALE EXAMPLE |
|---|---|
| 70 years old | 85 years old |
| 3067 kcals | 2403 kcals |
| Subtract 10 kcals/d for each year >19 | Subtract 7 kcals/d for each year >19 |
| 70 y − 19 y = 51 y | 85 y − 19 y = 66 y |
| 3067 − 510 = 2557 kcal | 2403 − 462 = 1941 kcal |

**TABLE 18.9** Comparing caloric intake of younger and older adults, by gender, with energy recommendations for sedentary adults, from the Dietary Guidelines for Americans, 2015

| | ACTUAL DAILY CALORIE INTAKE | | RECOMMENDED CALORIE INTAKE | |
|---|---|---|---|---|
| AGE | MALES | FEMALES | MALES | FEMALES |
| 20–29 | 2764 | 2019 | 2400 | 2000 |
| 60–69 | 2302 | 1663 | 2000 | 1600 |
| age 70+ | 2023 | 1555 | 2000 | 1600 |

SOURCE: *What We Eat in America*, NHANES, 2011–2012, Table 1.[65]

TABLE 18.10 Daily energy nutrient and cholesterol intakes of adults 70+ during NHANES 2011–2012, compared to nutrient intake recommendations

| NUTRIENT | ACTUAL INTAKE[a, b] MALES | FEMALES | RECOMMENDED INTAKE[c] MALES/FEMALES |
|---|---|---|---|
| Protein, g | 80 | 59 | 0.8 grams/kg/day (RDA)<br>56/46 grams/day (RDA)<br>10–35% of calories (AMDR) |
| Carbohydrate, g | 248 | 202 | 45–65% of calories (AMDR) |
| Total sugars, g | 108 | 93 | Part of SoFAS |
| Dietary fiber, g | 18 | 15 | 28/22 gm/day (AI)<br>14 gm fiber/1000 calories(IOM) |
| Total fat, g | 76 | 57 | 20–35% of calories (AMDR) |
| Saturated fat, g | 24 | 18 | <10% of calories |
| Monounsaturated fat, g | 28 | 20 | Up to 20% calories |
| Polyunsaturated fat, g | 18 | 15 | Up to 10% calories |
| Cholesterol, mg | 281 | 196 | <300 mg |
| Alcohol, g | 17 | 8 | Moderation (12–15 g = 1 drink) |

[a]Actual intake amounts, except for alcohol, from *What We Eat in America,* NHANES, 2011–2012, Table 1, individuals aged 70+. Available at http://www.ars.usda.gov/Services/docs.htm?docid=18349, accessed 6/09/15.

[b]Alcohol amounts for adults 20 and over [65] [Table 4].

[c]Recommended intake data are based on Dietary Reference Intake (DRI), Institute of Medicine of the National Academies. *Dietary Reference Intakes: Energy, carbohydrate, fiber, fat, fatty acids, cholesterol, protein, and amino acids.* Washington, D.C.: National Academies Press, 2002. Acceptable Macronutrient Distribution Range (AMDR), Institute of Medicine.

TABLE 18.11 Selected micronutrient intakes of male and female adults aged 70 and older compared with recommendations, 2011–2012 NHANES

| NUTRIENT, UNIT OF MEASURE | DAILY INTAKE MALES | FEMALES | DIETARY REFERENCE INTAKES MALES/FEMALES |
|---|---|---|---|
| Vitamin A, mcg RAE | 710 | 626 | 900/700 = RDA |
| Vitamin D, mcg | 5.60 | 4.70 | 20 = RDA |
| Vitamin E, mg alpha tocopherol | 9.20 | 6.60 | 15 = RDA |
| Vitamin K, mcg | 114 | 111 | 120/90 = AI |
| Thiamin, mg | 1.67 | 1.26 | 1.2/1.1 = RDA |
| Riboflavin, mg | 2.29 | 1.74 | 1.3/1.1 = RDA |
| Niacin, mg | 26.1 | 18.0 | 16/14 = RDA |
| Vitamin $B_6$, mg | 2.30 | 1.63 | 1.7/1.5 = RDA |
| Folate, mcg DFE | 582 | 444 | 400 mcg = RDA |
| Choline, mg | 344 | 250 | 550/425 = AI |
| Vitamin $B_{12}$, mcg | 6.03 | 4.14 | 2.4 = RDA |
| Added Vitamin $B_{12}$, mcg | 1.45 | 0.87 | |
| Vitamin C, mg | 82.2 | 80.8 | 90/75 = RDA |
| Sodium, mg | 3328 | 2526 | 1200 = AI |
| Potassium, mg | 2810 | 2345 | 4700 = AI |
| Calcium, mg | 881 | 809 | 1200 = RDA |
| Phosphorus, mg | 1350 | 1060 | 700 = RDA |
| Magnesium, mg | 301 | 249 | 420/320 = RDA |
| Iron, mg | 17.3 | 12.6 | 8 = RDA |
| Zinc, mg | 11.9 | 8.60 | 11/8 = RDA |
| Copper, mg | 1.40 | 1.10 | 0.9 = RDA |
| Selenium, mcg | 111 | 80.9 | 55 = RDA |

SOURCES: Actual consumption from "What we eat in America,"[65] Available at http://www.ars.usda.gov/Services/docs.htm?docid=18349, accessed 6/09/2015. Recommended intake data are Dietary Reference Intake (DRI) Institute of Medicine of the National Academies, Otten, J. J., Hellwig, J. P., and Meyers, L. D., eds. Institute of Medicine of the National Academies. DRI Dietary Reference Intakes: The Essential Guide to Nutrient Requirements. Washington, D.C.: The National Academies Press, 2006[63] and IOM.edu, for 2010 updates on calcium and Vitamin D.

to measure BMR. These measurements show that BMR ranged from 1004 kcal/day to 2060 kcal/day in older individuals with normal BMI.[63] Such a wide range of energy use reflects the heterogeneity of older adult populations and the need for individualized nutrition planning.

Traditionally, the Harris-Benedict equation has been used to estimate individual calorie needs. However, validation was done with mostly young adults. The Mifflin–St. Jeor formula most closely predicts energy requirements of healthy adults in general, and validation did include individuals up to age 80, but it was not specifically developed for older adults.

Arcerio and colleagues developed formulas for use with older adults.[67,68] The equation used with older adult females includes a factor for hormonal status (e.g., menopause). For males, they completed the Minnesota Leisure Time Activity survey as well as a set of three chest skinfold measurements.[69] Using these formulas requires training; they are not in common use.

Energy calculations and weight status are topics that illustrate the dangers of generalizing from populations to individuals, or the reverse. It is difficult to meet vitamin and mineral needs at caloric levels below 1600, and older adults are at greater risk for consuming less than 1600 calories. Older adults who are active enough to meet the physical activity recommendations are likely to eat more than 1600 calories.

## Nutrient Recommendations for Older Adults: Energy Sources

Some nutrients are potentially problematic for older adults to consume in adequate amounts (Tables 18.10 and 18.11). Several of the listed nutrients are consumed in amounts different from the recommended level. The following nutrients are most often potentially problematic for older adult populations.

**Carbohydrate and Fiber** Carbohydrate intake between 45 and 65 percent of calories (the acceptable macronutrient distribution range, AMDR) is generally not a problem.[65] However, older adults could improve the nutrient density of their carbohydrate intake by eating more fiber-rich food. Following the MyPlate recommendations ensures that the carbohydrate quantity and quality is adequate and that fiber guidelines are met. For example, individuals who need 2000 calories/day would need to eat 250 grams of carbohydrate per day to meet 50 percent of calories from carbohydrate sources (Table 18.12). Selecting whole grains and vegetables brings dietary fiber levels closer to recommended levels (14 grams/1000 calories) (Table 18.13). These foods would also help to raise nutrients that are underconsumed such as magnesium and vitamin E. Dietary fiber reduces the risk of coronary heart disease,[63] but older adults are more often concerned with the role of fiber for gastrointestinal health; this is discussed in Chapter 19. A slow increase of dietary fiber allows intestinal microflora to adapt to added substrate.

**TABLE 18.12** Using the MyPlate groups to estimate adequate carbohydrate (46% of kcal) and fiber portions (14 gm/1000 kcal) for a 2000-calorie diet

| NUMBER OF SERVINGS/GRAMS OF CARBOHYDRATE PER SERVING | CARBOHYDRATE, GRAMS | APPROXIMATE TOTAL FIBER CONTENT, GRAMS |
|---|---|---|
| BASIC FOOD GROUPS | | |
| 6 ounces of grain at 15 g each | 90 | 12 |
| 2 cups of fruit at 20 g each | 40 | 6 |
| 3 cups of dairy at 12 g each | 36 | 0 |
| 2.5 cups vegetable at 8 g each | 20 | 10 |
| **Total grams from basic groups** | 186 | 28 |
| OTHER CARBOHYDRATE-CONTAINING FOODS | | |
| 1 Tbsp sugar for coffee or tea | 12 | 0 |
| 3 Fig Newton cookies | 33 | 1 |
| **Total grams, including "other" group** | 231 | 29 |

NOTE: Mixed dishes such as soups, sandwiches, and salads count as partial servings from their contributing food groups.



**TABLE 18.13** An example of fiber-containing foods that might comprise one day's intake

| FOOD ITEM | GRAMS OF FIBER |
|---|---|
| Oatmeal (½ cup) with wheat germ (¼ cup) | 8 |
| Banana | 2 |
| Peanut butter (2 Tbsp)/whole-wheat bread (2 slices) | 6 |
| Orange | 3 |
| Baked potato with skin | 4 |
| Green beans (½ cup) | 3 |
| Bran muffin (1 med) | 2 |
| Pear | 4 |
| **Total dietary fiber** | 32 |

NOTE: Meat, poultry, fish, eggs, milk, sugar, and oils do not contain dietary fiber.



**Protein** On average, older adults in North America meet or exceed the Recommended Dietary Allowance (RDA) for protein.[65] Older adults who are living alone, living in poverty, who are obese, or who have functional limitations are vulnerable to inadequate protein intake; this contributes to muscle wasting (sarcopenia), weak bones, a weakened immune status, and delayed wound healing. Evidence about the beneficial role of protein and alkaline diets on muscle mass[70] suggests that vulnerable seniors can benefit from individualized dietary advice.

It is not clear what constitutes an optimal amount of protein for individual older adults, although current protein guidelines are consistent for adults across all age groups. Results of studies are conflicting. A meta-analysis of nitrogen balance studies and a more recent study[71,72] showed that age alone does not alter protein requirements. However, other studies indicated that protein intake between 1.0 and 1.5 g per kg body weight per day might provide health benefits to older adults beyond the 0.8 g protein per kg current RDA.[73]

Nitrogen-balance studies used to determine current recommendations of 0.8 gram per kilogram (or 0.36 gram per pound) were done primarily with young adults, who have proportionately more muscle mass than older adults, male or female, and are more efficient at maintaining nitrogen balance. Nitrogen balance is also easier to achieve when an individual is doing resistance training, when protein is ingested with adequate calories, and when the protein eaten is of high quality (such as meat, milk, and eggs; see Table 18.14). However, for older adults who are following modified diets, who are cutting back on meat because they can't afford it or lack energy to prepare it, or who may eat too few calories, protein quality can make the difference between a good and a poor diet.

Despite adequate protein-intake levels of older adults on average, individual elders may be at risk for protein malnutrition. The following questions help to determine protein adequacy for older individuals:

- Based on total energy requirements, how much protein will meet the individual need?
- Are enough calories eaten so that protein does not have to be used for energy?
- If marginal amounts of protein are eaten, is the protein of high quality?

TABLE 18.14 Protein sources and protein quality measures: examples of protein scores used by the Institute of Nutrition of Central America and Panama (INCAP)

| PROTEIN SOURCE | CHEMICAL QUALITY SCORE* | TRUE DIGESTIBILITY IN HUMANS |
|---|---|---|
| Meat, eggs, milk | 100 | 95 |
| Beans | 80 | 78 |
| Soy protein isolate | 97 | 94 |
| Rice | 73 | 88 |
| Oats, oatmeal | 63 | 86 |
| Lentils | 60 | Not available |
| Corn | 50 | 85 |
| Wheat | 44 | Refined, 96; whole wheat, 86 |

SOURCE: Data from Torun, B., Menchu, M. T., and Elias, L. G. *Recomendaciones dieteticas diarias del INCAP*. Guatemala: INCAP, 1994; and Shils, M. E., Olson, J. A., M. Shike, M., et al. *Modern Nutrition in Health and Disease*. Philadelphia: Lippincott, Williams & Wilkin, 1999.

*Amino acid score relative to amino acid score of egg, the reference protein.

- Are there additional needs—wound healing, tissue repair, surgery, fracture, infection?
- Is the individual exercising? It is harder to achieve nitrogen balance while sedentary.

Consuming a low-calorie diet, as many older adults do, leads to a proportionately greater need for protein. Instead of consuming 10 percent of total calories in protein, needs might be better met near the 35 percent end of the AMDR as set by the Institute of Medicine. Furthermore, the protein is more effective when distributed evenly throughout the day, which can be difficult for someone who has gotten used to a cup of tea and a piece of toast in the morning.

Decreasing muscle mass does not lead to lower protein requirements. In fact, someone who is losing muscle due to inactivity requires higher protein intake. Knowledge of the protein needs of older adults continues to evolve. The current approach, although still untested, is to optimize protein intake at specific meals and eating opportunities by consuming protein at intake levels slightly above the RDA (or at the higher end of the AMDR), and distributed evenly throughout the day. This may stimulate muscle synthesis and minimize the risk of sarcopenia in aging adults.[74,75]

**Fats and Cholesterol** The role of dietary fat does not seem to change with age; high saturated fat and *trans* fatty acid intake continue to be a risk factor for chronic disease. Minimizing the amount of saturated fat in the diet and keeping total fat between 20 and 35 percent of calories is a reasonable goal for older adults to maintain a beneficial blood cholesterol ratio. Cholesterol intake for older adults is within current recommended levels (see Table 18.10). However, there is lack of evidence linking dietary intake of cholesterol to LDL cholesterol. The 2013 AHA/ACC Guideline on Lifestyle Management to Reduce Cardiovascular Risk did not issue a recommendation to limit cholesterol intake.[76] Additionally, the 2015 Dietary Guidelines no longer include a recommendation to limit cholesterol intake because the current available evidence does not show a relationship between its consumption and serum cholesterol. Eggs, which have a high cholesterol content, are a nutrient-dense, convenient, and safe food for most people.

**Recommendations for Fluid** The water portion of total body weight decreases with age, indicating a shrinking water reservoir and resulting in a smaller safety margin for hydration maintenance. The DRIs for water are constant after age 19 (see inside cover pages). Drinking six or more glasses of fluid per day prevents dehydration (and subsequent confusion, weakness, and altered drug metabolism) in individuals whose thirst mechanism has grown less sensitive. Dehydration is discussed further in Chapter 19.

To individualize fluid recommendations, provide 1 milliliter (mL) of fluid per calorie eaten, with a minimum of 1500 mL. For a 2000-calorie diet, that would be 2000 mL or 2 liters of fluid, roughly 8 cups. Foods such as stews, puddings, fruits, and vegetables contribute significant amounts of fluid to the diet. The Tufts food guide (see Illustration 18.4) shows eight fluid sources, including a bowl of soup. This amount is adequate for a 2000-calorie diet. Individuals who need additional calories can use milk, juice, shakes, and low-salt soups as nutrient-dense fluids.

## Age-Associated Changes: Nutrients of Concern

The nutritional health of older adults depends on dietary habits that accommodate age-associated absorption and metabolism changes. The nutrients discussed in the following sections are of special concern for older adults because of age-associated metabolic changes or low dietary intake.

**Vitamin A** Diet surveys before the year 2000 reported that older adults were more likely to overdose on vitamin A than to be deficient in the nutrient, but the latest NHANES survey[65] showed dietary intake below the RDAs of 900 mcg and 700 mcg REA (retinol activity equivalents) for males and females, respectively (see Table 18.11). Plasma levels and liver stores of vitamin A increase with age. This may be due to increased absorption but is more likely due to decreased clearance of vitamin A metabolites (retinyl esters) from the blood. Kidney disease further elevates serum vitamin A levels because retinol-binding protein, another vitamin A metabolite, can no longer be cleared from blood. This makes older adults more vulnerable to vitamin A toxicity and possible liver damage. The UL for vitamin A is 3000 mcg (3 mg) for adults aged 19 and older, which could be reached if fish liver oils are taken in addition to daily vitamin supplements.

Vitamin A's plant precursor, beta-carotene, will not damage the liver, although supplements used as antioxidants to prevent cardiovascular disease have been linked to higher all-cause mortality.[77] Excess dietary beta-carotene, because it is water-soluble, may give old skin a yellow-orange tint, but it will not lead to hair loss, dry skin, nausea, irritability, blurred vision, or weakness as excess vitamin A would.

**Vitamin D, Calciferol** Age-associated metabolic changes affect vitamin D status, independent of dietary intake, primarily due to a four-fold decrease in the ability of aged skin to synthesize vitamin D.[78,79] In addition, older adults use more medications. Some of them, such as barbiturates, cholestyramine (bile acid sequestrant), phenytoin (Dilantin), and laxatives, interfere with vitamin D metabolism. Declining photochemical production ability may also be compounded by limited sunlight exposure due to wearing more clothes to stay comfortable, institutionalization or being homebound, and sunscreen use. Furthermore, in northern regions (above 42° north, the latitude of Boston and Chicago) between November and February, ultraviolet (UV) light is not powerful enough to synthesize vitamin D in exposed skin.[80] The sun's rays are even weaker in Edmonton, Canada (at 52° N latitude), so that previtamin $D_3$ is not synthesized between mid-October and mid-April. Dietary recommendations for vitamin D are higher for older adults than for any other population group (see inside cover), so individuals who live in these northern latitudes are at especially high risk for vitamin D deficiency. How far south does one have to go for the winter sun to convert vitamin D precursors? Tests in Los Angeles, at 34° N, showed vitamin D production in skin even in January. The sun's rays in Puerto Rico (latitude of 18° N) were even more effective.[80] Although humans store vitamin D, reaching and maintaining adequate serum 25 hydroxy vitamin D levels of 30 ng/mL (see Chapter 1) is likely to require supplements for people living at northern latitudes. Holick and Chen's review found that 800–1000 IU of vitamin D are needed to maintain adequate vitamin D serum levels, and this was especially so for nursing home residents.[79]

NHANES surveys of vitamin D intake[65] report significant dietary shortfalls (see Table 18.11), which are reflected in lower serum vitamin D levels of older adults, especially older women. Levels of 30 ng/mL (75 nmol/L) or higher are needed for improving muscle strength, for dental health (including reduced periodontal disease), and to reduce risk of colorectal cancer.[81] A vitamin D level of 80 nmol/L optimizes intestinal calcium absorption.[79] Vitamin D's main role is in the maintenance of blood calcium levels and in keeping bones strong and healthy. This is addressed in the section on osteoporosis in Chapter 19.

The UL for vitamin D was increased from 50 mcg to 100 mcg (4000 IU) in 2010. Symptoms of toxicity are hypercalcemia (high blood calcium levels), anorexia, nausea, vomiting, general disorientation, muscular weakness, joint pains, bone demineralization, and calcification (calcium deposits) of soft tissues. Toxicity is rare from food sources. Cod liver contains medicinal levels of vitamin D (about 21 mcg, or 840 IU, per teaspoon; check the label for amount) and may also contain Vitamin A.

**Vitamin E** Also known as tocopherol, vitamin E is a potent antioxidant. Dietary intake is usually well below the recommended 15 mg or 15 IU alpha-tocopherol (Table 18.11) in the general population. Vitamin E plays a special role in the health of older adults due to its interaction with vitamin K and its antioxidant functions in maintaining cell membranes. Vitamin E is associated with enhanced immune function and cognitive status, although not with reduced cardiovascular disease risk.[77,82,83] The UL is 1000 mg of alpha-tocopherol equivalent, which is obtained from supplements, fortified foods, or a combination of the two. Some research indicates that doses below the 1000 IU (mg) level are safe; a meta-analysis reported safe levels at up to 400 IU.[84] At higher doses, vitamin E may increase all-cause mortality and is linked to longer blood-clotting times and tendency to hemorrhage. Aspirin, anti-coagulants, and fish-oil supplements also increase blood-clotting times and are incompatible with high vitamin E intake.

**Vitamin K** Interest in vitamin K is increasing because, in addition to its blood coagulation role, vitamin K–dependent proteins have been found in bone, vascular, and central nervous system tissues.[85] Supplementation has been linked to reduced bone fractures.[86] On average, vitamin K intake is below the AI (see Table 18.11), although it is difficult to diagnose deficiency without blood tests, as bacteria in the large intestine synthesize vitamin K. However, for older populations, the concern is to maintain consistent intake levels that do not interfere with warfarin (a vitamin K antagonist used as a blood thinner) therapy.[87] Additional vitamin K information is provided in Chapter 19, including a table showing vitamin K content of foods.

**Vitamin $B_{12}$** Vitamin $B_{12}$ blood levels decrease with age even in healthy adults. Population intakes of total vitamin $B_{12}$ are higher than the RDA of 2.4 mcg (see Table 18.11), although intake of the synthetic form is below the RDA. Why does this matter? Many older adults are unable to use $B_{12}$ efficiently. Up to 30 percent of older adults suffer from atrophic gastritis and decreased absorption of $B_{12}$. In atrophic gastritis, a bacterial overgrowth of the stomach leads to inflammation and decreased secretion of hydrochloric acid and pepsin and subsequent inability to split vitamin $B_{12}$ from its food protein carrier (see Chapter 19). It takes years to develop a $B_{12}$ deficiency; but once developed, the neurological symptoms are irreversible. Symptoms include deterioration of mental function, change in personality, and loss of physical coordination.

"Food first" is usually sound advice regarding nutritional needs, but $B_{12}$ is one of the two vitamins better absorbed in synthetic or purified form. Folic acid is the other one. Synthetic, not protein-bound, vitamin $B_{12}$ is found in fortified foods such as cereals and soy products. NHANES now tracks "added vitamin $B_{12}$" (Table 18.11). Protein-bound $B_{12}$ is found in all animal products, although poultry is a surprisingly poor source (0.25 mcg of $B_{12}$ in 3 ounces of chicken compared to 2.0 mcg in 3 ounces of ground beef).

**Folate, Folic Acid** Fortification of grain products with folic acid has led to intakes well above the RDA (see Table 18.11). Absorption of folate, like vitamin $B_{12}$, may be impaired by atrophic gastritis. Moreover, alcoholism is associated with folate deficiency and subsequent pernicious anemia. Medications commonly used by older adults—such as antacids, diuretics, phenytoin (Dilantin), sulfonamides, and anti-inflammatory drugs—affect folate metabolism. For persons with low serum folate levels, dietary increases of folic acid (100–400 mcg) can lower serum homocysteine levels and subsequent risk of heart disease.[88] However, in the presence of vitamin $B_{12}$ deficiency, high folic acid intake may mask the blood symptoms of vitamin $B_{12}$ deficiency, which is more common in older adults than folic-acid deficiency, and can lead to neurological damage.

**Iron** Women's iron needs decrease after menopause, and older men and women eat more iron than the RDA of 8 mg (see Table 18.11). Like vitamin A, iron is stored more readily in the old than in the young. Excess iron contributes to oxidative stress, increasing the need for antioxidants to deal with oxidant overload. Fortunately, vitamin C intake, which increases iron absorption, also serves as an antioxidant.

Not every older person has adequate iron stores. Reasons for inadequate iron status include blood loss from disease or medication (e.g., aspirin), poor absorption due to antacid interference or decreased stomach acid secretion, and low caloric intake.

**Calcium** Research on calcium has led to several changes in recommendations over a relatively short time. A 1994 consensus conference sponsored by the National Institutes of Health[89] recommended calcium intake for women depending on estrogen status; namely, 1500 mg for women aged 50–64 not taking supplementary estrogen and 1000 mg calcium per day for postmenopausal women taking estrogen. It was recommended that all men and women consume 1500 mg calcium per day after age 65. This recommendation of 1500 mg was lowered in 1997, when the National Academy of Sciences set the AI for adults aged 51 and older at 1200 mg daily. Recommended levels are met by a small portion of the population; on average, calcium intake of older men and women ranges from 800 to 900 mg per day.

Most of calcium's role is bone and tooth building and maintenance, but a fraction of the remaining calcium plays a role in nerve transmission, transport across cell membranes, and regulating heart and skeletal muscle. Absorption declines with age. Low calcium levels have been linked to risk of colon cancer, overweight, and hypertension. An example of the protective effects of calcium intake in the development of hypertension comes from work by Appel.[90] For example, Appel and the DASH Collaborative Research Group found that the subgroup of hypertensive individuals with higher calcium intake also had the greatest decrease in blood pressure. On average, participants who adhered to the Dietary Approaches to Stop Hypertension (DASH) diet reduced their blood pressure. The diet includes two or more servings of low-fat dairy products (1265 mg calcium from food in the experimental group); 10 servings of fruits and vegetables; and limited fat, saturated fat, and cholesterol.

When it changed the RDAs for calcium in older adults, the National Academy of Sciences reduced the UL for calcium to 2000 mg per day, which is less than twice the RDA. An old guideline about nutrition was that up to 10 times the RDA was a safe intake amount. Excess calcium has a much lower bar for safety. An explosion of calcium-fortified foods and supplements presents the possibility of adverse effects of excess calcium. These adverse effects include kidney damage and calcium deposits in soft tissues and outside the bone matrix, such as bone spurs on the spine. High calcium intake may interfere with zinc, iron, and magnesium absorption, and it may result in elevated urinary excretion of calcium, leading to new kidney stones in individuals with a history of kidney stones. Low blood calcium levels lead to muscle cramps and twitches (tetany).

**Magnesium** Adequate magnesium intake (see Table 18.11) is needed for bone and tooth formation, nerve activity, glucose utilization, and synthesis of fat and proteins. An indication of the wide-ranging functions of magnesium is that it plays a part in over 300 enzyme systems. Age does not seem to affect magnesium metabolism, and the RDA is constant at 420 mg for males and 320 mg for females after age 31. The UL is 350 mg from nonfood (supplementary) sources. Older adult intake is below the RDA (see Table 18.11). Magnesium deficiency can result not only from low intake but also from malabsorption due to gastrointestinal disorders, chronic alcoholism, and diabetes. Signs of deficiency include personality changes (irritability, aggressiveness), vertigo, muscle spasms, weakness, and seizures.

Drugs used by older adults, such as magnesium hydroxide or citrate laxatives, may lead to magnesium overdose. Signs of magnesium toxicity are diarrhea, dehydration, and impaired nerve activity. Food sources including milk, yeast breads, coffee, ready-to-eat cereals, beef, and potatoes do not result in toxicity.

**Potassium** Meeting the ambitious sodium guidelines will be especially difficult for older adults. At the 1200 mg sodium level, foods need be prepared without added salt or sodium compounds. Even foods that do not taste salty can be too high in sodium. For example, a bowl of regular cornflakes, 2 slices of whole wheat bread, 2 ounces of deli roast beef and 3 cups of milk add up to 1500 mg sodium, but only 665 calories. One thing that would help to balance extra sodium intake is an adequate potassium intake (4700 mg/day). Current intakes are 50–60 percent of that (see Table 18.11). Beverages alone could contribute nearly half of the day's potassium. The following frequently consumed beverages and their potassium content per 8 fluid ounces shows that fluids can contribute nearly half of the day's potassium: coffee (115 mg), tea (90 mg), milk (365 mg), orange juice (445 mg), grape juice (200 mg), and lemonade (63 mg). Fruits and vegetables are excellent sources, especially potatoes, sweet potatoes, greens, beans, bananas, and tomatoes.

Potassium and sodium are the two electrolytes responsible for water balance in humans. The DASH diet, with its abundant fruits and vegetables, helped to reduce blood pressure even when sodium intake was above 1200 mg.

## Nutrient Supplements: When, Why, Who, What, and How Much?

Most people don't tell their health-care provider about the supplements they take, unless asked. Despite inconsistent evidence of benefit combined with growing evidence of risk,[91,92] the dietary supplement industry is booming with sales that reached $32.5 billion in 2012, $13.1 billion of which is from all vitamin-mineral-containing supplements.[93]

**When to Consider Supplements** When do older adults benefit from taking nutrient supplements? It depends on the circumstances and on the nutrient.[94] Recovery from illness and trauma is definitely aided by supplemental formulas, including vitamins, minerals, and energy nutrients such as protein and fatty acids. This section deals with multivitamin and mineral supplements. These can decrease infection,[95,96] but the evidence is weak and conflicting.[97] Supplements have not been shown to have a preventive benefit when taken by well-nourished aged populations. Here's what an NIH panel concluded after reviewing the role of vitamins and minerals in the prevention of chronic disease in 2006, long before the market spiked:[98]

> Multivitamin/mineral supplement use may prevent cancer in individuals with poor or suboptimal nutritional status. The heterogeneity in the study populations limits generalization to United States population. Multivitamin/mineral supplements conferred no benefit in preventing cardiovascular disease or cataract, and may prevent advanced age-related macular degeneration only in high-risk individuals. The overall quality and quantity of the literature on the safety of multivitamin/mineral supplements is limited.

This statement has not slowed growth of the multibillion-dollar supplement industry, even though this NIH panel conclusion still holds, and evidence about negative outcomes is accumulating. Health-conscious adults take supplements as insurance, even as the outdated consensus of "it can't hurt" is being replaced by knowledge of potential problems of excess. Nutrient research is complicated, as in the case of vitamins A, E, and beta-carotene, where the pill forms of a nutrient turned out to be harmful while food forms promoted health.[94] Nutrient contributions of enriched, fortified, and functional foods blur the lines of what counts as a supplement. How does one count the cereal that supplies 100 percent of the Daily Value of vitamins and minerals in one bowl? Is calcium-fortified orange juice a food or a dietary supplement? Calcium-enriched foods are good examples to use in calculating how close one's intake is to the UL of a nutrient. Calcium's UL of 2000 mg is less than twice the RDA of 1200 for adults over age 70, making the margin of error in reaching potentially toxic amounts very slim indeed. If supplements no longer serve as insurance for well-nourished older adults, when is it worth taking nutrient supplements?

Vitamin $B_{12}$ and folic acid may be one instance. For a significant part of the population, these two vitamins are better absorbed in a synthetic form than in their protein-bound food form—but this becomes important only when normal metabolic processes fail.

It is possible for older adults to live well without dietary supplements. However, population surveys show that diets of many older persons fall short of meeting recommended nutrient levels (see Table 18.11), and appropriately used supplements fill nutritional gaps.[99] Some age-associated circumstances make an individual vulnerable to malnutrition and more likely to benefit from dietary supplements. Such nutritional risk factors include the following:

- Lack of appetite resulting from illness, loss of taste or smell, or depression

- Diseases or bacterial overgrowths in the gastrointestinal tract that prevent absorption
- Poor diet due to loss of function, dieting, or disinterest in food
- Avoidance of specific food groups such as meats, milk, or vegetables
- Use of substances that affect diet, absorption, or metabolism: tobacco, alcohol, drugs

**Who Takes Supplements and Why?** Nearly half of individuals aged 71 and older (47.6 percent of males, 47.4 percent of females) took multivitamin/mineral supplements during the NHANES 2007–2010.[100] Adults' usage increases with age. The individuals most likely to take supplements are White, female, with more education and with higher incomes.[91,92,98] They eat fruits and vegetables and are less likely to be obese, to smoke, or to have preexisting illnesses. Older adults are motivated by wellness and want to take responsibility for their own health. They use vitamin and mineral supplements to make them feel better, to have more energy, to improve health, and to prevent or treat disease.[98]

**What to Take?** The first consideration when asking, "What should I take?" is safety. Is there a chance that taking this supplement is harmful? Supplements are not tested and regulated like medicines, even if consumers use them to promote health and wellness or to ward off disease. The Food and Drug Administration requires label and package inserts be accurate. But press about a product is governed by the Federal Trade Commission and is considered free speech. Articles or media messages about dietary supplements can make unsubstantiated claims (Lose pounds! Perform all night! Erase wrinkles!). Unlike drugs, a dietary supplement may promise medicinal effects, but it is up to the buyer to look into proof of safety and efficacy. A systematic review and meta-analysis of primary prevention trials were undertaken in 2015 and results should provide much needed information on the safety and effectiveness of dietary supplements and mortality and morbidity outcomes.[101]

Considerations that guide supplement choices are especially important for older adults, who use more medications than younger adults, and these are addressed by the following four questions:

1. Does the supplement supply the missing nutrients?
2. Are there unwanted nutrients, and if so, can you live with them?
3. Is the dose safe when all supplements and fortified foods are combined?
4. Does the supplement carry a ***USP*** (U.S. Pharmacopeia, a mark that indicates that the manufacturer followed recognized standards when making the product) or ***NSF*** (NSF.org; NSF International tests consumer products, including dietary supplements) code to assure potency and purity?

**How Much to Take?** In general, multivitamin/mineral supplements are developed for use in physiologic rather than high-potency doses. Physiologic dose formulas unique to older adults are available without iron, with less Vitamin A, and with additional vitamins $B_{12}$ and D.

Generously fortified breakfast cereals, "power" bars, and fortified beverages count as vitamin or mineral supplements. On average, dietary intakes of older adults lack sufficient choline, calcium, magnesium, potassium, and vitamins A, D, E, and K, but are adequate in the rest. Additional vitamins and minerals are superfluous and possibly unsafe (e.g., beta-carotene supplements) (Table 18.15).

**USP (United States Pharmacopeia)** A nongovernmental, nonprofit organization (since 1820); establishes and maintains standards of identity, strength, quality, purity, processing, and labeling for health care products.

**NSF** International, a nongovernmental, nonprofit that also tests dietary supplements.

TABLE 18.15 ▸ Selected dietary supplements used by older adults for selected conditions

| CONDITION OR HEALTH STATUS | SUPPLEMENT |
|---|---|
| Poor appetite or dieting, leading to intake below 1200–1600 calories | Multivitamin/mineral |
| Weight loss, chronic underweight | Add high-calorie/protein foods/fats as oils |
| Vegetarian or vegan | Vitamins $B_{12}$, D, calcium, zinc, iron |
| Age-related macular degeneration | AREDS formulation (high levels of C, E, A, Zn, Cu) for high-risk and current AMD; no evidence for preventing AMD incidence |
| Constipation | Fiber (cellulose, bran, psyllium), together with fluid; strengthening of gut and core muscle |
| Diarrhea | Fluid, multivitamin/mineral |
| Energy boosters | Evaluate total nutrient intake, adequate calories, iron if blood levels are low; guard against excess stimulant (caffeine and guarana) |
| Osteoporosis | Vitamins D, calcium, fluoride, magnesium |
| Sleep aids | Milk and carbohydrate at bedtime; possibly melatonin, secretion of this biorhythm regulator decreases with age<br>Avoid guarana, caffeine, and alcohol near bedtime |

Cengage Learning 2014

## Dietary Supplements, Functional Foods, and Complementary Medicine

Complementary and alternative medicine (CAM) therapies often involve herbs, stimulants, functional foods, and ***nutraceuticals.*** Adults use hundreds of nonvitamin and nonmineral products (e.g., energy shots, glucosamine chondroitin, CoQ10, melatonin, plant stanols), including some that have toxic effects at normal doses (e.g., blue cohosh, chaparral). A commentary in the journal Evidence-Based Complementary and Alternative Medicine estimated that only 7 percent of complementary medicine is based on sound evidence.[102] Furthermore, this estimate may be optimistic. Considering the explosion of functional foods in the market place, and the desire for natural treatments and cures, older adults are especially vulnerable. They eat fewer calories, are less resilient physically, take more medicines that might interact with supplements, and they have a smaller tolerance for mistakes in supplement use.

In some cases, the growing availability of functional foods can benefit nutrient-deficient older adults. They may appreciate the convenience of nutrient-dense foods such as calcium-fortified breads and orange juice, fortified high-fiber cereals, prebiotics such as inulin in fiber bars, probiotics in yogurt with live cultures, soy milks, breakfast powders with whey protein, and various fortified chews, bars, and drinks. However, regular users of functional foods, no matter what age, need to track all sources of their dietary vitamin and mineral intake in order to avoid potentially toxic nutrient levels (Table 18.16). Advice that "you can't overdose on nutrients from food" does not apply to fortified foods.

## Nutrient Recommendations: Using the Food Label

The Nutrition Facts panel on food packages is structured to provide nutrient content information relative to a 2000 kcal diet and in relation to nutrient needs.

Several of the recommended nutrient levels for older adults (aged 70 years and older) differ from those used as reference values (DV) for the nutrition label (see Table 18.16). For example, older adults need more vitamin C and calcium and less iron and zinc than the daily values used in labeling. Values also differ for vitamins D, E, and $B_{12}$. The UL shows upper limits that are considered safe. ULs range from $<2$ to $>60$ times the RDA, making it impossible to generalize about the safety of excess nutrients. Older adults can use the DV percentages on food labels for dietary guidance if they adjust them to get more than 100 percent of calcium and vitamins D and C and less than 100 percent of vitamin A, iron, and zinc. For example, the calcium DV is 1000 mg but the RDA for 71-year-olds is 1200 mg, so a food serving containing 20 percent of the DV (200 mg) provides 16.6 percent of the day's RDA of 1200 mg. Iron is important to track because it has a low UL compared to the DV (factor of 2.5). The DV is more than twice the RDA (18/8 mg) of an older adult. For a 51+ adult, the 8-mg RDA is only 44 percent of the DV, which might easily be consumed in a single serving of cereal. Using the DV for the needs of older adults can be cumbersome; it requires vision to read the label and dexterity and mental acuity to do the math and track it. It also requires motivation. On the other hand, older adults are motivated to guard their health.

The vitamin $B_{12}$ label recommendation is higher than the DRI, but poor absorption in older adults makes unsafe intake from food products unlikely. The Nutrition Facts panel information underscores that "one size does not fit all" in dietary guidance, especially when it comes to older adults!

## Cross-Cultural Considerations in Making Dietary Recommendations

Food habits develop in cultural contexts, and we can learn about them in various ways. Travel through North America would allow us to observe cultures that make up our society. Visiting ethnic restaurants, stores, and farmer's markets can be another way to get a glimpse of cultural food diversity. Cookbooks, films, talking with individuals about their food history, and participating in ethnic celebrations are other sources of insight into food patterns of various cultures. Each new immigrant wave adds unique food traditions to the country's mix. Older adults may be stronger advocates for upholding traditional food patterns than young people are. In working with them on food issues, it is useful (and interesting) to determine the cultural history of their food and lifestyle habits.

National food-monitoring programs survey the population with proportionately larger samples drawn from minority groups in order to develop a balanced picture of the whole population. North America is home to rapidly growing Hispanic, Asian, Russian, Middle-Eastern, and African immigrant groups. The U.S. Census tracks minority groups, but it is completed only once every 10 years. The local Area Agencies on Aging and Nutrition Programs also track population trends, and these are likely to yield greater insight about some of the smaller ethnic population groups in their unique communities and regions.

Cultural differences are reflected in approaches to dietary guidance. For example, Chile has separate guidelines for older and younger adults. In New Zealand, older adults are encouraged to socialize at mealtimes to improve appetite. In France, South Korea, and Japan, people of all ages are encouraged to enjoy mealtimes and take pleasure in eating. Other unique guidelines are those of China, which suggest people eat 20–25 grams (nearly an ounce) of fish daily. Guatemala uses a bean pot as a nutritional icon. India has developed one set of guidelines for the rich (i.e., overall energy intake should be restricted to

**nutraceutical** Combination of words *nutrient* and *pharmaceutical* to indicate a food-derived compound that can act as a drug, such as red yeast rice, a statin-like compound.

TABLE 18.16 ▸ Vitamin and mineral levels for nutrition labeling (Daily Reference Values or DV) compared with Dietary Reference Intakes (DRI) and Tolerable Upper Intake Levels (UL) for older adults

| | VITAMIN AND MINERAL COMPONENTS OF THE NUTRITION LABEL | | | |
|---|---|---|---|---|
| | | DRI FOR ADULTS OVER 70 | | |
| MANDATORY NUTRIENTS | DAILY VALUES (1993, 1995) ALL ADULTS | MALES | FEMALES | UPPER LIMIT (UL) |
| Vitamin A, IU or RE (5 IU = 1 RE = 1 RAE, Retinol Activity Equivalent) | 5000 IU | 900 RE | 700 RE | 3000 RE |
| Vitamin C, mg | 60 | 90 | 75 | 2000 |
| Sodium, mg | 2400 | 1200 | 1200 | 2300 |
| Calcium, mg | 1000 | 1200 | 1200 | 2000 |
| Iron, mg | 18 | 8 | 8 | 45 |
| VOLUNTARY VITAMIN AND MINERAL COMPONENTS OF THE NUTRITION LABEL | | | | |
| Vitamin D, mcg (1 mcg = 40 IU) | 400 IU | 15 mcg | 15 mcg | 50 mcg |
| Vitamin E, mg (1 mg = 1 TE = 1 IU) | 30 IU | 15 mg | 15 mg | 1000 mg |
| Vitamin K, mcg | 80 | 120 | 90 | – |
| Thiamin, mg | 1.5 | 1.2 | 1.1 | – |
| Riboflavin, mg | 1.7 | 1.3 | 1.1 | – |
| Niacin, mg | 20 | 16 | 14 | 35 |
| Vitamin $B_6$, mg | 2.0 | 1.7 | 1.5 | 100 |
| Folic acid, mcg | 400 | 400 | 400 | 1000[a] |
| Vitamin $B_{12}$, mcg | 6.0 | 2.4 | 2.4 | – |
| Biotin, mcg | 300 | 30 | 30 | – |
| Pantothenic acid, mg | 10 | 5.0 | 5.0 | – |
| Phosphorus, mg | 1000 | 700 | 700 | 3000 |
| Iodine, mcg | 150 | 150 | 150 | 1100 |
| Magnesium, mg | 400 | 420 | 320 | 350[b] |
| Zinc, mg | 15 | 11 | 8 | 40 |
| Selenium, mg | 70 | 55 | 55 | 400 |
| Copper, mcg | 2000 | 900 | 900 | 10,000 |
| Manganese, mg | 2.0 | 2.3 | 1.8 | 11 |
| Chromium, mcg | 120 | 30 | 20 | – |
| Molybdenum, mcg | 75 | 45 | 45 | 2000 |
| Chloride, mg | 3400 | 2300 | 2300 | – |
| Potassium, mg | 3500 | 4700 | 4700 | – |
| Choline, mg | – | 550 | 425 | 3500 |
| Fluoride, mg | – | 4.0 | 3.0 | 10 |

SOURCES: http://www.fda.gov/Food/GuidanceRegulation/GuidanceDocumentsRegulatoryInformation/LabelingNutrition/ucm064928.htm Accessed 6/9/15

[a]synthetic.

[b]nonfood sources.

levels commensurate with the sedentary occupations of the affluent, so that obesity is avoided; total fat intake is not to exceed 20 percent of total energy; and use of clarified butter, a prized Indian culinary ingredient, should be restricted to special occasions) and one for the poor (addressing the fact that at least one-third of the households in India are not able to afford even the minimum nutritional requirements, even though they are spending 80 percent of their income on food). These recommendations identify food combinations that are most likely to meet recommended dietary intakes.

Listening carefully, communicating effectively, and avoiding misinterpretation in intercultural settings is probably the most important thing a nutritionist can learn to do when working with older adults from various cultures. Cultural competence requires skill in transferring information, developing and maintaining relationships, and gaining compliance. Developing individual skills takes time, commitment, and practice. On the other hand, nutrition education and guidance tools have been developed in many languages and for diverse cultures, although not typically for elders of ethnic groups. Culturally appropriate resources can be found through local extension services, cross-cultural education centers, diabetes education programs, public health agencies, and some commodity groups.

# Food Safety Recommendations

LO 18.8 Explain how good food safety practices contribute to the health of older adults, and how increasing functional decline can be accommodated.

Older adults with a compromised immune status are particularly vulnerable to foodborne illness. No one knows exactly how widespread this problem is because many foodborne illnesses are not reported when individuals think they have the flu.

Poor food-handling practices leading to microorganism growth are generally to blame for foodborne illnesses. Impaired functioning may result in impaired food handling practices. Signs and symptoms of foodborne illness include gastrointestinal distress, diarrhea, vomiting, and fever and may appear within half an hour of eating a contaminated food or may not develop for up to three weeks.

Leading practices that put an older person at risk are as follows:

- Improper holding temperatures of foods
- Poor personal hygiene
- Contaminated food-preparation equipment (cutting boards, knives)
- Inadequate cooking time

Limited vision, decreased sense of smell, or forgetfulness may get in the way of actions that keep food nourishing by keeping it safe. To combat this, the recommendations are to:

- Wash hands and surfaces often.
- Separate raw, cooked, and ready-to-eat foods while shopping, preparing, and storing.
- Cook foods—especially raw meat, poultry, fish, and eggs—to a safe temperature.
- Refrigerate or freeze perishable or prepared foods within 2 hours.
- Follow the label for food-safety preparation and storage instructions.
- Serve hot foods hot (140°F or above) and cold foods cold (40°F or below).
- When in doubt, throw it out!

# Physical Activity Recommendations

LO 18.9 Appreciate the heterogeneity of older adults populations and suggest two or more reasons to tailor health promotion.

Exercise is a true fountain of youth. Physical activity (PA) builds lean body mass, helps to maintain balance and flexibility, contributes to aerobic capacity and to overall fitness, improves cognitive performance in previously sedentary older adults, and is associated with overall psychological well-being.[7] Older people benefit from PA even more than younger people do because strength training is the only way to maintain and build muscle mass. In addition to strength gains, increased muscle mass increases caloric needs. Higher caloric intake increases the chances of optimal nutrient intake. Low activity levels as well as deteriorating strength, endurance, and sense of balance are associated with, but not caused by, increasing age.

Age does not hinder training effects, as shown in Appendix A, from the American College of Sports Medicine. This research synopsis and position statement describes the effects of exercise and physical activity on older adults and includes recommended exercise prescriptions made collaboratively with the American Heart Association.[7]

## Physical Activity Guidelines

How can one predict whether PA will exacerbate existing medical conditions? Physician screening or assessment by completing a questionnaire like the one in Table 18.17 can identify potential contraindications or problem areas. A more detailed assessment to evaluate cardiovascular fitness, strength, function, balance, flexibility, body composition, and bone density can be made by an interdisciplinary team. Individuals, including those with physical limitations such as heart disease or inability to stand, can be cleared for participation.

The 2015 Dietary Guidelines[62] include key recommendations for physical activity for various age groups from the 2008 Physical Activity Guidelines for Americans. Adults aged 65 and older are encouraged to follow the adult guidelines as conditions allow, and to include exercises that maintain or improve balance if at risk of falling. Level of fitness and chronic conditions determine the frequency, intensity, and duration of exercise sessions for older adults:

- Muscle strengthening that involves all major muscle groups on 2 or more days per week
- At least 150 minutes per week of moderate intensity aerobic activity (episodes of 10 minutes or more, spread through the week)
- Drink water when exercising because thirst may be blunted
- Ensure adequate protein for muscle building throughout the day[75]

Appendix A lists the health improvements that older adults can achieve through exercise and training. Because bed rest and inactivity lead to bone and muscle wasting, everyone, including institutionalized individuals, can benefit from exercise. William Evans has shown that exercise can be adapted to nursing home residents, concluding that "there is no segment of the population that can benefit more from exercise than the elderly."[103] See Case Study 18.1 for an instance where exercise can be an integral part of treatment.

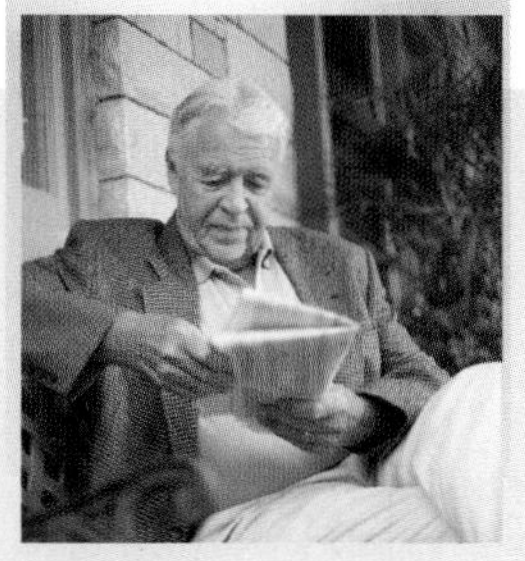
Masterfile

# CASE STUDY 18.1

## JT—Spiraling Out of Control?

JT, a retired computer company executive, eats out four times a week since his wife died last year. Meals at home consist of microwave dinners or supreme pizza. He belongs to a health club, which he visits three times a week, and where he has many friends. Occasionally, JT and his friends go out for beers after their workout. Shortly after his 69th birthday (2 years ago), he was diagnosed with type 2 diabetes. Last week, he visited the clinic for his annual checkup. He was measured at 5 feet 9 inches (1.75 m) and weighed 235 pounds (106.8 kg). His doctor is worried about JT's family history of heart disease.

### *Questions*

1. What would you ask JT about his food and fitness routine?
2. Calculate JT's BMI. How does it compare to guidelines? He wants to know whether BMI is an accurate measure of his body fat. How might you answer?
3. As his nutritionist, what nutrition remedies would you explore to help JT?
4. What fluid recommendation would you make?
5. What sort of monitoring and evaluation plan could you and JT devise to track his weight management?

# Nutrition Policy and Intervention for Risk Reduction

LO 18.10 Summarize the heterogeneity of older adult populations and suggest two or more reasons to tailor health promotion.

Nutrition policy promotes health by combining nutrition education for individuals and population interventions. The ultimate goal of nutrition intervention is to improve health outcomes.

## Nutrition Education

Contrary to some beliefs, older people do learn and change. Someone born in 1930 has seen the invention of microwaves, television and TV dinners, and a whole host of computer-controlled kitchen appliances, not to mention computers, smartphones, and online anything. To age is to adapt. Learning new nutrition habits is part of aging.

TABLE 18.17 ▸ Keep moving: fitness after 50 chart

A. Do I get chest pains while at rest and/or during exercise?
B. If the answer to question A is yes: Is it true that I have not had a physician diagnose these pains yet?
C. Have I ever had a heart attack?
D. If the answer to question C is yes: Was my heart attack within the last year?
E. Do I have high blood pressure?
F. If you do not know the answer to question E, answer this: Was my last blood pressure reading more than 150/100?
G. Am I short of breath after extremely mild exertion, and sometimes even at rest or at night in bed?
H. Do I have any ulcerated wounds or cuts on my feet that do not seem to heal?
I. Have I lost 10 pounds or more in the past 6 months without trying and to my surprise?
J. Do I get pain in my buttocks or the back of my legs—my thighs and calves—when I walk? (This question is an attempt to identify persons who suffer from intermittent claudication. Exercise training may be extremely painful; however, it may also provide relief from pain experienced when performing lower-intensity exercise.)
K. When at rest, do I frequently experience fast, irregular heartbeats, or, at the other extreme, very slow beats? (Although a low heart rate can be a sign of an efficient and well-conditioned heart, a very low rate can also indicate a nearly complete heart block.)
L. Am I currently being treated for any heart or circulatory condition, such as vascular disease, stroke, angina, hypertension, congestive heart failure, poor circulation to the legs, valvular heart disease, blood clots, or pulmonary disease?
M. As an adult, have I ever had a fracture of the hip, spine, or wrist?
N. Did I have a fall more than twice in the past year (no matter what the reason)? (Many older persons have balance problems, and at the initiation of a walking program will have a high chance of falling. These persons may benefit from balance training and resistance exercise before beginning a walking program.)
O. Do I have diabetes?

SOURCE: From Evans, W. J., and Cyr-Campbell, D. *Nutrition, Exercise, and Healthy Aging*. JADA 1997; 97:632–8. Copyright: American Dietetic Association. Reprinted by permission from the author.

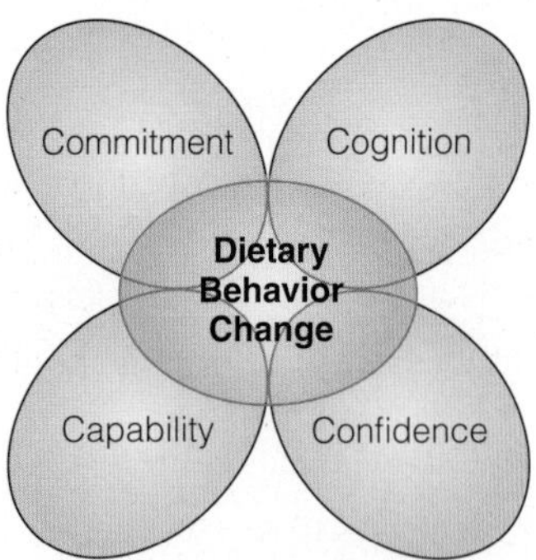


ILLUSTRATION 18.6 ▸ Four essential elements to achieve and maintain individual dietary behavior change.

SOURCE: Based on Krinke, U. B. Effective Nutrition Education Strategies to Reach Older Adults. in Watson, R. R., ed. *Handbook of Nutrition in the Aged*. Boca Raton, FL: CRC Press, 2001.

Nutrition education is different from education in general because its goal is changed dietary behaviors. Nutrition education consists of a set of learning experiences to facilitate voluntary adoption of nutrition-related behaviors that are conducive to health and well-being. Several requirements must be met for nutrition education—that is, behavior change—to occur (see Illustration 18.6). Think of them as the 4 Cs of nutrition education.[104]

1. *Commitment.* Commitment means being motivated to adopt health-promoting behaviors and intending to adopt and maintain a new food behavior.
2. *Cognitive processing.* Understanding how a food behavior contributes to health and planning how it will fit into your life constitutes cognitive processing.
3. *Capability.* Acquiring the skills to practise new food behaviors is part of nutrition education. An example is learning to identify whole-grain breads or to prepare vegetables when intending to adopt a high-fiber diet.
4. *Confidence.* "Nothing breeds success like success!" The best predictor that someone will practice new dietary habits is their personal confidence in being able to do so.

Educational sessions for older learners are best designed around their potential limitations, such as declines in visual acuity and hearing loss.[104] Adaptation for written material includes:

- Larger type size
- Serif ("with feet") lettering (Arial is a typeface with no serifs; Times Roman has serifs)
- Bold type
- High contrast (black on white)
- Non-glossy paper to decrease glare
- Avoidance of blue, green, and violet (paper and print color) due to decreased ability to discriminate among these colors
- Reading level of fifth to eighth grade for general audiences

Educational strategies can result in better diets for individuals, but these alone are not sufficient to enhance the dietary patterns of populations. Nutrition policies reflect community environments. Cultural environments support, ignore, or punish desired behavior change. An example of a culturally supportive environment is a peer group that values health and fitness; group members will help each other to achieve and maintain health-promoting behaviors. For instance, members may belong to a biking group, share in farmers' market trips, and serve healthful foods when entertaining. The 80-year-long Terman study, reported in The Longevity Project,[105] describes many examples of structuring one's environment to support longevity.

Food and nutrition policies arise from public values, beliefs, and opinions that define the cultural context in which dietary behaviors exist. Policies can be overt or unspoken. Public policies supporting the health of older adults in the United States are evident in the Social Security program, which provides financial support for post-retirement living, including health care and nutrition counseling.

# Community Food and Nutrition Programs

**LO 18.11** Describe one or more nutrition programs serving older adults.

Governmental programs for older adults include the USDA's Supplemental Nutrition Assistance Program (SNAP), Farmers Market Nutrition Programs, the Commodity Supplemental Foods, the Child and Adult Care Food Program, and the Ryan White Comprehensive AIDS Resources Emergency Act.[106] The U.S. Department of Health and Human Services (HHS) administers the Older Americans Act Nutrition Programs (OAANP), which includes a whole array of nutrition and community services. Home-delivered and congregate meal programs, with nutrition screening and counseling are provided to older adults nationally through a network of state units on aging, area agencies on aging and tribal and Native American organizations. HHS also administers Social Security programs that provide basic living expenses for older adults and health-care coverage through Medicare.

Nongovernmental programs may also provide food and nutrition services as part of a broader range of screening and assessment, nursing, and other support services. For instance, home health agencies provide staff who can offer nutritional counseling or aides who will shop for and prepare food, and clean up the kitchen afterward. Home care services allow individuals to receive the necessary support to stay in their homes for as long as they wish. Remaining in one's home indefinitely is sometimes referred to as "aging in place." Aging in place does not necessarily mean living in one home for a lifetime. Ideally, it means having the choice to grow old in one's preferred community. Livable communities offer a spectrum of options for residents of all ages. Supportive services customized to accommodate those who are fully active and have no impairments, those who require limited assistance, and those with more severe impairments who require care in long-term care facilities are basic to creating livable communities. In April 2012, the secretary of Health and Human Services announced the creation of an Administration for Community Living (ACL), bringing together the Administration on Aging, the Office of Disability, and the Administration on Developmental Disabilities into one agency that will enable individuals to live in their chosen communities. Food and nutrition programs help to meet the most basic human needs in a continuum of care.

Other food and nutrition programs that contribute to the continuum of nutrition services include food pantries, soup kitchens, cooperative buying groups such as Fare for All, and screening and referral services.

## Store-to-Door: A Nongovernmental Service that Supports Aging in Place

Store-to-Door is an example of a small program that was begun by one person who made a big difference. After retiring in the 1980s, Dr. David Berger surveyed his community to see where he might do some good. Many older adults told him that getting to the grocery store was impossible, and that even when they could get to the store, bringing the bags home was difficult. Winter ice and snow made things worse, for people feared falling. The community's grocery delivery service had closed because profits were not meeting shareholder expectations. So Dr. Berger joined forces with his wife, Fran, volunteer coordinator Judy Madaj, friends, colleagues, and many volunteers to start up the nonprofit Store-to-Door, a home-delivered grocery program for older people and those who are disabled. Volunteers will shop for and deliver your groceries. They buy items that discount grocers offer: food, of course, and also greeting cards, medicines, paper goods, and cleaning supplies. Customers can get credit for coupons. After starting Store-to-Door in the Midwest, Dr. Berger started other home-delivered grocery programs in Portland, Oregon, and Ventura, California. Does the program work? Yes: the first Store-to-Door celebrated its 30th anniversary in 2014, the Portland group is now over 25 years old, and the Ventura Shop Ahoy has expanded to several communities. That's no small feat for programs that depend on hundreds of volunteers and funding sources to help older and disabled adults live at home. And it all started with someone asking community members what they needed and acting on their answers.

## OAANP: Promoting Socialization and Improved Nutrition

Congress first appropriated funds under Title VII of the Older Americans Act of 1965 to begin the OAANP (previously called the Elderly Nutrition Program). The OAANP was created to alleviate poor nutritional intake and reduce social isolation among older adults. It was based on evidence that older adults do not eat adequately because of the following:

1. Lack of income limits ability to purchase food.
2. Lack of skills limits ability to select and prepare nourishing meals.
3. Limited mobility affects shopping and meal preparation.
4. Feelings of isolation and loneliness decrease the incentive to eat well.

Title IIIC of the Older Americans Act, is a community-based nutrition program that provides meals (congregate and home-delivered), increased social contact, nutrition screening and education, and information and linkages to other support programs and services, as well as volunteer opportunities. Anyone who is 60 or more years of age (and in some cases, their spouses or caregivers regardless of age) is eligible to participate in the congregate dining program; home-delivered meal clients must be homebound and unable to prepare their own meals. Although the OAANP is not means tested and individuals do not need to be of low socioeconomic status to participate, congregate meal sites are targeted to neighborhoods where older, frail, impoverished seniors live. Meal sites are located in community centers, senior centers, civic buildings, subsidized housing units, schools, and other accessible locations. Home-delivered meals are especially targeted to low-income minorities, rural older adults, those with limited English proficiency or those at risk of institutional care. Individuals contribute toward the cost of the meal according to their means and based on a suggested donation. The last major national evaluation of the OAANP completed in 1996 showed that for every $1.00 of Title III funds spent on congregate services it is supplemented by an additional $1.70 from other sources; the average cost of a congregate meal was $5.17, and a home-delivered one was $5.31.[107] A national study is ongoing that will provide updated information on the cost of the meals and the funds leveraged through the program. Title VI grant programs are similar to Title III programs and were established to help deliver social and nutrition services to older American Indians, Alaskan Natives, and Native Hawaiians. Other service variations to meet the needs of frail older seniors include multiple meals, weekend meals, take-home snacks, liquid supplements, nutrition screening and education, and one-to-one nutrition counseling. Also available are diets adapted for medical, religious, and cultural reasons.

Nutrition programs for older adults have successfully brought together millions of people to socialize and enjoy nutritious meals. In FY 2009, about 240 million congregate and home-delivered meals were served to approximately 2.6 million older adults.[108] The Older Americans Act 2000 Amendment, Section 339 (Nutrition) (H.R. 782), states that nutrition projects shall use a dietitian (or person with compatible expertise), provide a minimum of one-third of the daily RDAs, and comply with the Dietary Guidelines for Americans. A review of the literature showed that the HDM program is well targeted, efficient, and well liked; it provides quality food to needy individuals; and helps individuals remain living independently. HDMs was also shown to decrease institutionalization of older adults and resulting health care expenditures.[109] Increasing socialization was one of the original program goals and continues to be one of the outcomes. Relative to the general older population, participants are older and more likely to be female, to belong to an ethnic minority, to live alone, and to have incomes well below poverty level.

## The Promise of Prevention: Health Promotion

Aging boomers who expect to enjoy an active adulthood are driving longevity and aging research. Lifelong caloric restriction may not find many converts, but emulating the habits of long-lived populations is gaining interest. Dan Buettner has been studying regions of the world inhabited by disproportionately high numbers of centenarians. In describing the lives of these healthy old residents of Okinawa, Sardinia, Costa Rica, and North America in a book called *The Blue Zones*,[110] Buettner compiled a list of nine habits and traits among these population groups:

1. Being active as a regular part of daily life
2. *Hara hachi bu*, which means to stop eating when one is 80 percent full
3. Eating more beans, whole grains, vegetables, nuts, and fruits while limiting meats and processed foods
4. Drinking red wine, in moderation
5. Having a reason to get up in the morning, a *plan de vida* or *ikigai*
6. Making time to relieve stress
7. Belonging to, and participating in, a spiritual community
8. Making family a priority and upholding rituals and traditions
9. Picking the right tribe, that is, surrounding yourself with people who share long-life values

Residents of places like Okinawa, Sardinia, and Loma Linda are supported by their culture throughout life. Although good nutritional habits make a greater impact when started early in life, sometimes individuals are not motivated to pursue these risk-reduction strategies until they retire or experience a health problem. Successful strategies to reach an older audience address specific population needs and interests. The wave of aging baby boomers is less accepting of the status quo. Should the myth that a 70-year-old is too old to learn and practice health-promotion strategies still exist when they themselves turn 70, they will certainly disprove it! Boomers believe the words of the poet Robert Browning: "Grow old along with me, the best is yet to be!"

## KEY POINTS

1. Functional ability (the demonstrated ability to carry out activities of daily living) is more important than chronological age in assessing the health status of older adults.
2. Good nutrition, good health habits, environment, access to health care, and genetics contribute to human life expectancy, which is still significantly shorter than the potential human life span. Theories of aging, such as wear-and-tear theories, help to explore which factors contribute most to a longer, disease-free life.
3. Of all the physiological changes associated with aging, loss of lean body mass and the concomitant gains of body fat may well be the most important in determining functional age.
4. "Use it or lose it" applies to both the body and the mind: keep learning to maintain acute brain function, stay active to build muscle and bone, eat well to maintain and repair tissue, and cultivate a positive approach to life to improve longevity.
5. The DETERMINE acronym is a reasonable summary of warning signs associated with poor nutritional health.
6. While adults in general consume more than enough calories and protein, clusters of older adults may be lacking in adequate dietary protein and energy.
7. The thirst mechanism of older adults is not as sensitive as that of younger adults, placing them at higher risk of dehydration.

8. Physiological changes that lead to malnutrition in older adults are decreased absorption of vitamins D and $B_{12}$ and increased storage of vitamin A and iron.
9. In general, older adults eat better than do younger adults, but they do not consume enough vitamin A, D, E, K (men), choline, calcium, magnesium, or potassium to meet recommended intake levels.
10. Vitamin and mineral supplements can be helpful for older adults who have lost their appetite; avoid certain food groups; have poor diets due to, loss of function, dieting or depression; or who have gastrointestinal bacterial overgrowth that prevents nutrient absorption.
11. Excellent food safety practices are especially important for older adults, who may be more vulnerable to infection for many reasons, such as a higher prevalence of chronic diseases, sensory and functional losses, lower immune system, and decreased resilience in healing and recovery from illness.
12. Older adults are often more interested in nutrition education and health promotion than are younger adults. The stereotype that older adults will not change is just that: an old stereotype.

## REVIEW QUESTIONS

1. Older adults have proportionately more illness than younger adults, and the two leading causes of death are heart disease and cancer.

   _____ True _____ False
2. The CDC suggests that longevity depends more on lifestyle factors than on genetics.

   _____ True _____ False
3. U.S. life expectancy at birth is the highest in the world.

   _____ True _____ False
4. Fat-free mass or lean body mass tends to shrink in old age. This results in significantly decreased need for calories, vitamins, and minerals.

   _____ True _____ False
5. The OAANP serves individuals aged 60 and older. The congregate meal program was established to increase socialization as well as to improve nutritional intakes of older adults.

   _____ True _____ False
6. DETERMINE, MUST, and the MNA are three tools to screen for nutritional risk. List five factors that place older adults at risk of malnutrition.
7. Food guidance for older adults is different from that for the general public. Cite two adjustments in food guidance that are particularly important for older adults.
8. The AMDR for protein is 10–35 percent of calories, and the RDA is 0.8 gm/kg body weight. If the average older adult meets the RDA, why is protein a nutrient of concern for older adults?
9. Using information from Question 8, how would you determine the protein needs of JT in Case Study 18.1? *Hint:* He weighs 235 pounds (107 kg).

Visit www.cengagebrain.com to access MindTap, a complete digital course that includes additional resources.

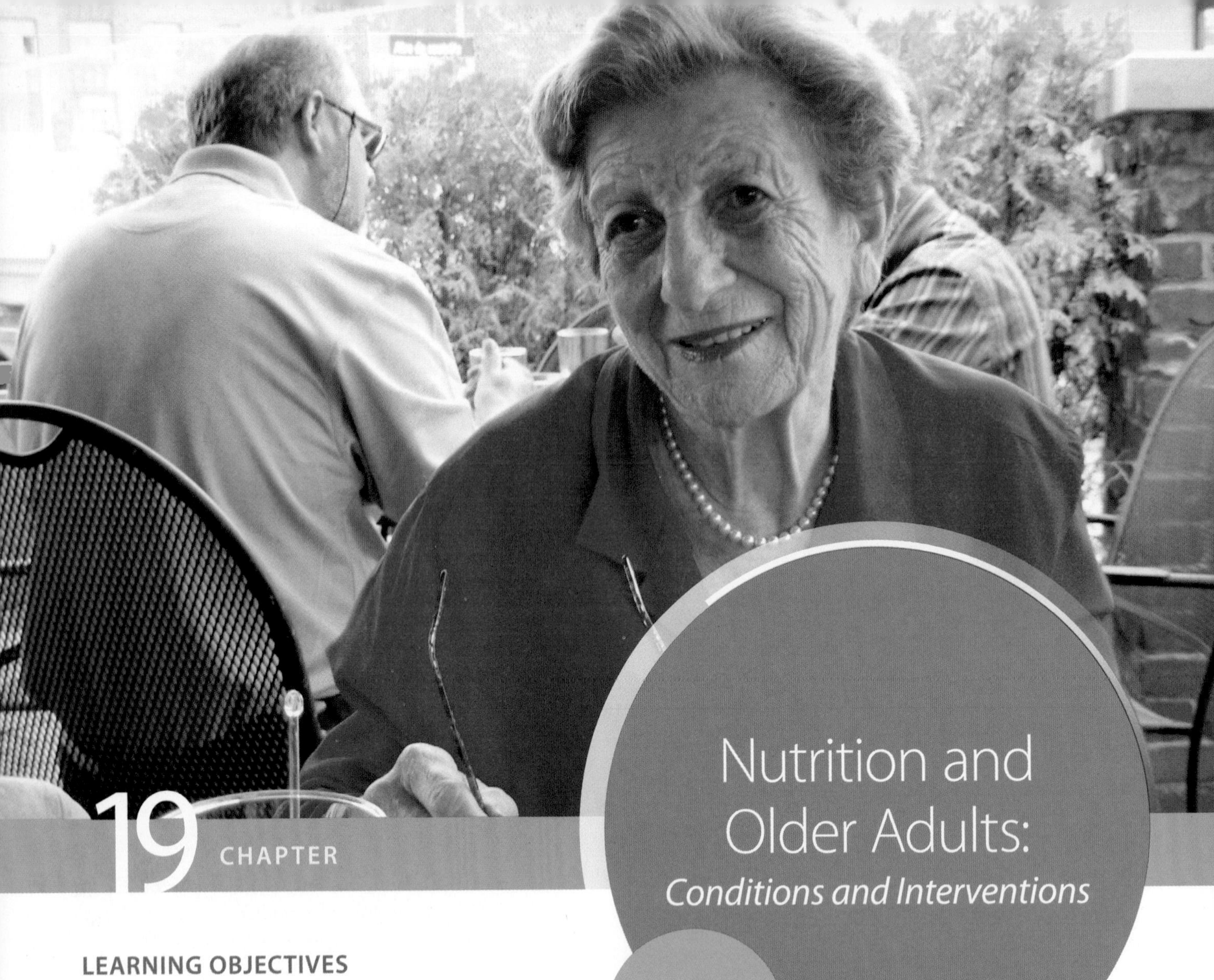

# Chapter 19: Nutrition and Older Adults: *Conditions and Interventions*

*Prepared by*
**Nadine R. Sahyoun**

## LEARNING OBJECTIVES

After studying the materials in this chapter you should be able to:

**19.1** Describe key nutritional approaches to the most prevalent chronic diseases of adults 65+, recognizing the heterogeneity of older populations.

**19.2** Describe key nutritional approaches to heart disease in adults 65+, recognizing the heterogeneity of older populations.

**19.3** Describe key nutritional approaches to addressing strokes and related diseases in adults 65+, recognizing the heterogeneity of older populations.

**19.4** Describe key nutritional approaches to hypertension in adults 65+, recognizing the heterogeneity of older populations.

**19.5** Describe key nutritional approaches to diabetes in adults 65+, recognizing the heterogeneity of older populations.

**19.6** Explain how sarcopenia combined with obesity affects fitness and weight management.

**19.7** Describe key nutritional approaches to osteoporosis in adults 65+, recognizing the heterogeneity of older populations.

**19.8** Identify three or more nutritional strategies that contribute to oral health.

**19.9** Describe the three most common GI problems of older adults, along with nutritional management strategies to ameliorate each condition.

**19.10** Describe key nutritional approaches to osteoarthritis in adults 65+, recognizing the heterogeneity of older populations.

**19.11** Describe key nutritional approaches to cognitive impairment, dementia, and Alzheimer's diseases of adults 65+, recognizing the heterogeneity of older populations.

**19.12** Understand how comorbidities and polypharmacy increase nutritional risk in older adults.

**19.13** Explain the challenges faced by underweight individuals and the consequences of sarcopenia on day-to-day functioning.

**19.14** List three or more signs of dehydration and explain why maintaining hydration status is important for the health of an older person.

**19.15** Explain how social support during bereavement can help the survivor to stay healthy.

Nadine Sahyoun

## Introduction: The Importance of Nutrition

The term ***healthspan*** is joining *lifespan* to focus on what really matters to older adults.[1] Aging adults want to stay ***healthy*** until death, and most (77 percent of adults aged 65 and over) rate their own health as *good, very good, or excellent.*[2] They believe this despite the increasing prevalence of chronic illness in old age. Having a chronic health problem (see Table 19.1) does not prevent someone from having the perception of being healthy. Still, self-perception of good health declines with age. By age 85, self-perceived health status of *good to excellent* decreases to 69 percent of Non-Hispanic Whites, 54 percent of Non-Hispanic Blacks, and 52 percent of Hispanic or Latino groups.[2] Good nutrition contributes to ***quality of life*** and ameliorates effects of illness. But illness often brings with it changes in eating pattern, either as a symptom of disease, such as the anorexia associated with depression, or as part of therapy, when avoidance of salt or fatty meats may leave individuals at a loss of how to replace their soup and sandwich lunch with a tasty, low-sodium, low-saturated fat version. ***Medical nutrition therapy (MNT)*** as part of a comprehensive treatment plan can encourage health-promoting food choices once diseases have been diagnosed. Outcome data regarding the effectiveness of MNT by registered dietitians (RD) have resulted in reimbursement provided to Medicare Part B beneficiaries with diabetes mellitus and kidney disease,[3] using nationally recognized nutrition protocols and evidence-based practice guidelines.[4] The most current Medicare rules can be found at the Center for Medicare and Medicaid Services (www.cms.hhs.gov).

Numerous studies have measured the health care utilization of older adults and found that better nutritional status is related to better health outcomes. The Lewin Group researchers estimated that covering medical nutrition therapy for older managed-care clients who had cardiovascular disease (CVD), diabetes, or renal disease would recover Medicare costs after 3 years and would begin to save system dollars by the fourth year.[5] Malnourished older patients have higher postoperative complication rates and longer hospital stays, therefore incurring greater health care costs.[6,7] In free-living older adults, nutritional risk status was found to be the most important predictor of total number of physician visits, visits to physicians in the emergency room, and hospitalization rates.[8] Aging adults use proportionately more health-care services and products than younger persons do; therefore, nutrition interventions can play a larger role in their health.

## Nutrition and Health

LO 19.1 Describe key nutritional approaches to the most prevalent chronic diseases of adults 65+, recognizing the heterogeneity of older populations.

The ancient Latin quotation "*Mens sana in corpore sano*" ("a sound mind in a sound body") is often used to emphasize a whole body approach to health. Public health professionals monitor health by measuring leading causes of mortality and morbidity in order to design interventions that improve the population's health. Leading health problems and disabilities become the focus of nutritional interventions.

Deaths from heart and ***cerebrovascular diseases*** have declined (Illustration 19.1), but they are still among the leading causes of death of older adults. Among persons aged 65 and older, more die from heart disease than any other cause (Table 19.2).

Lifestyle interventions have a huge potential to affect premature deaths. The prevalence of multiple chronic conditions increases with age. If you sum the percentages in Table 19.1, you'll note that the total

**healthspan** Illness-free life span.

**healthy** More than the absence of disease, health is a sense of well-being. Even individuals with a chronic condition may properly consider themselves to be healthy. For instance, a person with diabetes mellitus whose blood sugar is under control can be considered healthy.

**quality of life** A measure of life satisfaction that is difficult to define, especially in an aging heterogeneous population. Quality-of-life measures include factors such as social contacts, economic security, and functional status.

**medical nutrition therapy (MNT)** Comprehensive nutrition services by registered dietitians to treat the nutritional aspects of acute and chronic diseases.

**cerebrovascular disease** Conditions caused by problems that affect the blood supply to the brain.

TABLE 19.1 ▸ Percentage of people aged 65 and older who reported selected chronic conditions, 2012–2013, by sex[a]

| SEX | HEART DISEASE | HYPERTENSION (2009–2012) | STROKE | CANCER (ANY) | DIABETES[b] (2009–2012) |
|---|---|---|---|---|---|
| Men | | | | | |
| 65–74 | 30 | 62 | 7 | 17 | |
| 75+ | 42 | 75 | 12 | 25 | |
| Women | | | | | |
| 65–74 | 21 | 67 | 6 | 15 | |
| 75+ | 33 | 79 | 11 | 19 | |
| | | | | | 27 (age 65+ both sexes) |

SOURCE: [a]Health, United States, 2014, Table 42 and [b]Table 44 (physician-diagnosed and undiagnosed diabetes)[14]

is greater than 100. Common comorbid conditions are hypertension, heart disease, diabetes, cancer, stroke, arthritis, and kidney disease. For example, 21 percent of adults over 65 have hypertension and heart disease; 15 percent have hypertension and diabetes, and 11 percent have hypertension and cancer.[10] Despite eating patterns that earn better HEI (Healthy Eating Index) scores than those of younger people, the diets of older adults contribute to the incidence and course of their diseases, especially heart disease, hypertension, and cancer. These diseases can, in turn, affect functional ability. For example, an overweight individual with heart disease may continue to overeat and become obese, further complicating arthritis management. In turn, arthritis can limit functioning. Weight loss of even 1 pound will reduce stress on the knees during daily activities and may lead to enhanced management of heart disease, as well.[11] Old age is not a reason to forgo health promotion. The Physician's Health Study examined modifiable risk factors contributing to survival and optimal functioning of men at age 90 and beyond. Good health habits (not smoking, moderate alcohol intake, not becoming obese, and regular physical exercise; see Appendix A) contributed to delayed mortality and to higher functional status in old age.[12] An analysis of the dietary habits of post-menopausal women with established heart disease (mean ages of study's three groups: 64.1, 66.3, and 66.6 years) assessed how closely food intake met the 2005 Dietary Guidelines for Americans. Using a scoring tool that was weighted for heart health risk showed that women with diets most closely resembling the dietary guidelines had a slower rate of atherosclerosis progression over the 3.3-year period of follow-up.[13] Much of the research literature deals with contributions of nutrition to heart health because that is the leading, modifiable, disease in older adults. Healthy People 2020 goals (see Table 18.2) that are especially applicable to older adults with medical conditions are: to maintain physical activity for muscle strength, to reduce obesity, and to increase total vegetable consumption. This chapter addresses the role of nutrition as a factor in disease prevention, treatment, and recovery of overall health in adults aged 65 and older.

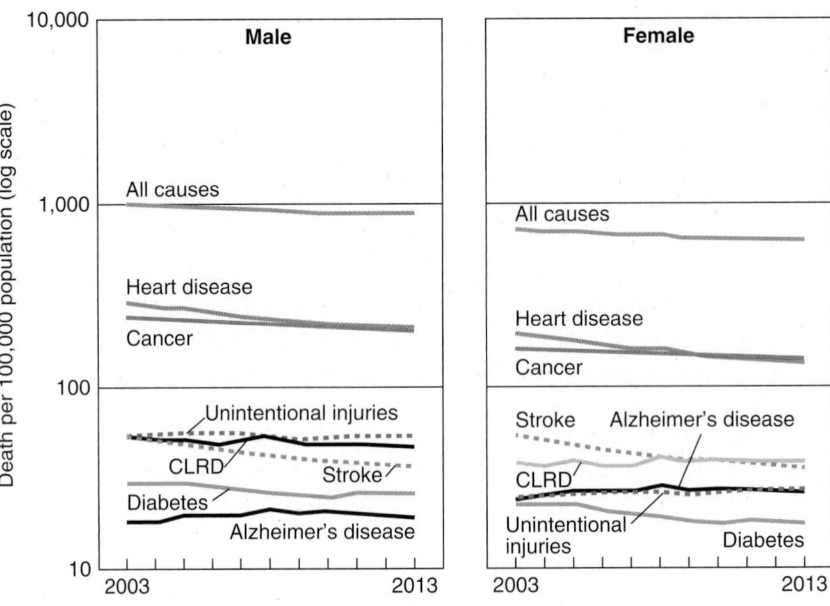


ILLUSTRATION 19.1 ▸ Selected causes of deaths.

SOURCE: CDC/NCHS, *Health, United States, 2014*, Figure 3 and Table 18. Data from the National Vital Statistics System (NVSS).[14]

TABLE 19.2 ▸ Number of deaths in the United States in 2013, by leading causes

| CAUSE OF DEATH | NUMBER OF DEATHS (2013) |
|---|---|
| Heart Disease | 488,156 |
| Malignant Neoplasm | 407,558 |
| Chronic Lower Respiratory Disease | 127,194 |
| Cerebrovascular Disease | 109,602 |
| Alzheimer Disease | 83,786 |
| Diabetes Mellitus | 53,751 |
| Influenza and Pneumonia | 48,751 |
| Unintentional Injury | 45,942 |
| Nephritis | 39,080 |
| Septicemia | 28,815 |

SOURCE: National Vital Statistics, National Center for Health Statistics, CDC.[9]

# Heart Disease

**LO 19.2** Describe key nutritional approaches to heart disease in adults 65+, recognizing the heterogeneity of older populations.

For a disease with modifiable risk factors, heart disease is still the leading cause of death in older adults and the leading cause of their hospitalizations. For example, for every 10,000 individuals aged 85 and older in year 2009–2010, 5,668 had short hospital stays, and when looking at their discharge diagnoses 1,055 were for heart disease, with the next highest number (525) for injuries (397 of those were for fractures; more on that under osteoporosis).[14] The adult risk factors and course of heart diseases were discussed in Chapter 17. Specifics for older adults are highlighted in this section, including stroke and hypertension.

## Prevalence

Cardiovascular disease (CVD), which includes coronary heart disease, heart failure, stroke, and hypertension, rises with age. Heart disease prevalence varies by age, race, and gender.[15] After age 80, less than 15 percent of men and 14 percent of women are free of heart disease.[16] It is more prevalent among men and Non-Hispanic Whites. The American Heart Association (AHA) publishes updated statistics on the prevalence of CVD.

## Risk Factors

Risk factors for CVD in old age remain the same as in younger adults, except that the factors have less predictive value in old age.[17] Results of a study by Odden and colleagues and supported by findings from other studies, indicated that elevated LDL cholesterol and obesity were not associated with cardiovascular events in persons older than 65 years. Also, elevated systolic blood pressure and low HDL cholesterol were associated with cardiovascular events only in persons <85 years. Other emerging risk factors such as kidney function, diabetes, inflammation and cardiac strain (cardiac contractility) were better predictors of cardiovascular events in older adults. The authors suggest that these risk factors may capture lifelong insults to the cardiovascular system and may be better measures of cardiovascular outcomes.[17] This is an ongoing and active area of research. Eating a Mediterranean-style diet is associated with lower CVD mortality, as is engaging in physical activity and not smoking. Fewer than 1 in 10 adults age 65 and over are current smokers.

## Nutritional Remedies for Cardiovascular Diseases

Assertive treatment can modify the course of heart disease at any age, although an older adult is more likely to have comorbid conditions that necessitate balancing multiple goals. Together, the older adult and his or her health care providers can develop a treatment plan that balances health and quality-of-life goals.

Basic questions address an individual's motivation to adopt and maintain heart-healthy routines. The individual may be wondering whether potential health gains are worth the necessary changes. Is the individual balancing quality of life with potential life expectancy? For individuals who are new to cooking or have become bored with it, are there classes that demonstrate how to prepare whole grains, cook new vegetables, or find ways to add fish into a meal plan? Will the budget support buying additional fruits and vegetables and eating at restaurants that offer more heart-healthy choices? If function is limited, what are the resources available to build a sustainable exercise routine? Is the person willing to ask for and accept assistance if needed to shop for groceries or to prepare meals? Can the individual maintain heart-healthy habits when eating with family and friends, at home, or in restaurants? The nutrition interventions that support heart health are not inherently different for an older adult than for a younger one. But the day-to-day context for adopting therapeutic lifestyle changes is likely different for an 80-year-old than for a 45-year-old. An individual's view of his or her own physical and emotional status is an integral part of how treatment will be pursued and how heart-healthy habits will be maintained. Nutritional habits alter the progression of atherosclerosis only if an individual adheres to the eating plan.

In 2013, the American College of Cardiology (ACC) and AHA, in collaboration with the National Heart, Lung, and Blood Institute (NHLBI) released four guidelines focused on the assessment of cardiovascular risk, lifestyle modifications to reduce cardiovascular risk and management of elevated blood cholesterol and body weight in adults. The 2013 AHA/ACC Guideline on Lifestyle Management to Reduce Cardiovascular Risk, which are based on thorough evidence-based review of the literature on CVD modifications, provided dietary and physical activity recommendations.[18] The guidelines emphasize a dietary pattern that is rich in fruit, vegetables, whole grains, fish, low-fat dairy, lean poultry, nuts, legumes, and nontropical vegetable oils consistent with the Mediterranean- and DASH (Dietary Approaches to Stop Hypertension)-type diet. Those diets are low in sweets, sugar-sweetened beverages, and red meats. The guidelines also specify a reduction in salt intake to 2300 mg and possibly lower to 1500 mg. The recommendations do not stress fat except to suggest restricting saturated fat to 5–6 percent of calories. The task force found insufficient evidence of a relationship between dietary cholesterol and LDL cholesterol to make a recommendation.[18] Some educational considerations in applying these interventions in older audiences are described in Table 19.3. The task force also recommend that "In general, advise adults to engage in aerobic physical activity to reduce LDL–C and non-HDL–C: three to four sessions a week, lasting on average 40 minutes per session, and involving moderate-to-vigorous intensity physical activity."[18]

Consumption of fish, fish oils, and omega-3 polyunsaturated fatty acids is also of interest to older adults because these are marketed to improve memory and alleviate depression as well as to reduce heart disease. A meta-analysis of omega-3 fatty acid (EPA and DHA) supplement use found insufficient evidence of reduced risk of all-cause mortality and of cardiovascular events in patients with a history of CVD. To reach this conclusion, the Korean Meta-analysis Study Group identified over 1,000 articles and selected the 14 that had used a randomized, double-blind, placebo-controlled design. Together, these 14 studies followed 20,485 participants, age 18 and older, all with history of CVD.[19] The authors cite two large randomized controlled trials that did show CVD risk reduction from omega-3 fatty acid use (the GISSI-Prevenzione trial and the JELIS trial). These were not included in the meta-analysis because the trials did not follow a single- or double-blind design, and hence were susceptible to bias. An earlier systematic review of randomized controlled trials on the effects of fish oil supplements on arrhythmias and mortality found that

TABLE 19.3 ▸ Treatment considerations for older adults with heart disease

| TARGET AREA | ADULTS (≥ 65 YEARS) |
|---|---|
| Promote healthy fats | Focus on 1–2 items to decrease saturated fat intake rather than change multiple items |
| • Use lean meats<br>• Substitute saturated fatty acids with PUFA & MUFA<br>• Decrease synthetic *trans*-fatty acids | Ensure adequate protein intake<br>Focus on oils currently using and suggest one to change.<br>Decrease synthetic *trans*-fatty acids.<br>Consider giving a brief description of *trans*-fatty acids and sources: hydrogenated oils and shortening, cookies, pastries, and other processed fats, based on mental awareness and readiness to change.<br>Discuss fats as calorie source if overweight. |
| Promote fruits & vegetables, encourage to suppress inflammation | Work with the fruits and vegetables that the individual can chew (e.g., if dentures, do they fit?).<br>Blend pureed fruits and vegetables into sauces, soups, smoothies.<br>Consider cooking classes and online videos for preparation techniques. |
| Healthy cooking | Goals: food safety, adequate nutrient intake, matched to skills. |
| Limit salt | Focus on "no added salt," and no salt shaker on the table.<br>Assess use of convenience products, fast foods, breads, cereals. |
| Label reading | May be difficult if eyesight is poor; consider financial limits; know bargain strategies; explain discrepancies between Daily Values and DRIs. |
| Medications, taste and smell | Check if sense of smell and taste is intact. Assess whether medications impair taste or affect appetite? |
| Maintain healthy weight | Strongly influenced by functional status of individual; emphasize adequate nutrient intake. |
| Begin with motivational interviewing | Determine individual's goals for health, nutrition, and exercise. |



"fish oil supplementation was associated with a significant reduction in deaths from cardiac causes but had no effect on arrhythmias or all-cause mortality."[20] The 2013 AHA/ACC Guidelines on Lifestyle Management to Reduce Cardiovascular Risk identified the relationship between omega-3 fatty acids, inflammation and CVD risk factors as a gap in our knowledge and suggested more research.[18] Similarly, the relationship between fish oil, memory, and depression are inconclusive. Until further information is available, two servings of fatty fish per week (cold-water or marine fish) are recommended, in part to replace red meat.[21]

# Stroke

**LO 19.3** Describe key nutritional approaches to addressing strokes and related diseases in adults 65+, recognizing the heterogeneity of older populations.

AHA and the American Stroke Association describe both stroke and ***transient ischemic attack (TIAs)*** as serious conditions involving reduced cerebral blood flow (brain ***ischemia***); both are markers for increased risk of disability and death.[22] TIAs, brief episodes of neurological dysfunction such as sudden confusion, trouble speaking or understanding, or sudden dizziness and difficulty in walking, often precede a stroke. During an ischemic stroke (about 85 percent of all strokes), an obstruction clogs a blood vessel and prevents oxygen and other nutrients from reaching part of the brain. A hemorrhagic stroke occurs when a weakened blood vessel breaks, such as the rupture of an ***aneurysm***. Leaking blood accumulates, putting pressure on the surrounding tissue and eventually destroying brain cells.

## Prevalence

Of adults aged 65 and older, 8 percent of females and 9 percent of males have had a stroke, but females have a greater lifetime risk.[2] At younger ages, incidence of stroke is higher for men than women, but by age 85, incidence is greater for women. Blacks are at much higher risk than other racial/ethnic groups, but risk depends somewhat on the type of stroke. For example, age-adjusted first-ever ischemic stroke rates per 1000 occur at the rate of 1.91 in Blacks, at 1.49 in Hispanics, and 0.88 in Whites.[2,16] But for

**transient ischemic attacks (TIAs)** Temporary and insufficient blood supply to the brain.

**ischemia** Blockage of blood vessel leading to lack of blood supply.

**aneurysm** Ballooning of the blood vessel wall.

intracranial atherosclerotic stroke, rates in Hispanics are five times those in Whites. Strokes have serious potential to affect the lifestyle and nutritional behaviors of survivors. Among individuals having a first stroke at age 65 or older, 13 percent die within one month. Six months after a stroke, 35 percent of survivors had depressive symptoms, 30 percent needed some assistance walking, 26 percent were institutionalized in a nursing home, and 19 percent had *aphasia (unable to speak).*

## Etiology

Factors that can lead to a stroke include blocked arteries (by a ***thrombus*** or ***cerebral embolism***), easily clotting blood cells, and weak heartbeats that are unable to keep blood circulating through the body, allowing pools of blood to form and clot. Hypertension contributes to strokes because the force of blood may break weak vessels.

## Effects of Stroke

Strokes deprive the brain of needed oxygen and other nutrients, causing brain and nerve cells to die. As a result, stroke leads to loss of function for parts of the body controlled by the oxygen-deprived cells. For example, stroke victims' bodies may become paralyzed in either the left or the right side, or they may become unable to speak (aphasia), walk, or swallow. Nutrition is likely to be affected in the stroke aftermath. Quick recognition of stroke results in faster treatment and better recovery. Although dead brain cells cannot be replaced, new nerve pathways can develop in the gray-matter reservoirs of the brain. The ability to develop new neural pathways provides hope for successful rehabilitation therapies. Relearning how to feed oneself, how to chew, and how to swallow may well be a part of the slow, arduous process of rehabilitation.

## Risk Factors

Geography seems to be a risk factor for increased mortality from stroke; the southeastern part of the country is considered the stroke belt, death rates are 20–40 percent higher here than in the rest of the country.[16] A study funded by the National Institute of Health named REasons for Geographic and Racial Differences in Stroke (REGARDS) is attempting to identify the reasons for this geographical disparity. Part of the answer is attributed to the usual risk factors such as hypertension, diabetes and the lifestyle factors, diet and smoking, however, these do not appear to completely explain the discrepancy. Research is ongoing to examine genetic and other lifestyle factors.[23] A strong predictor for incurring a stroke is age. Young adults rarely have strokes. In the 20- to 39-year-old age group, 0.2 percent of males and 0.7 percent of females had a stroke per year.[16] Stroke prevalence rose to 15.8 percent for males and 14.0 percent for females aged 80 and older. The risk of having a stroke rises sharply after midlife. Prevalence of stroke in adults age 80 and older is approximately twice that of adults aged 60–79 years. The additional presence of multiple chronic conditions complicates stroke prevention. The following factors place an individual at higher risk for stroke:

- Long-term high blood pressure (either systolic or diastolic)
- Family history
- African American, Asian, and Hispanic ethnicity
- Physical inactivity
- Cigarette smoking (doubles the risk of ischemic strokes)
- Comorbid conditions, including diabetes mellitus, ***carotid artery disease***, ***atrial fibrillation***, TIAs, sickle cell anemia, and depression
- Living in poverty
- Excessive use of alcohol; use of cocaine and illicit intravenous drugs

The role of alcohol is complex and controversial. Moderate amounts of any type of alcohol can be protective against stroke, while excessive amounts increase stroke risk significantly. In Japan, a 10.5-year prospective study with nearly 3,000 men aged 40 to 69 years (only 5 percent of women drank in Japan at that time) found the least risk at 42 grams of alcohol per day (a typical drink contains 12–15 grams of alcohol).[24] Men who consumed more than 70 grams of alcohol per day were 2.5 times more likely to have a stroke than the low-risk group. In a Framingham study of alcohol use and ischemic strokes in older adults, up to two drinks (or 24–30 grams of alcohol) per day counted as "moderate."[25] Moderate intake was protective, but public health advice for nondrinkers is not to start.

## Nutritional Remedies

Stroke prevention programs for older adults tend to be secondary or tertiary rather than primary. In the United States, not enough resources are allocated to prevention programs and the emphasis has been on treatment and rehabilitation. However, this is slowly changing. A review of dietary patterns resulting in reduced risk of stroke found increasing fruit and vegetable intake (especially cruciferous ones) to be an effective strategy of primary stroke prevention.[26] These dietary eating patterns—which include the Prudent Pattern, the DASH diet, and the Mediterranean Diet—were all correlated with reduced

**aphasia** Difficulties in self-expression, including inability to speak, finding the right words or understanding print or spoken words.

**thrombus** Blood clot.

**cerebral embolism** Piece of a blood clot formed elsewhere that travels to the brain.

**carotid artery disease** Arteries that supply blood to the brain and neck becoming damaged.

**atrial fibrillation** Degeneration of the heart muscle causing irregular contractions.

stroke incidence. The focus of dietary advice in stroke prevention is to normalize blood pressure and follow healthy lifestyle habits, which is discussed with hypertension. Individualized medical nutritional therapy is used to promote rehabilitation after a stroke.[26]

# Hypertension

LO 19.4 Describe key nutritional approaches to hypertension in adults 65+, recognizing the heterogeneity of older populations.

High blood pressure (HBP) is a risk factor for CVD and stroke. There is currently no consensus on the definition of HBP in older adults. In the "2014 Evidence-Based Guideline for the Management of High Blood Pressure in Adults" report, the blood pressure treatment initiation and goal attainment threshold for individuals aged 60 years and older, without diabetes or chronic kidney disease, was raised to 150 mm Hg systolic blood pressure and 90 mm Hg diastolic blood pressure.[27] However, the AHA released a statement indicating that there is insufficient evidence to change the AHA current guidelines and recommends initiating treatment starting with lifestyle changes and then medication, if necessary, at blood pressure 140/90 mm Hg.[28] An individual who controls high blood pressure with medication is still considered to have hypertension, because a controlled disease is still there.

## Prevalence

Hypertension (HBP) is the only chronic condition that has higher prevalence in older adults than arthritis (see Table 19.1). In Western societies, prevalence rises with age. Before age 45, a higher proportion of men than women have HBP; then the percentages are similar until age 64, when HBP becomes more common in women. Death rates from high blood pressure are much higher for Blacks than for Whites. For example, in 2011, mortality rates were 47.1 for Black and 17.6 for White males, and 35.1 for Black and 15.2 for White females. Rates for Hispanics are similar to or lower than those for Whites.[16] There has been considerable improvement in awareness, treatment, and control of hypertension; however, undiagnosed and uncontrolled hypertension among minority groups remains a challenge. In 2011–2012, 82.7 percent of hypertensives were aware of their hypertension, 75.6 percent reported currently taking prescribed medication to lower their blood pressure, and 51.8 percent had their blood pressure controlled.[29]

## Etiology

For most adults, blood pressure tends to develop over many years, and there are no identifiable causes. Family history and ethnic background increase the risk of hypertension; African Americans are most likely to have hypertension. Salt intake is a major contributor to hypertension.[30]

## Effects of Hypertension

Prolonged high blood pressure puts extra tension on blood vessels and organs in the body, wearing them out before the natural aging process. Damaged kidneys are a common sign of uncontrolled hypertension. HBP also increases the risk of CVD for millions of people worldwide.

## Risk Factors

A number of factors increase blood pressure, such as drinking too much alcohol, high salt intake, obesity, high–saturated-fat diets leading to dyslipidemia and atherosclerosis, physical inactivity, smoking, and a diet low in calcium and potassium.[31]

## Nutritional Remedies

Nutritional strategies to normalize blood pressure include weight management, moderation of alcohol intake for those who drink, and limiting sodium intake while maintaining adequate potassium, magnesium, and calcium intakes. Also, the consumption of dietary patterns such as the DASH diet (see Table 19.4 and Table 19.5) is effective in decreasing blood pressure.[32] Researchers found beneficial effects of lifestyle modifications including the

TABLE 19.4 ▸ DASH effectiveness increases as sodium decreases, but it's not easy to consume <1500 mg

| FOOD GROUP | | MG SODIUM |
|---|---|---|
| 6 grains | Raisin bran cereal (1 cup = 2 svgs) | 217 |
| | Whole wheat bread (2 slices = 2 svgs) | 270 |
| | Pasta, cooked without salt (1 cup = 2 svgs) | 4 |
| 4 Vegetables | Steamed asparagus (1 cup = 2 svgs) | 5 |
| | Lettuce (1 cup) | 10 |
| | Cherry tomatoes and baby carrots (5 each) | 46 |
| 4 Fruits | Dried cherries (¼ cup) | 0 |
| | Mixed fresh fruit (1 cup = 2 svgs) | 10 |
| | Banana or apple (1 med) | 1 |
| 2–3 Dairy | One-percent milk (1 cup) | 107 |
| | Plain Greek yogurt (6 oz) | 71 |
| | Cheese (1 oz) | 176 |
| Meats, fish | Fried catfish, 3 oz | 240 |
| Nuts | Pecans (20 halves) or 24 almonds | 0 |
| 2 Fats, Oils | Unsalted butter (1 tsp) | 1 |
| | Salad dressing (2 Tbsp regular Italian) | 292 |

SOURCE: Food composition data, SR25 Reports by Single Nutrients; Nutrient Data Lab, National Agricultural Library, FNIC, accessed 2.8.2013 at USDA.gov

TABLE 19.5 ▸ The DASH eating plan for blood-pressure control in older adults

| | SERVINGS PER DAY | SERVING SIZES OF FOODS WITHIN THE FOOD GROUP |
|---|---|---|
| **Grains and Grain Products**<br>Especially whole-grain[a] | 6–8 | Breads: 1 slice or 1 oz<br>Cereal: ½ cup cooked or dry<br>Rice, pasta: ½ cup cooked |
| **Vegetables**<br>Fresh, frozen, no-salt-added canned | 4–5 | Raw, 1 cup; cooked, ½ cup |
| **Fruits**<br>Fresh, frozen, or canned in juice | 4–5 | Juice: 6 oz<br>Fresh: 1 med piece<br>Mixed or cut: ½ cup<br>Juice: 6 oz<br>Dried: ¼ cup |
| **Dairy Foods**<br>Skim or 1% milk, fat-free dairy products | 2–3 | Milk: 8 oz<br>Yogurt: 1 cup<br>Cheese: 1½ oz |
| **Meats, Poultry, and Fish** | Up to 2 | 3 oz, cooked |
| **Nuts, Seeds, Dry Beans** | 4–5 per week | ⅓ cup or 1½ oz nuts<br>2 Tbsp or ½ oz seeds<br>2 Tbsp nut butter<br>½ cup cooked beans (legumes) |
| **Fats and Oils**[b]<br>Select olive, canola, corn, and safflower oils | 2–3 | 1 tsp soft margarine, oils, mayonnaise<br>2 Tbsp salad dressing |
| **Sweets** | Up to 5 per week | 1 Tbsp jam, jelly, syrup, or sugar<br>½ cup sorbet, gelatin |

SOURCE: Adapted from 2000-calorie DASH eating plan, Your guide to lowering your blood pressure with DASH. National Heart, Lung, and Blood Institute, revised April 2006.

[a]Whole grain is the entire edible part of wheat, corn, rice, oats, barley, and other grains. Whole-grain bread has the words *whole grain* before the type of flour that is listed; whole-grain breakfast cereals include the word *whole* or *whole-grain* before the grain name (e.g., *whole-grain wheat*).

[b]One serving is equivalent to 5 grams of fat.

DASH diet on blood pressure, particularly in individuals over age 50.[32,33] Other nondrug interventions such as using weight reduction and/or sodium restriction of 1500–1800 mg per day over 30 months have successfully lowered the blood pressure.[33,34] This sodium level is well below average intakes (see Table 18.11).

In the DASH sodium study, the greatest overall blood pressure reduction occurred in the subjects with the strictest sodium intake limit (1500 mg a day).[34] Blood pressure reduction occurred whether individuals were normo- or hypertensive. Choosing foods with less processing can help to limit sodium intake, because approximately 75 percent of dietary sodium is attributable to manufacturing and preservation processes, with salt at the table contributing the rest. For instance, the sodium in a plain potato averages 10–15 mg, compared to 150–200 mg sodium in a serving of potato chips.

Effectiveness of the DASH eating plan continues to be tested in various settings. For example, a cardiovascular health-center team, including a dietitian, used a modified DASH approach combined with exercise to help patients in an outpatient, office-based counseling program.[35] The team saw patients (aged 55, plus or minus 12 years) for CVD and weight loss. Patients had significant weight loss (5.3 percent of body weight) that was maintained for the 2.6 years of study follow-up. Diastolic blood pressure reduction was also significant, although systolic pressure reduction was not. Several DASH-adherence scoring systems are available and useful to compare research that use DASH eating patterns as intervention. Folsom's study of CVD mortality and hypertension in nearly 21,000 women found no statistically significant outcomes using a DASH concordance score.[36] In contrast to Folsom's study, Levitan and colleagues compared four scoring methods and found that following the DASH diet led to decreased heart failure for middle-aged and older women (48–83 years old).[37] The women most closely following the DASH diet (the top quartile of diet scores) had a 37 percent lower rate of heart failure than the lowest-scoring quartile in the 7-year-long study.

The DASH diet is one of the meal plan options in dietary guidance materials because it is considered to be health promoting for the general public as well as for people with hypertension. Dietary and lifestyle changes that address hypertension are also likely to have a beneficial effect on atherosclerosis.

# Diabetes: Special Concerns for Older Adults

LO 19.5 Describe key nutritional approaches to diabetes in adults 65+, recognizing the heterogeneity of older populations.

In the National Health and Nutrition Examination Survey (NHANES) 2009–2012, more than 1 in 4 adults aged 65 years and older reported having diabetes, primarily type 2 (see Table 19.1). Native American, Latino, African American, Asian American, and Pacific Islander adults face higher risks for diabetes than do Caucasians.[38]

Individuals with diabetes are at greater risk for heart disease and its complications; diabetes itself is an independent risk factor for atherosclerosis. Of individuals with comorbid conditions, 4 out of 5 have diabetes as one of the conditions. This complicates diabetes management.

Diabetes diagnosis criteria and management goals are the same for older as for younger adults, using individualized treatment plans that include assessment of functional status, cognitive capacities, and motivation.[38] However, the 2015 standards of medical care issued by the American Diabetes Association (ADA) recommend that ***glycosylated hemoglobin A1C (HbA1c)***, the measure of glycemic control, vary according to the health status of older adults. While HbA1c of <7.0 percent is the recommended level for healthy younger adults, the recommendation is to relax the guidelines to fit older individuals who can't achieve tight control with simple measures. A reasonable HbA1c goal for healthy adults aged 65 and older is <7.5 percent; however, for those older adults with advanced diabetes complications, life-limiting comorbid illness, or substantial cognitive or functional impairment, a less-intensive glycemic target goal of HbA1c <8.0–8.5 percent is recommended.[38] Factors that may prevent an individual from achieving tight control are use of medications that increase risk of hypoglycemia, declining cognitive function or capacity for self-care, and lack of a strong support system.[39] However, old age alone is no reason to curtail care; the ADA guidelines emphasize that risk of complications from hyperglycemia should be avoided in all patients."[38]

## Effects of Diabetes

Diabetes leads to a tenfold greater risk of amputations, macular degeneration, visual loss, cataracts, glaucoma, and neuropathies (nerve damage, pain, or tingling) of the hands and feet. Hyperglycemia may lead to sodium depletion and dehydration, trace mineral depletion (zinc, chromium, magnesium), insomnia, nocturia, blurred vision, increased platelet adhesiveness related to atherosclerosis, increased infection and decreased wound healing, and aggravated peripheral vascular disease. In older adults, diabetes may exacerbate declining organ functions, making them less resilient.

Alcohol and drugs such as salicylates (aspirin) contribute to drops in blood sugar. Hypoglycemia in older adults may lead to weakness, confusion, and possible falls and fractures. Other reasons for falls include declining vision and nerve function. For example, in the Health, Aging, and Body Composition[40] study of older adults with diabetes, 22–31 percent of participants reported falling in a 12-month span. Mean age at study enrollment was 73.6 years and falls increased as participants aged. In each subsequent year of the study, the percentage of participants who self-reported falls increased (from 22 percent, to 26 percent, 30 percent, and 31 percent at study end). Individuals were at higher risk of falling if they had reduced peripheral nerve function, renal function, and vision; all are diabetes complications.

## Nutritional Interventions

One outcome of increased life spans is that older adults with diabetes now have more years to maintain desired quality of life and avoid complications. Therefore, self-management education and support are critical to preventing complications. Diabetes self-management training, to the extent that the individual is able to manage his or her own regimen, works in tandem with medical nutrition therapy and lifestyle modifications to achieve glycemic control. Special concerns for older adults include the following:

1. *Carbohydrate and fiber recommendations do not change for old age.* The primary goal is to maintain a consistent carbohydrate intake (Table 19.6).[41] There is no ideal carbohydrate intake level for persons with diabetes. For adults with type 2 diabetes, the average (but not the ideal) carbohydrate intake is 45 percent of total energy.[41] A high-carbohydrate diet might contain 58–60 percent of calories from carbohydrates. Some individuals benefit from carbohydrates with low glycemic index scores, but the most effective glycemic control at any age begins with an individualized meal plan. Carbohydrates from vegetables, fruits, whole grains, legumes, and dairy products are advisable. Individuals could benefit from following the Mediterranean, DASH, or Prudent pattern-type diet.
2. *For people with diabetic kidney disease*, "reducing the amount of dietary protein below the recommended daily allowance of 0.8 g/kg/day (based on ideal body weight) is not recommended because it does not alter glycemic measures, cardiovascular risk measures, or the course of GFR decline."[41]
3. *Assess dietary adequacy and supplement with vitamins and minerals to meet age-appropriate nutrient Dietary Reference Intake (DRI).* Routine antioxidant supplementation (vitamins E, C, and beta-carotene) is not

**glycosylated hemoglobin A1C (HbA1c)** A blood test that measures how well the blood sugar level has been maintained over the last 2 to three months.

TABLE 19.6 ▸ Comparison of cereal grain nutrients, including glycemic index, ½ cup cooked portion

| GRAIN, ½ CUP COOKED | KCAL | G CARB | G FIBER | G PRO | G FAT | MG CALCIUM | MG MAGNESIUM | GLYCEMIC INDEX |
|---|---|---|---|---|---|---|---|---|
| Amaranth | 129 | 23 | 2.3 | 4.7 | 2.4 | 58 | 87 | 74 |
| Barley | 96 | 21 | 4.3 | 2.7 | 0.3 | 9 | 22 | 35 |
| Brown rice | 108 | 22 | 2.8 | 2.5 | 0.9 | 10 | 42 | 50 |
| Corn/grits/polenta | 75 | 16 | 0.8 | 1.4 | 0.3 | 4 | 8 | 68 |
| Farina, cream of wheat | 61 | 13 | 0.6 | 1.7 | 0.2 | 105 | 6 | 51 |
| Oatmeal, steel-cut | 101 | 18 | 2.7 | 3.5 | 1.7 | 21 | 39 | 49 |
| Quinoa | 113 | 20 | 2.1 | 4.3 | 1.8 | 16 | 61 | 53 |
| Teff | 126 | 25 | 2.7 | 4.5 | 0.8 | 64 | 64 | 45 |
| Rolled Wheat | 69 | 15 | 1.9 | 2.3 | 0.4 | 11 | 26 | 45 |
| Wild rice | 83 | 17 | 1.5 | 3.3 | 0.3 | 2 | 26 | 50 |
| **Compare protein:** | | | | | | | | |
| Small egg | 59 | .4 | 0 | 4.8 | 4 | 19 | 4 | 0 |
| Peanut Butter, 1Tbsp | 95 | 3 | 1 | 4.0 | 8.1 | 7 | 25 | 35 |

G = gram

Mg = milligram

Glycemic index: Glucose = 100

SOURCE: Nutrition Data System for Research 2011, University of Minnesota.



recommended due to a lack of evidence of efficacy and concerns about potential harm.[41]

4. *Monitor functional status and modify the care plan as appropriate for the psychosocial and physical needs of an aging individual.* For example, based on 2008–2012 pooled data of the American Community Service, 52 percent of males and 32 percent of females aged 65 and over had trouble hearing, so eliciting feedback about a client's understanding during a counseling session is worth the extra time required.[42] Also, many older adults have trouble seeing; 18 percent of males and 20 percent of females aged 65 and over reported trouble seeing (even with glasses or contacts).[42] Carbohydrate counting requires vision to read labels and cognitive ability to track carbohydrate grams. Glycemic management in older adults may be harder to achieve due to altered senses; decreased mobility; difficulty in buying, preparing, or eating food; and depression, all of which may result in muscle loss from missed exercise or increased sedentary behaviors.
5. *Ask about special foods and alternative and complementary therapies.* Complementary medicine has a long history among Mexican American and Native American populations. Evening primrose oil, milk thistle, fenugreek seeds, bitter melon, and prickly pear cactus leaves (nopales) are foods used as botanical treatments. Safe complementary nutritional remedies can enhance the standard nutritional therapies. However, there is insufficient evidence to support the use of certain herbs and supplements in treating diabetes.[41] These must be clarified with the individual.
6. *Sugar alcohols (e.g., xylitol, sorbitol) in candies and gums are sweeter than sucrose and fructose and have fewer calories per gram.* Use of non-nutritive sweeteners (stevia, sucralose, saccharin, aspartame) can help to reduce total energy intake and aid in weight management.[43] Although these polyols provide fewer calories, they are not totally calorie-free foods and the food labels should be checked. High doses of some of these sweeteners often lead to diarrhea.

# Obesity

LO 19.6 Explain how sarcopenia combined with obesity affects fitness and weight management in older adults.

## Definition

The National Heart, Lung, and Blood Institute guidelines[44] and the World Health Organization[45] define obesity as a BMI of 30.0 or higher, and extreme obesity as a BMI of 40 or higher. These definitions are intended for adults of all ages. However, the underlying research for BMI cut-points relied primarily on young and middle-aged populations.[46] In older adults, BMI alone is not an adequate indicator of excess body fat associated with morbidity and mortality.

TABLE 19.7 ▸ Percent obesity (BMI > 30) in older adults in 1999–2002 and 2009–2012 NHANES data

| AGE | MALES | | FEMALES | |
|---|---|---|---|---|
| | 1999–2002 | 2009–2012 | 1999–2002 | 2009–2012 |
| 65–74 | 31.9 | 36.4 | 39.3 | 44.2 |
| 75+ | 18.0 | 27.4 | 23.6 | 29.8 |

SOURCE: Health US 2014[14], Table 64.

## Prevalence

Body composition changes with age. Population mean body weight and BMI tend to peak around age 60 and decline after age 70,[44] although the girth of the average older adult has grown along with that of the rest of the country (see Table 19.7).[14] Age-related changes in weight and BMI can mask fat gain and muscle loss. Fat-free mass decreases with age while body fat increases. Body fat is redistributed with an accumulation in the visceral (intra-abdominal) region, especially in men and intramuscularly, weakening the structure of the muscles. Therefore, determining what is healthy weight or body composition in older adults is very complex.

## Etiology, Effects, and Risk Factors of Obesity

The relationship between obesity, morbidity, and mortality in older adults is complicated. Overweight and obesity are associated with functional decline, higher disability, and higher risk of chronic conditions such as diabetes, hypertension, and stroke.[47] However, the relationship between obesity and mortality is inconclusive. This is, in part, because BMI, which does not reflect the proportion of lean muscle mass and body fat, has been used to assess body composition of older adults. Optimum BMI cut-points for older adult populations are in a U-shaped curve, and the range of BMIs associated with good health and functional status aren't necessarily the same as those for lowered mortality risk. Recent studies and meta-analysis showed that the body mass index associated with the lowest mortality falls within the overweight range and mortality increased at BMI 35 and higher[48] or at BMI over 33.[49] For older adults, extra weight during illness episodes, especially hospitalizations, seems to be protective.

Using BMI to define obesity in older adults comes with so many caveats (difficulty in measuring height, shrinking height, shifts in body composition from youth, hydration status) that assessment will be more meaningful when using BMI in conjunction with more reliable measures of excess body fat. Two large longitudinal studies that followed populations consisting of[50] or including[51] older adults suggested that abdominal obesity is a better measure of premature death than BMI. An exploration of obesity as a risk factor for stroke and transient ischemic attacks found that markers of waist circumference, waist-to-stature ratio, and

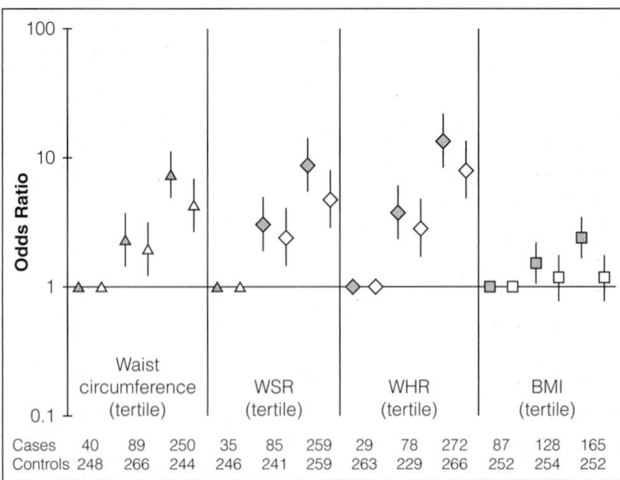


ILLUSTRATION 19.2 ▸ Association of markers of obesity with risk of stroke and TIA.

SOURCE: Yaroslav Winter, Sabine Rohrmann, Jakob Linseisen, Oliver Lanczik, Peter A. Ringleb, Johannes Hebebrand, Tobias Back, "Contribution of Obesity and Abdominal Fat Mass to Risk of Stroke and Transient Ischemic Attacks," Stroke, 2008 39(12): 3148. Reprinted with permission from Wolters Kluwer Health.

NOTE. WSR. Waist-to-Stature Ratio; WHR: Waist to Hip Ratio; TIA: Transient Ischemic Attack; Vertical bars indicate 95% Confidence Interval.

waist-to-hip ratio predicted stroke cases better than BMI (see Illustration 19.2).[52] Unintended weight loss is also a good predictor of higher mortality. Weight gain or loss as measured by changes in BMI often serve as an initial estimate for health and fitness, awaiting elaboration with a more detailed nutrition assessment. Therefore, interpretation of BMI should be in the context of health status and functional capacity. There have been also controversies on determination of the lower BMI cut-points. The results of a 2014 meta-analysis showed that the risk of mortality in older adults increased with a BMI of <23.0 and the lowest risk of mortality was BMI 24.0–30.9.[49] In younger adults, BMI <18.5 is considered underweight.[44] See Table 19.8 for a compilation of BMI ranges suggested for use with older adults.

In older populations' health, fitness plays an essential role. One can maintain weight while losing muscle and organ tissue, resulting in ***sarcopenia*** and declining function. Approximately one-fourth of adults aged 65 and over found it difficult or impossible to walk a quarter of a mile or to climb up 10 steps without resting.[2] Feeling weak is likely to contribute to reduction in aerobic and strength-building activities. An example of how cardiorespiratory fitness contributes to longevity comes from the Aerobics Center Longitudinal Study, in which 2,603 adults with a mean age of 64 years were followed for 12 years.[53] Fit individuals, even with a BMI of 30–34.9, had greater longevity.

A consensus is still lacking on the definition of obesity in older adults and criteria for evaluating and treating obesity. High values of waist circumference alone or in conjunction with BMI may be a better definition of obesity in this

**sarcopenia** Muscle wasting

TABLE 19.8 ▸ BMI values suggested for use with older adults

| SCREENING/ASSESSMENT TOOL OR RESEARCHER | BMI ($KG/M^2$) THAT REPRESENTS SMALLEST RISK OF MALNUTRITION | COMMENT |
|---|---|---|
| Mini Nutritional Assessment (MNA), see Illustration 18.3 | ≥23.0 | "Obese" does not generate higher risk scores; tool developed by Nestle Nutrition Institute |
| Malnutrition Universal Screening Tool (MUST), www.bapen.org.uk | >20.0 and no recent weight loss | A BMI of 30.0 or greater does not generate a higher risk score; developed for use in communities and long-term care settings |
| Nutrition Screening Initiative (NSI), Physician's Guide to Nutrition in Chronic Disease Management | 22.0–27.0 | Developed by American Academy of Family Physicians, the NSI and ADA; partly funded by Ross Products, Abbott Laboratories |
| G.M. Price et al.[50] | Assess diet and health status when BMI <23.0 in men and <22.3 in women | At age 75 or older, use waist-to-hip ratio |
| K.M. Flegal et al.[48] | 18.5 to <35.0 | Body mass index associated with lowest mortality |
| J.E. Winter [49] | 24.0 to 30.9<br>Monitor weight status at BMI <23.0 | Body mass index associated with lowest mortality<br>Mortality started to increase at BMI 33.0 |



population, however, waist circumference cut-off points also need to be further evaluated. The 2013 task force for the management of overweight and obesity in adults determined that there were not enough data available to make a recommendation on healthy BMI in older adults or even on strategies and prescriptions for weight loss.[44]

### Nutritional Remedies

Weight loss in obese older adults can improve functional status and chronic disease symptoms, but it needs to occur while maintaining muscle and organ tissue.

***Sarcopenic obesity*** may complicate intentional weight loss in older adults. Body weight lost contains more lean tissue than body weight regained, resulting in ever-increasing levels of body fat. In a study of post-menopausal women, 0.26 kilogram (kg) lean was lost for every kg of fat; regained weight was composed of 0.12 kg lean for each kg of fat.[54] Weight loss to ameliorate obesity can be harmful if there is no plan for preventing regain or for maintaining muscle and organ mass. A healthy eating program is based on sufficient nutrient-dense calories to support a gradual loss of fat and minimize bone or muscle tissue loss. Weight management was discussed in earlier chapters; a balance of servings from basic food groups, such as outlined in the MyPlate, the DASH eating patterns or the Mediterranean diet, can promote health in older as well as younger adults. Comorbidities in older adults may require the help of a registered dietitian to balance various nutrition priorities, such as sodium, protein, and saturated fat restrictions when high blood pressure and kidney disease complicate diabetes in an obese individual.

Physical activity promotes functional independence. Physical activity, especially resistance exercise or strength training, is the only way to prevent muscle loss.[55] Functional limitations need not be barriers to exercise. Physical therapists and community and seniors' centers can be helpful resources to develop and promote special routines using chairs, a pool, and adaptive tools. Generally, the best approach is to prevent weight gain from middle-age to older age. Also, recent recommendations suggest that obese older adults should focus on weight maintenance rather than weight loss and participation in a combination of aerobic and resistance exercise to improve function.[56]

## Osteoporosis

LO 19.7 Describe key nutritional approaches to osteoporosis in adults 65+, recognizing the heterogeneity of older populations.

### Definition

*Osteoporosis* means "porous bone." Disruption of bone architecture and reduced bone mass can result from an imbalance of available nutrients, shifts in hormones, or both. Osteoporosis progression depends on the homeostatic mechanism involved. An accelerated phase of bone loss occurs due to estrogen or testosterone loss. Bone mass loss is greater for women, who can lose up to 20 percent in the 5–7 years past menopause.[57] However, after age 65, the rate of loss slows to less than 1 percent per year. Men develop osteoporosis later than women because they have larger frames, and their testosterone levels fall more slowly. However, in males with prostate cancer, bone mass losses double when androgen deprivation is initiated.

**sarcopenic obesity** Low lean body mass combined with excessive fat stores.

World Health Organization criteria for bone mass density (BMD, based on measures such as dual-energy x-ray absorptiometry or DXA scans) are used worldwide to diagnose osteoporosis. BMD that falls 2.5 or more standard deviations below values for healthy young adults denotes osteoporosis.[58] BMD that is 1–2.5 standard deviations below the adult normal is diagnosed as low bone density (osteopenia) and increases fracture risk.

A DXA measures bone mass or density. However, bone tissue is not static. In order to measure the effect various nutrients or medications have on the constant remodeling of bone, researchers are developing biochemical markers to predict age- and menopause-related bone turnover and the risk for fracture. For example, two bone resorption measures involve cross-linked ***telopeptides*** of type 1 collagen (the major collagen of bone and tendons). These molecules split carbon and nitrogen terminals from collagen chains, resulting in elevated levels of serum C-telopeptide and urinary N-telopeptide. Telopeptide excretion is reported as a ratio to creatinine. Both serum and urine telopeptides are elevated in osteoporosis, rheumatoid arthritis, and bone cancer. Levels decline after treatment with antiresorptive medications. Bone formation can be measured by serum bone-specific alkaline phosphatase or osteocalcin tests.[59]

## Prevalence

Prevalence of osteoporosis varies by age and ethnicity. For every one man diagnosed with osteoporosis, four women have the disease. The prevalence of osteoporosis ranged in men from 3 percent (age 50–59) to 10 percent (age 80+) and in women 7 percent (age 50–59) to 35 percent (age 80+).[60] Blacks have greater BMD and therefore lower overall rates of osteoporosis than Caucasians. When compared with the age-adjusted prevalence of osteoporosis in Non-Hispanic White women (15 percent), the age-adjusted prevalence of osteoporosis is higher in Mexican-American women (26 percent) and lower in Non-Hispanic Black women (9 percent).[60] Prevalence rates for osteoporosis are elusive because osteoporosis has no symptoms, such as feeling one's bones becoming weaker. Diagnosis relies on BMD measurement or fracture. The chance that an adult over age 50 will have an osteoporosis-related fracture during the remainder of his or her life span is approximately 1 in 2 for women and 1 in 4 to 5 for men.[61]

## Etiology

Bone mass is gained primarily during growth periods, with peak bone density reached between age 18 and 30. Subsequently, bone mass remains stable until about age 40–50 for women (menopause) and about age 60 for men. Inadequate building of peak bone mass coupled with significant bone loss leads to low bone density.

**Inadequate Bone Mass** Although osteoporosis is seen most often in the elderly, the risk for developing osteoporosis in later years begins during childhood and adolescence. Development of osteoporosis is delayed when an individual develops bigger, denser bones during youth.[61] For example, an epidemiological study in Yugoslavia showed that higher calcium intake in youth led to higher peak bone mass, independent of exercise and other factors. Higher bone mass is associated with slower decline in later life.[62] Studies in the United States have also shown that getting enough calcium during growth spurts (ages 11–17) reduces the risk of osteoporosis. In an intervention study, girls aged 11–12 years who received calcium supplements (500 mg calcium citrate-malate) gained an additional 1.3 percent bone mineral density per year compared to controls.[63]

Inactivity, including bed rest and a sedentary lifestyle, leads to loss of bone and muscle tissue. Bone mass develops in response to weight-bearing or resistance exercises because bone grows in response to pressure on the bone tissue. The more often and the harder you push on the bone (not enough to break it, of course), the more the body will respond by depositing minerals (calcium, magnesium, phosphorus, fluoride, and boron) into the bone matrix. For instance, tennis players have significantly higher bone mass in their playing arm than do nonathletic counterparts. Individuals have greater bone mass in their dominant arm than in the less-used one. Exercise also stimulates growth hormone, which in turn stimulates bone development. "Use it or lose it" applies here. Adults who are frail may fear falling and fracture to the degree that it prevents them from getting much-needed exercise, contributing to a vicious circle.

**Increased Bone Loss** The skeleton acts as structural support and as a calcium reservoir for the body. Bone tissue includes jawbones and teeth. Bones and teeth contain about 99 percent of the calcium in an adult. The remaining 1 percent of calcium is found linked with protein in blood, soft tissues, and extracellular fluids. This reservoir is used for nerve transmission, muscle contraction, and enzyme systems such as those controlling blood clotting. Maintaining nerve transmissions takes physiologic priority over maintaining bone structure. In order for calcium to be consistently available, it is tightly regulated by hormone systems. Parathyroid hormone (PTH) levels are increased by low blood 25-hydroxy vitamin D levels, by high phosphate levels, and by low calcium levels. When calcium levels in the blood fall, the body responds by secreting more PTH. PTH acts to raise blood calcium levels by increasing dietary calcium absorption, decreasing urinary excretion, and by releasing calcium from bone. People with hypoparathyroidism take calcium supplements because there is not enough PTH to stimulate release of calcium from the bone reservoir in order to raise calcium levels to normal. The hormone calcitonin

**telopeptides** Molecules that degrade the major collagen of tendon and bone and leave carbon and nitrogen fragments in blood and urine.

slows release of stored calcium. Calcitonin secretion is stimulated when blood calcium levels are high.

Bone mineral reserves are dissolved (resorption) and rebuilt continuously. A consistent dietary supply of bone-building minerals (i.e., calcium, magnesium, phosphorus, fluoride, boron, zinc, copper, and manganese) and vitamins (primarily D) coupled with regular weight-bearing exercise helps maintain the skeletal mineral reserves. When a portion of this build-dissolve-rebuild cycle is malfunctioning, the body's first priority is to maintain blood calcium levels for nerve, muscle, and enzyme functions.

Osteoporosis can develop from a shortage of phosphorus during bone mineralization. A varied diet provides a balanced calcium–phosphate ratio and allows both nutrients to be used by the osteoblasts (cells that build bone). Lack of sufficient phosphorus promotes release of calcium from the skeleton. Although phosphorus is abundant in the food supply, some antacids bind with phosphorus, making it unusable by the body and delaying bone formation until more phosphate is available. Shortage of vitamin D also delays bone mineralization.

Finally, the process of normal aging results in a slow increase of PTH as well as a decrease in the skin's ability to make vitamin D; both lead to bone loss.

## Effects of Osteoporosis

**Falls and Fractures** Not everyone who falls sustains a fracture. However, unintentional falls were the leading cause of deaths from injury among adults aged 65 and older in 2013.[64] Fractures and the resulting injuries may make it impossible for an older adult to remain independent. Ten to 20 percent of older persons who break a hip die within a year.[65] Death is not due to the fracture itself but to complications resulting from the break. One of these complications is impaired mobility, complicating all the activities of daily living (including eating and exercising). If an older adult has also had a stroke, impaired mobility becomes the leading cause of institutionalization in the United States. Furthermore, 50 percent of older individuals who fracture a hip have permanent functional disabilities. Falls generate fear in older adults; these feared events are largely preventable.

**Shrinking Height, Kyphosis** In contrast to hip fractures, most vertebral fractures (67 percent) are asymptomatic. Postmenopausal women with compression and/or a bone fracture in the spinal column have a condition known as "shrinking height," leading to dowager's hump (also known as *kyphosis*, meaning a bent upper spine). Shrinking in height is slow and usually not painful. For example, a woman who was 5 feet 6 inches tall at age 30 may measure 5 feet tall at age 83. She may not notice the gradual height loss until someone comments or until she notices that clothes no longer fit. Compression of vertebrae can be a reason for increasing lumbar vertebrae bone mass in DXA scans, making wrist and hip scores better predictors of osteoporosis.

**Risk Factors** A typical osteoporosis patient is a petite, elderly White female. Brittle bones develop from a complex array of physiological factors, including poor nutrition and lack of exercise (Table 19.9). The World Health Organization (WHO) developed an online calculator that generates a 10-year probability of fracture based on several risk factors, such as age, height, weight, smoking, having had a previous fracture, and bone mass density score based on the type of DXA machine used (FRAX™ algorithm available at http://www.shef.ac.uk/FRAX/tool.jsp?locationValue=9).

## Nutritional Remedies

**Calcium** On average, older Americans are consuming 300–450 mg less calcium than the DRI, which is 1200 mg per day (see Table 18.11). The goal is to provide enough available calcium and vitamin D through diet or supplements so that bone loss is minimized despite declining absorption rates. Many foods are good sources of calcium, and a sample meal plan that provides the DRI for calcium is shown in Table 19.10.

Adhering to a calcium supplementation routine may not be any easier than eating a healthful diet every day. In a five-year, double-blind, placebo-controlled study with nearly 1,500 women, mean age 75 years, the authors concluded that supplementation with 1200 mg of calcium

**TABLE 19.9** Risk factors associated with osteoporosis in older adults

| Not Modifiable |
|---|
| Female, multiple pregnancies, intervals between pregnancies |
| Age at which pregnancy(ies) occurred, breastfeeding |
| Family history of osteoporosis, maternal history of hip fracture |
| Caucasian, Asian |
| Thin, small-boned rather than large-boned |
| History of amenorrhea, premature menopause |
| Hypogonadism, low levels of testosterone |
| Extensive steroid use |
| **Potentially Modifiable** |
| Muscle wasting, sarcopenia |
| Cigarette smoking |
| Long-term dietary phosphorus deficiency (e.g., use of phosphorus-binding antacid) |
| Heavy alcohol consumption |
| Malnourished |
| Inadequate dietary calcium, vitamin D intake |
| **Still Controversial or Not Yet Clear** |
| Diet high in sweetened carbonated beverages |
| Inadequate fluoride, boron, and magnesium in diet |
| Renal acid load from excessive protein and/or low fruit and vegetable intake |

TABLE 19.10 ▸ An example of one day's food that provides at least 1200 mg calcium

| FOOD | AMOUNT OF CALCIUM (MG) |
|---|---|
| Oatmeal made with milk 1 cup total | 266 |
| Banana, one medium | 6 |
| Coffee, 10 oz with 1 oz (2 Tbsp) evaporated milk | 87 |
| Turkey sandwich on whole-wheat bread, lettuce, mayonnaise | 54 |
| Cheese added to sandwich, 1 oz cheddar | 148 |
| Canned fruit cocktail, ½ cup | 9 |
| Iced tea, plain | 0 |
| Orange juice, calcium-fortified, 8 oz | 289 |
| Roasted almonds, 2 Tbsp | 33 |
| Pasta with chicken, 1½ cup | 54 |
| Tomato slices, 2 | 2 |
| Sugar cookie, 1 medium | 5 |
| Chocolate milk, 8 oz | 287 |



TABLE 19.11 ▸ Dietary components that contribute to calcium in urine

| | CALCIUM LOST IN URINE |
|---|---|
| Salt: for 1 gram salt (NaCl) (approximately 400 mg sodium) | ~26 mg |
| Protein: for 1 gram dietary protein | ~1 mg |
| Protein amount in 1 oz of meat, fish, poultry, or egg | ~7 mg |
| Quarter-pound hamburger | ~25–30 mg |
| Caffeine: 6 oz of regular coffee | ~40 mg |



carbonate per day "is effective in those patients who are compliant."[66] The problem in recommending calcium supplementation to prevent clinical fractures was "poor long-term compliance."

**Balancing Nutrients for Bone Health** While calcium is the best-known nutrient when it comes to bone health, other dietary components contribute to the complex relationships among hormones, muscles, and bones. Depending on level of intake, some nutrients interfere with calcium metabolism (see Table 19.11). High protein levels lead to greater calcium excretion, although losses are small. In the Nurses Health Study, women (aged 35 to 59, followed for 12 years) who ate more than 95 grams protein per day suffered more osteoporotic forearm (but not hip) fractures.[67] On the other hand, Heaney and Layman reviewed the role of protein in sarcopenia and bone health and concluded that "higher protein diets are actually associated with greater bone mass and fewer fractures when calcium intake is adequate."[68] They found that high-protein diets (30 percent of energy) did not lead to excess calcium excretion in urine. Instead, low protein intakes were associated with lowered intestinal calcium absorption and increased PTH levels.

To promote the effective daily remodeling of bone, several nutritional habits can improve calcium intake and absorption:

- Consume calcium-rich beverages like milk and kefir or yogurt drinks with a meal: food slows intestinal transit time and allows more calcium to be absorbed from the gut; protein from dairy products becomes substrate for new bone matrix.
- Increase fruit and vegetable intake for their alkalinizing effect; the alkaline environment improves calcium balance by inhibiting bone resorption.[68,69,70]
- Consume foods that are rich in bone-building vitamins and minerals at recommended levels. This balance will promote bone synthesis of the collagen matrix, into which minerals are deposited during bone mineralization.
- Vitamin D stimulates active calcium transport in the small intestine and colon; for residents of locales with seasonally ineffective sun exposure, supplemental vitamin D can maintain blood levels to suppress PTH and increase calcium absorption. Aim for 800–1000 IU per day.[59]
- High sodium intake leads to higher levels of urinary calcium.
- Caffeine to equal 2–3 cups of coffee daily (in postmenopausal women), consumed in conjunction with a low calcium intake, has been associated with bone loss.
- If taking supplements, divide dosage throughout the day for greater absorption. Carbonate is better absorbed with food, while citrate is well absorbed with or without food. Take calcium at a different time than antacids, because stomach acidity enhances absorption. In cases where stomach acidity is decreased, calcium citrate is more soluble than calcium carbonate.

**Exercise** Weight-bearing exercise builds bones and muscle, which work in tandem to enhance balance and prevent falls. Bed rest and immobilization lead to rapid loss of bone mass; patients who are institutionalized will not stay strong without concerted effort.

## Other Issues Affecting Nutritional Remedies

**Hormones** Hormones direct the dynamic system of bone remodeling. Estrogen, testosterone, growth hormone, and insulin-like growth factor-1 (IGF-1) increase intestinal calcium absorption. Hormone replacement, with or without additional calcium, can effectively increase bone mineral density in postmenopausal women. However, in 2002, the

Women's Health Initiative reported increased rates of breast cancer, coronary heart disease, stroke, and venous thromboembolism in addition to decreased rates of hip fracture and colorectal disease from estrogen replacement.[71]

**Medications** Serotonin reuptake inhibitors (SSRIs) such as Prozac are frequently prescribed for depression; they are associated with bone loss. Serotonin produced in the duodenum suppresses osteoblast proliferation. There are intricate links between the skeleton, gut, and brain.[72] It seems easy to accept that blood cells and taste buds are renewed in a matter of days, but it is not so easy to picture bones as a dynamic tissue that is being remodeled continuously, even in old age. The remodeling systems of older adults are just not quite as efficient and resilient as those of younger adults.

In summary, the best osteoporosis prevention strategy is an adequate diet and exercise in young people when bones are first growing. For older individuals who have brittle bones, a nutrient-dense diet, potentially supplemented with calcium and vitamin D, coupled with appropriate exercise, strengthens bones. Bone-building medications require a physician's care.

TABLE 19.12 ▸ Proportion of older people who reported having no natural teeth, by age, race, and poverty

| AGE AND RACE[a] | NO NATURAL TEETH IN 2011–2012 (%) |
|---|---|
| Age 65–74 | 13.0 |
| Age 75 and older | 26.0 |
| White | 16.9 |
| Black or African American | 29.2 |
| Hispanic | 14.9 |
| **For ages 65 and older, by economic status,[b]** | |
| Near poor (100 to 200% of poverty) | 31.8 |
| Poor (<100% poverty) | 38.2 |
| Not poor (<200% of poverty) | 16.4 |

[a]SOURCE: CDC/NCHS, CDC/NCHS, National Health and Nutrition Examination Survey, 2011–2012, Data Brief, No. 197, May 2015, available at: http://www.cdc.gov/nchs/data/databriefs/db197_table.pdf#4, accessed 6/16/15.

[b]SOURCE: CDC/NCHS, National Health Interview Survey, 2011–2013, interactive data warehouse, "Trends in Health and Aging." Available at http://www.cdc.gov/nchs/hdi.htm, accessed 6/16/15.

# Oral Health

LO 19.8 Identify three or more nutritional strategies that contribute to oral health.

It is possible to be well nourished without a full set of teeth, or even without any teeth at all (edentulous). However, the ability to bite and chew facilitates fruit and vegetable intake, which is linked to better health. Fortunately, more people are keeping their teeth as a result of better dental care. At the turn of the century, about one-third of all adults had no natural teeth; now that number has dropped to less than one-fourth of older adults who have no natural teeth. Edentulousness differs by race and is twice as likely among the poor and near poor (Table 19.12). Chewing is more effective with natural teeth; individuals who wear complete dentures have approximately 20 percent of the chewing ability of those having all natural teeth.[73] Foods can be cut, sliced, chopped, grated, and made into smoothies and soups to ensure a varied diet when chewing ability is impaired. Lack of natural teeth does not have to result in a poor diet, however, this requires more effort. Nutrition education may be essential to assist in planning healthy diets. Studies have shown associations between edentulousness and inadequate intake of certain vitamins and minerals.[74,75]

Changes in oral health are most likely to be a result of disease, medical treatment, or medications rather than aging itself. ***Xerostomia*** (known as dry mouth) and periodontal disease (PD) are two conditions that can interfere with food tolerance and with enjoyment of food. Xerostomia is a symptom of Sjogren's syndrome, however, medications and other treatments are the most likely causes of dry mouth in the older population. For example, diuretic treatment for hypertension leads to decreased salivary secretion; other medications associated with dry mouth include anti-anxiety drugs, antidepressants, sedatives, and antihistamines. Head and neck cancer treatment can also lead to xerostomia when the salivary glands are involved. Lack of saliva for any reason gives bacteria a better environment to build plaque and damage teeth. Saliva helps to recoat the teeth with minerals and slow down infections. Xerostomia is often accompanied by loss of taste (dysgeusia) and pain of the tongue (glossodynia), factors that further interfere with the enjoyment of food.

The key treatment of xerostomia is good oral hygiene, especially after meals, plus stimulating saliva with sugar-free candy, frozen fruit bits, chewing sugar-free gums (xylitol, maltitol), and frequent sips of water. Artificial saliva and specialized mouth washes can also help to keep the oral cavity moist.

PD results from bacterial infections of the ***gingiva***, leading to destruction of the ligaments attaching teeth to the jawbone and to receding gums. Plaque builds up in the resultant pockets, contributing to further infection and eventual tooth loss. Over the years 2009 to 2012, 46 percent of U.S. adults had periodontitis.[76] PD increases with age, is higher in males than females, highest in Hispanics and Non-Hispanic Blacks and lowest in Non-Hispanic Whites. Persons whose overall health and immune system are compromised are at greater risk for periodontal disease. PD is associated with atherosclerotic vascular disease (ASVD),

**xerostomia** Dry mouth can be a side effect of medications (especially antidepressants), of head and neck cancer treatments, of diabetes, and also a symptom of Sjogren's syndrome, which is an autoimmune disorder for which no cure is known.

**gingiva** Gum tissue.

although treatment that reduces PD and systemic inflammation has not yet been shown to prevent ASVD[77] Prevention of PD emphasizes strict oral hygiene to remove plaque, enhance immune status, and ensure optimal nutrition. Evidence from an observational study using NHANES data found that DHA and EPA intakes at modest levels were associated with lower prevalence of PD in adults.[78] Additionally, intervention studies with omega-3 fatty acids showed an improvement in certain periodontal disease indicators compared to control subjects. It is hypothesized that omega-3 fatty acids may reduce chronic inflammation and hence reduce the symptoms of periodonditis.[79] However, more research is needed before recommending these omega-3 fatty acids for oral health. Besides deficiencies of vitamin C and zinc that are associated with PD, correcting potential deficiencies of calcium, vitamin D, and magnesium will help postmenopausal women keep their bones, including the jaw, strong. Ensuring optimal nutrition includes management of diabetes. High blood sugar raises glucose in saliva, leading to caries and accelerated periodontal disease. It can also make the mouth more susceptible to yeast infection (candidiasis). Diabetes control translates into better oral health.

Good oral health for older adults also includes caries prevention. Brushing, flossing, and dietary recommendations for older adults match those of younger ones.

# Gastrointestinal Diseases

LO 19.9 Describe the three most common GI problems of older adults, along with nutritional management strategies to ameliorate each condition.

The gastrointestinal (GI) system serves so many functions that it should not be surprising to learn that by late adulthood, it occasionally malfunctions. It seems miraculous that we so consistently eat what we like, without much thought, and our body converts that food to energy for daily living. Parts of the GI system most likely to malfunction in old age are:

1. The esophageal-stomach juncture: weakened muscle results in *gastroesophageal reflux disease* (GERD)
2. The stomach: decreased acidity leading to *changes in nutrient absorption*
3. The intestines: *altered motility* resulting in constipation, diarrhea, and some specific food intolerances

Often these problems are secondary to other diseases. No matter what the cause, older adults are at higher risk for the GI conditions discussed next, any of which might impair older adults' activities.

## Gastroesophageal Reflux Disease (GERD)

**Definition** GERD is a chronic disorder that results when stomach contents flow back into the esophagus, causing troublesome symptoms and/or complications. Difficulty in diagnosis led to a global consensus called the Montreal 2006 definition; it is patient centered rather than relying on endoscopic findings.[80] Contrary to earlier theories that GERD was part of a spectrum of diseases, it is now considered to be a set of discrete syndromes, with nonerosive reflux disease being the most common.

**Prevalence** Not all individuals with GERD symptoms seek medical care, so prevalence estimations can range widely. Gastroesophageal reflux disease is the most common GI-related diagnosis given in clinic visits. Prevalence statistics range from 10 percent of Americans having daily episodes of heartburn to an estimated 25–35 percent of the U.S. population being affected with GERD.[80]

**Etiology and Effects** It is not clear whether acid in the esophagus leads to a weakened ***lower esophageal sphincter (LES)*** or whether a weakened sphincter leads to GERD. The main symptoms of GERD are heartburn and acid regurgitation. Stomach contents, which are highly acidic, spill back into the esophagus, resulting in irritation, belching, hoarseness, and substernal pain. Ulceration and swallowing disorders are symptoms of severe cases of GERD. *Helicobacter pylori (H. pylori)*, a cause of peptic ulcer disease, does not cause GERD.[81] A review of the impact of gut macrobiota on human health suggests that in old age, the symbiotic bacterial mix of the gut changes due to medication usage (e.g., antibiotics), resulting in decreased anti-inflammatory protection from H-pylori strains.[82]

**Nutritional Risk Factors** Excess alcohol, obesity, and smoking are consistently linked to GERD episodes. In addition, both regular and decaffeinated coffee are associated with heartburn.

**Nutritional Remedies** The main dietary remedy is to omit foods that are chemically or mechanically irritating. Variation in symptoms among individuals has contributed to making the diagnosis of GERD reliant on a patient-centered approach rather than on straightforward lab values or measurements. However, general guidelines are to choose a low-fat diet, avoid large meals, and to take advantage of gravity by remaining upright for several hours after eating. High-fat meals and alcohol both lower LES pressure. Fermented beverages (wine, beer) and caffeine stimulate gastric acid, so reducing them may give some relief. Protein also stimulates gastric acid, so consuming the necessary protein throughout the day rather than in one or two sittings will help to minimize reflux. Spicy foods, caffeine, chocolate, peppermint, citrus, and tomato products are among potentially reflux–pain inducing foods.[80]

**lower esophageal sphincter (LES)** The muscle enabling closure of the junction between the esophagus and stomach.

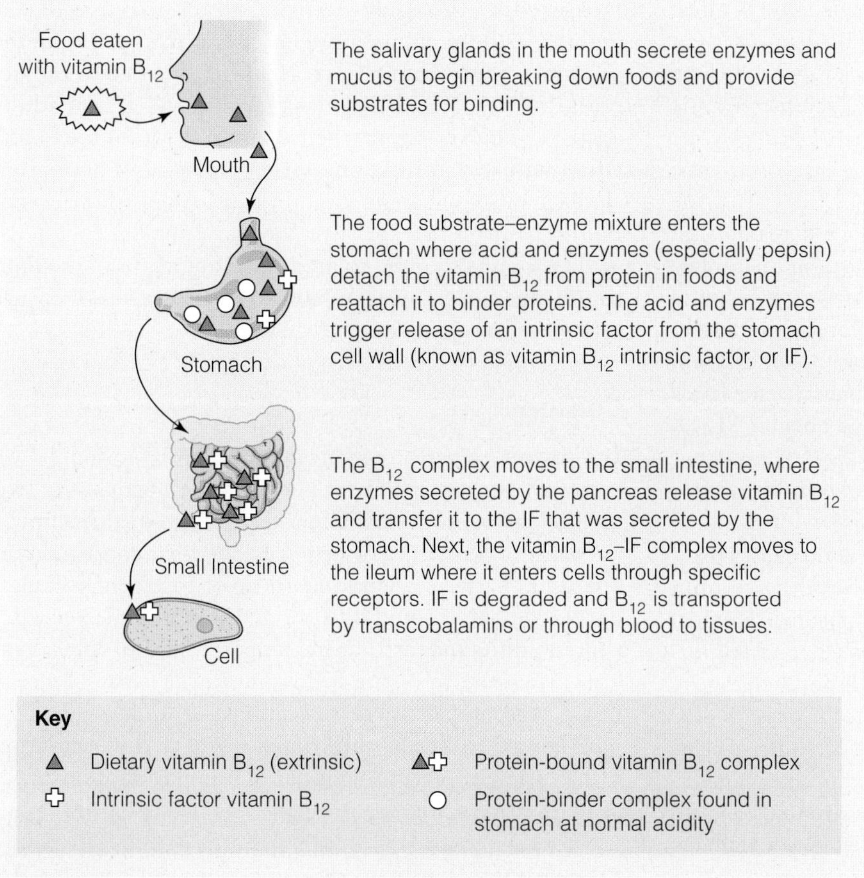


ILLUSTRATION 19.3 ▸ Overview of vitamin $B_{12}$ absorption.



## Stomach Conditions Affect Nutrient Availability: Vitamin $B_{12}$ Malabsorption

**Definition and Etiology** Absorption of vitamin $B_{12}$ from foods requires stomach acidity, enzymes (especially pepsin), and intrinsic factor (IF). Stomach acids and enzymes split off and transfer vitamin $B_{12}$ from foods to carrier proteins (mostly secreted by the salivary gland in the mouth). Then the vitamin $B_{12}$-carrier protein complex moves into the small intestine, where the vitamin $B_{12}$ will again be broken off and bound to the IF (produced in the stomach and migrated to the small intestine). The vitamin $B_{12}$–IF linked complex then binds to a specific site in the lining of the small intestine, is transported across it, and released into blood serum to be taken to tissue cells (Illustration 19.3).

Pernicious anemia and atrophic gastritis are two conditions that result in vitamin $B_{12}$ deficiency. Pernicious anemia (macrocytic megaloblastic anemia), which is due to lack of intrinsic factor (IF) being released from the stomach cell wall, is rare in individuals under 35. It is also uncommon even in older adults. The most common cause of vitamin $B_{12}$ deficiency in older adults is related to abnormal stomach function. Prolonged inflammation, followed by the atrophied stomach mucosa secreting less acid, leads to atrophic gastritis. Older adults with atrophic gastritis still absorb some dietary vitamin $B_{12}$, but they will become deficient over time. Finally, antacid treatment neutralizes stomach acid and raises stomach pH, preventing vitamin $B_{12}$ from being split from its protein carrier, even though the intrinsic vitamin $B_{12}$ factor is present. Symptoms of vitamin $B_{12}$ deficiency begin to appear after 3–6 years of poor absorption.

**Prevalence and Detection** *Cobalamin* (vitamin $B_{12}$) deficiency may be an underrecognized problem in older adults because the criteria used to assess $B_{12}$ status is not consistent. Estimations of deficiency range from under 1 percent to 46 percent of the population, depending on the criteria used for diagnosis.[83] In a national study among a representative sample of the United States population, the prevalence of low serum vitamin $B_{12}$ ranged from 3–26 percent depending on the cut-off levels used.[84] Low serum vitamin $B_{12}$ was higher in women than men and depending on the criteria used, tended to be higher

**cobalamin** Another name for vitamin $B_{12}$. Important roles of cobalamin are fatty-acid metabolism, synthesis of nucleic acid (i.e., DNA, a complex protein that controls the formation of healthy new cells), and formation of the myelin sheath that protects nerve cells.

for adults aged 60 and over and in Non-Hispanic Whites. In the United States, intake of vitamin $B_{12}$ is more than adequate (see Table 18.11), so low blood levels need to be evaluated in relation to other conditions such as atrophic gastritis, anemia, osteoporosis and CVD.

Vitamin $B_{12}$ status is dependent on two other nutrients: vitamin $B_6$ and folic acid. Blood levels of the coenzyme ***homocysteine*** could reflect a deficiency of dietary intake in one of any of the three nutrients. In contrast, another intermediate product, ***methylmalonic acid (MMA)***, is only found in a vitamin $B_{12}$–specific pathway. Therefore, rising blood levels of MMA occur when adequate amounts of vitamin $B_{12}$ are unavailable. Elevated MMA and homocysteine levels confirm a vitamin $B_{12}$ deficiency whereas normal MMA together with elevated homocysteine levels indicates that folic acid deficiency or another cause should be investigated.

**Effects** Vitamin $B_{12}$ is needed to make blood cells, DNA, and for normal brain function. Deficiency of the vitamin leads to anemia and potentially to irreversible neurological damage, walking and balance disturbances, and cognitive impairment (including confusion and mood changes). High levels of homocysteine are known to be a risk factor for heart and peripheral vascular disease. If vitamin $B_{12}$ is deficient in the presence of high folic acid intake, this latter can prevent anemia but not cognitive dysfunction and the impact of vitamin $B_{12}$ deficiency on neurologic damage can proceed undetected.

**Risk Factors** Risk factors for vitamin $B_{12}$ malabsorption include gastrointestinal disorders, genetic family patterns, medications, and (to some extent) inadequate food intake particularly, among strict vegetarians and vegans. Gastrointestinal disorders that affect vitamin $B_{12}$ absorption include atrophic gastritis, which increases with age, partial stomach removal, and *H. pylori* infection. Medications that suppress stomach acid secretion or impair absorption are associated with the risk of deficiency. Examples of these types of medicines are oral biguanides (e.g., metformin used to treat type 2 diabetes mellitus), modified-release potassium preparations, hydrogen-receptor antagonists (e.g., Cimetidine® or Tagamet®), and proton pump inhibitors (e.g., omeprazole/Prilosec® given for gastroesophageal reflux disease).

**Nutritional Remedies** The DRI of vitamin $B_{12}$ for adults of all ages is 2.4 mcg/day, and the tolerable upper intake level has not been determined. However, oral pharmacological doses for vitamin $B_{12}$-deficient patients are 0.2–2 mg (200–2000 mcg) per day and are above the DRI because roughly 1–2 percent is absorbed through passive diffusion in the small intestine.[85] A dose-finding study tested vitamin $B_{12}$ doses from 2.5 mcg to 1000 mcg with healthy, free-living adults over age 70 and found that mild deficiencies can be normalized with doses of 500–1000 mcg of cyanocobalamin, depending on the blood indicator measured.[86] Although the primary food source of vitamin $B_{12}$ is from animal proteins, the bioavailability of the protein-bound vitamin decreases with age due to the decrease in stomach acidity. It is recommended that adults aged 51 and over obtain their vitamin $B_{12}$ from foods fortified with crystalline or synthetic vitamin $B_{12}$ or from supplements containing vitamin $B_{12}$, because they are not bound to protein and, therefore, are not dependent on acidity for absorption. Folate is now abundant in the food supply due to fortification and so it is essential to ensure that vitamin $B_{12}$ intake is adequate.[87]

## Constipation

**Definition** There are many definitions of "normal bowel pattern." Normal patterns of defecation can consist of two or three bowel movements per day to two or three bowel movements per week. To help sort out what constitutes an abnormal pattern, a working group of gastroenterologists developed the Rome III criteria.[88] Functional constipation in adults means that in the past year, an individual had two or more of the following for at least 12 weeks (in 25 percent or more of defecations): straining, lumpy or hard stools, sensation of incomplete evacuation, sensation of blockage in rectum, manual manipulation, and fewer than three defecations per week.

**Prevalence** Constipation is quite prevalent, and depending on its definition can affect around 12–19 percent of the general population. Its prevalence increases with age and is more frequently reported in female patients; it affects 26 percent of women and 16 percent of men age 65 and over, and this increases to 34 and 26 percent of women and men, respectively, age 84 and over.[89] These rates are much lower than the percentage of the older population concerned about the regularity of their bowel movements. For example, of people aged 65 years and older living in a Midwestern community, 40 percent reported having had some type of constipation.[90]

**Etiology and Effects** Medications and diseases such as diabetes, cancer, Parkinson's, and irritable bowel and other gastric diseases are associated with constipation. There is also a public perception that "being regular" means having a bowel movement each morning. Enthusiastic publicity for celebrities' cleansing diets further contributes to perceptions that stool should be cleared from the colon

**homocysteine** Another intermediate product that depends on vitamin $B_{12}$ for complete metabolism. However, both vitamin $B_{12}$ and folate (another B vitamin) are coenzymes in the breakdown of certain protein components in this pathway. Thus, elevated homocysteine levels can result from vitamin $B_{12}$, folate, or pyridoxine deficiencies.

**methylmalonic acid (MMA)** An intermediate product that needs vitamin $B_{12}$ as a coenzyme to complete the metabolic pathway for fatty-acid metabolism. Vitamin $B_{12}$ is the only coenzyme in this reaction; when it is absent, the blood concentration of MMA rises.

TABLE 19.13 ▸ Misconceptions about chronic constipation

| COMMON MYTH | WHAT THE EVIDENCE SHOWS |
|---|---|
| Stool that remains in the colon for a long time causes "autointoxication"; this theory gave rise to colonic cleansing, enemas. | There is no evidence that toxins are absorbed from the colon. |
| An elongated colon may cause constipation because too much water is reabsorbed from stool, making it hard, and there is danger of kinking. | Calculated normal colon lengths in human adults ranged from ++95 to 180 cm in 6 studies reported; length depends on methodology. No studies link colonic length with transit time. |
| Hormones lead to constipation. | Some do; in a very small percentage of older adults, hypothyroidism is associated with constipation, hyperthyroidism with diarrhea. |
| Constipation is due to a diet low in fiber and is best treated with dietary fiber. | Fiber has various functions and is not digested uniformly; this complicates studies. Yes, fiber increases stool bulk. Wheat bran and psyllium reduce transit time. A low-fiber diet may be a contributor to constipation, but some cases of severe constipation are exacerbated by additional dietary fiber. |
| Low fluid intake causes hard stool. | Interviews with older adults showed no association between estimated fluid intake and constipation; drinking mineral water may have a slight laxative effect due to magnesium content. Except in cases of dehydration, "available data do not suggest that stools can be manipulated to a clinically relevant extent by modifying fluid ingestion." |
| A sedentary life style and inactivity leads to constipation. | Bowel-management programs in nursing homes (fiber, fluid, exercise) have reduced laxative consumption. "Intervention programs to increase physical activity as part of a broad rehabilitation program may help." |
| Laxative intake causes electrolyte disturbances and abdominal complaints. | Abdominal complaints occur with constipation and with laxative use; stimulant laxatives (senna, bisacodyl) may cause cramping; bulk-forming or osmotic agents may increase pressure that feels like bloating. Laxatives can cause electrolyte disturbances, but these can be managed. |
| Laxative use induces habituation and tolerance. | Limited studies of laxative tolerance suggest that tolerance is uncommon "in the majority of users." Those with severe cases using stimulant laxatives may need increasingly large doses. |

SOURCE: Table content compiled from summary information in References 90 and 91.

daily. Older adults are not immune to these promotions. Writing about the widely held myths and misconceptions surrounding normal bowel movements, Müller-Lissner and three international gastroenterologist colleagues introduced their paper with an observation that could fit other conditions: "As with any widespread disorder that has been incompletely understood, there are many strongly held beliefs, which are often not evidence-based. . . ."[91] (Table 19.13). Stool transit times, weights, and consistencies vary greatly among healthy adults of all ages. This is understandable when considering the main functions of the colon, which are water conservation, serving as a place where bacterial action can digest food remnants to usable nutrients, and acting as a site for waste storage until suitable times and places for a bowel movement. Lower levels of stomach secretions and potentially less muscle strength affect peristalsis. Animal studies indicate that aging intestinal muscles become less responsive and that the brain–muscle transmitters are either faulty or less responsive. Also, older adults' thirst mechanisms become blunted. There is a potential for avoiding fiber-rich foods due to chewing problems; such low-fiber diets can also exacerbate ***diverticulitis***. Declining cognitive function may become so severe that the individual may not recognize the urge to defecate; this can also lead to constipation or fecal incontinence.

**Risk Factors** Consistent evidence that exercise relieves constipation in older adults is lacking, although epidemiologic studies have found that higher levels of regular physical activity were associated with a lower risk for constipation.[92] Nutritional risk factors for constipation include:

- Dehydration
- Medications, such as opioid and nonsteroidal anti-inflammatory drugs
- Calcium and other mineral supplements and antacids
- Diets low in fiber

**Nutritional Remedies** Traditional remedies are to encourage increased dietary fiber in tandem with increased fluid. Fiber, fluid, and muscle tone together promote bowel movements; one needs all three.[93] In the presence of dehydration, adding fluid improves constipation. There are no studies available to suggest

**diverticulitis** Infected "pockets" within the large intestine.

Power Pudding, also known as Behm's Special Recipe[92]
1 cup applesauce
1 cup unprocessed bran, all-bran, or bran buds
½ cup prune juice

Mix all ingredients and refrigerate or freeze.
Serve 2 tablespoons at supper, follow by extra fluid such as 1 cup of water.

You can even find Power Pudding online:

1½ cups pitted prunes
1 cup unsweetened applesauce
½ cup All-Bran
¾ cup prune juice
Put all ingredients into blender and puree until smooth.
Serve ¼ cup daily, followed by a glass of water.

ILLUSTRATION 19.4 ▸ High-fiber recipes as alternative to laxatives.



the minimum fluid intake that will maintain the normal bowel routine of an older adult. In healthy adults, fluid intake can vary widely while maintaining regular bowel movements.[91] Optimizing food and fiber intake will help create stool mass; on average, older adults fall far short of the recommended fiber intake. Insoluble fiber sources include bran and cellulose in fruits and vegetables; these fibers are fermented by the colonic bacteria, producing gas (leading to flatulence). Bacterial type and food residue determine gas production. Sugar alcohols are fermented in the colon, as are stachyose and raffinose, two of the carbohydrates in legumes. Bran in breads and cereals is one way to add to fecal bulk that stimulates peristalsis to move wastes through the colon. The fiber section of Chapter 18 offers suggestions for incorporating dietary fiber (see Tables 18.12 and 18.13). Long-term-care nutrition services have devised special recipes to wean residents off laxatives, such as incorporating psyllium fiber, applesauce, and juice into fruit-flavored gelatin. One particularly popular method is called Behm's Special Recipe, or Power Pudding (see Illustration 19.4).[93] There is one caution before increasing fiber: Determine if there is potential for fecal impaction due to disease such as colon cancer. Integrating activity and exercise training can improve peristalsis and alleviate constipation; it may also relieve bloating and flatulence.

# Inflammatory Diseases: Osteoarthritis

LO 19.10 Describe key nutritional approaches to osteoarthritis in adults 65+, recognizing the heterogeneity of older populations.

Inflammatory diseases include periodontal disease, osteoarthritis, rheumatoid arthritis, celiac disease (***gluten*** intolerance), irritable bowel disease, diverticulitis (an infection in the large intestine), atrophic gastritis, and asthma. Of these conditions, arthritis affects the greatest number of older individuals.

Osteoarthritis (OA) is the focus of this section because it is the most common form of arthritis. Approximately 12.4 million (33.6 percent of) adults aged 65 and over are affected by OA, most often involving knee, spine, hand or hip joints.[94] Incidence increases with age, but levels off around age 75–80. OA is among the leading causes of disability in community-dwelling adults; of patients with OA, 80 percent have some limitations of movement. Women are at higher risk of OA than men (see Case Study 19.1).

## Etiology

OA has no known cause, although genetic triggers have been linked to its development. It is characterized by degeneration of bone and cartilage in joints, bone hypertrophy, changes in the synovial membrane, hardening of soft tissues, and inflammation leading to tissue damage. Variability in occurrence and progression of knee, hip, and hand osteoarthritis suggests that the disease may be a group of different and unique conditions. In contrast to osteoarthritis, rheumatoid arthritis is an autoimmune collagen disease, also characterized by inflammation.

## Effects of Osteoarthritis

Osteoarthritis inflammation causes pain, stiffness and swelling. Currently, there is no cure. OA is among the most disabling conditions of older adults. Although functional decline does not have to affect nutritional status, it is likely to complicate one or more of the steps needed to eat well: food procurement, safe preparation, cleanup, and simple enjoyment. Pain colors activities of everyday living, leaving individuals exhausted and frustrated. Treatment goals are to control pain, improve joint function, maintain a normal body weight, and achieve a healthy lifestyle. Treatment can include a combination of physical therapy, weight control, use of medications, and eventually total joint replacement.

## Risk Factors

Obesity, joint injuries, and muscle weakness are modifiable risk factors for developing osteoarthritis.[94] Possible risk factors include continuous overexposure to oxidants, and possibly low vitamin D levels. The relationship between vitamin D and progression of OA and/or pain reduction is inconclusive. In one study, individuals with low serum vitamin D had

**gluten** A protein found in wheat, spelt, kamut, dinkel, and triticale (genus Triticum), barley, and rye. Spelt, dinkel, and kamut are ancestral forms of today's wheat. Oats appear on some "gluten" lists; oats are inherently gluten free, but they may be contaminated by gluten-containing grains during processing.

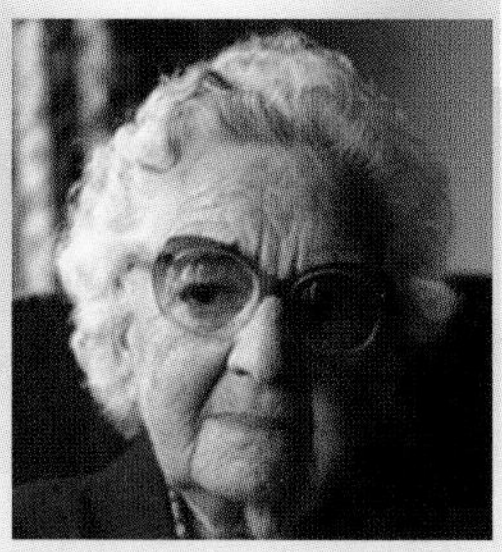
Photodisc

# CASE STUDY 19.1

## Bridget Doyle Remembers Laura

Just because she lives at Lenoir Manor, a continuing-care retirement facility, Laura, a petite (4 ft. 8 in., 97 pounds) widow of the local college dean, does not consider herself as old. She is 87. She has had no major nutritional or health problems and her appetite is good. She had been a good cook and entertained graciously, but in the residential care facility, meals are prepared for her. Because she has had slight fluid retention over the past year, she no longer adds salt to her meals. She tells Bridget Doyle, her nutritionist, that yes, occasionally she does not like her meals and misses cooking for herself.

One Monday morning, Laura is found in bed with her left side paralyzed. The diagnosis is a right-sided stroke, resulting in three weeks of hospitalization. Back at the skilled-care wing of Lenoir, Laura needs a nasogastric tube for feeding. She is alert and knows people but is limited in speech. Overnight, Laura's care has changed from an individual needing routine nutritional monitoring to someone with many interrelated problems:

- Inability to communicate her overall medical and nutritional concerns clearly
- Weight loss of 9 pounds during the three-week hospital stay
- Intense dislike of the nasal tube, as demonstrated by repeated attempts to pull it out, leading to restraint of her hands

### *Questions*

**Assessment**

1. What nutritional parameters should be assessed and monitored now that Laura is back at Lenoir Manor?

**Diagnosis**

2. What disciplines should be involved in Laura's care plan, and why?
3. The interdisciplinary care team wants to meet Laura's needs in a dignified and respectful manner. How can the care team address both clinical and ethical concerns?
4. What are strategies young adults can adopt to reduce their risk of stroke?

**Monitoring and Evaluation**

5. How could Bridget ensure that Laura's nutritional needs are met?

elevated risk of knee OA progression compared to those with higher vitamin D concentrations.[95] However, a clinical trial did not show reduced symptoms or progression of osteoarthritis with vitamin D supplementation over 2 years.[96] Osteoporosis has been inversely linked to OA. Obesity may have two detrimental effects. One is the weight stressing the joint, and the other is due to secretion of cytokines in adipose tissue. Fat, a metabolically active tissue, secretes signaling molecules that can trigger inflammation.

**Nutritional Remedies** A painful, incurable disease with high prevalence but with unknown causes is likely to generate great public interest and experimentation in its treatment. Treatments used in OA far exceed the evidence of effectiveness. Overall, weight loss and certain exercises have a positive impact on decreasing pain and improving physical function and health.[11,94] Messier and associates[11] found that weight loss of as little as 1 pound reduces the load exerted on the knees. Herbal medicinal products are frequently used in the treatment of OA; however, at this time, there is insufficient evidence of the effectiveness of these products.[97] Other popular nutritional approaches to symptom reduction have small or no evidence of benefit. For example, anti-inflammatory diets have become popular. However, a healthy diet following the Dietary Guidelines, the DASH, or Mediterranean eating patterns, is the recommended approach.[98]

**Chondroitin and Glucosamine** These two substances naturally occur in the body as substrate for cartilage repair. Clinical trials of their use, separately and together, demonstrate significant pain reduction when knee pain is moderate to severe.[99] Joint space in the knee improved and hip progression was slowed. A caution: Product tests have shown that quality and levels of active compound display surprisingly great variation. Not all products contain the specified levels of active compound. Check with the FDA or go to www.consumerlab.com to find out how specific brands rate.

**Other Treatments** There is no conclusive evidence currently to recommend vitamin intake to relieve OA symptoms or to prevent its progression. Balancing specific fatty acids and oils has potential to reduce inflammation, but there is no solid intervention data to show that it reduces symptoms of either osteo- or rheumatoid arthritis. Other treatments such as borage seed and evening primrose oils contain GLA or gamma-linolenic acid, which plays a role in prostaglandin synthesis (GLA competes with other fatty acids, limiting the production of inflammatory omega-6 fatty acids) and are popular even though not proven in clinical studies. Flaxseed and purslane also contain a form of omega-3 fatty acid. Traditional Native American medical therapy used echinacea (three varieties) for pain relief, rheumatism, and arthritis; ginseng for asthma and rheumatism; garlic for asthma; and evening primrose oil for obesity.[100] There are not enough studies to assess the efficacy of for many of these treatments.[97] Disease treatment claims can't be made on the container unless they are backed by evidence, but dietary supplements typically don't undergo drug testing. Marketing for the botanicals used by many older adults is often driven by tradition and personal testimonials (blogs, articles, books, websites). Echinacea and ginseng are said to boost immune function, and evening primrose oil serves as an antioxidant— customers often leap to the assumption that these will treat inflammatory diseases such as OA.

# Cognitive Impairment, Dementia and Alzheimer's Disease

LO 19.11 Describe key nutritional approaches to cognitive impairment, dementia, and Alzheimer's diseases of adults 65+, recognizing the heterogeneity of older populations.

## Definition

One of the dreaded aspects of "getting old" is becoming dependent on others. ***Memory impairment*** and ***mild cognitive impairment (MCI)*** are steps in the loss of independence. Serious losses of memory and cognitive function are frequently grouped under the term *dementia*. Dementia is a condition of progressive cognitive decline, typically characterized by impaired memory, thinking, decision making, and linguistic ability. Dementia is not a disease itself, but rather the manifestation of various forms of physiological damage. Diseases associated with dementia include Alzheimer's disease (AD), Parkinson's disease, alcoholism, and vascular diseases (see Table 19.14).

Alzheimer's disease is the most common cause of dementia and accounts for an estimated 60–80 percent of cases.[101] Revised diagnostic criteria published in 2011,[102] define dementia as the last of three stages in the AD progression. Dementia may, but does not necessarily follow a symptomatic, pre-dementia phase labeled MCI. Mild cognitive impairment may include reduced ability to learn and retain new information, but it does not interfere significantly with day-to-day activities or the ability to live independently. A pre-clinical asymptomatic phase measured by change in biomarkers is defined for research purposes. The current thinking is that AD pathology has a genetic component, becoming more pronounced with age. Cognitive decline results from accumulation of beta-amyloid plaques and synaptic dysfunction, formation of neurofibrillary tau protein tangles, and neuronal death.[102]

## Prevalence

AD ranks fifth in leading causes of death for adults aged 65 and older in the United States. About 11 percent of people age 65 and older and 32 percent age 85 and older have AD in the United States. The numbers are expected to increase as the population is aging.[100,103] Approximately 14 percent of older (≥ 71 years) adults have dementia.[100,104] In 2002, an estimated 22 percent of the United States

**memory impairment** Moderate or severe impairment is when 4 or fewer words can be recalled from a list of 20.

**mild cognitive impairment (MCI)** MCI Subtle loss of memory, thinking and/or reasoning skills beyond expectations of normal but not serious enough to be classified as dementia.

TABLE 19.14 ▸ Conditions associated with cognitive impairment and dementia

| CONDITION | CHANGES LEADING TO COGNITIVE IMPAIRMENT |
|---|---|
| Vascular dementia | "Mini-strokes" and vascular obstructions deprive brain of oxygen and other nutrients. |
| Degenerative diseases (Alzheimer's and Parkinson's) | Neurological changes eventually affect memory and ability to think. |
| Physical trauma and infection | Brain injuries may impair physical and/or cognitive function. |
| Depression | Change in brain chemistry can affect ability to maintain high-level functioning. |
| Chronic substance, alcohol abuse | Neurological damage may become irreversible. |
| Malnutrition, including $B_{12}$ deficiency and dehydration | Confusion resulting from dehydration is reversible<br>Neurological damage of $B_{12}$ deficiency is permanent.<br>Chronic hunger keeps brain from focusing on life beyond acquiring food. |
| Deficiencies of niacin, thiamin, folic acid, biotin, iron, and selenium | Decreased ability to learn and depression are among the effects of these vitamin and mineral deficiencies. |

population aged 71 and older had cognitive impairment without dementia.[105]

## Etiology of Cognitive Impairment

Dementia can be caused by a variety of conditions resulting in traumatic physiologic changes (see Table 19.14). The symptoms of dementia may be completely or partially reversible in some conditions, including reduction of cerebrovascular risk factors, early treatment of drug abuse, metabolic disorders such as a vitamin $B_{12}$ deficiency and hypoglycemia, and medical interventions such as surgery to remove tumors or change of medications.

Nontreatable forms of dementia include those associated with degenerative diseases such as Alzheimer's, Huntington's, and Parkinson's. Searches for a cause of AD (leading to treatment) are ongoing. Aluminum, copper, carnitine, vitamin $B_6$, and choline have been examined as possible causes of AD due to their role in neurological function, but have not been demonstrated to be causal.

Deficiencies of vitamin $B_{12}$ and folate are related to high concentrations of homocysteine, an amino acid associated with the promotion of poor vascular health and cognitive decline. In order to prevent the buildup of homocysteine in the blood and neural tissue, vitamin $B_{12}$ and folate are needed to convert it to the amino acid methionine. Methionine contributes to the synthesis of S-adenosylmethionine, which is widely distributed throughout the central nervous system for use in methylation reactions. Primary examples of methylation reactions include vitamin $B_{12}$ in the production of myelin (the insulation cover on nerves) and folate in the DNA cycle (cell replication). Excess homocysteine in brain tissue is thought to contribute to the development of Alzheimer's disease either through vascular mechanisms or as a neurotoxin. High-dose vitamin B supplementation has decreased homocysteine levels but has not slowed progression of cognitive decline in people with AD.[106]

To discover dietary habits that may prevent cognitive decline, and especially AD, researchers are reviewing dietary patterns and physical activity. There is accumulating evidence that aerobic exercise and the Mediterranean diet have positive impact on improving cognitive ability and prolonging longevity. A systematic review of studies up to May 2014 that examined the role of dietary patterns in relation to cognitive decline or dementia show that better adherence to a Mediterranean diet is associated with less cognitive decline, dementia, or Alzheimer's disease.[107] For example, researchers of a prospective cohort study in Bordeaux, France, developed an adherence score and assessed the dietary patterns of 1,410 adults aged 65 and older.[108] After adjustment for cardiovascular risk factors, higher adherence to the Mediterranean diet was associated with slowed cognitive decline in one of the four cognitive function tests (the Mini-Mental State Exam). Also, a prospective cohort study of 1,880 older adults in New York showed that the Mediterranean-type diet and physical activity were independently related to lower AD risk.[109] Comparisons of adults with better diet scores and higher levels of physical activity to those with low scores on both showed that a dose–response relationship in risk reduction may exist. Intervention studies with long follow-up are needed to support these findings.

Other promising research into the mechanisms of cognition in aging deals with the theory of caloric restriction and inflammation.[110] A small intervention study in humans (29 healthy women, mean age 60.5 years) showed that a reduced-calorie diet (30 percent below normal intake, not to drop below 1200 kcal) improved insulin sensitivity, inflammatory response (tumor necrosis factor-alpha), and memory performance on the Rey Auditory Verbal Learning Task test. Both obesity and long-term underweight were associated with lower cognitive scores in the larger Whitehall Cohort Study.[111]

The term *cognitive disorders* describes a range of brain malfunctions. The etiology of AD may be elusive, but any progress into elucidating contributors to cognitive health will find an appreciative audience, both in individuals with the disorder and, perhaps more so, in their caregivers.

## Effects of Cognitive Impairment

Confusion, anxiety, agitation, loss of oral muscular control, impairment of hunger and appetite regulation, changes in smell and taste, chewing and swallowing difficulties, and dental problems are all aspects of Alzheimer's disease that make it difficult to maintain good nutritional habits. As the disease advances, individuals with AD will require more and more assistance with meal preparation and eating. In later stages of the disease, wandering and restless movements expend energy and increase caloric need. Behavioral, physical, or neurologic problems may impede adequate food intake. Consequently, individuals with late-stage AD suffer from unintentional weight loss (this is discussed in the "Low Body Weight/Underweight" section).

## Nutrition Interventions for Cognitive Impairment

After examination of 25 systematic reviews and 250 primary research studies, an independent panel concluded its 727-page report into the research of protective factors for Alzheimer's disease, saying that evidence is inadequate "to confidently assess their [the factors'] association with AD or cognitive decline."[112] The panel did find that cognitive engagement and physical activities were associated with decreased risk of AD. However, this panel did not address the many different types of cognitive impairment (see Table 19.14).

The search for hope includes food: Researchers at a 2012 presentation at the International Alzheimer's Association Congress reported on a medical food supplement that has led to modest memory improvement during a

24 weeks follow-up and up to 48 weeks on a subsample of patients with mild AD. The supplement was designed to support the formation and function of nerve synapses. Ingredients include fish oil components, antioxidants, and B vitamins.[113] The supplement is marketed in several countries but is currently undergoing clinical testing at several health centers to verify its effectiveness so that it can be marketed in the United States as a medical food.

In the meantime, ensuring food safety and safe use of kitchen tools and equipment are primary considerations for good nutrition; many dangers lurk in the kitchens of cognitively impaired persons who are trying to maintain an independent life at home. Involving a caretaker can ensure adequate intake while preventing foodborne illness or injuries related to food preparation.

Since there is no cure for AD, the dietary focus is to maintain a nutrient-dense diet that is acceptable to the individual, maintains hydration, and supplies needed energy. Additional calories may be needed for increased energy expended by individuals who pace and wander. Persons with dementia can benefit from meals offered in a calm dining environment, free of loud noise and confusion (no highly patterned tableware, nothing extraneous on the table). Additional strategies caregivers might use to promote food and fluid intake are to (1) maintain the focus on eating, (2) provide plenty of time to eat, (3) serve finger foods, and (4) encourage regular drinks between bites. In cases of decreased physical coordination, adaptive eating utensils, such as slip-resistant placemats, mugs or cups without saucers and spoons, and silverware with built-up handles, may promote independent eating.

# Polypharmacy: Prescription and Over-the-Counter Medications

LO 19.12 Understand how comorbidities and polypharmacy increase nutritional risk in older adults.

Prescription medicines are those ordered by a physician or other licensed health care provider, and do not include vitamins, herbal medicines, or over-the-counter (OTC) medicines. OTC medications are any pills, liquids, salves, creams, and supplements that are purchased at a pharmacy, discount, or food store without prescription. Complementary medicines such as botanicals and herbs are typically sold as OTCs.

Several terms have been used to describe multiple medication usage. Polypharmacy and hyperpharmacotherapy refer to use of multiple and/or inappropriate medications. Use of multiple medications increases the risk of adverse drug reactions, hospitalization, and death.[114] Using three or more medications per day (prescription or OTC) constitutes nutritional risk on the Nutrition Screening Initiative DETERMINE tool (Illustration 18.2). On the MNA long form (assessment, not screen), nutritional risk is defined as more than three prescription drugs per day.

How many drugs does the average older person take, assuming that there is an average old person? It is difficult, maybe impossible, to find a meaningful number; the emphasis of prescribers is on *appropriate* medications. Both the Beers criteria (Chapter 18) and a 2012 Cochrane review[115] reinforce appropriate medication usage, whether OTC or prescription. In 2009–2010, 39 percent of adults age 65 and older used five or more prescription medications. From 1988 to 2009–2010, there were substantial increases in cardioprotective and antidepressant medication use. Cardioprotective medications constituted about 52 percent of the prescriptions in 2009–2010.[116]

## Medication Effects on Physical, Mental and Financial Status

The potential for medication errors increases with disease progression, drug side effects, functional limitations such as poor eyesight or impaired memory, and number of drugs used. Taking multiple medications is inevitable for an individual with multiple illnesses, and it can affect mental, physical, and financial security. Worry about tracking and taking drugs properly, perhaps while having undesired side effects like dry mouth, decreased taste sensation, and sleepiness, can lead to periodic "forgetting" to take a pill. Budget shortfalls can add to the worry: Shall I buy food for the cat, fresh fruit for me, or blood pressure medicine? In the absence of money or insurance coverage, older adults have been known to divide pills and take half doses.

Older patients taking multiple prescribed drugs tend to be frail. In the Australian CHAMP study of nearly 3,000 free-living males aged 70 and older, the group taking 10 or more prescribed medications (compared to 5 or more) was older and experienced proportionately greater weight loss (19 percent of the group compared to 10 percent), weakness (56 percent compared to 43 percent), and low activity (51 percent compared to 32 percent).[114]

## Medication Effects on Food Consumption

Medications may require dietary restrictions and can interfere with appetite, digestion, metabolism, and general alertness. For example, the blood-thinning drug warfarin requires a stable vitamin K intake (see Table 19.15). Other medications alter the senses of taste and smell. Eliminating the pleasure of a meal is an obvious loss, but unforeseen circumstances include injuries from falls. For an example, take the case report of drug-related taste disturbance from two Canadian physicians. They describe the case of an 85-year-old fully functioning woman, admitted to the ER with fractures and intracranial hemorrhages after taking a misstep during her nightly trip to the bathroom.[117] She had started taking eye drops for glaucoma. These drops left her with a bitter taste, which she

TABLE 19.15 ▸ Amounts of vitamin K in selected fruits and vegetables (DRI for ages 51 and older is 120 mcg/day for males, 90 mcg/day for females)

|  |
|---|
| **Less than 5 mcg vitamin K:** |
| 1 cup servings of applesauce, cherries, corn, mushrooms, navy and baked beans, onions, pineapple, potatoes, strawberries<br>1 each apple, banana, orange, nectarine, peach, pear, tangerine; 5 dried apricots, 5 dates |
| **5 to 10 mcg vitamin K:** |
| 1 cup canned apricots, chickpeas, lima beans, fruit cocktail, fresh raspberries, papaya, all varieties of squash, stewed tomatoes, sweet potatoes |
| **>10 and <50 mcg vitamin K:** |
| 1 cup blueberries, raw red cabbage, carrots, cauliflower, celery, cucumber with and without peel, iceberg lettuce, roasted peppers, canned plums, grapes, string beans<br>½ cup cooked chard, prunes or dried plums<br>1 kiwi, 2 sprigs parsley, 1 Tbsp raw green onion |
| **>50 mcg vitamin K (1 cup cooked unless specified):** |
| Beet greens, turnip greens (529–851)<br>Broccoli (183–220)<br>Cabbage, (27–58)<br>Collards (836–1059)<br>Kale (1062–1147)<br>Mustard greens (419)<br>Okra (64)<br>Rhubarb (71)<br>Cooked spinach (1027)<br>1 cup raw: green leaf lettuce (97), Romaine (57), spinach (145) |

SOURCE: www.nal.usda.gov/fnic/foodcomp/Data/SR18/nutrlist/sr18a430.pdf; and NDSR, University of Minnesota, accessed 8/31/09.

tried to wash away with a glass or two of water, resulting in nocturia, which is waking up at night to urinate. On the night of the tumble down seven steps, she had mistaken the stairwell for the adjacent bathroom door, resulting in a trip to the emergency department. Bitter taste is likely to be listed as one of the side effects on the eye drop package insert, but the potential consequences of trying to eliminate bitter taste are not. It may take some creative probing to assess medication compliance and potential nutritional implications.

Some medications lead to unintentional weight loss, while others, such as steroids lead to undesired weight gain. Table 19.16 describes nutritional implications associated with medications used to treat diseases that are prevalent in older adults.

# Low Body Weight/ Unintentional Weight Loss

LO 19.13 Explain the challenges faced by underweight individuals and the consequences of sarcopenia on day-to-day functioning.

## Definition

There is no consensus or universal definition for underweight in frail older adults. Individuals with weights falling at the lowest percentiles of this age group can be defined as *underweight*. Individuals who have been thin and healthy for a lifetime face increased health risks when they lose muscle or other lean tissue.

Body mass index (BMI) scores allow characterization of underweight across populations. A BMI falling into the lowest percentile of a reference standard in a comparable population can help to identify nutritional risks. NHLBI defines underweight as a BMI $< 18.5$ kg/meter squared for all adults,[118] while WHO further defines levels of underweight as grades of "thinness."[119]

BMI 17.0–18.49 indicates grade 1 thinness
BMI 16.0–16.99 indicates grade 2 thinness
BMI $< 16.00$ indicates grade 3 thinness

As discussed in the section on obesity, there is disagreement on what constitutes the lower BMI cut-points in older adults. Many national and international organizations and researchers have defined underweight with BMI. The results of a 2014 meta-analysis showed that the risk of mortality in older adults increased with a BMI of $< 23.0$.[49] Although BMI remains an anthropometric measurement tool for assessing health status, unintentional weight loss is a validated indicator of malnutrition and has been associated with increased mortality. There is no consensus in clinical definition of unintended weight loss; however, studies have used a weight loss of 5 percent or more of body weight within the previous 3–6 months.[120]

TABLE 19.16 ▸ Medications associated with chronic conditions in older adults: nutritional implications

**Coronary Heart Disease**

Cardiac glycosides (e.g., digitalis) may result in anorexia and/or nausea.

Statins may result in elevated liver enzymes.

High doses of niacin may be associated with flushing, hyperglycemia, hypotension, hypoalbuminemia, upper GI distress, and liver enzyme elevation.

**Hypertension**

Diuretics may result in depletion of sodium, calcium, magnesium, and/or potassium.

Centrally acting anti-hypertensives may result in a decline in food intake due to sedation, confusion, and depression.

Medications such as beta-blockers may cause constipation and delayed gastric emptying.

Potential related side effects are dizziness, dry mouth, or mouth pain.

**Diabetes Mellitus**

Medications to treat diabetes may cause hypoglycemia, especially if nutritional intake is erratic and/or if there is increased or decreased appetite or diarrhea.

Oral hypoglycemics (e.g., sulfonylureas such as glipizide) may cause heartburn, nausea, hypoglycemia, decreased appetite; biguanides (such as Glucophage) may cause decreased appetite, diarrhea, and vomiting.

**Depression**

Antipsychotic/antidepressants with anticholinergic side effects may lead to dry mouth, delayed stomach emptying, and constipation.

Antidepressants may enhance appetite in depressed patients, but Selective Serotonin Reuptake Inhibitors may cause a decrease in appetite.

**Congestive Heart Failure**

Diuretics may lead to electrolyte abnormalities, especially sodium and potassium and/or thiamin deficiency (e.g., Furosemide, chlorothiazide).

**Cancer**

Radiation, chemotherapy, and/or surgery can negatively affect nutritional status and metabolism.

**Chronic Obstructive Pulmonary Disease (COPD)**

Xanthine derivatives (e.g., theophylline) may result in anorexia and nausea.

**Lower Respiratory Infections**

Antibiotics (e.g., amoxicillin) may result in nausea, anorexia, diarrhea, and stomatitis.

**Pain**

Low dose aspirin

SOURCE: Based on American Academy of Family Physicians, Nutrition Screening Initiative, American Dietetic Association. *A physician's guide to nutrition in chronic disease management for older adults*. Waldorf, MD: 2002.

## Etiology and Effects

Unintentional weight loss may be an indicator of underlying, undiagnosed disease that alters biochemical and physiologic mechanisms, which, in turn, affect functional status and appetite. Underlying causes of unplanned weight loss and low body weight may include protein–calorie malnutrition, illness, poverty, and functional decline. (See Case Study 19.2.) Changes in taste and smell, whether due to aging or medication use, can turn eating into a chore. Restrictive diets (low salt, low cholesterol, diabetic) have also been linked to malnutrition.[121] Anorexia (no appetite) and cachexia (chronically lacking appetite) lead to sarcopenia (muscle loss).

Weight loss after 65 or 70 may be due in part to the blunted appetite and satiety signals of older adults. Just as the thirst mechanism becomes less sensitive to dehydration, the response to eat after caloric deprivation is less acute. Older adults have lower circulating levels of ghrelin, the signaling protein that stimulates appetite.[122] Fat tissue accumulates as muscle is lost in sedentary older populations. Fat contains ***adipocytokines*** such as leptin, which suppress appetite. Circulating levels of leptin correspond to the amount of adipose tissue, so that someone with high body fat may have reduced appetite.

For older adults, underweight is much more serious than overweight. Being thin has been related to increased incidence of diseases, but it is impossible to tell from the data whether thinness precedes or follows incidence of disease. Chronic malnutrition reduce immune response, muscle and respiratory function, and wound healing.

## Nutrition Interventions

Avoiding unintentional weight loss is desirable but not always possible. Weight loss is associated with diseases that alter biochemical and physiologic mechanisms, which, in turn, affect functional status and appetite. A first step is to determine what caused the weight loss so that proper intervention is administered.

In a systematic review of studies, which evaluated the effect of nutrition therapy in protein–energy malnutrition connected with multiple disorders in the elderly, 20 studies noted an improvement in anthropometric or biochemical measures, and 10 studies reported an improvement in function. In contrast, there was insufficient evidence to determine how nutrition therapy should be formulated due to inconsistent or uncertain treatment adherence.[123] In a systematic review of 22 studies reported by the Cochrane Library, protein and energy supplementation appears to produce a small but consistent weight

**adipocytokines** Adipose tissue secretes several signaling proteins, including the appetite suppressants adiponectin, leptin, and resitin.

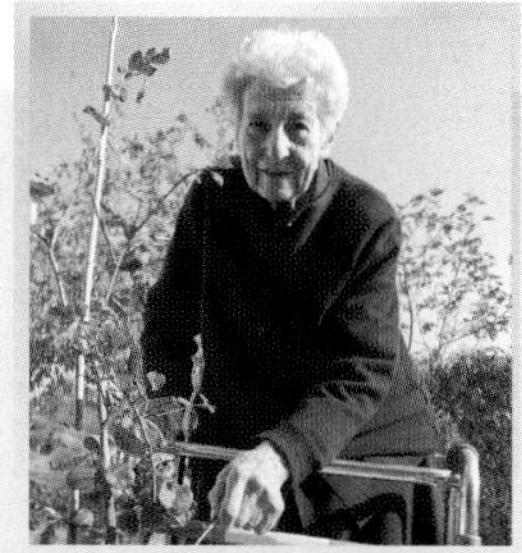
burnel1/Shutterstock.com

# CASE STUDY 19.2

## Ms. Wetter: A Senior Suffering Through a Bad Stretch

About to turn 81, Elizabeth Wetter is 5 feet 6 inches tall and weighs 106 pounds. She has had Parkinson's disease for 5 years, but that is not what concerns her. Her problem is pain from arthritis and lack of energy. She saw an ad on television for a vitamin–mineral supplement with ginseng that promises "more energy." Her son also told her to take a liquid dietary supplement to "feel better." Eighteen months ago, she had successful surgery for colon cancer, which was followed by chemotherapy treatments. She is now free of cancer. After the cancer treatment, she fell and broke a hip. This healed well, but serious leg pains started shortly afterward. There seems to be no cause for the pain, and a cure is unavailable. She is no longer able to take her walks through the neighborhood or tend her prize-winning garden. She would like to weigh 118 pounds again (her "usual") and is seeking nutritional counseling to try to regain some of her energy.

### Questions

1. What are some of the nutritional issues faced by Ms. Wetter? (*Hint:* Calculate her current weight compared to her usual body weight as a percentage.)
2. How would you prioritize these in a nutritional care plan?
3. Calculate her energy needs and suggest strategies she might use to regain some energy.
4. What other information would you want to know in order to counsel Ms. Wetter?

gain (2–4 percent), reduced mortality, and shorter length of hospital stays.[124] Supplementation was associated with nausea, diarrhea, and other gastrointestinal disturbances. Overall, medical nutrition therapy for a frail, malnourished person should occur in consultation with an experienced registered dietitian. Refeeding and rehydration are done gradually:

- *Calories:* Eat and exercise to build muscle mass, strength. A meta-analysis indicated that Harris–Benedict formula significantly underestimates daily needs in frail older adults with pressure ulcers[125] and supported the international recommendations for 30–35 kcal per kilogram body weight per day.[126]
- *Protein:* 1.0–1.5 grams of protein per kilogram body weight is adequate; 1.5–2.0 g/kg/day in cases of severe depletion, balanced throughout the day. Exceptions are patients with renal or liver failure, who may need a protein restriction.
- *Fluid:* Drink 1 mL per kcal; rehydrate slowly (see the "Dehydration" section).

### Connection: Fluid

8 ounces = 1 cup = 240 mL (milliliters) = 240 cc (cubic centimeters)

A super-sized soda (32 ounces) equals approximately 4 cups (or 4 × 240 = 960 mL). A 2-liter bottle of soda provides a little more than 8 cups of fluid. Some foods also count as fluid. For example, soup, gelatin products, and sherbet are considered fluids.

# Dehydration

LO 19.14 List three or more signs of dehydration and explain why maintaining hydration status is important for the health of an older person.

## Definition

Dehydration is the physiological state in which cell fluid loss interferes with metabolic processes. Normal urination does not cause dehydration. Phillips and colleagues[127] defined dehydration as losing nearly 2 percent of initial body weight; this can occur after avoiding all fluid and eating only dry foods for 24 hours. There is currently no acceptable biomarkers of hydration status at the population level. Serum osmolality, hypertonicity and urine osmolality are usually measured but they are weak indicators of hydration status especially among older adults.[128] The clinical signs of dehydration come from a review of 38 potential indicators of dehydration in older adults (61–98 years old, median age 82; $n$ = 55; half were free-living; half were admitted to the hospital emergency department from extended care).[129] Seven signs and symptoms were strongly related to dehydration, although *not* to patient age:

1. Upper-body muscle weakness
2. Speech difficulty
3. Confusion
4. Dry mucous membranes in nose and mouth
5. Longitudinal tongue furrows
6. Dry tongue
7. Sunken appearance of eyes in their sockets

TABLE 19.17 ▸ Percent of initial weight lost due to dehydration and physiological signs

| PERCENT LOST | PHYSIOLOGICAL SIGNS |
|---|---|
| 1% | Thirst (true for young people, not necessarily in older men or women) |
| 4–6% | Economy of movement, flushed skin, sleepiness, apathy, nausea, tingling in arms, hands, feet, headache, heat exhaustion in fit men, increases in body temperature, pulse rate, respiratory rate |
| 8% | Dizziness, slurred speech, weakness, confusion |
| 12% | Cognitive signs: wakefulness, delirium |
| 20% | Bare survival limit |
| For someone who normally weighs 160 lb:<br>1% loss means weight down to 158.4 lb<br>4% loss means weight down to 153.6 lb<br>6% loss means weight down to 150.4 lb<br>20% loss means weight down to 128.0 lb | |

SOURCE: Adapted from Briggs and Calloway, originally NASA, 1967.[131]

These signs were also confirmed in a systematic review of maintaining oral hydration in older people.[130] In older adults, thirst and skin turgor (pinch a skin fold on the forearm, forehead, or over the breastbone, and watch it fall back) are not good indicators of dehydration.[129] Although regulation of body temperature is one of the functions of the body's water compartment, fever or elevated temperature did not identify dehydration status in Gross's study of individuals admitted to emergency rooms. However, fever or elevated temperature may be an indicator of impending dehydration.

Dehydration can be measured as percentage of body weight lost when normal body weight is known. In a continuum of dehydration shown by Briggs and Calloway (Table 19.17),[130] originally designed for the National Aeronautics Space Administration (NASA), the indicators are somewhat different from the indicators that Gross found.[129] The NASA continuum shows how the human body responds to water losses.

Weight loss of 4 percent normal weight would be hard to ignore unless the individual had a compromised mental or cognitive status. Flushed skin, nausea, and apathy or lack of energy occur when 4 percent body weight is lost due to dehydration. Prevalence data are hard to gather because dehydration is usually temporary, and there is no simple or commonly used standard definition for diagnosing dehydration in the elderly. For example, patients coming to a nursing home from a hospital may have IV tubes, and chart notes may simply say, "The patient looks well-hydrated."

## Etiology

Aging itself does not cause dehydration, even though the percentage of total body water shrinks from infancy to old age. Dehydration occurs more often in the elderly as a result of illness or other problems. Older people are less sensitive in detecting thirst than are younger people, and they therefore may not think to drink.[127] Once fluids are consumed, aging kidneys may lose the ability to concentrate urine, and ***antidiuretic hormone*** may become less effective. Swallowing problems, depression, or dementia may cause individuals to avoid food or drink. Decreased mobility impairs older adults' access to water and subsequent ability to reach the bathroom. Fear of incontinence, in general, is another reason leading to decreased fluid intake and subsequent dehydration.

## Effects of Dehydration

Dehydration increases the resting heart rate and susceptibility to urinary tract infection, pneumonia, and pressure ulcers; it also leads to confusion, disorientation, and dementia.[132] Because confusion and delirium are signs of—as well as risk factors for—dehydration, consuming adequate fluids can become a vicious circle for someone at risk for cognitive decline.

## Nutritional Interventions

The Institute of Medicine's DRI for water does not change as adults get older: "The AI for total water (drinking water, beverages, and foods) for the elderly is set based on median total water intake of young adults."[132] Some health professionals suggest fluid levels to be 1 mL per calorie eaten, with a minimum of 1500 mL per day (approximately 6 cups). The ultimate beverage is *water*—tap or flavored, *not* sugared. Water is generally accessible, adds no calories to the diet, provides traces of minerals needed for metabolism, and is very low in sodium, even when softened. Pure water does not provide energy, but lacking water to the point of dehydration dramatically reduces an individual's energy.

Many beverages contribute nutrients as well as fluid:

1. Tea, especially green tea, contains flavonoids that have been linked to heart health.[133]
2. Coffee (115 mg/8 fl oz) and black tea (90 mg/8 fl oz) contain potassium for electrolyte balance. The DRI for older adults is 4700 mg, but small contributions add up.
3. Milk provides much-needed high quality protein, calcium, riboflavin, and vitamin D. Low-fat milk enhances hypertension treatment and weight maintenance. Other protein drinks might be made from fruit blended with yogurt, whey powder, or nut butters.
4. Regular use of cranberry juice reduces urinary tract infection in women.[134]
5. Fruit and vegetable juices count as part of the recommended fruit and vegetable servings.

**antidiuretic hormone** Causes kidneys to absorb more water from urine, resulting in increased blood volume.

### Rehydrate Slowly

To treat dehydration in older adults, replace fluids slowly. Guidelines are to provide roughly one-fourth to one-third of the overall fluid deficit each day in the form of water or a 5 percent glucose solution (when the individual's blood values are stable).[130] For individuals with swallowing problems, or dysphagia, thickened liquids count as fluid. When bedridden older adults are offered fluids hourly and also with medication, they achieve higher levels of hydration.[130]

### Dehydration at End of Life

Dehydration can occur in people with terminal illness or who are near death. Some individuals stop eating and/or drinking hours, days, or even weeks before death. Dehydration at the end of life contributes to an overall slowing of body systems, including decreased production of body fluids, resulting in less congestion, less edema and ascites, and less gastrointestinal action together with increasing levels of drowsiness. An individual may experience slight thirst, although many dying patients do not report being thirsty. They may experience dry mouth that can be alleviated by ice chips or artificial saliva. Decreased urine output can be a benefit because there is less need to go to the toilet. It is not known whether medically assisted hydration (provided via intubation) improves quality of life.[135] A survey of hospice nurses found that patients who stopped food and fluids usually died a "good" death within two weeks of refusing nourishment.[136] "Good" was measured on a nine-point scale that included variables for suffering, pain, peacefulness, and overall quality of death and based on the nurses' perceptions.

## Bereavement

LO 19.15 Explain how social support during bereavement can help the survivor to stay healthy.

Bereavement is the loss felt when someone who is personally significant dies. Losses of friends and family members happen more often in the lives of older persons. Grief, a very powerful emotion, is a natural response to bereavement. The grieving process, with its stages of shock and denial, disorganization, volatile reactions, guilt, loss and loneliness, relief, and reestablishment,[137] diverts attention from normal activities. Shopping and food preparation, eating, and drinking may be ignored in the grieving process. Any loss of long-shared relationships through death, dementia, or moving brings about lack of interest in activities surrounding meal planning, preparation, shopping, and eating. People who are in mourning are vulnerable to malnutrition.

Widowhood has been shown to trigger disorganization and changes in daily routine, especially related to food preparation and eating.[138] Widowed persons who are able to enjoy mealtimes, have good appetites, have higher-quality diets, and receive social support work through the grieving process with fewer health consequences (Illustration 19.5).

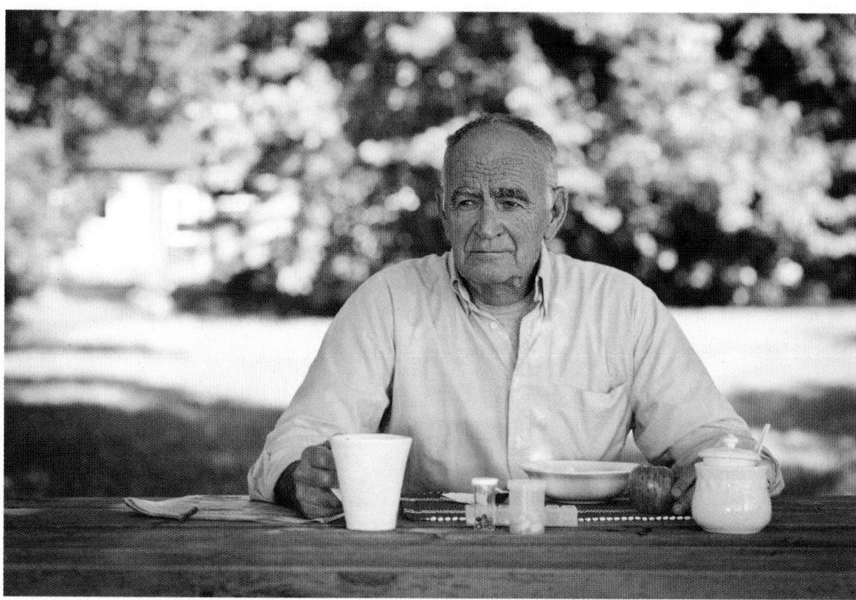

Nadino/Shutterstock.com

ILLUSTRATION 19.5 ▸ Grief can have a negative impact on diet.

## KEY POINTS

1. Nearly three of four older adults consider their health to be good, very good, or excellent, despite the high prevalence of chronic disease in older adults.
2. Hypertension, which affects about two-thirds of older adults, can be moderated with the DASH diet; further blood pressure reductions can be achieved by restricting sodium intake in addition to following the DASH eating pattern.
3. Of adults over age 65, about one in four has diabetes, primarily type 2, which has an impact on many other conditions and suggests the importance of lifestyle and diet modifications.
4. Body Mass Index should be combined with other measures such as waist circumference to assess weight status in older adults; a BMI range of 23–27 seems reasonable for older adults.
5. Bed rest and inactivity is detrimental to strong bones. Exercise combined with good nutrition—including adequate calcium and vitamins D, C, and $B_6$—helps to maintain bone mass density.
6. Polypharmacy is a risk factor for malnutrition and may contribute to poor oral health; dry mouth and the associated gingival disease can result from medications (such as antihistamines, antidepressants, sedatives, and anti-anxiety drugs).
7. Despite adequate dietary intake of vitamin $B_{12}$, older adults may still have low blood levels due to malabsorption. Monitoring $B_{12}$ blood levels in vulnerable populations can help to prevent the irreversible nerve damage caused by $B_{12}$ deficiency. Vitamin $B_{12}$ is one instance when the synthetic version of a vitamin is better absorbed than the food-bound version.
8. Osteoarthritis is the most common inflammatory disease of older adults. Weight loss helps to reduce the load exerted on knees and also reduces risk of developing osteoarthritis (as does adequate intake of vitamin D).
9. Dementia associated with old age can be due to vascular and degenerative diseases, physical trauma and infection, depression, and malnutrition. However, most of the dementia in older adults in the United States is associated with Alzheimer's disease. Nutritional efforts focus on treatment of underlying causes and maintaining quality of life.
10. Weight loss in an older adult signals potential illness and malnutrition; an individual who is losing weight without trying needs a thorough assessment.
11. Confusion and muscle weakness related to dehydration is avoidable. Adequate fluid intake prevents dehydration and can also contribute needed nutrients to the diet of an older adult, such as calcium, vitamin D, protein, and riboflavin from milk, antioxidants from tea and coffee, and vitamins, minerals, and fiber from juices. Socializing over a beverage may add to quality of life. Some long-term care institutions have implemented "happy hour" programs to encourage fluid intake.

## REVIEW QUESTIONS

1. What are the three most common chronic conditions affecting **men** over age 65?
2. What are the three most common chronic conditions affecting **women** over age 65?
3. BMI is a less effective predictor of morbidity and mortality in older than younger adults. Why is BMI a less reliable tool in older adults?

In questions 4–8, determine whether the statement is true or false.

4. The DASH diet has been shown to reduce HBP; additional sodium restrictions have led to further reductions in blood pressure.

   _____ True _____ False
5. Even a small loss of body weight can improve osteoarthritis.

   _____ True _____ False
6. Vitamin K levels present in dark green vegetables may interfere with warfarin (anti-coagulant) therapy.

   _____ True _____ False
7. Eating a Mediterranean-style diet is associated with lower CVD mortality in older adults.

   _____ True _____ False
8. Older adults who suffer from sarcopenia may benefit from high-protein diets. High protein intake will also help to keep their bones strong.

   _____ True _____ False
9. Vitamin $B_{12}$ deficiency can cause irreversible neurological damage. List at least three reasons why an older adult might have low vitamin $B_{12}$ levels.
10. Dehydration can result in confusion. List three or more strategies that can help to restore hydration and provide nutrients an older adult might be missing.

Visit www.cengagebrain.com to access MindTap, a complete digital course that includes additional resources.

# Answers to Review Questions

## Chapter 1

1. True
2. False
3. False
4. False
5. True
6. Answers consist of pregnant women, breastfeeding women, infants, growing children, frail elderly, ill persons, and people recovering from illness.
7. True
8. False
9. True
10. False
11. a
12. True
13. False
14. False
15. True
16. True
17. True
18. d
19. a
20. c

## Chapter 2

1. b
2. True
3. False
4. True
5. d
6. a
7. i
8. b
9. c
10. h
11. f
12. e
13. g
14. False
15. True
16. False
17. d
18. True
19. True
20. False
21. True
22. False
23. True
24. False
25. False
26. False
27. False
28. True
29. c

## Chapter 3

1. True
2. False
3. True
4. False
5. False
6. False
7. True
8. True
9. True
10. False
11. False
12. True
13. True
14. False
15. True
16. True
17. True
18. True
19. True
20. True
21. False
22. True
23. False
24. False

## Chapter 4

1. c
2. True
3. 4 lb 10 oz
4. False
5. False
6. a
7. d
8. a
9. b
10. True
11. False
12. True
13. True
14. False
15. False
16. True
17. False
18. True

19. True
20. c
21. False
22. a
23. 130 nmol/L
24. 193 pmol/L
25. 911nmol/L
26. True
27. False
28. False
29. c
30. True
31. False
32. True
33. False

## *Chapter 5*

1. True
2. True
3. False
4. False
5. False
6. True
7. False
8. d
9. True
10. False
11. True
12. True
13. False
14. False
15. False
16. False

## *Chapter 6*

1. d
2. a
3. c
4. b
5. c
6. b
7. c
8. a
9. c
10. Lactogenesis 1: the first stage of milk production which extends into the first few postpartum days when suckling is not needed for milk production. Lactose and protein content of milk increases.

    Lactogenesis II: begins 2-5 days postpartum and continues to about 10 days of postpartum. This is when milk comes in, the lactose and fat composition are increasing, the protein content decreases, and the volume of milk produced is increasing.

    Lactogenesis III: begins about 10 days postpartum and milk composition becomes stable.
11. Correct answers include:
    - The balance of nutrients in human milk matches human infant requirements for growth and development closely; no other animal milk or HMS meets infant needs as well.
    - Human milk is isosmotic (of similar ion concentration; in this case human milk and plasma are of similar ion concentration) and therefore meets the requirements for infants without other forms of food or water.
    - The relatively low protein content of breast milk compared to cow's milk meets the infant's needs without overloading the immature kidneys with nitrogen.

    Minerals including iron and zinc are provided in a form that is highly available.

## *Chapter 7*

1. Trauma from poor positioning, poor latch, improper release of suction after a feeding, infection, thrush, incorrect flange size during pumping or too much pressure while pumping and disorganized or dysfunctional suck.
2. d
3. Development after cracked or sore nipples, missing a feeding or mom sleeping through the night, restrictive clothing or a tight bra.
4. True
5. True
6. True
7. False
8. Jaundice observed in the first 24 hours of life, blood group incompatibility or haemolytic disease, gestational age 35–36 weeks, previous siblings received phototherapy, significant bruising, exclusive breastfeeding when not going well and/or excessive weight loss, east Asian race.
9. d
10. d

## Chapter 8

1. b
2. c
3. d
4. c
5. a
6. Correct answers include: increase gastrointestinal distress, increase gastroesophageal reflux, stifle infant hunger and fullness cues, increase spitting up.
7. c
8. a
9. The correct answers include: responding appropriately to the infant's hunger and satiety cues, recognizing the infants developmental abilities and feeding skills, fostering the infant's abilities to initiate and guide feeding and mealtime interactions, and providing pleasant eating environments.

## Chapter 9

1. c
2. a
3. False
4. True
5. False
6. False
7. The correct answers include: cleft lip and palate, congenital anomalies, and chromosomal disorders.
8. The correct answers include: disorders that impact brain growth, side effects of medications, altered body composition, increased or decreased energy expediture.
9. Correct answers include: nasogastric feeding, orogastric feeding, parenteral feeding, and gastrostomy tube feeding.

## Chapter 10

1. c
2. d
3. e
4. a
5. True
6. d
7. Whole-grain breads and cereals.
   - Fruits and vegetables.
   - Low-fat dairy products.
   - Lean meats, fish, and beans.
   - Limited amount of sweetened beverages and sweets.
8. Physical activity plays a role in maintaining energy balance.

   Physical activity helps to build muscle strength.

   Being physically active is a healthy lifestyle behavior that is important to establish at a young age.

   Appropriate activities for children include riding a tricycle or bicycle, walking, skipping, running, and active play.

   Limiting screen time and moving screens from young children's bedrooms is also recommended.

## Chapter 11

1. c
2. d
3. c
4. a
5. True
6. True
7. False
8. Correct answers include: to identify a decreasing rate of head growth, because any change in brain growth can impact weight and height (or length) growth, conditions such as spastic quadriplegia, cerebral palsy, Rett syndrome, Prater-Willi syndrome, or Down syndrome.
9. Correct answers include: offering food textures that make the child a successful eater, allowing a monotonous diet if required for limited oral feeding skills, allowing a bottle longer than expected due to developmental delays requiring it.
10. Correct answers include: when a child has to have a restricted diet, such as a result of allergies; when medications cause side effects that lower appetite; when a child has behaviors that limit food choices, such as autism, Prader-Willi syndrome; treatment with a calorie-restricted diet.

## Chapter 12

Timothy, in Case Study 12.1, returns to his pediatrician 6 months later at 7½ years of age for a weight check. He has gained 10 kg in 6 months and now weighs 90 pounds (41 kg). His height has increased to 51 inches (130 cm).

1. BMI = weight in kg divided by height in meters squared; 41 kg divided by 1.69 = 24.26 kg/m$^2$.
2. >99$^{th}$ % for his age and gender.
3. e
4. Timothy would enter the Prevention Plus approach to treatment for 3–6 months. If he maintains his weight or his BMI-for-age percentile is deflecting down, he would continue the Prevention Plus. If he gains weight, the next approach would be a structured weight management program. If he has weight loss or his BMI-for-age percentile deflects down, he would continue the structured weight management program. If he continues to gain weight, then he would enter a comprehensive multidisciplinary intervention.
5. d
6. Find a safe route for walking or biking to school.

   Encourage at least 60 minutes of active play per day.

   Work within the community to maintain parks and other safe places for children to play.

   Child can participate in organized sports that are appropriate for his stage of development and physical abilities.
7. Decrease "screen time" to less than 2 hours per day.

   Remove televisions, video games, and computers from children's bedrooms.

   Be active as a family.
8. c

## Chapter 13

1. c (the other conditions are not known to impact growth directly).
2. b (because this child would have a change in body composition).
3. c (as this is the only answer having to do with limited activity).
4. b
5. True
6. True
7. False
8. Examples of support services for families are maternal and child health services, school nutrition programs, and school educational programs.
9. Correct answers include medication side effects and ability to concentrate or attend to meals.
10. An IEP is a school educational plan that could include feeding or eating assistant, access to snacks or meals at set times at school, and selection of foods appropriate for the child's abilities or condition.

## Chapter 14

1. a
2. False
3. d
4. False
5. b
6. b
7. Biological age is based on sexual maturation rating. It assesses the degree of physical development, which can vary greatly among individuals of the same gender and age, thus is a better indicator of the nutrient needs of individuals as it provides a physiological estimate of needs based on growth velocity, body composition, and reproductive capacity.
8. d
9. d

## Chapter 15

1. True
2. c
3. d
4. c
5. c
6. While both conditions include eating large amounts of food in a short period of time, a diagnosis of bulimia nervosa requires frequent purging methods to compensate for the calories consumed while the diagnosis of binge-eating disorder does not include a criteria for purging.
7. Energy intake that results from the consumption of alcohol may displace energy intake from food. Because alcohol does not provide micronutrients, the overall dietary quality would be reduced in an individual who consumed alcohol frequently. The use of tobacco increases vitamin C requirements. The use of recreational drugs may result in increased intakes of snack foods and other highly refined simple carbohydrates which are high in sodium and fat and low in micronutrients.

## Chapter 16

1. Individual factors—Things individuals are primarily responsible for, including food and nutrient intake and nutritional adequacy, physical activity and other lifestyle habits; and the results of individual behavior on weight status and chronic disease risk factors. These are monitored at the individual level using standard indicators, summarized across population groups, and compared to national Healthy People 2020 objectives.

   External or environmental factors—Things that are the result of decisions made by planners, retailers, employers and healthcare providers and others that affect the environments in schools, worksites, and the community; as well as the social environment (support systems, income, education, discrimination), physical environment (housing, transportation, location of retail stores and restaurants), and availability and quality of health and nutrition services. These are monitored at the local community, state and federal levels and compared to Healthy People 2020 objectives.

2. Bone density and muscular strength peak by age 30. By middle adulthood there is a loss in muscle mass and an increase and redistribution of body fat. With the decline of estrogen production bone loss is accelerated, abdominal fat increases and blood cholesterol and triglyceride levels raise. Risk for hypertension, insulin resistance, diabetes, stroke, gallbladder disease and coronary artery disease increase with the accumulation of additional body fat. These changes shift the person from resilient and healthy with metabolic homeostasis to observable physiologic and metabolic alteration and the development of clinical conditions and chronic diseases.

3. Caloric needs can be determined by using reference tables (Table 16.4), measured through indirect calorimetry, and calculated using the Mifflin-St. Jeor formula or the simple method of 15 calories per pound of body weight. Factors that decrease calorie needs are sedentary lifestyle, and aging with declines in metabolic rate and loss of muscle mass. Calorie needs are increased by physical activity, and by increases in weight and muscle mass.

4. Males consume too much total and saturated fat, cholesterol, sugar and sodium and not enough fiber, vitamins A, D, E, K (for young men), choline, magnesium and potassium. Females have too much total and saturated fat, and sodium and low intakes of fiber, vitamins A and E, choline, calcium, iron, magnesium and potassium. Inadequacies and excesses alter substrate availability, cause imbalances at the cellular and subcellular levels, and result in changes in tissues such as bone, blood vessels, skin and mucosal membranes.

5. Considerations include: Priority health issues and nutrient needs of young adults and older faculty and staff, and current Dietary Guidelines for Americans. The challenge on college campuses is to provide nutrient-dense foods, minimize solid fats and added sugars, and offer appropriate serving sizes while taking into account product availability, cultural and taste preferences, convenience and cost. Education messages should include guidance on what and how much to eat, and could incorporate components of the Eating Competence Model. You might consider environmental changes and policies to support healthful food choices and opportunities for physical activity.

6. Compare your current level of activity with the national guidelines on Table 16.9. Being more physically active increases muscle strength, balance and endurance, support physical and mental health, improves cognitive function, helps manage weight and combat weight gain, reduces blood cholesterol and blood pressure, and helps prevent the onset or progression of several chronic diseases. Sedentary lifestyle results in the loss of these benefits.

7. Individuals—Education and counseling to increase knowledge and encourage behavior change, primary care providers assessing and talking about BMI, eating habits, and physical activity.

   Organizations—Health promotion programs, sponsored events, community gardens, food shelves, and policies about types of foods served in cafeteria and events.

   Environmental Changes—Increased access to grocery stores, farmers markets and community gardens, healthful food and beverage choices vending machines, point of purchase signage about calories and fat content.

   Product Development and Marketing—functional foods, front-of-package food rating symbols, smaller package and serving sizes.

   Policies—Enrichment of foods, food labelling and health claims, and nutrition programs to improve food security.

## Chapter 17

1. Essential components of cognitive behavioral change programs include:
   - Long duration—programs are 12–16 weeks long to build knowledge, modify beliefs and attitude, and integrate new behaviors.
   - Combination of skills training and analysis of behavior and thought processes.
   - Two key features are helping the client recognize and replace automatic and irrational thoughts and beliefs (cognitive restructuring) and increasing awareness and control of cues associated with eating (stimulus control).
   - Strategies include setting realistic goals, calorie deficit if needed for weight loss, individualized meal plan that includes variety of enjoyed foods and fits lifestyle and budget, skills development, problem solving, self-management, cognitive restructuring, stress management, having a support system, and regular exercise, followed by maintenance support—all directed to long-term effectiveness.
2. Differences between recommendations to reduce risk of the population and treatment of high risk individuals:
   - Population messages vs. individualized behavioral counseling and on-going intervention with health care providers to help make therapeutic lifestyle changes.
   - Cardio-protective diet that emphasizes plant foods and is similar to Dietary Guidelines for Americans vs. tighter restrictions on dietary fats and cholesterol intake and higher amounts of fiber with emphasis on viscous fiber.
   - Pharmacotherapy is often added for high risk individuals to lower LDL cholesterol and reduce plaque formation on the lining of arterial walls.
3. Abdominal obesity, high blood pressure, elevated fasting glucose, dyslipidemia with elevated LDL cholesterol, low HDL and high triglycerides. Three are needed for a diagnosis of metabolic syndrome. Waist circumference is a simple screening method.
4. There is a long pre-symptomatic phase with marginally elevated glucose during which vascular changes occur. Intervention in the prediabetes phase can prevent conversion to diabetes and reduce cardiovascular risk factors.
5. Diet flexibility within an individualized plan. This includes a target calorie level based on current weight and weight goal, with a defined distribution of calories among carbohydrate, protein and fat. A meal plan including snacks that provides relatively stable carbohydrate intake throughout the day. A variety of food to meet basic nutrient needs (RDA and DRI) and is consistent with healthy eating/ cardio-protective diet (Dietary Guidelines for Americans).
6. Prevention—Healthy diet with caloric intake adjusted to achieve or maintain weight within normal ranges.

   Treatment—Medical nutrition therapy to restore nutrient shortages, maintain nutritional health, and prevent or manage complications of cancer and the side effects of treatment.

   Remission—Healthy diet with caloric intake adjusted to achieve or maintain weight within normal ranges.

   Advanced Stages of Cancer—Food and fluid intake adjusted to meet patient wishes and manage symptoms and improve quality of life.
7. HIV raises energy requirements by 10%. Macro and micro nutrient needs increase during periods of high viral load, decline of immune function, secondary infections and altered absorption and metabolism. Changes in gut and gastrointestinal pathogens can lead to nutrient malabsorption. Weight maintenance is associated with a person's ability to survive HIV disease. Adults with HIV have high rates of metabolic syndrome and are at risk for cardiovascular disease and type 2 diabetes. Often guidelines for CVD and diabetes and other comorbidities must be added to HIV nutrition considerations. Medication regimens require careful meal spacing. In later stages of the disease oral lesions, nausea, and diarrhea make eating difficult. Substance abuse, economic issues and food insecurity may also be complicating factors.
8. True
9. True
10. False
11. False
12. Total cholesterol, smoking status, and blood pressure.
13. Reduce caloric intake, while emphasizing foods that are compatible with a cardio-protective diet, and increase physical activity to lose weight. She should get 30 minutes of moderate physical activity most days of the week and work up to longer duration or greater intensity as she is able.
14. Common themes:
    - Maintain a healthy weight—if overweight, this means a weight loss of 5–10% of body weight. For HIV disease, the focus is on maintaining weight and maintaining lean body mass.
    - Avoid or reduce central or abdominal adiposity, because this is associated with insulin resistance and hyperglycemia, hyperlipidemia,

metabolic syndrome, cardiovascular disease, and type 2 diabetes.

- A healthy, cardio-protective diet emphasizes plant foods (vegetables, fruit, whole grains, legumes), healthy fats, low fat dairy products and lean meats. *Trans* fat is avoided and saturated fat is limited to 5-6% of calories; and intake of sweets and red meats is minimized.
- Choosing a "healthy diet," being physically active, and maintaining a healthy weight can help prevent the development of chronic disease and delay complications.
- Regular physical activity at a moderate or vigorous level is important because it aids weight loss and maintenance and improves insulin/glucose profile, as well as reducing lipids and blood pressure.
- Be screened and "know your numbers" (BMI, waist circumference, blood lipid levels, blood glucose, and blood pressure) to be aware of risk level and perhaps be motivated to take action.
- Lifestyle changes often require intensive, on-going intervention.

## *Chapter 18*

1. True
2. True, lifestyle factors are estimated to account for 51% of longevity compared to a 19% contribution from genetics.
3. False
4. False. [It's a trick question] While energy needs decrease with age, some vitamins (Vitamins $B_6$, C, D) and minerals (Mg, Ca) increase with age while iron and chromium decrease.
5. True
6. Here are seven factors that put older adults at risk of malnutrition: 1) food insecurity or low income, 2) eating fewer than two meals per day, 3) illness or a condition that has affected dietary intake, 4) lost or gained more than 10 pounds in the last 6 months, 5) polypharmacy, 6) BMI below 19 and 7) physical limitations to shop, cook, and feed self.
7. Here are three adjustments of generic food-guides to make for older adults: 1) Greater risk of dehydration requires fluid assessment and recommendations, 2) lower caloric intake needs to be balanced with greater nutrient density, especially when activity level is low, and 3) guidance needs to ensure adequate protein intake when caloric intake is marginal.
8. Reasons might include: Lack of money may affect ability to buy high quality protein, compromised ability to chew, inability to cut meats once cooked, cognitive impairment that leads to forgetting to eat.
9. Multiply 107 kg by 0.8–1.3 gm protein per kg body weight; distribute the 86–139 gm of protein that would be adequate for JT throughout the day in a way that he would consume as food and beverages; use heart-healthy protein sources.
10. True

## *Chapter 19*

1. Hypertension, arthritis and heart diseases.
2. Hypertension, arthritis and heart diseases, in other words, older men and women face the same chronic diseases.
3. The BMI is calculated using height and weight. Getting an accurate height may be more difficult in older adults who have compressed vertebrae or kyphosis which has reduced normal height. On average, older adults have lost muscle tissue which has been replaced with fat tissue and BMIs were developed with measurements of younger adults. Dehydration can introduce further errors into the interpretation of a BMI in an older individual. Thus, less weight may be due to less muscle and body water.
4. True, adherence to the DASH diet reduces blood pressure. An additional dose-response effect on blood pressure reduction results from sodium restriction.
5. True
6. True. Approximately 11% of men above age 65 and 4.5% of women over age 65 take warfarin and must keep their vitamin K levels stable for effective blood-thinning effect.
7. True
8. True
9. $B_{12}$ deficiency may result from malabsorption due to atrophic gastritis, GI infections such as H. pylori, lack of animal products in the diet, family history of pernicious anemia, and medications.
10. Push fluids by structuring reminders to drink (such as a water jug in the refrigerator that should be empty at day's end), drinking liberal amounts of water when taking medications, offering nutritious beverages to increase nutrients, observing "happy hour" as a time to socialize and consume fluids, and perhaps most importantly for many older women, deal with fears related to incontinence by fixing underlying structural problems and doing exercise (Kegels).

APPENDIX A

# Measurement Abbreviations and Equivalents

| METRIC OR SI UNIT | |
|---|---|
| UNIT | ABBREVIATION |
| Kilogram | kg |
| Gram | g |
| Milligram | mg |
| Microgram | $\mu g$, mcg |
| Nanogram | ng |
| Meter | m |
| Centimetre | Cm |
| Millimetre | Mm |
| Liter | L |
| Decilitres | dL |
| Millilitre | mL |
| Millimole | mmol |
| Micromole | $\mu$mol |
| Picomole | pmol |

| NONMETRIC | |
|---|---|
| UNIT | ABBREVIATION |
| Ounce | Oz |
| Pound | Lb |
| Tablespoon | Tbsp |
| Teaspoon | Tsp |
| Cup | cup |
| Pint | Pt |
| Quart | Qt |
| Gallon | Gal |
| Inch | in. |
| Foot | Ft |
| Yard | Yd |

**EQUIVALENTS**

| WEIGHT: METRIC | | |
|---|---|---|
| 1 kilogram | = | 2.2 pounds; 1000 grams |
| 1 gram | = | 0.035 ounce; 1000 milligrams |
| 1 milligram | = | 1000 micrograms |
| 1 microgram | = | 1000 nanograms |

| WEIGHT: NONMETRIC | | |
|---|---|---|
| 1 ounce | = | 28.35 grams |
| 1 pound | = | 0.45 kilograms; 454 grams |

| LINEAR | | |
|---|---|---|
| 1 millimeter | = | 0.039 inch |
| 1 centimeter | = | 0.01 meter; 0.39 inch |
| 1 meter | = | 100 centimeters; 39.4 inches; 3.28 feet |
| 1 inch | = | 2.54 centimeters; 0.025 meter |
| 1 foot | = | 30.5 centimeters; 0.31 meter |
| 1 yard | = | 3 feet; 0.91 meters |

| FLUID VOLUME | | |
|---|---|---|
| 1 teaspoon | = | 5 mL |
| 1 tablespoon | = | 15 mL; 0.5 ounce; 3 teaspoons |
| 1 ounce | = | 30 mL; 29.57 grams; 6 teaspoons; 2 tablespoons |
| 1 cup | = | 240 mL; 8 ounces; 48 teaspoons; 16 tablespoons |
| 1 pint | = | 480 mL; 2 cups; 16 ounces; 1 pound ("A pint is a pound the whole world round.") |
| 1 quart | = | 0.95 liter; 2 pints; 4 cups; 32 ounces; 2 pounds |
| 1 liter | = | 1.06 quarts; 1000 mL |
| 1 gallon | = | 3.79 liters; 4 quarts; 8 pints; 16 cups; 8 pounds ("Two cups in a pint, two pints in a quart, four quarts in a gallon.") |

| CONVENTIONAL UNITS AND SI UNITS[a] | | | |
|---|---|---|---|
| a. To convert conventional units to SI units, multiply by the conversion factor.<br>b. To convert from SI units to conventional units, divide by the conversion factor. | | | |
| | CONVENTIONAL UNITS | CONVERSION FACTOR | SI UNIT |
| Calcium | mg/dL | 0.25 | mmol/L |
| Cholesterol | mg/dL | 0.0259 | mmol/L |
| HDL cholesterol | mg/dL | 0.0259 | mmol/L |
| Ferritin | ng/mL | 2.247 | pmol/L |
| Folate | ng/mL | 2.266 | nmol/L |
| Glucose | mg/dL | 0.0555 | mmol/L |
| Hematocrit | % | 0.01 | Proportion of 1.0 |
| Hemoglobin | g/dL | 10.0 | g/L |
| Homocysteine | mg/L | 7.397 | μmol/L |
| Insulin | μIU/mL | 6.945 | pmol/L |
| Iron | μg/dL | 0.179 | μmol/L |
| LDL cholesterol | mg/dL | 0.0259 | mmol/L |
| Lipoprotein (a) | mg/dL | 0.0357 | μmol/L |
| Triglycerides | mg/dL | 0.0113 | mmol/L |
| Vitamin A (retinol) | μg/dL | 0.0349 | μmol/L |
| Vitamin E | μg/dL | 0.0232 | μmol/L |
| Vitamin $B_6$ | ng/mL | 4.046 | nmol/L |
| Vitamin $B_{12}$ | pg/mL | 0.738 | nmol/L |
| Vitamin C | mg/dL | 56.78 | pmol/L |
| Vitamin D | ng/mL | 2.5 | nmol/L |

[a] "SI" stands for *le Système International d'unités*. SI values are based on decades of international cooperation in developing a universal system of measurement.

# APPENDIX B Body Mass Index (BMI)

| | 18 | 19 | 20 | 21 | 22 | 23 | 24 | 25 | 26 | 27 | 28 | 29 | 30 | 31 | 32 | 33 | 34 | 35 | 36 | 37 | 38 | 39 | 40 |
|---|---|---|---|---|---|---|---|---|---|---|---|---|---|---|---|---|---|---|---|---|---|---|---|
| **Height** | | **Body Weight (pounds)** | | | | | | | | | | | | | | | | | | | | | |
| 4'10" | 86 | 91 | 96 | 100 | 105 | 110 | 115 | 119 | 124 | 129 | 134 | 138 | 143 | 148 | 153 | 158 | 162 | 167 | 172 | 177 | 181 | 186 | 191 |
| 4'11" | 89 | 94 | 99 | 104 | 109 | 114 | 119 | 124 | 128 | 133 | 138 | 143 | 148 | 153 | 158 | 163 | 168 | 173 | 178 | 183 | 188 | 193 | 198 |
| 5'0" | 92 | 97 | 102 | 107 | 112 | 118 | 123 | 128 | 133 | 138 | 143 | 148 | 153 | 158 | 163 | 168 | 174 | 179 | 184 | 189 | 194 | 199 | 204 |
| 5'1" | 95 | 100 | 106 | 111 | 116 | 122 | 127 | 132 | 137 | 143 | 148 | 153 | 158 | 164 | 169 | 174 | 180 | 185 | 190 | 195 | 201 | 206 | 211 |
| 5'2" | 98 | 104 | 109 | 115 | 120 | 126 | 131 | 136 | 142 | 147 | 153 | 158 | 164 | 169 | 175 | 180 | 186 | 191 | 196 | 202 | 207 | 213 | 218 |
| 5'3" | 102 | 107 | 113 | 118 | 124 | 130 | 135 | 141 | 146 | 152 | 158 | 163 | 169 | 175 | 180 | 186 | 191 | 197 | 203 | 208 | 214 | 220 | 225 |
| 5'4" | 105 | 110 | 116 | 122 | 128 | 134 | 140 | 145 | 151 | 157 | 163 | 169 | 174 | 180 | 186 | 192 | 197 | 204 | 209 | 215 | 221 | 227 | 232 |
| 5'5" | 108 | 114 | 120 | 126 | 132 | 138 | 144 | 150 | 156 | 162 | 168 | 174 | 180 | 186 | 192 | 198 | 204 | 210 | 216 | 222 | 228 | 234 | 240 |
| 5'6" | 112 | 118 | 124 | 130 | 136 | 142 | 148 | 155 | 161 | 167 | 173 | 179 | 186 | 192 | 198 | 204 | 210 | 216 | 223 | 229 | 235 | 241 | 247 |
| 5'7" | 115 | 121 | 127 | 134 | 140 | 146 | 153 | 159 | 166 | 172 | 178 | 185 | 191 | 198 | 204 | 211 | 217 | 223 | 230 | 236 | 242 | 249 | 255 |
| 5'8" | 118 | 125 | 131 | 138 | 144 | 151 | 158 | 164 | 171 | 177 | 184 | 190 | 197 | 203 | 210 | 216 | 223 | 230 | 236 | 243 | 249 | 256 | 262 |
| 5'9" | 122 | 128 | 135 | 142 | 149 | 155 | 162 | 169 | 176 | 182 | 189 | 196 | 203 | 209 | 216 | 223 | 230 | 236 | 243 | 250 | 257 | 263 | 270 |
| 5'10" | 126 | 132 | 139 | 146 | 153 | 160 | 167 | 174 | 181 | 188 | 195 | 202 | 209 | 216 | 222 | 229 | 236 | 243 | 250 | 257 | 264 | 271 | 278 |
| 5'11" | 129 | 136 | 143 | 150 | 157 | 165 | 172 | 179 | 186 | 193 | 200 | 208 | 215 | 222 | 229 | 236 | 243 | 250 | 257 | 265 | 272 | 279 | 286 |
| 6'0" | 132 | 140 | 147 | 154 | 162 | 169 | 177 | 184 | 191 | 199 | 206 | 213 | 221 | 228 | 235 | 242 | 250 | 258 | 265 | 272 | 279 | 287 | 294 |
| 6'1" | 136 | 144 | 151 | 159 | 166 | 174 | 182 | 189 | 197 | 204 | 212 | 219 | 227 | 235 | 242 | 250 | 257 | 265 | 272 | 280 | 288 | 295 | 302 |
| 6'2" | 141 | 148 | 155 | 163 | 171 | 179 | 186 | 194 | 202 | 210 | 218 | 225 | 233 | 241 | 249 | 256 | 264 | 272 | 280 | 287 | 295 | 303 | 311 |
| 6'3" | 144 | 152 | 160 | 168 | 176 | 184 | 192 | 200 | 208 | 216 | 224 | 232 | 240 | 248 | 256 | 264 | 272 | 279 | 287 | 295 | 303 | 311 | 319 |
| 6'4" | 148 | 156 | 164 | 172 | 180 | 189 | 197 | 205 | 213 | 221 | 230 | 238 | 246 | 254 | 263 | 271 | 279 | 287 | 295 | 304 | 312 | 320 | 328 |
| 6'5" | 151 | 160 | 168 | 176 | 185 | 193 | 202 | 210 | 218 | 227 | 235 | 244 | 252 | 261 | 269 | 277 | 286 | 294 | 303 | 311 | 319 | 328 | 336 |
| 6'6" | 155 | 164 | 172 | 181 | 190 | 198 | 207 | 216 | 224 | 233 | 241 | 250 | 259 | 267 | 276 | 284 | 293 | 302 | 310 | 319 | 328 | 336 | 345 |
| | **Under-weight** (<18.5) | **Healthy Weight** (18.5–24.9) | | | | | | **Overweight** (25–29.9) | | | | | **Obese** (≥30) | | | | | | | | | | |

Find your height along the left-hand column and look across the row until you find the number that is closest to your weight. The number at the top of that column identifies your BMI. The area shaded in blue-green represents healthy weight ranges. The figures below present silhouettes of various BMI.

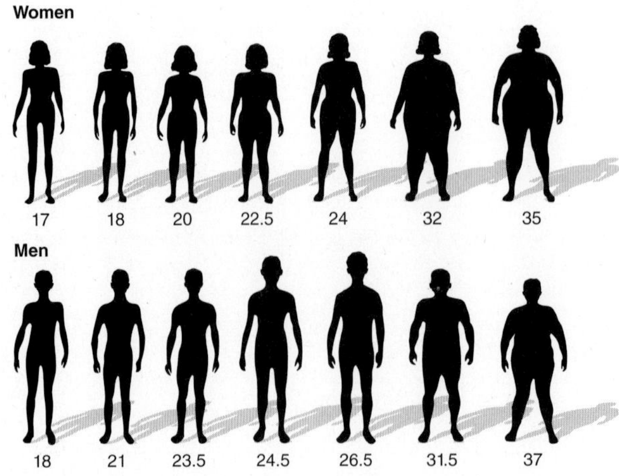


SOURCE: Reprinted from material of the Dietitians of Canada.

# References


## *Chapter 1*

1. What is food security? www.ers.usda.gov/topics/food-nutrition-assistance/food-security-in-the-us/measurement.aspx#insecurity, accessed10/18/14.

2. Coleman-Jensen, A., et al. Economic Household Food Security in the United States in 2013. Research Report No. (ERR-173) 41 pp., September 2014. Available at: www.ers.usda.gov/publications/err-economic-research-report/err173.aspx#.VAiu7ChWz6F, accessed 9/4/14.

3. Edge, J., et al. Enough for All: Household Food Security in Canada, The Conference Board of Canada, Aug 2103, www.conferenceboard.ca/e-library/abstract.aspx?did=5723, accessed 10/20/14.

4. *Summary Report on Application of the DRIs for Dietary Assessment*. Washington, DC: National Academy of Sciences, 2000.

5. Grabitske, H. A., et al. Low-digestible carbohydrates in practice. *J Am Diet Assoc* 2008; 108:1677–1681.

6. Glycemic Index and Diabetes, available at: www.diabetes.org/food-and-fitness/food/what-can-i-eat/understanding-carbohydrates/glycemic-index-and-diabetes.html, May 14, 2014, accessed 12/14/14.

7. *Dietary Reference Intakes: Energy, Carbohydrate, Fiber, Fat, Fatty Acids, Cholesterol, Protein, and Amino Acids*. Washington, DC: National Academies Press, 2002.

8. Brand-Miller, J. C., et al. Glycemic index, postprandial glycemia, and the shape of the curve in healthy subjects: Analysis of a database of more than 1000 foods. *Am J Clin Nutr* 2009; 89:97–105.

9. Data extracted from Foster-Powell, K., et al. International table of glycemic index and glycemic load values. *Am J Clin Nutr* 2002; 76:5–56.

10. Jonnalagadda, S. S., et al. Putting the whole grain puzzle together: health benefits associated with whole grains—Summary of American Society for Nutrition 2010 Satellite Symposium. *J Nutr* 2011; 141:1011S–22S.

11. 2015 Dietary Guidelines Advisory Committee. Advisory report to the Secretary of Health and Human Services and Secretary of Agriculture. Published February 2015. http://www.health.gov/dietaryguidelines/2015-scientific-report/PDFs/Scientific-Report-of-the-2015-Dietary-Guidelines-Advisory-Committee.pdf, accessed 3/12/15.

12. Harris, W. S., et al. Omega-6 fatty acids and risk for cardiovascular disease. *Circulation* 2009. Available at http://circ.ahajournals.org. Accessed 1/09.

13. Position of the American Dietetic Association and Dietitians of Canada: Dietary fatty acids. *J Am Diet Assoc* 2007; 107:1599–1611.

14. Hansel, B. Why dietary cholesterol is no longer enemy number one. *Medscape Diabetes & Endocrinology*. March 19, 2015. www.medscape.com/viewarticle/841486?nlid=78597_1521&src=wnl_edit_medp_wir&uac=61213SX&spon=17.

15. Ordovas, J. M. Genetic influences on blood lipids and cardiovascular disease risk: Tools for primary prevention. *Am J Clin Nutr* 2009; Suppl: 1509S–17S.

16. Bao, Y., Fenwick, R. *Phytochemicals in Health and Disease*. Boca Raton, FL: CRC Press, 2004.

17. Liu, R. H. Health benefits of fruit and vegetables are from additive and synergistic combinations of phytochemicals. *Am J Clin Nutr* 2003; 78:517S–520S.

18. Wolfe, K. L., et al. Cellular antioxidant activity of common fruits. *J Agric Food Chem* 2008; 56:8418–8426.

19. Halvorsen, B. L., et al. Content of redox-active compounds in foods consumed in the United States. *Am J Clin Nutr* 2006; 84:95–135.

20. *Dietary Reference Intakes: Water and Electrolytes*. Washington, DC: National Academies Press, 2004.

21. Kolasa, K. M. Water: The recommendations we give—Are they scientifically accurate? (Conference paper.) Food and Nutrition Conference and Exhibition, Oct. 2002; American Dietetic Association.

22. Corte, C., et al. People with marginal vitamin C status are at high risk of developing vitamin C deficiency. *J Am Diet Assoc* 1994; 99:854–856.

23.Vitamin C (Ascorbic acid). www.nlm.nih.gov/medlineplus/druginfo/natural/1001.html.

24. Lee, C., et al. Structural genomic variation and personalized medicine. *N Engl J Med* 2008; 358:740–741.

25. Bookman, E. B., et al. Gene-environment interplay in common complex diseases: Forging an integrative model—Recommendations from an NIH Workshop. *Genet Epidemiol Publ*, doi: 10.1002/gepi.20571, accessed 2/22/15.

26. Williams, R. A., et al. Phenylketonuria: An Inborn Error of Phenylalanine Metabolism. *Clin Biochem Rev* 2008; 29:31–41.

27. Galactosemia. ghr.nlm.nih.gov/condition=galactosemia. Published 3/17/12.

28. Hemochromatosis. digestive.niddk.nih.gov/ddiseases/pubs/hemochromatosis, April 2007, accessed 3/17/12.

29. Barker, D. J. Developmental origins of chronic disease. *Pub Health* 2012; 126:185–189.

30. Cornelis, M. C., et al. TCF7L2, dietary carbohydrate, and risk of type 2 diabetes in U.S. women. *Am J Clin Nutr* 2004; 89:1256–1262.

31. May P. A., et al. Maternal risk factors for fetal alcohol spectrum disorders: Not as simple as it might seem. *Alcohol Res Health*, 2011. Available at: pubs.niaaa.nih.gov/publications/arh341/15-26.htm.

32. Adhami, V. M., et al. Molecular targets for green tea in prostate cancer prevention. *J Nutr* 2003; 133(7 Suppl): 2417S–2424S.

33. Paez, K. More Americans getting multiple chronic illnesses. *Medscape Diabetes & Endocrinology.* Retrieved from www.medscape.com/view article/586363. Accessed 1/09.

34. Mortality in the United States, 2012, www.cdc.gov/nchs/data/databriefs/db168.htm. NCHS Data Brief, Number 168, October 2014.

35. World Cancer Research Fund/American Institute for Cancer Research. *Food, Nutrition, Physical Activity, and the Prevention of Cancer. A Global Perspective*. Washington, DC: AIRC, 2007.

36. Sievenpiper, J. L., et al. Are sugar-sweetened beverages the whole story? *Am J Clin Nutr* 2013; 98:261–263.

37. Bauer U. E., et al. Prevention of chronic disease in the 21st century: Elimination of the leading preventable causes of premature death and disability in the USA. *The Lancet*, July 5, 2014; 384; 9937: 45–52, doi:10.1016/S0140-6736(14)60648-6. Published Online 5/2/14.

38. Graudal, N., et al. Compared with usual sodium intake, low- and excessive-sodium diets are associated with increased mortality: a meta-analysis. *Am J Hyperten* 2014; 27:1129–1137, doi: 10.1093/ajh/hpu028.

39. Oyebode, O., et al. Fruit and vegetable consumption and all-cause, cancer and CVD mortality: Analysis of Health Survey for England data. *J Epidemiol Community Health* doi:10.1136/jech-2013-203500, accessed 5/20/14.

40. Wang, X., et al. Fruit and vegetable consumption and mortality from all causes, cardiovascular disease, and cancer: systematic review and dose-response meta-analysis of prospective cohort studies. *BMJ* July 29, 2014; 349:g4490. doi: 10.1136/bmj.g4490.

41. Cho, S. S., et al. Consumption of cereal fiber, mixtures of whole grains and bran, and whole grains and risk reduction in type 2 diabetes, obesity, and cardiovascular disease. *Am J Clin Nutr* August 2013; doi: 10.3945/ajcn.113.067629.

42. Inflammation in Chronic Disease. Mar 2015, www.cihr-irsc.gc.ca/e/43625.html, accessed 4/16/15.

43. Hiza, HAB., et al. Position of the Academy of Nutrition and Dietetics: Total diet approach to healthy eating. *J Am Acad Nutr Diet* 2013; 113:307–317.

44. Factsheet on the New Proposed Nutrition Facts Label. www.fda.gov/Food/GuidanceRegulation/GuidanceDocumentsRegulatoryInformation/LabelingNutrition/ucm387533.htm, 2/27/14, accessed 10/27/14.

45. Park, Y. K., et al. History of cereal-grain product fortification in the United States. *Nutr Today* 2001; 36:23–36.

46. Gutierrez-Castrellon, P., et al. *Probiotics* March 2104; doi: 10.1542/peds.2013–0652.

47. Boyle, R. J., et al. Risks of probiotic treatment. *Am J Clin Nutr* 2006; 83:1254–1264.

48. Douglas, D. C., et al. Probiotics and prebiotics in dietetics practice. *J Am Diet Assoc* 2008; 108:510–521.

49. Blackmore, K. M., et al. Early vitamin D intake and future risk of breast cancer. *Am J Epidemiol* 2008; 168:915–924.

50. Kittler, P. G., et al. Diet counseling in a multicultural society. *Diabetes Educator* 1989; 16: 127–132.

51. Freeland-Graves, J., et al. Position of the American Dietetic Association Total Diet Approach to Communicating Food and Nutrition Information. *J Am Diet Assoc* 2002; 102:100–108.

52. Conti, K. The four winds nutrition model: A new culturally specific food guide and nutrition approach for the Northern Plains Indians. (Seminar presentation.) Minneapolis: University of Minnesota, Oct 28, 2002.

53. Dirks, R. T. et al. African American dietary patterns at the beginning of the 20th century. *J Nutr* 2001; 131:1881–1889.

54. McCaffree, J. Dietary restrictions of other religions. *J Am Diet Assoc* 2003; 103:912.

55. Dwyer, J. Dietary assessment. In Shils, M. E., ed. *Modern Nutrition in Health and Disease*. Philadelphia: Lippincott, Williams & Wilkins: 1998. 937–962.

56. Horner, N. K., et al. Participant characteristics associated with errors in self-reported energy intake from the Women's Health Initiative food-frequency questionnaire. *Am J Clin Nutr* 2004; 76:766–773.

57. Kirkpatrick, S., et al. Performance of the Automated Self-Administered 24-hour Recall relative to a measure of true intakes and to an interviewer-administered 24-h recall. *Am J Clin Nutr*. 2014;100:233–240.

58. Automated self-administered 24-hour recall. Jan 2015, appliedresearch.cancer.gov/asa24, accessed 4/17/15.

59. Guenther, P. M., et al. The Healthy Eating Index-2010 is a valid and reliable measure of diet quality according to the 2010 Dietary Guidelines for Americans. *J Nutr.* 2014; 144:399–407.

60. Selhub, J., et al. The use of blood concentrations of vitamins and their respective functional indicators to define folate and vitamin $B_{12}$ status. *Food Nutr Bull* 2008; 29(2Suppl): S67–73.

61. Kranz, A., et al. Laboratory reference values. *N Engl J Med* 2004; 351:1548–1563.

62. Greer, J. P. et al. *Wintrobe's Clinical Hematology*, 11th ed. Philadelphia, PA: Lippincott Williams and Wilkins, 2004.

63. Second National Report on Biochemical Status Indicators of Diet and Nutrition in the U.S. Population. CDC, National Center for Environmental Health, Division of Laboratory Sciences, Mar. 27, 2012.

64. National Nutrition Monitoring System. Available at www.cdc.gov/nchs/nhanes.htm, accessed 8/06.

65. Food and Nutrition Assistance. Available at www.ers.usda.gov/Browse/FoodNutritionAssistance, accessed 11/08.

66. WIC Income Eligibility Guidelines. March 2015, www.fns.usda.gov/wic/wic-income-eligibility-guidelines, accessed 4/16/15.

67. Position of the American Dietetic Association: Child and adolescent food and nutrition programs. *J Am Diet Assoc* 2003; 103:887–892.

68. Healthy People *2020.* Available at: www.healthypeople.gov. Accessed September 23, 2011.

69. A Series of Systematic Reviews on the Relationship Between Dietary Patterns and Health Outcomes, www.nel.gov/vault/2440/web/files/DietaryPatterns/DPRptFullFinal.pdf, March 2014.

70. Nowson, C. A. et al. Blood pressure response to dietary modifications in free-living individuals. *J Nutr* 2004; 134:2322–2329.

71. Brand-Miller, J. C. et al. Glycemic index, postprandial glycemia, and the shape of the curve in healthy subjects: Analysis of a database or more than 1000 foods. *Am J Clin Nutr* 2009; 89:97–105.

72. Data extracted from Foster-Powell, K. et al. International table of glycemic index and glycemic load values. *Am J Clin Nutr* 2002; 76:5–56.

73. Wolfe, K. L., et al. Cellular antioxidant activity of common fruits. *J Agric Food Chem* 2008; 56:8418–8426.

74. Halvorsen, B. L., et al. Content of redoxactive compounds in foods consumed in the United States. *Am J Clin Nutr* 2006; 84:95–135.

75. Williams, R. A., et al. Phenylketonuria: An inborn error of phenylalanine metabolism. *Clin Biochem Rev* 2008; 29:31–41.

76. Galactosemia. ghr.nlm.nih.gov/condition=galactosemia. Published 3/12/12.

77. Hemochromatosis. digestive.niddk.nih.gov/ddiseases/pubs/hemochromatosis, April 2007, accessed 3/17/12.

78. Graudal, N., et al. Compared with usual sodium intake, low- and excessive-sodium diets are associated with increased mortality: A meta-analysis. *Am J Hyperten* 2014; 27:1129–1137, doi: 10.1093/ajh/hpu028.

79. Oyebode, O., et al. Fruit and vegetable consumption and all-cause, cancer and CVD mortality: Analysis of Health Survey for England data. *J Epidemiol Community Health*.

80. Wang, X., et al. Fruit and vegetable consumption and mortality from all causes, cardiovascular disease, and cancer: systematic review and dose-response meta-analysis of prospective cohort studies. *BMJ* July 29, 2014; 349:g4490. doi: 10.1136/bmj.g4490.

81. Cho, S. S., et al. Consumption of cereal fiber, mixtures of whole grains and bran, and whole grains and risk reduction in type 2 diabetes, obesity, and cardiovascular disease. *Am J Clin Nutr* August 2013; doi: 10.3945/ajcn.113.067629.

82. Hiza, H. A. B., et al. Position of the Academy of Nutrition and Dietetics: Total diet approach to healthy eating. *J Am Acad Nutr Diet*. 2013; 113:307–317.

83. Ollberding, N. J., et al. Within- and between-individual variation in nutrient intake in children and adolescents. *J Acad Nutr Diet*. 2014; 114:1749–1758.

84. Andreyeva T., et al. The positive effects of the revised milk and cheese allowances in the special supplemental nutrition program for women, infants, and children. *J Acad Nutr Diet*. 2014; 114:622–630.

85. Dietary Guidelines for Americans, 2015-2020. health.gov/dietaryguidelines/2015/guideline, accessed 1/1/16

## Chapter 2

1. Louis, G.M.B., et al. Periconception window: Advising the pregnancy planning couple. *Fertil Steril. 2008; 89(2 Suppl): e119–e121.*

2. Kauffman, A. S., et al. Critical periods of susceptibility to short-term energy challenge during pregnancy: impact on fertility and offspring development. *Physiol Behav.* 2010; 99: 100–108.

3. Ramírez-Vélez, R. In Utero Fetal Programming and Its Impact on Health in Adulthood. *Endocrinol Nutr*. 2012 Apr 5.

4. Jensen, T. K., et al. Does moderate alcohol consumption affect fertility? Follow- up study among couples planning first pregnancy *BMJ*. 1998 Aug 22; 317(7157): 505–510.

5. Births and Natality. Feb 6, 2015, www.cdc.gov/nchs/fastats/births.htm, accessed 3/9/15.

6. Herbert, D. L., et al. Birth outcomes after spontaneous or assisted conception among

infertile Australian women aged 28 to 36 years: A prospective, population-based study. *Fertil Steril* 2012; 97:603–608.

7. Dunson, D. B. Increased infertility with age in men and women. *Obstet Gynecol* 2004; 103:51–56.

8. Van Voorhis, B. J. *In vitro* fertilization. *N Engl J Med* 2007; 356:379–386.

9. Kovac, P. Recurrent pregnancy loss. Available at www.medscape.com /viewprogram/5293, accessed 4/06.

10. Age-Related Factors That Influence Fertility, Nov 2012. www.nichd.nih.gov/health /topics/infertility/conditioninfo/Pages/age .aspx, accessed 4/30/15.

11. Wong, W. Y., et al. Male factor subfertility: Possible causes and the impact of nutritional factors. *Fertil Steril* 2000; 73:435–442.

12. Drakh, A., et al. Low Energy Availability in Female Athletes. emedicine.medscape.com /article/312312-overview.1/16/14.

13. Afeiche, M. C., et al. Processed meat intake is unfavorably and fish intake favorably associated with semen quality indicators among men attending a fertility clinic. *J Nutr.* 2014; 144:1091–1098.

14. Chavarro, J. E., et al. Diet and lifestyle in the prevention of ovulatory disorder infertility. *Obstet Gynecol* 2007; 110(5):1050–1058.

15. Homan, G. F., et al. The impact of lifestyle factors on reproductive performance in the general population and those undergoing infertility treatment: A review. *Hum Reprod Update* 2007; 13:209–223.

16. Trent, M., et al. Adverse adolescent reproductive health outcomes after pelvic inflammatory disease. *Arch Pediatr Adolesc Med* 2011; 165:49–54.

17. Giudice, L. C. Endometriosis. *N Engl J Med* 2010; 362:2389–2398.

18. Puscheck, E. E., et al. Infertility. Nov. 2014. emedicine.medscape.com /article/274143-overview?src=wnl_ref _clinfo&uac=61213SX, accessed 2/13/15.

19. Robker, R., et al. Are changes in ovarian environment linked to obesity and infertility? *J Clin Endocrinol Metab* 2009; March 12.

20. Pesant. M-H., et al. The lack of effect of insulin on luteinizing hormone pulsatility in healthy male volunteers provides evidence of a sexual dimorphism in the metabolic regulation of reproductive hormones. *Am J Clin Nutr* 2012; 96:283—288.

21. Bongaarts, J. Does malnutrition affect fecundity? A summary of evidence. *Science* 1980; 208:564–569.

22. Gordon, C. M. Functional hypothalamic amenorrhea. *N Engl J Med* 2010; 363, 365–371.

23. Bellver, J. Impact of body weight and lifestyle in IVF outcome. *Expert Rev Obstet Gynceol* 2008; 3:607–625.

24. The Practice Committee of the American Society for Reproductive Medicine, Obesity and Reproduction: An educational bulletin. *Fertil Steril* 2008; 90:S21–29.

25. Chavarro, J. E., et al. Body mass index in relation to semen quality, sperm DNA integrity, and serum reproductive hormone levels among men attending an infertility clinic. *Fertil Steril* 2009; Mar 2.

26. Chavarro, J. E., et al. Body mass index in relation to semen quality, sperm DNA integrity, and serum reproductive hormone levels among men attending an infertility clinic. *Fertil Steril* 2009; Mar 2.

27. Overweight and Obesity. Sept. 2014, www.cdc.gov/obesity/data/adult.html, accessed 11/19/14.

28. Reichlin, S. Female fertility and the body fat connection (review). *N Engl J Med* 2003; 348:869–870.

29. Bolúmar, F., et al. Body mass index and delayed conception: A European Multicenter Study on Infertility and Subfecundity. *Am J Epidemiol* 2000; 151:1072–1079.

30. Keys, A., et al. *The biology of human starvation.* Minneapolis: University of Minnesota Press, 1950.

31. Williams, N. L., et al. Evidence for a causal role of low energy availability in the induction of menstrual cycle disturbances during strenuous exercise training. *J Clin Endocrinol Metab* 2001; 86:5184–5193.

32. Ruder, E. H., et al. Oxidative stress and antioxidants: Exposure and impact on female fertility. *Hum Reprod Update* 2008; 14:345–357.

33. Agarwal, A., et al. Clinical relevance of oxidative stress in male factor infertility: An update. *Am J Reprod Immunol* 2008; 59:2–11.

34. Tremellen, K., et al. Oxidative stress and male infertility: A clinical perspective. *Hum Reprod Update* 2008; 14:243–258.

35. Agarwal, A. Oxidative stress and its implications in female infertility: A clinician's perspective. *Reprod Biomed Online* 2005; 11:641–650.

36. Mendiola, J., et al. A low intake of antioxidant nutrients is associated with poor semen quality in patients attending fertility clinics. *Fertil Steril* 2009; Jan 13.

37. Eskenazi, B., et al. Antioxidant intake is associated with semen quality in healthy men. *Hum Reprod* 2005; 20:1006–1012.

38. Showell, M. G., et al. Antioxidant vitamins and minerals for male subfertility, Dec 2014. www.cochrane.org/CD007411 /MENSTR_antioxidant-vitamins-and-minerals -for-male-subfertility, accessed 4/30/15.

39. Mendiola, J., et al. A low intake of antioxidant nutrients is associated with poor semen quality in patients attending fertility clinics. Fertil Steril. 2010; 93:1128–1133. doi: 10.1016/j.fertnstert.2008.10.075.

40. Agarwal, A., et al. Utility of antioxidants during assisted reproductive techniques: an evidence based review. *Reprod Biol Endocrinol.* 2014; 12: 112. doi: 10.1186/1477-7827-12-112.

41. Walczak–Jedrzejowska., et al. The role of oxidative stress and antioxidants in male fertility. *Cent European J Urol.* 2013; 66(1): 60–67.

42. Tian, X., et al. Acute dietary zinc deficiency before conception compromises oocyte epigenetic programming and disrupts embryonic development. *Dev Biol.* 2013 Apr 1; 376(1): 51–61.

43. Yuyan, L., et al. Are serum zinc and copper levels related to semen quality? *Fertil Steril* 2008; 89:1008–1011.

44. Colagar, A. H., et al. Zinc levels in seminal plasma are associated with sperm quality in fertile and infertile men. *Nutr Res* 2009; 29:82–88.

45. Abbasi, A. A., et al. Experimental zinc deficiency in man. Effect on testicular function. *J Lab Clin Med* 1980; 96:544–550.

46. Mumford, S. L., et al. Higher urinary lignan concentrations in women but not men are positively associated with shorter time to pregnancy. J Nutr. 2014 Mar; 144(3):352–358.

47. Griffith, J. Association between vegetarian diet and menstrual problems in young women: A case presentation and brief review. *J Pediatr Adolesc Gynecol* 2003; 16:319–323.

48. Jacobsen, B. K., et al. Soy isoflavone intake and the likelihood of ever becoming a mother: the Adventist Health Study-2. *Int J Womens Health.* 2014 Apr 5; 6:377–384.

49. Setchell, K. D. R. Absorption and metabolism of soy isoflavones—from food to dietary supplements and adults and infants. *J Nutr* 2000; 130:654S–5S.

50. Dietary Guidelines for Americans, 2010. www.dietaryguidelines.gov.

51. Second National Report on Biochemical Status Indicators of Diet and Nutrition in the U.S. Population. CDC, National Center for Environmental Health, Division of Laboratory Sciences, March 27, 2012. Available at www.cdc.gov/nutritionreport.

52. Chavarro, et al. Iron consumption and the risk of infertility. *Obstet Gynecol* 2006; 108:1145–1152.

53. Taylor, K. C., et al. Alcohol, smoking, and caffeine in relation to fecundability, with effect modification by *NAT2*. *Ann Epidemiol.* 2011 Nov; 21(11): 864–872. doi: 10.1016/ j.annepidem.2011.04.011.

54. Chavarro, J. E., et al. Caffeinated and alcoholic beverage intake in relation to ovulatory disorder infertility. *Epidemiology* 2009; 20:374–381.

55. Hatch, E. E., et al. Caffeinated beverage and soda consumption and time to pregnancy. *Epidemiol.* 2012;23:393–401.

56. Bolumar, F., et al. Caffeine intake and delayed conception: A European multicenter study on infertility and subfecundity. European study group on infertility subfecundity. *Am J Epidemiol* 1997; 145:324–334.

57. Hatch, E. E., and Bracken, M. B. Association of delayed conception with

caffeine consumption. *Am J Epidemiol* 1993; 138:1082–1092.

58. Jensen, T. K., et al. Does moderate alcohol consumption affect fertility? Follow-up study among couples planning first pregnancy. *BMJ* 1998; 317:505–510.

59. Tolstrup, J. S., et al. Alcohol use as predictor for infertility in a representative population of Danish women. *Acta Obstet Gynecol Scand* 2003; 82:744–749.

60. Benoff, S., et al. Blood lead levels and infertility in males. *Hum Reprod* 2003; 18: 374–383.

61. Lamb, E. J., et al. Epidemiologic studies of male factors in infertility. *Ann NY Acad Sci* 1994; 709:165–178.

62. Queiroz, E. K., et al. Occupational exposure and effects on the male reproductive system. *Cad Saude Publica* 2006; 22:485–493.

63. Wirth, J. J., et al. Adverse Effects of Low Level Heavy Metal Exposure on Male Reproductive Function. *Syst Biol Reprod* Med 2010; 56:147–167.

64. Meeker, J. D., et al. Cadmium, lead, and other metals in relation to semen quality: Human evidence for molybdenum as a male reproductive toxicant. *Environ Health Perspect* 2008; 116:1473–1479.

65. Queiroz, E. K., et al. Occupational exposure and effects on the male reproductive system. *Cad Saude Publica* 2006; 22:485–493.

66. Loucks, A. B., et al. The female athlete triad: Do female athletes need to take special care to avoid low energy availability? *Med Sci Sports Exerc* 2006; 38:1694–1700.

67. Soleimany, G., et al. Bone Mineral Changes and Cardiovascular Effects among Female Athletes with Chronic Menstrual Dysfunction. *Asian J Sports Med* 2012; 3:53–58.

68. Carmichael, S. L., et al. Maternal periconceptional alcohol consumption and risk for conotruncal heart defects. *Clin Molecular Teratol* 2003; 67:875–878.

69. Kim, M. H., et al. Factors associated with a positive intake of folic acid in the periconceptional period among Korean women. *Public Health Nutr* 2009 Apr. ; 12(4):468.

70. Position of the Academy of Nutrition and Dietetics: Nutrition and Lifestyle for a Healthy Pregnancy Outcome. *J Acad Nutr Diet.* 2014;114:1099–1103.

71. Langley-Evans, S. C. Nutrition in early life and the programming of adult disease. *J Human Nutr Diet* Jan 2104; doi: 10.1111/jhn.12212.

72. Occurrence prevention, Dec. 2014, www.cdc.gov/ncbddd/folicacid/recommendations.html, accessed 4/29/15.

73. Greenberg, J. A., et al. Folic acid supplementation and pregnancy: More than just neural tube defect prevention. *Rev Obstet Gynecol* 2011; 4:52–59.

74. Dunlap, B., et al. Folic acid and human reproduction—Ten important issues for clinicians. *J Exp Clin Assist Reprod.* 2011; 8: 2. Published online 2011 August 10: www.ncbi.nlm.nih.gov/pmc/articles/PMC3183498/?tool=pmcentrez.

75. Poretti, A., et al. Neural tube defects in Switzerland from 2001 to 2007: Are periconceptual folic acid recommendations being followed? *Swiss Med Wkly* 2008; 138:608–613.

76. Williams, J., et al. Updated estimates of neural tube defects prevented by mandatory folic acid fortification—United States, 1995–2011. MMR*Weekly*, January 16, 2015; 64(01);1–5, available at: www.cdc.gov/mmwr/preview/mmwrhtml/mm6401a2.htm?s_cid=mm6401a2_w#fig.

77. Nutrient Intakes from Food and Beverages: Mean Amounts Consumed per Individual, by Gender and Age, What We Eat in America, NHANES 2011-2012. Agricultural Research Service. 2014, www.ars.usda.gov/SP2UserFiles/Place/80400530/pdf/1112/Table_1_NIN_GEN_11.pdf, accessed 3/25/15.

78. Chen, L. W., et al. Maternal folate status, but not that of vitamins $B_{12}$ or $B_6$, is associated with gestational age and preterm birth risk in a multiethnic Asian population. *J Nutr.* 2015 Jan; 145(1):113–120. doi: 10.3945/jn.114.196352.

79. Hodgetts, V. A., et al. Effectiveness of folic acid supplementation in pregnancy on reducing the risk of small-for-gestational age neonates: a population study, systematic review and meta-analysis, *BJOG* Nov. 26, 2014; doi:10.1016/S0140-6736(14)61368.

80. Greenberg, J. A., et al. Folic acid supplementation and pregnancy: More than just neural tube defect prevention. *Rev Obstet Gynecol* 2011; 4:52–59.

81. Botto, L. D., et al. 5,10-Methylenetetrahydrofolate reductase gene variants and congenital anomalies: A HuGE Review. *Am J Epidemiol.* 2000; 151: 862–877.

82. Anderson, P. Less than half of young women with epilepsy take folic acid. Dec 2013. www.medscape.com/viewarticle/817559, accessed 5/3/15.

83. Arth, A, et al. Supplement use and other characteristics among pregnant women with a previous pregnancy affected by a neural tube defect—United States, 1997–2009. *Weekly.* January 16, 2015/; 64(01);6–9. available at: www.cdc.gov/mmwr/preview/mmwrhtml/mm6401a3.htm?s_cid=mm6401a3_w.

84. Dunlap, B., et al. Folic acid and human reproduction—Ten important issues for clinicians. *J Exp Clin Assist Reprod.* 2011; 8: 2. Published online 2011 August 10: www.ncbi.nlm.nih.gov/pmc/articles/PMC3183498/?tool=pmcentrez.

85. Hamner, H. C., et al. Fortification of corn masa flour with folic acid in the United States: an overview of the evidence. *Ann N Y Acad Sci.* 2014; 1312:8–14.

86. Duffy, M. E., et al. Biomarker response to folic acid intervention in healthy adults: a meta-analysis of randomized controlled trials. *Am J Clin Nutr.* 2014; 99:96–106.

87. West, A. S., et al. Folate-status response to a controlled folate intake in nonpregnant, pregnant, and lactating women. *Am J Clin Nutr* 2012; 96:789–800.

88. Micronutrient deficiencies: Iron deficiency anemia, 2015. www.who.int/nutrition/topics/ida/en, accessed 5/1/15.

89. Allen, L. H. Biological mechanisms that might underlie iron's effects on fetal growth and preterm birth. *J Nutr.* 2001;131:581S–589S.

90. Vandevijvere, S., et al. Iron status and its determinants in a nationally representative sample of pregnant women. *J Acad Nutr Diet.* 2013; 113:659–666.

91. *Dietary Reference Intakes for Vitamin A through Zinc, Food and Nutrition Board, Institute of Medicine.* Washington, DC: National Academy Press, 2001.

92. Dietary Reference Intakes. Food and Nutrition Board, Institute of Medicine, National Academy of Sciences, 12/10/10. Access through www.nap.edu.

93. Gardiner, P. M., et al. The clinical content of preconception care: nutrition and dietary supplements. *Am J Obstet Gynecol*, Dec. 2008, doi: 10.1016/j.ajog.2008.10.049.

94. 2015 Dietary Guidelines Advisory Committee. Advisory report to the Secretary of Health and Human Services and Secretary of Agriculture. Published February 2015. http://www.health.gov/dietaryguidelines/2015-scientific-report/PDFs/Scientific-Report-of-the-2015-Dietary-Guidelines-Advisory-Committee.pdf, accessed 3/12/15.

95. Grieger, J. A., et al. Preconception dietary patterns in human pregnancies are associated with preterm delivery. *J Nutr* 2014; 144:1075–1080.

96. Gardiner, P. M., et al. The clinical content of preconception care: nutrition and dietary supplements. *Am J Obstet Gynecol*, Dec. 2008, doi: 10.1016/j.ajog.2008.10.049.

97. Oral contraception and combination hormonal methods. health.nytimes.com/health/guides/specialtopic/birth-control-and-family-planning/oral-contraception-and-combination-hormonal-methods.html, 6/11/12.

98. Petitti, D. B. Hormonal contraceptives are arterial thrombosis—Not risk-free but safe enough. *N Engl J Med* 2012; 366:2316–2318.

99. Agren, U. M., et al. Effects of a monophasic combined oral contraceptive containing nomegestrol acetate and 17β-oestradiol compared with one containing levonorgestrel and ethinylestradiol on haemostasis, lipids and carbohydrate metabolism. *Eur J Contracept Reprod Health Care.* 2011; 16:444–457.

100. Winner, B., et al. Effectiveness of long-acting reversible contraception. *N Engl J Med* 2012; 366:1998–1908.

101. Effect of birth control pills and patches on weight, Jan. 2014, www.cochrane.org/CD003987/FERTILREG_effect-of-birth-control-pills-and-patches-on-weight, accessed 4/30/15.

102. Beksinska, M. E., et al. Weight change and hormonal contraception: fact and

fiction. *Expert Rev Obstet Gynecol* 2011; 6:45–56.

103. Lopez, L. M., et al. Effects of progestin-only birth control on weight. July 2013, www.cochrane.org/CD008815/FERTILREG_effects-of-progestin-only-birth-control-on-weight, accessed 4/30/15.

104. Wiegratz, I., et al. Hormonal contraception—What kind, when, and for whom? *Dtsch Arztebl Int.* 2011 July; 108(28–29): 495–506.

105. Lidegaard, O., et al. Thrombotic stroke and myocardial infarction with hormonal contraception. *N Engl J Med* 2012; 366:2257–66.

106. Berenson, A. B., et al. Effect of injectable and oral contraceptives on glucose and insulin levels. *Obstet Gynecol* 2011; 117: 41–47.

107. Roth, M. Y., et al. Pharmacologic development of male hormonal contraceptive agents. *Clin Pharmacol Ther 2011;* 89:133–136.

108. Harrison, G. G., et al. WIC infant and toddler feeding practices study: protocol design and implementation. *Am J Clin Nutr* 2014; 99(suppl):742S–746S.

109. The Role of the WIC Program in Improving Periconceptional Nutrition: A Small-Grants Research Program. www.ph.ucla.edu.

110. Caan, B., et al. Benefits associated with WIC supplemental feeding during the interpregnancy interval. *Am J Clin Nutr* 1987; 45:29–41.

111. Jus'at, I., et al. Reaching young Indonesian women through marriage registries: An innovative approach for anemia control. *J Nutr* 2000; 130:456S–8S.

112. Lu, M. C., et al. Recommendations for Preconception Care. *Am Fam Physician* 2007; 76:397–400.

113. Kohnle, D. Health tip: Talk to your doctor before you are pregnant. April 11, 2012.

114. Recommendations to improve preconception health and health care, United States. *MMWR* April 21, 2006.

115. *Summary of the Nutrition Care Process Steps for Nutrition Assessment (Pocket Guide for International Dietetics & Nutrition Terminology), Reference Manual*, 2nd ed. Chicago: American Dietetic Association, 2009.

116. Healthy People 2020. Maternal, Infant and Child Health: Preconception Health and Behaviors. www.healthypeople.gov/2020/topicsobjectives2020/objectiveslist.aspx?topicId=26, accessed 6/8/12.

117. Cereals that Contain 100% of the Daily Value (DV) of Folic Acid. Apr 2012, www.cdc.gov/ncbddd/folicacid/cereals.html, accessed 4/15/15.

118. USDA Nutrient Data Bank. ndb.nal.usda.gov/ndb/nutrients/report?nutrient1=431&nutrient2=&nutrient3=&fg=&max=25&subset=0&offset=425&sort=c&totCount=6501&measureby=m, accessed 4/29/15.

## Chapter 3

1. Obesity and overweight, Apr 2015.www.cdc.gov/nchs/fastats/obesity-overweight.htm, accessed 5/7/15.

2. Fryar, C. D., et al. Prevalence of Underweight Among Adults Aged 20 and Over: United States, 1960–1962 Through 2011–2012, Sep 2014. www.cdc.gov/nchs/data/hestat/underweight_adult_11_12/underweight_adult_11_12.htm, accessed 5/7/15.

3. Pasquali, R., et al. Metabolic effects of obesity on reproduction. *Reprod Biomed Online* 2006; 12:542–51.

4. Treating as a disease, Jan 2015. www.heart.org/HEARTORG/GettingHealthy/WeightManagement/Obesity/Treating-Obesity-as-a-Disease_UCM_459557_Article.jsp, accessed 5/7/15.

5. Can obesity and overweight affect fertility? Sept 2013. www.nichd.nih.gov/health/topics/obesity/conditioninfo/pages/faqs_fertility.aspx, accessed 5/7/15.

6. Wise, L. A., et al. Body size and time-to-pregnancy in black women. *Hum Reprod.* 2013; 28:2856–2864.

7. Suren, P., et al. Parental Obesity and Risk of Autism Spectrum Disorder. *Pediatrics*, published online April 7, 2014, doi:10.1542/peds.2013-3664.

8. Garcia-Bailo, B., et al. Vitamins D, C, and E in the prevention of type 2 diabetes mellitus: modulation of inflammation and oxidative stress. *Biologics.* 2011; 5:7–19.

9. Chavarro, J. E., et al. Body mass index in relation to semen quality, sperm DNA integrity and serum reproductive hormone levels among men attending an infertility clinic. *Fertil Steril* 2010; 93:2222–2231.

10. MaRoth, M. Y., et al. Treatment of male infertility secondary to morbid obesity. Nat *Clin Pract Endocrinol Metab* 2008; 4:415–419.

11. Kasturi, S. S., et al. The metabolic syndrome and male infertility. *J Androl* 2008; 29:251–259.

12. Tobias, D. K., et al. Prepregnancy adherence to dietary patterns and lower risk of gestational diabetes mellitus. *Am J Clin Nutr* 2012; 96:289–295.

13. Travers, R. L., et al. The impact of adiposity on adipose tissue-resident lymphocyte activation in humans. International Journal of Obesity. 2015; 39:762–769.

14. Kauffman, A. S., et al. Critical periods of susceptibility to short-term energy challenge during pregnancy: impact on fertility and offspring development. *Physiol Behav* 2010; 99:100–108.

15. Fairley, D. A., et al. Anovulation. *BMJ* 2003; 327:546.

16. Jensen, T. K., et al. Body mass index in relation to semen quality and reproductive hormones among 1,558 Danish men. *Fertil Steril* 2004; 82:863–870.

17. Bozorgmanesh, M., et al. No obesity paradox—BMI incapable of adequately capturing the relation of obesity with all-cause mortality: An Inception Diabetes Cohort Study. *Int J Endocrin* 2014, doi.org/10.1155/2014/282089.

18. Hamer, M., et al. Obesity not always tied to higher heart risk: Study. http://bit.ly/JI0aUn *The Journal of Clinical Endocrinology & Metabolism*, online April 16, 2012.

19. Physical Activity and Health, Feb 2011. www.cdc.gov/physicalactivity/everyone/health/index.html?s_cid=tw_ob279, accessed 5/9/15.

20. Gene linked to male hormones in female infertility disorder, Apr 2014. www.nih.gov/news/health/apr2014/nichd-15.htm, accessed 5/9/15.

21. Zain, M. M., et al. Impact of obesity on female fertility and fertility treatment. *Women's Health* (Lond Engl) 2008; 4:183–194.

22. Vaughan, E., et al. Weight loss versus behavioral change as the primary goal in clinical practice. *Am J Lifestyle Med* 2015: doi:10.1177/1559827615579166.

23. Irresponsible messages from the Physicians Committee for Responsible Medicine? Medscape, Apr 3, 2012, boards.medscape.com/forums?128@173.j9bHaIJfgtf@.2a309794!comment=1.

24. Willis, K., et al. Bariatric surgery and pregnancy outcome—The ultimate solution? *Am J Obstet Gynecol* 2014; doi:10.1016/j.bpobgyn.2014.04.015.

25. Mingrone, G., et al. Bariatric surgery versus conventional medical therapy for type 2 diabetes. *N Engl J Med* 2012; 366:1577–1585.

26. Gadgil, M. D., et al. Laboratory testing for and diagnosis of nutritional deficiencies in pregnancy before and after bariatric surgery. *J Womens Health (Larchmt).* 2014; 23:129–137.

27. Mingrone, G., et al. Bariatric surgery versus conventional medical therapy for type 2 diabetes. *N Engl J Med* 2012; 366:1577–1585.

28. Bariatric surgery in women of reproductive age: Special concerns for pregnancy. Agency for Healthcare Research and Quality, 11/9/08. Available at ww.ahrq.gov/clinic/tp/babarireptp.htm.

29. The Practice Committee of the American Society for Reproductive Medicine, Obesity and Reproduction: An educational bulletin. *Fertil Steril* 2008; 90:S21–29.

30. Gordon, C. M. Functional hypothalamic amenorrhea. *N Engl J Med* 2010; 363:365–371.

31. Katz, M. G., et al. The reproductive endocrine consequences of anorexia nervosa. BJOG 2000; 107:707–713.

32. Hoffman, E. R., et al. Reproductive issues in anorexia nervosa. *Expert Rev Obstet Gynecol* 2011; 6:403–414.

33. Maxwell, M., et al. Life beyond the eating disorder: Education, relationships, and reproduction. *Int J Eat Disord* 2011; 44:225–232.

34. Drakh, A., et al. Low energy availability in female athletes. Medscape. emedicine .medscape.com/article/312312-overview, 1/16/14.

35. Joy, E., et al. Physician lack of knowledge of the female athlete triad. American College of Sports Medicine 57th Annual Meeting, Abs. 793, presented 5/28/09.

36. Soleimany, G., et al. Bone mineral changes and cardiovascular effects among female athletes with chronic menstrual dysfunction. *Asian J Sports Med* 2012; 3:53–58.

37. Lorber, D. L. Preconception counseling of women with diabetes. *Pract Diabetol* 1995; 14:12–16.

38. Carr, S. R. Effect of maternal hyperglycemia on fetal development. American Dietetic Association Annual Meeting and exhibition, Kansas City, MP\O, Oct. 10, 1998.

39. Neff, L. M. Evidence-based dietary recommendations for patients with type 2 diabetes mellitus. *Nutr Clin Care* 2003; 6:51–61.

40. O'Connor, L., et al. Prospective associations and population impact of sweet beverage intake and type 2 diabetes, and effects of substitutions with alternative beverages. *Diabetologia* 2015; doi: 10.1007/s00125-015-3572-1.

41. Bantle, J. P., et al. American Diabetes Association updated guidelines for Medical Nutrition Therapy to prevent diabetes, manage existing diabetes, and prevent or slow the rate of development of diabetes complications. *Diabetes Care* 2008; 31(Suppl):S61–78.

42. Astrup A., et al. The role of higher protein diets in weight control and obesity-related comorbidities. *Int J Obes* 2015; 39:721–726.

43. Liu, A. G., et al. Reducing the glycemic index or carbohydrate content of mixed meals reduces postprandial glycemia and insulinemia over the entire day but does not affect satiety. *Diabetes Care*. June 11, 2012; doi: 10.2337/dc12-0329.

44. Post, R. E., et al. Dietary fiber for the treatment of type 2 diabetes mellitus. J *Am Board Fam Med* 2012; 25:16–23.

45. American Dietetic Association. Evidence-based Nutrition Practice Guidelines. Available at www.adaevidencelibrary.com /topic.cfmf?cat=3731, accessed 2/09.

46. Peters, A. L., et al. Simple Strategy Triples Patient Weight Loss. American Diabetes Association (ADA) 72nd Scientific Sessions®, June 8–12, 2012; Philadelphia, www .medscape.com/viewarticle/766223?src =mp&spon=38, 7/15/12.

47. Marcason, W. A. What is the appropriate distribution of macronutrients for a patient with diabetes? *J Acad Nutr Diet* 2012; 112:776.

48. Diabetes risk after Gestational Diabetes. National Diabetes Education Program, ndep .nih.gov/media/fs_post-gdm.pdf, accessed 8/6/12.

49. Standards of Medical Care in Diabetes—2015 Abridged for Primary Care Providers, American Diabetes Association. Available at: clinical.diabetesjournals.org/content/33/2/97 .full.pdf.

50. Institute of Medicine, National Academy of Sciences, *Weight Gain During Pregnancy: Re-examining the Guidelines*. Washington, DC: National Academies Press, 2009.

51. Tobias, D. K., et al. Prepregnancy adherence to dietary patterns and lower risk of gestational diabetes mellitus. *Am J Clin Nutr* 2012; 96:289–295.

52. Diabetes Prevention Program Research Group. Reduction in the incidence of type 2 diabetes with lifestyle intervention or metformin. *N Engl J Med* 2002; 346:393–403.

53. Zhang, C., et al. Effect of dietary and lifestyle factors on the risk of gestational diabetes: review of epidemiology evidence. *Am J Clin Nutr* 2011; 94(suppl):1975S–9S.

54. Psaltopoulou, T., et al. The role of diet and lifestyle in primary, secondary, and tertiary diabetes prevention: A review of meta-analyses. *Rev Diabet Stud* 2010; 7:26–35.

55. Cooper, A. J., et al. A prospective study of the association between quantity and variety of fruit and vegetable intake and incident type 2 diabetes. *Diabetes Care*. 2012; 35:1293–1300.

56. Barr, S., et al. An isocaloric low glycemic index diet improves insulin sensitivity in women with polycystic ovary syndrome. *J Acad Nutr Diet*. 2013;113:1523–1531.

57. Polycystic ovary syndrome. Feb 2014, www.nlm.nih.gov/medlineplus/ency /article/000369.htm, accessed 5/9/15.

58. Cascella, T., et al. Visceral fat is associated with cardiovascular risk in women with polycystic ovary syndrome. *Human Reprod* 2008; 23:153–159.

59. ESHRE Capri Workshop Group. Health and fertility in World Health Organization group 2 anovulatory women. *Hum Reprod Update*, 2012 May 30.

60. Azziz, R. Diagnostic criteria for polycystic ovary syndrome: A reappraisal. *Fertil Steril* 2004; 83:1343–6.

61. Tolstoi, L. G., et al. Weight loss and medication in polycystic ovary syndrome therapy. *Nutr Today* 2002; 37:57–62.

62. Asagami, T., et al. Differential effects of insulin sensitivity on androgens in obese women with polycystic ovary syndrome or normal ovulation. *Metab* 2008; 57:1355–1360.

63. Stein, K. Polycystic ovary syndrome: What it is and why registered dietitians need to know. *J Am Diet Assoc* 2006; 106:1738–1741.

64. Nieuwenhuis-Ruifrok, A. E., et al. Insulin-sensitizing drugs for weight loss in women of reproductive age who are overweight or obese: Systematic review and meta-analysis. *Human Reprod Update* 2009; 15:57–68.

65. McKittrick, M. Diet and polycystic ovary syndrome. *Nutr Today* 2002; 37: 63–69.

66. Moran, L. J., et al. Dietary composition in the treatment of polycystic ovary syndrome: a systematic review to inform evidence-based guidelines. *J Acad Nutr Diet*. 2013; 113:520–545.

67. Goss, AM., et al. Effects of a eucaloric reduced-carbohydrate diet on body composition and fat distribution in women with PCOS. *Metabol-Clin Experimental* 2014; 63:1257–1264.

68. Thomson, R. L., et al. The effect of diet and exercise on markers of endothelial function in overweight and obese women with polycystic ovary syndrome. *Hum Reprod* 2012; 27:2169–2176.

69. Marsh, K. A., et al. Effect of a low glycemic index compared with a conventional healthy diet on polycystic ovary syndrome. *Am J Clin Nutr* 2010; 92:83–92.

70. Giovannini, M., et al. Phenylketonuria: nutritional advances and challenges. *Nutr Metab (Lond)*. 2012; 9: 7. Published online 2012 February 3; doi:10.1186/1743-7075-9-7.

71. Michals-Matalon, K., et al. Maternal phenylketonuria, low protein intake, and congenital heart defects. *Am J Obstet Gynecol* 2002; 187:221–224.

72. Waisbren, S. E., et al. Outcome at age 4 years in offspring of women with maternal phenylketonuria: The Maternal PKU Collaborative Study. *JAMA* 2000; 283:756–62.

73. Friedman, E. G., et al. The International Collaborative Study on maternal phenylketonuria: Organization, study design and description of the sample. *Eur J Pediatr* 1996; 155(Suppl)1:S158–161.

74. de Baulny, H. O., et al. Management of phenylketonuria and hyperphenylalaninemia. *J Nutr* 2007; 137(6 Suppl 1):1561S–1563S.

75. Simon, E., et al. Evaluation of quality of life and description of the sociodemographic state in adolescent and young adult patients with phenylketonuria (PKU). *Health Qual Life Outcomes* 2008; 6:25.

76. Isaacs, J. Metabolic dietician. Personal communication, 12/10/03.

77. Arnold, G. L., et al. Phenylketonuria treatment & management. *Medscape*, April, 2014. emedicine.medscape.com /article/947781-treatment, accessed 4/28/15.

78. Committee on Genetics, American Academy of Pediatrics. Maternal phenylketonuira. *Pediatrics* 2008; 122:445–449.

79. Giovannini, M., et al. Phenylketonuria: nutritional advances and challenges. *Nutr Metab (Lond)*. 2012; 9:7. Published online 2012 February 3; doi:10.1186/1743-7075-9-7.

80. Prick, B. W., et al. Maternal phenylketonuria and hyperphenalainemia in pregnancy: pregnancy complications and neonatal sequelae in untreated pregnancies. *Am J Cln Nutr* 2012; 95:374–382.

81. Pellicano, R., et. al. Women and celiac disease: Association with unexplained infertility. *Minerva Med* 2007; 98:217–219.

82. Rapaport L. Celiac disease linked to miscarriages and preterm deliveries, *Ann Gastroenterol* 2015. Available at: www.medscape.com/viewarticle/843296?nlid=80164_2826&src=wnl_edit_medn_fmed&uac=61213SX&spon=34, accessed 5/6/15.

83. Stazi, A. V., et al. Reproductive aspects of celiac disease. *Ann Ital Med Int* 2005; 20:143–57.

84. Hadziselimovic, F., et al. Celiac disease, pregnancy, small for gestational age: Role of extravillous trophoblast. *Fetal Pediatr Pathol* 2007; 26:125–134.

85. Neumann, J. Celiac disease showing up in many forms and at all ages. December 01, 2014, www.medscape.com/viewarticle/835567?src=wnl_edit_medn_wir&uac=61213SX&spon=34.

86. Choi, J. M., et al. Increased Prevalence of Celiac Disease in Patients with Unexplained Infertility in the United States: A Prospective Study. *J Reprod Med* 2011 May–Jun; 56(5–6):199–203.

87. Ludvigsson, J. F., et al. Celiac disease and risk of adverse fetal outcome: A population-based cohort study. *Gastroenterology* 2005; 129:454–463.

88. American Dietetic Association's Evidence-Based Library, Celiac. Available at www.adaevidencelibrary.com/topic.cfm?cat=3726, accessed 6/09.

89. Mansueto, P., et al. Non-Celiac Gluten Sensitivity: Literature Review. *J Am Coll Nutr.* 2014; 33:39–54.

90. Rubio-Tapia, A., et al. The prevalence of celiac disease in the United States. *Am J Gastroenterol* 31 July 2012; doi:10.1038/ajg.2012.219.

91. Fox, S. Celiac disease: Not so rare, mostly undiagnosed. *Medscape,* www.medscape.com/viewarticle/768473, posted Aug 1, 2012.

92. Premenstrual syndrome (PMS) fact sheet. Dec 2014. www.womenshealth.gov/publications/our-publications/fact-sheet/premenstrual-syndrome.html, accessed 5/6/15.

93. O'Brien, P. M., et al. Towards a consensus on diagnostic criteria, measurement and trial design of the premenstrual disorders: the ISPMD Montreal consensus. *Arch Womens Ment Health* 2011; 14:13–21.

94. Managing Premenstrual Symptoms, Jun 2008, www.arhp.org/Publications-and-Resources/Quick-Reference-Guide-for-Clinicians/PMS/signs, accessed 5/7/15.

95. Rapkin AJ., et al. Treatment of premenstrual dysphoric disorder. Womens Health (Lond Engl). 2013;9:537–556.

96. Htay, T. T., et al. Premenstrual dysphoric disorder. emedicine.medscape.com/article/293257, updated May 14, 2012.

97. Freeman, E. W., et al. Clinical subtypes of premenstrual syndrome and responses to sertraline treatment. *Obstet Gynceol* 2011; 118:1293–1230.

98. Yonkers, K. A., et al. Premenstrual syndrome. *Lancet* 2008; 5:1200–1210.

99. Ebrahimi, E., et al. Effects of Magnesium and Vitamin B6 on the Severity of Premenstrual Syndrome Symptoms. J Caring Sci. 2012; 1:183–189.

100. Rapkin AJ., et al. Treatment of premenstrual dysphoric disorder. *Womens Health (Lond Engl).* 2013; 9:537–556.

101. Dennehy, C. E. The use of herbs and dietary supplements in gynecology: An evidence-based review. *J Midwifery Womens Health* 2006; 51:402–409.

102. Whelan, A. M., et al. Herbs, vitamins and minerals in the treatment of premenstrual syndrome: a systematic review. *Can J Clin Pharmacol.* 2009; 16:e407–429.

103. Alberti, K. G., et al. Harmonizing the metabolic syndrome. A joint statement of the International Diabetes Federation Task Force on Epidemiology and Prevention; National Heart, Lung, and Blood Institute; American Heart Association; World Heart Federation; International Atherosclerosis Society; and the International Association for the Study of Obesity. *Circulation* 2009; 120:1640–1645.

104. Riediger, N. D., et al. Prevalence of metabolic syndrome in the Canadian adult population. *CMAJ* 2011; 183:e1127–e1134.

105. Can obesity and overweight affect fertility? Sept 2013. www.nichd.nih.gov/health/topics/obesity/conditioninfo/pages/faqs_fertility.aspx, accessed 5/7/15.

106. Azadbakht, L., et al. Beneficial effects of a Dietary Approaches to Stop Hypertension Eating Plan on Features of the Metabolic Syndrome. *Diabetes Care* 2005; 28:2823–2831.

107. Das, S. K., et al. Adipose tissue gene expression and metabolic health of obese adults. *Int J Obes* 2015; 39:869–873.

108. Serralde-Zúñiga, A. E., et al. Omental adipose tissue gene expression, gene variants, branched-chain amino acids, and their relationship with metabolic syndrome and insulin resistance in humans. *Genes Nutr.* 2014; 9:431, doi:10.1007/s12263-014-0431-5.

109. Diagnosis of diabetes. diabetes.niddk.nih.gov/dm/pubs/diagnosis, Dec. 5, 2011.

110. DeSisto, C. L., et al. Prevalence Estimates of Gestational Diabetes Mellitus in the United States, Pregnancy Risk Assessment Monitoring System (PRAMS), 2007–2010. *Prev Chronic Dis* 2014. Available at: www.cdc.gov/pcd/issues/2014/13_0415.htm.

111. National diabetes statistics report. 2014. Available at: www.cdc.gov/diabetes/pubs/statsreport14/national-diabetes-report-web.pdf.

112. Schenk, S., et al. Insulin sensitivity: Modulation by nutrients and inflammation. *J Clin Invest* 2008; 118:2992–3002.

113. Romao, I., et al. Genetic and environmental interactions in obesity and type 2 diabetes. *J Am Diet Assoc* 2008; 108:S24–S28.

114. Warwick, H., Anderson, W. H., et al. Gut reactions—From celiac affection to autoimmune model. *N Engl J Med* 2014; 371:6–7.

115. Rashtak, S., et al. Review article: Coeliac disease, new approaches to therapy. *Alimentary Pharmacology & Therapeutics.* 2012; 35(7):768–781.

116. Lionetti, E., et al. Introduction of gluten, HLA status, and the risk of celiac disease in children. *N Engl J Med* 2014; 371:1295–1303.

117. Lehman, L. More evidence for rise, and race difference, in U.S. celiac disease. Reuters. March 19, 2015. www.reuters.com/article/2015/03/18/us-health-race-celiac-gluten-idUSKBN0ME2SY20150318, accessed 3/13/15.

118. Rashtak, S., et al. Review article: Coeliac disease, new approaches to therapy. *Alimentary Pharmacology & Therapeutics.* 2012; 35(7):768–781.

119. Rewers, M., et al. Rotavirus infections and the development of celiac disease. *Am J Gastroenterol* 2006; 101:2333–2340.

120. Polycystic ovary syndrome, Feb 2014, www.nlm.nih.gov/medlineplus/ency/article/000369.htm, accessed 5/9/15.

121. Margaret, Doll. Retrieved from www.savebabies.org/familystories/photos/MargaretDollPKU.jpg, accessed 7/09.

122. Ford, A. C., et al. Relationships between celiac disease and irritable bowel syndrome. *Arch Intern Med* 2009; 169:651–658.

123. Catassi, C., et al. Celiac disease. *Curr Opin Gastroenterol* 2008; 24:687–691.

124. American Dietetic Association's Evidence-Based Library, Celiac. Available at www.adaevidencelibrary.com/topic.cfm?cat=3726, accessed 6/09.

125. Harding, C. Progress toward cell directed therapy for phenylketonuria. *Clin Genet* 2008; 74:97–104.

126. Sapone, A., et al. Spectrum of gluten-related disorders: consensus on new nomenclature and classification. *BMC Med.* 2012; 10:13. Published online 2012 February 7; doi:10.1186/1741-7015-10-13.

127. Waldrop, J. Early identification and interventions for female athlete triad. *J Pediatr Health Care* 2005; 19:213–220.

128. Cristine M. Trahms Program for Phenylketonuria. The essentials of PKU. depts.washington.edu/pku/resources/essentials.html, accessed 4/28/15.


## Chapter 4


1. Heisler, E. J., et al. The U.S. Infant Mortality Rate: International Comparisons, Underlying Factors, and Federal Programs. Congressional Research Service, April 4, 2012; www.fas.org/sgp/crs/misc/R41378.pdf.

2. Wegman, M. E. Infant mortality in the 20th century, dramatic but uneven progress. *J Nutr* 2001; 131:401S–408S.

3. Infant Mortality, 2013. mchb.hrsa.gov/chusa13/perinatal-health-status-indicators/p/infant-mortality.html, accessed 5/11/15.

4. The World Fact Book, Central Intelligence Agency, www.cia.gov/library/publications /the-world-factbook/rankorder/2091rank .html. Accessed 3/10/15. Figure of 56th based on estimate report for the U.S. in 2014.

5. Krisberg, K. U. S. lagging behind many other nations on infant mortality rates: Healthy behavior, healthier babies. Nation Health 2/27/2009; available at www .medscape.com/viewarticle/587840.

6. MacDorman, M. NCHS Data Brief No, 23, Oct. 2006, www.medscape.com /viewarticle/711795, accessed 11/17/09.

7. Collins, J. W., et al. Very Low Birthweight in African American Infants: The Role of Maternal Exposure to Interpersonal Racial Discrimination. *Am J Public Health* 2004 December; 94(12): 2132–2138.

8. CDC Fastats, A to Z. Available at www .cdc.gov/nchs/fastats/births.htm, accessed 7/09.

9. Kirkegaard, I., et al. Size at birth and later school performance. *Pediatrics* 2006; 118:1600–1606.

10. Langley-Evans SC. Nutrition in early life and the programming of adult disease. *J Human Nutr Diet* Jan 2104; doi: 10.1111/ jhn.12212.

11. King, J. C. Physiology of pregnancy and nutrient metabolism. *Am J Clin Nutr* 2000; 71:1218S–1225S.

12. Mshelia, D. S., et al. The importance of lipid and lipoprotein ratios in interpretations of hyperlipidemia of pregnancy. 2012; dx.doi .org/10.5772/46064.

13. Gernand, A. D., et al. Maternal nutritional status in early pregnancy is associated with body water and plasma volume changes in a pregnancy cohort in rural Bangladesh. *J Nutr* 2012; 142:1109–1115.

14. Hytten, F. E., and Leitch, I. *The Physiology of Human Pregnancy.* Oxford: Blackwell Scientific Publications, 1971.

15. Krisberg, K. U. S. lagging behind many other nations on infant mortality rates: Healthy behavior, healthier babies. *Nation Health* 2/27/2009; available at www.medscape .com/viewarticle/587840.

16. Mshelia, D. S., et al. The importance of lipid and lipoprotein ratios in interpretations of hyperlipidemia of pregnancy. 2012; dx.doi .org/10.5772/46064.

17. Butte, N. F. Carbohydrate and lipid metabolism in pregnancy: Normal compared with gestational diabetes mellitus. *Am J Clin Nutr* 2000; 71:1256S–1261S.

18. Duggleby, S. L., et al. Higher weight at birth is related to decreased amino acid oxidation during pregnancy. *Am J Clin Nutr* 2002; 76:852–857.

19. Godfrey, K. M. Maternal regulation of fetal development and health in adult life. *Eur J Obstet Gynecol* 1998; 78:141–150.

20. Wiznitzer, A., et al. Association of lipid levels during gestation with preeclampsia and gestational diabetes mellitus: a population-based study. *Am J Obstet Gynecol* 2009; 201: 482.e1–482.e8.

21. Saarelainen, H., et al. Pregnancy-related hyperlipidemia and endothelial function in healthy women. *Circ J* 2006; 70:768–772.

22. Khoury, J., et al. Effect of a cholesterol-lowering diet on maternal, cord, and neonatal lipids, and pregnancy outcome: A randomized clinical trial. *Am J Obstet Gynecol* 2005; 193:1292–1301.

23. Martin, U., et al. Is normal pregnancy atherogenic? *Clin Sci* (Colch) 1999; 96:421–425.

24. King, J. C. Effect of reproduction on the bioavailability of calcium, zinc and selenium. *J Nutr* 2001; 131:1355S–1358S.

25. Nickens, M.A., et al. Cardiovascular disease in pregnancy. *South Med J* 2013; 106:624–630.

26. Best Practices: Overview of pregnancy complications, Salt restriction. 14 Feb 2011, bestpractice.bmj.com/best-practice /monograph/494/overview/evidence /intervention/1402/0/sr-1402-i10.html, accessed 8/20/12.

27. American College of Obstetricians and Gynecologists. Nutrition during pregnancy. *ACOG Technical Bulletin No. 179* 1993:1–7.

28. Desoye, G., et al. Placental transport in pregnancy pathologies. *Am J Clin Nutr* 2011; 95(suppl):1895S–1902S.

29. Kourtis, A. P., et al. Pregnancy and infection. *N Engl J Med* 2014; 370:2211–2218.

30. Gude, N. M., et al. Growth and function of the normal human placenta. *Thromb Res.* 2004; 114:397–407.

31. Gluckman, P. D. Fetal origins of adult disease: Insulin resistance. *Medscape Ob/Gyn & Women's Health* 2003; 8:4–5.

32. Trahair, J. F., et al. Ultrastructural anomalies in the fetal small intestine indicate that fetal swallowing is important for normal development: An experimental study. *Virchows Arch A Pathol Anat Histopathol* 1992; 420:305–312.

33. Rosso, P. *Nutrition and metabolism in pregnancy.* New York: Oxford University Press, 1990; 117–118, 125, 150–151.

34. Scholl, T. O., et al. Leptin and maternal growth during adolescent pregnancy. *Am J Clin Nutr* 2000; 72:1542–7.35.

35. Georgieff, M. K. Nutrition and the developing brain: Nutrient priorities and measurement. *Am J Clin Nutr* 2007; 85(Suppl):614S–620S.

36. Smith, D. W. Growth and its disorders: Basics and standards, approach and classifications, growth deficiency disorders, growth excess disorders, obesity. In Schaeffer, A. J. and Markowitz, M., eds. *Major problems in clinical pediatrics*, Vol. 15. Philadelphia: W. B. Saunders Company, 1979; 134–169.

37. Winick, M. Malnutrition and brain development. *J Pediatr* 1969; 74:667–679.

38. Rosso, P., et al. Intrauterine growth retardation: A new systematic approach based on the clinical and biochemical characteristics of this condition. *J Perinat Med* 1974; 2:147–160.

39. Godfrey, K. M., et al. Fetal nutrition and adult disease. *Am J Clin Nutr* 2000; 71:1344S–1352S.

40. Hogeveen, M., et al. Maternal homocysteine and small-for-gestational-age offspring: systematic review and meta-analysis. *Am J Cin Nutr* 2012; 95:130–136.

41. Hediger, M. L., et al. Growth of infants and young children born small or large for gestational age: Findings from the Third National Health and Nutrition Examination Survey. *Arch Pediatr Adolesc Med* 1998; 152:1225–1231.

42. Dearden, L., et al. The road between early growth and obesity: new twists and turns. *Am J Clin Nutr* 2014; 100:6–7.

43. Jolly, M. C., et al. Risk factors for macrosomia and its clinical consequences: A study of 350,311 pregnancies. *Eur J Obstet Gynecol Repro Biol* 2003; 111:9–14.

44. Stotland, N. E., et al. Gestational Weight Gain and Adverse Neonatal Outcome Among Term Infants. *Obstet Gynecol* 2006; 108:635–643.

45. Luo, Z. C., et al. Length and body mass index at birth and target height influences on patterns of postnatal growth in children born small for gestational age. *Pediatrics* 1998; 102:E72.

46. Branch, D. W., et al. Recurrent miscarriage. *N Engl J Med* 2010; 363:1740–1747.

47. Kwak-Kim, J., et al. Managing women with recurrent pregnancy losses and antiphospholipid syndrome. *Am J Repro Immunol* 2013; 69:595–607.

48. National Academy of Sciences. *Nutrition during Pregnancy. I. Weight gain. II. Nutrient supplements*. Washington, DC: National Academy Press, 1990.

49. Maconochile, N., et al. Underweight and the risk of miscarriage. Online edition of *BJOG: An International Journal of Obstetrics and Gynecology*, available at www.medicinenet.com/script/main/art .asp?articlekey=77914, accessed 12/06.

50. Benammar A., et al. Nutrition and miscarriages: a literature review. *Gynecol Obstet Fertil.* 2012 March; 40:162–169.

51. Catov, J. M., et al. Inflammation and dyslipidemia related to risk of spontaneous preterm birth. *Am J Epidemiol* 2007; 166:1312–1319.

52. Shamin, A. A., et al. First-trimester plasma tocopherols are associated with the risk of miscarriage in rural Bangladesh. Am J Clin Nutr 2015;101: 294–301.

53. Hand, L. Misconceptions about cause, frequency of miscarriage common, Oct 2013. www.medscape.com/viewarticle/813084, accessed 5/15/15.

54. Williams, Z. Inducing tolerance to pregnancy. *N Engl J Med* 2012; 367:1159–1162.

55. Hudson, K. L., et al. In support of SUPPORT—A view from the NIH. *N Engl J Med* 2013; 368:2349–2352.

56. Elizabeth, K. E., et al. Umbilical cord blood nutrients in low birth weight babies

in relation to birth weight & gestational age. *Indian J Med Res* 2008; 128:128–133.

57. Kramer, M. S., et al. The contribution of mild and moderate preterm birth to infant mortality. Fetal and Infant Health Study Group of the Canadian Perinatal Surveillance System. *JAMA* 2000; 284:843–849.

58. Chery, C., et al. Hyperhomocysteinemia is related to a decreased level of vitamin $B_{12}$ in the second and third trimesters of pregnancy. *Clin Chem Lab Med* 2002; 40:1105–1108.

59. Ortega, R. M., et al. Riboflavin levels in maternal milk: The influence of vitamin $B_2$ status during the third trimester of pregnancy. *J Am Coll Nutr* 1999; 18:324–329.

60. Sommer, A., et al. Assessment and control of vitamin A deficiency: The Annecy Accords. *J Nutr* 2002; 132:2845S–50S.

61. Siega-Riz, M., et al. Second trimester folate status and preterm birth. *Am J Obstet Gynecol* 2004; 191:1851–1857.

62. Bukowski, R., et al. Preconceptional folate supplementation and the risk of spontaneous preterm birth: A cohort study. *PLoS Med* 2009; 6(5): e1000061. doi:10.1371/journal .pmed.1000061.

63. Haugen, M., et al. Mediterranean-type diet and risk of preterm birth among women in the Norwegian Mother and Child Cohort Study (MoBa): A prospective cohort study. *Acta Obstet Gynecol Scand.* 2008;87(3):319–324.

64. Klebanoff, M., et al. Fish consumption, erythrocyte fatty acids, and preterm birth. *Obstet Gynecol* 2011; 117:1071–1077.

65. Grieger, J. A., et al. Preconception dietary patterns in human pregnancies are associated with preterm delivery. *J Nutr.* 2014;144:1075–1080.

66. Englund-Ögge, L., et al. Association between intake of artificially sweetened and sugar-sweetened beverages and preterm delivery: A large prospective cohort study. *Am J Clin Nutr.* 2012; 96:552–559.

67. Saunders, L., et al. Effect of a Mediterranean diet during pregnancy on fetal growth and preterm delivery: Results from a French Caribbean Mother-Child Cohort Study (TIMOUN). *Paediatr Perinat Epidemiol.* 2014 May; 28(3):235–244.

68. Castro, L. C., et al. Maternal obesity and pregnancy outcomes. *Curr Opin Obstet Gynecol* 2002; 14:601–606.

69. Juhl, M., et al. Physical exercise during pregnancy and the risk of preterm birth: A study within the Danish national birth cohort. *Am J Epidemiol* 2008; 167:859–856.

70. Catov, J. M., et al. Early pregnancy lipid concentrations and spontaneous preterm birth. *Am J Obstet Gynecol* 2007; 197:610.e1–7.

71. Chen, X., et al. Association of elevated free fatty acids during late pregnancy with preterm delivery. *Obstet Gynecol* 2008; 112:297–303.

72. Susser, M., et al. Timing in prenatal nutrition: A reprise of the Dutch Famine Study. *Nutr Rev* 1994; 52:84–94.

73. Melter, H. M., et al. Effect of dietary factors in pregnancy on risk of pregnancy complications: results from the Norwegian Mother and Child Cohort Study, *Am J Clin Nutr* 2011; 94(suppl):1970S–4S.

74. Zeisel, S. H. Diet–gene interactions underlie metabolic individuality and influence brain development: Implications for clinical practice derived from studies on choline metabolism. *Ann Nutr Metab* 2012; 60(suppl 3):19–25.

75. Ma, R. C. W., et al. Maternal diabetes, gestational diabetes and the role of epigenetics in their long-term effects on offspring. *Progress in Biophysics and Molecular Biology*, available online 16 March 2015, doi:10.1016/j.pbiomolbio.2015.02.010.

76. Gluckman, P. D., et al. Effect of *in utero* and early-life conditions on adult health and disease. *N Engl J Med* 2008; 359:61–73.

77. Rich-Edwards, J. W., et al. Birth weight and risk of cardiovascular disease in a cohort of women followed up since 1976. *BMJ* 1997; 315:396–400.

78. Vivian, E. M. Type 2 diabetes in children and adolescents—The next epidemic? *Curr Med Res Opin* 2006; 22:297–306.

79. Robinson, S. M., et al. Combined effects of dietary fat and birth weight on serum cholesterol concentrations: The Hertfordshire Cohort Study. *Am J Clin Nutr* 2006; 84:237–244.

80. Kuzawa, C. W., et al. Lipid profiles in adolescent Filipinos: Relation to birth weight and maternal energy status during pregnancy. *Am J Clin Nutr* 2003; 77:960–966.

81. Gabory A., et al. Developmental programming and epigenetics. *Am J Clin Nutr.* 2011;94(6 Suppl):1943S-1952S.

82. Vickers, M. H. Developmental programming of the metabolic syndrome—critical windows for intervention. *World J Diabetes*. 2011; 15; 2:137–148.

83. Stein, A. D. Nutrition in early life and cognitive functioning. *Am J Clin Nutr* 2014; 99:1–2.

84. To, W. W., et al. The relationship between weight gain in pregnancy, birthweight and postpartum weight retention. *Aust N Z J Obstet Gynaecol* 1998; 38:176–179.

85. Villar, J., et al. Nutritional factors associated with low birth weight and short gestational age. *Clin Nutr* 1986; 5:78–85.

86. Eastman, N. J. *Expectant motherhood.* Boston: Little, Brown and Company, 1947: 198.

87. Rassmussen, K. M., et al. Weight gain during pregnancy: Reexamining the guidelines. Institute of Medicine, 2009. Available at www.nap.edu/catalog/12584.html.

88. Nohr, E. A., et al. Combined associations of prepregnancy body mass index and gestational weight with the outcome of pregnancy. *Am J Clin Nutr.* 2008; 87:1750–1759.

89. Pregnancy Nutrition Surveillance, www.cdc.gov/pednss/pdfs/PNSS_2009.pdf, accessed 8/21/12.

90. Siega-Riz, A. M. A systematic review of outcomes of maternal weight gain according to the Institute of Medicine recommendations: birthweight, fetal growth, and postpartum weight retention. *Am J Obstet Gynecol* 2009; 201:339.e1–14.

91. Parker, J. D., et al. Prenatal weight gain advice: An examination of the recent prenatal weight gain recommendations of the Institute of Medicine. *Obstet Gynecol* 1992; 79:664–669.

92. Stotland, N. E., et al. Excess gestational weight gain associated with adverse neonatal outcomes. *Obstet Gynecol* 2006; 108:635–643.

93. Starling, A. P., et al. Associations of maternal BMI and gestational weight gain with neonatal adiposity in the Healthy Start Study. *Am J Clin Nutr* 2015; 101:302–309.

94. Lau, E.Y., et al. Maternal Weight Gain in Pregnancy and Risk of Obesity among Offspring: A Systematic Review. *J Obesity.* 2014; doi.org/10.1155/2014/524939.

95. Skidmore, P. M. L., et al. An obesogenic postnatal environment is more important than the fetal environment for the development of adult adiposity: A study of female twins. *Am J Clin Nutr* 2009; 90:401–406.

96. Nohr, E. A., et al. Combined associations of prepregnancy body mass index and gestational weight with the outcome of pregnancy. *Am J Clin Nutr.* 2008; 87:1750–1759.

97. Andersson, E. S., et al. No association of maternal gestational weight gain with offspring blood pressure and hypertension at age 18 years in male sibling-pairs: A prospective register-based cohort study. *PLOS One*, Published: March 20, 2015, doi: 10.1371/ journal.pone.0121202.

98. Brown, J. E., et al. Variation in newborn size by trimester weight change in pregnancy. *Am J Clin Nutr* 2002; 76:205–209.

99. Carmichael, S. L., et al. A critical review of the relationship between gestational weight gain and preterm delivery. *Obstet Gynecol* 1997; 89:865–873.

100. To, W. W., et al. The relationship between weight gain in pregnancy, birthweight and postpartum weight retention. *Aust N Z J Obstet Gynaecol* 1998; 38:176–179.

101. Keppel, K. G., et al. Pregnancy-related weight gain and retention: Implications of the 1990 Institute of Medicine guidelines. *Am J Public Health* 1993; 83:1100–1103.

102. Nehring, I., et al. Gestational weight gain and long-term postpartum weight retention: a meta-analysis. *Am J Clin Nutr* 2011; 94:1225–1231.

103. Gunderson, E. P., et al. Does the pattern of postpartum weight change differ according to pregravid body size? *Int J Obes* 2001; 25:853–862.

104. Rode, L., et al. Association between gestational weight gain according to body mass index and postpartum weight in a large cohort of Danish women. *Matern Child Health J* 2011 Mar 24.

105. Streuling, I., et al. Can gestational weight gain be modified by increasing physical activity and diet counseling? A meta-analysis of interventional trials. *Am J Clin Nutr* 2010; 92:678–87.

106. Shangaratinam, S., et al. Effects of interventions in pregnancy on maternal weight and obstetric outcomes: meta-analysis of randomized evidence. *BMJ* 2012; 344:e2088.

107. 2015 Dietary Guidelines Advisory Committee. Advisory report to the Secretary of Health and Human Services and Secretary of Agriculture. Published February 2015. http://www.health.gov/dietaryguidelines/2015-scientific-report/PDFs/Scientific-Report-of-the-2015-Dietary-Guidelines-Advisory-Committee.pdf, accessed 3/12/15.

108. Mussey, R. D. Nutrition and human reproduction: an historical review. *Am J Obstet Gynecol* 1949; 58:1037–1048.

109. Stein, A. D., et al. Famine, third-trimester pregnancy weight gain, and intrauterine growth: The Dutch Famine Birth Cohort Study. *Hum Biol* 1995; 67:135–150.

110. Smith, C. A. Effects of maternal undernutrition upon the newborn infant in Holland (1944–1945). *J Pediatr* 1947; 30:229–243.

111. Antonov, A. N. Children born during the siege of Leningrad in 1942. *J Pediatr* 1947; 30:250–259.

112. Gruenwald, P., et al. Influence of environmental factors on fetal growth in man. *Lancet* 1967; I:1026–1028.

113. United Nations Live births, deaths, and infant mortality rate, unstats.un.org/unsd/demographic/products/vitstats/serATab3.pdf, accessed 4/1/12.

114. Huang, C., et al. Early life exposure to the 1959–1961 Chinese famine has long-term health consequences. *J. Nutr* 2010; 140; 1874–1878.

115. Simic, S., et al. Nutritional effects of the siege on newborn babies in Sarajevo. *Eur J Clin Nutr* 1995; 49(Suppl., 2):S33–6.

116. Lumey, L. H., et al. Prenatal famine and adult health. *Annual Review of Public Health* 2011; 32:237–262.

117. Burke, B. S. Nutritional needs in pregnancy in relation to nutritional intakes as shown by dietary histories. *Obstetr Gynecol Survey* 1948; 3:716–730.

118. Burke, B. S., et al. Nutrition studies during pregnancy. IV. Relation of protein content of mother's diet during pregnancy to birth length, birth weight, and condition of infant at birth. *J Pediatr* 1943; 23:506–515.

119. Position of the Academy of Nutrition and Dietetics: Nutrition and Lifestyle for a Healthy Pregnancy Outcome. *J Acad Nutr Diet* 2014;114:1099–1103.

120. Carmichael, S. L., et al. Reduced Risks of Neural Tube Defects and Orofacial Clefts With Higher Diet Quality. *Arch Pediatr Adolesc Med*, published online October 3, 2011, doi:10.1001/archpediatrics.2011; 185.

121. Rodríguez-Bernal, C. L., et al. Diet quality in early pregnancy and its effects on fetal growth outcomes: the Infancia y Medio Ambiente (Childhood and Environment) Mother and Child Cohort Study in Spain. *Am J Clin Nutr.* 2010; 91:1659–1666.

122. Butte, N. F. Energy requirements during pregnancy and consequences of deviations from requirement on fetal outcome. *Nestle Nutr Workshop Ser Pediatr Program* 2005; 55:49–67.

123. Brown, J. E., et al. Maternal nutrition and the outcome of pregnancy: A renaissance in research. *Clin Perinatol* 1997; 24:433–449.

124. Nutrient Intakes from Food and Beverages: Mean Amounts Consumed per Individual, by Gender and Age, What We Eat in America, NHANES 2011–2012. Agricultural Research Service. 2014, www.ars.usda.gov/SP2UserFiles/Place/80400530/pdf/1112/Table_1_NIN_GEN_11.pdf, accessed 3/25/15.

125. Deierlein, A. L., et al. Dietary energy density but not glycemic load is associated with gestational weight gain. *Am J Clin Nutr* 2008; 88:693–699.

126. Suez J., et al. Artificial sweeteners induce glucose intolerance by altering the gut microbiota. *Nature*. 2014; 514:181–186.

127. Denny, C. H., et al. Pattern of alcohol use during pregnancy since 1991. *MMWR* 2009; 58:529–532.

128. Preidt, R. Many women still smoke during pregnancy. http://www.nlm.nih.gov/medlineplus/news/fullstory_125046.html, released 11 May 2012.

129. Keuhn, D., et al. A prospective cohort study of the prevalence of growth, facial, and central nervous system abnormalities in children with heavy prenatal alcohol exposure. *Alcohol Clin Experiment Res*, first published online: 23 Jul 2012; doi: 10.1111/j.1530-0277.2012.01794.x.

130. Barker D., et al. Developmental biology: Support mothers to secure future public health. *Nature*. 2013; 504:209–211.

131. Chambers, C., et al. Prenatal alcohol exposure patterns and alcohol-related birth defects and growth deficiencies: A prospective study. Alcoholism. *Clin Exper Res*, Article first published online: 17 Jan 2012, doi: 10.1111/j.1530-0277.2011.01664.x.

132. Duggleby, S. L., et al. Protein, amino acid and nitrogen metabolism during pregnancy: How might the mother meet the needs of her fetus? *Curr Opin Clin Nutr Metab Care* 2002; 5:503–509.

133. Nutrient Intakes from Food and Beverages: Mean Amounts Consumed per Individual, by Gender and Age, What We Eat in America, NHANES 2011–2012. Agricultural Research Service. 2014, www.ars.usda.gov/SP2UserFiles/Place/80400530/pdf/1112/Table_1_NIN_GEN_11.pdf, accessed 3/25/15.

134. *Dietary Reference Intakes: Energy, Carbohydrate, Fiber, Fat, Fatty Acids, Cholesterol, Protein, and Amino Acids*. Washington, DC: National Academies Press, 2002.

135. Moore, V. M., et al. Dietary composition of pregnant women is related to size of the baby at birth. *J Nutr* 2004; 134: 1820–1826.

136. Williams, C. M., et al. Long-chain n-3 PUFA: Plant v. marine sources. *Proc Nutr Soc* 2006 Feb; 65(1):45–50.

137. Kolanowski, W., et al. Possibilities of fish oil application for food products enrichment with omega-3 PUFA. *Int J Food Sci Nutr* 1999; 50:39–49.

138. Williams, C. M., et al. Long-chain n-3 PUFA: Plant v. marine sources. *Proc Nutr Soc* 2006; 65:42–50.

139. Position of the American Dietetic Association and Dietitians of Canada: Dietary fatty acids. *J Am Diet Assoc* 2007; 107:1599–1611.

140. Harris, W. S., et al. Towards establishing dietary reference intakes for EPA and DHA. *J Nutr* 2009; 139:804S–19S.

141. Swanson, D., et al. Omega-3 fatty acids EPA and DHA: Health benefits throughout life. *Adv Nutr* 2012; 3: 1–7.

142. Swanson, D., et al. Omega-3 fatty acids EPA and DHA: Health Benefits Throughout Life. *Adv Nutr* 2012; 3: 1–7.

143. Steer, C. D., et al. Maternal fatty acids in pregnancy, FADS polymorphisms, and child intelligence quotient at 8 y of age. *Am J Clin Nutr.* 2013; 98:1575–1582.

144. Jingjing, Jiao., et al. Effect of n–3 PUFA supplementation on cognitive function throughout the life span from infancy to old age: a systematic review and meta-analysis of randomized controlled trials. First published October 15, 2014, *Am J Clin Nutr*, doi: 10.3945/ajcn.114.095315.

145. Leventakou V., et al. Fish intake during pregnancy, fetal growth, and gestational length in 19 European birth cohort studies. Am J Clin Nutr. 2014;99:506-16.

146. Harris, W. S., et al. Towards establishing dietary reference intakes for eicosapentaenoic and docosahexaenoic acids. *J Nutr.* 2009; 139:804S–19S.

147. What We Eat in America, NHANES, 2007–2008. www.ars.usda.gov/Services/docs.htm?docid=13793, accessed 2/25/11.

148. Position of the American Dietetic Association: Vegetarian diets. *J Am Diet Assoc* 2009;109:1266–82.

149. FDA Issues Guidelines on Maternal Fish Consumption. www.medscape.org/viewarticle/827731?nlid=62707_2707&src=cmemp, 7/21/14, accessed 8/20/14.

150. Strain, J. J., et al. Prenatal exposure to methyl mercury from fish consumption and polyunsaturated fatty acids: associations with child development at 20 mo of age in an observational study in the Republic of Seychelles. *Am J Clin Nutr* 2015; 101:530–537.

151. Lumley, J., et al. Periconceptional supplementation with folate and/or multivitamins for preventing neural tube defects. *Cochrane Database Syst Rev* 2000; 2.

152. Suitor, C. W., et al. Dietary folate equivalents: Interpretation and application. *J Amer Diet Assoc* 2000; 100:88–94.

153. Anthony, A. C. *In utero* physiology: role of folic acid in nutrient delivery and fetal development. *Am J Clin Nutr* 2007; 85 (suppl):598S–603S. 168:2020–2023.

154. Yang, Q., et al. Prospective study of methylenetetrohydratefolate reductase (MTHFR) variant C677T and risk of all-cause cardiovascular mortality among 6000 US adults. *Am J Clin Nutr* 2012; 95:1245–1253.

155. Greenberg, J. A., et al. Folic acid supplementation and pregnancy: More than just neural tube defect prevention. *Rev Obstet Gynecol* 2011; 4:52–59.

156. Warkany, J. Production of congenital malformations by dietary measures. *JAMA* 1958;168:2020–2023.

157. Smithells, R. W. Availability of folic acid. *Lancet* 1984; 1:508.

158. Eskes, T. K. A. B. From birth to conception, open or closed. *Eur J Obstet Gynecol Reprod Biol* 1998; 78:169–177.

159. Folic acid. *MMWR Morb Mortal Wkly Rep* 2001; 50:185–9.

160. Folate status in women of childbearing age—United States, 1999. *MMWR Morb Mortal Wkly Rep* 2000; 49:962–965.

161. Guo, T., et al. Methylenetetrahydrofolate Reductase Polymorphisms C677T and Risk of Autism in the Chinese Han Population. Genet Test Mol Biomarkers. 2012 Jul 9.

162. Dunlap, B., et al. Folic acid and human reproduction—Ten important issues for clinicians. *J Exp Clin Assist Reprod.* 2011; 8:2. Published online 2011 August 10: www.ncbi.nlm.nih.gov/pmc/articles/PMC3183498/?tool=pmcentrez.

163. Daly, L. E., et al. Folate levels and neural tube defects. *JAMA* 1995; 274:1698–702.

164. Duffy ME., et al. Biomarker response to folic acid intervention in healthy adults: a meta-analysis of randomized controlled trials. *Am J Clin Nutr* 2014;99:96–106.

165. Pfeiffer, C. M., et al. Estimation of trends in serum and RBC folate in the U.S. population from pre- to postfortification using assay-adjusted data from the NHANES 1988–2010. *J Nutr* 2012; 142:886–893.

166. Shane, B. Folate-responsive birth defects: of mice and women. *Am J Clin Nutr* 2012.95:1–2.

167. Occurrence prevention, Dec. 2014, www.cdc.gov/ncbddd/folicacid/recommendations.html, accessed 4/29/15.

168. Rosenberg, I. Getting folic acid nutrition right. *Am J Clin Nutr* 2010; 91:3–4.

169. Yang Q., et al. Prospective study of methylenetetrahydrofolate reductase (MTHFR) variant C677T and risk of all-cause and cardiovascular disease mortality among 6000 US adults. *Am J Clin Nutr.* 2012; 95:1245–1253.

170. Velzing-Aarts, F. V., et al. Plasma choline and betaine and their relation to plasma homocysteine in normal pregnancy. *Am Clin Nutr* 2005; 81:1383–1389.

171. Yan J., et al. Pregnancy alters choline dynamics: results of a randomized trial using stable isotope methodology in pregnant and nonpregnant women. *Am J Clin Nutr.* 2013;98:459–467.

172. Caudill, M. A. Pre- and postnatal health: evidence of increased choline needs. *J Am Diet Assoc* 2010; 110:1198–1206.

173. Signore, C., et al. Choline concentrations in human maternal and cord blood and intelligence at 5 y of age. *Am J Clin Nutr* 2008; 87:896–902.

174. Zile, M. H. Function of vitamin A in vertebrate embryonic development. *J Nutr* 2001; 131:705–708.

175. Werner, C. A., et al. Women's experiences with isotretinoin risk reduction counseling. *JAMA Dermatol.* Published online November 20, 2013, doi:10.1001/jamadermatol.2013.6862.

176. Lott, I. T., et al. Fetal hydrocephalus and ear abnormalities associated with maternal use of isotretinion. *J Pediatr* 1984; 105:597–600.

177. Mathews-Roth, M. M., et al. Lack of genotoxicity with beta-carotene. *Tox Letters* 1988; 41:185–191.

178. Thielitz, A., et al. Topical retinoids in acne vulgaris: update on efficacy and safety. *Am J Clin Dermatol* 2008; 9:369–81.

179. McCullough, M. L. Vitamin D deficiency in pregnancy: Bringing the issue to light, *J Nutr* 2007; 137:305–306.

180. Dror, D. K., et al. Vitamin D inadequacy in pregnancy: biology, outcomes, and interventions. *Nutr Rev* 2010; 68:465–477.

181. Schroth, R., et al. Influence of maternal vitamin D status on infant oral health, Abs. no. 1646, International Association for Dental Research, July 4, 2008.

182. Hart P H., et al. Vitamin D in Fetal Development: Findings from a Birth Cohort Study. *Pediatrics*, published online December 15, 2014, doi: 10.1542/peds.2014-1860.

183. Ota K., et al. Vitamin D deficiency may be a risk factor for recurrent pregnancy losses by increasing cellular immunity and autoimmunity. *Hum Reprod.* 2014; 29:208–219.

184. Bodnar, L. M., et al. High prevalence of vitamin D insufficiency in black and white women residing in the northern United States and their neonates. *J Nutr* 2007; 137:447–452.

185. Schneuer, F. J., et al. Effects of maternal serum 25-hydroxyvitamin D concentrations in the first trimester on subsequent pregnancy outcomes in an Australian population. *Am J Clin Nutr.* 2014; 99:287–295.

186. Hollis, B. W., et al. Vitamin D supplementation during pregnancy: Double-blind, randomized clinical trial of safety and effectiveness. *J Bone Min Res* 2011; June 27, 2011, doi: 10.1002/jbmr.463.

187. Kovacs, C. S. Vitamin D in pregnancy and lactation: Maternal, fetal, and neonatal outcomes from human and animal studies. *Am J Clin Nutr* 2008; 88(Suppl): 520S–8S.

188. Hollis, B. W., et al. Vitamin D supplementation during pregnancy: Double-blind, randomized clinical trial of safety and effectiveness. *J Bone Min Res* 2011; June 27, 2011, doi: 10.1002/jbmr.463.

189. Macones, G. A., et al. Vitamin D: Screening and supplementation during pregnancy. *Obstet Gynecol* 2011; 118:197–198.

190. Tangpricha, V. Vitamin D in food and supplements. *Am J Clin Nutr* 2012; 95:1299–1300.

191. O'Brien, K. O., et al. Serum 1,25-dihydroxyvitamin D and calcium intake affect rates of bone calcium deposition during pregnancy and the early postpartum period. *Am J Clin Nutr* 2012; 96:64–72.

192. O'Brien, K. O., et al. Serum 1,25-dihydroxyvitamin D and calcium intake affect rates of bone calcium deposition during pregnancy and the early postpartum period. *Am J Clin Nutr* 2012; 96:64–72.

193. Stefanie, L. Exploring potential pathways between parity and tooth loss among American women. *Am J Public Health* 2008; 98:1263–1270.

194. Olausson, H., et al. Changes in bone mineral status and bone size during pregnancy and the influence of body weight and calcium intake. *Am J Clin Nutr* 2008; 8:1032–1039.

195. Gedalia, I., et al. Effect of prenatal and postnatal fluoride on the human deciduous dentition: A literature review. *Adv Dent Res* 1989; 3:168–176.

196. Stefanie, L. Exploring potential pathways between parity and tooth loss among American women. *Am J Public Health* 2008; 98:1263–1270.

197. Essential Nutrition Actions Improving Maternal–Newborn–Infant and Young Child Health and Nutrition Draft, May 2011. www.who.int/nutrition/EB128_18. _background paper2_A_reviewofhealthinterventions withaneffectonnutrition.pdf, accessed 4/16/12.

198. Fairbanks, V. F. Iron in medicine and nutrition. In Shils, M. E., et al., eds. *Modern Nutrition in Health and Disease*, 9th ed. Philadelphia: Lippincott, Williams & Wilkins, 1999: 193–221.

199. Cantor, A. G., et al. Routine iron supplementation and screening for iron deficiency anemia in pregnancy: A systematic review for the U.S. Preventive Services Task Force. *Ann Intern Med.* Published online 30 March 2015 doi:10.7326/M14-2932.

200. Mei, Z., et al. Assessment of iron status in US pregnant women from the National Health and Nutrition Examination Survey (NHANES), 1999–2006. *Am J Clin Nutr* 2011; 93:1312–20.

201. Tamura, T., et al. Cord serum ferritin concentrations and mental and psychomotor development of children at five years of age. *J Pediatrics*, 2002; 140:165–170.

202. Allen, L. H. Biological mechanisms that might underlie iron's effects on fetal growth and preterm birth. *J Nutr* 2001; 131:581S–9S.

203. Tamura, T., et al. Cord serum ferritin concentrations and mental and psychomotor development of children at five years of age. *J Pediatrics*, 2002; 140:165–170.

204. Allen, L. H. Anemia and iron deficiency: Effects on pregnancy outcome. *Am J Clin Nutr* 2000; 71:1280S–4S.

205. Recommendations to prevent and control iron deficiency in the United States. Centers for Disease Control and Prevention. *MMWR Morb Mortal Wkly Rep* 1998; 47:1–29.

206. Hinderaker, S. G., et al. Anemia in pregnancy in the highlands of Tanzania. *Acta Obstet Gynecol Scand* 2001; 80:18-26.207 .205.

207. Recommendations to prevent and control iron deficiency in the United States. Centers for Disease Control and Prevention. *MMWR Morb Mortal Wkly Rep* 1998; 47:1–29.

208. National Academy of Sciences. *Nutrition during Pregnancy. I. Weight gain. II. Nutrient supplements*. Washington, DC: National Academy Press, 1990.

209. Allen, L. H. Multiple micronutrients in pregnancy and lactation: An overview. *Am J Clin Nutr* 2005; 81:1206S–1212S.

210. Casanueva, E., et al. Iron and oxidative stress in pregnancy. *J Nutr* 2003; 133:1700S–1708S.

211. Cogswell, M. E., et al. Iron supplement use among women in the United States: Science, policy, and practice. *J Nutr* 2003; 133:1974S–7S.

212. Vilke, G. M., et al. Pediatric poisonings in children younger than five years responded to be paramedics, *J Emerg Med* 2011; 41:265–269.

213. Roberfroid D., et al. Randomized controlled trial of 2 prenatal iron supplements: Is there a dose-response relation with maternal hemoglobin? *Am J Clin Nutr.* 2011; 93:1012–1018.

214. Ribot, B., et al. Depleted iron stores without anaemia early in pregnancy carries increased risk of lower birthweight even when supplemented daily with moderate iron. *Hum Reprod.* 2012; 27:1260-6. doi: 10.1093/humrep/des026.

215. Peña-Rosas, J. P., et al. Daily oral iron supplementation during pregnancy. Cochrane Database Syst Rev. 2012; 12: CD004736. Published online 2012 Dec 12. doi: 10.1002/14651858.CD004736.pub4.

216. Gautam, C. S., et al. Iron Deficiency in Pregnancy and the Rationality of Iron Supplements Prescribed During Pregnancy. *Medscape J Med.* 2008; 10(12): 283.

217. Young, M. F., et al. Utilization of iron from an animal-based iron source is greater than that of ferrous sulfate in pregnant and nonpregnant women. *J Nutr* 2010; 140:2162–2166.

218. Zimmerman, M. B. The adverse effects of mild-to-moderate iodine deficiency during pregnancy and childhood: A review. *Thyroid* 2007; 17:829–835.

219. Xue-Yi, C., et al. Timing of vulnerability of the brain to iodine deficiency in endemic cretinism. *N Eng J Med* 1994; 331:1739–1744.

220. Mahomed, K., et al. Maternal iodine supplements in areas of deficiency (Cochrane Review). The Cochrane Library. Issue 3. Oxford: Update Software, 1999.

221. Shah, P. S., et al. Knowledge Synthesis Group on Determinants of Low Birth Weight and Preterm Births. Effects of prenatal multi-micronutrient supplementation on pregnancy outcomes: A meta-analysis. *CMAJ* 2009; 180:E99–108.

222. Caldwell, K. L., et al. Urinary iodine concentration: United States National Health and Nutrition Examination Survey 2001–2002. *Thyroid*, 2005; 15:692–699.

223. Becker, D. V., et al. Iodine supplementation for pregnancy and lactation, United States and Canada: Recommendations from the American Thyroid Association. *Thyroid* 2006; 16:959–951.

224. WHO/UNIFEC. Researching optimal iodine nutrition in pregnant and lactating women and young children. Geneva, Switzerland: World Health Organization, 2007, doi: 10.1017/S1368980007361004.

225. Leung, A. M., et al. Iodine content of prenatal multivitamins in the United States. *N Engl J Med* 2009; 360:939–940.

226. Pike, R. L., et al. Further evidence of deleterious effects produced by sodium restriction during pregnancy. *Am J Clin Nutr* 1970; 23:883–889.

227. Duley, L., et al. Altered dietary salt for preventing preeclampsia, and its complications. *Cochrane Database of Syst Rev* 2005; Issue 4, Art. No. CD005548, doi 10.1002/14651858.CD005548.

228. Meydani, M., et al. Diabetes risk: Antioxidants or lifestyle? *Am J Cli Nutr* 2009; 90:253–254.

229. Mistry, H. D., et al. The importance of antioxidant micronutrients in pregnancy. *Oxid Med Cell Longev.* 2011; 2011: 841749.

230. Litonjua, A. A., et al. Maternal antioxidant intake in pregnancy and wheezing illnesses in children at 2 y of age. *Am J Clin Nutr* 2006; 84:903–911.

231. Devereux, G., et al. Low intake of vitamin E during pregnancy may increase risk for childhood asthma. *Am J Respir Grit Care Med* 2006; 174:499–507.

232. Nehlig, A., et al. Consequences on the newborn of chronic maternal consumption of coffee during gestation and lactation: A review. *J Am Coll Nutr* 1994; 13:6–21.

233. Hinds, T. S., et al. The effect of caffeine on pregnancy outcome variables. *Nutr Rev* 1996; 54:203–207.

234. Christian, M. S., et al. Teratogen update: Evaluation of the reproductive and developmental risks of caffeine. *Teratol* 2001; 64:51–78.

235. Crippa A., et al. Coffee consumption and mortality from all causes, cardiovascular disease, and cancer: A dose-response meta-analysis. *Am J Epidemiol.* 2014; 180: 763–775.

236. Bakker, R., et al. Maternal caffeine intake from coffee and tea, fetal growth, and the risks of adverse birth outcomes: The Generation R Study. *Am J Clin Nutr* 2010; 91:1691–1698.

237. Pittman, G. Some caffeine okay during pregnancy: obstetricians. Released Jul 21, 2010, www.medscape.com /viewarticle/725562, accessed 7/27/10.

238. Maslova, E., et al. Caffeine consumption during pregnancy and risk of preterm birth: a meta-analysis. *Am J Clin Nutr* 2010; 92:1120–1132.

239. Jahanfar, S., et al. Effects of restricted caffeine intake by mother on fetal, neonatal and pregnancy outcome. *Cochrane Database Syst Rev* 2009; 15:CD006965.

240. Brent, R. L., et al. Evaluation of the reproductive and developmental risks of caffeine. *Birth Defects Res B Dev Reprod Toxicol.* 2011; 92:152–187.

241. Bech, B. H., et al. Effect of reducing caffeine intake on birth weight and length of gestation: Randomized controlled trial. *BMJ* 2007; 334:409–414.

242. Pittman, G. Some caffeine okay during pregnancy: Obstetricians. Released Jul 21, 2010, www.medscape.com /viewarticle/725562, accessed 7/27/10.

243. Ershow, A. G., et al. Intake of tapwater and total water by pregnant and lactating women. *Am J Public Health* 1991; 81:328–834.

244. Hook, E. B. Dietary cravings and aversions during pregnancy. *Am J Clin Nutr* 1978; 31:1355–62.

245. Brown, J. E., et al. Taste changes during pregnancy. *Am J Clin Nutr* 1986; 43:412–416.

246. Johns, T., et al. Detoxification and mineral supplementation as functions of geophagy. *Am J Clin Nutr* 1991; 53:448–456.

247. Rainville, A. J. Pica practices of pregnant women are associated with lower maternal hemoglobin level at delivery. *J Amer Diet Assoc* 1998; 98:293–296.

248. 2015 Dietary Guidelines Advisory Committee. Advisory report to the Secretary of Health and Human Services and Secretary of Agriculture. Published February 2015. http://www.health.gov /dietaryguidelines/2015-scientific-report /PDFs/Scientific-Report-of-the-2015 -Dietary-Guidelines-Advisory-Committee.pdf, accessed 3/12/15.

249. Piccoli, G. B., et al. Vegan-vegetarian diets in pregnancy: danger or panacea? A systematic narrative review. *BJOG* 2015;122:623–633.

250. Neurologic impairment in children associated with maternal dietary deficiency of

cobalamin—Georgia, 2001. *MMWR* 2003; 52(04):61–64.

251. Position of the American Dietetic Association and Dietitians of Canada: Vegetarian diets. *J Am Diet Assoc* 2003; 103:748–765.

252. Leitzman, C. Vegetarian nutrition: past, present, future. *Am J Clin Nutr* 2014; 100(suppl):496-502S.

253. White, N. D. Lifestyle and Complementary Medicine for Common Gastrointestinal Disorders in Pregnancy. *J Lifestyle Med*. 2014; 8:97–99.

254. Ural SH., et al. Prenatal Nutrition. emedicine.medscape.com/article/259059-overview#aw2aab6b2, accessed 5/20/15.

255. American Academy of Pediatrics, American College of Obstetricians and Gynecologists. *Guidelines for Perinatal Care*. 6th ed. Elk Grove Village, IL: AAP; Washington, DC: ACOG, 2007. p.103, 284–286, 323–325, 352.

256. Picciano, M. F., et al. Use of dietary supplements by pregnant and lactating women in North America. *Am J Clin Nutr* 2009; 89(Suppl):663S–7S.

257. Zeisel, S. H. Is maternal diet supplementation beneficial? Optimal development of infant depends on mother's diet. *Am J Clin Nutr* 2009; 89:685S–7S.

258. Shah, P. S., et al. Knowledge Synthesis Group on Determinants of Low Birth Weight and Preterm Births. Effects of prenatal multimicronutrient supplementation on pregnancy outcomes: A meta-analysis. *CMAJ* 2009; 180:E99–108.

259. Shah, P. S., et al. Knowledge Synthesis Group on Determinants of Low Birth Weight and Preterm Births. Effects of prenatal multimicronutrient supplementation on pregnancy outcomes: A meta-analysis. *CMAJ* 2009; 180:E99–108.

260. Dog, L. T. The use of botanicals during pregnancy and lactation. *Altern Ther Health Med* 2009; 15:54–58.

261. Marcus, D. M. Do no harm: Avoidance of herbal medicines during pregnancy. *Obstet Gynecol* 2005; 105(5 Pt. 1):1119–1122.

262. FDA statement concerning structure/function rule and pregnancy claims. HHS Statement, U.S. Department of Health and Human Services; 65 FR 1000; January 6, 2000; Docket No. 98N-0044.

263. Meisler, J. G. Toward optimal health: The experts discuss the use of botanicals by women. *J Women's Health* 2003; 12:847–852.

264. Jones, F. A. Herbs: Useful plants. *J R Soc Med* 1996; 89:717–719.

265. Dugoua, J. J., et al. Safety and efficacy of ginkgo (Ginkgo biloba) during pregnancy and lactation. *Can J Clin Pharmacol* 2006; 13:e277–84 (Epub Nov. 3, 2006).

266. Vutyavanich, T., et al. Ginger for nausea and vomiting in pregnancy: Randomized, double-masked, placebo-controlled trial. *Obstet Gynecol* 2001; 97:577–582.

267. Food safety for pregnant women. www.fda.gov/downloads/Food/ResourcesForYou/Consumers/SelectedHealthTopics/UCM312787.pdf, accessed 4/3/15.

268. *Summary of the Nutrition Care Process Steps for Nutrition Assessment* (Pocket Guide for International Dietetics & Nutrition Terminology Reference Manual), 2nd ed. Chicago: American Dietetic Association, 2009.

269. Larsson, A., et al. Reference values for clinical chemistry tests during normal pregnancy. *BJOG* 2008; 115:874–881.

270. Hayes L., et al. Change in level of physical activity during pregnancy in obese women: findings from the UPBEAT pilot trial. *BMC Pregnancy and Childbirth* 2015, 15:52.

271. Artal, R., et al. Exercise during pregnancy—Safe and beneficial for most. *Physician and Sports Medicine* 1999; 27:51–56.

272. Dempsey, J. C., et al. No need for a pregnant pause: Physical activity may reduce the occurrence of gestational diabetes mellitus and preeclampsia. *Exerc Sport Sci Rev* 2005; 33:141–149.

273. Physical Activity Guidelines for Americans, 2008, U.S. Department of Health & Human Services. Available at http://www.health.gov/PAGuidelines.

274. Clapp, J. F., et al. Exercise during pregnancy may improve perimenopauseal fitness. *Am J Obstet Gynecol* 2008; 199:489.e1–489.e6.

275. Clapp, J. F., et al. Beginning regular exercise in early pregnancy: Effect on fetoplacental growth. *Am J Obstet Gynecol* 2000; 183:1484–8.

276. The spectrum of gastrointestinal disorders during pregnancy. *Nat Clin Pract Gastroenterol Hepatol*, 2008. Available at medscape.comCME, www.medscape.com, accessed 4/09.

277. White, ND. Lifestyle and complementary medicine for common gastrointestinal disorders in pregnancy. *J Lifestyle Med*. 2014;8:97–99.

278. Badell, M. L., et al. Treatment options for nausea and vomiting during pregnancy. *Pharmacotherapy* 2006; 26:1273–1287.

279. Gross, S., et al. Maternal weight loss associated with hyperemesis gravidarum: A predictor of fetal outcome. *Am J Obstet Gynecol* 1989; 160:906–909.

280. Salli, A. Revived focus on treatment for morning sickness. *Medscape Wire* 2000.

281. Brown, J. E., et al. Profets, profits and proof: Do nausea and vomiting of early pregnancy protect women from "harmful" vegetables? *Am J Obstet Gynecol* 1997; 176:179–181.

282. Koren, G., et al. Effectiveness of delayed-release doxylamine and pyridoxine for nausea and vomiting of pregnancy: a randomized placebo controlled trial. *Am J Obstet Gynecol* 2010; 203:571.e1–571.e7.

283. Keller, J., et al. The spectrum and treatment of gastrointestinal disorders during pregnancy. *Nat Clin Pract Gastroenterol Hepatol* 2008; 5:430–443.

284. Higgins, A. C., et al. Impact of the Higgins Nutrition Intervention Program on birth weight: A within-mother analysis. *J Amer Diet Assoc* 1989; 89:1097–1103.

285. Dubois, S., et al. Ability of the Higgins Nutrition Intervention Program to improve adolescent pregnancy outcome. *J Amer Diet Assoc* 1997; 97:871–878.

286. Duquette, M. P., Director of the Montreal Diet Dispensary. Personal communication, 2000.

287. USDA Finalizes Changes to the WIC Program, Expanding Access to Healthy Fruits and Vegetables, Whole Grains, and Low-Fat Dairy for Women, Infants, and Children. www.fns.usda.gov/pressrelease/2014/003114, 2/28/14.

288. CDC Fastats A to Z. Available at www.cdc.gov/nchs/fastats/births.htm, accessed 7/09.

289. Kassenaum NJ., et al. Global, regional, and national levels and causes of maternal mortality during 1990–2013: a systematic analysis for the Global Burden of Disease Study 2013. Lancet. 2014 Sep 13; 384(9947): 980–1004. Available at: www.ncbi.nlm.nih.gov/pmc/articles/PMC4255481/?report=classic.

290. Gregory, E. C. W., et al. Trends in Fetal and Perinatal Mortality in the United States, 2006–2012, 2014. NCHS data brief, no 169. Hyattsville, MD: National Center for Health Statistics. 2014, available; at: www.cdc.gov/nchs/data/databriefs/db169.htm, accessed 5/11/15.

291. Williams, R. L., et al. Fetal growth and perinatal viability in California. *Obstet Gynecol* 1982; 59:624–632.

292. Leading Causes of Neonatal and Postneonatal Deaths—United States, 2002. *MMWR Weekly Report* September 30, 2005; 54:966. 7. Health United States, 2000, Vol. 2001.

293. Martin, A., et al. Births: Final Data for 2013, Jan 2015. Available at: www.cdc.gov/nchs/data/nvsr/nvsr64/nvsr64_01.pdf.

294. Cruikshank, D. P., et al. Maternal physiology in pregnancy, In Gabbe, S. G., et al., eds. *Obstetrics: Normal and problem pregnancies*. New York: Churchill Livingstone, 1996; 91–109.

295. Fazleabas, A. T. Update and advances in reproductive biology. Experimental Biology Annual Meeting, San Diego, April 11, 2003.

296. van Stiphout, W. A. H. J., et al. Serum lipids in young women before, during, and after pregnancy. *Am J Epidemiol* 1987; 126:922–928.

297. Roseboom, T. J., et al. Plasma lipid profiles in adults after prenatal exposure to the Dutch famine. *Am J Clin Nutr* 2000; 72:1101–1106.

298. Ziegler, E. E., et al. Body composition of the reference fetus. *Growth* 1976; 40:329–41.

299. Messina, V., et al. A new food guide for North American vegetarians. *J Am Diet Assoc* 2003; 103:771–775.

300. Susser, M., et al. Timing in prenatal nutrition: A reprise of the Dutch Famine Study. *Nutr Rev* 1994; 52:84–94.

301. Roseboom, T. J., et al. Plasma lipid profiles in adults after prenatal exposure to the Dutch famine. *Am J Clin Nutr* 2000; 72:1101–1106.

302. United States Department of Agriculture (USDA), Agricultural Research Service (ARS), Nutrient Data Laboratory. Available at www.ars.usda.gov/nutrientdata.

303. Ulven, S. M., et al. Metabolic effects of krill oil are essentially similar to those of fish oil but at lower dose of EPA and DHA, in healthy volunteers. *Lipids* 2011; 46:37–46.

304. Dawson, E. B., et al. Iron in prenatal multivitamin/multimineral supplements. Bioavailability. *J Reprod Med* 1998; 43:133–40.

305. Singh, K., et al. A comparison between intravenous iron polymaltose complex (ferrum jausmann) and oral ferrous fumarate in the treatment of iron deficiency anemia in pregnancy. *Eur J Haematol* 1998;60:119-24.


## Chapter 5


1. Tenenbaum-Gavish, K., et al. Impact of maternal obesity on fetal health. *Fetal Diagn Ther.* 2013; 34:1–7.

2. Johansson, K., et al. Outcomes of pregnancy after bariatric surgery. *N Engl J Med* 2015; 372:814–824.

3. Hackethal, V., et al. High maternal BMI linked with stillbirths. *Medscape* 6/18/14,/ www.medscape.org/viewarticle/826036?nlid=61043_2707&src=cmemp.

4. Leddy, M. A., et al. The impact of maternal obesity on maternal and fetal health. *Rev Obstet Gynecol.* 2008; 1:170–178.

5. Chu, S. Y., et al. Association between obesity during pregnancy and increased use of health care. *N Engl J Med* 2008; 358:1444–1453.

6. Bartha, J. L., et al. Ultrasound evaluation of visceral fat and metabolic risk factors during early pregnancy. *Obesity* (Silver Springs) 2007; 15:2233–2239.

7. Heerwagen, M. J. R., et al. Maternal obesity and fetal metabolic programming: A fertile epigenetic soil. *Am J Physiol Regul Integr Comp Physiol* 2010; 299: R711–R722.

8. Wildman, R. P., et al. The obese without cardiometabolic risk factor clustering and the normal weight with cardiometabolic risk factor clustering: Prevalence and correlates of 2 phenotypes among the US population: (NHANES 1999–2004). *Arch Intern Med* 2008; 168:1617.

9. Krakoff, L. R. Adiposity and Risk for Hypertension: Does Location Matter? *J Am Coll Cardiol.* 2014; 64:1003–1004.

10. Bozorgmanesh, M., et al. No Obesity Paradox—BMI Incapable of Adequately Capturing the Relation of Obesity with All-Cause Mortality: An Inception Diabetes Cohort Study. *Int J Endocrin* 2014; doi.org/10.1155/2014/282089.

11. Adult obesity facts. Sep 2014. www.cdc.gov/obesity/data/adult.html, accessed 5/26/15.

12. Ogden, C. L., et al. Prevalence of childhood and adult obesity in the United States, 2011–2012. *JAMA* 2014; 26; 311:806–814.

13. Bombak, A. Obesity, health at every size, and public health policy. *Am J Public Health* 2014; 104:e60–67.

14. Jou, C. The biology and genetics of obesity—A century of inquiries. *N Engl J Med.* 2014; 370:1874–1877.

15. Obstetrics & Gynecology: Committee Opinion No. 600: Ethical Issues in the Care of the Obese Woman. *Obstet Gynecol.* June 2014. Available at: www.acog.org/Resources-And-Publications/Committee-Opinions/Committee-on-Ethics/Ethical-Issues-in-the-Care-of-the-Obese-Woman.

16. Ma, D., et al. Association between gestational weight gain according to prepregnancy body mass index and short postpartum weight retention in postpartum women. *Clin Nutr,* available online 4/24/14, doi:10.1016/j.clnu.2014.04.010.

17. Vesco, K. K., et al. Efficacy of a group-based dietary intervention for limiting gestational weight gain among obese women: a randomized trial. *Obesity* (Silver Spring). 2014; 22:989–996.

18. Nainggolan L. Intervene early in pregnancy to limit weight gain in obese, June 21, 2014. Joint Meeting of the International Society of Endocrinology and the Endocrine Society: ICE/ENDO 2014, Available at www.medscape.com/viewarticle/827170.

19. Bloomberg, M., et al. Maternal and Neonatal Outcomes Among Obese Women With Weight Gain Below the New Institute of Medicine Recommendations. *Obstet Gynecol* 2011; 117:1065–1070.

20. Rasmussen, K. M., et al. Recommendations for Weight Gain During Pregnancy in the Context of the Obesity Epidemic. *Obstet Gynecol* 2010; 116:1191–1195.

21. Maggard, M. A., et al. Pregnancy and Fertility Following Bariatric Surgery: A Systematic Review. *JAMA* 2008; 300:2286–2296.

22. Aasheim, E. T., et al. Vitamin status after bariatric surgery: A randomized study of gastric bypass and duodenal switch. *Am J Clin Nutr* 2009; 90:15–22.

23. Malinowski, S. S. Nutritional and metabolic complications of bariatric surgery. *Am J Med Sci* 2006; 331:219–225.

24. Kominiarek, M. A., et al. Guidelines on managing obesity in pregnancy. American College of Obstetrics and Gynecology. *Obstet Gynecol* 2009; 113:1405–1413.

25. Mechanick, J. I., et al. Clinical Practice Guidelines for the Perioperative Nutritional, Metabolic, and Nonsurgical Support of the Bariatric Surgery Patient—2013 Update. *Obesity* 2013; 21:S1–S27.

26. Maggard, M. A., et al. Pregnancy and fertility following bariatric surgery: A systematic review. *JAMA* 2008; 300:2286–2296.

27. Redman, C. W. G., et al. *Hypertension* in Pregnancy. The NICE Guidelines. *Heart* 2011; 97:1967–1969.

28. Mustafa, R., et al. Comprehensive Review of Hypertension in Pregnancy. *J Pregnancy.* 2012 May 23; doi:10.1155/2012/105918.

29. Moussa, H. N., et al. Management of Hypertensive Disorders in Pregnancy: Definitions & Classifications. CME Released: 09/26/2014, www.medscape.org/viewarticle/831994. accessed 11/12/14.

30. Mustafa, R., et al. Comprehensive Review of Hypertension in Pregnancy. *J Pregnancy.* 2012 May 23; doi:10.1155/2012/105918.

31. Report of the National High Blood Pressure Education Program Working Group on High Blood Pressure in Pregnancy. *Am J Obstet Gynecol* 2000; 183:S1–S22.

32. Moussa, H. N., et al. Management of Hypertensive Disorders in Pregnancy: Definitions & Classifications. CME Released: 09/26/2014, www.medscape.org/viewarticle/831994, accessed 11/12/14.

33. Sibai, B. M., et al. Risk factors for preeclampsia, abruptio placentae, and adverse neonatal outcomes among women with chronic hypertension. National Institute of Child Health and Human Development Network of Maternal–Fetal Medicine Units. *N Engl J Med* 1998; 339:667–671.

34. Report of the National High Blood Pressure Education Program Working Group on High Blood Pressure in Pregnancy. *Am J Obstet Gynecol* 2000; 183:S1–S22.

35. Haddad, B., et al. Chronic hypertension in pregnancy. *Ann Med* 1999; 31:246–252.

36. Mustafa, R., et al. Comprehensive Review of Hypertension in Pregnancy. *J Pregnancy* 2012 May 23; doi:10.1155/2012/105918.

37. Mosca, L., et al. Effectiveness-based guidelines for the prevention of cardiovascular disease in women—2011 update. *Circulation* 2011; 123:1243–1262.

38. Thadhani, R., et al. Preclampsia—A glimpse into the future? *N Engl J Med* 2008; 359:858–860.

39. Germain, A. M., et al. Endothelial dysfunction: A link among preeclampsia, recurrent pregnancy loss, and future cardiovascular events? *Hypertension* 2007; 43:90–95.

40. Ciantar, E., et al. Pre-eclampsia, severe pre-eclampsia and hemolysis, elevated liver enzymes and low platelets syndrome. What Is New? *Women's Health* 2011; 7(5):555–569.

41. Redman, C. W. G., et al. *Hypertension* in pregnancy. The NICE Guidelines. *Heart* 2011; 97:1967–1969.

42. Al-Safi, Z., et al. Preeclampsia and eclampsia may occur days to weeks after delivery. *Obstet Gynecol* 2011; 118:1102–1107.

43. Prevent recurrent eclamptic seizures with magnesium sulfate, an unconventional anticonvulsant. *Drug Ther Perspect* 2000; 16:6–8.

44. Hernandez-Diaz, S., et al. Risk of preeclampsia in first and subsequent pregnancies: Prospective cohort study. *BMJ* 6/26/09.

Available at www.medscape.com/viewarticle/704801.

45. Xiong, X., et al. Association of preeclampsia with high birth weight for age. *Am J Obstet Gynecol* 2000; 183:148–155.

46. Klebanoff, M. A., et al. Maternal size at birth and the development of hypertension during pregnancy: A test of the Barker hypothesis. *Arch Intern Med* 1999; 159:1607–1612.

47. Davis, E. F., et al. Cardiovascular risk factors in children and young adults born to preeclamptic pregnancies: A systematic review. *Pediatrics*, published online 2012 May 21; doi: 10.1542/peds.2011–3093.

48. Zhou, S. J., et al. Fish-oil supplementation in pregnancy does not reduce the risk of gestational diabetes or preeclampsia. *Am J Clin Nutr*. 2012; 95:1378–1384.

49. Rumbold, A., et al. Antioxidants for preventing preeclampsia. *Cochrane Database Syst Rev* 2008; 23(1):CD004227.

50. Scholl, T. O., et al. Vitamin D, secondary hyperparathyroidism, and preeclampsia. *Am J Clin Nutr* 2013; 98:787–793.

51. Hofmeyr, G. J., et al. Calcium supplementation during pregnancy for preventing hypertensive disorders and related problems. *Cochrane Database Syst Rev* 2006; 3:CD001059.

52. Bodnar, L. M., et al. Periconceptional multivitamin use reduces the risk of preeclampsia. *Am J Epidemiol* 2006; 164:470–477.

53. Catov, J. M., et al. Association of periconceptional multivitamin use with reduced risk of preeclampsia among normal-weight women in the Danish National Birth Cohort. *Am J Epidemiol* 2009; 169:1304–1311.

54. Brantsaeter, A. L., et al. A dietary pattern characterized by high intake of vegetables, fruits, and vegetable oils is associated with reduced risk of preeclampsia in nulliparous pregnant Norwegian women. *J Nutr* 2009; 139:1162–1168.

55. Adiga, U., et al. Antioxidant activity and lipid peroxidation in preeclampsia. *J Chin Med Assoc* 2007; 70:435–438.

56. Qui, C., et al. Dietary fiber intake early in pregnancy and risk of subsequent preeclampsia. *Am J Hyperten* 2008:21:903–909.

57. Duley, L., et al. Altered dietary salt for preventing pre-eclampsia, and its complications. *Cochrane Database of Syst Rev* 2005; Issue 4. Art. No. CD005548, doi 10.1002/14651858.CD005548.

58. Rayman, M. P., et al. Iron supplementation in preeclampsia. *Am J Obstet Gynecol* 2002; 187:412–418.

59. Hopkins, S. A., et al. The role of exercise in reducing the risks of gestational diabetes mellitus. *Women's Health* 2013; 9:569–581.

60. Mathieu, C. Gestational diabetes: A worldwide controversial topic. *Chantal.* August 01, 2014, www.medscape.com/viewarticle/827645, accessed 5/28/15.

61. Rosenberg, T. J., et al. Maternal obesity and diabetes as risk factors for adverse pregnancy outcomes: Differences among 4 racial/ethnic groups. *Am J Public Health* 2005; 95:1545–1551.

62. Magon, N., et al. Gestational diabetes mellitus: Non-insulin management. *Indian J Endocrinol Metab* 2011; 15:284–293.

63. 2011 National Diabetes Fact Sheet. www.cdc.gov/diabetes/pubs/factsheet11.htm, accessed 9/12/12.

64. American Diabetes Association. Management of diabetes in pregnancy. In: *Standards of Medical Care in Diabetes—2015*. Diabetes Care 2015; 38(Suppl. 1):S77–S79.

65. Curry A. Avoiding diabetes in pregnancy: Tailoring treatment plans for different Asian ethnic groups. *Diabetes Forecast* 2014 Feb; 71,73.

66. Zhang, C., et al. Effect of dietary and lifestyle factors on the risk of gestational diabetes: review of epidemiology evidence. *Am J Clin Nutr* 2011; 94 (suppl):1975S–9S.

67. Landon, M. B. Diabetes mellitus and other endocrine disorders. In Gabbe, S. G., et al., eds. Obstetrics, normal and problem pregnancies. New York: Churchill-Livingstone, 1996: 1037–1081.

68. Pettitt, D. J., et al. *In utero* exposure to diabetes and type 2 diabetes risk later in life. *Diabetes Care* 2008; 31:2126–2130.

69. Lindsay, R. S., et al. Secular trends in birth weight, BMI, and diabetes in the offspring of diabetic mothers. *Diabetes Care* 2000; 23:1249–1254.

70. MacNeill, S., et al. Rates and risk factors for recurrence of gestational diabetes. *Diabetes Care* 2001; 24:659–662.

71. Kitzmiller, J. L., et al. Managing preexisting diabetes for pregnancy. *Diabetes Care* 2008; 31:1060–1079.

72. Xiao, R. S., et al. Diet Quality and History of Gestational Diabetes Mellitus Among Childbearing Women, United States, 2007–2010. *Prev Chronic Dis*. 2015; www.medscape.com/viewarticle/840902?nlid=78803_905&src=wnl_edit_medp_obgy&uac=61213SX&spon=16, accessed 4/5/15.

73. Tobias, D. K., et al. Prepregnancy adherence to dietary patterns and lower risk of gestational diabetes mellitus. *Am J Clin Nutr* 2012; 96:289–295.

74. Chang, C. L., et al. Identification of metabolic modifiers that underlie phenotypic variations in energy-balance regulation. *Diabetes* 2011; 60:726–734.

75. Zhang, C., et al. Dietary fiber intake, dietary glycemic load, and the risk for gestational diabetes mellitus. *Diabetes Care* 2006; 29:2223–2230.

76. McMahon, M. J., et al. Gestational diabetes mellitus: Risk factors, obstetric complications and infant outcomes. *J Reprod Med* 1998; 43:372–378.

77. American College of Obstetricians and Gynecologists (ACOG): Gestational diabetes mellitus. *Obstet Gynecol* 2013; 122:406–416.

78. Diabetes in pregnancy: Management of diabetes and its complications from preconception to the postnatal period. National Institute for Health Care and Health Care Excellence. Feb 2015, www.nice.org.uk/guidance/ng3/chapter/1-recommendations, accessed 3/23/15.

79. Peters, A. L., et al. Simple Strategy Triples Patient Weight Loss. American Diabetes Association (ADA) 72nd Scientific Sessions.June 8–12, 2012; Philadelphia, www.medscape.com/viewarticle/766223?src=mp&spon=38, 7/15/12.

80. Buhling, K. J., et al. No influence of high- and low-carbohydrate diet on the oral glucose tolerance test in pregnancy. *Clin Biochem* 2004; 37:323–327.

81. American Diabetes Association. Standards of Medical Care in Diabetes—2012. *Diabetes Care* 2012; 35:S11–S63.

82. Coad, S., et al. Understanding urinalysis, clues for the obstetrician-gynecologist. *Expert Rev of Obstet Gynecol* 2012; 7:269–279.

83. Artal, R. The role of exercise in reducing the risks of gestational diabetes mellitus in obese women. *Best Pract Res Clin Obstet Gynaecol*. 2014; S1521-6934:00174-6.

84. Reader, D. M. Medical nutrition therapy and lifestyle interventions. *Diabetes Care* 2007; 30 (Supplement 2): S188–S193.

85. Menato, G., et al. Current management of gestational diabetes mellitus. *Expert Rev Obstet Gynecol* 2008; 3:73–91.

86. Lashen, H. Role of metformin in the management of polycystic ovary syndrome. *Ther Adv Endocrinol Metab*. 2010; 1:117–128.

87. de Barros, M. C., et al. Resistance exercise and glycemic control in women with gestational diabetes mellitus. *Am J Obstet Gynecol* 2010; 203:556.e1–6.

88. Executive summary of the American Dietetic Association's recommendations for evidence-based practice guidelines for gestational diabetes. Available at www.adaevidencelibrary.com/topic.cfm?cat=3731, accessed 6/09.

89. Latif L., et al. Metformin Effects on Treatment Satisfaction and Quality of Life in Gestational Diabetes. *Brit J Diabetes Vascular Dis*. 2013; 13:178–182.

90. Evert, A.B., et al. Nutrition therapy recommendations for the management of adults with diabetes. *Diabetes Care*, October 9, 2013, doi: 10.2337/dc13-2042, accessed 7/21/14.

91. Marcason, W. A. What is the appropriate distribution of macronutrients for a patient with diabetes? *J Acad Nutr* Diet 2012; 112:776.

92. Astrup, A., et al. The role of higher protein diets in weight control and obesity-related comorbidities. *International Journal of Obesity* 2015; 39:721–726.

93. Butte, N. F. Dieting and exercise in overweight, lactating women [editorial]. *N Engl J Med* 2000; 342:502–503.

94. Bao W et al. Physical activity and sedentary behaviors associated with risk

of progression from gestational diabetes mellitus to type 2 diabetes mellitus: A prospective cohort study. *JAMA Intern Med.* Published online May 19, 2014. doi:10.1001/jamainternmed.2014.1795.

95. Hopkins, S. A., et al. The role of exercise in reducing the risks of gestational diabetes mellitus. *Women's Health* 2013; 9:569–581.

96. Negrato, C. A., et al. Adverse pregnancy outcomes in women with diabetes. *Diabetol Metab Syndr* 2012; 4:41.

97. ter Braak, E. W. M., et al. Maternal hypoglycemia during pregnancy in type 1 diabetes: maternal and fetal consequences. *Diabetes Metab Res Rev* 2002; 18:96–105.

98. Metzger, B. E., et al. Summary and Recommendations of the Fifth International Workshop-Conference on Gestational Diabetes Mellitus. *Diabetes Care* 2007; 30: Supplement 2, S251–S260.

99. Gestational diabetes: What you need to know. Oct 2013. www.diabetes.niddk.nih.gov/dm/pubs/gestational_es, accessed 5.25/15.

100. Raychaudhuri, K., et al. Glycemic control throughout pregnancy and fetal growth in insulin-dependent diabetes. *Obstet Gynecol* 2000; 95:190–194.

101. Mello, G., et al. What degree of maternal metabolic control in women with type 1 diabetes is associated with normal body size and proportions in full-term infants? *Diabetes Care* 2000; 23; 1494–1498.

102. Timar, B. et al. Predictors for pregnancy outcomes in Romanian women with Type 1 Diabetes Mellitus: a prospective study. Diabetol Metab Synd, Published online 2014 Nov 22, doi:10.1186/1758-5996-6-125.

103. Kalkwarf, H. J., et al. Dietary fiber intakes and insulin requirements in pregnant women with type 1 diabetes. *J Am Diet Assoc* 2001; 101:305–310.

104. Artificial pancreas could help pregnant diabetic women. Jan 31, 2011. diabetes.webmd.com/news/20110131/artificial-pancreas-pregnant-diabetic-women, accessed 9/12/12.

105. Martin, A., et al. Births: Final data for 2013, Jan 2015. Available at: www.cdc.gov/nchs/data/nvsr/nvsr64/nvsr64_01.pdf.

106. Skora, D., et al. Adverse Perinatal Events Associated With ART. *Semin Reprod Med* 2012; 30:84–91.

107. Brown, J. E., et al. Prepregnancy weight status, prenatal weight gain, and the outcome of term twin gestations. *Am J Obst Gynecol* 1990; 162:182–186.

108. Kulkarni, A. D., et al. Fertility treatments and multiple births in the United States. *N Engl J Med* 2013; 369:22118–22125.

109. Martin, J. A., et al. Three Decades of Twin Births in the United States, 1980–2009, www.cdc.gov/nchs/data/databriefs/db80.htm, accessed 8/16/12.

110. Martin, J. A., et al. Births: Final data for 2009. www.cdc.gov/nchs/data/nvsr/nvsr60/nvsr60_01.pdf, accessed 8/16/12.

111. Hoskins, R. E. Zygosity as a risk factor for complications and outcomes of twin pregnancy. *Acta Genet Med Gemellol* 1995; 44:11–23.

112. Redline, R. W. Non-identical twins with a single placenta—Disproving dogma in perinatal pathology. *N Engl J Med* 2003; 349:111–114.

113. Imaizumi, Y. A comparative study of twinning and triplet rates in 17 countries, 1971–1996. *Acta Genet Med Gemellol* 1998; 47:101–114.

114. Czeizel, A. E., et al. Higher rate of multiple births after periconceptional vitamin supplementation. *New Engl J Med 1994*; 330:1687–1688.

115. Kogan, M. D., et al. Trends in twin birth outcomes and prenatal care utilization in the United States, 1981–1997. *JAMA* 2000; 284:335–341.

116. Ellings, J. M., et al. Reduction in very low birth weight deliveries and perinatal mortality in a specialized, multidisciplinary twin clinic. *Obstet Gynecol* 1993; 81:387–391.

117. Ventura, S. J., et al. Births: Final data for 1999. Vol. 2001, available at www.cdc.gov/nchs.

118. Kogan, M. D., et al. Trends in twin birth outcomes and prenatal care utilization in the United States, 1981–1997. *JAMA* 2000; 284:335–41.

119. Ellings, J. M., et al. Reduction in very low birth weight deliveries and perinatal mortality in a specialized, multidisciplinary twin clinic. *Obstet Gynecol* 1993; 81:387–391.

120. Dubois, S., et al. Twin pregnancy: The impact of the Higgins Nutrition Intervention Program on maternal and neonatal outcomes. *Am J Clin Nutr* 1991; 53:1397–1403.

121. National Academy of Sciences. Nutrition during pregnancy. I. Weight gain. II. Nutrient supplements. Washington, DC: National Academy Press, 1990.

122. Rassmussen, K. M., et al. Weight gain during pregnancy: Reexamining the guidelines. Institute of Medicine, 2009. Available at www.nap.edu/catalog/12584.html.

123. Brown, J. E., et al. Nutrition and multifetal pregnancy. *J Am Diet Assoc* 2000; 100:343–348.

124. Konwinski, T., et al. Maternal pregestational weight and multiple pregnancy duration. *Acta Genet Med Gemellol* 1973; 22:44–47.

125. Zeijdner, E. E., et al. Essential fatty acid status in plasma phospholipids of mother and neonate after multiple pregnancy. *Prostaglandins Leukotrienes and Essential Fatty Acids* 1997; 56:395–401.

126. Rich, K. C., et al. Maternal and infant factors predicting disease progression in human immunodeficiency virus type 1–infected infants. Women and Infants Transmission Study Group. *Pediatrics* 2000; 105:E8.

127. Baarouch, D. H. The quest for an HIV-1 vaccine—Moving forward. *N Engl J Med* 2013; 369:2073–2076.

128. Report on advances in HIV research. *The Scientist*, Aug 2010; pp. 33–25.

129. Fields-Gardner, C., et al. Position of the American Dietetic Association and Dietitians of Canada: Nutrition intervention in the care of persons with human immunodeficiency virus infection. *J Am Diet Assoc* 2000; 100:708–717.

130. Shapiro, R. L., et al. Antiretroviral regimes in pregnancy and breastfeeding in Botswana. *N Engl J Med* 2010; 362:2282–2294.

131. Report on advances in HIV research. *The Scientist*, Aug 2010; pp. 33–25.

132. Zulling, L., et al. Nutrition for HIV positive women: practical guidelines. *Women's Health and Reproductive Nutrition Report.* 2005 Winter; 1, 4,14–16.

133. Fields-Gardner, C., et al. Position of the American Dietetic Association and Dietitians of Canada: Nutrition intervention in the care of persons with human immunodeficiency virus infection. *J Am Diet Assoc* 2000; 100:708–717.

134. Raiten, D. J., et al. Executive summary: nutritional care of HIV-infected adolescents and adults, including pregnant and lactation, *Am J Clin Nutr* 2011; 94(suppl):1667S–76S.

135. Position of the American Dietetic Association: Nutrition intervention and human immunodeficiency virus infection. *J Am Diet Assoc* 2012; 110:105–119.

136. Morrill, E. S., et al. Bulimia nervosa during pregnancy: A review. *J Am Diet Assoc* 2001; 102:448–454.

137. Becker, A. E., et al. Eating disorders. *N Engl J Med* 1999; 340:1092–1098.

138. Hoffman, E. R., et al. Reproductive Issues in Anorexia Nervosa. *Expert Rev of Obstet Gynecol* 2011; 6:403–414.

139. Little, L., et al. Midwifery. Love of women with eating disorders. *Women's Health* 2000; 45:301–307.

140. Linna MS., et al. Pregnancy, obstetric and perinatal health outcomes in eating disorders. *Am J Obstet Gynceol* 2014 April 7; doi:10.1016/j.ajog.2014.03.067.

141. Pregnancy treatment and prevention of IUGR, an email discussion among clinical dietitians on eating disorders in pregnancy, *Women's Health* DPG, 2010 May.

142. Chambers, C., et al. Prenatal Alcohol Exposure Patterns and Alcohol-Related Birth Defects and Growth Deficiencies: A Prospective Study. Alcoholism: *Clin Exper Res*, Article first published online: 17 Jan 2012, doi: 10.1111/j.1530–0277.2011.01664.x.

143. Denny, C. H., et al. Pattern of alcohol use during pregnancy since 1991. *MMWR* 2009; 58:529–532.

144. Shankar, K., et al. Physiologic and genomic analyses of nutrition ethanol interactions during gestation: Implications for fetal ethanol toxicity. *Exp Biol Med* (Maywood). 2006; 231:1379–1397.

145. May, P. A., et al. Prevalence and characteristics of fetal alcohol spectrum disorders. *Pediatrics* 2014; 134:855–866.

146. Fetal alcohol spectrum disorder. www .cdc//gov/ncbdd/fasd/index.html, accessed Jan 18 2012.

147. Wang, L. L., et al. Ethanol exposure induces differential microRNA ad target gene expression and teratogenic effects which can be suppressed by folic acid supplementation. *Hum Repro* 2009; 24:562–579.

148. Keuhn, D., et al. A prospective cohort study of the prevalence of growth, facial, and central nervous system abnormalities in children with heavy prenatal alcohol exposure. *Alcohol Clin Experiment Res*, first published online: 23 Jul 2012; doi: 10.1111/j.1530-0277.2012.01794.x.

149. Kesmodel, U., et al. The effect of different alcohol drinking patterns in early to mid pregnancy on the child's intelligence, attention, and executive function. *BJOG* 20 June 2012; doi: 10.1111/j.1471-0528.2012.03393.x.

150. Baker, P. N., et al. A prospective study of micronutrient status in adolescent pregnancy. *Am J Clin Nutr* 2009; 89:1114–1124.

151. Anderson, A. E., et al. Women's perceptions of information about alcohol use during pregnancy: A qualitative study. *BMC Public Health*. 2014; 14(1048). Available at: www .medscape.com/viewarticle/834709?nlid=73424_905&src=wnl_edit_medp_obgy&uac =61213SX&spon=16, accessed 1/9/15.

152. O'Leary, C. M., et al. Guidelines for pregnancy: What's an acceptable risk, and how is the evidence (finally) shaping up? *Drug Alcohol Rev* 2012; 31:170–183.

153. Barker, D., et al. Developmental biology: Support mothers to secure future public health. *Nature*. 2013; 504:209–211.

154. Sexual experiences and contraceptive use among female teens—United States, 1995, 2002, and 2006–2010. *MMWR* May 4 2012; 61(7):297–301.

155. Baker, P. N., et al. A prospective study of micronutrient status in adolescent pregnancy. *Am J Clin Nutr* 2009; 89:1114–1124.

156. Iannotti, L. L., et al. Iron deficiency anemia and depleted body iron reserves are prevalent among pregnant African-American adolescents. *J Nutr* 2005; 135:2572–2577.

157. Lee, S., et al. Nutrient Inadequacy Is Prevalent in Pregnant Adolescents, and Prenatal Supplement Use May Not Fully Compensate for Dietary Deficiencies. *Infant Child Adol Nutr* 2014; 6:152–159.

158. Scholl, T. O., et al. Maternal growth during pregnancy and the competition for nutrients. *Am J Clin Nutr* 1994; 60:183–188.

159. Wallace, J. M., et al. Nutritionally mediated placental growth restriction in the growing adolescent: consequences for the fetus. *Biol Reprod* 2004; 71:1055–1062.

160. Scholl, T. O., et al. Leptin and maternal growth during adolescent pregnancy. *Am J Clin Nutr* 2000; 72:1542–1547.

161. Thame, M. M., et al. Comparing the glucose kinetics of adolescent girls and adult women during pregnancy. *Am J Clin Nutr* 2010; 91:604–609.

162. Sukalich, S., et al. Obstetric outcomes in overweight and obese adolescents. *Am J Obstet Gynecol* 2006; 195:851–855.

163. Young, B. E., et al. Maternal vitamin D status and calcium intake interact to affect fetal skeletal growth *in utero* in pregnant adolescents. *Am J Clin Nutr* 2012; 95:1103–1112.

164. Nielsen, J. N., et al. Interventions to improve diet and weight gain among pregnancy adolescents and recommendations for future research. *J Am Diet Assoc* 2006; 106:1825–1840.

165. Berkowitz, K. M. Insulin resistance and preeclampsia. *Clin Perinatol* 1998; 25:873–885.

166. Adams, K. M., et al. Sequelae of unrecognized gestational diabetes. *Am J Obstet Gynecol* 1998; 178:1321–1332.

167. Martin, J. A., et al. Births: Final data for 2006. *National Vital Statistics Report* 2009 Jan. 7; 57(7).

168. Position of the Academy of Nutrition and Dietetics: Nutrition and Lifestyle for a Healthy Pregnancy Outcome. *J Acad Nutr Diet*. 2014; 114:1099–1103.

169. Gilbert, W., et al. Birth outcomes in teenage pregnancies. *J Mat Fetal Neonat Med* 2004; 16:265–270.

170. American Diabetes Association. Diagnosis and classification of diabetes mellitus. *Diabetes Care* 2012; 35 Suppl 1:S64–71.

171.Trends in Teen Pregnancy and Childbearing, Mar 2015. www.hhs.gov/ash/oah /adolescent-health-topics/reproductive-health /teen-pregnancy/trends.html, accessed 5/13/15.

## *Chapter 6*

1. Hartmann, P. E., Changes in the composition and yield of the mammary secretion of cows during the initiation of lactation. *J Endocrinol* 1973; 59(2):231–247.

2. Brownell, E., et al. Delayed onset lactogenesis II predicts the cessation of any or exclusive breastfeeding. *J Pediatr* 2012; 161(4):608–614.

3. Vorherr, H., Human lactation and breastfeeding., in The mammary gland/human lactation/milk synthesis, B. L. Larson, Editor. 1978, New York: Academic Press.

4. Lawrence, R. A., et al. Breastfeeding: A Guide for the Medical Professional. 6th ed. 2005, Minneapolis: Mosby.

5. Cox, D. B., et al. Blood and milk prolactin and the rate of milk synthesis in women. *Exp Physiol* 1996; 81(6):1007–1020.

6. Neville, M. C., The physiological basis of milk secretion. Part I. Basic physiology 1990;5861–5868. *Ann NY Acad Sci* 1990; 5:861–868.

7. Jensen, R. G., The Lipids of Human Milk. 1989, Boca Raton, FL: CRC Press.

8. Ballard, O., et al. Human milk composition: nutrients and bioactive factors. *Pediatr Clin North Am* 2013; 60(1):49–74.

9. Prentice, A., Food and Nutrition Bulletin, in Consistuents of Human Milk. 1996, The United Nations University Press.

10. Koletzko, B., et al. Global standard for the composition of infant formula: recommendations of an ESPGHAN coordinated international expert group. *J Pediatr Gastroenterol Nutr* 2005; 41(5):584–599.

11. Lima, M. S., et al. Vitamin E concentration in human milk and associated factors: a literature review. *J Pediatr (Rio J)* 2014; 90(5):440–448.

12. Williams, H. G., 'And not a drop to drink'—Why water is harmful for newborns. *Breastfeed Rev* 2006; 14(2):5–9.

13. Axelson, I., et al. Protein and energy intake during weaning: I. Effects on growth. *Acta Paediatrica Scandinavica* 1987; 76(2):321–327.

14. Butte, N. F., et al. Longitudinal changes in milk composition of mothers delivering preterm and term infants. *Early Hum Dev* 1984; 9(2):153–162.

15. Hediger, M. L., et al. Early infant feeding and growth status of US-born infants and children aged 4–71 mo: analyses from the third National Health and Nutrition Examination Survey 1988–1994; *Am J Clin Nutr* 2000; 72(1):159–167.

16. Innis, S. M., Impact of maternal diet on human milk composition and neurological development of infants. *Am J Clin Nutr* 2014; 99(3):734S–41S.

17. Nishimura, R. Y., et al. Dietary polyunsaturated fatty acid intake during late pregnancy affects fatty acid composition of mature breast milk. *Nutrition* 2014; 30(6):685–689.

18. Insull, W., et al. The fatty acids of human milk from mothers on diets taken ad libitum. *Biochem J* 1959; 72:27.

19. Meier, P. P., et al. Mothers' milk feedings in the neonatal intensive care unit: accuracy of the creamatocrit technique. *J Perinatol* 2002; 22(8):646–649.

20. Scholtz, S. A., et al. Clinical overview of effects of dietary long-chain polyunsaturated fatty acids during the perinatal period. Nestle Nutr Inst Workshop Ser 2013; 77:145–54.

21. Kovacs, A., et al. Fatty acids in early human milk after preterm and full-term delivery. *J Pediatr Gastroenterol Nutr* 2005; 41(4):454–459.

22. Helland, I. B., et al. Maternal supplementation with very-long-chain n–3 fatty acids during pregnancy and lactation augments children's IQ at 4 years of age. *Pediatrics* 2003; 111(1):e39–44.

23. Mosley, E., et al. Trans fatty acids in milk produced by women in the United States. *Am J Clin Nutr* 2005; 82(6):1292–1297.

24. Ratnayake, W. N., et al. Mandatory trans fat labeling regulations and nationwide product reformulations to reduce trans fatty acid content in foods contributed to lowered concentrations of trans fat in Canadian women's breast milk samples collected in 2009–2011. *Am J Clin Nutr* 2014; 100(4):1036–1040.

25. Scopesi, F., et al. 7-ketocholesterol in human and adapted milk formulas. *Clin Nutr* 2002; 21(5):379–384.

26. Kamelska, A. M., et al. Variation of the cholesterol content in breast milk during 10 days collection at early stages of lactation. *Acta Biochim Pol* 2012; 59(2):243–247.

27. Wong, W. W., et al. Effect of dietary cholesterol on cholesterol synthesis in breast-fed and formula-fed infants. *J Lipid Res* 1993; 34(8):1403–1411.

28. Rosen, J. M., et al. Regulatory sequences involved in the hormonal control of casein gene expression. *Ann N Y Acad Sci* 1986; 464:87–99.

29. Phadke, S. M., et al. Antimicrobial peptides in mucosal secretions: the importance of local secretions in mitigating infection. *J Nutr* 2005; 135(5):1289–1293.

30. Velona, T., et al. Protein profiles in breast milk from mothers delivering term and preterm babies. *Pediatr Res* 1999; 45(5 Pt 1):658–663.

31. Lonnerdal, B., et al. Nitrogenous components of milk, in Handbook of Milk Composition, R. G. Jensen, Editor. 1995, San Diego: Academic Press, 351–368.

32. Newburg, D. S., et al. Carboyhdrates in milks: analysis, quantities, and signficance., in Handbook of Milk Composition, R. G. Jensen, Editor. 1995, San Diego: Academic Press, 273–349.

33. Morrow, A. L., et al. Human-milk glycans that inhibit pathogen binding protect breast-feeding infants against infectious diarrhea. *J Nutr* 2005; 135(5):1304–1307.

34. Bode, L., Recent advances on structure, metabolism, and function of human milk oligosaccharides. *J Nutr* 2006; 136(8):2127–2130.

35. Newburg, D. S., et al. Recent advances in human milk glycobiology. *Pediatr Res* 2014. 75(5):675–679.

36. Food and Nutrition Board Institute of Medicine, Dietary Reference Intakes for Vitamin A, Vitamin K, Arsenic, Boron, Chromium, Copper, Iodine, Iron, Manganese, Molybdenum, Nickel, Silicon, Vanadium, and Zinc. Washington, DC: National Academy Press, 2001.

37. Oliveira-Menegozzo, J. M., et al. Vitamin A supplementation for postpartum women. *Cochrane Database Syst Rev* 2010; (10):CD005944.

38. Thiele, D. K., et al. Maternal vitamin D supplementation to meet the needs of the breastfed infant: a systematic review. *J Hum Lact* 2013; 29(2):163–170.

39. Ala-Houhala, M., et al. 25-Hydroxyvitamin D and vitamin D in human milk: Effects of supplementation and season. *Am J Clin Nutr* 1988; 48(4):1057–1060.

40. Dawodu, A., et al. Mother-child vitamin D deficiency: an international perspective. *Arch Dis Child* 2007; 92(9):737–740.

41. Lammi-Keefe, C. J., et al. Fat-soluble vitamins in human milk. *Nutr Rev* 1984; 42(11):365–71.

42. Haug, M., et al. Vitamin E in human milk from mothers of preterm and term infants. *J Pediatr Gastroenterol Nutr* 1987; 6(4):605–609.

43. Chappell, J. E., et al. Vitamin A and E content of human milk at early stages of lactation. *Early Hum Dev* 1985; 11(2):157–167.

44. Allen, L. H., B vitamins in breast milk: relative importance of maternal status and intake, and effects on infant status and function. *Adv Nutr* 2012; 3(3):362–369.

45. Food and Nutrition Board Institute of Medicine, Dietary Reference Intakes for Thiamin Riboflavin, Niacin, Vitamin B6, Folate, Vitamin B12, Pantothenic Acid, Biotin, and Choline. Washington, DC: National Academy Press, 1998.

46. Dror, D. K., et al. Effect of vitamin B12 deficiency on neurodevelopment in infants: current knowledge and possible mechanisms. *Nutr Rev* 2008; 66(5):250–255.

47. Butte, N. F., et al. Macro- and trace-mineral intakes of exclusively breast-fed infants. Am *J Clin Nutr* 1987. 45(1):42–48.

48. Fransson, G. B., et al. Zinc, copper, calcium, and magnesium in human milk. *J Pediatr* 1982. 101(4):504–508.

49. Atkinson, S. A., et al. Abnormal zinc content in human milk. Risk for development of nutritional zinc deficiency in infants. *Am J Dis Child* 1989; 143(5):608–611.

50. Duncan, B., et al. Iron and the exclusively breast-fed infant from birth to six months. *J Pediatr Gastroenterol Nutr* 1985; 4(3):421–425.

51. Pisacane, A., et al. Iron status in breast-fed infants. J Pediatr 1995; 127(3):429–421.

52. Krebs, N. F., et al. Zinc requirements and zinc intakes of breast-fed infants. *Am J Clin Nutr* 1986; 43(2):288–292.

53. Severi, C., et al. Zinc in plasma and breast milk in adolescents and adults in pregnancy and pospartum: a cohort study in Uruguay. *Nutr Hosp* 2013; 28(1):223–8.

54. Food and Nutrition Board Institute of Medicine, Dietary Reference Intakes for Calcium, Phosphorus, Magnesium, Vitamin D, and Fluoride. Washington, DC: National Academy Press, 1999, 448.

55. McDowell, M. M., et al. Breastfeeding in the United States: findings from the national health and nutrition examination surveys 1999–2006. *NCHS Data Brief* 2008; (5):1–8.

56. Palmer, C., et al. Position of the American Dietetic Association: the impact of fluoride on health. J Am Diet Assoc 2005; 105(10):1620–1628.

57. McDowell, M. M., et al. Breastfeeding in the United States: Findings from the national health and nutrition examination surveys 1999–2006. NCHS Data Brief 2008; (5):1–8.

58. McDaniel, M. R., et al. Sensory characterization of human milk. *J Dairy Sci* 1989; 72(5):1149–1158.

59. Menella, J. A., Mother's Milk: a medium for early flavor experiences. *J Hum Lactation* 1995; 11(39–45).

60. Hausner, H., et al. Differential transfer of dietary flavour compounds into human breast milk. *Physiol Behav* 2008; 95(1–2):118–124.

61. Menella, J. A., et al. Experience with a flavor in mother's milk modifies the infants acceptance of flavored cereal. *Developmental Psychobiol* 1999; 34:197–203.

62. Gerrish, C. J., et al. Flavor variety enhances food acceptance in formula-fed infants. *Am J Clin Nutr* 2001; 73(6):1080–1085.

63. Schwartz, C., et al. Breast-feeding duration: influence on taste acceptance over the first year of life. *Br J Nutr* 2013; 109(6):1154–1161.

64. Lessen, R., et al. Position of the academy of nutrition and dietetics: promoting and supporting breastfeeding. *J Acad Nutr Diet* 2015; 115(3):444–449.

65. Kuzela, A. L., et al. Breastfeeding and mother-infant interactions1990;8:185–194. *J Reprod Infant Psychol* 1990; 8:185–194.

66. Karlson, E. W., et al. Do breast-feeding and other reproductive factors influence future risk of rheumatoid arthritis? Results from the Nurses' Health Study. *Arthritis Rheum* 2004; 50(11):3458–3467.

67. Labbok, M. H., et al. Breastfeeding: maintaining an irreplaceable immunological resource. *Nat Rev Immunol* 2004; 4(7):565–572.

68. Keeney, S. E., et al. Activated neutrophils and neutrophil activators in human milk: increased expression of CD11b and decreased expression of L-selectin. *J Leukoc Biol* 1993; 54(2):97–104.

69. German, J. B., et al. Composition, structure and absorption of milk lipids: a source of energy, fat-soluble nutrients and bioactive molecules. *Crit Rev Food Sci Nutr* 2006; 46(1):57–92.

70. Sprong, R. C., et al. Bactericidal activities of milk lipids. *Antimicrob Agents Chemother* 2001; 45(4):1298–1301.

71. Pickering, L. K., et al. Modulation of the immune system by human milk and infant formula containing nucleotides. *Pediatrics* 1998; 101(2):242–249.

72. World Health Organization, Global Strategy for Infant and Young Child Feeding. 2003: Geneva, Switzerland.

73. Hauck, F. R., et al. Breastfeeding and reduced risk of sudden infant death syndrome: a meta-analysis. Pediatrics 2011; 128(1):103–110.

74. American Academy of Pediatrics, Section on Breastfeeding, Breastfeeding and the use of human milk. *Pediatrics* 2012; 129(3):e827–841.

75. Ip, S., et al. Breastfeeding and maternal and infant health outcomes in developed countries. *Evid Rep Technol Assess (Full Rep)* 2007; (153):1–186.

76. Greer, F. R., et al. Effects of early nutritional interventions on the development of atopic disease in infants and children: the role of maternal dietary restriction, breastfeeding,

timing of introduction of complementary foods, and hydrolyzed formulas. *Pediatrics* 2008; 121(1):183–91.

77. Dewey, K. G., et al. Growth of breast-fed and formula-fed infants from 0 to 18 months: the DARLING Study. *Pediatrics* 1992; 89(6 Pt 1):1035–1041.

78. Evenhouse, E., et al. Improved estimates of the benefits of breastfeeding using sibling comparisons to reduce selection bias. *Health Serv Res* 2005; 40(6 Pt 1): 1781–1802.

79. Andres, A., et al. Developmental status of 1-year-old infants fed breast milk, cow's milk formula, or soy formula. *Pediatrics* 2012; 129(6):1134–1140.

80. Smith, M. M., et al. Initiation of breastfeeding among mothers of very low birth weight infants. *Pediatrics* 2003; 111(6 Pt 1):1337–1342.

81. Rao, M. R., et al. Effect of breastfeeding on cognitive development of infants born small for gestational age. *Acta Paediatr* 2002; 91(3):267–274.

82. Ors, R., et al. Comparison of sucrose and human milk on pain response in newborns. Eur *J Pediatr* 1999; 158(1):63–66.

83. Shah, P. S., et al. Breastfeeding or breast milk for procedural pain in neonates. *Cochrane Database Syst Rev* 2006; 3:CD004950.

84. Bartick, M., et al. The burden of suboptimal breastfeeding in the United States: a pediatric cost analysis. *Pediatrics* 2010; 125(5):e1048–1056.

85. Ma, P., et al. A case study on the economic impact of optimal breastfeeding. *Matern Child Health J* 2013; 17(1):9–13.

86. Tuttle, C. R., et al. Establishing the business case for breastfeeding. *Breastfeed Med* 2009. 4 Suppl 1:S59–62.

87. Institute of Medicine, Nutrition During Lactation. Washington, DC: National Academy Press, 1991, 303.

88. Dewey, K. G., et al. Infant self-regulation of breast milk intake. *Acta Paediatr Scand* 1986; 75(6):893–898.

89. Daly, S. E. J., et al. Infant demand and milk supply. Part 2: The short-term control of milk synthesis in lactating women. *J Hum Lactation* 1995; 11:27–37.

90. Daly, S. E., et al. Infant demand and milk supply. Part 1: Infant demand and milk production in lactating women. *J Hum Lact* 1995; 11(1):21–6.

91. Daly, S. E., et al. The short-term synthesis and infant-regulated removal of milk in lactating women. *Exp Physiol* 1993; 78(2):209–20.

92. Saint, L., et al. Yield and nutrient content of milk in eight women breastfeeding twins and one woman breastfeeding triplets. *Br J Nutr* 1986; 56:49–58.

93. Hill, P. D., et al. Breastfeeding experience and milk weight in lactating mothers pumping for preterm infants. *Birth* 1999; 26(4).

94. Niefert, M., et al. Practical aspects of breastfeeding the premature infant. *Perinatol Neonatol* 1988; 12:24.

95. Souto, G. C., et al. The impact of breast reduction surgery on breastfeeding performance. *J Hum Lact* 2003; 19(1):43–9; quiz 66–9 120.

96. Hurst, N., Breastfeeding after breast augmentation. *J Hum Lact* 2003; 19(1):70–71.

97. Brown, S. L., et al. Breast implant surveillance reports to the U. S. Food and Drug Administration: maternal-child health problems. *J Long Term Eff Med Implants* 2006. 16(4):281–290.

98. Semple, J. L., et al. Breast milk contamination and silicone implants: preliminary results using silicon as a proxy measurement for silicone. *Plast Reconstr Surg* 1998; 102(2):528–533.

99. Morland-Schultz, K., et al. Prevention of and therapies for nipple pain: a systematic review. *J Obstet Gynecol Neonatal Nurs* 2005; 34(4):428–437.

100. Wooldrige, M. S., et al. Colic, "overfeeding" and symptoms of lactose malabsorption in the breast-fed baby. *Lancet* 1988; 2:382–384.

101. Butte, N. F., et al. Feeding patterns of exclusively breast-fed infants during the first four months of life. *Early Hum Dev* 1985; 12(3):291–300.

102. Brams, M., et al. "Nursing bottle caries" in breast-fed children. *J Pediatr* 1983; 103:415–416.

103. Palmer, B., The influence of breastfeeding on the development of the oral cavity: a commentary. *J Hum Lact* 1998; 14(2):93–98.

104. American Academy of Pediatrics, Controversies concerning vitamin K and the newborn. American Academy of Pediatrics Committee on Fetus and Newborn. *Pediatrics* 2003; 112(1 Pt 1):191–192.

105. Ross, A. C., et al. The 2011 Dietary Reference Intakes for Calcium and Vitamin D: what dietetics practitioners need to know. *J Am Diet Assoc* 2011. 111(4):524–527.

106. Wagner, C. L., et al. Prevention of rickets and vitamin D deficiency in infants, children, and adolescents. *Pediatrics* 2008; 122(5):1142–1152.

107. Institute of Medicine Food and Nutrition Board, Dietary Reference Intakes for Calcium and Vitamin D. Washington, DC: National Academy Press.

108. United States Department of Agriculture. Human Nutrition Information Service. Dietary Guidelines Advisory Committee., et al. Report of the Dietary Guidelines Advisory Committee on the dietary guidelines for Americans 2010: To the Secretary of Agriculture and the Secretary of Health and Human Services. Washington, DC: United States Dept. of Agriculture: United States Dept. of Health and Human Services, 2010, vi, 445.

109. Institute of Medicine Food and Nutrition Board, Dietary Reference Intakes for Energy, Carbohydrate, Fiber, Fat, Fatty Acids, Cholesterol, Protein, and Amino Acids (Macronutrients). Washington, DC: National Acadmies Press, 2002.

110. Institute of Medicine. Dietary reference intakes for energy, carbohydrate, fiber, fat, fatty acids, cholesterol, protein, and amino acids. Washington, DC: National Academies Press, 2005, xxv 1331.

111. Goldberg, G. R., et al. Longitudinal assessment of energy expenditure in pregnancy by the doubly labeled water method. *Am J Clin Nutr* 1993; 57:494–505.

112. Roberts, S., et al. Lactational performance in relation to energy intake in the baboon. Am J Clin Nutr 1985; 41:1270–76.

113. Endres, L. K., et al. Postpartum weight retention risk factors and relationship to obesity at 1 year. *Obstet Gynecol* 2015; 125(1):144–152.

114. Neville, C. E., et al. The effectiveness of weight management interventions in breastfeeding women—a systematic review and critical evaluation. *Birth* 2014. 41(3):223–236.

115. Strode, M. A., et al. Effects of short-term caloric restriction on lactational performance of well-nourished women. *Acta Paediatr Scand* 1986; 75(2):222–9.

116. Dusdieker, L. B., et al. Is milk production impaired by dieting during lactation? *Am J Clin Nutr* 1994; 59(4):833–840.

117. Lovelady, C. A., et al. The effects of dieting on food and nutrient intake of lactating women. *J Am Diet Assoc* 2006; 106(6):908–12.

118. Mohammad, M. A., et al. Effect of dietary macronutrient composition under moderate hypocaloric intake on maternal adaptation during lactation. *Am J Clin Nutr* 2009; 89(6):1821–1827.

119. Lovelady, C. A., et al. Lactation performance of exercising women. *Am J Clin Nutr* 1990; 52(1):103–109.

120. Intsitute of Medicine, Dietary Reference Intakes for Water, Potassium, Sodium, Chloride, and Sulfate, I. o. Medicine, Editor. Washington, DC: National Academies Press, 2005.

121. Lust, K. D., et al. Maternal intake of cruciferous vegetables and other foods and colic symptoms in exclusively breast-fed infants. *J Am Diet Assoc* 1996; 96(1):46–48.

122. Hill, D. J., et al. A low allergen diet is a significant intervention in infantile colic: results of a community-based study. *J Allergy Clin Immunol* 1995; 96(6 Pt 1):886–892.

123. Partty, A., et al. Gut microbiota and infant distress—The association between compositional development of the gut microbiota and fussing and crying in early infancy. *Microb Ecol Health Dis* 2012; 23.

124. Sung, V., et al. Probiotics to prevent or treat excessive infant crying: systematic review and meta-analysis. *JAMA Pediatr* 2013; 167(12):1150–1157.

125. Ziegler, E. E., et al. Cow milk feeding in infancy: Further observations on blood loss from the gastrointestinal tract. *J Pediatr* 1990; 116:11–18.

126. Institute of Medicine. Committee on Leading Health Indicators for Healthy People 2020., Leading health indicators for healthy people 2020: Letter report. Washington, DC: National Academies Press, 2011, xiii, 84.

127. Centers for Disease Control. Breastfeeding Among U. S. Children Born 2001–2011, CDC National Immunization Survey. 2014.

128. National Center for Health Statistics. National Immunization Survey 2011 Births. NCHS CD-ROM number 8 2002; 1 CD-ROM.

129. U. S. Department of Health and Human Services, HHS Blueprint for Action on Breastfeeding. Washington, DC: U. S. Department of Health and Human Services, Office on Women's Health, 2000.

130. Bryant, C., et al. Best Start's Three Step Counseling Strategy. 1997, Tampa, FL: Best Start, Inc.

131. Dyson, L., et al. Interventions for promoting the initiation of breastfeeding. *Cochrane Database Syst Rev* 2005; (2):CD001688.

132. McCamman, S., et al. Breastfeeding success: You can make the difference. *Perinatal Nutr Report* 1998; 4(Winter):2–4.

133. Bentley, M. E., et al. Sources of influence on intention to breastfeed among African-American women at entry to WIC. *J Hum Lact* 1999; 15(1):27–34.

134. Barron, S. P., et al. Factors influencing duration of breast feeding among low-income women. *J Am Diet Assoc* 1988; 88(12):1557–1561.

135. Renfrew, M. J., et al. Support for healthy breastfeeding mothers with healthy term babies. *Cochrane Database Syst Rev* 2012; 5:CD001141.

136. Baxter, R. J. Kaiser Permanente's commitment to breastfeeding. *Breastfeed Med* 2014. 9(7):345–346.

137. Pisacane, A., et al. A controlled trial of the father's role in breastfeeding promotion. *Pediatrics* 2005; 116(4):e494–498.

138. Asiodu, I. V., et al. Breastfeeding and use of social media among first-time African american mothers. *J Obstet Gynecol Neonatal Nurs* 2015; 44(2):268–278.

139. Perez-Escamilla, R., et al. Infant feeding policies in maternity wards and their effect on breast- feeding success: an analytical overview. *Am J Public Health* 1994; 84(1):89–97.

140. World Health Organization, Protecting, promoting, and supporting breastfeeding. The special role of maternity services (a joint WHO/UNICEF statement). 1989, WHO/ UNICEF: Geneva, Switzerland.

141. Merten, S., et al. Do baby-friendly hospitals influence breastfeeding duration on a national level? *Pediatrics* 2005; 116(5):e702–708.

142. Shealy, K. R., et al. The CDC Guide to Breastfeeding Intervention. Atlanta: U.S. Department of Health and Human Services, Centers for Disease Control and Prevention, 2005.

143. Petrova, A., et al. Effectiveness of Exclusive Breastfeeding Promotion in Low-Income Mothers: A Randomized Controlled Study. *Breastfeed Med* 2009.

144. Bryant, C., et al. A strategy for promoting breastfeeding among economically disadvantaged women and adolescents. NAACOG's *Clin Issu Perinat Women's Health Nurs* 1992; 3(4):723–730.

145. Guendelman, S., et al. Juggling work and breastfeeding: effects of maternity leave and occupational characteristics. *Pediatrics* 2009; 123(1):e38–46.

146. Mirkovic, K. R., et al. Maternity leave duration and full-time/part-time work status are associated with US mothers' ability to meet breastfeeding intentions. *J Hum Lact* 2014; 30(4):416–419.

147. Meehan, K., et al. The association between an electric pump loan program and the timing of requests for formula by working mothers in WIC. *J Hum Lact* 2008; 24(2):150–158.

148. Splett, P. L., et al. The economic benefits of breastfeeding an infant in the WIC program twelve month follow-up study. Washington, DC: Food and Consumer Service, US Department of Agriculture, 1998.

149. Ortiz, J., et al. Duration of breast milk expression among working mothers enrolled in an employer-sponsored lactation program. *Pediatr Nurs* 2004; 30(2):111–119.

150. Healthy Mothers Healthy Babies Coalition, Workplace Models of Excellence 2000: Outstanding programs supporting working women that breastfeed. 2000, Alexandria, VA: National Healthy Mothers, Healthy Babies coalition.

151. Rinker, B., et al. The effect of breastfeeding on breast aesthetics. *Aesthet Surg J* 2008; 28(5):534–7.

152. Lewin, S. A., et al. Lay health workers in primary and community health care. *Cochrane Database Syst Rev* 2005; (1):CD004015.

153. Khoury, A. Social Marketing Institute Success Stories: National WIC breastfeeding promotion project. http://www.social-marketing.org/success/cs-nationalwic.html. 2001, Mississippi WIC Program.

154. Stremler, J., et al. Insight from a breastfeeding peer support pilot program for husbands and fathers of Texas WIC participants. *J Hum Lact* 2004; 20(4):417–422.

155. Cricco-Lizza, R. The milk of human kindness: environmental and human interactions in a WIC clinic that influence infant-feeding decisions of Black women. *Qual Health Res* 2005; 15(4):525–538.

156. Ahluwalia, I. B., et al. Why do women stop breastfeeding? Findings from the Pregnancy Risk Assessment and Monitoring System. *Pediatrics* 2005; 116(6):1408–1412.

## Chapter 7

1. From the association: Position of the American Dietetic Association: Promotion and Supporting Breastfeeding *J Am Diet Assoc* 2009; 109:1926–1942.

2. Buck, M. L., Amir, L. H., Cullinane, M., and Donath. S. M. Nipple Pain, Damage, and Vasospasm in the First 8 Weeks Postpartum. *Breastfeed Med.* 2014; 9(2):56–62.

3. Mass, S. Breast pain: engorgement, nipple pain and mastitis. *Clin Obstet Gynecol* 2004; 47:676–682.

4. Inch, S. Breastfeeding problems: prevention and management. *Community Pract* 2006; 79:165–167.

5. Smith, J. W., and Tully, M. R. Midwifery management of breastfeeding: using the evidence. *J Midwifery Womens Health* 2001; 46:423–438.

6. Martin, C., and Krebs, N. F. *The nursing mother's problem solver.* New York: Simon and Schuster, 2000.

7. Walker, M. Conquering Common Breast-feeding Problems. J *Perinat Neonat Nurs* 2008; (22)267–274.

8. Kvist, L.J. Re-examination of old truths: Replication of a study to measure the incidence of lactational mastitis in breastfeeding women. *International Breastfeeding J* 2013; 8:2.

9. Mangesi, L., and Dowswell, T. Treatments for breast engorgement during lactation. *Cochrane Database Syst Rev* 2014 (9); doi:10.1002/14651858.CD006946.pub2.

10. Academy of Breastfeeding Medicine. Clinical Protocol 20: Engorgement. *Breastfeed Med* 2009; 4(2):111–113.

11. Walker, M. *Breastfeeding Management for the Clinician: Using the Evidence.* MA: Jones and Bartlett Publishers, 2nd Ed. 2011; 550–551.

12. Amir, L. H., and the Academy of Breastfeeding Medicine. Clinical Protocol #4: Mastitis. *Breastfeed Med* 2014; 9(5):239–243.

13. Lau, C. The Effects of Stress on Lactation. *Pediatr Clin North Am* 2001; (48):1; 221–234.

14. Matheson, I., et al. Bacteriological findings and clinical symptoms in relation to clinical outcome in puerperal mastitis. *Acta Obstet Gynecol Scand* 1988; 67:723–726.

15. Academy of Breastfeeding Medicine: Clinical Protocol #9: Use of Galactogogues in Initiating or Augmenting Maternal Milk Secretion, *Breastfeed Med* 2011; (6):1,41–49.

16. Hale, T. W., and Hartmann, P. E. Hale & *Hartmann's Textbook of Human Lactation,* 1st ed. Hale Publishing, 2007: 479.

17. USLCA Press Release: Orphan drug designation obtained for Domerpidone in the US. Available at breastfeeding.org, accessed 8/12.

18. Lawrence, R. A., and Lawrence, R. M. *Breastfeeding: a guide for the medical profession,* 7th ed. St Louis: Mosby, Inc., 2011.

19. Hale, T. W. *Medications and Mother's Milk,* 16th ed. Amarillo, TX: Pharmasoft Medical Publishing, 2014.

20. Lagoy, C. T., et al. Medication use during pregnancy and lactation: An urgent call for public health action. *J Womens Health* 2005; 14:104–109.

21. Berlin, C. M., and Briggs, G. G. Drugs and chemicals in human milk. *Semin Fetal Neonatal Med* 2005; 10:149–159.

22. Begg, E. J., et al. Studying drugs in human milk: Time to unify the approach. *J Hum Lact* 2002; 18:323–332.

23. Amir, L. H., Rirotta, M. V., and Raval, M. Breastfeeding—Evidence-based guidelines for the use of medicines. Aust Fam Physician 2011; 40(9):684–690.

24. Sachs, H. C., and the AAP Committee on Drugs. Clinical Report: The Transfer of Drugs and Therapeutics Into Human Milk: An Update on Selected Topics. Pediatrics 2013; 132:e796-e809.

25. Committee on Nutrition, American Academy of Pediatrics. *Pediatric Nutrition Handbook*, 1st ed. Elk Grove Village, IL: American Academy of Pediatrics, 2004.

26. Chung, A. M., Reed, M. D., and Blumer, J. L. Antibiotics and breast-feeding: A critical review of the literature. *Paediatr Drugs* 2002; 4:817–837.

27. Guthmann, R. A., Bang, J., and Nashelsky, J. Combined oral contraceptives for mothers who are breastfeeding. *Am Fam Physician* 2005; 72:1303–1304.

28. Diaz, S. Contraceptive implants and lactation. *Contraception* 2002; 65:39–46.

29. Nice, F. J., Snyder, J. L., and Kotansky, B. C. Breastfeeding and over-the-counter medications. *J Hum Lact* 2000; 16:319–31.

30. Department of Child and Adolescent Health. Breastfeeding and Maternal Medication: Recommendations for Drugs in the Eleventh WHO Model List of Essential Drugs, 2003. UNICEF World Health Organization, 2003.

31. The complete German Commission E monographs: *Therapeutic guide to herbal medicines*. Boston: Integrative Medicine Communications, 1998.

32. Hardy, M. L. Herbs of special interest to women. *J Am Pharm Assoc* (Wash.) 2000; 40:234–242.

33. Scott, C. R., and Jacobson, H. A. Selection of international nutritional & herbal remedies for breastfeeding concerns. *Midwifery Today* 2005; 38–39.

34. Mortel, M., and Mehta, S. D. Systematic Review of the Efficacy of Herbal Galactogogues. *J Hum Lact* 2013; 29(2): 154–162.

35. Humphrey, S. L., and McKenna, D. J. Herbs and breastfeeding. *Breastfeeding Abstracts* 1997; 17:11–12.

36. Conover, E., and Buehler, B. A. Use of herbal agents by breastfeeding women may affect infants. *Pediatr Ann* 2004; 33:235–240.

37. Woolf, A. D. Herbal remedies and children: do they work? Are they harmful? *Pediatrics* 2003; 112:240–246.

38. Humphrey, S. Sage advice on herbs and breastfeeding. *LEAVEN* 1998; 34:43–47.

39. Leung, A., and Foster, S. *Encyclopedia of common natural ingredients used in* foods, drugs, and cosmetics. New York: John Wiley & Sons, 1996.

40. Cunningham, E. and Hansen, K. Question of the month: Where can I get information on evaluating herbal supplements? *J Am Diet Assoc* 1999; 99:1240.

41. The American Botanical Council. The ABC Clinical Guide to Herbs. American Botanical Council, 2005.

42. Cartwright, M. M. Herbal use during pregnancy and lactation: A need for caution. American Dietetic Association Public Health/Community Nutrition Practice Group. *The Digest (Summer)* 2001; 1–3.

43. Klier, C. M., et al. St. John's wort (*Hypericum perforatum*) and breastfeeding: Plasma and breast milk concentrations of hyperforin for 5 mothers and 2 infants. *J Clin Psychiatry* 2006; 67(2):305–309.

44. Lee, A., et al. The safety of St. John's wort (*Hypericum perforatum*) during breastfeeding. *J Clin Psychiatry* 2003; 64(8):966–968.

45. Gabay, M. P. Galactogogues: Medications that induce lactation. *J Hum Lact* 2002; 18:274–279.

46. Betzold, C. M. Galactagogues. *J Midwifery Womens Health* 2004; 49:151–154.

47. American Academy of Pediatrics Policy Statement: Breastfeeding and the use of Human Milk. *Pediatrics* 2012; 129:e827–841.

48. Haastrup, M. B., Potteg, A., and Damkier, P. Alcohol and Breastfeeding. Basic & Clinical Pharmacology & Toxicology 2014; 114:168–173.

49. Giglia, R., and Binns, C. Alcohol and lactation: A systematic review. *Nutrition and Dietetics* 2006; 63:103.

50. Ho, E., et al. Alcohol and breast-feeding: Calculation of time to zero level in milk. *Biol Neonate* 2001; 80:219–222.

51. Mennella, J. A., Pepino, M. Y., and Teff, K. L. Acute alcohol consumption disrupts the hormonal milieu of lactating women. *J Clin Endocrinol Metab* 2005; 90:1979–1985.

52. Mennella, J. A. Regulation of milk intake after exposure to alcohol in mothers' milk. *Alcohol Clin Exp Res* 2001; 25:590–593.

53. Mennella, J. A., and Gerrish, C. J. Effects of exposure to alcohol in mother's milk on infant sleep. *Pediatrics* 1998; 101:E2.

54. Mennella, J. A., and Garcia Comez, P. L. Sleep disturbances after acute exposure to alcohol in mother's milk. *Alcohol Int Biomed J* 2001; 25:153–158.

55. Gunzerath, L., et al. National Institute on Alcohol Abuse and Alcoholism report on moderate drinking. *Alcohol Clin Exp Res* 2004; 28:829–847.

56. Little, R. E., et al. Maternal alcohol use during breast-feeding and infant mental and motor development at one year. *N Engl J Med* 1989; 321:425–430.

57. Mohrbacher, N., and Stock, J. *The Breastfeeding Answer Book*. Schaumburg, IL: La Leche League International, 2003.

58. Subcommittee on Nutrition During Lactation, Committee on Nutritional Status During Pregnancy and Lactation. *Food and Nutrition Board Institute of Medicine National Academy of Sciences. Nutrition During Lactation: Summary, Conclusions, and Recommendations*. Washington, DC: National Academy Press, 1991.

59. Howard, C. R., and Lawrence, R. A. Xenobiotics and breastfeeding. *Pediatr Clin North Am* 2001; 48:485–504.

60. Dempsey, D. A., and Benowitz, N. L. Risks and benefits of nicotine to aid smoking cessation in pregnancy. *Drug Saf* 2001; 24:277–322.

61. Amir, L. H., and Donath, S. M. Does maternal smoking have a negative physiological effect on breastfeeding? The epidemiological evidence. *Birth* 2002; 29:112–123.

62. Ilett, K. F., et al. Use of nicotine patches in breast-feeding mothers: Transfer of nicotine and cotinine into human milk. *Clin Pharmacol Ther* 2003; 74:516–524.

63. Chapman, D. J. Short-term Effects of Smoking on Breastfed Infants. *J Hum Lact* 2008; (24):1, 92–93.

64. Dahlstrom, A., et al. Nicotine and cotinine concentrations in the nursing mother and her infant. *Acta Paediatr Scand* 1990; 79:142–147.

65. Gaffney, K. F. Postpartum smoking relapse and becoming a mother. *J Nurs Scholarsh* 2006; 38:26–30.

66. Nickerson, K. Environmental contaminants in breast milk. *J Midwifery Womens Health* 2006; 51:26–34.

67. Baeza-Lova, S., Viswanath, H., Carter, A., Molfese, D. L., Velasquez, K. M., Baldwin, P. R., Thompson-Lake, D.,G., Y., Sharp, C., Fowler, J. C., De La Garza, R., and Salas, R. Perceptions about e-cigarette safety may lead to e-smoking during pregnancy. *Bull Menninger Clin.* 2014 Summer; 78(3):243–252.

68. Fernandez-Ruiz, J., et al. Cannabinoids and gene expression during brain development. *Neurotox Res* 2004; 6:389–401.

69. Hill. M., and Reed, K. Pregnancy, breastfeeding, and marijuana: a review article. *Obstet Gynecol Surv.* 2013 Oct; 68(10):710–718. doi: 10.1097/01.ogx.0000435371.51584.d1.

70. Norman, R. J., and Nisenblat, V. The effects of caffeine on reproductive outcomes in women. UpToDate. Updated Feb 23, 2015, accessed April, 6, 2015.

71. Rivera-Calimlim, L. The significance of drugs in breast milk. Pharmacokinetic considerations. *Clin Perinatol* 1987; 14:51–70.

72. World Health Organization. Safe food: Crucial for child development. Available at www.who.int/ceh/publications/en/poster15new.pdf, accessed 10/06.

73. Massart, F., et al. Human breast milk and xenoestrogen exposure: A possible impact on human health. *J Perinatol* 2005; 25:282–288.

74. Condon, M. Breast is best, but it could be better: What is in breast milk that should not be? *Pediatr Nurs* 2005; 31:333–338.

75. Wang, R. Y., et al. Human milk research for answering questions about human health. *J Toxicol Environ Health* 2005; 68:1771–1801.

76. Haddad, S., Ayotte, P., and Verner, M. A. D. Derivation of exposure factors for infant lactational exposure to persistent organic pollutants (POPs). *Regulatory Toxicology and Pharmacology* 2015; 71:135–140.

77. Schreiber, J. S. Parents worried about breast milk contamination. What is best for baby? *Pediatr Clin North Amer* 2001 Oct; 48(5):11113–11127, viii.

78. Centers for Disease and Control and Prevention. Breastfeeding: Exposure to Environmental Toxins. Updated April 2010. Accessed from http://www.cdc.gov/breastfeeding/disease/environmental_toxins.htm.

79. World Health Organization. Report of the WHO working group on the assessment of health risks for human infants from exposure to PCDDs, PCDFs, PCBs. *Chemosphere* 1998; 57:1627–1643.

80. Pronczuk, J., et al. Global perspectives in breast milk contamination: Infectious and toxic hazards. *Environ Health Perspect* 2002; 110:A349–A351.

81. American Academy of Pediatrics Subcommittee on Hyperbilirubinemia. Management of hyperbilirubinemia in the newborn infant 35 or more weeks of gestation. *Pediatrics* 2004; 114:297–316.

82. Academy of Breastfeeding Medicine: Clinical Protocol #22: Guidelines for Management of Jaundice in the Breastfeeding Infant Equal to or Greater Than 35 weeks' Gestation. *Breastfeeding Med* 2010; (5):2:87–93.

83. Cohen, S. M. Jaundice in the full-term newborn *Pediatr Nurs* 2006; 32:202–208.

84. Stokowski, L. A. Early recognition of neonatal jaundice and kernicterus. *Adv Neonatal Care* 2002; 2:101–114.

85. Watchko, J. F. Vigintiphobia revisited. *Pediatrics* 2005; 115:1747–1753.

86. Bhutani, V. K., and Johnson, L. Kernicterus in the 21st Century: Frequently asked questions. *J Perinatol* 2009; 29:S20–24.

87. Seagraves, K., Brulte, A., McNeely, K., and Pritham, U. Nursing for Women's Health 2013; 17(6):498–508.

88. Joint Commission on Accreditation of Healthcare Organizations. Kernicterus threatens healthy newborns. *Sentinel Event Alert* April 2001, Issue 18. Joint Commission on Accreditation of Healthcare Organizations, 2001.

89. Stark, A. R. and Lannon, C. M. System changes to prevent severe hyperbilirubinemia and promote breastfeeding: pilot approaches. *J Perinatol* 2009; 29:S.53–57.

90. Gartner, L. M., and Herschel, M. Jaundice and breastfeeding. *Pediatr Clin North Am* 2001; 48:389–399.

91. Reiser, D. J. Neonatal jaundice: physiologic variation or pathologic process. *Crit Care Nurs Clin North Am* 2004; 16:257–269.

92. Moerschel, S. K., Clanciaruso, L. B., and Tracy, L. R. A Practical Approach to Neonatal Jaundice. *Amer Fam Phys* 2008; (77):9.

93. Reiser, D. J. Hyperbilirubinemia. AWHONN. *Lifelines* 2001; 5:55–61.

94. AAP Subcommittee on Neonatal Pediatrics: Neonatal jaundice and kernicterus. *Pediatrics* 2001; 108:763–765.

95. Gartner, L. M. Breastfeeding and jaundice. *J Perinatol* 2001; 21(Suppl.)1:S25–S29.

96. Gourley, G. R. Breast-feeding, neonatal jaundice and kernicterus. *Semin Neonatol* 2002; 7:135–141.

97. Willis, S. K., Hannon, P. R., and Scrimshaw, S. C. The impact of the maternal experience with a jaundiced newborn on the breastfeeding relationship. *J Fam Pract* 2002; 51:465.

98. Geraghty, S. R., et al. Breast milk feeding rates of mothers of multiples compared to mothers of singletons. *Ambul Pediatr* 2004; 4:226–231.

99. Flidel-Rimon, O., and Shinwell, E. S. Breast-feeding multiples. *Semin Neonatol* 2002; 7:231–239.

100. Gromada, K. K., and Spangler, A. K. Breastfeeding twins and higher-order multiples. *J Obstet Gynecol Neonatal Nurs* 1998; 27:441–449.

101. Gromada, K. K. Breastfeeding more than one: Multiples and tandem breastfeeding. NAACOGS. *Clin Issu Perinat Womens Health Nurs* 1992; 3:656–666.

102. Auer, C., and Gromada, K. K. A case report of breastfeeding quadruplets: Factors perceived as affecting breastfeeding. *J Hum Lact* 1998; 14:135–141.

103. Palmer, G. *The Politics of Breastfeeding*, 2nd ed. London: Pandora Press/Harper Collins, 1993: 32.

104. Saint, L., Maggiore, P., and Hartmann, P. E. Yield and nutrient content of milk in eight women breast-feeding twins and one woman breast-feeding triplets. *Br J Nutr* 1986; 56:49–58.

105. Hattori, R., and Hattori, H. Breastfeeding twins: guidelines for success. *Birth* 1999; 26:37–42.

106. Geraghty, S. R., Khoury, J. C., and Kalkwarf, H. J. Comparison of feeding among multiple-birth infants. *Twin Res* 2004; 7:542–547.

107. Zeiger, R. S., and Friedman, N. J. The relationship of breastfeeding to the development of atopic disorders. *Nestle Nutr Workshop Ser Pediatr Program* 2006; 57:93–105.

108. O'Connell, E. J. Pediatric allergy: A brief review of risk factors associated with developing allergic disease in childhood. *Ann Allergy Asthma Immunol* 2003; 90:53–58.

109. Greer, F. R., Sicherer, S. H., Burks, A. W., and the Committee on Nutrition and Section on Allergy and Immunology. Effects of Early Nutritional Interventions on the Development of Atopic Disease in Infants and Children: The Role of Maternal Dietary Restriction, Breastfeeding, Timing of Introduction of Complementary Foods, and Hydrolyzed Formulas. AAP Clinical Report. *Pediatrics* 2008; (121)1:183–191.

110. Burks, et al. NIAID-Sponsored 2010 Guidelines for Managing Food Allergy: Applications in the Pediatric Population. *Pediatrics* 2011; 128:(5):955–965.

111. Guidelines for the diagnosis and management of food allergy in the United States: Report of the NIAID sponsored expert panel. *J Allergy & Clin Immunol* 2010; 126:(6):S1–S58.

112. Hill, D. J., et al. Effect of a low-allergen maternal diet on colic among breastfed infants: A randomized, controlled trial. *Pediatrics* 2005; 116:e709–e715.

113. Mennella, J. A., and Beauchamp, G. K. The effects of repeated exposure to garlic-flavored milk on the nursling's behavior. *Pediatr Res* 1993; 34:805–808.

114. Mennella, J. A., and Beauchamp, G. K. Maternal diet alters the sensory qualities of human milk and the nursling's behavior. *Pediatrics* 1991; 88:737–744.

115. Cooper, R. L., and Cooper, M. M. Red pepper-induced dermatitis in breast-fed infants. *Dermatology* 1996; 193:61–62.

116. Zeretzke, K. Allergies and the breastfeeding family. *New Beginnings* 1998; 15(4):100.

117. Davidoff, M. J., et al. Changes in the gestational age distribution among U.S. singleton births: Impact on rages of late preterm birth, 1992–2002. *Semin Perinatol* 2006; 30(1):8–15.

118. Meier, P., Patel, A. L., Wright, K., Engstrom, J. L. Management of Breastfeeding During and After the Maternity Hospitalization for Late Preterm Infants,. *Clin Perinatol.* 2013 December; 40(4): 689–705.

119. Engle, W. A., Tomashed, K. M., Wallman, C. and the Committee on Fetus and Newborn. "Late-Preterm" Infants: A Population at Risk. AAP Clinical Report. *Pediatrics* 2007; 120:(6):1390–1401.

120. Academy of Breastfeeding Medicine: Clinical Protocol #10: Breastfeeding the Late Preterm Infant. *Breastfeed Med* 2011; 6:(3):151–156.

121. Shulman, R. J., et al. Early feeding, feeding tolerance, and lactase activity in preterm infants. *J Pediatr* 1998; 133:645–649.

122. Spatz, D. L. State of the science: Use of human milk and breast-feeding for vulnerable infants. *J Perinat Neonatal Nurs* 2006; 20:51–55.

123. Callen, J., and Pinelli, J. A review of the literature examining the benefits and challenges, incidence and duration, and barriers to breastfeeding in preterm infants *Adv Neonatal Care* 2005; 5:72–88.

124. Rodriguez, N. A., Miracle, D. J., and Meier, P. P. Sharing the science on human milk feedings with mothers of very-low-birth-weight infants. *JOCNN* 2005; 34:109–119.

125. Schanler, R. J., Shulman, R. J., and Lau, C. Feeding strategies for premature infants: Beneficial outcomes of feeding fortified human milk versus preterm formula. *Pediatrics* 1999; 103:1150–1157.

126. Spatz, D. L. Ten steps for promoting and protecting breastfeeding for vulnerable infants. *J Perinat Neonatal Nurs* 2004; 18:385–396.

127. Sisk, P. M., et al. Lactation counseling for mothers of very low birth weight infants: Effect on maternal anxiety and infant intake of human milk. *Pediatrics* 2006; 117:67–75.

128. Lawrence, R. M., and Lawrence, R. A. Breast milk and infection. *Clin Perinatol* 2004; 31:501–528.

129. Lawrence, R. M., and Lawrence, R. A. Given the benefits of breastfeeding, what contraindications exist? *Pediatr Clin North Am* 2001; 48:235–251.

130. Newell, M. L. Current issues in the prevention of mother-to-child transmission of HIV-1 infection. *Trans R Soc Trop Med Hyg* 2006; 100:1–5.

131. Dorosko, S. M. Vitamin A, mastitis, and mother-to-child transmission of HIV-1 through breast-feeding: Current information and gaps in knowledge. *Nutr Rev* 2005; 63:332–346.

132. Jackson, D. J., et al. HIV and infant feeding: Issues in developed and developing countries. *J Obstet Gynecol Neonatal Nurs* 2003; 32:117–127.

133. American Academy of Pediatrics, Section on Breastfeeding. Breastfeeding and the use of human milk. *Pediatrics* 2005; 115:496–506.

134. World Health Organization. HIV and Infant Feeding: Principles and Recommendations for Infant Feeding in the Context of HIV and Summary of Evidence. Geneva, Switzerland: World Health Organization: 2010.

135. Coutsoudis, A. Breastfeeding and the HIV-positive mother: the debate continues. *Early Hum Dev* 2005; 81:87–93.

136. International Lactation Association: Position Paper on HIV and Infant Feeding, 2006. Available at www.Ilca.org, accessed 8/2012.

137. Academy of Breastfeeding Medicine. Clinical Protocol #8. Human Milk Storage Information for Home Use for Full-Term Infants. *Breastfeed Med* 2010; 5:(3):127–129.

138. Jones, F. Best Practice for Expressing, Storing and Handling Human Milk in Hospitals, Homes and Child Care Settings, 3rd ed. 2011.

139. Mohrbacher, N., and Kendall-Tackett, K. *Breastfeeding Made Simple: Seven Natural Laws for Nursing Mothers*. Oakland, CA: New Harbinger Publications, Inc., 2005.

140. Lang, S. *Breastfeeding Special Care Babies*. China: Elsevier Health, 2002.

141. Jones, F. History of North American donor milk banking: One hundred years of progress. *J Hum Lact* 2003; 19:313–318.

142. HMBANA.org. Accessed 8/2012.

143. Paxson, C. I. Survival of human milk leukocytes. *J Pediatr* 1979; 94:61–64.

144. Keim, S. A., Hogan, J. S., McNamara, K. A., Gudimetla, V., Dillon, C. E., Kwiek, J. J., and Geraghty, S. R. Microbial contamination of human milk purchased via the Internet. *Pediatrics* 2013 Nov 1; (5):e1227–e1235.

145. Prolacta. Accessed at http://www.prolacta.com/.

146. Meier, P. P., et al. The Rush Mother's Milk Club: Breastfeeding interventions for mothers with very low birth weight infants. *JOGNN* 2004; 33:164–174.

## Chapter 8

1. Ziegler, E. E. The term infant. In Duggan, C., Watkins, J. B., Walker, W. A. (eds.). *Nutrition in Pediatrics*, 4th ed. (pp. 403–410). Hamilton, ON: BC Decker Inc., 2008.

2. Zlotkin, S. Neonatal Nutrition. In Linder M. A. (ed.). *Nutritional Biochemistry and Metabolism with Clinical Applications* (pp. 349–371). New York: Elsevier Science Publishing Co., Inc., 1991.

3. Prado, E. L., Dewey K. G. Nutrition and brain development in early life. *Nutrition Reviews* 2014; 72(4):267–284.

4. American Academy of Pediatrics, American College of Obstetrics and Gynecology. Guidelines for Perinatal Care, 6th ed. Elk Grove Village, IL: American Academy of Pediatrics, 2007.

5. Chumlea, W. C., LaMonte M. Physical Growth and Maturation. In Samour P. Q., King K. (eds.). *Pediatric Nutrition* (pp. 23–34). Sudbury, MA: Jones & Bartlett Learning, 2012.

6. Healthy People 2020 Objectives. 2015, April 24; Retrieved from Healthy People 2020: http://www. healthypeople.gov/.

7. Martin, J. A., et al. Births: Final Data for 2013, National Vital Statistics Report, vol. 64, no. 1. Hyattsville, MD: U.S. Department of Health and Human Services, Centers for Disease Control and Prevention, National Center for Health Statistics, 2015.

8. MacDorman, M. F., Matthews T. J. The challenge of infant mortality: Have we reached a plateau? *Public Health Rep* 2009; 670–681.

9. MacDorman, M. F., et al. Recent Declines in Infant Mortality in the United States, 2005–2011. National Center for Health Statistics Data Brief, No 120, April 2013.

10. MacDorman, M. F., et al. International comparisons of infant mortality and related factors: United States and Europe, 2010. Hyattsville, MD: National Vital Statistics Reports, U.S. Department of Health and Human Services, Centers for Disease Control and Prevention, 2014.

11. Mathews, T. J., MacDorman M. F. Infant mortality statistics from the 2006 period linked birth/infant death data set. *Natl Vital Stat Rep* 2010; 58:17.

12. Oestergaard, M. Z., et al. Neonatal Mortality Levels for 193 Countries in 2009 with Trends Since 1990: A systematic analysis of progress, projections, and priorities. *PLoS Med* 2011; 8(8):e1001080.

13. Centers for Medicare & Medicaid Services. Children's Health Insurance Program. Retrieved from medicaid.gov, accessed 5/10/15.

14. Hagan, J. F., et al. *Bright Futures: Guidelines for Health Supervision of Infants, Children and Adolescents*, 3rd ed. Elk Grove Village, IL: American Academy of Pediatrics, 2008.

15. Holt, K., et al. *Bright Futures Nutrition*, 3rd ed. Elk Grove Village, IL: American Academy of Pediatrics, 2011.

16. Fanaroff, A. A., et al. Very low birth weight outcomes of the National Institute of Child Health and Human Development Neonatal Research Network. *Am J Obstet Gyn* 1995; 167:1499–1505.

17. Barker, D. Human growth and disease in later life. In Duggan, C., Watkins, J. B., Walker, W. A. (eds.). *Nutrition in Pediatrics*, 4th ed. (pp. 305–309). Hamilton, ON: BC Decker Inc., 2008.

18. Kail, R. V., Cavanaugh J. C. *Human Development: A Lifespan View*, 2nd ed. Belmont, CA: Wadsworth/Thomson Learning, 2000.

19. March of Dimes. Understanding the Behavior of Term Infants. 2003. http://amygilliland.com/documents/MofDInfantStateHO.pdf

20. Agostoni C., et al. Complementary feeding: A commentary by the ESPGHAN Committee on Nutrition. *J Pediatr Gastroenterol Nutr* 2008; 46(1):99–110.

21. Santrock, J. *Life-Span Development*, 7th ed. New York: McGraw Hill, 1999.

22. Nardella, M. T., Owens-Kuehner A. Feeding and Eating. In Lucas B (ed.). *Children with Special Health Care Needs: Nutrition Care Handbook* (pp. 59–87), Chicago: American Dietetic Association, 2004.

23. Shelton, T. L., et al. Principles of Child Development and Developmental Assessment. In Osborne L., et al. *Pediatrics* (pp. 41–57). St Louis: Mosby, 2005.

24. Gardner, J. M., et al. Zinc supplementation and psychosocial stimulation: Effects on the development of undernourished Jamaican children. *Am J Clin Nutr* 2005; 82:399–405.

25. Hobbie, C., et al. Parental understanding of basic infant nutrition: Misinformed feeding choices. *J Pediatr Health Care* 2000; 14:26–31.

26. American Academy of Pediatrics. Development of Gastrointestinal Function. In Kleinman, R. E., and Greer, F. R. *Pediatric Nutrition*, 7th ed. (pp. 15–40). Elk Grove Village, IL: American Academy of Pediatrics, 2014.

27. Thomas, D. W., and Greer, F. R. Clinical Report: Probiotics and prebiotics in pediatrics. *Pediatrics* 2010; 126:1217–1231.

28. Faith, M. S., and Hittner, J. B. Infant temperament and eating style predict change in standardized weight status and obesity risk at 6 years of age. *Int J Obes* 2010; 34:1515–1523.

29. Dietary Guidelines for Americans. Retrieved from www.dietaryguidelines.gov, accessed 4/25/15.

30. Institute of Medicine, Food and Nutrition Board. Dietary Reference Intakes for Energy, Carbohydrate, Fiber, Fat, Fatty Acids, Cholesterol, Protein and Amino Acids. Washington, DC: National Academies Press, 2005.

31. American Academy of Pediatrics. Protein. In Kleinman, R. E., and Greer, F. R. *Pediatric Nutrition*, 7th ed. (pp. 369–386). Elk Grove Village, IL: American Academy of Pediatrics, 2014.

32. Milner, J. A., and Allison, R. G. The role of dietary fat in child nutrition and development: Summary of an ASNS workshop. *J Nutr* 1999; 129: 2094–2105.

33. Krohn, K., et al. Macronutrient Requirements for Growth: Fats and Fatty Acids. In Duggan C., Watkins, J. B., Walker, W. A. (eds). *Nutrition in Pediatrics*, 4th ed. (pp. 59–65). Hamilton, ON: BC Decker Inc., 2008.

34. Lawrence, R. A., Lawrence, R. M. *Breastfeeding: A Guide for the Medical Profession*, 7th ed. Maryland Heights, MO: Elsevier Mosby, 2011.

35. American Academy of Pediatrics. *Fats and Fatty Acids.* In Kleinman, R. E., and Greer, F. R. (eds). *Pediatric Nutrition, 7th ed.* (pp. 407–434). Elk Grove Village, IL: American Academy of Pediatrics, 2014.

36. American Academy of Pediatrics. Nutrition and oral health. In Kleinman, R. E., and Greer, F. R. *Pediatric Nutrition,* 7th ed. (pp. 1167–1183). Elk Grove Village, IL: American Academy of Pediatrics, 2014.

37. Esala, S., et al. Effect of fluorine intake on breast milk fluorine content. *Br J Nutr* 1982; 48:201–204.

38. American Academy of Pediatric Dentistry. Guidelines on fluoride therapy, updated 2014. www.aapd.org/media/Policies?Guidelines /G_FluorideTherapy.pdf, accessed 10/22/15.

39. 2012 Water Fluoridation Statistics. 2015, April 25; Retrieved from Centers for Disease Control and Prevention. www.cdc.gov// fluoridation/statistics/2012stats.htm.

40. Institute of Medicine, Food and Nutrition Board. *Dietary Reference Intakes for Calcium, Phosphorus, Magnesium, Vitamin D, and Fluoride.* Washington, DC: National Academies Press, 1997.

41. Kupka, R., et al. Vitamins. In Duggan, C., Watkins, J. B., and Walker, W. A. (eds.). *Nutrition in Pediatrics* (pp. 99–114). Hamilton, ON: BC Decker Inc., 2008.

42. Hollis, B. W., et al. Vitamin D and its metabolites in human and bovine milk. *J Nutr* 1981; 111:1240–1248.

43. Wagner, C. L., and Greer, F. R. Prevention of rickets and vitamin D deficiency in infants, children and adolescents. *Pediatrics* 2010; 126:1040–1050.

44. Institute of Medicine Food and Nutrition Board. *Dietary Reference Intakes: Water, Potassium, Sodium, Chloride and Sulfate.* Washington, DC: National Academies Press, 2004.

45. Khambalia, A. Z., and Zlotkin, S. Iron. In Duggan, C., Watkins, J. B., Walker, W. A. (eds.). *Nutrition in Pediatrics*, 4th ed. (pp. 83–98). Hamilton, ON: BC Decker Inc., 2008.

46. Lozoff, B., et al. Long-lasting neural and behavioral effects of iron deficiency in infancy. *Nutr Rev*, 2006; 64:S34–S91.

47. Rao, R., and Georgieff, M. K. Perinatal aspects of iron metabolism. *Acta Paediatr Suppl*, 2002; 91:124–129.

48. Smith, N. J., Rios, E. Iron metabolism and iron deficiency in infancy and childhood. *Adv Pediatr*, 1974; 21:239–280.

49. Baker, R., and Greer, F. R. Clinical Report: Diagnosis and prevention of iron deficiency and iron-deficiency anemia in infants and young children (0–3 years of age). *Pediatrics* 2010; 126:1040–1050.

50. Centers for Disease Control. Preventing Lead Poisoning in Young Children. Retrieved from Centers for Disease Control and Prevention, Division of Emergency and Environmental Health Services. 2005. www.cdc.gov /nceh/lead/publications/PrevLeadPoisoning.pdf.

51. Black, M. M., and Ackerman, J. P. *Neuropsychological Development.* In Duggan, C., Watkins, J. B., Walker, W. A. (eds.). *Nutrition in Pediatrics,* 4th ed. (pp. 273–282); Hamilton, ON: BC Decker Inc., 2008.

52. Wang, H., et al. Association of blood lead with calcium, iron, zinc and hemoglobin in children aged 0–7 years: a large population-based study. *Biol Trace Elem Res* 2012; 149(2):143–147.

53. Bright Futures/American Academy of Pediatrics. Recommendations for Preventive Pediatric Health Care. www.pediatriccare .solutions.aap.org.

54. WHO Multicentre Growth Reference Study Group. *WHO Child Growth Standards.* Geneva, Switzerland: World Health Organization, 2006.

55. Turck, D., et al. World Health Organization 2006 child growth standards and 2007 reference charts: A discussion paper by the committee on Nutrition of the European Society for Pediatric Gastroenterology, Hepatology, and Nutrition. *J Pediatr Gastroenterol Nutr* 2013; 57(2):258–264.

56. American Academy of Pediatrics. Policy Statement: Breastfeeding and the use of human milk. *Pediatrics* 2012; 129:e827–e841.

57. Academy of Nutrition and Dietetics. Practice paper of the Academy of Nutrition and Dietetics: Promoting and supporting breastfeeding. *J Acad Nutr Diet* 2015.

58. Brown, K. H. Complementary Feeding. In Duggan, C., Watkins, J. B., Walker, W. A. *Nutrition in Pediatrics*, 4th ed. (pp. 411–416). Hamilton, ON: BC Decker Inc., 2008.

59. Department of Health and Human Services. Current Good Manufacturing Practices, Quality Control Procedures, Quality Factors Notification Requirement, and Records and Reports for Infant Formula. Washington, DC: *Federal Register*. 2014; Vol. 79, No. 111.

60. Corkins, M. *Pediatric Nutrition Support Handbook*. Silver Springs, MD: American Society for Parenteral and Enteral Nutrition, 2011.

61. American Academy of Pediatrics. Formula Feeding of Term Infants. In Kleinman, R. E., and Greer, F. R. (eds). *Pediatric Nutrition*, 7th ed. (pp. 61–81). Elk Grove Village, IL: American Academy of Pediatrics, 2014.

62. Amorde-Spalding, K., Nieman, L. (eds.). *Pediatric Manual of Clinical Dietetics*. Chicago, IL: Academy of Nutrition and Dietetics, 2008.

63. Tervo, R. Parent's reports predict their child's developmental problems. *Clin Pediatr* 2005; 44:601–611.

64. American Academy of Pediatric Dentistry, American Academy of Pediatrics. Policy on Early Childhood Caries (EEC): Classifications, Consequences, and Preventive Strategies. Chicago: Oral Health Policies, 2014.

65. Chapin, M.M. et al. Nonfatal choking on food among children 14 years or younger in the United States, 2001–2009. *Pediatrics* 2013; 132(2):275–281.

66. American Academy of Pediatrics. Policy Statement on Prevention of Choking Among Children. *Pediatrics* 2010; 125:601–607.

67. Institute of Medicine, Food and Nutrition Board. Dietary Reference Intakes: Water, Potassium, Sodium, Chloride and Sulfate. Washington, DC: National Academies Press, 2004.

68. Faith, M.S., Hittner, J.B. Infant temperament and eating style predict change in standardized weight status and obesity risk at 6 years of age. Int J Obes 2010; 34(10):1515–1523.

69. Ventura, A. K., and Worobey, J. Early influences on the development of food preferences. Curr Biol 2013; 23(9):R401–408.

70. Menella, J. A., Beachamp, G. Maternal diet alters the sensory qualities of human milk and the nursling' behavior. *Pediatrics* 1991; 88:737–744.

71. Birch, L. L., Fisher, J.O. Development of eating behaviors among children and adolescents. *Pediatrics* 1998; 101:539–549.

72. Llewellyn, C. H., et al. Nature and nurture in infant appetite: Analysis of the Gemini twin birth cohort. *Am J Clin Nutr* 2010; 91(5):1172–1179.

73. Zero to Three. www.zerotothree.org, accessed 4/20/15.

74. U.S. Department of Health and Human Services National Heart, Lung and Blood Institute. Expert Panel on Integrated Guidelines for Cardiovascular Health and Risk Reduction in Children and Adolescents: Summary Report, 2011. Retrieved from U.S. Department of Health and Human Services, National Heart, Lung and Blood Institute: www.nhlbi.nih.gov.

75. American Academy of Pediatrics. Policy Statement: Media use by children younger than 2 years. *Pediatrics* 2011; 128:1040–1045.

76. American Academy of Pediatrics. Policy Statement: Infant exercise programs. *Pediatrics* 1998; 82:800.

77. Krebs, N. F., et al. Meat as a first complementary food for breastfed infants: Feasibility and impact on zinc intake and status. *J Pediatr Gastroenterol Nutr* 2006; 42(2):207–214.

78. Mangels, A. R., and Messina, V. Considerations in planning vegan diets: Infants. *J Am Diet Assoc* 2001; 101:670–677.

79. Academy of Nutrition and Dietetics. Position of the American Dietetic Association:

Vegetarian diets. *J Am Diet Assoc* 2009; 109:1266–1282.

80. Donaldson, M. Metabolic vitamin $B_{12}$ status on a mostly raw vegan diet with follow-up using tablets, nutritional yeast, or probiotic supplements. *Ann Nutr Metab* 2000; 44:229–234.

81. Cohen-Silver J, Ratnapalan S. Management of infantile colic: A review. *Clinical Pediatr* 2009; 48(1):14–17.

82. Hill, D. J., and Hosking, C. S. Infantile colic and food hypersensitivity. *J Pediatr Gastroenterol Nutr* 2000; 30(1):S67–76.

83. Metcalf, T. J., et al. Simethicone in the treatment of infant colic. *Pediatrics* 1994; 94:29–34.

84. Savino F., et al. Lactobacillus reuteri versus simethicone in the treatment of infantile colic: a prospective randomized study. *Pediatrics* 2007; 119(1):124–130.

85. Hill, D. J., et al. Effect of a low-allergen maternal diet on colic among breastfed infants: A randomized controlled trial. *Pediatrics* 2005; 116:e709–715.

86. Centers for Disease Control and Prevention. The management of acute diarrhea in children: oral rehydration, maintenance, and nutritional therapy. *MMWR* 1992; 41(RR-16).

87. Burpee, T., and Duggan, C. Diarrheal Diseases. In Duggan, C., Watkins, J. B., Walker W. A. (eds). *Nutrition in Pediatrics*, 4th ed. (pp. 631–640). Hamilton, ON: BC Decker Inc., 2008.

88. American Academy of Pediatrics. Oral Therapy for Acute Diarrhea. In Kleinman R. E., Greer F. R. (eds). *Pediatric Nutrition* (pp. 717–726). Elk Grove Village, IL: American Academy of Pediatrics, 2014.

89. Isaacs, J. S. Fluid and bowel problems. In Lucas B. (ed), *Children with Special Health Care Needs: Nutrition Care Handbook* (pp. 103–118). Chicago, IL: American Dietetic Association, 2004.

90. American Academy of Pediatrics. Policy Statement: The use and misuse of fruit juice in pediatrics. *Pediatrics* 2001; 107(5):1210–1213.

91. DiSanto, C.; Duggan, C. Gastrointestinal Diseases. In Hendricks K. M., Duggan C. *Manual of Pediatric Nutrition*, 4th ed. (pp. 531–568). Hamilton, ON: BC Decker, 2005.

92. Loening-Baucke, V. Constipation in early childhood: Patient characteristics, treatment, and long term follow up. *Gut* 1993; 34:1400–1404.

93. Tabbers, M. M., et al. Evaluation and treatment of functional constipation in infants and children: Evidence-based recommendations from ESPGHAN and NASPGHAN. *J Pediatr Gastroenterol Nutr* 2014; 58:258–274.

94. American Academy of Pediatric Dentistry, American Academy of Pediatrics. Policy on Early Childhood Carries (EEC): Classifications, Consequences, and Preventive Strategies. Chicago: Oral Health Policies, 2014.

95. U.S. Department of Health and Human Services, National Institutes of Health, National Institute of Allergy and Infectious Diseases. *Guidelines for the Diagnosis and Management of Food Allergy in the United States*. Washington, DC: U.S. Government Printing Office, 2010.

96. Greer, F. R., et al. Clinical Report: Effects of early nutritional interventions on the development of atopic disease in infants and children: The role of maternal dietary restriction, breastfeeding, timing of introduction of complementary foods, and hydrolyzed formulas. *Pediatrics* 2008; 121:183–191.

97. Sicherer S.H. and Wood, R.A. Allergy testing in childhood: Using allergen-specific IgE tests. *Pediatrics* 2012; 129:193–197.

98. American Academy of Pediatrics. Food Allergy. In Kleinman R. E., Greer, F. R. *Pediatric Nutrition*, 7th ed. (pp. 845–862). Elk Grove Village, IL: American Academy of Pediatrics, 2014.

99. American Academy of Pediatrics. Carbohydrate and Dietary Fiber. In Kleinman, R. E., and Greer, F. R. *Pediatric Nutrition*, 7th ed. (pp. 387–406). Elk Grove Village, IL: American Academy of Pediatrics, 2014.

100. VanWinckel, M., et al. Clinical Practice: Vegetarian infant and child nutrition. *Eur J Pediatr* 2011; 170(12):1489–1494.

101. Rosello, M., et al. Height, age at menarche, body weight and body mass index in life-long vegetarians. *Public Health Nutrition* 2005; 8:870–875.

102. Sanders, T. A. B., and Reddy, S. The influence of a vegetarian diet on the fatty acid composition of human milk and the essential fatty acid status of the infant. *J Pediatr* 1992; 120(suppl):S71–S77.

103. Child Nutrition. 2015, April 12. Retrieved from Head Start: http://eclkc.ohs.acf.hhs.gov/hslc/standards/hsspps/104/1304:23.

## Chapter 9

1. Gilliam J., Laney S. Nutrition Screening and Assessment. In Yang Y., Lucas B., Feucht S. (eds) *Nutrition Interventions for Children with Special Health Care Needs*, 3rd ed. (pp. 1–11). Olympia, WA: Washington State Department of Health, 2010.

2. McPherson M., et al. A new definition of children with special health care needs. *Pediatrics*, 1998; 102(1)1:137–140.

3. Lichtenwalter, L., et al. Providing nutrition services to children with special needs in a community setting. *Topics in Clin Nutr* 1993; 8(4):75–78.

4. Bayerl, C. T., Ries J. Nutrition issues of children in early intervention programs: Primary care team approach. *Semin Pediatr Gastroenterol Nutr*, 1993; 4:11–15.

5. Koletzko, B., Uauy R. Defining the Nutritional Needs of Preterm Infants. In Koletzko, B., Poindexter B., Uauy R. (eds). *Nutritional Care of Preterm Infants* (pp. 110:4–10). Basel, Switzerland: Karger, 2014.

6. Singh, G. K., et al. Infant mortality in the United States, 1935–2007:Over seven decades of progress and disparities. Rockville, MD: U.S. Department of Health and Human Services, Health Resources and Services Administration, Maternal and Child Health Bureau, 2010.

7. MacDorman, M. F., et al. Recent Declines in Infant Mortality in the United States, 2005–2011. National Center for Health Statistics Data Brief, No 120, April 2013.

8. Saigal, S., et al. Physical growth and current health status of infants who were of extremely low birth weight and controls at adolescence. *Pediatrics* 2001; 108:407–415.

9. Ehrenkranz, R.A., et al. Growth in the neonatal intensive care unit influences neurodevelopmental and growth outcomes of extremely low birth weight infants. *Pediatrics* 2006; 117:1253–1261.

10. Raju, T.N., et al. Optimizing care and outcome for late-preterm (near term) infants: A summary of the workshop sponsored by the National Institute of Child Health and Human Development. *Pediatrics* 2006; 118(3):1207–1214.

11. Engle, W. A., et al. "Late-Preterm" infants: A population at risk. *Pediatrics* 2007; 120(6):1390–1401.

12. Bright Futures. Children and Adolescents With Special Health Care Needs. In Holt K., Wooldridge N., Story M., Sofka D. *Bright Futures: Nutrition* (pp. 123–129). Elk Grove Village, IL: American Academy of Pediatrics, 2011.

13. O'Bryan, A. M. Prematurity. In Hendricks, K. M., Duggan, C. (eds). *Manual of Pediatric Nutrition*, 4th ed. (pp. 690–709). Hamilton, ON: B.C. Decker, 2005.

14. American Academy of Pediatrics. Nutritional Needs of the Preterm Infant. In Kleinman R.E. (ed.), *Pediatric Nutrition Handbook*, 6th ed. (pp. 79–112). Elk Grove Village, IL: American Academy of Pediatrics, 2009.

15. Zemel, B., Stallings V. Developmental Disabilities. In Duggan, C., Watkins, J. B., Walker, W.A. (eds). *Nutrition in Pediatrics*, 4th ed. (pp. 497–504). Hamilton, ON: BC Decker, Inc., 2008.

16. Institute of Medicine, Food and Nutrition Board. *Dietary References for Energy, Carbohydrate, Fiber, Fat, Fatty Acids, Cholesterol, Protein and Amino Acids (Macronutrients)*. Washington, DC: National Academies Press, 2002.

17. Cloud, H. H. Developmental Disabilities. In Samour, P. Q., and King, K. (eds). *Pediatric Nutrition*, 4th ed. (pp. 219–238). Sudbury, MA: Jones & Bartlett Learning, 2012.

18. American Academy of Pediatrics. Nutritional Needs of the Preterm Infant. In Kleinman, R. E., Greer, F. R. (eds.). *Pediatric Nutrition*, 7th ed. (pp. 83–121). Elk Grove Village, IL: American Academy of Pediatrics, 2014.

19. Agostoni, C., et al. Enteral nutrient supply for preterm infants: Commentary from the European Society of Paediatric Gastroenterology, Hepatology and Nutrition. *J Pediatr Gastroenterol Nutr* 2010; 50(1):85–91.

20. Tudehope, D., et al. Nutritional needs of the micropreterm infant. *J Pediatr* 2013; 162:S72–80.

21. Ramel, S. E., and Georgieff, M. K. Preterm Nutrition and the Brain. In Koletzko, B., Poindexter B., and Uauy R. (eds). *Nutritional Care of Preterm Infants* (pp. 190–200). Basel, Switzerland: Karger, 2014.

22. Ramel, S. E., et al. The relationship of poor linear growth velocity with neonatal illness and two year neurodevelopment in preterm infants. *Neonatology* 2012; 102:19–24.

23. Pongcharoen, T., et al. Influence of prenatal and postnatal growth on intellectual functioning in school aged children. *Arch Pediatr Adolesc Med* 2012; 166:411–416.

24. Mehta N. M., Jaksic T. The Critically Ill Child. In Duggan, C., Watkins, J. B., Walker, W. A. (eds.). *Nutrition in Pediatrics,* 4th ed. (pp. 663–673). Hamilton, ON: BC Decker Inc., 2008.

25. Dewey, K. G., et al. Protein requirements of infants and children. *Eur J Clin Nutr* 1996; 50(suppl 1):S119–S147.

26. American Academy of Pediatrics. Formula Feeding of Term Infants. In Kleinman, R. E., Greer, F. R. (eds). *Pediatric Nutrition*, 7th ed. (pp. 61–81). Elk Grove Village, IL: American Academy of Pediatrics, 2014.

27. Acosta, P. B. Genetic Screening and Nutritional Management. In Samour, P.Q., King, K. (eds). *Pediatric Nutrition*, 4th ed. (pp. 179–217). Sudbury, MA: Jones & Bartlett Learning, 2012.

28. Krohn K., et al. Macronutrient Requirements for Growth: Fats and Fatty Acids. In Duggan, C., Watkins, J. B., Walker, W. A. (eds). *Nutrition in Pediatrics*, 4th ed. (pp. 59–65). Hamilton, ON: BC Decker Inc., 2008.

29. Picciano, M. F. Nutrient composition of human milk. *Pediatr Clin North Am* 2001; 48:53–67.

30. Lapillonne, A. Enteral and Parenteral Lipid Requirements for Preterm Infants. In Koletko B., Poindexter B., Uauy R. (eds.). *Nutritional Care of Preterm Infants* (pp. 110: 82–98). Basel, Switzerland: Karger, 2014.

31. Gura, K. M., and Chan, L. Drug Therapy and the Role of Nutrition. In Duggan, C., Watkins, J. B., Walker, W. A. (eds.). *Nutrition in Pediatrics*, 4th ed (pp. 191–208). Hamilton, Ontario, Canada: BC Decker Inc., 2008.

32. American Academy of Pediatrics. Inborn Errors of Metabolism. In Kleinman, R. E., Greer, F. R. (eds.). *Pediatric Nutrition*, 7th ed. (pp. 727–739). Elk Grove Village, IL: American Academy of Pediatrics, 2014.

33. Baker, R. D., Greer, F. Clinical Report—Diagnosis and prevention of iron deficiency and iron–deficiency anemia in infants and young children (0–3 years of age). *Pediatrics* 2010; 126; No 5:1040–1050.

34. Redding, E., Despino, S. Pulmonary Diseases. In Samour, P. Q., King, K. (eds.). *Pediatric Nutrition* (pp. 239–274). Sudbury, MA: Jones & Bartlett Learning, 2012.

35. Ziegler, E. E. Human Milk and Human Milk Fortifiers. In Koletzko, B., Poindexter B., and Uauy R. (eds.). *Nutritional Care of Preterm Infants* (pp. 215–227). Basel, Switzerland: Karger, 2014.

36. Fenton, T. R., Kim, J. A systematic review and meta–analysis to revise the Fenton growth chart for preterm infants. *BMC Pediatrics* 2013; 13:59.

37. Olsen, I. E., et al. New intrauterine growth curves based on United States data. *Pediatrics* 2010; 125:e214–e224.

38. Olsen I. E., et al. BMI curves for preterm infants. *Pediatrics* 2015; 135:e572–e581.

39. Adamkin, D. H. *Nutritional Strategies for the Very Low Birthweight Infant*. New York: Cambridge University Press, 2009.

40. Anderson, D. M. Nutrition for Preterm Infants. In Samour P. Q., King, K. (eds). *Pediatric Nutrition*, 4th ed. (pp. 53–69). Sudbury, MA: Jones & Bartlett Learning, 2012.

41. Hay, W. W., et al. Workshop summary: Nutrition of the extremely low birth weight infant. *Pediatrics* 1999; 104:1360–1368.

42. Longo, S., et al. Short–term and long–term sequelae in intrauterine growth retardation (IUGR). *J Matern Fetal Neonatal Med* 2013; 26(3):222–225.

43. American Congress of Obstetricians and Gynecologists. IUGR (FGR)—Detection and Surveillance. 2015, June 28. Retrieved from American Congress of Obsetricians and Gynecologists: www.acog/org.

44. Barker, D. The developmental origins of adult disease. *J Am Coll Nutr* 2004; 23(6 suppl):588S–595S.

45. Chyi, L. J., et al. School outcomes of later preterm infants: Special needs and challenges for infants born 32 to 36 weeks gestation. *J Pediatr* 2008; 153:25–31.

46. Hintz, S..R., et al. Changes in neurodevelopmental outcomes at 18 to 22 months corrected age among infants of less than 25 weeks gestational age born in 1993–1999. *Pediatrics* 2005; 115(6):1645–1651.

47. Franz, A. R., et al. Intrauterine, early neonatal, and postdischarge growth and neurodevelopmental outcome at 5.4 years in extremely preterm infants after intensive neonatal nutrition support. *Pediatrics* 2009; 123:e101–e109.

48. Clark, R. H., et al. Extrauterine growth restriction remains a serious problem in prematurely born neonates. *Pediatrics* 2003; 111:986–990.

49. Hans, D. M., et al. Nutritional practices in the neonatal intensive care unit: Analysis of a 2006 neonatal nutrition survey. *Pediatrics* 2009; 123:51–57.

50. Weaver, L. Rapid growth in infancy: Balancing the interests of the child. *J Pediatr Gastroenterol Nutr* 2006; 43:428–432.

51. Baylor College of Medicine, Department of Pediatrics, Section on Neonatology. *Guidelines for Acute Care of the Neonate,* 19th ed. Houston, TX: Baylor College of Medicine, 2012.

52. Eicher, P. S. Feeding. In Batshaw, M.L., Roizen, N. J., and Lotrecchiano, G. R. (eds). *Children with Disabilities* (pp. 479–498). Baltimore, MD: Paul H. Brookes, 2007.

53. Persson, B., et al. Screening for infants with developmental deficits and/or autism. *J Pediatr Nurs* 2006; 21:313–324.

54. Hayes, D., et al. Pulmonary function outcomes in bronchopulmonary dysplasia through childhood and into adulthood: Implications for primary care. *Prim Care Respir J* 2011; 20(2):128–133.

55. Glass, R. P., Wolf, L. Oral-Motor Feeding Problems. In Yang Y., Lucas B., Feucht S. (eds). *Nutrition Interventions for Children with special Health Care Needs, 3rd ed.* (pp. 93–99). Olympia: Washington State Department of Health, 2010.

56. American Dietetic Association. Position of the American Dietetic Association: Providing nutrition services for infants, children, and adults with developmental disabilities with Special Health care needs. *J Am Diet Assn* 2004; 104(1):97–107.

57. Academy of Nutrition and Dietetics. *International Dietetics and Nutrition Terminology Reference Manual*. Chicago, IL: Academy of Nutrition and Dietetics, 2012.

58. Parker, S.E., et al. Updated national birth prevalence estimates for selected birth defects in the United States, 2004–2006. *Birth Defects Res A Clin Mol Teratol* 2010; 82(12):1008–1016.

59. Barker, D. Human Growth and Disease in Later Life. In Duggan, C., Watkins, J., and Walker, W. A. (eds.). *Nutrition in Pediatrics,* 4th ed. (pp. 305–309). Hamilton, ON: BC Decker Inc., 2008.

60. Aamoudse–Moens, C. S., et al. Meta–analysis of neurobehavioral outcomes in very preterm and/or very low birth weight children. *Pediatrics* 2009; 124(2)717–728.

61. Ehrenkranz, R. A. Nutrition, Growth and Clinical Outcomes. In Koletzo B., Poindexter B., Uauy R. *Nutritional Care of Preterm Infants* (pp. 110:11–26). Basel, Switzerland: Karger, 2014.

62. Bankhead, R., et al. ASPEN Enteral Nutrition Practice Recommendations. *J Parenter Enteral Nutr* 2009; 33(2):122–167.

63. Bhatia, J. Human milk and the premature infant. *Ann Nutr Metab* 2013; 62 (suppl) 3:8–14.

64. Human Milk Banking of North America. *Guidelines for the Establishment and Operation of a Donor Human Milk Bank*. Fort Worth, TX: Human Milk Banking Association of North America, 2013.

65. Schanler, R. J. et al. Randomized trial of donor human milk versus preterm formula as substitutes for mothers' own milk in the feeding of extremely premature infants. *Pediatrics* 2005; 116:400–406.

66. Forchielli, M. L., Bines, J. Enteral nutrition. In Duggan, C., Watkins, J. B., Walker, W. A. (eds). *Nutrition in Pediatrics*, 4th ed. (pp. 765–775). Hamilton, ON: BC Decker Inc., 2008.

67. Robbins, S. T., Meyers, R. *Infant Feedings: Guidelines for Preparation of Human Milk and Formula in Health Care Facilities*, 2nd ed. Chicago: Academy of Nutrition and Dietetics, 2011.

68. Groh–Wargo, S. Gastrointestinal Development. In Groh–Wargo, S., Thompson, M., Cox, J. H. (eds). *Nutritional Care for High–Risk Newborns*, 3rd ed. (pp. 209–230). Chicago: Precept Press, Inc., 2000.

69. Lawrence, R.A. and Lawrence, R.M. *Breastfeeding: A Guide for the Medical Professional*. Maryland Heights, MO: Elsevier Mosby, 2011.

70. Pinelli, J and Symington, A. Non–nutritive sucking for promoting physiologic stability and nutrition in preterm infants. *Cochrane Database Syst Rev* 2005; 19(4):CD001071.

71. Levy, R. J., et al. Birth weight of infants with congenital heart disease. *Am J Dis Child* 1978; 1:249–254.

72. Jones, F. *Best Practice for Expressing, Storing and Handling Human Milk*, 3rd ed. Fort Worth, TX: Human Milk Banking Association of North America, 2011.

73. Thoyre, S. M., et al. The early feeding skills assessment for preterm infants. *Neonatal Netw* 2005; 24(3):7–16.

74. Kucik, J. E., et al. Racial/ethnic variations in the prevalence of selected major birth defects, metropolitan Atlanta, 1994–2005. *Public Health Rep* 2012; 127(1):52–61.

75. Centers for Disease Control and Prevention. *Data and Statistics: Spina Bifida*. 2014.

76. AAP Council on Children with Disabilities, Section on Developmental Behavioral Pediatrics. Policy Statement: Identifying infants and young children with developmental disorders in the medical home: An algorithm for developmental surveillance and screening. *Pediatrics* 2006; 118(1):405–420.

77. American Academy of Pediatrics. Complementary foods. In Kleinman, R. E., and Greer, F. R. (eds). *Pediatric Nutrition*, 7th ed., pp. 123–139. Elk Grove Village, IL: American Academy of Pediatrics, 2014.

## Chapter 10

1. Center on Hunger, Poverty and Nutrition Policy. *Statement on the link between nutrition and cognitive development in children*. Tufts University: School of Nutrition Science and Policy, 1998.

2. The Annie E. Casey Foundation. *2011 KIDS COUNT Data Book*. Baltimore, MD: The Annie E. Casey Foundation, 2011.

3. U.S. Department of Health and Human Services, Health Resources and Services Administration, Maternal and Child Health Bureau. *Child Health USA 2011*. Rockville, MD: U.S. Department of Health and Human Services, 2011.

4. Jiang, Y., Ekono, M., and Skinner, C. Basic facts about low-income children: Children under 6 years, 2013. *National Center for Children in Poverty* January 2015. www.nncp.org/publications/pub_1097.html, accessed 5/2015.

5. U.S. Department of Health and Human Services. *Healthy People 2020* Washington, DC: U.S. Department of Health and Human Services, December 2010; Available at www.HealthyPeople.gov, accessed 06/15.

6. Kliegman, R. M., Stanton, B. F., St. Geme, J. W., Schor, N. F., and Behrman, R. E. *Nelson's Textbook of Pediatrics*, 20th ed. Philadelphia, PA: Elsevier/Saunders, 2015.

7. Centers for Disease Control and Prevention, National Center for Health Statistics. *CDC growth charts: United States*. Available at www.cdc.gov//growthcharts/cdc_charts.htm, accessed 06/15

8. Barlow, S. E., and the Expert Committee. Expert Committee Recommendations regarding the prevention, assessment, and treatment of child and adolescent overweight and obesity: Summary report. *Pediatrics* 2007; 120(S4):S164–S192.

9. WHO Multicentre Growth Reference Study Group. *WHO Child Growth Standards: Length/height-for-age, weight-for-age, weight-for-length, weight-for-height and body mass index-for-age: Methods and development*. Geneva: World Health Organization, 2006. Available at http://www.who.int/childgrowth/standards/technical_report/en/index.html, accessed 07/12.

10. Holt, K., Wooldridge, N., Story, M., and Sofka, D., eds. *Bright Futures Nutrition*. Elk Grove Village, IL: American Academy of Pediatrics, 2011.

11. United States Department of Agriculture, MyPlate. Available at www.MyPlate.gov.

12. Satter, E. The feeding relationship: Problems and interventions. *J Pediatr* 1990; 117:181–189.

13. Birch, L. L. Children's food acceptance patterns. *Nutr Today* 1996; 31:234–240.

14. Birch, L. L., et al. The variability of young children's energy intake. *N Eng J Med* 1991; 324:232–235.

15. Story, M., and Brown, J. E. Do young children instinctively know what to eat? The studies of Clara Davis revisited. *New Eng J Med* 1987; 316:103–106.

16. Van den Bree, M. B. M., et al. Genetic and environmental influences on eating patterns of twins ages >50 years. *Am J Clin Nutr* 1999; 70:456–465.

17. Chess, S., and Thomas, A. Dynamics of individual behavioral development. In Levine, M. D., Carey, W. B., and Crocker, A. C., eds. *Developmental-behavioral pediatrics*. Philadelphia, PA: WB Saunders Co., 1992:84–94.

18. Birch, L. L., and Fisher, J. O. Development of eating behaviors among children and adolescents. *Pedatrics* 1998; 101:539–49(S).

19. Birch, L. L., and Fisher, J. A. Appetite and eating behavior in children. *Pediatr Clinic N Amer* 1995; 42:931–953.

20. Fisher, J. O., et al. Parental influences on young girls' fruit and vegetable, micronutrient, and fat intakes. *J Amer Diet Assoc* 2002; 102:58–64.

21. Fisher, J. O., and Birch, L. L. Restricting access to palatable foods affects children's behavioral response, food selection, and intake. *Am J Clin Nutr* 1999; 69:1264–1272.

22. Connor, S. M. Food-related advertising on preschool television: Building brand recognition in young viewers. *Pediatrics* 2006; 118:1478–1485.

23. Birch, L. L., and Fisher, J. O. Food intake regulation in children, fat and sugar substitutes and intake. *Ann NY Acad Sci* 1997; 819:194–220.

24. Rolls, B. J., Engell, D., and Birch, L. L. Serving portion size influences 5-year-old but not 3-year-old children's food intake. *J Amer Diet Assoc* 2000; 100:232–234.

25. Fisher, J. O., Rolls, B. J., and Birch, L. L. Children's bite size and intake of an entrée are greater with large portions than with age-appropriate or self-selected portions. *Am J Clin Nutr* 2003; 77:1164–1170.

26. Fisher, J. O., and Birch, L. L. Parents' restrictive feeding practices are associated with young girls' negative self-evaluation of eating. *J Amer Diet Assoc* 2000; 100:1341–1346.

27. Davison, K. K., and Birch, L. L. Weight status, parent reaction, and self-concept in five-year-old girls. *Pediatrics* 2001; 107:46–53.

28. Abramovitz, B. A., and Birch, L. L. Five-year-old girls' ideas about dieting are predicted by their mothers' dieting. *J Amer Diet Assoc* 2000; 100:1157–1163.

29. Satter, E. Feeding dynamics: Helping children to eat well. *J Pediatr Health Care* 1995; 9:178–184.

30. Davis, M. M., et al. Recommendations for prevention of childhood obesity. *Pediatrics* 2007; 120(S4):S229–253.

31. National Academy of Sciences. Institute of Medicine. Food and Nutrition Board. Dietary Reference Intakes for energy, carbohydrate, fiber, fat, protein, and amino acids. Washington, DC: National Academy Press, 2005.

32. National Academy of Sciences. Institute of Medicine. Food and Nutrition Board. Dietary reference intakes for calcium, and vitamin D. Washington, DC: National Academy Press, 2010.

33. National Academy of Sciences. Institute of Medicine. Food and Nutrition Board. Dietary reference intakes for vitamin A, vitamin K, arsenic, boron, chromium, copper, iodine, iron, manganese, molybdenum, nickel, silicon, vanadium, and zinc. Washington, DC: National Academy Press, 2001.

34. Centers for Disease Control and Prevention. Recommendations to prevent and control iron deficiency in the United States. *Morbidity and Mortality Weekly Report* April 3, 1998; 47 (RR-03):1–29.

35. Baker, R. D., and Greer, F. R. American Academy of Pediatrics Committee on Nutrition. Diagnosis and prevention of iron deficiency and iron deficiency anemia in infants and young children (0 to 3 years). *Pediatrics* 2010; 126(5): 1040–1050.

36. Dye, B. A., Thornton, Evans G., Li, X., and Iafolla, T. J. Dental caries and sealant prevalence in children and adolescents in the United States 2011–2012. NCHS Data Brief,No 191. Hyattsville, MD: National Center for Health Statistics, 2015. www.cdc.gov/nchs/data/databriefs/db191.htm.

37. American Academy of Pediatric Dentistry. Policy on early childhood caries (ECC): Classifications, consequences, and preventive strategies, 2011; available at http://www.aapd.org/media/Policies_Guidelines/P_ECCClassification.pdf, accessed 07/12.

38. Casamassimo, P. *Bright Futures in Practice: Oral Health*. Arlington, VA: National Center for Education in Maternal and Child Health, 1996.

39. American Academy of Pediatrics, *Committee on Nutrition. Pediatric Nutrition Handbook*, 6th ed. Kleinman, R. E., ed. Elk Grove Village, IL: American Academy of Pediatrics, 2009.

40. McClung, H. J., Boyne, L., and Heitlinger, L. Constipation and dietary fiber intake in children. *Pediatrics* 1995; 96:999–1001(S).

41. Centers for Disease Control and Prevention. Blood lead levels—United States, 1999–2002. *MMWR Morb Mortal Wkly Rep*. 2005; 54(20):513–516.

42. American Academy of Pediatrics, Committee on Environmental Health. Lead exposure in children: Prevention, detection, and management. *Pediatrics* 2005; 116:1036–1046.

43. U.S. Preventive Services Task Force. Screening for elevated blood lead levels in children and pregnant women: recommendation statement. Rockville, MD: Agency for Healthcare Research and Quality, 2006. Available at www.uspreventiveservicestaskforce.org, accessed 06/15.

44. Centers for Disease Control and Prevention Advisory Committee on Childhood Lead poisoning Prevention. Interpreting and managing blood lead levels <10 microg/dl in children and reducing childhood exposures to lead: recommendations of CDC's Advisory Committee on Childhood Lead Poisoning Prevention. *MMWR Recomm Rep*. 2007; 56(RR-8): 1–16.

45. Ballew, C., et al. Blood lead concentration and children's anthropometric dimensions in the Third National Health and Nutrition Examination Survey (NHANES III), 1988–1994. *J Pediatr* 1999; 134:623–630.

46. Binns, H. J., et al. Interpreting and managing blood lead levels of less than 10 mcg/dL in children and reducing childhood exposure to lead: Recommendations of the Centers for Disease Control and Prevention Advisory Committee on Childhood Lead Poisoning Prevention. *Pediatrics* 2007; 120:e1285–1298.

47. Advisory Committee on Childhood Lead Poisioning Prevention. Low Level Lead Exposure Harms Children: A Renewed Call for Primary Prevention. Available at http://www.cdc.gov/nceh/lead/acclpp/final_document_030712.pdf, accessed 6/2015.

48. Coleman-Jensen, A., Nord, M., Andrews, M., Carlson, Sl Household food security in the United States in 2010. Economic Research Report No. (ERR-125) 37 pp., September 2011. Available at www.ers.usda.gov/Publications/err-economic-research-report/err 125.aspx, accessed 06/15.

49. Kleinman, R. E., et al. Hunger in children in the United States: Potential behavioral and emotional correlates. *Pediatrics* [serial online] 1998; 101:E3. Available at www.pediatrics.org/cgi/content/full/101/1/e3, accessed 06/15.

50. Centers for Disease Control and Prevention, National Center for Infectious Diseases, U.S. Department of Health and Human Services. Foodborne Illness. Available at www.cdc.gov/ncidod/diseases/food/index.htm, accessed 06/15.

51. Partnership for Food Safety Education: FightBAC™. Available at www.fightbac.org, accessed 06/15.

52. U.S. Department of Health and Human Services and U.S. Department of Agriculture. Dietary Guidelines for Americans, 2010, 7th ed. Washington, DC: U.S. Government Printing Office, December 2010.

53. Kavey, R. W., et al. American Heart Association guidelines for primary prevention of atherosclerotic cardiovascular disease beginning in childhood. *Circulation* 2003; 107:1562–1566.

54. Ogden, C. L., Carroll, M. D., Kit, B. K., Flegal, K. M. Prevalalence of childhood and adult obesity in the United States, 2011–2012. JAMA 2014:311(8):806–814.

55. Krebs, N. F., et al. Assessment of child and adolescent overweight and obesity. *Pediatrics* 2007; 120(S4):S193–S228.

56. Spear, B. A., et al. Recommendations for treatment of child and adolescent overweight and obesity. *Pediatrics* 2007; 120(S4):S254–S288.

57. Dietz, W. H., and Gortmaker, S. L. Preventing obesity in children and adolescents. *Annu Rev Public Health* 2001; 22:337–353.

58. Whitaker, R. C., et al. Early adiposity rebound and the risk of adult obesity. *Pediatrics* [serial online] 1998; 101:E5. Available at www.pediatrics.org/cgi/content/full/101/3/e5, accessed 6/15.

59. Gidding, S. S., et al. Implementing American Heart Association pediatric and adult nutrition guidelines: A scientific statement from the American Heart Association Nutrition Committee of the Council on Nutrition, Physical Activity and Metabolism, Council on Cardiovascular Disease in the Young, Council on Arteriosclerosis, Thrombosis and Vascular Biology, Council on Cardiovascular Nursing, Council on Epidemiology and Prevention, and Council for High Blood Pressure Research. *Circulation* 2009; 119:1161–1175.

60. Gidding, S. S., et al. Dietary recommendations for children and adolescents: A guide for practitioners. Consensus statement from the American Heart Association. *Circulation* 2005; 112:2061–2075.

61. American Heart Association, Gidding, S. S., et al. Dietary recommendations for children and adolscents: A guide for practitioners. *Pediatrics* 2006; 117:544–559.

62. Lichtenstein, A. H., et al. Diet and lifestyle recommendations revision 2006: A scientific statement from the American Heart Association Nutrition Committee. *Circulation* 2006; 114:82–96.

63. Rask-Nissila, L., et al. Prospective, randomized, infancy-onset trial of the effects of a low-saturated-fat, low-cholesterol diet on serum lipids and lipoproteins before school age: The special turku coronary risk factor intervention project (STRIP). *Circulation* 2000; 102:1477–1483.

64. Daniels, S. R., et al. Lipid screening and cardiovascular health in childhood. *Pediatrics* 2008; 122:198–208.

65. Expert Panel on Integrated Guidelines for Cardiovascular health and Risk Reduction in Children and Adolescents. Expert panel on integrated guidelines for cardiovascular health and risk reduction in children and adolescents: summary report. *Pediatrics* 2011; 128:S213–256.

66. Ervin, R. B., Wright, J. D., Reed-Gillette, D. Prevalence of leading types of dietary supplements used in the Third National Health and Nutrition Examination Survey, 1988–1994. *Advance Data from Vital Health Statistics*. No. 349, November 9, 2004.

67. Bailey, R. L., Gachche, J. J., Lenino, C. V., Dwyer, J. T., Engel, J. S., Thomas, P. R., Betz, J. M., Sempos, C. T., Picciano, M. F. Dietary Supplement Use in the United States, 2003–2006. J Nutr.doi:10.3945/jn.110.133025.

68. Lohse, B., Stotts, J. L., and Priebe, J. R. Survey of herbal use by Kansas and Wisconsin WIC participants reveals moderate, appropriate use and identifies herbal education needs. *J Amer Diet Assoc* 2006; 106:227–237.

69. Buck, M. L., and Michael, R. S. Talking with families about herbal products. *J Pediatr* 2000; 136:673–678.

70. FDA and EPA issue updated advice for fish consumption, U.S. Food and Drug Administration, news release, June 20, 2014, http://www.fda.gov/NewsEvents/Newsroom/PressAnnouncements/ucm397929.htm.

71. American Dietetic Association. Position of the American Dietetic Association: Dietary guidance for healthy children aged 2 to 11 years. *J Amer Diet Assoc* 2008; 108:1038–1047.

72. A summary of conference recommendations on dietary fiber in childhood: Conference on Dietary Fiber in Childhood, New York, May 24, 1994. *Pediatrics* 1995; 96:1023–1028.

73. Hampl, J. S., Betts, N. M., and Benes, B. A. The "age + 5" rule: Comparisons of dietary fiber intake among 4- to 10-year-old children. *J Amer Diet Assoc* 1998; 98:1418–1423.

74. Wagner, C. L., Greer, F. R., and the Section on Breastfeeding and Committee on Nutrition. Prevention of rickets and vitamin D deficiency in infants, children, and adolescents. *Pediatrics* 2008; 122:1142–1152.

75. Greer, F. R., Krebs, N. F., and Committee on Nutrition. Optimizing bone health and calcium intakes of infants, children, and adolescents. *Pediatrics* 2006; 117:578–585.

76. Wang, Y. C., Bleich, S. N., and Gortmaker, S. L. Increasing caloric contribution from sugar-sweetened beverages and 100% fruit

juices among U.S. children and adolescents, 1988–2004. *Pediatrics* 2008; 121:e1604–614.

77. Siega-Riz, A. M., et al. Food consumption patterns of infants and toddlers: where are we now? *J Am Diet Assoc* 2010; 110:S38–S51.

78. Harnack, L., Stang, J., and Story, M. Soft drink consumption among U.S. children and adolescents: Nutritional consequences. *J Amer Diet Assoc* 1999; 99:436–441.

79. American Academy of Pediatrics. Committee on Nutrition. The use and misuse of fruit juices in pediatrics. *Pediatrics* 2001; 107:1210–1213.

80. U.S. Department of Agriculture, Agricultural Research Service. 2012. *What We Eat in America.* NHANES 2009–2010. Energy Intakes: Percentages of energy from protein, carbohydrate, fat, and alcohol, by gender and age in the United States, 2009–2010; Nutrient Intakes from Food: Mean amounts consumed per individual by gender and age, in the United States, 2009–2010. Available at www.ars.usda.gov/ba/bhnrc.fsrg, accessed 09/12.

81. Butte, N. F. Nutrient intakes of US infants, toddlers, and preschoolers meet or exceed dietary reference intakes. *J Amer Diet Assoc* 2010; 110:S27–S37.

82. Skinner, J. D., et al. Longitudinal study of nutrient and food intakes of white preschool children aged 24 to 60 months. *J Amer Diet Assoc* 1999; 99:1514–1521.

83. Picciano, M. F., et al. Nutritional guidance is needed during dietary transition in early childhood. *Pediatrics* 2000; 106:109–114.

84. Bowman, S. A., et al. Effects of fast-food consumption on energy intake and diet quality among children in a national household survey. *Pediatrics* 2004; 113:112–118.

85. Kranz, S., et al. Adverse effect of high added sugar consumption on dietary intake in American preschoolers. *J Pediatr* 2005; 146:105–111.

86. McConaby, K. L., et al. Food portions are positively related to energy intake and body weight in early childhood. *J Pediatr* 2002; 140:340–347.

87. Sanders, T. A. B. Vegetarian diets and children. *Pediatr Clinic N Amer* 1995; 42:955–965.

88. American Dietetic Association. Position of the American Dietetic Association: Vegetarian diets. *J Amer Diet Assoc* 2009; 109: 1266–1282.

89. American Dietetic Association. Position of the American Dietetic Association: Benchmarks for nutrition programs in child-care settings. *J Amer Diet Assoc* 2005; 105:979–986.

90. American Academy of Pediatrics, American Public Health Association, Health Resources and Services Administration, Maternal and Child Health Bureau. *Caring for our children, national health and safety performance standards: Guidelines for out-of-home child care programs,* 2nd ed. Elk Grove Village, IL: American Academy of Pediatrics, 2002.

91. American Academy of Pediatrics, Council on Sports Medicine and Fitness and Council on School Health. Active healthy living: Prevention of childhood obesity through increased physical activity. *Pediatrics* 2006; 117:1834–1842.

92. Hagan, J. F., Shaw, J., and Duncan, P. M., eds. *Bright Futures: Guidelines for Health Supervision of Infants, Children, and Adolescents,* 3rd ed. Elk Grove Village, IL: American Academy of Pediatrics, 2008.

93. U.S. Department of Agriculture. Food and Nutrition Services, WIC. Available at www.usda.gov, accessed 05/15.

94. Women, Infants and Children (WIC)WIC Racial-Ethnic Group Enrollment Data 2012 http://www.fns.usda.gov/wic/wic-racial-ethnic-group-enrollment-data-2012, accessed 5/2015.

95. Food Research and Action Center. Impact of the revised wic food packages on nutrition outcomes and the retail food environment, 9/2014; http://frac.org/pdf/frac_brief_revised_wic_food_package_impact_nutrition_retail.pdf, accessed 5/2015.

96. Rose, D., Habicht, J. P., and Devaney, B. Household participation in the food stamp and WIC programs increases the nutrient intakes of preschool children. *J Nutr* 1998; 128:548–555.

97. U.S. Department of Health and Human Services. Administration for Children and Families. Office of Head Start. Available at www.dhhs.gov, accessed 07/12.

98. U.S. Department of Agriculture. Supplemental Nutrition Assistance Program (SNAP), http://www.fns.usda.gov/pd/supplemental-nutrition-assistance-program-snap, accessed 5/15.

99. Ratcliffe, C., McKennan, S. M., Zhang, S. How much does the Supplemental Nutrition Assistance Program reduce food insecurity? *Am J Agr Econ.* 2011; 93:1082–1098.

## Chapter 11

1. Healthy People 2020 Objectives. Available at http://www.healthypeople.gov/2020/topicsobjectives2020, accessed 6/15.

2. Dietary Guidelines for Americans, 2010. Available at www.dietaryguidelines.gov, accessed 6/15.

3. United States Department of Labor. What does disability.gov do? Available at https://www.disability.gov/home/about_us, accessed 6/15.

4. United States Department of Education. National Center for Education Statistics. Children and youth with disabilities. Indicator 9-2012. Available at http://nces.ed.gov/programs/coe/indicator_ope.asp, accessed 6/15.

5. Yeargin-Allsopp, M., Drews-Botsch, C., and Van Naarden, B. Epidemiology of developmental disabilities. In Batshaw, M. L., Pellegrino, L., and Roizen, N. J., eds. *Children with disabilities,* 6th ed. Baltimore, MD: Paul H. Brookes, 2007:231–243.

6. Staiano, A. Food refusal in toddlers with chronic diseases. *J Ped Gastro Nutr* 2003; 37:225–227.

7. Council on Children With Disabilities, Section on Developmental Behavioral Pediatrics, Bright Futures Steering Committee, and Medical Home Initiatives for Children With Special Needs Project Advisory Committee. Identifying infants and young children with developmental disorders in the medical home: An algorithm for developmental surveillance and screening. *Pediatrics* 2006; 118:405–420.

8. Hagan, J. F., Shaw, J. S., and Duncan, P. M., eds. *Bright Futures: Guidelines for Health Supervision of Infants, Children and Adolescents.* Elk Grove Village, IL: American Academy of Pediatrics, 2008.

9. National Information Center for Children and Youth with Disabilities. General information about disabilities. Available at www.nichcy.org/general.htm, accessed 6/15.

10. Prader-Willi Syndrome. Updated 2011. Available at http://www.mayoclinic.com/health/prader-willi-syndrome/DS00922, accessed 6/15.

11. Trumbo, P., et al. Dietary reference intakes: Vitamin A, vitamin K, arsenic, boron, chromium, copper, iodine, iron, manganese, molybdenum, nickel, silicon, vanadium, and zinc. *J Amer Diet Assoc* 2001; 101:294–301.

12. Institute of Medicine Food and Nutrition Board. Dietary Reference Intakes for energy, carbohydrate, fiber, fat, fatty acids, cholesterol, protein, and amino acids. Washington, DC: National Academy Press, 2002.

13. Kleinman, R. E., ed. *Pediatric Nutrition Handbook 7th* ed. Chicago, IL: American Academy of Pediatrics, 2013.

14. Academy of Nutrition and Dietetics. Nutrition Terminology Reference Manual (eNCPT): Dietetics Language for Nutrition Care. http://ncpt.webauthor.com, accessed 6/01/2015.

15. DeVore, J., and Shotton, A., eds. *Pocket Guide to Children with Special Health Care and Nutritional Needs.* Chicago, IL: Academy of Nutrition and Dietetics, 2012.

16. Bull, M. J., and the Committee on Genetics. Clinical Report: Health supervision for children with Down Syndrome. *Pediatrics* 2011; 128 (2):393–406.

17. TEIS (Therapeutic Early Intervention Services in Pennsylvania). What are nutrition services in Early Intervention? Available at http://www.earlyinterventionsupport.com/parentingtips/feeding/ei-nutrition.aspx, accessed 6/15.

18. Greenwood Genetics Center. *Growth References* 3rd ed. Greenwood, SC: Greenwood Genetics Center, 2011.

19. Holt, K., Wooldridge, N. H., Story M., Sofka, D. eds. *Bright Futures Nutrition,* 3rd ed. Elk Grove Village, IL: American Academy of Pediatrics, 2011.

20. Centers for Disease Control and Prevention. Use of World Health Organization and CDC growth charts for children aged 0–59 months in the United States. *MMWR*2010; 59 (No. RR-9):1–15.

21. National Center for Health Statistics. *NCHS growth curves for children 0–19 years*. U.S. Vital and Health Statistics, Health Resources Administration. Washington, DC: U.S. Government Printing Office, 2000.

22. Nellhaus, G. Composite international and interracial graphs. *Pediatrics* 1968; 41:106–114.

23. Isaacs, J. S., et al. Eating difficulties in girls with Rett syndrome compared with other developmental disabilities. *J Amer Diet Assoc* 2003; 103(2):224–230.

24. Elias, E. R., Murphy, N. A. and the Council on Children with Disabilities. Home care of children and youth with complex health care needs and technology dependencies. *Pediatrics* 2012; 129:996–1005.

25. American Academy of Pediatrics. The use and misuse of fruit juice in pediatrics. *Pediatrics* 2001; 107:1210–1213.

26. Ruottinen, S., Niinikoski, H., Lagström, H., Rönnemaa, T., Hakanen, M., Viikari, J., et al. High sucrose intake is associated with poor quality of diet and growth between 13 months and 9 years of age: The Special Turku Coronary Risk Factor Intervention Project. *Pediatrics* 2008; 121:e1676–e1685.

27. Council on Children With Disabilities. Role of the medical home in family centered early intervention services. *Pediatrics* 2007; 120:1153–1158.

28. Ficicioglu, C. and An Haack, K. Failure to thrive: When to suspect inborn errors of metabolism. *Pediatrics* 2009; 124:3 972–979.

29. Kellogg, N. D., and the Committee on Child Abuse and Neglect. Evaluation of suspected child physical abuse. *Pediatrics* 2007; 119:1232–1241.

30. Berkovitch, M., et al. Copper and zinc blood levels among children with nonorganic failure to thrive. *J Clin Nutr* 2003; 22(2):183–186.

31. Boyle, E. M., Poulsen, G., Field D. J., Kurinczuk, J. J., Wolke, D., Alfirevic, Z., Quigley, M. A. Effects of gestational age at birth on health outcomes at 3 and 5 years of age: Population-based cohort study. *BMJ* 2012; 344:e896.

32. Niewinski, M. M. Advances in celiac disease and gluten-free diet. *J Amer Diet Assoc* 2008; 108:661–672.

33. Autism and Developmental Disabilities Monitoring Network Surveillance Year 2008 Principal Investigators. Prevalence of autism spectrum disorders—Autism and developmental monitoring network, 14 sites, United States, 2008. *MMWR* 2012; 61(SS03):1–19.

34. Johnson, C. P., Myers, S. M., and Council on Children with Disabilities. American Academy of Pediatrics Policy Clinical Report: Identification on evaluation of children with autism spectrum disorder. *Pediatrics* 2007; 120:1183–1215.

35. About ASD. http://www.cdc.gov/ncbddd/autism/facts.html, accessed 6/15.

36. Marí-Bauset, S., Zazpe, I., Mari-Sanchis, A., Llopis-González, A., and Morales-Suárez-Varela, M.. Evidence of the gluten-free and casein-free diet in autism spectrum disorders: a systematic review. *J Child Neurol.* 2014 Dec; 29(12):1718–1727.

37. Bell KL, Samson-Fang L. Nutritional management of children with cerebral palsy. *Eur J Clin Nutr.* 2013 Dec; 67 Suppl 2:S13–16.

38. United States Public Health Service. Asthma prevalence, health care use, and mortality: United States, 2005–2009. *PHS* 2011; No. 32:1250.

39. Thiara, G., Goldman, R. D. Milk consumption and mucus production in children with asthma. *Can Fam Physician* 2012 Feb; 58:165–166.

40. Lang, J. E. Obesity and asthma in children: Current and future therapeutic options. *Pediatric Drugs* 2014; 16: 179–188.

41. Strueby, L., and Thébaud B. Advances in bronchopulmonary dysplasia. *Expert Rev Respir Med.* 2014 Jun; 8(3):327–338.

42. Hayes, D. Jr., Meadows, J. T. Jr., Murphy, B. S., Feola, D. J., Shook, L. A., and Ballard, H. O. Pulmonary function outcomes in bronchopulmonary dysplasia through childhood and into adulthood: Implications for primary care. *Prim Care Respir J* 2011; 20 (2):128–133.

43. Stroustrup, A., and Trasande, L. Epidemiological characteristics and resource use in neonates with bronchopulmonary dysplasia: 1993–2006. *Pediatrics* 2010; 125:291–297.

44. American Association on Intellectual and Developmental Disabilities (AAIDD). FAQ on Intellectual Disability. Available at http://aamr.org/content_104.cfm, accessed 7/12.

45. U.S. Department of Health and Human Services. National Institutes of Health, National Institute of Allergy and Infectious Diseases. *Guidelines for the diagnosis and management of food allergy in the United States.* Washington, DC: U.S. Government Printing Office, 2010. NIH Publication No. 11-7700.

46. Thomas, D. W., and Greer, F. R., American Academy of Pediatrics Committee on Nutrition Section on Gastroenterology, Hepatology, and Nutrition. Clinical report Probiotics and prebiotics in pediatrics. *Pediatrics* 2010; 126:1217–1231.

47. Ball, S. D., Kertesz, D., Laurie, J., and Moyer-Mileur, L. J. Dietary supplement use is prevalent among children with a chronic illness. *J Amer Diet Assoc* 2005; 105:78–84.

48. National Institutes of Medicine, National Center of Complementary and Alternative Medicine. Patterns of Complementary and Alternative Medicine Use in Children. Available at http://nccam.nih.gov/health/children#patterns, accessed 6/15.

49. National Down Syndrome Society. Alternative therapies. Available at http://www.ndss.org/en/Healthcare/Alternative-Therapies, accessed 6/15.

50. Maternal and Child Health Bureau, Health and Human Services. LEND program. Available at http://mchb.hrsa.gov/html/drte.html, accessed 6/15.

51. Public Law 109-416, 109th Congress. http://www.gpo.gov/fdsys/pkg/PLAW-109publ416/pdf/PLAW-109publ416.pdf, accessed 6/2015.


## *Chapter 12*


1. Holt, K., Wooldridge, N., Story, M., and Sofka, D., eds. *Bright Futures Nutrition.* Elk Grove Village, IL: American Academy of Pediatrics, 2011.

2. Adolphus, K., Lawton, C. L., Dye, L. The effects of breakfast on behaviour and academic performance in children and adolescents. *Front Hum Neurosci.* 2013; 7:425.

3. U.S. Department of Health and Human Services, Health Resources and Services Administration, Maternal and Child Health Bureau. *Child Health USA 2012.* Rockville, MD: U.S. Department of Health and Human Services, 2012.

4. The Annie E. Casey Foundation. *2014 KIDS COUNT Data Book.* Baltimore, MD: The Annie E. Casey Foundation, 2014.

5. Ogden, C. L., et al. Prevalence of obesity and trends in body mass index among US adolescents, 1999–2010. *JAMA* 2012; 307(5):483–490.

6. U.S. Department of Health and Human Services. *Healthy People 2020* Washington, D.C.: U.S. Department of Health and Human Services, December 2012. Available at www.HealthyPeople.gov, accessed 07/12.

7. Kliegman, R. M., Stanton, B. M. D., St. Geme J. W., Schor, N. F. Behrman, R. E. eds. *Nelson Textbook of Pediatrics*, 19th ed. Philadelphia: Elsevier/Saunders, 2011.

8. Centers for Disease Control and Prevention, National Center for Health Statistics. CDC growth charts: United States. Available at http://www.cdc.gov/growthcharts/cdc _charts.htm, accessed 07/12.

9. Troiano, R. P., and Flegal, K. M. Overweight children and adolescents: Description, epidemiology, and demographics. *Pediatrics* 1998; 101:497–504.

10. Barlow, S. E. Expert committee recommendations regarding the prevention, assessment, and treatment of child and adolescent overweight and obesity: Summary report. *Pediatrics* 2007; 120:S164–S192.

11. Krebs, N. F., et al. Assessment of child and adolescent overweight and obesity. *Pediatrics* 2007; 120:S193–S228.

12. de Oris, M., et al. Development of a WHO growth reference for school-aged children and adolescents. *Bulletin of the World Health Organization* 2007; 85:660–667.

13. Dietz, W. H. Critical periods in childhood for the development of obesity. *Am J Clin Nutr* 1994; 59:955–959.

14. Rolland-Cachera, M. F., et al. Early adiposity rebound: causes and consequences of obesity in children and adults. *International Journal of Obesity* 2006; 30:S11–S17.

15. Satter, E. Feeding dynamics: Helping children to eat well. *J Pediatr Health Care* 1995; 9:178–184.

16. Hammons, A. J., and Fiese, B. H. Is frequency of shared family meals related to the nutrition health of children and Adolescents? *Pediatrics* 2001; 127(6):e1565–e1574.

17. Scalioni, S., et al. Determinants of children's eating behavior. *Am J Clin Nutr.* 2011; 94(6suppl):2006S–2011S.

18. Gillman, M. W., et al. Family dinner and diet quality among older children and adolescents. *Arch Fam Med* 2000; 9:235–240.

19. Batada, A., et al. Nine out of 10 food advertisements shown during Saturday morning children's television programming are for foods high in fat, sodium, or added sugars, or low in nutrients. *J Amer Diet Assoc* 2008; 108:673–678.

20. U.S. Department of Agriculture. *MyPlate.* Available at www.MyPlate.gov, accessed 07/12.

21. Academy of Nutrition and Dietetics. Nutrition guidance for healthy children (2–11 yrs) project. 2013. http://andevidence library.com/topic. cfm?cat=4314, accessed April 28, 2015.

22. Moore, E., and the Kaiser Family Foundation. *It's child play: Advergaming and the online marketing of food to children.* Menlo Park, CA: Henry J. Kaiser Family Foundation, 2006.

23. Federal Trade Commission. *A review of Food Marketing to Children and Adolescents: Follow-Up Report.* Washington, DC: Office US Government Printing Office; 2012.

24. Cheyne, A., et al. *Food and Beverage Marketing to Children and Adolescents: Limited Progress by 2012.* Minneapolis, MN: Healthy Eating Research; 2013.

25. Duffey, K. J., and Popkin, B. M. Causes of increased energy intake among children in the US, 1977–2010. *Am J Prev Med.* 2013; 44(2):e1–e8.

26. Piernas, C., and Popkin, B. M. Food portion patterns and trends among US children and ther realtionsihp to total eating occasion size, 1977–2006. *J Nutr.* 2011; 141(6):1159–1164.

27. Birch, L. L., and Fisher, J. O. Food intake regulation in children, fat and sugar substitutes and intake. *Ann NY Acad of Sci* 1997; 819:194–220.

28. Rodgers, R. F., et al. Maternal feeding practices predict weight gain and obesogenic eating behaviors in young children: A prospective study. *Int J Behav Nutr Phys Act.* 2013; 10:24.

29. Bergmeier, H., et al. Associations between child termperament, maternal feeding practices and child body mass index during the preschool years: A systematic review of the literature. *Obes Rev.* 2014; 15(1):9–18.

30. Anzman, S. L., and Birch, L. L. Low inhibitory control and restrictive feeding practices predict weight outcomes. *J Pediatr.* 2009; 155(5):651–656.

31. Birch, L. L., and Fisher, J. O. Mothers' child-feeding practices influence daughters' eating and weight. *Amer J Clin Nutr* 2000; 71:1054–1061.

32. Birch, L. L., and Fisher, J. A. Appetite and eating behavior in children. *Pediatr Clinic N Amer* 1995; 42:931–953.

33. Birch, L. L. Psychological influences on the childhood diet. *J Nutr* 1998; 128:407S–10S.

34. Fisher, J. O., and Birch, L. L. Parents' restrictive feeding practices are associated with young girls' negative self evaluation of eating. *J Amer Diet Assoc* 2000; 100:1341–1346.

35. Birch, L. L., and Fisher, J. O. Development of eating behaviors among children and adolescents. *Pediatrics* 1998; 101:539–49(s).

36. Cachelin, F., et al. Does ethnicity influence body-size preference? A comparison of body image and body size. *Obesity Research* 2002; 10:158–166.

37. National Academy of Sciences, Institute of Medicine, Food and Nutrition Board. Dietary Reference Intakes for energy, carbohydrate, fiber, fat, protein, and amino acids. Washington, DC: National Academy Press, 2005.

38. U.S. Department of Health and Human Services and U.S. Department of Agriculture. Dietary Guidelines for Americans, 2010, 7th ed. Washington, DC: U.S. Government Printing Office, December 2010.

39. National Academy of Sciences, Institute of Medicine, Food and Nutrition Board. Dietary Reference Intakes for calcium, and vitamin D. Washington, DC: National Academy Press, 2010.

40. National Academy of Sciences, Institute of Medicine, Food and Nutrition Board. Dietary Reference Intakes for vitamin A, vitamin K, arsenic, boron, chromium, copper, iodine, iron, manganese, molybdenum, nickel, silicon, vanadium, and zinc. Washington, DC: National Academy Press, 2001.

41. Centers for Disease Control and Prevention. Iron deficiency. United States, 1999–2000. *Morbidity and Mortality Weekly Review* 2002; 51:897–899.

42. American Academy of Pediatrics, Committee on Nutrition. *Pediatric Nutrition Handbook*, 7th ed. Kleinman, R. E., ed. Elk Grove Village, IL: American Academy of Pediatrics, 201.

43. Centers for Disease Control and Prevention. Recommendations to prevent and control iron deficiency in the United States. *Morbidity and Mortality Weekly Report* April 3, 1998; 47:RR-03, 1–29.

44. Casamassimo, P., and Holt K, eds. *Bright Futures in Practice: Oral Health— Pocket Guide (2nd ed.).* Washington, DC: National Maternal and Child Oral Health Resource Center, 2014.

45. Slining, M. S., et al. Trends in food and beverage sources among US children and adolescents: 1989–2010. *J Acad Nutr Diet.* 2013; 113:1683–1694.

46. Freedman, D. S., et al. The relation of overweight to cardiovascular risk factors among children and adolescents: The Bogalusa Heart Study. *Pediatrics* 1999; 103:1175–1182.

47. Hoelscher, D. M., et al. Position of the Academy of Nutrition and dietetics: Interventions for the prevention and treatment of pediatric overweight and obesity. *J Acad Nutr Diet.* 2013; 113:1375–1394.

48. Ogden, C. L., et al. Prevalence of childhood and adult obesity in the United States, 2011–2012. *JAMA* 2014; 311(8):806–814.

49. Freedman, D. S., et al. Cardiovascular risk factors and excess adiposity among overweight children and adolescents: The Bogalusa Heart Study. *J Pediatr* 2007; 150:12–17.

50. Dietz, W. H. Health consequences of obesity in youth: Childhood predictors of adult disease. *Pediatrics* 1998; 101:518S–25S.

51. Dabelea, D., et al. Prevalence of type 1 and type 2 diabetes among children and adolescents from 2001 to 2009. *JAMA.* 2014; 311(17):1778–1786.

52. American Diabetes Association. Type 2 diabetes in children and adolescents. *Pediatrics* 2000; 105:671–80.

53. Dietz, W. H. Childhood weight affects adult morbidity and mortality. *J Nutr* 1998; 128:411S–14S.

54. Freedman, D. S., et al. BMI rebound, childhood height and obesity among adults: the Bogalusa Heart study. *Int J Obes Relat Metab Disord.* 001; 25:543–549.

55. Strauss, R. S., and Knight, J. Influence of the home environment on the development of obesity in children. *Pediatrics* [serial online] 1999; 103:e85. Available at http://www.aap .publications.org, accessed 07/12.

56. Whitaker, R. C., et al. Predicting obesity in young adulthood from childhood and parental obesity. *New Eng J Med* 1997; 337:869–873.

57. Dowda, M., Ainsworth, B. E., and Addy, C. L. Environmental influences, physical activity, and weight status in 8- to 16-year-olds. *Arch Pediatr Adolesc Med* 2001; 155:711–717.

58. U.S. Department of Health and Human Services. Health Indicators Warehouse. www .healthindicators.gov, accessed 05/15.

59. American Academy of Pediatrics, Council on Communications and Media. Policy Statement—Children, adolescents, obesity and the media. *Pediatrics* 2011; 128:201–208.

60. Klesges, R. C., Shelton, M. L., and Klesges, L. M. Effects of television on metabolic rate: Potential implications for childhood obesity. *Pediatrics* 1993; 91:281–286.

61. Wiecha, J. L., Peterson, K. E., Ludwig, D. S., Kim, J., Sobol, A., and Gortmaker, S. L. When children eat what they watch; impact of television viewing on dietary intake in youth. *Arch Pediatr Adolesc Med* 2006; 160(4):436–442.

62. Spear, B. A., et al. Recommendations for treatment of child and adolescent overweight and obesity. *Pediatrics* 2007; 120:S254–S288.

63. Davis, M. M., et al. Recommendations for prevention of childhood obesity. *Pediatrics* 2007; 120:S229–S253.

64. Hoelscher, D. M., Kirk, S., Ritchie, L., Cunningham-Sabo, L. Position of the Academy of Nutrition and Dietetics: Interventions for the prevention and treatment of pediatric overweight and obesity. *J Acad Nutr Diet* 2013; 113:1375–1394.

65. American Heart Association. Gidding, S. S., et al. Dietary recommendations for children and adolescents: A guide for practitioners. *Pediatrics* 2006; 117:544–59.

66. Lichtenstein, A. H., et al. Diet and lifestyle recommendations revision 2006: A scientific statement from the American Heart Association Nutrition Committee. *Circulation* 2006; 114:82–96.

67. Daniels, S. R., Greer F. R. American Academy of Pediatrics, Committee on Nutrition. Lipid screening and cardiovascular health in childhood. *Pediatrics*. 2008; 122(1):198–208.

68. Gidding, S. S., et al. Implementing American Heart Association pediatric and adult nutrition guidelines: A scientific statement from the American Heart Association Nutrition Committee of the Council on Nutrition, Physical Activity and Metabolism, Council on Cardiovascular Disease in the Young, Council on Arteriosclerosis, Thrombosis and Vascular Biology, Council on Cardiovascular Nursing, Council on Epidemiology and Prevention, and Council on High Blood Pressure Research. *Circulation* 2009; 119:1161–1175.

69. Expert Panel on Integrated Guidelines for Cardiovascular Health and Risk Reduction in Children and Adolescents. Expert panel on integrated guidelines for cardiovascular health and risk reduction in children and adolescents: summary report. *Pediatrics* 2011; 128:S213–256.

70. Black, L. I., Clarke, T. C., Barnes, P. M., Stussman, B. J., Nahin R. L. Use of complementary health approaches among children aged 4–17 years in the United States: National Health Interview Survey, 2007–2012. *Natl Health Stat Rep* 2015; Number 78.

71. Kranz, S., Brauchia, M., Slavin, J. L., Miller, K. B., What do we know about dietary fiber intake in children and health? The effects of fiber intake on constipation, obesity, and diabetes in children. *Adv Nutr* 2012; 3(1):47–53.

72. Dwyer, J. T. Dietary fiber for children: How much? *Pediatrics* 1995; 96:1019S–22S.

73. Golden, N. H., Abrams, S. A., and American Academy of Pediatrics, Committee on Nutrition. Optimizing bone health in children and adolescents. *Pediatrics* 2014; 134:e1229–e1243.

74. Heyman, M. B., and American Academy of Pediatrics, Committee on Nutrition. Lactose intolerance in infants, children, and adolescents. *Pediatrics* 2006; 118:1279–1286.

75. American Academy of Pediatrics. Committee on Nutrition and the Council on Sports Medicine and Fitness. Sports drinks and energy drinks for children and adolescents: are they appropriate? *Pediatrics* 2011; 127:1182–1189.

76. American College of Sports Medicine, Sawka, M. N., et al. American College of Sports Medicine position statement: Exercise and fluid replacement. *Medicine and Science in Sports and Exercise* 2007; 39:377–390.

77. Wang, V. C., et al. Increasing caloric contribution from sugar-sweetened beverages and 100% fruit juices among U.S.children and adolescents, 1988–2004. *Pediatrics* 2008; 121:e1604–e1614, accessed 07/12.

78. Ludwig, D. S., Peterson, K. E., and Gortmaker, S. L. Relation between consumption of sugar-sweetened drinks and childhood obesity: A prospective, observational analysis. *Lancet* 2001; 357:505–508.

79. Mrdjenovic, G., and Levitsky, D. A. Nutritional and energetic consequences of sweetened drink consumption in 6- to 13-year-old children. *J Pediatr* 2003; 142:604–610.

80. Rampersaud, G. C., et al. National survey beverage consumption data for children and adolescents indicate the need to encourage a shift toward more nutritive beverages. *J Am Diet Assoc* 2003; 97–100.

81. Bowman, S. A., et al. Effects of fast-food consumption on energy intake and diet quality among children in a national household survey. *Pediatrics* 2004; 113:112–118.

82. American Dietetic Association. Position of the American Dietetic Association: Use of nutritive and nonnutritive sweeteners. *J Acad Nutr Diet* 2012; 112:739–758.

83. U.S. Department of Agriculture, Agricultural Research Service, 2014. *What We Eat in America,* NHANES 2011–2012. Available at http://www.ars.usda.gov/Services/docs. htm?docid=18349, accessed 05/15.

84. Guenther, P. M., Casavale, K. O., Reedy, J., Kirkpatrick, S. I., Hiza, H. A. B., Kuczynski, K. J., Kahle, L. L, Krebs-Smith, S. M. Update of the Healthy Eating Index: HEI-2010. *J Acad Nutr* Diet 2013; 113(4):569–580.

85. United States Department of Agriculture, Center for Nutrition Policy and Prevention. Diet quality of children age 2–17 years as measured by the Healthy Eating Index-2010. 2013. Available at: http://www.cnpp.usda.gov/sites/default/files/nutrition_insights_uploads/Insight52.pdf, accessed 05/15.

86. Kittler, P. G., Sucher, K. P., and Nelms, M. *Food and culture*, 6th ed. Belmont, CA: Wadsworth/Thomson Learning, 2011.

87. Cullum-Dugan, D., Pawlak, R. Position of the Academy of Nutrition and Dietetics: Vegetarian Diets. *J Acad Nutr Diet.* 2015; 115:801–810.

88. Messina, V., and Mangel, A. R. Considerations in planning vegan diets: Children. *J Amer Diet Assoc* 2001; 101:661–669.

89. American Academy of Pediatrics, Council on Sports Medicine and Fitness and Council on School Health. Active healthy living: prevention of childhood obesity through increased physical activity. *Pediatrics* 2006; 117:1834–1842.

90. American Academy of Pediatrics, Committee on Environmental Health. The built environment: Designing communities to promote physical activity in children. *Pediatrics* 2009; 123:1591–1598.

91. Department of Health and Human Services *2008 Physical Activitiy Guidelines for Americans.* Available at www.health.gov/paguidelines/, accessed 07/12.

92. Kohl, H. W., and Hobbs, K. E. Development of physical activity behaviors among children and adolescents. *Pediatrics* 1998; 101:549–554.

93. American Academy of Pediatrics, Committee on Sports Medicine and Fitness and Committee on School Health. Organized sports for children and preadolescents. *Pediatrics* 2001; 107:1459–1462.

94. American Academy of Pediatrics, Committee on Nutrition and Council on Sports Medecine and Fitness. Clinical report-sports drinks and energy drinks for children and adolescents: are they appropriate? *Pedaitrics* 2011; 127(6):1182–1189.

95. American Dietetic Association. Join Position of ADA, Society for Nutrition Education, and School Nutrition Association: Comprehensive school nutrition services. *J Amer Diet Assoc* 2010; 110:1738–1749.

96. Celebuski, C., Farris, E. Nutrition education in public elementary school classrooms, K–5. Washington, D. C: US Department of Education, Office of Educational Research and Improvement; 2000. NCES 2000–040. Available at: http://nces. ed.gov/surveys/frss/publications/2000040/, accessed 05/15.

97. United States Department of Agriculture, Team Nutrition. Local School Wellness Policy. 2015. Available at: http://www.fns.usda.gov/tn/local-school-wellness-policy, accessed 05/15.

98. American Dietetic Association. Position of the American Dietetic Association: Local support for nutrition integrity in schools. *J Amer Diet Assoc* 2010; 110:1244–1254.

99. Fox, M. K., Gordon, A., Nogales, R., Wilson, A. Availability and consumption of competitive foods in US public schools. *J Amer Diet Assoc.* 2009; 109:S57–S66.

100. Finkelstein, D. M., et al. School food environments and policies in US public schools. *Pediatrics* 2008; 122:e251–e359.

101. American Academy of Pediatrics, Committee on School Health. Soft drinks in schools. *Pediatrics* 2004; 113:152–154.

102. American Academy of Pediatrics, Council on School Health and Committee on Nutrition. Policy Statement: snacks, sweetened beverages, added sugars, and schools. *Pediatrics* 2015; 135:575–583.

103. Centers for Disease Control and Prevention. School Health Index: A self-assessment and planning guide, elementary school version. Atlanta, GA: 2014. Available at http://www.cdc.gov/Healthyyouth/SHI/pdf/Elementary-Total-2014-Tagged_508.pdf, accessed 05/15.

104. Hagan, J. F., Shaw, J. S., and Duncan, P. M., eds. *Bright Futures: Guidelines for Health Supervision of Infants, Children, and*

*Adolescents*, 3rd ed. Elk Grove Village, IL: American Academy of Pediatrics, 2008.

105. Centers for Disease Control and Prevention, National Fruit and Vegetable Program. *Fruits & Veggies—More Matters.* Available at www.fruitsandveggiesmorematters.org, accessed 05/15.

106. American Dietetic Association. Position of the American Dietetic Association: Child and adolescent nutrition assistance programs. *J Amer Diet Assoc* 2010; 110:791–799.

107. United States Department of Agriculture, Economic Research Service. Ralston, K., et al. The National School Lunch Program: Background, trends, and issues. *Economic Research Report* Number 61, July 2008. Available at http://www.ers.usda.gov/publications/err-economic-research-report/err61.aspx, accessed 05/15.

108. U.S. Department of Agriculture, Food and Nutrition Service. 7 CFR Parts 210 and 220. Nutrition Standards in the National School Lunch and School Breakfast Programs; Final Rule. *Federal Register* 77 (17): January 26, 2012.

109. U.S. Department of Agriculture, Food and Nutrition Service. *Team Nutrition.* Available at http://www.fns. usda.gov/tn/team-nutrition, accessed 05/15.

## Chapter 13

1. United States Department of Education, Office of Special Education Services. Center for Parent Information and Resources. Newark, NJ: U.S. Government Printing Office. Available at http://www.parentcenterhub.org/resources/, accessed 05/15.

2. U.S. Department of Education, Office of Special Education Programs Individualized Education Plans. Available at idea.ed.gov, accessed 05/15.

3. Autism and Developmental Disabilities Monitoring Network Surveillance Year 2010 Principal Investigators. Prevalence of autism spectrum disorders among children aged 8 years—Autism and developmental disabilities monitoring network, 11 sites, United States, 2010. *MMWR* 2014; 63(SS02):1–21.

4. United States Department of Education. National Center for Education Statistics. Children and youth with disabilities. Students with disabilities. Available at https://nces.ed.gov/fastfacts/display.asp?id=64, accessed 05/15.

5. United States Department of Health and Human Services, Health resources and Services Administration, Maternal and Child Health Bureau. *The National Survey of Children with Special Health Care Needs 2009-2010.* Rockville, MD: U.S. Department of Health and Human Services, 2012. Available at http://childhealthdata.org/learn/NS-CSHCN, accessed 05/15.

6. United States Department of Health and Human Services, Health resources and Services Administration, Maternal and Child Health Bureau. *The Mental and Emotional Well-Being of Children: a Portrait of State and the Nation 2007.* Rockville, MD: U.S. Department of Health and Human Services, 2010.

7. Perrin, J. M., Bloom, S. R., and Gorkmaker, S. L. The increase of childhood chronic conditions in the United States. *J Am Med Assoc* 2007; 297(24):2755–2759.

8. Brooks, J., Day, S., Shavelle, R., and Strauss, D. Low weight, morbidity and mortality in children with cerebral palsy: New clinical growth charts. *Pediatrics* 2011; 128 (9):e299–e307.

9. Stevenson, R. D., Conaway, M. R. Weight and mortality rates: "Gómez classification" for children with cerebral palsy? *Pediatrics* 2011; 128(2):e436–437.

10. Isaacs, J. S., and Zand, D. Single-gene autosomal recessive disorders and Prader-Willi syndrome: An update for food and nutrition professionals. *J Am Diet Assoc* 2007; 107(3):466–478.

11. Institute of Medicine Food and Nutrition Board. Dietary reference intakes for energy, carbohydrate, fiber, fat, fatty acids, cholesterol, protein, and amino acids, 2002.

12. Kleinman, R. E., ed. *Pediatric nutrition handbook*, 6th ed. Chicago: American Academy of Pediatrics, 2009: 821–842.

13. DeVore, J., and Shotton, A., eds. *Pocket Guide to Children with Special Health Care and Nutritional Needs.* Chicago: Academy of Nutrition and Dietetics, 2012.

14. Healthy People 2020 Objectives. Available at http://www.healthypeople.gov/2020/topicsobjectives2020, accessed 8/12.

15. Dietary Guidelines for Americans, 2010. Available at www.dietaryguidelines.gov, accessed 8/12.

16. Bankhead, R., Boullata, J., Brantley, S., Corkins, M., Guenter, P., Krenitsky, J., et al., A.S.P.E.N. Enteral Nutrition Practice Recommendations. *JPEN J Parenter Enteral Nutr* 2009; 33: 122–167.

17. Prader-Willi Syndrome. Updated 2011. Available at http://www.mayoclinic.com/health/prader-willi-syndrome/DS00922, accessed 7/12.

18. Schertz, M., et al. Predictors of weight loss in children with attention deficit hyperactivity disorder treated with stimulant medication. *Pediatrics* 1996; 98:763–769.

19. Yang Y., Lucas B., Feucht S., editors. *Nutrition Interventions for Children with Special Health Care Needs,* 3rd ed. Washington State Department of Health; 2010.

20. Dodge, J. A., and Turck, D. Cystic fibrosis: Nutritional consequences and management. *Best Practice & Research in Clinical Gastroenterology* 2006; 20:531–46.

21. Lefebvre, D. E., et al. Dietary proteins as environmental modifiers of type 1 diabetes mellitus. *Annu Rev Nutr* 2006; 26:175–202.

22. Parrish, C. R. Nutritional assessment and intervention in cerebral palsy. *Nutrition Issues in Gastroenterology* 2011; series 92.

23. U.S. Department of Health and Human Services. National Institutes of Health, National Institute of Allergy and Infectious Diseases. *Guidelines for the diagnosis and management of food allergy in the United States.* Washington, DC: U.S. Government Printing Office, NIH Publication No 11-7700, 2010.

24. Trumbo, P., et al. Dietary reference intakes: Vitamin A, vitamin K, arsenic, boron, chromium, copper, iodine, iron, manganese, molybdenum, nickel, silicon, vanadium, and zinc. *J Am Diet Assoc* 2001; 101:294–301.

25. Greer, F. R., and Krebs, N. F. Committee on Nutrition. Optimizing bone health and calcium intakes of infants, children, and adolescents. *Pediatrics* 2006; 117:578–585.

26. Hagan, J. F., Shaw, J. S., and Duncan, P. M., eds. *Bright Futures: Guidelines for Health Supervision of Infants, Children and Adolescents.* Elk Grove Village, IL: American Academy of Pediatrics, 2008.

27. Food and Nutrition Board, Institute of Medicine. *Report Brief: Dietary Reference Intakes for Calcium and Vitamin D.* Washington, DC: National Academies Press; 2010. Available at http://tinyurl.com/2b5ych3, accessed 8/12.

28. Brown, T. Critically ill children often are deficient in Vitamin D. Medscape Education 2012. Available at www.medscape.org, accessed 8/12.

29. Centers for Disease Control and Prevention. National Center for Health Statistics. *NCHS growth curves for children 0–19 years.* U.S. Vital and Health Statistics, Health Resources Administration. Washington, DC: U.S. Government Printing Office, 2000.

30. D'Amico, A., Mercuri, E., Tiziano, F. D., and Bertini, E. Spinal muscular atrophy. *Orphanet J Rare Dis.* 2011; 6:71.

31. Lucas, A., Fewtrell, M. S., and Cole, T. J. Fetal origins of adult disease—The hypothesis revisited. *Br Med J* 1999; 319(7204):245–249.

32. Dewey, K. G., Begum, K. Long-term consequences of stunting in early life. *Matern Child Nutr* 2011; 7, Supple s3:5–18.

33. Duijts, L. Fetal and infant origins of asthma. *Eur J Epidemiol.* 2012; 27(1): 5–14.

34. Bull MJ; American Academy of Pediatrics Committee on Genetics. Clinical report—Health supervision for children with Down syndrome. *Pediatrics* 2011; 128:393–406.

35. Frisancho, A. R. Triceps skinfold and upper arm muscle size norms for assessment of nutritional status. *Am J Clin Nutr* 1974; 27:1052–1157.

36. Fomon, S., et al. Body composition of reference children from birth to age 10 years. *Am J Clin Nutr* 1982; 35:1169–1175.

37. Carel, J. C., Ecosse, E., Landier, F., et al. Long-term mortality after recombinant growth hormone treatment for isolated growth hormone deficiency or childhood short stature: preliminary report of the French SAGhE study. *J Clin Endocrinol Metab.* 2012; 97(2):416–425.

38. Nellhaus, G. Composite international and interracial graphs. *Pediatrics* 1968; 41:106–114.

39. Batshaw, M. L. Chromosomes and heredity. In Batshaw, M. L., Pellegrino, L., and Roizen, N. J., eds. *Children with disabilities*, 6th ed. Baltimore, MD: Paul H. Brookes, 2007: 3–26, 770.

40. *Growth references: Third trimester to adulthood*, 3rd ed. Clinton, SC: Greenwood Genetic Center, 2011.

41. Elias E. R., Murphy N. A., and the Council on Children with Disabilities. Home care of children and youth with complex health care needs and technology dependencies. *Pediatrics* 2012; 129:996–1005.

42. Mahant, S., Jovcevska, V., and Cohen, E. Decision-making around gastrostomy—Feeding in children with neurologic disabilities *Pediatrics* 2011; 127(6):e1471–1481.

43. Mahant, S., Pastor, A. C., Deoliveira, L., Nicholas, D. B., and Langer, J. C. Well-being of children with neurologic impairment after fundoplication and gastrojejunostomy tube feeding. *Pediatrics* 2011; 128(2):e395–403.

44. World Health Organization. Nutrition for HIV-infected infants and children. In: *Antiretroviral Therapy for HIV Infections in Infants and Children: Towards Universal Access Recommendations for a Public Health Approach*. 2010; 69–75.

45. Shingadia, D., et al. Gastrostomy tube insertion for improvement of adherence to highly active antiretrovial therapy in pediatric patients with human immunodeficiency virus. *Pediatrics* 2000; 105:1–5. Available at www.pediatrics.org/cgi/content/full/105/6/e80, accessed 8/12.

46. Stallings, V. A., Stark, L. J., Robinson, K. A., Feranchak, A. P., Quinton, H., and Clinical Practice Guidelines on Growth and Nutrition Subcommittee; Ad Hoc Working Group. Evidence-Based Practice Recommendations for Nutrition-Related Management of Children and Adults with Cystic Fibrosis and Pancreatic Insufficiency: Results of a Systematic Review. *J Am Diet Assoc* 2008; 108(5):832–839.

47. American Diabetes Association. Position Statement. Standards of Medical Care in Diabetes—2012. *Diabetes Care* 2012; 35 Suppl 1 S11–S63, 48.

48. Crowther, N. J., Cameron, N., Trusler, J., Toman, M., Norris, S. A., and Gray, I. P. Influence of catch-up growth on glucose tolerance and β-cell function in 7-year-old children: Results from the birth to twenty study. *Pediatrics* 2008; 121:e1715–e1722.

49. National Institutes of Health. National Institute of Diabetes, and Digestive and Kidney Diseases. National Diabetes Information Clearinghouse. National diabetes statistics—2011. New cases of diagnosed diabetes among people younger than 20 years of age, United States, 2002–2005. Available at http://www.diabetes.niddk.nih.gov/dm/pubs/statistics/#NewCasesDDY20, accessed 8/12.

50. Kossoff, E. H., Zupec-Kania, B. A, Rho, J. M. Ketogenic diets: An update for child neurologists. *J Child Neurol.* 2009; 24(8):979–988.

51. Pellegrino, L. Cerebral palsy. In Batshaw, M. L., Pellegrino, L., and Roizen, N. J., eds. *Children with disabilities*, 6th ed. Baltimore, MD: Paul H. Brookes, 2007: 387–408.

52. Burlina, A., and Blau, N. Effect of BH(4) supplementation on phenylalanine tolerance. *J Inherit Metab Dis* 2009; 32(1):40–45.

53. Perrin, J. M., Friedman, R. A., and Knilans, T. K. Black Box Working Groups, Section on Cardiology and Cardiac Surgery. Cardiovascular Monitoring and Stimulant Drugs for Attention-Deficit/Hyperactivity Disorder. *Pediatrics* 2008; 122:451–453.

54. Zachor, D. A., et al. Effects of long-term psychostimulant medication on growth of children with ADHD. *Res Dev Disabil* 2006; 27:162–174.

55. Kemper, K. J., Vohra, S., and Walls, R. Task Force on Complementary and Alternative Medicine. The use of complementary and alternative medicine in pediatrics. *Pediatrics* 2008; 122:1374–1386.

56. Ball, S. D., Kertesz, D., and Moyer-Mileur, L. J. Dietary supplement use is prevalent among children with a chronic illness. *J Am Diet Assoc* 2005; 105(1):78–84.

57. Weber, W., Vander Stoep, A., McCarty, R. L., et al. Hypericum perforatum (St. John's Wort) for attention-deficit/hyperactivity disorder in children and adolescents. *JAMA* 2008; 299(22):2633–2641.

58. Steele, R., Gibson, P., Anderson, R., Day, A., Cameron, D., Hogan, C., et al. Diagnosis and management of coeliac disease in children. *Postgrad Med J.* 2011; 87(1023):19–25.

59. National Institutes of Health. National Institute of Diabetes, and Digestive and Kidney Diseases. Celiac Awareness Campaign. Available at http://celiac.nih.gov, accessed 8/12.

60. National Down Syndrome Society. Alternative therapies. Available at http://www.ndss.org/en/Healthcare/Alternative-Therapies, accessed 8/12.

61. Maternal and Child Health Bureau, Health and Human Services. Available at http://mchb.hrsa.gov/html/drte.html, accessed 8/12.

62. Murphy, N. A., Carbone, P. S., and the Council on Children with Disabilities. Clinical Report. Parent–provider–community partnerships: optimizing outcomes for children with disabilities. *Pediatrics* 2011; 128(4):795–802.

## Chapter 14

1. Tanner, J. Growth at adolescence, Oxford: Blackwell Scientific Publications, 1962.

2. Rosenfield, R. L., et al.: Thelarche, pubarche and menarche attainment in children with normal and elevated body mass index, Pediatrics 123(1):84, 2009.

3. Unknown from old version.

4. Poulton, A. S., et al. Growth and pubertal development of adolescent boys on stimulant medication for attention deficit hyperactivity disorder. *Med J Aust* 198(1):29, 2013.

5. Frisch, R. E. Fatness, puberty, and fertility: The effects of nutrition and physical training on menarche and ovulation. In Brooks-Gunn, J., and Peterson, A. C., eds. Girls at Puberty: Biological and Psychosocial Perspectives. New York: Plenum Press, 1983, 29–49.

6. Frisch, R. E., and McArthur, J. W. Menstrual cycles: Fatness as a determinant of minimum weight for height necessary for their maintenance or onset. *Science* 1974; 185:949–951.

7. Bonjour, J-P., Gueguen, L., Palcios, C., Shearer, M. J., Weaver, C. M. Minerals and vitamins in bone health: The potential value of dietary enhancement. *British Journal Nutrition* 2009;101:1581–1596.

8. Blakemore, S-J., Robbins, T. W. Decision-making in the adolescent brain, *Nat Neurosci* 2012; 15(9):1184.

9. Steinberg, L. *Adolescence,* 9th ed. New York: McGraw-Hill Higher Education, 2010.

10. Tremblay, L., and Lariviere, M. The influence of puberty onset, body mass index and pressure to be thin on disordered eating behaviors. *Eat Behav* 2009; 10(2):75–83.

11. Bratberg, G. H., Nilesen, T. I., Holmen, T. L., and Vatten, L. J. Perceived pubertal timing, pubertal status and the prevalence of alcohol drinking and cigarette smoking in early and late adolescence: A population-based study of 8950 Norwegian boys and girls. *Acta Paediatr* 2007; 96(2):292–295.

12. Gellar, L., et al. Exploratory research to design a school nurse-delivered intervention to treat adolescent overweight and obesity. *J Nutr Educ Behav* 2012; 44:46.

13. Berge, J. M., et al. Healthful eating and physical activity in the home environment: results from multi-family focus groups. *J Nutr Educ* 2012; 44:123.

14. Cusatis, D. C., et al. Longitudinal nutrient intake patterns of U.S. adolescent women: The Penn State Young Women's Health Study. *J Adolesc Health* 2000; 26:194–204.

15. US Department of Agriculture, Agricultural Research Service. 2014. Snacks: Distribution of snack occasions, by gender and age. *What we eat in America*, 2011–2012.

16. Larson, N., and Story, M. A review of snacking patterns among U.S. children and adolescents: What are the implications of snacking for weight status? *Child Obes* 2013; 9:104.

17. Sebastian, R. S., Goldman, J. D., and Wilkinson, Enns C. Snacking patterns of U.S. adolescents. *What we eat in America.* NHANES 2005–2006 Food Surveys Research Group Dietary Data Brief No. 2. September 2010.

18. Sebastian, R. S., Cleveland, L. E., and Goldman, J. D. Effect of snacking frequency on adolescents' dietary intakes and meeting national recommendations. *J Adolesc Health* 2008; 42:503–511.

19. US Department of Agriculture, Agricultural Research Service. 2014. Snacks: Percentages of selected nutrient contributed by food and beverages consumed at snack occasions,

by gender and age, *What we eat in America,* NHANES 2011–2012.

20. Reedy, J., and Krebs-Smith, S. M. Dietary sources of energy, solid fats, and added sugars among children and adolescents in the United States. *J Am Diet Assoc* 110(10):1477–1484. 2010.

21. Han, E., and Powell, L. M. Consumption patterns of sugar-sweetened beverages in the United States. *J Acad Nutr Diet* 2013; 113:343.

22. Centers for Disease Control and Prevention. Youth Risk Behavior Surveillance—United States, 2013. *MMWR* 2014; 63(4):17–42.

23. Moore, L.L., et al. Food group intake and micronutrient adequacy in adolescent girls. *Nutrients* 2012; 4:1692.

24. Woodruff, S. J., Hanning, R. M., Lambraki, I., Storey, K. E., and McCarger, L. Healthy Eating Index-C is compromised among adolescents with body weight concerns, weight loss dieting and meal skipping. *Body Image* 2008; 5:404–408.

25. Timlin, M. T., Pereira, M. A., Story, M., and Neumark-Sztainer, D. Breakfast eating and weight change in a 5-year prospective analysis of adolescents: Project EAT. *Pediatrics* 2008; 121:e638–e645.

26. Larson, N. I., Nelson, M. C., Neumark-Sztainer, D., Story, M., and Hannan, P. J. Making time for meals: Meal structure and associations with dietary intake in young adults. *J Am Diet Assoc* 2009; 109:72–79.

27. US Department of Agriculture, Agricultural Research Service. 2014. Away from home: Percentages of selected nutrients contributed by food and beverages, by gender and age. *What We Eat in America,* NHANES 2011–2012.

28. Poti, J. M., Slining, M. M., and Popkin, B. M. Where are kids getting their empty calories? Stores, school and fast-food restaurants each played an important role in empty calorie intake among US children during 2009–2010. *JAND* 2014;114:908–917.

29. USDA http://www.fns.usda.gov/sites/default/files/pd/slsummar.pdf.

30. Fox, M. K., et al. *School Nutrition Dietary Assessment Study IV, Volume I: School Foodservice Operations, School Environments, and Meals Offered and Served.* Alexandria, VA: U.S. Department of Agriculture, Food and Nutrition Service, Office of Research and Analysis, 2012.

31. US Department of Agriculture, Food and Nutrition Service. 7 CFR Parts 210 and 220. Local School Wellness Policy Implementation under the Healthy, Hunger-Free Kids Act of 2010. Federal Register, Feb 26, 2014. http://federalregister.gov/a/2014-04100.

32. Child Trends. Family meals: indicators on children and youth, 2013. http://www.childtrends.org/wp-content/uploads/2012/09/96_Family_Meals.pdf, accessed 12/13.

33. Larson, N., et al. Eating breakfast and dinner together as a family: associations with sociodemographic characteristics and implications for diet quality and weight status. *J Acad Nutr Diet* 2013; 113:1601.

34. Fulkerson, J. A., et al. A review of associations between family or shared meal frequency and dietary and weight status outcomes across the lifespan. *J Nutr Educ Behav.* 2014; 46:2.

35. Neumark-Sztainer, D., et al. Family meals and adolescents: what have we learned from Project EAT (Eating Among Teens), *Public Health Nutr* 2010; 13:1113.

36. Robinson-O'Brien, R., Perry, C. L., Wall, M. M., Story, M., and Neumark-Sztainer, D. Adolescent and young adult vegetarianism: Better dietary intake and weight outcomes but increased risk of disordered eating behaviors. *J Am Diet Assoc* 2009; 109(4): 648–655.

37. Rosell, M., Appleby, P., and Key, T. Height, age at menarche, body weight and body mass index in life-long vegetarians. *Public Health Nutr* 2005; 8(7):870–875.

38. Winston, C. J. Health effects of vegan diets. *Am J Clin Nutr* 2009; 89(suppl):1627S1633S.

39. Office of Disease Prevention and Health Promotion, U.S. Department of Health and Human Services, 2008. Physical Activity Guidelines for Americans. Available at www.health.gov/guidelines, accessed 6/30/2009.

40. Bielemann RM, Martinez-Mesa J, Petrucci Gigante D. Physical activity during life course and bone mass: a systemati review of methods and findings from cohort studies with young adults. *BMC Musculoskeletal Disorders* 2013;14:77.

41. Stanley, R. M., Ridley, K., and Dollman, J. Correlates of children's time-specific physical activity: A review of the literature. *International Journal of Behavior Nutrition and Physical Activity* 2012;9:50.

42. Food and Nutrition Board, Institute of Medicine. Otten, J. J., Hellwig, J. P., and Meyers, L. D., eds. Dietary Reference Intakes: The essential guide to nutrient requirements. Washington, DC: National Academies Press, 2006.

43. Community Nutrition Research Group, Beltsville Human Nutrition Research Center, Agricultural Research Service, USDA. Pyramid serving intakes in the U.S. 1999–2002, 1 day. Available at www.ba.urs.usda.gov/cnrg.

44. US Department of Agriculture, Agricultural Research Service. 2014. Energy intakes: Percentages of energy from protein, carbohydrate, fat and alcohol, by gender and age, *What we eat in America,* NHANES 2011–2012.

45. Weaver, C. M. Vitamin D, calcium homeostasis and skeletal accretion in children. *Journal of Bone and Mineral Research* 2007; 22(2).

46. U.S. Department of Agriculture, Agricultural Research Service. 2014. Nutrient intakes from food and beverages: mean amounts consumed per individual, by gender and age. *What we eat in America,* NHANES 2011–2012.

47. Gao, X., et al. Meeting adequate intake for dietary calcium without dairy foods in adolescents aged 9 to 18 years (National Health and Nutrition Examination Survey 2001–2022). *J Amer Diet Assn* 2006; 106:1759–1765.

48. Rajeshwari, R., Nicklas, T. A., Yang, S. J., and Berenson, G. S. Longitudinal changes in intake and food sources of calcium from childhood to young adulthood: The Bogalusa Heart Study. *J Am Coll Nutr* 2004; 23:341–350.

49. Hearney, R. P., and Rafferty, K. The settling problem in calcium-fortified soybean drinks. *J Amer Diet Assoc* 2006; 106:1753.

50. Centers for Disease Control and Prevention. Recommendations to prevent and control iron deficiency anemia in the United States. *Morb Mortal Wkly Rep* 2002; 51(40):897–899.

51. Ginde, A. A., Liu, M. C., and Camargo, C. A. Demographic differences and trends of vitamin D insufficiency in the U.S. population, 1988–2004. *Arch Intern Med* 2009; 169(6):626–632.

52. Wagner, C. L., and Greer, F. R. American Academy of Pediatrics Section on Breastfeeding and Committee on Nutrition. Prevention of rickets and vitamin D de-ficiency in children. *Pediatrics* 2008; 122:1142–1152.

53. Reis, J. P., von Muhlen, D., Miller, E. R. III, Michos, E. D., and Appel, L. J. Vitamin D Status and Cardiometabolic Risk Factors in the US Adolescent Population. *Pediatrics* 2009; 124:e371–e379.

54. Institute of Medicine: Dietary reference intakes for calcium and vitamin D. Washington, DC: The National Academies Press, 2011.

55. Holick, M. F., et al. Evaluation, treatment, and prevention of vitamin D deficiency: an Endocrine Society clinical practice guidelines. *J Clin Endocrinol Metab* 2011; 96:1911.

56. Wagner, C. L., and Greer, F. R. American Academy of Pediatrics Section on Breastfeeding and Committee on Nutrition. Prevention of rickets and vitamin D de-ficiency in children. *Pediatrics* 2008; 122:1142–1152.

57. McDowell, M. A., Lacher, D. A., Pfeiffer, C. M., Mulinare, J., Picciano, M. F., Rader, J. L., Yetley, E. A., Kennedy-Stephenson, J., and Johnson, C. L. Blood folate levels: The latest NHANES results. NCHS Data Brief. 2008; 6:1–8. Available at http://www.cdc.gov/nchs/data/databriefs/db06.htm.

58. Centers for Disease Control and Prevention, National Center for Environmental Health. Second National Report on Biochemical Indicators of Diet and Nutrition in the U.S. Population. 2012. Available at http://www.cdc.gov/nutritionreport/, accessed online July 31, 2012.

59. U.S. Department of Agriculture, Agricultural Research Service, 2008. Nutrient Intakes from Food: Mean Amounts Consumed per Individual, One Day, 2005–2006. Available at www.ars.usda.gov/ba/bnnrc/fsrg.

60. Barlow, S. E. Expert Committee recommendation regarding the prevention, assessment and treatment of child and adolescent

overweight and obesity: Summary report. *Pediatrics* 2007; 120:S164–S192.

61. National Cancer Institute. Automated Self-Administered 24-hour Dietary Recall. Available at https://asa24.westat.com/.

62. Olson, A. L., Gaffney, C. A., Hedberg, V. A., and Gladstone, G. R. Use of inexpensive technology to enhance adolescent health screening and counselling. *Arch Pediatr Adolesc Med* 2009; 163(2):172–177.

63. Leverton, R. M. The paradox of teen-age nutrition. *J Amer Diet Assoc* 1968; 53:13–16.

64. Larson, N., Lask, M. N., Story, M., Neumark-Sztainer, D. Predictors of fruit and vegetables intake in young adulthood. *J Academy Nutrition Dietetics* 2012; 112:1216–1222.

65. Cutler, G. J., Flood, A., Hannan, P., Neumark-Sztainer, D. Multiple sociodemographic and socioenvironmental characteristics are correlated with major patterns of dietary intake in adolescents. *J American Dietetic Assn.* 2011; 111:230–240.

66. Arcan, C., Neumark-Sztainer, D., Hannan, P., von den Berg, P., Story, M., and Larson, N. Parental eating behaviours, home food environment and adolescent intakes of fruits, vegetables and dairy foods: Longitudinal findings from Project EAT. *Public Health Nutr* 2007; 10(11):1257–1265.

67. O'Dougherty, M., Story, M., and Lytle, L. Food choices of young African-American and Latino adolescents: Where do parents fit in? *J Am Diet Assoc* 2006; 106:1846–1850.

68. Centers for Disease Control and Prevention. School Health Guidelines to Promote Healthy Eating and Physical Activity. *Morb Mortal Wkly Rep.* September 16, 2011; 60(RR05); 1–71.

69. Centers for Disease Control and Prevention. School Health Index: A Self-Assessment and Planning Guide. Middle school/high school version. Atlanta, Georgia. 2012.

70. Centers for Disease Control and Prevention. Strategies to Improve the Quality of Physical Education. Atlanta, Georgia. 2010. Available at http://www.cdc.gov/healthyyouth/physicalactivity/pdf/quality_pe.pdf.

71. Centers for Disease Control and Prevention. Results from the School Health Policies and Practices Study, 2012. Atlanta, Georgia. 2013.

72. Demissie, Z., Brener, N. D., McManus, T., Shanklin, S. L., Hawkins, J., and Kann, L. Results from the School Health Profiles, 2012: Characteristics of Health Programs Among Secondary Schools. Centers for Disease Control and Prevention. Atlanta, Georgia; 2013. Available at http://www.cdc.gov/healthyyouth/profiles/index.htm.

73. US Department of Agriculture, Food and Nutrition Service. National School Lunch Program Fact Sheet. September 2013. Available at http://www.fns.usda.gov/sites/default/files/NSLPFactSheet.pdf.

74. US Department of Agriculture, Food and Nutrition Service. Smart Snacks in School: USDA's "All Foods Sold in Schools" Standards. USDA 2014. Available at http://www.fns.usda.gov/sites/default/files/allfoods_flyer.pdf.

75. Federal Register. Volume 77, No. 17, Part II. 7 CFR Parts 210 and 220. Nutrition Standards in the National School Lunch and School Breakfast Programs; Final Rule. January 26, 2012.

76. Hanks, A. S., Just, D. R., Wansink, B. Smarter lunchrooms can address new school lunchroom guidelines and child obesity. *J Pediatr* 2013; 162:867–869.

77. Wansink, B., Just, D. R., Payne, C. R., and Klinger, M. Z. Attractive names sustain increased vegetable intake in schools. *Preventive Medicine* 2012; 55:330–332.

78. Urban Roots, Annual Report: September 2011–August 2012. Available at http://urbanrootsmn.org/annual-report/.

## *Chapter 15*

1. Nader, P. R., et al. National Institute of Child Health and Human Development, Early Child Care Research Network. Identifying risk for obesity in early childhood. *Pediatrics* 2006 Sept.; 118(3):e594–601.

2. Barlow, S. E. Expert Committee recommendation regarding the prevention, assessment and treatment of child and adolescent overweight and obesity: Summary report. *Pediatrics* 2007; 120:S164–S192.

3. Rutman, S., Park, A., Castor, M., et al. "Urban American Indian and Alaska Native Youth: Youth Risk Behavior Survey 1997–2003." *Maternal and Child Health Journal* 2008; 12(S1):S76–S81.

4. Zephier, E., Himes, J. H., Story, M., and Zhou, X. Increasing Prevalences of Overweight and Obesity in Northern Plains American Indian Children. *Arch Pediatr Adolesc Med* 2006; 160:34–39.

5. Singh, A. S., Mulder, C., Twisk, J. W. R., van Mechelsen, W., and Chinapaw, M. J. Tracking of childhood overweight into adulthood: A systematic review of the literature. *Obes Rev* 2008; 9:474–488.

6. Kelly, A. S., et al. Severe obesity in children and adolescents: identification, associated health risks, and treatment approaches: a scientific statement from the American Heart Association. *Circulation* 2013; 128:1689.

7. Reilly, J. J., Kelly, J. Long-term impact of overweight and obesity in childhood and adolescence on morbidity and premature mortality in adulthood: systematic review. *Int J Obes* 2011; 35:891.

8. Spear, B. A., Barlow, S. E., Ervin, C., et al. Recommendations for treatment of child and adolescent overweight and obesity. *Pediatrics* 2007; 120:S254–S288.

9. August, G. P., Caprio, S., Fennoy, I., et al. Prevention and Treatment of Pediatric Obesity: An Endocrine Society Clinical Practice Guidelines Based on Expert Opinion. *J Clin Endocrinol Metab.* 2008; 93(12):4576–4599.

10. Matson, K. L., Fallon, R. M. Treatment of Obesity in Children and Adolescents. *J Pediatr Pharmacol Ther* 2012; 17(1):45–57.

11. Pratt, J. S. A., Lenders, C. M., Dionne, E. A., et al. Best practice updates for pediatric/adolescent weight loss surgery. *Obesity* 2009; 17:901–910.

12. Ibele, A. R., Mattar, S. G. Adolescent Bariatric Surgery. *Surg Clin N Am* 2011; 91:1339–1351.

13. Treadwell, J. R., Sun, F., Schoelles, K. Systematic review and meta-analysis of bariatric surgery for pediatric obesity. *Ann Surg.* 2008; 248:763–776.

14. Lawson, M. L., et al. One-year outcomes of Roux-en-Y gastric bypass for morbidly obese adolescents: A multicenter study from the Pediatric Bariatric Study Group. *J Ped Surg* 2006; 41:137–143.

15. Fullmer, M. A., Abrams, S. H., Hrovat, K., Mooney, L., et al. Nutritional strategy for adolescents undergoing bariatric surgery: Report of a working group of the nutrition committee of the NASPGHAN/NACHRI. *JPGN* 2012; 54: 125–135.

16. Dwyer, J., et al. Prevalence and predictors of children's dietary supplement use: the 2007 National Health Interview Survey. *Am J Clin Nutr* 2013; 97:1331.

17. Bell, A., et al. A look at nutritional supplement use in adolescents. *J Adol Health* 2004; 34:508–516.

18. Stang, J., et al. Relationships between vitamin and mineral supplement use, dietary intake, and dietary adequacy among adolescents. *J Am Diet Assoc* 2000; 100:905–910.

19. Wu, C-H, et al. The prevalence of herb and dietary supplement use among children and adolescents in the United States: results from the 2007 National Health Interview Survey. *Complement Ther Med* 2013; 21:358.

20. Yussman, S. M., Wilson, K. M., and Klein, J. D. Herbal products and their association with substance use in adolescents. *J Adolescent Health* 2006; 38(4):395–400.

21. Centers for Disease Control and Prevention. Youth Risk Behavior Surveillance—United States, 2013. *MMWR.* 2014; 63(4):17–42.

22. Eisenberg, M. E., et al. Muscle-enhancing behaviors among adolescent girls and boys. *Pediatrics* 2012; 130:1019.

23. Diehl, K., Thiel, A., Zipfel, S., Mayer, J., Schnell, A., and Schneider, S. Elite adolescent athletes' use of dietary supplements: Characteristics, opinions and sources of supply and information.

24. Calfee, R., and Fadale, P. Popular ergogenic drugs and supplements in young athletes. *Pediatrics* 2006; 117:e577–e589.

25. Castillo, E. M., and Comstock, R. D. Prevalence of performance-enhancing substances among United States adolescents. *Pediatr Clin N Am* 2007; 54:663–675.

26. Lattavo, A., Kipperud, A., and Rogers, P. D. Creatine and other supplements. *Pediatr Clin N Am* 2007; 45:735–760.

27. Position of the American Dietetic Association, Dietitians of Canada and the American college of Sports Medicine: Nutrition and

athletic performance. *J Am Diet Assoc* 2009; 109:509–527.

28. Bright Futures Nutrition. 3rd ed. K. Holt, N. Wooldridge, M. Story, D. Sofka, eds. Elk River, IL: American Academy of Pediatrics, 2011.

29. Pisetsky, E. M., Chao, Y. M., Dierker, L. C., et al. Disordered eating and substance use in high-school students: Results from the Youth Risk Behavior Surveillance System. *Int J Eat Disord* 2008; 41(5):464–470.

30. Centers for Disease Control and Prevention. Recommendations to prevent and control iron-deficiency anemia in the United States. *Morb Mortal Wkly Rep* 2002; 51(40):897–899.

31. U.S. Department of Health and Human Services, National Institutes of Health, National Heart, Lung and Blood Institute: Expert panel on integrated guidelines for cardiovascular health and risk reduction in children and adolescents. Summary report. NIH Publication No 12-7486A, October 2012.

32. Centers for Disease Control and Prevention: National diabetes fact sheet: national estimates and general information on diabetes and prediabetes in the United States, 2011. Accessed February 2014 from http://www.cdc.gov/diabetes/pubs/pdf/ndfs_2011.pdf.

33. Neumark-Sztainer, D., et al. Obesity, disordered eating, and eating disorders in a longitudinal study of adolescents: How do dieters fare 5 years later? JADA 2006; 106(4):559–568.

34. Halvarsson-Edlund, K., Sjödén, P.-O., and Lunner, K. Prediction of disturbed eating attitudes in adolescent girls: A 3-year longitudinal study of eating patterns, self-esteem and coping. *Eating Weight Disord* 2008; 13:87–94.

35. Neumark-Sztainer, D., et al. Secular trends in weight status and weight-related attitudes and behaviors in adolescents from 1999 to 2010. *Prep Med* 54:77, 2012.

36. Abraham, S., Boyd, C., and All, M., et al. Time since menarche, weight gain and body image awareness among adolescent girls: Onset of eating disorders? *J Psychoso Obstet Gynaecol* 2009; 30:89–94.

37. Neumark-Sztainer, D., et al. Weight related concerns and behaviors among over-weight and non-overweight adolescents: Implications for preventing weight-related disorders. *Arch Ped Adolesc Med* 2002; 156(2):171–178.

38. Herpetz-Dahlmann, B. Adolescent eating disorders: Definitions, symptomatology, epidemiology and co-morbidity. *Child Adolesc Psychiatr Clin N Am* 2009; 18(1):31–47.

39. American Psychiatric Association: Diagnostic and Statistical Manual of Mental Disorders, Fifth Edition. Arlington, VA, 2013, American Psychiatric Association. Accessed 10 January 2015 from www.dsm.psychiatryonline.org.

40. Steinhausen, H.-C. Outcome of Eating Disorders. *Child Adolesc Psychiatric Clin N Am* 2008; 18:225–242.

41. Mazzeo, S. E., and Bulik, C. M. Environmental and genetic risk factors for eating disorders: What the clinician needs to know. *Child Adolesc Psychiatr Clin N Am* 2008; 18:67–82.

42. Herpetz-Dahlmann, B., and Slaback-Andrae, H. Overview of treatment modalities in adolescent anorexia nervosa. *Child Adolesc Psychiatr Clin N Am* 2008; 18:131–145.

43. Campbell, K., Peebles, R. Eating disorders in children and adolescents: State of the art review. *Pediatrics* 2014; 134:582–592.

44. Shaw, H., Stice, E., and Becker, C. B. Preventing eating disorders. *Child Adolesc Psychiatr Clin N Am* 2008; 18:199–207.

## Chapter 16

1. Ford, E. S., et al. Healthy living is the best revenge. Findings from the European Prospective Investigation into cancer and nutrition—Potsdam Study. *Arch Intern Med* 2009; 169:1355–1362.

2. Fraser, G. E., et al. Ten years of life: Is it a matter of choice? *Arch Intern Med* 2001; 161:1645–1652.

3. Ogden, C. L., et al. Prevalence of childhood and adult obesity in the United States, 2011–2012. *JAMA* 2014; 311:806–814.

4. Behavioral Risk Factor Surveillance System, Prevalence and Data Trends. Available at cdc.gov/brfss/data_tools.htm, accessed 4/10/15.

5. Mozaffarian, D., et al. Population approaches to improve diet, physical activity, and smoking habits: A scientific statement from the American Heart Association *Circulation* 2012; 126: 1514–1563.

6. Supplemental data systems and social determinants of health. *Special Issue of Public Health Reports* 2011; 126 (supplement 3).

7. Source for Social Determinants of Health. Available at: www.healthypeople.gov/2020/topics-objectives/topic/social-determinants-health, accessed 4/11/15.

8. U.S. Department of Health and Human Services, Office of Disease Prevention and Health Promotion. *Healthy People 2020.* Washington, DC, 2011. Available at http://healthypeople.gov/2020, accessed 4/10/15.

9. Mozaffaruan, D., et al. Heart disease and stroke statistics—2015 update: a report from the American Heart Association. *Circulation* 2015; 131:e29-e322. Doi: 10.1161/CIR.0000000000000152.

10. *Promoting health equity: A resource to help communities address social determinants of health.* Atlanta: U.S. Department of Health and Human Services, Centers for Disease Control and Prevention, 2008.

11. Braveman, P. A., et al. Health disparities and health equity: The issue is justice. *Am J Public Health* 2011; 101(Suppl 1):S149-55. Epub 2011 May 6.

12. Slentz, C. A., et al. Exercise, abdominal obesity, skeletal muscle and metabolic risk: evidence of dose response. *Obesity* 2009; 17(Suppl):S27–S33.

13. Favero, G., et al. Endothelium and its alterations in cardiovascular diseases: life style intervention. *Biomed Res Int* 2014; 801896. doi: 10.1155/2014/801896. Epub 2014 Feb 26.

14. Sipila, S. Body composition and muscle performance during menopause and hormonal replacement therapy. *J Endocrinol Invest* 2003; 26:893–901.

15. Kling, J. M. Osteoporosis prevention, screening, and treatment: a review. *J Womens Health* 2014; 23(7):563–572. doi: 10.1089/jwh.2013.4611. Epub 2014 Apr 25.

16. Britten, K. A., et al. Ectopic fat deposits and cardiovascular disease. Circulation 2011; 124:e837–841. doi 10.1161/CIRCULATIONAHA.111.077602.

17. Xu, Z., et al. Dietary effects on human gut microbiome diversity. *Br J Nutr* 2015; 113(Suppl):S1–5. Doi: 10.1017/S0007114514001 27 Epub 2014 Dec 11.

18. Hansen, T. H., et al. The gut microbiome in cardio-metabolic health. Genome Med 2015; 7:33. doi: 10.1186/s1307-015-0157-z.

19. World Cancer Research Fund/American Institute for Cancer Research. *Food, nutrition, physical activity, and the prevention of cancer: A global perspective.* Washington, DC: AICR, 2007 Available at dietandcancerreport.org, accessed 4/10/15.

20. Arroyave, G. Genetic and biologic variability in human nutrient requirements. *Am J Clin Nutr* 1979; 32:486–500.

21. Leyse-Wallace, R. *Linking nutrition to mental health: A scientific exploration.* Lincoln, NE: iUniverse, Inc., 2008.

22. Food and Nutrition Board, Institute of Medicine. *Dietary reference intakes for energy, carbohydrate, fiber, fat, fatty acids, cholesterol, protein, and amino acids.* Washington, DC: National Academy Press, 2002.

23. *Human energy requirements.* Report of a Joint FAO/WHO/UNU Expert Consultation. FAO Food and Nutrition Technical Report Series 1, Rome 2004 Available at www.fao.org/docrep/007/y5686e/y5686e00.htm, accessed 4/10/15.

24. Harper, E. J. Changing perspectives on aging and energy requirements: Aging and energy intakes in humans, dogs and cats. *J Nutr* 1998; 128:2623S–2626S.

25. McGandy, R. B., et al. Nutrient intakes and energy expenditure of men of different ages. *J Gerontol* 1966; 21:581–587.

26. US Department of Agriculture and US Department of Health and Human Services. *Dietary Guidelines for Americans 2010*, 7th Edition, Washington, DC: US Government Printing Office, January 2011. Available at health.gov/dietaryguidelines/2010.asp, accessed 4/10/15.

27. Ravussin, E. and Bogardus, C. Relationship of genetics, age, and physical fitness to daily energy expenditure and fuel utilization. *Am J Clin Nutr* 1989; 49:968–975.

28. Ravussin, E., et al. Twenty-four hour energy expenditure and resting metabolic rate in obese, moderately obese and control subjects. *Am J Clin Nutr* 1982; 35:566–573.

29. Mifflin, M. C., et al. A new predictive equation for resting energy expenditure in healthy individuals. *Am J Clin Nutr* 1990; 51:241–247.

30. Harris, J. A., and Benedict, F. G. *Standard basal metabolism constants for physiologists and clinicians: A biometric study of basal metabolism in man.* Washington, DC: Carnegie Institute of Washington, 1919.

31. Resting metabolic rate: Best ways to measure it—And best ways to raise it, too. American Council on Exercise. *Certified News* October 2012. Available at: www .acefitness.org/ceertifiednewsletterarticle /2882/resting-metabolic-rate-best-ways-to -mesaure-it-and-best-ways-to-raise-it-too, accessed 3/19/15.

32. Hamwi, G. J. Therapy: Changing dietary concepts. Chapter 17 in *Diabetes Mellitus: Diagnosis and Treatment.* T. S. Danowski ed. New York: American Diabetes Association, 1964, 73–78.

33. Swinburn, B. A., et al. Estimating change in the energy flux that characterizes the obesity prevalence. *Am J Clin Nutr* 2009; 89:1723–1728.

34. Souza, R. J. Effects of 4 weight-loss diets differing in fat, protein, and carbohydrate on fat mass, lean mass, visceral adipose tissue, and hepatic fat: results from the POUNDS LOST trial. *Am J Clin Nutr* 2012; 26(3):481–491.

35. Pennington, J. A., and Hubbard, V. S. Derivation of daily values used for nutrition labeling. *J Am Diet Assoc* 1997; 97:1407–1412.

36. Nutrient intakes from food and beverages: Mean amounts consumed per individual, by gender and age. *What we eat in America*, NHANES, 2011–2012. U.S. Department of Agriculture, Agriculture Research Service, 2014. Available at www.ars.usda.gov, accessed 4/13/15.

37. Maldonado-Contreras, A. L, and McCormick, B. A. Intestinal epithelial cells and their role in innate mucosal immunity. *Cell Tissue Res* 2011; 343(1):5–12.

38. Brownawell, A. M., et al. Prebiotics and the health benefits of fiber: current regulatory status, future research, and goals. *J Nutr* 2012; 142(5):962–974.

39. Ross, C. A., et al., eds. *Dietary reference intakes for calcium and vitamin D.* Institute of Medicine. 2011. Available at www.nap.edu, accessed 4/11/15.

40. Bailey, R. L., et al. Estimates of total and usual vitamin D intakes in the United States. *J Nutr* 2010; 140:817–822.

41. Vitamin D and calcium: A systematic review of health outcomes (update) Sept 15, 2014. Evidence Report/Technology Assessment No. 217. Effectivehealthcare.ahrq.gov /ehc/products, accessed 3/24/15.

42. Collins, A. A. Carotenoids and DNA damage. *Mutat Res* 2012; 733(1-2):4–13.

43. Wintergerst, E. S., et al. Contribution of selected vitamins and trace elements to immune function. *Ann Nutr Metab* 2007; 51(4):301–323.

44. Ueland, P. M. Choline and betaine in health and disease. *J Inherit Metab Dis* 2011; 34:3–15.

45. Anderson. O. S., et al. Nutrition and epigenetics: interplay of dietary methyl donors, one-carbon metabolism and DNA methylation. *J Nutr Biochem* 2012; 23:853–859.

46. Mente, A., et al. Association of urinary sodium and potassium excretion with blood pressure. *N Engl J Med* 2014; 371(7):601–611.

47. Eckel, R. H., et al. AHA/ACC guideline on lifestyle management to reduce cardiovascular risk: a report of the American College of Cardiology/American Heart Association Task Force on Practice Guidelines. *J Am Coll Cardiol* 2014; 63(25 Pt B):2960–2984.

48. Dibaba, D.T., et al. Dietary magnesium intake is inversely associated with serum C-reactive protein. *Eur J Clin Nutr* 2014; 68(4):510–516. doi: 10.1038/ejcn.2014.7. Epub 2014 Feb12.

49. Algner, E., et al. Obesity as an Emerging Risk Factor for Iron Deficiency. *Nutrients* 2014; 6:3587–3600.

50. Scientific Report of the 2015 Dietary Guidelines Advisory Committee. Available at health,gov/dietaryguidelines/2015 -scientific-report, accessed 4/11/15.

51. USDA. MyPlate. Available at www .choosemyplate.gov, accessed 4/10/15.

52. Kushi, L. H., et al. American Cancer Society Guidelines on Nutrition and Physical Activity for Cancer Prevention: reducing the risk of cancer with healthy food choices and physical activity. *CA: A Cancer J Clin* 2012; 62:30–67.

53. Lichtenstein, A. H., et al. Diet and lifestyle recommendations revision 2012: A scientific statement from the American Heart Association Nutrition Committee. *Circulation* 2006; 114:82–96. Updates on website but not new publication.

54. Nitzke, S., Freeland-Graves, J. Total diet approach to communicating food and nutrition information. *J Amer Diet Assoc* 2007; 107(7):1224–1232.

55. Rowe S, et al. Translating the Dietary Guidelines for Americans 2010 to bring about real behavior change. *J Am Diet Assoc* 2011; 11(1):28–39.

56. Britten P, et al. Impact of typical rather than nutrient-dense food choices in the US Department of Agriculture Food Patterns. *J Acad Nutr Diet.* 2012; 112:1560–1569.

57. Wansink, B., and Van Ittersun, K. Portion size me: Downsizing our consumption norms. *J Amer Diet Assoc* 2007; 107:1103–1106.

58. Rolls, B. J. What is the role of portion control in weight management? *Int J Obes (Lond).* 2014; 38 Suppl 1:S1-8. doi: 10.1038/ ijo.2014.82.

59. Food and Nutrition Board, Institute of Medicine of the National Academy of Sciences. *Dietary reference intakes for water, potassium, sodium, chloride, and sulfate.* Washington, DC: The National Academies Press, 2005.

60. Kant, A. K., et al. Intakes of plain water, moisture in foods and beverages, and total water in the adult U.S. population—Nutritional, meal pattern, and body weight correlates: National Health and Nutrition Examination Surveys 1999–2006. *Am J Clin Nutr* 2009; 90:655–663.

61. McCrickerd, K., et al. Fluid or fuel? The context of consuming a beverage is important for satiety. PLoS One. 2014; 9(6):e100406. doi: 10.1371/journal.pone.0100406.

62. *Rethink Your Drink* Available at cdc.gov /healthyweight/healthy_eating/drinks.html, accessed 4/10/15.

63. Grandjean, A. C., et al. The effect of caffeinated, non-caffeinated, caloric and non-caloric beverages on hydration. *J Am Coll Nutr* 2000; 19:591–600.

64. Iziar, A. L., et.al. Coffee: biochemistry and potential impact on health. *Food & Function* 2014; 5(8):1695–1717. DOI: 10.1039/ c4fo00042k [www.rsc.org/foodfunction] Aug 2014, accessed 3/26/15.

65. Health behaviors of adults, United States 2002–2004; Chapter 3, "Alcohol use," in *CDC Reports* Series 10, Number 230:8–9, published September 2006.

66. Bailey, R. L., et al. Dietary supplement use in the United States, 2003–2006. *J Nutr.* 2011; 141(2):261–266.

67. Nicoletti, M. Nutraceuticals and botanicals: Overview and perspectives. *Int J Food Sci Nutr.* 2012; 63(Suppl 1):2–6.

68. Hasler, C. M., et al. Position of the American Dietetic Association: Functional foods. *J Am Diet Assoc* 2009; 109:735–746.

69. Satter, E. Eating competence: Definition and evidence for the Satter Eating Competence Model. *J Nutr Educ Behav* 2007; 39(Suppl.):S142–153.

70. Satter, E. Eating competence: Nutrition education with the Satter Eating Competence Model. *J Nutr Educ Behav* 2007; 39(Suppl.):S189–194.

71. Physical Activity Guidelines Advisory Committee Report to the Secretary of Health and Human Services, 2008. U.S. Department of Health and Human Services website. Available at http://www.health.gov/paguidelines, accessed 4/10/15.

72. World Health Organization. *Global strategy on physical activity and health.* Geneva: WHO, 2011. Available at www.who .int/dietphysicalactivity/en, accessed. 4/10/15.

73: *Be Active Your Way: A Guide for Adults.* Available at health.gov/paguidlines. [OR is extension needed pdf/adultguide.pdf] Accessed 3/23/15. ODPHP Publ. No. U0037, October 2008.

74. CDC. Early Release of Selected Estimates Based on the National Health Interview Survey, January-September 2014. Available at www.cdc.gov/nchs/data/nhis/earlyrelease /earlyrelease201503_07.pdf, accessed 4/10/15.

75. Swift, D. L., et al, Physical activity, cardiorespiratory fitness, and exercise training in primary and secondary coronary prevention. *Circ J.* 2013; 77:281–292.

76. Rodrigues, N. R., et al. Position paper of the American Dietetic Association and the Canadian Dietetic Association: Nutrition and athletic performance. *J Am Diet Assoc* 2009; 109:509–527.

77. S. E., et al. The influence of menu labeling on calories selected or consumed: a systematic review and meta-analysis. *J Acad Nutr Diet.* 2014; 114(9):1375–1388e15.

78. *Sisters Together Program Guide.* Weight-control Information Network (WIN), National Institute of Diabetes and Digestive and Kidney Diseases (NIDDK). Available at http://win.niddk.nih.gov/publications /SisPrmGuide2.pdf, accessed 3/28/15.

79. *Household Food Security in the United States in 2013.* Economic Research Report No. (ERR-173) Economic Research Service, USDA.

80. DeNavas-Walt, C., et al. *Income, poverty in the United States: 2013.* Current Population Reports, P60-249, Washington, DC: U.S. Census Bureau, 2014. Available at www .census.gov/content/dam/Census/library /publications/2014/demo/p60-249.pdf, accessed 4/11/15.

81. Poverty Definition. Available at http:// aspe.hhs.gov/poverty/faq.cfm, accessed 4/11/15.

82. Supplemental Food and Nutrition Programs. Available at FNS.usda.gov, accessed 3/19/15.

## Chapter 17

1. National Center for Health Statistics. Deaths: Final Data for 2013, Tables 9 and 11. Available at cdc.gov/nchs/data/nvsr/nvsr64 /nvsr64_02.pdf, accessed 4/15/15.

2. Garvey, W. T., et al. AACE/ACE Consensus Conference on Obesity: building an evidence base for comprehensive action. *Endocrine Practice* 2014; 20:956–976.

3. Shah, A., et al. Adipose inflammation, insulin, and cardiovascular disease. *J Parenter Enteral Nutr* 2008; 32(6):638–644.

4. World Health Organization. Obesity: Preventing and managing the global epidemic. Report of a WHO Consultation. *World Health Organ Tech Rep Ser* 2000; 894:1–253.

5. Adult Obesity Facts. Available at www .cdc.gov/nccdphp/dnpa/obesity/trend/maps/, accessed 5/16/15.

6. Levi, J., et al. *F as in Fat: How obesity threatens America's future 2012.* Robert Wood Johnson Foundation September 2012. Available at healthyamericans.org/assets /files/TFAH2012FasInFatfinal.pdf, accessed 5/12/15.

7. Yu, Y-H., et al. Metabolic vs. hedonic obesity: a conceptual distinction and its clinical implications. *Obesity Reviews* 2015; 16:234–247.

8. Rudkowsha, I., et al. Individualized weight management: what can be learned from nutrigenomics and nutrigenetics? *Prog Mol Biol Tranl Sci* 2012; 108:347–382.

9. Waalen, J. The genetics of human obesity. *Transl Res.* 2014 Oct; 164(4):293-301. doi: 10.1016/j.trsl.2014.05.010. Epub 2014 May 23.

10. Clusky, M., and Grobe, D. College weight gain and behavior transitions: Male and female differences. *J Amer Diet Assoc* 2009; 109:325–329.

11. Report of the 2015 Dietary Guidelines Advisory Committee. Available at health,gov /dietaryguidelines/2015-scientific-report, accessed 4/11/15.

12. Egger, G., & Dixon, J. Beyond obesity and lifestyle: a review of 21st century chronic disease determinants. *BioMed Res International* 2014. doi: 10.1155/2017/731685.

13. Puhl, R. M., and Heuer, C. A. Obesity stigma: important considerations for public health. *Am J Public Health* 2010; 100:1019–1028.

14. Grover, S. A. Years of life lost and healthy life-years lost from diabetes and cardiovascular disease in overweight and obese people: a modelling study. *Lancet: Diabetes & Endocrinology* 2015; 3:114–122.

15. Fontana, L., et al. Optimal body weight for health and longevity: bridging basic, clinical, and population research. *Aging Cell* 2004; 13:391–400.

16. Lohman, T., et al. *Anthropometric Standardization Reference Manual.* Champaign, IL: Human Kinetics, 1991.

17. Kushner, R. F. Clinical assessment and management of adult obesity. *Circulation* 2012; 126:2870–2877.

18. Shananhan, J. F., et al. Eds. *Smith's Patient Centered Interviewing*, 3rd ed. Philadelphia: Lippincott Williams & Wilkins, 2012.

19. Forbes, D. L. Toward a unified model of human motivation. *Rev Gen Psych* 2011; 15(2): 85–98.

20. Dombrowski, S. U., et al. Behavioural interventions for obese adults with additional risk factors for morbidity: systematic review of effects on behaviour, weight and disease risk factors. *Obes Facts* 2010; 3(6):377–396. Epub 2010 Dec 14.

21. US Preventive Services Task Force. Obesity in adults: screening and management. June 2012. Available at www.uspreventive servicestaskforce.org, accessed 4/16/15.

22. Kirk, S. F., et al. Effective weight management practice: a review of the lifestyle intervention evidence. *Int J Obes (Lond)* 2012; 36(2):178–185.

23. Wadden, T. A., et al. Lifestyle modification for obesity: new developments in diet, physical activity, and behavior therapy. *Circulation.* 2012; 125:1157–1170.

24. Jull, S. D. Middle-aged women's decisions about body weight management: Needs assessment and testing of a knowledge translation tool. *Menopause.* 2015 Apr; 22(4):414–422. doi: 10.1097/ GME.0000000000000326.

25. Robertson, C., et al. Systematic reviews of and integrated report on the quantitative, qualitative and economic evidence base for the management of obesity in men. *Health Technol Assess* 2014 May; 18(35):v–vi, xxiii–xxix, 1–424. doi: 10.3310/hta18350.

26. Adult weight management guideline (2014). Academy of Nutrition and Dietetics Evidence Analysis Library. Available at: andeal.org, accessed 5/12/15.

27. Saks, F. M., et al. Comparison of weight-loss diets with different compositions of fat, protein, and carbohydrates. *N Engl J Med* 2009 Feb; 360(9):859–873.

28. Cooper, Z., et al. *Cognitive-Behavioral Treatment of Obesity: A Clinician's Guide.* New York: The Guilford Press, 2003.

29. Corbalan, M. D., et al. Effectiveness of cognitive-behavioral therapy based on the Mediterranean diet for the treatment of obesity. *Nutrition* 2009; 25:861–869.

30. Physical Activity Guidelines Advisory Committee Report to the Secretary of Health and Human Services, 2008. U.S. Department of Health and Human Services website. Available at http://www.health.gov/paguidelines, accessed 4/10/15.

31. Clark, J. E. Diet, exercise or diet with exercise: comparing the effectiveness of treatment options for weight-loss and changes in fitness for adults (18-65 years old) who are overfat, or obese; systematic review and meta-analysis. *J Diabetes Metab Disord.* 2015 Apr 17;14:31. doi: 10.1186/s40200-015-0154-1. eCollection 2015.

32. Hill, J., et al. Weight Maintenance: What's Missing? *J Amer Diet Assoc* 2005; 105:63–66.

33. Jones, L. R., et al. Lifestyle modification in the treatment of obesity: An educational challenge and opportunity. *Clin Pharmacol Ther* 2007; 81:776–779.

34. Greenway, F. L. Physiological adaptations to weight loss and factors favouring weight regain. *Int J Obes (Lond).* 2015 Apr 21; doi: 10.1038/ijo.2015. [Epub ahead of print]

Wing, R. R., and Phelan, S. Long-term weight loss maintenance. *Am J Clin Nutr* 2005; 82 (Suppl. 1):222S–225S.

35. Burke, L. E., et al. Self-monitoring in weight loss: a systematic review of the literature. *J Am Diet Assoc* 2011; 111:92–102.

36. Manon, S., et al. The use of web-based interventions to prevent excess weight gain. *J Telemed Telecare* 2012 Nov 18; 18:37–41, Epub 2011.

37. Kakkar, A. K., et al. Drug treatment of obesity: Current status and future prospects. *Eur J Intern Med.* 2014 Jan 6; doi:10.1016/j. ejim2015.01.005. Epub.

38. Poddar, K. Nutraceutical supplements for weight loss: A systematic review. *Nutr Clin Pract* 2011; 26(5):539–552.

39. Office of Dietary Supplements. Dietary Supplements for Weight Loss. Fact Sheet of Health Professionals. http://ods.od.nih.gov /factsheets/WeightLoss-HealthProfessional, accessed 4/16/15.

40. Mechanick, J. I., et al. AACE/TOS/ASMBS medical guidelines for clinical practice for the perioperative nutritional, metabolic, and

nonsurgical support of the bariatric surgery patient. Obesity 2009; 17(Suppl):S1–S70.

41. Shankar, P., et al. Micronutrient deficiencies after bariatric surgery. *Nutrition* 2010; 26(11–12):1031–1037.

42. U.S. Department of Health and Human Services, Office of Disease Prevention and Health Promotion. *Healthy People 2020* Washington, D.C. 2011. Available at http://healthypeople.gov/2020, accessed 5/3/15.

43. Heart Disease and Stroke Statistics 2014 Update: A report from the American Health Association Statistics Committee and Stroke Statistics Subcommittee. *Circulation* 2014; 125:e28–e292.

44. Mosca, L., et al. Effectiveness-Based Guidelines for the Prevention of Cardiovascular Disease in Women—2011 Update: A Guideline from the American Heart Association. *Circulation.* 2011; 123:1243–1262.

45. Lee, C. D., et al. Abdominal obesity and coronary artery calcification in young adults: The Coronary Artery Risk Development in Young Adults (CARDIA) Study. *Am J Clin Nutr* 2007; 86:48–54.

46. Willerson, J. T., and Ridker, P. M. Inflammation as a cardiovascular risk factor. *Circulation* 2004; 109:2–10.

47. Jeppesen, P., et al. Insulin resistance, the metabolic syndrome, and risk of incident cardiovascular disease: A population-based study. *J Am Coll Cardiol* 2007; 49(21):2112–2129.

48. Eckel, R. H., et al. AHA/ACC Guidelines on lifestyle management to reduce cardiovascular risk. *Circulation* 2014; 129: S76-S99 Published online before print November 12, 2013, doi: 10.1161/01.cir.0000437740.48606.d1.

49. Kuivenhoven, J. A., et al. Beyond the genetics of HDL: Why is HDL cholesterol inversely related to cardiovasculardisease? *Handb Exp Pharmacol.* 2015; 224:285–300. doi: 10.1007/978-3-319-09665-0_8.

50. Goff, D. C., et al. ACC/AHA Guidelines on the assessment of cardiovascular risk. *J Am Coll Cardiol.* 2014 Jul 1; 63(25 Pt B):2935-59. doi: 10.1016/j.jacc.2013.11.005. Epub 2013 Nov 12.

51. The Emerging Risk Factors Collaboration. C-reactive protein, fibrinogen, and cardiovascular prediction. *NEJM*; 2012:1310–1320.

52. Upadhyay, R. Y. Emerging risk biomarkers in cardiovascular diseases and disorders. *J Lipids.* 2015; 2015:97 1453. doi: 10.1155/2015/97 1453. Epub 2015 Apr 8.

53. *Academy of Nutrition and Dietetics E evidence-based practice guideline and toolkit: Disorders of lipid metabolism.* Chicago: Academy of Nutrition and Dietetics. 2012.

54. Lichtenstein, A. H., et al. Diet and lifestyle recommendations revision 2006: A scientific statement from the American Heart Association Nutrition Committee. *Circulation* 2006; 114:82–96.

55. Mozaffarian, D., et al. Population approaches to improve diet, physical activity and smoking habits: a scientific statement of the American Heart Association. *Circulation* 2012; 126:1514–1563.

56. Hooper, L., et al. Reduced or modified dietary fat for preventing cardiovascular disease. *Cochrane Database Syst Rev* 2012 May 16; 5:CD002137.

57. Delgado-Lista, J., et al. Long chain omega-3 fatty acids and cardiovascular disease: A systematic review. *B J Nutr* 2012; 107 (Suppl2):S201–213.

58. Position of the American Dietetic Association: Health implications of dietary fiber. *J Am Diet Assoc* 2008; 108:1716–1731.

59. Ramprasath, V. R., et al. Consumption of a dietary portfolio of cholesterol lowering foods improves blood lipids without affecting concentrations of fat soluble compounds *Nutr J.* 2014; 13: 101. Published online 2014 Oct 18. doi: 10.1186/1475-2891-13-101.

60. Weingartner, O., et al. Controversial role of plant sterols in the management of hypercholesterolemia. *European Heart Journal* 2009; 30, 404–409.

61. Shamliyan, T. A., et al. Are your patients with risk of CVD getting the viscous soluble fiber they need? Few patients eat the right amount of fiber known to reduce CVD risks and events. *Journal of Family Practice* Sept. 2006.

62. Stone, N. J., et al. 2013 ACC/AHA guideline on the treatment of blood cholesterol to reduce atherosclerotic cardiovascular risk in adults: a report of the American College of Cardiology/American Heart Association Task Force on practice guidelines. 2013 Nov 7. http://dx.doi.org/10.1016/j.jacc.2013.11.002. pii: S0735-1097(13)06028-2.

63. Alberti, K. G. M. M., et al. Harmonizing the Metabolic Syndrome A Joint Interim Statement of the International Diabetes Federation Task Force on Epidemiology and Prevention; National Heart, Lung, and Blood Institute; American Heart Association; World Heart Federation; International Atherosclerosis Society; and International Association for the Study of Obesity. *Circulation* 2009; 120:1650–1645.

64. Beltrán-Sánchez, H., et al. Prevalence and Trends of Metabolic Syndrome in the Adult U.S. Population, 1999–2010. *J Am Coll Cardiol.* 2013; 62(8):697–703. doi:10.1016/j.jacc.2013.05.064

65. Durward, C. M., et al. All-cause mortality risk of metabolically healthy obese individuals in NHANES III. *J Obes.* 2012; 2012:460321.

66. Russell, M., et al. The metabolic syndrome in American Indians: The Strong Heart Study. *JCMS* 2007; 2:283–287.

67. Sumner, A., and Cowie, C. C. Ethnic differences in the ability of triglyceride levels to identify insulin resistance. *Atherosclerosis* 2008; 196:696–703.

68. Tota-Maharaj, R., et al. A practical approach to the metabolic syndrome: review of current concepts and management. *Curr Opin Cardiol.* 2010; 25:502–512.

69. Higgins, S. P., et al. Acanthosis nigricans: A practical approach to evaluation and management. *Dermatology Online J* 2008; 19(9): 2.

70. Misra, A., et al. Novel phenotype markers and screening score for the metabolic syndrome in adult Asian Indians. *Diabetes Res Clin Pract* 2008; 79:E1–E5.

71. Kastorini, C. M., et al. The effect of Mediterranean diet on metabolic syndrome and its components: a meta-analysis of 50 studies and 534,906 individuals. *J Am Col Cardio* 2011; 57:1299–1313.

72. Phelan, S., et al. Impact of weight loss on the metabolic syndrome. *Int J Obs* (Lond) 2007; 9:1442–1448.

73. Joshua, D., et al. Prediabetes: A prevalent and treatable, but often unrecognized clinical condition. *J Acad Nutr Diet.* 2013 Feb; 113(2): 213–218.

74. Hamman, R. F., et al. Effect of weight loss with lifestyle intervention on risk of diabetes. *Diabetes Care* 2006; 29: 2102–2107.

75. American Diabetes Association. *National Diabetes Statistics Report, 2014.* Available at www.diabetes.org/diabetes-basics/statistics, accessed 5/7/15.

76. Peek, M. E., et al. Diabetes health disparities: a systematic review of health care interventions. *Med Care Res Rev* 2007 October; 64(5 Suppl): 101S–156S.

77. Al-Goblan, A. S., et al. Mechanism linking diabetes mellitus and obesity. *Diabetes Metab Syndr Obes.* 2014; 7:587–591. doi: 10.2147/DMSO.S67400. eCollection 2014.

78. Dokken, B. B. The pathophysiology of cardiovascular disease and diabetes: beyond blood pressure and lipids. *Diabetes Spectrum* 2008; 21(3):160–165.

79. American Diabetes Association. Standards of medical care in diabetes—2015. *Diabetes Care* 2015; 38(Suppl.1):S1–S93.

80. Franz, M. J., et al. Evidence-based diabetes nutrition therapy recommendations are effective: the key is individualization. Diabetes, Metabolic Syndrom and Obesity: Targets and Therapy 2014; 7:65–72.

81. Academy of Nutrition and Dietetics. Prevention of type 2 diabetes (PDM) guideline 2013. Available at andeal.org, accessed 4/24/15.

82. Delahanty, L. M., et al. Association of diet with glycated hemoglobin during intensive treatment of type 1 diabetes in the Diabetes Control and Complications Trial. *Am J Clin Nutr* 2009; 89:518–524.

83. Haas, L., et al. National standards for diabetes self-management education and support. *Diabetes Care* November 2012; 35: 2393–2240.1.

84. Inzucchi, S. E., et al. Management of hyperglycemia in type 2 diabetes: A patient-centered approach: position statement of the American Diabetes Association (ADA) and the European Association for the Study of Diabetes (EASD). *Diabetes Spectrum* 2012; 25:154–171.

85. Colberg, S. R., et al. Exercise and Type 2 Diabetes: The American College of Sports Medicine and the American Diabetes Association: Joint Position Statement. Diabetes Care 2010; 33:1395–1402.

86. Katzmarzyk, P. T., et al. Sitting time and mortality from all causes, cardiovascular disease, and cancer. *Med Sci Sports Exerc* 2009; 41:998–1005.

87. Geil, P., and Shane-McWhorter, L. Dietary supplements in the management of diabetes: Potential risks and benefits. *J Am Diet Assoc* 2008; 108(Suppl.): S59–S65.

88. World Cancer Research Fund/American Institute for Cancer Research. The cancer process. Chapter 2 in *Nutrition, Physical Activity and the Prevention of Cancer: A Global Perspective*. Washington, DC: AICR, 2007.

89. Rowland, J. H., et al. Cancer survivorship: A new challenge in delivering quality cancer care. *J Clin Oncology* 2006; 24:5101–5104.

90. Kohler, B. A., et al. Annual Report to the Nation on the Status of Cancer, 1975–2011, Featuring Incidence of Breast Cancer Subtypes by Race/Ethnicity, Poverty, and State. *J Natl Ca Inst*. Online March 30, 2015. DOI: 10.1093/jnci.j/djv048.

91. Zoderman, A. B., et al. The influence of health disparities on targeting cancer prevention efforts. *Am J Prev Med* 2014; 46(3S1):S87–S97.

92. Eheman, C., et al. Annual Report to the Nation on the Status of Cancer, 1975–2008, Featuring Cancers Associated with Excess Weight and Lack of Sufficient Physical Activity. *Cancer*. 2012 May 1; 118(9):2338–2366. Epub 2012, Mar 28.

93. Renehan, A. G., et al. Obesity and cancer: Pathophysiological and biological mechanisms. *Arch Physiol Biochem* 2008; 114:71–83.

94. O'Rourke, R. W., et al. Obesity and cancer: the crossroads of cellular metabolism and proliferation. *Surgery for Obesity and Related Diseases*. 2014; 10:1208–1219.

95. Romaquera, D., et al. Is concordance with the World Cancer Research Fund/American Institute for Cancer Research guidelines for cancer prevention related to subsequent risk of cancer? Results from the EPIC study. *Am J Clin Nutr* 2012; 96:150–163.

96. Parekh, N., et al. Obesity, insulin resistance, and cancer prognosis: Implications for practice for providing care among cancer survivors. *J Amer Diet Assoc* 2009; 109:346–1353.

97. Kushi, L. H., et al. The American Cancer Society guidelines on nutrition and physical activity for cancer prevention: Reducing the risk of cancer with healthy food choices and physical activity. *CA Cancer J Clin* 2012; 62:30–67. Available at: http://onlinelibrary.wiley.com/doi/10.3322/caac.20140/pdf, accessed 5/15/15.

98. Nutrition in Cancer Care (PDQ) Tumor-Induced Effects on Nutritional Status. Available at www.cancer.gov/cancer topics/pdq/supportive care/nutrition/HelthProfessional/Page2#_4, accessed 5/7/2015.

99. National Cancer Institute. Nutrition in Cancer Care (PDQ). Available at www.cancer.gov/cancertopics/pdq/supportivecare/nutrition/HealthPatient/page1, accessed 5/15/15.

100. Zick, S. M., et al. Phase II trial of encapsulated ginger as a treatment for chemotherapy-induced nausea and vomiting. *Support Care Cancer*. 2009; 17:563-72. doi: 10.1007/s00520-008-0528-8. Epub 2008 Nov 13.

101. Chastain, D. B., et al. Epidemiology and Management of Antiretroviral-Associated Cardiovascular Disease. *Open AIDS J*. 2015; 9: 23–37. Published online 2015 Mar 31. doi: 10.2174/1874613601509010023.

102. Centers for Disease Control and Prevention. HIV Surveillance Report, 2013, vol. 25. http://www.cdc.gov/hiv/library/reports/surveillance. Published Feb 2015, accessed 5/8/2015.

103. Kosmiski, L. Energy expenditure in HIV infection. *Am J Clin Nutr* 2011; 94(6):1677S–1682S. Epub 2011 Nov 16.

104. Carter, G. M. Micronutrients in HIV: A Bayesian Meta-Analysis. *PLoS One*. 2015; 10(4): e0120113. Published online 2015 Apr 1. doi:10.1371/journal.pone.0120113.

105. Shivakoti R. Prevalence and risk factors of micronutrient deficiencies pre- and post-antiretroviral therapy (ART) among a diverse multicountry cohort of HIV-infected adults. *Clin Nutr*. 2015 Feb 10. pii: S0261-5614(15)00045-X. doi: 10.1016/j.clnu.2015.02.002.

106. Position of the American Dietetic Association and the Dietitians of Canada: Nutrition intervention in the care of persons with human immunodeficiency virus infection. *J Am Diet Assoc* 2004; 104:1425–1441.

107. Srinivasa, S., et al. Metabolic and body composition effects of newer antiretrovirals in HIV-infected patients. *Eur J Endocrinol*. 2014 Apr 10; 170(5):R185-202. doi: 10.1530/EJE-13-0967. Print 2014 May.

108. Warriner, A. H. Bone alterations associated with HIV. *Curr HIV/AIDS Rep*. 2014 Sep;11(3):233-40. doi: 10.1007/s11904-014-0216-x.

109. Grodensky, C., et al. Systematic review: Effect of alcohol on adherence to outpatient medication regimens for chronic disease. *J Stud Alcohol Drugs* 2012; 73:899–910.

110. Mankal, P. K., & Kotler, D. T. From Wasting to Obesity, Changes in Nutritional Concerns in HIV/AIDS. *Endocrinaol Metab Clin N Am* 2014; 43:647–663.

111. Beraldo, R. A., et al. Proposed ratios and cutoffs for the assessment of lipodystrophy in HIV-seropositive individuals. *Eur J Clin Nutr*. 2015 Feb; 69(2):274–278. doi: 10.1038/ejcn.2014.149. Epub 2014 Jul 30.

112. Tang, A. M., et al., Nutrition assessment, counseling, and support interventions to improve health-related outcomes in people living with HIV/AIDS: a systematic review of the literature. *J Acquir Immune Defic Syndr*. 2015 Apr 15; 68 Suppl 3:S340–349. doi: 10.1097/QAI.0000000000000521.

## *Chapter 18*

1. U.S. Census Bureau. P23-212, 65+ in the United States: 2010. Washington, DC: U.S. Government Printing Office, 2014.

2. Barrett, L. L. Healthy @ Home, AARP Knowledge Management. 2008. Available at http://assets.aarp.org/rgcenter/il/healthy_home.pdf, accessed 7/1/15.

3. Position of the Academy of Nutrition and Dietetics: Food and nutrition for older adults: Promoting health and wellness. *J Acad Nutr Diet* 2012; 112:1255–1277.

4. Anderson, A. L., et al. Dietary patterns and survival of older adults. *J Am Diet Assoc*. 2011; 111: 84–91.

5. Trichopoulou, A., et al. Anatomy of health effects of Mediterranean diet: Greek EPIC prospective cohort study. *Br Med J* 2009; 338:b2337.

6. King, D. E., et al. Turning back the clock: Adopting a healthy lifestyle in middle age. *Am J Med* 2007; 120:598–603.

7. American College of Sports Medicine, Position Stand. Exercise and physical activity for older adults. *Med Sci. Sports Exerc* 2009; 41: 1510–1530.

8. National Center for Injury Prevention and Control. *10 Leading Causes of Death by Age Group, United States, 2013*. Available at http://www.cdc.gov/injury/wisqars/leading causes.html, accessed 6/12/15.

9. National Center for Health Statistics. Health, United States, 2014: With Special Feature on Adults Aged 55–64. Hyattsville, MD. 2015.

10. Taylor, P., et al. Pew Research Center. Growing Old in America: Expectations vs. Reality. June 29, 2009. Available at http://www.pewsocialtrends.org/2009/06/29/growing-old-in-america-expectations-vs-reality/, accessed 6/17/15.

11. U.S. Census Bureau. QuickFacts Beta. Available at http://www.census.gov/quickfacts/map/AGE775213/00, accessed 6/11/15.

12. Vincent, G. K., and Velkoff, V. A. The next four decades. The older population in the United States: 2010 to 2050 Population Estimates and Projections. Current Population Reports, P25–1138. Washington, DC: U.S. Census Bureau, 2010.

13. 1995 White House Conference on Aging. The road to aging policy for the 21st Century. Washington, DC: U.S. National Commission on Libraries, 1996.

14. Hayflick, L. How and why we age. *Exp Gerontol* 1998; 33:639–653.

15. Gerontology Research Group. Official Tables from the International Committee on Supercentenarians. Available at http://www.grg.org/Adams/C.HTM, accessed 6/5/2015.

16. *Healthy People 2020: Improving the Health of Americans*. Available at http://www.healthypeople.gov/2020/default.aspx, accessed 6/12/15.

17. Capri, M., et al. The genetics of human longevity. *Ann NY Acad Sci* 2006; 1067:252–263.

18. Forbes, G. B. *Human body composition: Growth, aging, nutrition, and activity.* New York: Springer-Verlag, 1987, 31.

19. Buys, C. H. Telomeres, telomerase, and cancer. *N Engl J Med* 2000; 342:1282–1283.

20. Weindruch, R., and Sohal, R. S. Seminars in medicine of the Beth Israel Deaconess Medical Center. Caloric intake and aging. *N Engl J Med* 1997; 337:986–994.

21. McCay, C., et al. The effect of retarded growth upon the length of life span and upon the ultimate body size. *J Nutr* 1935; 10:63–79.

22. Colman, R. J., et al. Caloric restriction delays disease onset and mortality in Rhesus monkeys. *Science* 2009; 325:201–204.

23. Mattison, J. A., et al. Impact of caloric restriction on health and survival in rhesus monkeys from the NIA study. *Nature* 2012; 489: 318–321.

24. Colman, R. J., et al. Caloric restriction reduces age-related and all-cause mortality in rhesus monkeys. *Nat. Commun* 2014; 5:3557. DOI: 10.1038/ncomms4557. Available at www.nature.com/naturecommunications, accessed 6/17/15.

25. Walford, R. L., et al. Calorie restriction in biosphere 2: Alterations in physiologic, hematologic, hormonal, and biochemical parameters in humans restricted for a 2-year period. *J Gerontol A Biol Sci Med Sci* 2002; 57:B211–224.

26. Fontana, L., et al. Effect of long-term calorie restriction with adequate protein and micronutrients on thyroid hormones. *J Clin Endocrine Metab* 2006; 91:3232–3235.

27. Willcox, B. J., et al. Caloric restriction, the traditional Okinawan diet, and healthy aging. The diet of the world's longest-lived people and its potential impact on morbidity and life span. *Ann NY Acad Sci* 2007; 1114:434–455.

28. Guo, S. S., et al. Aging, body composition, and lifestyle: The Fels Longitudinal Study. *Am J Clin Nutr* 1999; 70:405–411.

29. Wilmore, J. H., et al. Alterations in body weight and composition consequent to 20 weeks of endurance training: The HERITAGE Family Study. *Am J Clin Nutr* 1999; 70:346–352.

30. Fiatarone, M. A., et al. High-intensity strength training in nonagenarians: Effects on skeletal muscle. *J Am Med Assoc* 1990; 263:3029–3034.

31. Villareal, D. T., et al. Obesity in older adults: Technical review and position statement of the American Society for Nutrition and NAASO, The Obesity Society. *Obes Res* 2005; 13:1849–1863.

32. Forbes, G. B. Longitudinal changes in adult fat-free mass: Influence of body weight. *Am J Clin Nutr* 1999; 70:1025–1031.

33. Elahi, V. K., et al. A longitudinal study of nutritional intake in men. *J Gerontol* 1983; 38:162–180.

34. DeVere, R., and Calvert M. Navigating smell and taste disorders. New York: Demos Medical Publishing, 2011.

35. Murphy, C., et al. Prevalence of olfactory impairment in older adults. *J Am Med Assoc* 2002; 288:2307–2312.

36. Schiffman, S. Changes in taste and smell: Drug interactions and food preferences. *Nutr Rev* 1994; 52:S11–14.

37. Dye, B. A., et al. Selected oral health indicators in the United States, 2005–2008. NCHS data brief, no 96. Hyattsville, MD: National Center for Health Statistics. 2012. Available at, http://www.cdc.gov/nchs/data/databriefs/db96.htm#Ref3, accessed 6/7/15.

38. Sahyoun, N. R., et al. Nutritional status of the older adult is associated with dentition status. *J Am Diet Assoc* 2003; 103: 61–66.

39. Holm-Pedersen, P., et al. Tooth loss and subsequent disability and mortality in old age. *J Am Geriatr Soc* 2008; 56:429–435.

40. American Dietetic Association. Position of the American Dietetic Association: Oral health and nutrition. *J Am Diet Assoc* 2007; 107:1418–1428.

41. Roberts, S. B., et al. Control of food intake in older men. *J Am Med Assoc* 1994; 272:1601–1606.

42. Rolls, B. J. Regulation of food and fluid intake in the elderly. *Ann N Y Acad Sci* 1989; 561:217–225.

43. Phillips, P. A., et al. Disturbed fluid and electrolyte homoeostasis following dehydration in elderly people. *Age Ageing* 1993; 22:S26–33.

44. Phillips, P. A., et al. Reduced thirst after water deprivation in healthy elderly men. *N Engl J Med* 1984; 311:753–759.

45. Hooper L., et al. Water-loss dehydration and aging. *Mech Ageing Dev.* 2014; 136-137:50–58.

46. Sebastian, R. S., et al. Monitoring Sodium Intake of the US Population: Impact and Implications of a Change in What We Eat in America, National Health and Nutrition Examination Survey Dietary Data Processing. *J Acad Nutr Diet* 2013 113:942–949.

47. White, J. V., et al. Nutrition screening initiative: Development and implementation of the public awareness checklist and screening tools. *J Am Diet Assoc* 1992; 92:163–167.

48. White, J. V., et al. Consensus of the Nutrition Screening Initiative: Risk factors and indicators of poor nutritional status in older Americans. *J Am Diet Assoc* 1991; 91:783–787.

49. Posner, B. M., et al. Nutrition and health risks in the elderly: The nutrition screening initiative. *Am J Public Health* 1993; 83:972–978.

50. Dixon, L. B., et al. Dietary intakes and serum nutrients differ between adults from food-insufficient and food-sufficient families: Third National Health and Nutrition Examination Survey, 1988–1994. *J. Nutr* 2001; 131:1232–1246.

51. Lee, J. S., and Frongillo, E. A. Nutritional and health consequences are associated with food insecurity among U.S. elderly persons. *J. Nutr* 2001; 131:1503–1509.

52. Bowman, S. A. Socioeconomic characteristics, dietary and lifestyle patterns, and health and weight status of older adults in NHANES 1999–2002: A comparison of Caucasians and African Americans. *J Nutr Elderly* 2009; 28:30–46.

53. Gu, Q., et al. Prescription drug use continues to increase: U.S. prescription drug data for 2007–2008. NCHS data brief, no 42. Hyattsville, MD: National Center for Health Statistics. 2010. Available at http://www.cdc.gov/nchs/data/databriefs/db42.pdf, accessed 6/7/15.

54. The American Geriatrics Society 2012 Beers Criteria Update Expert Panel. American Geriatrics Society updated Beers criteria for potentially inappropriate medication use in older adults. *J Am Geriatr Soc* 2012; 60:616–631.

55. Sahyoun, N. R., and Zhang X. L. Dietary quality and social contact among a nationally representative sample of the older adult population in the United States. *J Nutr Health Aging* 2005; 9: 177–183.

56. De Castro, J. M. Social facilitation of food intake: People eat more with other people. *Food Nutr News* 1994; 66:29–30.

57. Gerrior, S. A., et al. How does living alone affect dietary quality? U.S. Department of Agriculture, ARS, Home Economics Research Report No. 51. *Fam Econ Nutr Rev* 1995; 8:44–46.

58. Sahyoun, N. R., et al. Nutrition Screening Initiative checklist may be a better awareness/educational tool than a screening one. *J Am Diet Assoc* 1997; 97:760–764.

59. Cereda, E., et al. The ability of the Geriatric Nutritional Risk Index to assess the nutritional status and predict the outcome of home-care resident elderly: A comparison with the Mini- Nutritional Assessment. *British J of Nutrition* 2009; 1–8.

60. Elia, M., Smith, R. M., and British Association for Parenteral and Enteral Nutrition. *Improving nutritional care and treatment: Perspectives and recommendations from population groups, patients and carers*, 2009. Available at http://www.bapen.org.uk/screening-for-malnutrition/must/introducing-must, accessed 6/9/15.

61. Phillips M. B., et al. Nutritional screening in community-dwelling older adults: A systematic literature review. *Asia Pac J Clin Nutr* 2010; 19:440–449.

62. U.S. Department of Agriculture and U.S. Department of Health and Human Services. Dietary Guidelines for Americans, 2010. 7th Edition, Washington, DC: U.S. Government Printing Office, December 2010.

63. Otten, J. J., et al., eds. Institute of Medicine of the National Academies. *DRI Dietary Reference Intakes: The Essential Guide to Nutrient Requirements.* Washington, DC: The National Academies Press, 2006.

64. Zizza, C. A., et al. Benefits of snacking in older Americans. *J Am Diet Assoc* 2007; 107:800–806.

65. USDA Food Surveys Research Group. Summary data tables on total nutrient intakes, meal patterns, and snack occasions for 2011–2012. *What we eat in America*, NHANES. Available at http://www.ars.usda.gov/Services/docs.htm?docid=18349, accessed 6/9/2015.

66. Ogden, C. L., et al. Prevalence of obesity among adults: United States, 2011–2012. NCHS Data Brief, No. 131, Hyattsville, MD: National Center for Health Statistics, 2013. Available at http://www.cdc.gov/nchs/data/databriefs/db131.pdf, accessed 6/13/15.

67. Arcerio, P. J., et al. A practical equation to predict resting metabolic rate in older men. *Metabolism* 1993; 42:950–957.

68. Arcerio, P. J., et al. A practical equation to predict resting metabolic rate in older females. *J Am Geriatric Soc* 1994; 41:389–395.

69. Taylor, H. L., et al. A questionnaire for the assessment of leisure-time physical activities. *J Chronic Dis* 1978; 31:741–755.

70. Dawson-Hughes, B., et al. Alkaline diets favour lean tissues in older adults. *Am J Clin Nutr* 2008; 87:662–665.

71. Campbell, W. W., et al. Dietary protein requirements of younger and older adults. *Am J Clin Nutri* 2008; 88:1322–1329.

72. Rand, W. M., et al. Meta-analysis of nitrogen balance studies for estimating protein requirements in healthy adults. *Am J Clin Nutr* 2003; 77:109–127.

73. Paddon-Jones, D., et al. Protein and health aging. *Am J Clin Nutr* 2015; 101:1339S–1345S.

74. Paddon-Jones, D., et al. Role of dietary protein in the sarcopenia of aging. *Am J Clin Nutr* 2008; 87(Suppl.):1562S–1566S.

75. Symons, T. B., et al. A moderate serving of high-quality protein maximally stimulates skeletal muscle protein synthesis in young and elderly subjects. *J Am Diet Assoc.* 2009; 109:1582–1586.

76. Eckel, R. H., et al. 2013 AHA/ACC guideline on lifestyle management to reduce cardiovascular risk: a report of the American College of Cardiology/American Heart Association Task Force on Practice Guidelines. *J Am Coll Cardiol* 2014; 63:2960–2984.

77. Vivekananthan, D. P., et al. Use of antioxidant vitamins for the prevention of cardiovascular disease: Meta-analysis of randomised trials. *Lancet* 2003; 361:2017–2023.

78. Weaver, C. M., and Fleet, J. C. Vitamin D requirements: Current and future. *Am J Clin Nutr* 2004; 80(Suppl.):1735S–1739S.

79. Holick, M. F., and Chen, T. C. Vitamin D deficiency: A worldwide problem with health consequences. *Am J Clin Nutri* 2008; 87(Suppl.):1080S–1086S.

80. Webb, A. R., et al. Influence of season and latitude on the cutaneous synthesis of vitamin $D_3$: Exposure to winter sunlight in Boston and Edmonton will not promote vitamin $D_3$ synthesis in human skin. *J Clin Endocrinol Metab* 1988; 67:373–378.

81. Bischoff-Ferrari, H. A., et al. Estimation of optimal concentrations of 25-hydroxyvitamin D for multiple health outcomes. *Am J Clin Nutr* 2006; 84:18–28.

82. Meydani, M. Effect of functional food ingredients: Vitamin E modulation of cardiovascular diseases and immune status in the elderly. *Am J Clin Nutr* 2000; 71:1665S–1668S.

83. Sano, M., et al. A controlled trial of selegiline, alpha-tocopherol, or both as treatment for Alzheimer's disease. The Alzheimer's Disease Cooperative Study. *N Engl J Med* 1997; 336:1216–1222.

84. Miller, E. R., et al. Meta-analysis: High-dosage vitamin E supplementation may increase all-cause mortality. *Ann Intern Med* 2005; 142:37–46.

85. Presse, N., et al. Validation of a semi-quantitative food frequency questionnaire measuring dietary vitamin K intake in elderly people. *J Am Diet Assoc* 2009; 109:1251–1255.

86. Cockayne, S., et al. Vitamin K and the prevention of fractures: Systematic review and meta-analysis of randomized controlled trials. *Arch Intern Med* 2006; 166:1256–1261.

87. Marcason, W. Vitamin K: What are the current dietary recommendations for patients taking Coumadin? *J Am Diet Assoc* 2007; 107:2022.

88. Malinow, M. R., et al. Reduction of plasma homocyst(e)ine levels by breakfast cereal fortified with folic acid in patients with coronary heart disease. *N Engl J Med* 1998; 338:1009–1015.

89. Optimal calcium intake. National Institutes of Health Consensus Statement. 1994; 12:1–31.

90. Appel, L. J., et al. A clinical trial of the effects of dietary patterns on blood pressure. DASH Collaborative Research Group. *N Engl J Med* 1997; 336:1117–1124.

91. Mursu, J., et al. Less is More: Dietary supplements and mortality rate in older women. The Iowa Women's Health Study. *Arch Intern Med.* 2011; 171:1625–1633.

92. Park, S-Y et al. Multivitamin use and the risk of mortality and cancer incidence The Multiethnic Cohort Study. *Am J Epidemiol.* 2011; 173:906–914.

93. Multivitamin/mineral supplements Fact Sheet for Health Professional. Available at http://ods.od.nih.gov/factsheets/MVMS-HealthProfessional, accessed 6/9/15.

94. Bjelakovic, G., Nikolova, D., Gluud, L. L., et al. Antioxidant supplements for prevention of mortality in healthy participants and patients with various diseases. *Cochran Db Syst Rev* 2008; Issue 2. Art. No.:CD007176. Doi:10.1002/14651858.CD007176.

95. Prasad, A. S., et al. Zinc supplementation decreases incidence of infections in the elderly: Effect of zinc on generation of cytokines and oxidative stress. *Am J Clin Nutr* 2007; 85:837–844.

96. Barringer, T. A., et al. Effect of a multivitamin and mineral supplement on infection and quality of life: A randomized, double-blind, placebo-controlled trial. *Ann Intern Med* 2003; 138:365–371.

97. El-Kadiki, A., and Sutton, A. J. Role of multivitamins and mineral supplements in preventing infection in elderly people: Systematic review and meta-analysis of randomised controlled trials. *Brit Med J* 2005; 330(7496):871. doi:10.1136/bmj.38399.495648.8F.

98. National Institutes of Health, State-of-the-Science conference statement. Multivitamin/mineral supplements and chronic disease prevention. *Ann Intern Med* 2006; 145.

99. Silver, H. J., Oral strategies to supplement older adults' dietary intakes: comparing the evidence. *Nutr Rev.* 2009; 67:21–31.

100. Nicastro, H.L., et al. Using 2 Assessment Methods May Better Describe Dietary Supplement Intakes in the United States. *J Nutr.* First published ahead of print May 27, 2015, doi: 10.3945/jn.115.211466.

101. Schwingshackl, L., et al. Dietary supplements and risk of cause-specific death, cardiovascular disease, and cancer: a protocol for a systematic review and network meta-analysis of primary prevention trials. *Syst Rev* 2015; 4:34.

102. Ernst, E. Commentary How much of CAM is based on research evidence? Evidence-Based Complementary and Alternative Medicine. Vol. 2011, Article ID 676490, 3 pages. Doi:10.1093/ecam/nep044.

103. Evans, W. J. Exercise training guidelines for the elderly. *Med Sci Sports Exerc* 1999; 31:12–17.

104. Krinke, U. B. Effective nutrition education strategies to reach older adults. In Watson, R. R., ed. *Handbook of nutrition in the aged.* Boca Raton, FL: CRC Press, 2001, 319–331.

105. Friedman, H. S., and Martin, L. R. The Longevity Project Surprising discoveries for health and long life from the landmark eight decade study. New York: Hudson Street Press, 2011.

106. Position of the American Dietetic Association, the American Society for Nutrition, and the Society for Nutrition Education. Food and Nutrition Programs for Community-Residing Older Adults: *J Nutr Educ Behav.* 2010; 42(2):72–82.

107. Wellman, N. S., et al. Thirty years of the Older Americans Nutrition Program. *J Am Diet Assoc* 2002; 102:348–350.

108. Senior Hunger and the Older Americans Act: Hearings before the Subcommittee on Primary Health and Aging, of the Senate Committee on Health, Education, Labor and Pensions, 106th Cong. (2011) (testimony of Kathy Greenlee). Available at http://www.hhs.gov/asl/testify/2011/06/t20110621a.html, accessed 6/13/15.

109. Sahyoun, N. R., and Vaudin, A. Home-delivered meals and nutrition status among older adults. *Nutr Clin Pract* 2014; 29:459–465.

110. Buettner, D. *The Blue Zone: Lessons for living longer from the people who've lived the longest.* Washington, DC: National Geographic Society, 2008.

## Chapter 19


1. Kagawa, Y. From clock genes to telomeres in the regulation of healthspan. *Nutrition Reviews* 2012; 70:459–471.

2. Federal Interagency Forum on Aging-Related Statistics. Older Americans 2012: Key indicators of well-being. Washington, DC: U.S. Government Printing Office, June 2012. Available at www.agingstats.gov, accessed 6/15/15.

3. Medicare Program; Revisions to Payment Policies and Five-Year Review of and Adjustments to the Relative Values Units Under the Physician Fee Schedule for Calendar Year 2002: Final Rule Subpart G—Medical Nutrition Therapy. Federal Register, 42 *CFR*, Part 405; 66(212), November 1, 2001: 55275–55281.

4. Lacey, K., and Pritchett, E. Nutrition care process and model: ADA adopts road map to quality care and outcomes management. *J Am Diet Assoc* 2003; 103(8):1061–1072.

5. American Dietetic Association Position Paper. Cost effectiveness of medical nutrition therapy. *J Am Diet Assoc* 1995; 95:88–91.

6. Chima, C. S., et al. Relationship of nutritional status to length of stay, hospital costs, and discharge status of patients hospitalized in the medicine service. *J Am Diet Assoc* 1997; 97:975–78; quiz 979–980.

7. Position of the American Dietetic Association: Integration of Medical Nutrition Therapy and Pharmacotherapy. *J Am Diet Assoc* 2010; 110:950–956.

8. Wolinsky, F. D., et al. Health services utilization among the noninstitutionalized elderly. *J Health Soc Behav* 1983; 24:325–337.

9. National Center for Injury Prevention and Control. *10 Leading Causes of Death, by Age Group, United States, 2013*. Available at http://www.cdc.gov/injury/wisqars/leadingcauses.html, accessed 6/12/15.

10. Freid, V. M., et al. Multiple chronic conditions among adults aged 45 and over: Trends in the past 10 years. NCHS data brief, No. 100 Hyattsville, MD: National Center for Health Statistics. 2012.

11. Messier, S. P., et al. Weight loss reduces knee-joint loads in overweight and obese older adults with knee osteoarthritis. *Arthritis & Rheumatism* 2005; 52:2026–2032.

12. Yates, L. B., et al. Exceptional longevity in men: Modifiable risk factors associated with survival and function to age 90 years. *Arch Intern Med* 2008; 168:284–290.

13. Imamura, F., et al. Adherence to 2005 Dietary Guidelines for Americans is associated with a reduced progression of coronary artery atherosclerosis in women with established coronary artery disease. *Am J Clin Nutr* 2009; 90:193–201.

14. National Center for Health Statistics. Health, United States, 2014: With Special Feature on Adults Aged 55–64. Hyattsville, MD, 2015.

15. Schoenborn, C. A., and Heyman, K. M. Health characteristics of adults aged 55 years and over: United States, 2004–2007. Centers for Disease Control and Prevention, NCHS: National Health Statistics Reports, Number 16, July 8, 2009.

16. Mozaffarian, D., et al. on behalf of the American Heart Association Statistics Committee and Stroke Statistics Subcommittee. Heart disease and stroke statistics—2015 update: a report from the American Heart Association. *Circulation*. 2015;131:e29–e322. Available at http://www.heart.org/HEARTORG/General/Heart-and-Stroke-Association-statistics_UCM_319064_SubHomePage.jsp#, accessed 6/18/2015.

17. Odden, M. C., et al. Risk factors for cardiovascular disease across the spectrum of older age: the Cardiovascular Health Study. *Atherosclerosis*. 2014; 237:336–342.

18. Eckel, R. H., et al. 2013 AHA/ACC guideline on lifestyle management to reduce cardiovascular risk: a report of the American College of Cardiology/American Heart Association Task Force on Practice Guidelines. J Am Coll Cardiol 2014; 63:2960–2984.

19. Kwak, S. M., et al. for the Korean Meta-analysis Study Group. Efficacy of Omega-3 fatty acid supplements (Eicosapentaenoic acid and docosahexaenoic acid) in the secondary prevention of cardiovascular disease. A meta-analysis of randomized, double-blind, placebo-controlled trials. *Arch Intern Med*. 2012; 172:686–694.

20. Leon, H., et al. Effect of fish oil on arrhythmias and mortality: Systematic review. *BMJ* 2009; 338:a2931.

21. Hu, F. B., and Manson, J. E. Omega-3 fatty acids and the secondary prevention of cardiovascular disease—Is it just a fish tale? (comment). *Arch Intern Med*. 2012; 172:694–696.

22. Easton, D., et al. Definition and evaluation of transient ischemic attack. *Stroke* 2009; 40:2276–2293.

23. Bhatt, H., et al. Coronary heart disease risk factors and outcomes in the twenty-first century: findings from the REasons for Geographic and Racial Differences in Stroke (REGARDS) Study. Curr Hypertens Rep. 2015; 17:541.

24. Hiroyasu I., et al. Alcohol intake and the risk of cardiovascular disease in middle-aged Japanese men. *Stroke* 1995; 26:767–773.

25. Sacco, R. L., et al. The protective effects of moderate alcohol consumption on ischemic stroke. *J Amer Med Assoc* 1999; 281:53–60.

26. Meschia, J. F., et al. Guidelines for the Primary Prevention of Stroke: A Statement for Healthcare Professionals from the American Heart Association/American Stroke Association. *Stroke*. 2014; 45:3754–3832.

27. James, P. A. 2014 Evidence-Based Guideline for the Management of High Blood Pressure in Adults. Report From the Panel Members Appointed to the Eighth Joint National Committee (JNC 8). *J Amer Med Assoc* 2014; 311:507–520.

28. American Heart Association. American Heart Association backs current BP treat-ments. Available at http://www.heart.org/HEARTORG/Conditions/HighBloodPressure/PreventionTreatmentofHighBloodPressure/American-Heart-Association-backs-current-BP-treatments_UCM_459129_Article.jsp, accessed 6/25/15.

29. Nwankwo, T., et al. Hypertension among adults in the United States: National Health and Nutrition Examination Survey, 2011–2012. NCHS data brief, no 133. Hyattsville, MD: National Center for Health Statistics, 2013.

30. Stamler J. The INTERSALT Study: background, methods, findings, and implications. *Am J Clin, Nutr* 1997; 65(suppl):626S–642S.

31. Appel, L. J., et al. Dietary approaches to prevent and treat hypertension. A scientific statement from the American Heart Association. *Hypertension* 2006; 47:296–308.

32. Svetkey, L. P., et al. Effect of lifestyle modifications on blood pressure by race, sex, hypertension status, and age. *J Hum Hypertens* 2005; 19:21–31.

33. Whelton, P. K., et al. Sodium reduction and weight loss in the treatment of hypertension in older persons: A randomized controlled trial of nonpharmacologic interventions in the elderly (TONE). TONE Collaborative Research Group. *J Am Med Assoc* 1998; 279:839–846.

34. Sacks, F. M., et al. Effects on blood pressure of reduced dietary sodium and the Dietary Approaches to Stop Hypertension (DASH) diet. DASH-Sodium Collaborative Research Group. *N Engl J Med* 2001; 344:3–10.

35. Welty, F. K., et al. Effect of onsite dietitian counseling on weight loss and lipid levels in an outpatient physician office. *Am J Cardiol* 2007; 100:73–75.

36. Folsom, A. R., et al. Degree of concordance with DASH diet guidelines and incidence of hypertension and fatal cardiovascular disease. Am J Hypertens 2007; 20:225–232.

37. Levitan, E. B., et al. Consistency with the DASH diet and incidence of heart failure. *Arch Intern Med* 2009; 169:851–857.

38. American Diabetes Association. Older adults. Sec. 10. In *Standards of Medical Care in Diabetes—2015*. Diabetes Care 2015; 38 (Suppl. 1).

39. Inzucchi, S. E., et al. Management of hyperglycemia in type 2 diabetes: A patient-centered approach. Position Statement of the American Diabetes Association (ADA) and the European Association for the study of diabetes (EASD). *Diabetes Care* 2012; 35:1364–1379.

40. Schwartz, A. V., et al. Diabetes-related complications, glycemic control, and falls in older adults. *Diabetes Care* 2008; 31:391–396.

41. American Diabetes Association. Foundations of care: Education, nutrition, physical activity, smoking cessation, psychosocial care, and immunization. Sec. 4. In *Standards of Medical Care in Diabetes 2015. Diabetes Care* 2015; 38(Suppl. 1):S20–S30.

42. Wan, H., and Larsen, L. J. U.S. Census Bureau, American Community Survey

Reports, ACS-29, Older Americans With a Disability: 2008–2012. Washington, DC: U.S. Government Printing Office, 2014.

43. Gardner, C., et al. Nonnutritive sweeteners: current use and health perspectives. A scientific statement from the American Heart Association and the American Diabetes Association. *Circulation* 2012; 126:509–519.

44. Jensen, M. D., et al. 2013 AHA/ACC/TOS guideline for the management of overweight and obesity in adults: a report of the American College of Cardiology/American Heart Association Task Force on Practice Guidelines and The Obesity Society. *J Am Coll Cardiol.* 2014; 63:2985–3023.

45. World Health Organization Consultation on Obesity. *Obesity: Preventing and managing the global epidemic.* Geneva, Switzerland: World Health Organization, 2000; WHO Technical Report Series 894.

46. Heiat, A., et al. An evidence-based assessment of federal guidelines for overweight and obesity as they apply to elderly persons. *Arch Intern Med* 2001; 161:1194–1203.

47. Osher, E., and Stern N. Obesity in elderly subjects: in sheep's clothing perhaps, but still a wolf! *Diabetes Care.* 2009; 32 Suppl 2:S398-402.

48. Flegal, K. M., et al. Association of All-Cause Mortality with Overweight and Obesity Using Standard Body Mass Index Categories: A Systematic Review and Meta-analysis. *J Amer Med Assoc* 2013; 309:71–82.

49. Winter J. E., et al. BMI and all-cause mortality in older adults: a meta-analysis. *Am J Clin Nutr* 2014; 99:875–890.

50. Price, G. M., et al. Weight, shape, and mortality risk in older persons: Elevated waist–hip ratio, not high body mass index, is associated with a greater risk of death. *Am J Clin Nutr* 2006; 84:449–460.

51. Pischon, T., et al. General and abdominal adiposity and risk of death in Europe. *N Eng J Med* 2008; 359:2105–2120.

52. Winter, Y., et al. Contribution of obesity and abdominal fat mass to risk of stroke and transient ischemic attacks. *Stroke* 2008; 39:3145–3151.

53. Sui, X., et al. Cardiorespiratory fitness and adiposity as mortality predictors in older adults. *J Amer Med Assoc* 2007; 298:2507–2516.

54. Beavers, K. M., et al. Is lost lean mass from intentional weight loss recovered during weight regain in postmenopausal women? *Am J Clin Nutr.* 2011; 94:767–774.

55. American College of Sports Medicine, Position Stand, "Exercise and Physical Activity for Older Adults." *Med Sci. Sports Exerc* 2009; 41: 1510–1530.

56. DeCaria, J. E., et al. Scoping review report: obesity in older adults. *Int J Obesity* 2012; 36: 1141–1150.

57. National Osteoporosis Foundation. *Bone Health Basics: Get the Facts.* Available at http://nof.org/learn/basics, accessed 6/22/15.

58. World Health Organization Scientific Group on the assessment of osteoporosis at primary health care level. Summary meeting report, Brussels, Belgium, 5–7 May 2004. Available at http://who.int/chp/topics/Osteoporosis.pdf?ua=1, accessed 6/22/15.

59. National Osteoporosis Foundation. Clinician's guide to prevention and treatment of osteoporosis. Washington, DC: National Osteoporosis Foundation, 2010.

60. Looker, A. C., et al. Osteoporosis or low bone mass at the femur neck or lumbar spine in older adults: United States, 2005–2008. NCHS data brief no 93. Hyattsville, MD: National Center for Health Statistics, 2012.

61. Rubin, L. A., et al. Determinants of peak bone mass: Clinical and genetic analyses in a young female Canadian cohort. *J Bone Miner Res* 1999; 14:633–643.

62. Matkovic, V., et al. Bone status and fracture rates in two regions of Yugoslavia. *Am J Clin Nutr* 1979; 32:540–549.

63. Lloyd, T., et al. Calcium supplementation and bone mineral density in adolescent girls. *J Am Med Assoc* 1993; 270:841–844.

64. National Center for Health Statistics, National Vital Statistics System. 10 leading causes of injury deaths by age group highlighting unintentional injury deaths, United States, 2013. Available at cdc.gov/injury/wisquars, accessed on 6/22/2015.

65. Bischoff-Ferrari, H. A., et al. Fracture prevention with vitamin D supplementation: A meta-analysis of randomized controlled trials. *J Amer Med Assoc* 2005; 293:2257–2264.

66. Prince, R. L., et al. Effects of calcium supplementation on clinical fracture and bone structure. *Arch Intern Med* 2006; 166:869–875.

67. Feskanich, D., et al. Protein consumption and bone fractures in women. *Am J Epidemiol* 1996; 143:472–479.

68. Heaney, R. P., and Layman, D. K. Amount and type of protein influences bone health. *Am J Clin Nutr* 2008; 87(Suppl.):1567S–1570S.

69. Burckhardt, P. The effect of the alkali load of mineral water on bone metabolism: Interventional studies. *J Nutr* 2008; 138:435S–437S.

70. Dawson-Hughes, B., et al. Alkaline diets favour lean tissue mass in older adults. *Am J Clin Nutr* 2008; 87:662–665.

71. Writing Group for the Women's Health Initiative Investigators. Risks and benefits of estrogen plus progestin in healthy postmenopausal women. Principal results from the Women's Health Initiative randomized controlled trial. *J Am Med Assoc* 2002; 288:321–333.

72. Rosen, C. J. Serotonin rising–the bone, brain, bowel connection. *N Engl J Med* 2009; 360:957–959.

73. National Health Interview Survey, 2010. National Center for Health Statistics. *Vital Health Statistics.* 2009; 10:240.

74. Sahyoun, N. R., et al. Nutritional status of the older adult is associated with dentition status. *J Am Diet Assoc.* 2003; 103: 61–66.

75. Academy of Nutrition and Dietetics. Position of the Academy of Nutrition and Dietetics: Oral Health and Nutrition. *J Acad Nutr Diet* 2013; 113: 693–701.

76. Eke, P. I., et al. Update on prevalence of periodontitis in adults in the United States: NHANES 2009 to 2012. *J Periodontol* 2015; 86:611–622.

77. Lockhart, P. B., et al. Periodontal disease and atherosclerotic vascular disease: does the evidence support independent association?: A scientific Statement from the American Heart Association. *Circulation* 2012; 125:2520–2544.

78. Naqvi, A. Z., et al. n-3 fatty acids and periodontitis in US adults. *J Am Diet Assoc* 2010; 110; 1669–1675.

79. Naqvi, A. Z., et al. Docosahexaenoic Acid and Periodontitis in Adults: A Randomized Controlled Trial. *J Dent Res* 2014; 93:767–773.

80. Vakil, N., et al. Global Consensus Group. The Montreal definition and classification of gastroesophageal reflux disease: a global evidence-based consensus. *Am J Gastroenterol* 2006; 101:1900–1920.

81. Scott, M., and Gehot, A. R. Gastroesophageal reflux disease: Diagnosis and management. *Am Fam Physician* 1999; 59:1161-69. Available at http://www.aafp.org/afp/1999/0301/p1161.html, accessed 6/26/15.

82. Ables, A. Z., et al. Update on *Helicobacter pylori* treatment. *Am Fam Physician* 2007; 75:351–358. Available at http://www.aafp.org/afp/2007/0201/p351.html, accessed 6/25/15.

83. Chatthanawaree, W. Biomarkers of cobalamin (vitamin B12) deficiency and its application. *J Nutr Health Aging.* 2011; 15:227–231.

84. Bailey, R. L., et al. Monitoring of vitamin B-12 nutritional status in the United States by using plasma methylmalonic acid and serum vitamin B-12. *Am J Clin Nutr.* 2011; 94:552–561.

85. Otten, J. J., et al., eds. Institute of Medicine of the National Academies. Dietary Reference Intakes: The Essential Guide to Nutrient Requirements. Washington, DC: The National Academies Press, 2006.

86. Eussen, S. J. P. M., et al. Oral Cyanocobalamin supplementation in older people with vitamin $B_{12}$ deficiency: A dose-finding trial. *Arch Intern Med* 2005; 165:1167–1172.

87. Bente, L. B., and Gerrior, S. A. Selected food and nutrient highlights of the 20th century: U.S. food supply series. *Family Econ Nutr Rev* 2002; 14:43–51.

88. Drossman, D. A. Rome III: the new criteria. *China J Dig Disease* 2006; 7:181–185.

89. Gallegos-Orozco, J. F., et al. Chronic constipation in the elderly. Am J Gastroenterol. 2012; 107:18–25.

90. Talley, N. J., et al. Constipation in an elderly community: A study of prevalence and potential risk factors. *Am J Gastroenterol* 1996; 91:19–25.

91. Müller-Lissner, S. A., et al. Myths and misconceptions about chronic constipation. *Am J Gastroenterol* 2005; 100:232–242.

92. Rao, S. S., and Go, J. T. Update on management of constipation in the elderly: New treatment options. *Clin Interv Aging* 2010; 5:163–171.

93. Behm, R. M. A special recipe to banish constipation. *Geriatr Nurs* 1985; 6:216–217.

94. Centers for Disease Control and Prevention. Osteoarthritis. Available at cdc.gov/arthritis/basics/osteoarthritis.htm, accessed 6/17/2015.

95. Zhang, F. F., et al. Vitamin D deficiency is associated with progression of knee osteoarthritis. *J Nutr* 2014; 144:2002–2008.

96. McAlindon, T., et al. Effect of vitamin D supplementation on progression of knee pain and cartilage volume loss in patients with symptomatic osteoarthritis. *J Amer Med Assoc* 2013; 309:155–162.

97. Cameron, M., et al. Evidence of effectiveness of herbal medicinal products in the treatment of arthritis. Part I: Osteoarthritis. *Phytother Res.* 2009; 23:1497–1515.

98. Marcason, W. What is the anti-inflammatory diet? Question of the month in *J Am Diet Assoc* 2010; 110:1780.

99. Clegg, D. O., et al. Glucosamine, chondroitin sulphate, and the two in combination for painful knee osteoarthritis. *N Engl J Med* 2006; 354:795–808.

100. Borchers, A. T., et al. Inflammation and Native American medicine: The role of botanicals. *Am J Clin Nutr* 2000; 72:339–347.

101. Alzheimer's Association, 2014 Alzheimer's Disease Facts and Figures, Alzheimer's & Dementia, Volume 10, Issue 2. http://www.alz.org/downloads/facts_figures_2014.pdf, Accessed 6/17/2015.

102. Jack Jr., C. R., et al. Introduction to the recommendations from the National Institute on Aging–Alzheimer's Association workgroups on diagnostic guidelines for Alzheimer's disease. *Alzheimers Dement* 2011; 7:257–262.

103. Hebert, L. E., et al. Alzheimer disease in the United States (2010–2050) estimated using the 2010 Census. *Neurology* 2013; 80:1778–1783.

104. Plassman, B. L., et al. Prevalence of dementia in the United States: The aging, demographics, and memory study. *Neuroepidemiology* 2007; 29:125–132.

105. Plassman, B. L., et al. Prevalence of cognitive impairment without dementia in the United States. *Ann Intern Med* 2008; 148:427–434.

106. Aisen, P. S., et al. High-dose B vitamin supplementation and cognitive decline in Alzheimer disease: A randomized controlled trial. *J Amer Med Assoc* 2008; 300:1774–1783.

107. van de Rest, O., et al. Dietary patterns, cognitive decline, and dementia: a systematic review. *Adv Nutr* 2015; 6:154–168.

108. Feart, C., et al. Adherence to a Mediterranean diet, cognitive decline, and risk of dementia. *J Amer Med Assoc* 2009; 302:638–648.

109. Scarmeas, N., et al. Physical activity, diet, and risk of Alzheimer's disease. *J Amer Med Assoc* 2009; 302:627–637.

110. Witte, A. V., et al. Caloric restriction improves memory in elderly humans. *P Natl Acad of Sci USA* 2009; 106:1255–1260.

111. Sabia, S., et al. Body mass index over the adult life course and cognition in late midlife: The Whitehall II Cohort study. *Am J Clin Nutr* 2009; 89:601–607.

112. Williams, J. W., et al. *Preventing Alzheimer's Disease and Cognitive Decline.* Evidence Report/Technology Assessment Number 193. AHRQ Publication No. 10-E005. April 2010.

113. Cassells, C. Medical food linked to memory improvement in mild Alzheimer's. Available at www.medscape.com/viewarticle/767960, accessed 6/18/2015.

114. Gnjidic, D., et al. High-risk prescribing and incidence of frailty among older community-dwelling men. *Clin Pharmacol Ther* 2012; 91:521–528.

115. Patterson, S. M., et al. Interventions to improve the appropriate use of polypharmacy for older people. *Cochrane Db Syst Rev* 2012; 5:CD008165.

116. Charlesworth, C. J., et al. Polypharmacy among adults aged 65 years and older in the United States: 1988–2010. *J Gerontol A Biol Sci Med Sci.* 2015; doi:10.1093/gerona/glv013.

117. Douglass, R., and Heckman, G. Drug-related taste disturbance. *Can Fam Physician* 2010; 56:1142–1147.

118. National Institutes of Health. Clinical guidelines on the identification, evaluation, and treatment of overweight and obesity in adults—The evidence report. *Obes Res* 1998; 6(Suppl 2):51S–209S.

119. The World Health Organization/Food and Agricultural Organization/United Nations University. *Physical status: The use and interpretation of anthropometry.* Report of a WHO Expert Committee. Geneva: World Health Organization, 1995.

120. Wong, C. J. Involuntary weight loss. *Med Clin North Am.* 2014; 98:625–643.

121. Zeanandin, G., et al. Impact of restrictive diets on the risk of undernutrition in a free-living elderly population. *Clin Nutr* 2012; 31:69–73.

122. Wernette, C. M., et al. Signaling proteins that influence energy intake may affect unintentional weight loss in elderly persons. *J Am Diet Assoc* 2011; 111:864–873.

123. Akner, G., and Cederholm, T. Treatment of protein-energy malnutrition in chronic nonmalignant disorders. *Am J Clin Nutr* 2001; 74:6–24.

124. Milne, A. C., et al. Protein and energy supplementation in elderly people at risk from malnutrition. *Cochrane Db Syst Rev* 2002; Issue 4:1–71.

125. Cereda, E., et al. Energy balance in patients with pressure ulcers: A systematic review and meta-analysis of observational studies. *J Am Diet Assoc.* 2011; 111:1868–1876.

126. National Pressure Ulcer Advisory Panel, European Pressure Ulcer Advisory Panel and Pan Pacific Pressure Injury Alliance. Prevention and Treatment of Pressure Ulcers: Quick Reference Guide. Emily Haesler (Ed.). Cambridge Media: Perth, Australia; 2014. Available at http://www.npuap.org/wp-content/uploads/2014/08/Updated-10-16-14-Quick-Reference-Guide-DIGITAL-NPUAP-EPUAP-PPPIA-16Oct2014.pdf, accessed 6/27/15.

127. Phillips, P. A., et al. Reduced thirst after water deprivation in healthy elderly men. *N Eng J Med* 1984; 311:753–759.

128. Popkin, B. M., et al. Water, Hydration and Health. *Nutr Rev.* 2010; 68: 439–458.

129. Gross, C. R., et al. Clinical indicators of dehydration severity in elderly patients. *J Emerg Med* 1992; 10:267–274.

130. Hodgkinson, B., et al. Maintaining oral hydration in older people, The Joanna Briggs Institute for Evidence Based Nursing and Midwifery. *Systematic Review* 2001; 12:1–66.

131. Briggs, G. M., and Calloway, D. H. *Bogert's nutrition and physical fitness.* New York: Holt, Rinehart and Winston, 1984.

132. Institute of Medicine of the National Academies. Dietary Reference Intakes for water, potassium, sodium, chloride, and sulfate. Washington, DC: The National Academies Press, 2005.

133. Cabrera, C., et al. Beneficial effects of green tea—a review. *J Am Coll Nutri* 2006; 25:79–99.

134. Wang, C-H., et al. Cranberry-containing products for prevention of urinary tract infections in susceptible populations A systematic review and meta-analysis of randomized controlled trials. *Arch Intern Med* 2012; 172:988–996.

135. Good, P., et al. Medically assisted hydration for adult palliative care patients. *Cochrane Library* Published online April 2014. Available at http://www.cochrane.org/CD006273/SYMPT_medically-assisted-hydration-to-assist-palliative-care-patients, accessed 6/26/15.

136. Ganzini, L., et al. Nurses' Experiences with Hospice Patients Who Refuse Food and Fluids to Hasten Death. *N Engl J Med* 2003; 349:359–365.

137. Leming, M. R., and Dickinson, G. E. *Understanding dying, death, and bereavement.* Fort Worth, TX: Holt, Rinehart, and Winston, 1990.

138. Stahl, S. T., and Schulz R. Changes in routine health behaviors following late-life bereavement: A systematic review. *J Behav Med.* 2014; 37:736–755.

# Glossary

**Acinus** Small sacs lined by cells that produce milk.

**active living movement** Building a culture where regular physical activity and healthy eating are the accepted norm for people of all ages, abilities and income levels. Involves partnerships of public and private entities and the local community to bring about changes.

**activity thermogenesis** Energy expended through physical activity and nonexercise activity such as fidgeting.

**adipocytokines** Adipose tissue secretes several signaling proteins, including the appetite suppressants adiponectin, leptin, and resitin.

**allele** A different version of the same gene. Alleles have a different arrangement of bases than the usual version of the gene.

**allergic diseases** Conditions resulting from hypersensitivity to a physical or chemical agent.

**Alveoli** A rounded or oblong-shaped cavity present in the breast.

**Alzheimer's disease** A brain disease that represents the most common form of dementia. It is characterized by memory loss for recent events that expands to more distant memories over the course of 5 to 10 years. It eventually produces profound intellectual decline characterized by dementia and personal helplessness.

**amenorrhea** Absence of menstrual cycle.

**amenorrhea** Absence of menstrual cycles.

**amino acids** The "building blocks" of protein. Unlike carbohydrates and fats, amino acids contain nitrogen.

**amniotic fluid** The fluid contained in the amniotic sac that surrounds the fetus in the uterus.

**amylophagia** Compulsive consumption of laundry starch or cornstarch.

**anaphylaxis** Sudden onset of a reaction with mild to severe symptoms, including a decrease in ability to breathe, which may be severe enough to cause a coma.

**androgens** Types of steroid hormones produced in the testes, ovaries, and adrenal cortex from cholesterol. Some androgens (testosterone, dihydrotestosterone) stimulate development and functioning of male sex organs.

**androgens** Types of steroid hormones produced in the testes, ovaries, and adrenal cortex from cholesterol. Some androgens (testosterone, dihydrotestosterone) stimulate development and functioning of male sex organs.

**anemia** A reduction below normal in the number of red blood cells per cubic mm in the quantity of hemoglobin, or in the volume of packed red cells per 100 mL of blood. This reduction occurs when the balance between blood loss and blood production is disturbed.

**anencephaly** Condition initiated early in gestation of the central nervous system in which the brain is not formed correctly, resulting in neonatal death.

**aneurysm** Ballooning of the blood vessel wall.

**anorexia nervosa** An eating disorder characterized by extreme weight loss, poor body image, and irrational fears of weight gain and obesity.

**anorexia nervosa** An eating disorder characterized by extreme weight loss, poor body image, and irrational fears of weight gain and obesity.

**anovulation** The absence of ovulation.

**anovulatory cycles** Menstrual cycles in which ovulation does not occur.

**Anthropometry** The science of measuring the human body and its parts.

**antidiuretic hormone** Causes kidneys to absorb more water from urine, resulting in increased blood volume.

**antioxidants** Chemical substances that prevent or repair damage to cells caused by exposure to oxidizing agents such as oxygen, ozone, and smoke and to other oxidizing agents normally produced in the body. Many different antioxidants are found in foods; some are made by the body.

**antioxidants** Chemical substances that prevent or repair damage to molecules and cells caused by oxidizing agents. Vitamins C (see Illustration 2.3) and E, selenium, and certain components of plants function as antioxidants.

**aphasia** Difficulties in self-expression, including inability to speak, finding the right words or understanding print or spoken words.

**appropriate for gestational age (AGA)** Weight, length, and head circumference are between the 10th and 90th percentiles for gestational age.

**assisted reproductive technology (ART)** An umbrella term for fertility treatments such as *in vitro* fertilization (IVF, a technique in which egg cells are fertilized by sperm outside the woman's body), artificial insemination, and hormone treatments.

**asthma** Condition in which the lungs are unable to exchange air due to lack of expansion of air sacs. It can result in a chronic illness and sometimes unconsciousness and death if not treated.

**atherogenic diet** A pattern of eating and food choices that promotes deposits of plaque in arterial walls and contributes to the development of cardiovascular disease.

**atherosclerosis** A disease of the arterial blood vessels (arteries) in which the walls of the blood vessels become thickened and hardened by cholesterol and calcium-containing plaque.

**atherosclerosis** A type of hardening of the arteries in which cholesterol is deposited in the arteries. These deposits narrow the coronary arteries and may reduce the flow of blood to the heart.

**athetosis** Uncontrolled movements of the large muscle groups as a result of damage to the central nervous system.

**atrial fibrillation** Degeneration of the heart muscle causing irregular contractions.

**attention deficit hyperactivity disorder (ADHD)** Condition characterized by low impulse control and short attention span, with and without a high level of overall activity.

**autism spectrum disorders (ASDs)** A group of developmental disorders characterized by deficits in communication, social interaction, and behaviors that meet diagnostic criteria in standardized testing, with onset generally before age 3.

**autoimmune disease** Diseases that result from a failure of an organism to recognize its own constituent parts as "self." The organism attempts to defend itself from the perceived foreign substance through actions of its immune system. These actions can damage molecules, cells, tissues, and organs. Type 1 diabetes, lupus, and rheumatoid arthritis are examples of autoimmune disease.

**B-lymphocytes** White blood cells that are responsible for producing immunoglobulins.

**basal metabolic rate (BMR)** Amount of energy required for cellular metabolic processes and function of organs. It is measured in an individual who has been awake less than 30 minutes and is still at absolute rest, has fasted for 10 hours or more, and is in a quiet room with normal, comfortable temperature.

**bilirubin Encephalopathy or Kernicterus** The chronic and permanent clinical sequelae that are the end result of very high untreated bilirubin levels. Excessive bilirubin in the system is deposited in the brain, causing toxicity to the basal ganglia and various brainstem nuclei.

**binge-eating disorder** An eating disorder characterized by periodic binge eating, which normally is not followed by vomiting or the use of laxatives. People must experience eating binges twice a week on average for over six months to qualify for this diagnosis.

**bioactive food components** Constituents in foods or dietary supplements other than those needed to meet basic human nutritional needs that are responsible for changes in health status.

**BMI rebound** A normal increase in body mass index that occurs after BMI declines and reaches its lowest point at 4–6 years of age.

**body mass index (BMI)** Weight in kg/height in $m^2$. BMIs $< 18.5$ are considered underweight, 18.5–24.9 normal weight, 25–29.9 overweight, and BMIs of 30 and higher obesity.

**body mass index** An index that correlates with total body fat content or percent body fat and is an acceptable measure of adiposity or body fatness in children and adults. It is calculated by dividing weight in kilograms by the square of height in meters ($kg/m^2$).

**bone age** Bone maturation; correlates well with stage of pubertal development.

**bronchopulmonary dysplasia (BPD)** Condition in which the underdeveloped lungs in a preterm infant are damaged so that breathing requires extra effort.

**bulimia nervosa** A disorder characterized by repeated bouts of uncontrolled, rapid ingestion of large quantities of food (binge eating) followed by self-induced vomiting, laxatives or diuretic use, fasting, or vigorous exercise in order to prevent weight gain.

**bulimia nervosa** An eating disorder characterized by recurrent episodes of rapid, uncontrolled eating of large amounts of food in a short period of time. Episodes of binge eating are followed by compensatory behaviors such as such as self-induced vomiting, dieting, excessive exercise, or misuse of laxatives, to prevent weight gain.

**calorie** A unit of measure of the amount of energy supplied by food. Also known as the "kilocalorie" (kcal), or the "large Calorie."

**calorie restriction** Decreasing the energy level of one's diet by 25–30 percent while meeting protein, vitamin, and mineral needs.

**carcinogenesis** The process by which normal cells are transformed into cancer cells. It includes activation, initiation, promotion, progression, and invasion and metastasis. Dietary constituents can modify the process at several points along the continuum.

**carcinogenic diet** A pattern of eating and food choices that increases the risk of some cancers.

**cardio-protective diet** A diet that emphasizes plant foods (vegetables, fruits, grains, especially whole grains, and legumes), appropriate fats, and fish, along with smaller amounts of lean meat and dairy.

**carotid artery disease** Arteries that supply blood to the brain and neck becoming damaged.

**catch-up growth** The accelerated growth of a premature or small infant, or malnourished infant or child that occurs during the first two years of life.

**centenarian** Person who reaches age 100 or more.

**cephalopelvic disproportion** A mismatch between the size of the fetal head and size of the maternal pelvis, resulting in "failure to progress" in labor for mechanical reasons.

**cerebral embolism** Piece of a blood clot formed elsewhere that travels to the brain.

**cerebral palsy** A group of disorders characterized by impaired muscle activity and coordination present at birth or developed during early childhood.

**cerebrovascular disease** Conditions caused by problems that affect the blood supply to the brain.

**children and youth with special health care needs (CYSHCN)** Infants, children and adolescents who have or are at increased risk for a chronic physical, developmental, behavioral, or emotional condition and who also require health and related services of a type or amount beyond that required by children generally.

**children with special health care needs** A general term for infants and children with, or at risk for, physical or developmental disabilities or chronic medical conditions from genetic or metabolic disorders, birth defects, premature births, trauma, infection, or prenatal exposure to drugs.

**cholesterol** A fat-soluble, colorless liquid primarily found in animals products.

**chronic condition** Disorder of health or development that is the usual state for an individual and unlikely to change, although secondary conditions may result over time.

**chronic disease** Slow-developing, long-lasting diseases that are not contagious (e.g., heart disease, cancer, diabetes). They can be treated but not always cured.

**chronic diseases** Slow-developing, long-lasting diseases that are not contagious (e.g., heart disease, cancer, diabetes).

**chronic inflammation** Low-grade inflammation that lasts weeks, months, or years. Inflammation is the first response of the body's immune system to infectious agents, toxins, or irritants. It triggers the release of biologically active substances that promote oxidation and other reactions to counteract the infection, toxin, or irritant. A side effect of chronic inflammation is that it also damages lipids, cells, and tissues.

**chronic inflammation** Low-grade inflammation that lasts weeks, months, or years. Inflammation is the first response of the body's immune system to infectious agents, toxins, or irritants. It triggers the release of biologically active substances that promote oxidation and other reactions to counteract the infection, toxin, or irritant. A side effect of chronic inflammation is that it also damages lipids, cells, and tissues.

**cleft lip and palate** Condition in which the upper lip and roof of the mouth are not formed completely and are surgically corrected, resulting in feeding, speaking, and hearing difficulties in childhood.

**climacteric change** Point in life where crucial changes occur; refers to the loss of reproductive activity, marked by menopause in women and reduction in testosterone production in men.

**cobalamin** Another name for vitamin $B_{12}$. Important roles of cobalamin are fatty-acid metabolism, synthesis of nucleic acid (i.e., DNA, a complex protein that controls the formation of healthy new cells), and formation of the myelin sheath that protects nerve cells.

**coenzymes** Chemical substances that activate enzymes.

**cognitive behavioral therapy** Programs designed to build knowledge, modify beliefs and attitudes, and integrate new behaviors through a combination of skills training and analysis of behavior and thought processes over a period of several weeks. Key features are cognitive restructuring and stimulus control.

**Cognitive function** The process of thinking.

**colic** A condition marked by a sudden onset of irritability, fussiness, or crying in a young infant between 2 weeks and 3 months of age who is otherwise growing and healthy.

**Colostrum** The milk produced in the first 2–3 days after the baby is born. Colostrum is higher in protein and lower in lactose than milk produced after a milk supply is established.

**commodity program** A USDA program in which food products are sent to schools for use in the child nutrition programs. Commodities are usually acquired for farm price support and surplus-removal reasons.

**comorbidity** The presence of one or more diseases or conditions in addition to the primary disease or disorder.

**competitive foods** Foods sold to children in food service areas during meal times that compete with the federal meal programs.

**compression of morbidity** Shortening the period of illness and decreased functional capabilities at the end of life.

**congenital abnormality** A structural, functional, or metabolic abnormality present at birth. Also called congenital anomalies. These may be caused by environmental or genetic factors, or by a combination of the two. Structural abnormalities are generally referred to as congenital malformations, and metabolic abnormalities as inborn errors of metabolism.

**congenital anomalies** Structural, functional, or metabolic abnormalities present at birth. Also called congenital abnormalities.

**congenital anomaly** Condition evident in a newborn that is diagnosed at or near birth, usually as a genetic or chronic condition, such as spina bifida or cleft lip and palate.

**congenital diaphragmatic hernia** Displacement of the intestines up into the lung area due to incomplete formation of the diaphragm *in utero*.

**Continuum of Nutritional Health** Stages of nutritional status that range from optimal to unable to sustain life. The stages are resilient and healthy, altered substrate availability, nonspecific signs and symptoms, clinical conditions, chronic conditions, and terminal illness and death.

**corpus luteum** (*corpus* = body, *luteum* = yellow) A tissue about 12 mm in diameter formed from the follicle that contained the ovum prior to its release. It produces estrogen and progesterone. The "yellow body" derivation comes from the accumulation of lipid precursors of these hormones in the corpus luteum.

**corrected age** A term also known as adjusted age; it is used with preterm infants. It is calculated by subtracting the number of weeks born before 40 weeks of gestation from the infant or child's chronological (actual) age.

**critical periods** Pre-programmed time periods during embryonic and fetal development when specific cells, organs, and tissues are formed and integrated, or functional levels established. Also called *sensitive periods*.

**daily values (DVs)** Scientifically agreed-upon standards for daily intakes of nutrients from the diet developed for use on nutrition labels.

**demographic transition** Transition from high birth and death rates to low birth and death rates.

**developmental delay** An impairment in the performance of tasks or achieving developmental milestones that an infant or child should achieve by a specific chronological age. The diagnosis is made with testing that assesses cognitive, physical, social and emotional development, communication and adaptive skills.

**developmental disabilities** A group of conditions related to impairment in physical, learning, language, or behavioral areas. These conditions have onset in the developmental period, may impact daily functioning, and usually last throughout a person's lifetime.

**developmental plasticity** The concept that development can be modified by particular environmental conditions experienced by a fetus or infant.

**development** Progression of the physical and mental capabilities of an organism through growth and differentiation of organs and tissues, and integration of functions.

**diabetes self-management education and support** An ongoing process of individualized education and support to facilitate the knowledge, skill, and ability necessary for prediabetes and diabetes self-care and quality of life.

**dietary fiber** Complex carbohydrates and lignins naturally occurring and found mainly in the plant cell wall. Dietary fiber cannot be broken down by human digestive enzymes.

**dietary folate equivalents (DFE)** A measure of folate availability used by the Reference Dietary Intakes. 1 DFE = 1 mcg food folate, which is equivalent to 0.6 mcg. folic acid.

**dietary guidance** Providing concise recommendations and consumer information to guide daily food choices.

**dietary guidance system** A comprehensive set of dietary and lifestyle recommendations, based on the latest scientific information, that are developed to promote heath and prevent disease or its complications, ensure adequate intake of nutrients of concern, and offer guidance on what and how much to eat.

**Dietary Guidelines** A report, including scientific information and rationale, on dietary information and guidelines for the general public or a defined subpopulation. The guidelines provide a cohesive set of recommendations that are adopted by the government or organization. They represent policy and are integrated into food, nutrition, and health programs.

**dietary pattern** The quantities, proportions, variety, or combination of different foods, drinks, and nutrients in diets, and the frequency with which they are habitually consumed.

**Dietary Reference Intakes (DRIs)** Quantitative estimates of nutrient intakes, used as reference values for assessing the diets of healthy people. DRIs include Recommended Dietary Allowances (RDAs), Adequate Intakes (AI), Tolerable Upper Intake Levels (UL), and Estimated Average Requirements (EAR).

**dietary supplements** Any product intended to supplement the diet, including vitamin and mineral supplements, proteins, enzymes, amino acids, fish oils, fatty acids, hormones and hormone precursors, and herbs and other plant extracts. In the United States, such products must be labeled "Dietary Supplement."

**differentiation** Cellular acquisition of one or more characteristics or functions different from that of the original cells.

**disproportionately small for gestational age (dSGA)** Newborn weight is less than 10th percentile of weight for gestational age; length and head circumference are normal. Also called *asymmetrical* SGA.

**diverticulitis** Infected "pockets" within the large intestine.

**DNA methylation** The modification of a replicated strand of DNA by addition of a methyl group ($CH_3$) to specific regions of the strand. Methylation can suppress the activity of certain genes in ways that affect metabolic processes and disease risk. It is a normal part of development and is needed for cellular differentiation and organ development but can also be influenced by nutritional and other environmental exposures.

**Doula** An individual who surrounds, interacts with, and aids the mother at any time within the period that includes pregnancy, birth, and lactation; may be a relative, friend, or neighbor and is usually but not necessarily female. One who gives psychological encouragement and physical assistance to a new mother.

**Down syndrome** Condition in which three copies of chromosome 21 occur, resulting in lower muscle strength, lower intelligence, and greater risk for overweight.

**dumping syndrome** A condition characterized by weakness, dizziness, flushing, nausea, and palpitation immediately or shortly after eating and produced by abnormally rapid emptying of the stomach, especially in individuals who have had part of the stomach removed.

**dyslipidemia** Abnormal blood levels of cholesterol and/or triglycerides resulting from altered lipid metabolism.

**early childhood caries (ECC)** The presence of one or more decayed (noncavitated or cavitated lesions), missing (due to caries), or filled tooth surfaces in any primary tooth in a child 71 months of age or younger.

**Early Intervention Program** Educational intervention for the development of children from birth up to 3 years of age.

**early intervention services** Federally mandated evaluation and therapy services for children in the age range from birth to 3 years under the Individuals with Disabilities Education Act.

**Eating Competence Model** A new paradigm for nutrition education and dietary guidance that considers four components: eating attitudes, food acceptance, regulation of food intake, and eating context. A competent eater is positive, comfortable, and flexible with eating and is matter-of-fact and reliable about getting enough to eat of enjoyable, nourishing food.

**eating plan** A plan for timing of meals and snacks and types and amount of foods eaten to achieve nutrition goals.

**edema** Swelling (usually of the legs and feet, but can also extend throughout the body) due to an accumulation of extracellular fluid.

**eicosanoids** Molecules synthesized from essential fatty acids. They exert complex control over many bodily systems, mainly in inflammation and immunity, and act as messengers in the central nervous system.

**embryo** The developing organism from conception through 8 weeks.

**empty-calorie foods** Foods that provide an excess of calories relative to their nutrient content.

**endocrine** A system of ductless glands, such as the thyroid, adrenal glands, ovaries, and testes, that produces secretions that affect body functions.

**endometriosis** A disease characterized by the presence of endometrial tissue in abnormal locations, such as deep within the uterine wall, in the ovary, or in other sites within the body. The condition is quite painful and is associated with abnormal menstrual cycles and infertility in 30–40 percent of affected women.

**endothelium** The layer of cells lining the inside of blood vessels.

**energy-dense foods** Food that have relatively high-calorie values per unit weight of the food.

**energy balance** An equilibrium state in which the number of calories consumed equals the number of calories expended.

**enrichment** The replacement of thiamin, riboflavin, niacin, and iron lost when grains are refined.

**enteral feeding** Method of delivering nutrients directly to the digestive system, in contrast to methods that bypass the digestive system.

**epididymis** Tissues on top of the testes that store sperm.

**epigenetic** (*epi* = over, above) Heritable changes in gene function that do not entail a change in DNA sequence. Epigenetic modifications play a crucial role in the silencing and expression of noncoding portions of genes.

**Epithelial cells** Cells that line the surface of the body.

**EPSDT** The Early Periodic Screening, Detection, and Treatment Program is a part of Medicaid and provides routine checkups for low-income families.

**ergogenic aids** Nutritional products that are purported to enhance performance. Examples range from caffeine and protein powders to sports drinks and energy gels and bars.

**essential amino acids** Amino acids that cannot be synthesized in adequate amounts by humans and therefore must be obtained from the diet. Also called *indispensible amino acids.*

**essential fatty acids** Components of fat that are a required part of the diet (i.e., linoleic and alpha-linolenic acids). Both contain unsaturated fatty acids.

**essential nutrients** Substances required for growth and health that cannot be produced, or produced in sufficient amounts, by the body. They must be obtained from the diet.

**estimated energy requirement (EER)** The average dietary energy intake for adults in good health, by age, gender, weight, height, and level of physical activity, that is predicted to maintain energy balance and is consistent with good health.

**exposure index** The average infant milk intake per kilogram body weight per day × (M/P ratio ÷ Rate of drug clearance) × 100. It is indicative of the amount of the drug in the breast milk that the infant ingests and is expressed as a percentage of the therapeutic (or equivalent) dose for the infant.

**extremely low-birthweight infant (ELBW)** An infant weighing $<$1000 g at birth.

**familial hyperlipidemia** A condition that runs in families and results in high levels of serum cholesterol and other lipids.

**fasting** Going 24 hours or more without eating.

**fat-free mass** Used interchangeably with lean body mass, comprising bone, muscle, water.

**fatty acids** The fat-soluble components of fats in foods.

**fecundity** Biological ability to bear children.

**female athlete triad** A condition marked by the simultaneous presence of an eating disorder, menstrual dysfunction, and osteoporosis in otherwise healthy female athletes. It is characterized by the interrelated factors of energy deficit, menstrual dysfunction, and loss of bone mineral density.

**fermentable fiber** Type of fiber that enters the large colon undigested, where it is acted on by the bacteria of the gut. Formerly called insoluble fiber.

**fertility** Actual production of children. The word best applies to specific vital statistic rates, but it is commonly taken to mean the ability to bear children.

**fetus** The developing organism from 8 weeks after conception to the moment of birth.

**fine motor skills** Development and use of smaller muscle groups demonstrated by stacking objects, scribbling, and copying a circle or square.

**fluorosis** Permanent white or brownish staining of the enamel of teeth caused by excessive ingestion of fluoride before teeth have erupted.

**follicle stimulating hormone (FSH)** A hormone produced by the pituitary gland that stimulates ovarian follicle growth and maturation, estrogen secretion, and endometrial changes characteristic of the first portion of the menstrual cycle in females. It stimulates sperm production in males.

**food allergy (hypersensitivity)** Abnormal or exaggerated immunologic response, usually immunoglobulin E (IgE) mediated, to a specific food protein.

**food insecurity** Limited or uncertain availability of safe, nutritious foods, or the ability to acquire them in socially acceptable ways.

**food intolerance** An adverse reaction involving digestion or metabolism but not the immune system.

**food security** Access at all times to a sufficient supply of safe, nutritious foods.

**food security** Access at all times to a sufficient supply of safe, nutritious foods.

**fortification** The addition of one or more vitamins or minerals to a food product.

**free radicals** Chemical substances (often oxygen-based) that are missing electrons. The absence of electrons makes the chemical substance reactive and prone to oxidizing nearby molecules by stealing electrons from them. Free radicals can damage lipids, cell membranes, DNA, and tissues by altering their chemical structure and functions. They also form as a normal part of metabolism. Over time, oxidative stress causes damage to lipids, cell membranes, DNA, cells, and tissues.

**full-term infants** Infants born at or after 37 weeks gestation.

**functional fiber** Isolated or purified undigestible carbohydrates that have beneficial physiological effects in humans.

**functional fiber** Nondigestible carbohydrates including plant, animal, or commercially produced sources that have beneficial effects in humans.

**functional foods** A food product that has a physiological benefit or reduces the risk of chronic disease beyond basic nutritional functions.

**functional status** Ability to perform daily activities to meet basic needs and live independently, including telephoning, grocery shopping, food preparation, and eating.

**galactogogue** A medicine or herbal substance taken with the belief to increase milk supply. It may also be taken to help with breastmilk initiation and maintenance.

**galactosemia** A rare genetic condition of carbohydrate metabolism in which a blocked or inactive enzyme does not allow breakdown of galactose, causing serious illness in infancy.

**galactosemia** A rare genetic condition of carbohydrate metabolism in which a blocked or inactive enzyme does not allow breakdown of galactose. It can cause serious illness if not identified and treated soon after birth.

**gastroesophageal reflux (GER)** Movement of the stomach contents backward into the esophagus due to stomach muscle contractions. The condition may require treatment depending on its duration and degree. Also known as *gastroesophageal reflux disease (GERD).*

**gastrostomy feeding** Form of enteral nutrition support for delivering nutrition by tube placement directly into the stomach, bypassing the mouth through a surgical procedure that creates an opening through the abdominal wall and stomach.

**gastrostomy** Form of enteral nutrition support for delivering nutrition by tube directly into the stomach, bypassing the mouth through a surgical procedure that creates an opening through the abdominal wall and stomach.

**gavage feeding** A procedure where a tube is passed through the nose or mouth into the stomach. This is used to feed preterm or newborn infants who are not yet able or have weak or uncoordinated ability to suck and swallow.

**gene variant** An alteration in the normal coding sequence of a gene. The different forms of the same genes are considered *alleles.*

**Gene variant** An alteration in the normal sequence of a gene. The different forms of the same genes are considered "alleles."

**geophagia** Compulsive consumption of clay or dirt.

**gestational diabetes** Carbohydrate intolerance with onset of, or first recognition in, pregnancy.

**gingiva** Gum tissue.

**glucogenic amino acids** Amino acids such as alanine and glutamate that can be converted to glucose.

**gluten** A protein found in wheat, spelt, kamut, dinkel, and triticale (genus Triticum), barley, and rye. Spelt, dinkel, and kamut are ancestral forms of today's wheat. Oats appear on some "gluten" lists; oats are inherently gluten free, but they may be contaminated by gluten-containing grains during processing.

**glycemic index (GI)** A measure of the extent to which blood glucose levels are raised by consumption of an amount of food that contains 50 grams of carbohydrate compared to 50 grams of glucose. A portion of white bread containing 50 grams of carbohydrate is sometimes used for comparison instead of 50 grams of glucose.

**glycemic index** A measure of the extent to which blood glucose levels are raised by consumption of an amount of food that contains 50 grams of carbohydrate compared to 50 grams of glucose. A portion of white bread containing 50 grams of carbohydrate is sometimes used for comparison.

**glycerol** A component of fats that is soluble in water. It is converted to glucose in the body.

**glycosylated hemoglobin A1C (HbA1c)** A blood test that measures how well the blood sugar level has been maintained over the last 2 to three months.

**gonadotropin releasing hormone (GnRH)** A hormone produced in the hypothalamus that is responsible for the release of follicle stimulating hormone and luteinizing hormone by the pituitary gland.

**gravida** Number of pregnancies a woman has experienced.

**gross motor skills** Development and use of large muscle groups as exhibited by walking alone, running, walking up stairs, riding a tricycle, hopping, and skipping.

**growth** Increase in an organism's size through cell multiplication (hyperplasia) and enlargement of cell size (hypertrophy).

**growth velocity** The rate of growth over time.

**gut dysbiosis** Breakdown in the balance of protective and harmful bacterial in the intestines.

**health disparity** Significant differences in the incidence, prevalence, mortality, and burden of disease and other adverse conditions that exist among specific population groups. Health disparity is closely linked to social and economic disadvantage.

**healthspan** Illness-free life span.

**healthy** More than the absence of disease, health is a sense of well-being. Even individuals with a chronic condition may properly consider themselves to be healthy. For instance, a person with diabetes mellitus whose blood sugar is under control can be considered healthy.

**healthy weight** A weight range compatible with normal function and long, healthy life.

**heart disease** The leading cause of death and a common cause of illness and disability in the United States. Coronary heart disease is the principal form of heart disease and is caused by buildup of cholesterol deposits in the coronary arteries, which feed the heart.

**hedonic obesity** Body weight maintained above set point due to sustained overeating.

**hematocrit** An indicator of the proportion of whole blood occupied by red blood cells. A decrease in hematocrit is a late indicator of iron deficiency.

**hemoglobin A1c** A form of hemoglobin used to identify blood glucose levels over the lifetime of a red blood cell (120 days). Glucose molecules in blood will attach to hemoglobin (and stay attached). The amount of glucose that attaches to hemoglobin is proportional to levels of glucose in the blood. The normal range of hemoglobin A1c is 4–5.9 percent. Also called glycosylated hemoglobin and glycated hemoglobin.

**hemoglobin** A protein that is the oxygen-carrying component of red blood cells. A decrease in hemoglobin concentration in red blood cells is a late indicator of iron deficiency.

**hemolytic uremic syndrome (HUS)** A serious, sometimes fatal complication associated with illness caused by *E. coli 0157:H7*, which occurs primarily in children under the age of 10 years. HUS is characterized by renal failure, hemolytic anemia, and a severe decrease in platelet count. Clean: Wash hands and surfaces often.

**HIV** Human immunodeficiency virus.

**homeostasis** Constancy of the internal environment. The balance of fluids, nutrients, gases, temperature, and other conditions needed to ensure ongoing, proper functioning of cells and, therefore, all parts of the body.

**homocysteine** Another intermediate product that depends on vitamin $B_{12}$ for complete metabolism. However, both vitamin $B_{12}$ and folate (another B vitamin) are coenzymes in the breakdown of certain protein components in this pathway. Thus, elevated homocysteine levels can result from vitamin $B_{12}$, folate, or pyridoxine deficiencies.

**hydrolyzed protein formula** Formula that contains enzymatically digested protein, or single amino acids, rather than protein as it naturally occurs in foods.

**hyperbilirubinemia** Elevated blood levels of bilirubin, a yellow pigment that is a byproduct of the breakdown of fetal hemoglobin.

**hyperbilirubinemia** Presence of an excess of bilirubin in the blood.

**hyperglycemia** Abnormally high levels of glucose in the blood.

**hyperinsulinemia** A state of excess levels of insulin circulating in the blood. It is common among persons with metabolic syndrome and type 2 diabetes and is caused by the pancreas trying to compensate for insulin resistance of cells.

**hypertension** High blood pressure. It is defined in adults as blood pressure exerted inside blood vessel walls that typically exceeds 140/90 mmHg (millimeters of mercury).

**hypertension** High blood pressure. It is defined in adults as blood pressure exerted inside blood vessel walls that typically exceeds 140/90 mmHg (millimeters of mercury).

**hypertonia** Condition characterized by high muscle tone, stiffness, or spasticity.

**hypoallergenic** Foods or products that have a low risk of promoting food or other allergies.

**hypothalamic amenorrhea** A condition characterized by cessation of menstruation due to changes in hypothalamic signals that maintain ovulation. Changes in hypothalamic function appear to be triggered by an energy deficit. Also called *functional hypothalamic amenorrhea* and *weight-related amenorrhea*.

**hypothalamus** A section of the brain responsible for the production of many hormones and other chemical substances that affect body functions such as temperature regulation, thirst, hunger, sleep, mood, reproduction, and the release of other hormones within the body.

**hypothyroidism** A condition characterized by growth impairment, intellectual disabilities, and deafness when caused by inadequate maternal intake of iodine during pregnancy. Used to be called *cretinism*.

**hypothyroidism** Condition in which thyroid hormone is not produced in sufficient quantities, interfering with growth and mental development if untreated in infants.

**hypotonia** Condition characterized by low muscle tone, floppiness, or muscle weakness.

**immunological** Having to do with the immune system and its functions in protecting the body from bacterial, viral, fungal, or other infections and from foreign proteins (i.e., those proteins that differ from proteins normally found in the body).

**infant mortality** Death that occurs within the first year of life.

**infant mortality rate** The number of infant deaths for every 1000 live births.

**infecundity** Biological inability to bear children after one year of unprotected intercourse.

**infertility** Involuntary absence of production of children.

**Innocenti Declaration** On the Protection, Promotion, and Support of Breastfeeding: Policy statement adopted by participants at the World Health Organization UNICEF policymakers' meeting on breastfeeding, a global initiative held in Italy in 1990. The policy established exclusive breastfeeding from birth to 4–6 months of age as a global goal for optimal maternal and child health.

**insulin** Hormone usually produced in the pancreas to regulate movement of glucose from the bloodstream into cells within organs and muscles.

**insulin resistance** A condition in which cell membranes have a reduced sensitivity to insulin so that more insulin than normal is required to transport a given amount of glucose into cells.

**insulin resistance** A condition in which cell membranes have reduced sensitivity to insulin so that more insulin than normal is required to transport a given amount of glucose into cells.

**insulin resistance** A condition in which cells "resist" the action of insulin in facilitating the passage of glucose into cells.

**intellectual disability** Substantially below-average intelligence and problems in adapting to the environment, which emerge before age 18 years.

**intra-abdominal fat** Fat located within the abdominal cavity around organs such as the liver, pancreas, and intestines. Intra-abdominal fat is referred to as visceral fat and is much more metabolically active than fat stored in other parts of the body.

**intrauterine growth retardation (IUGR)** Fetal undergrowth from any cause, resulting in a disproportionality in weight, length, or weight-for-length percentiles for gestational age. Sometimes called *intrauterine growth restriction*.

**longevity** Length of life, measured in years.

**iron-deficiency anemia** A condition often marked by low hemoglobin level. It is characterized by the signs of iron deficiency plus paleness, exhaustion, and a rapid heart rate.

**iron deficiency** A condition marked by depleted iron stores. It is characterized by weakness, fatigue, short attention span, poor appetite, increased susceptibility to infection, and irritability.

**ischemia** Blockage of blood vessel leading to lack of blood supply.

**ischemia** Inadequate blood supply to a local area due to partial or complete blockage of a blood vessel.

**Isotonic** Similar salt concentration as the blood.

**juvenile rheumatoid arthritis** Condition in which joints become enlarged and painful as a result of the dysfunction of the immune system; generally occurs in children or teens.

**ketogenic diet** High-fat, low-carbohydrate meal plan in which ketones are made from metabolic pathways used in converting fat as a source of energy.

**ketones** Metabolic byproducts of the breakdown of fatty acids in energy formation. b-hydroxybutyric acid, acetoacetic acid, and acetone are the major ketones, or *ketone bodies*.

**ketones** Metabolic byproducts of the breakdown of fatty acids in energy formation. Beta-hydroxybutyric acid, acetoacetic acid, and acetone are the major ketones, or "ketone bodies."

**Kwashiorkor** A severe form of protein-energy malnutrition in young children. It is characterized by swelling, fatty liver, susceptibility to infection, profound apathy, and poor appetite. The cause of kwashiorkor is unclear.

***L. monocytogenes*, or listeria** A foodborne bacterial infection that can lead to preterm delivery and stillbirth in pregnant women. Listeria infection is commonly associated with the ingestion of soft cheeses, unpasteurized milk, ready-to-eat deli meats, and hot dogs.

**lactation consultant** Health care professional whose scope of practice is focused on providing education and management to prevent and solve breastfeeding problems and to encourage a social environment that effectively supports the breastfeeding mother–infant dyad. Those who successfully complete the International Board of Lactation Consultant Examiners (IBLCE) certification process are entitled to use the IBCLC (International Board Certified Lactation Consultant) after their names (www.iblee.org).

**Lactogenesis** Another term for human milk production.

**lactose** A form of sugar or carbohydrate composed of galactose and glucose.

**La Leche League** International, nonprofit, nonsectarian organization dedicated to providing education, information, support, and encouragement to women who want to breastfeed. Founded in 1956 by seven women who had learned about successful breastfeeding while nursing their own babies, it currently has approximately 7,100 accredited lay leaders to facilitate more than 3,000 monthly mother-to-mother breastfeeding support group meetings around the world (www.lalecheleague.org).

**large for gestational age (LGA)** Weight for gestational age exceeds the 90th percentile for gestational age. Also defined as birthweight greater than 4500 g (10 lb) and referred to as *excessively sized for gestational age,* or *macrosomic.*

**LDL cholesterol** Low-density lipoprotein cholesterol, the lipid most associated with atherosclerotic disease. Diets high in saturated fat, *trans* fatty acids, and dietary cholesterol have been shown to increase LDL cholesterol levels.

**lean body mass** Sum of fat-free body tissue: muscle, mineral (as in bone), and water.

**lean body mass** Sum of fat-free body tissues: muscle, mineral as in bone, and water.

**leptin** A protein secreted by fat cells that, by binding to specific receptor sites in the hypothalamus, decreases appetite, increases energy expenditure, and stimulates gonadotropin secretion. Leptin levels are elevated by high, and reduced by low, levels of body fat.

**life span** Maximum number of years someone might live; human life span is projected to range from 110 to 120 years.

**life expectancy** Average number of years of life remaining for persons in a population cohort or group; most commonly reported as life expectancy from birth.

**liveborn infant** A liveborn infant is the outcome of delivery when a completely expelled or extracted fetus breathes, or shows any sign of life such as beating of the heart, pulsation of the umbilical cord, or definite movement of voluntary muscles, whether or not the cord has been cut or the placenta is still attached.

**Lobes** Rounded structures of the mammary gland.

**low-birthweight infant (LBW)** An infant weighing <2500 g at birth.

**lower esophageal sphincter (LES)** The muscle enabling closure of the junction between the esophagus and stomach.

**luteal phase** The second half of the menstrual cycle (usually days 14 to 28) that occurs after ovulation.

**luteinizing hormone (LH)** A hormone produced by the pituitary gland that stimulates ovulation, the development of the corpus luteum (which secretes progesterone), and the production of testosterone in males.

**macrobiotic diet** This diet falls between semivegetarian and vegan diets and includes foods such as brown rice, other grains, vegetables, fish, dried beans, spices, and fruits.

**macrocephaly** Abnormally large head size for age and gender.

**Macrophages** A white blood cell that acts mainly through phagocytosis.

**macrosomia** A newborn with an excessive birth weight (macro = big, somia = body). Newborn macrosomia has been defined in several different ways, including birth weight of 4000–4500 grams (8 lb 13 oz to 9 lb 15 oz) or greater than the 90th percentile of weight for gestational age.

**malnutrition** The cellular imbalance between the supply of nutrients and energy and the body's demand for them to ensure growth, maintenance, and specific functions.

**Mammary gland** The source of milk for offspring, also commonly called the breast. The presence of mammary glands is a characteristic of mammals.

**maple syrup urine disease** Rare genetic condition of protein metabolism in which breakdown byproducts build up in blood and urine, causing coma and death if untreated.

**meal replacement** A nutritionally balanced beverage, meal bar, or packaged meal used to replace a meal in weight management.

**meconium** Dark green mucilaginous material in the intestine of the full-term fetus.

**medical neglect** Failure of parent or caretaker to seek, obtain, and follow through with a complete diagnostic study or medical, dental, or mental health treatment for a health problem, symptom, or condition that, if untreated, could become severe enough to present a danger to the child.

**medical nutrition therapy (MNT)** Comprehensive nutrition services by registered dietitians to treat the nutritional aspects of acute and chronic diseases.

**Medicare** Federal health insurance for all people age 65 and older, and for younger individuals with certain disabling conditions.

**medicinal herbs** Plants used to prevent or remedy illness.

**memory impairment** Moderate or severe impairment is when 4 or fewer words can be recalled from a list of 20.

**menarche** The occurrence of the first menstrual cycle.

**meningitis** Viral or bacterial infection in the central nervous system that is likely to cause a range of long-term consequences in infancy, such as intellectual disability, blindness, and hearing loss.

**menopause** Cessation of the menstrual cycle and reproductive capacity in females.

**menses** The process of menstruation.

**menstrual cycle** An approximately 4-week interval in which hormones direct a build up of blood and nutrient stores within the wall of the uterus and ovum maturation and release. If the ovum is fertilized by a sperm, the stored blood and nutrients are used to support the growth of the fertilized ovum. If fertilization does not occur, they are released from the uterine wall over a period of 3 to 7 days. The period of blood flow is called the *menses*, or the menstrual period.

**metabolic obesity** Body weight set point shifts to a higher level due to alterations of the energy balance system.

**metabolic syndrome** A constellation of metabolic abnormalities that increases the risk of type 2 diabetes and cardiovascular diseases. It is characterized by insulin resistance, abdominal obesity, high blood pressure and triglyceride levels, low HDL cholesterol, and elevated fasting glucose or impaired glucose tolerance. Also called Syndrome X, insulin-resistance syndrome, and the dysmetabolic syndrome.

**metabolic syndrome** A constellation of metabolic abnormalities that increase the risk of heart disease, hypertension, type 2 diabetes, and other disorders. Metabolic syndrome is characterized by insulin resistance, abdominal obesity, high blood pressure and triglycerides levels, low levels of HDL cholesterol, and impaired glucose tolerance. It is also called *insulin resistance syndrome.*

**metabolism** The chemical changes that take place in the body. The conversion of glucose to energy or body fat is an example of a metabolic process.

**methylmalonic acid (MMA)** An intermediate product that needs vitamin $B_{12}$ as a coenzyme to complete the metabolic pathway for fatty-acid metabolism. Vitamin $B_{12}$ is the only coenzyme in this reaction; when it is absent, the blood concentration of MMA rises.

**microcephaly** Abnormally small head size for age and gender.

**middle childhood** Children between the ages of 5 and 10 years; also referred to as "school-age."

**mild cognitive impairment (MCI)** MCI Subtle loss of memory, thinking and/or reasoning skills beyond expectations of normal but not serious enough to be classified as dementia.

**milk-to-plasma drug concentration ratio (M/P ratio)** The ratio of the concentration of drug in milk to the concentration of drug in maternal plasma. Since the ratio varies over time, a time-averaged ratio provides more meaningful information than data obtained at a single time point. It is helpful in understanding the mechanisms of drug transfer and should not be viewed as a predictor of risk to the infant, as it is the concentration of the drug in milk, and not the M/P ratio, that is critical to the calculation of infant dose and assessment of risk.

**miscarriage** Generally defined as the loss of a conceptus in the first 20 weeks of pregnancy. Also called spontaneous abortion.

**monounsaturated fats** Fats in which only one pair of adjacent carbons in one or more of its fatty acids is linked by a double bond (e.g., –C–C=C–C–).

**Monovalent ion** An atom with an electrical charge of +1 or −1.

**Morbidity** The rate of illnesses in a population.

**Mortality** Rate of death.

**Myoepithelial cells** Specialized cells that line the alveoli and that can contract to cause milk to be secreted into the duct.

**necrotizing enterocolitis (NEC)** Condition with inflammation or damage to a section of the intestine, with a grading from mild to severe.

**neural tube defects (NTDs)** A group of birth defects that are caused by incomplete development of the brain, spinal cord, or their protective coverings. Spina bifida is one of the most common types of neural tube defects.

**neurobehavioral** Pertains to control of behavior by the nervous system.

**neuromuscular disorders** Conditions of the nervous system characterized by difficulty with voluntary or involuntary control of muscle movement.

**neuromuscular** Term pertaining to the central nervous system's control of muscle coordination and movement.

**Neutrophils** Class of white blood cells that are involved in the protection against infection.

**non-nutritive sucking** The sucking by newborns and young infants on items that do not provide fluid or nutrition.

**nonessential amino acids** Amino acids that can be readily produced by humans from components of the diet. Also referred to as *dispensable amino acids.*

**nonessential nutrients** Nutrients required for growth and health that can be produced by the body from other components of the diet.

**NSF** International, a nongovernmental, nonprofit that also tests dietary supplements.

**nutraceutical** Combination of words *nutrient* and *pharmaceutical* to indicate a food-derived compound that can act as a drug, such as red yeast rice, a statin-like compound.

**nutrient-dense food** A food that provides substantial amounts of vitamins, minerals, and other biologically active food components with relatively few calories. Also called nutrient-rich.

**nutrient-dense foods** Foods that contain relatively high amounts of nutrients compared to their caloric value.

**nutrients** Chemical substances in foods that are used by the body for growth and health.

**nutrigenomics** The study of diet- and nutrient-related functions and interactions of genes and their effects on health and disease.

**nutrition monitoring** Assessment of dietary or nutrition status at intermittent times with the aim of detecting changes in the dietary or nutritional status of a population.

**nutrition support** Provision of nutrients by methods other than eating regular foods or drinking regular beverages, such as directly accessing the stomach by tube or placing nutrients into the bloodstream.

**nutrition surveillance** Continuous assessment of nutritional status for the purpose of detecting changes in trend or distribution in order to initiate corrective measures.

**obesity** BMI-for-age greater than or equal to the 95th percentile.

**obesogenic diet** A pattern of eating and food choices that leads to excessive energy intake and accumulation of body fat.

**obesogenic environment** The sum of influences that promote overeating and minimize physical activity and lead to weight gain and hinder weight loss.

**oral-gastric (OG) feeding** A form of enteral nutrition support for delivering nutrition by tube placement from the mouth to the stomach.

**Osmolality** A measure of the concentration of particles in solution.

**osmolarity** Measure of the number of particles in a solution, which predicts the tendency of the particles to move from high to low concentration. Osmolarity is a factor in many systems, such as in fluid and electrolyte balance.

**osteoporosis** Condition in which low bone density or weak bone structure leads to an increased risk of bone fracture.

**ova** Eggs of the female produced and stored within the ovaries (singular is *ovum*).

**overweight** Body mass index-for-age between the 85th and 94th percentiles.

**oxidative stress** A condition that occurs when cells are exposed to more oxidizing molecules (such as free radicals) than to antioxidant molecules that neutralize them. Over time, oxidative stress causes damage to lipids, DNA, cells, and tissues. It increases the risk of heart disease, type 2 diabetes, cancer, and other diseases.

**oxidative stress** A condition that occurs when cells are exposed to more oxidizing molecules (such as free radicals) than to antioxidant molecules that neutralize them and help repair cell damage. Over time, oxidative stress causes damage to lipids, DNA, cells, and tissues.

**Oxytocin** A hormone produced during letdown that causes milk to be ejected into the ducts.

**pagophagia** Compulsive consumption of ice or freezer frost.

**parenteral feeding** Delivery of nutrients directly to the bloodstream.

**parity** The number of previous deliveries experienced by a woman; *nulliparous* = no previous deliveries, *primiparous* = one previous delivery, *multiparous* = two or more previous deliveries. Women who have delivered infants are considered to be *parous.*

**patient-centered care** An approach to care that is respectful of and responsive to the patient's preferences, needs, and values and ensures that the patient's values guide all clinical decisions.

**pelvic inflammatory disease (PID)** A general term applied to infections of the cervix, uterus, fallopian tubes, or ovaries. Occurs predominantly in young women and is generally caused by infection with a sexually transmitted disease, such as gonorrhea or Chlamydia.

**periconceptional period** The time period around conception, variously measured in weeks or months, depending on the pregnancy outcomes of interest.

**periconceptional period** The time period around conception, variously measured in weeks or months depending on the pregnancy outcomes of interest.

**perimenopause and menopause** An approximately 4-year period of decreasing estrogen production followed by the end of menstruation; a marking point for increased risk of cardiovascular disease and other chronic conditions for women.

**persistent organic pollutants (POPs)** A family of chemicals manufactured either for a specific purpose (e.g., pesticides or flame retardants in electrical equipment or furniture) or produced as byproducts of incinerated waste. The POP family includes dioxins, polychlorinated biphenyuls (PCBs), polybrominated didphenyl ether (PBDE), and organochlorine pesticides.

**pharmacotherapy** Treatment of disease through the use of drugs.

**phenylketonuria (PKU)** An inherited error in phenylalanine metabolism most commonly caused by a deficiency of phenylalanine hydroxylase, which converts the essential amino acid phenylalanine to the nonessential amino acid tyrosine. Also called hyperphenylalaninemia.

**phytochemicals** (phyto = plants) Chemical substances in plants, some of which affect body processes in humans that may benefit health. Also called phytonutrients.

**pica** An eating disorder characterized by the compulsion to eat substances that are not food.

**pituitary gland** A pea-sized gland located at the base of the brain. It is connected to the hypothalamus and produces and secretes growth hormone, prolactin, oxytocin, follicle-stimulating hormone, luteinizing hormone, and other hormones in response to signals from the hypothalamus.

**placenta abruption** The separation of the placenta from its attachment to the uterus wall before the baby is delivered. Also called abruptio placenta. Consequences of this condition range from mild to severe for the mother and fetus depending on blood loss, extent of fetal distress, gestational age of the fetus, and other factors.

**placenta** A disk-shaped organ of nutrient and gas interchange between mother and fetus. At term, the placenta weighs about 15 percent of the weight of the fetus.

**Polycystic ovary syndrome (PCOS)** (polycysts = many cysts; i.e., abnormal sacs with membranous linings). A condition in females generally characterized by insulin resistance, high blood insulin levels, obesity, polycystic ovaries, menstrual dysfunction, amenorrhea, infertility, hirsutism (excess body hair), and acne.

**polyunsaturated fats** Fats in which more than one pair of adjacent carbons in one or more of its fatty acids are linked by two or more double bonds (e.g., –C–C=C–C=C–).

**postictal state** Time of altered consciousness after a seizure; appears to be like a deep sleep.

**pouring rights** Contracts between schools and soft-drink companies, whereby the schools receive a percentage of the profits of soft-drink sales in exchange for the school offering only that soft-drink company's products on the school campus.

**Prader-Willi syndrome** Condition in which partial deletion of chromosome 15 interferes with control of appetite, muscle development, and cognition.

**preadolescence** The stage of development immediately preceding adolescence; 9–11 years of age for girls and 10–12 years of age for boys.

**prebiotics** Certain fiberlike forms of indigestible carbohydrates that support the growth of beneficial bacteria in the lower intestine. Nicknamed "intestinal fertilizer."

**prediabetes** A condition in which blood glucose levels are higher than normal but not high enough for the diagnosis of diabetes. It is characterized by impaired glucose tolerance, or fasting blood glucose levels between 100 and 125 mg/dL.

**preloads** Beverages or food such as yogurt in which the energy/macronutrient content has been varied by the use of various carbohydrate and fat sources. The preload is given before a meal or snack and subsequent intake is monitored. This study design has been employed by Birch et al. in their studies of appetite, satiety, and food preferences in young children.

**premenstrual syndrome** (*premenstrual* = the period of time preceding menstrual bleeding; *syndrome* = a constellation of symptoms). A condition occurring among women of reproductive age that includes a group of physical and psychological symptoms with onset in the luteal phase and subsiding with menstrual bleeding. Premenstrual dysphoric disorder (PMDD) is a severe form of PMS.

**preschool-age children** Children between the ages of 3 and 5 years who are not yet attending kindergarten.

**preterm infants** Infants born before 37 weeks of gestation.

**primary malnutrition** Malnutrition that results directly from inadequate or excessive dietary intake of energy or nutrients.

**probiotics** Strains of lactobacillus and bifidobacteria that have beneficial effects on the body. Also called "friendly bacteria."

**Prolactin** A hormone necessary for milk production.

**proportionately small for gestational age (pSGA)** Newborn weight, length, and head circumference are less than 10th percentile for gestational age. Also called *symmetrical* SGA.

**prostacyclin** A potent inhibitor of platelet aggregation and a powerful vasodilator and blood pressure reducer derived from n-3 fatty acids.

**prostacyclins** Biologically active substances produced by blood vessel walls that inhibit platelet aggregation (and therefore blood clotting), dilate blood vessels, and reduce blood pressure.

**prostaglandins** A group of physiologically active substances derived from the essential fatty acids. They are present in many tissues and perform such functions as the constriction or dilation of blood vessels and stimulation of smooth muscles and the uterus.

**prostaglandins** A group of physiologically active substances derived from the essential fatty acids. They are present in many tissues and perform such functions as the constriction or dilation of blood vessels and stimulation of smooth muscles and the uterus.

**psychostimulant** Classification of medication that acts on the brain to improve mental or emotional behavior.

**puberty** The period in life during which humans become biologically capable of reproduction.

**puberty** The time frame during which the body matures from that of a child to that of a young adult.

**pulmonary** Related to the lungs and their movement of air for exchange of carbon dioxide and oxygen.

**quality of life** A measure of life satisfaction that is difficult to define, especially in an aging heterogeneous population. Quality-of-life measures include factors such as social contacts, economic security, and functional status.

**Recommended Dietary Allowances (RDAs)** The average daily dietary intake levels sufficient to meet the nutrient requirements of nearly all (97–98%) healthy individuals in a population group. RDAs serve as goals for individuals.

**recumbent length** Measurement of length while the child is lying down. Recumbent length is used to measure toddlers <24 months of age and those between 24 and 36 months who are unable to stand unassisted.

**reflex** An automatic (unlearned) response that is triggered by a specific stimulus.

**registered dietitian nutritionist (RDN)** An individual who has acquired food and nutrition knowledge and skills necessary to pass a national registration examination and who participates in continuing professional education.

**resilience** Ability to bounce back, to deal with stress, and recover from injury or illness.

**resting energy expenditure (REE)** Measured or estimated energy expenditure in an individual at rest.

**resting energy expenditure** The amount of energy needed by the body in a state of rest.

**Rett syndrome** Condition in which a genetic change on the X chromosome results in severe neurological delays, causing children to be short, thin-appearing, and unable to talk.

**root reflex** Action that occurs if one cheek is touched, resulting in the infant's head turning toward that cheek and the infant opening his mouth.

**rotavirus** A virus that is the most common cause of severe diarrhea among children. Diarrhea caused by rotavirus generally lasts 2 days, and recovery is full in otherwise healthy children. The rotavirus is generally spread from an infected person's stools to food.

**sandwich generation** Refers to middle-aged adults, usually women, who are multigenerational caregivers dealing with the complex roles of wife, mother, daughter, caregiver, and employee.

**sarcopenia** Age-associated loss of skeletal muscle mass and function.

**sarcopenia** Muscle wasting

**sarcopenic obesity** Low lean body mass combined with excessive fat stores.

**saturated fats** Fats in which adjacent carbons in the fatty acid component are linked by single bonds only (e.g., –C–C–C–C–).

**scoliosis** Condition in which the vertebral bones in the back show a side-to-side curve, resulting in a shorter stature than expected if the back were straight.

**secondary condition** Common consequence of a condition, which may or may not be preventable over time.

**secondary malnutrition** Malnutrition that results from a condition (e.g., disease, surgical procedure, medication use) rather than primarily from dietary intake.

**secondary sexual characteristics** Physiological changes that signal puberty, including enlargement of the testes, penis, and breasts and the development of pubic and facial hair.

**Secretory cells** Cells in the acinus (milk gland) that are responsible for secreting milk components into the ducts.

**Secretory immunoglobin A** A protein found in secretions that protect the body's mucosal surfaces from infections. The mode of action may be by reducing the binding of a microorganism with cells lining the digestive tract. It is present in human colostrum but not transferred across the placenta.

**seizures** Condition in which electrical nerve transmission in the brain is disrupted, resulting in periods of loss of function that vary in severity.

**semen** The penile ejaculate containing a mixture of sperm and secretions from the testes, prostate, and other glands. It is rich in zinc, fructose, and other nutrients. Also called seminal fluid.

**senescence** The condition or process of deterioration with age.

**sensorimotor** An early learning system in which the infant's senses and motor skills provide input to the central nervous system.

**serotonin** A neurotransmitter derived from the amino acid tryptophan that affects nerve cell activities that excite or inhibit various behaviors and body functions. It plays a role in mood, appetite regulation, food intake, respiration, pain transmission, blood vessel constriction, sleep, and other body functions.

**serum iron, plasma ferritin, and transferrin saturation** Measures of iron status obtained from blood plasma or serum samples.

**sex hormone binding globulin (SHBG)** A protein that binds with the sex hormones testosterone and estrogen. These hormones are inactive when bound to SHBG, but are available for use when needed. Low levels of SHBG are related to increased availability of testosterone and estrogen in the body.

**shoulder dystocia** Blockage or difficulty of delivery due to obstruction of the birth canal by the infant's shoulders.

**small for gestational age (SGA)** Newborn weight is less than 10th percentile for gestational age. Also called *small for date* (SFD).

**small for gestational age** Newborn weight is less than 10th percentile for gestational age.

**social determinants of health** Socioeconomic and environmental factors that are powerful determinants of health and are largely outside of the control of individuals and groups.

**spastic quadriplegia** A form of cerebral palsy in which brain damage interferes with voluntary muscle control in both arms and legs.

**spinal muscular atrophy** Condition in which muscle control declines over time as a result of nerve loss, causing death in childhood.

**stature** Standing height.

**steroid hormones** Hormones such as progesterone, estrogen, and testosterone produced primarily from cholesterol.

**stroke** An event that occurs when a blood vessel in the brain ruptures or becomes blocked. Stroke is often associated with "hardening of the arteries" in the brain. Also called cerebral vascular accident.

**subfertility** Reduced level of fertility characterized by unusually long time to conception (over 12 months) or repeated pregnancy losses.

**suckle** A reflexive movement of the tongue moving forward and backward; earliest feeding skill.

**supercentenarian** Person who has reached age 110 or more, validated.

**T-lymphocyte** A white blood cell that is active in fighting infection. (May also be called T-cell; the t in T-cell stands for thymus.) These cells coordinate the immune system by secreting hormones that act on other cells.

***T. Gondii*, or toxoplasmosis** A parasitic infection that can impair fetal brain development. The source of the infection is often hands contaminated with soil or the contents of a cat litter box; or raw or partially cooked pork, lamb, or venison.

**telomere** A caplike structure that protects the ends of chromosomes; it erodes during replication.

**telopeptides** Molecules that degrade the major collagen of tendon and bone and leave carbon and nitrogen fragments in blood and urine

**teratogenic** Exposures that produce malformations in embryos or fetuses.

**testes** Male reproductive glands located in the scrotum. Also called testicles.

**testes** One of the two male reproductive glands located in the scrotum.

**therapeutic lifestyle change (TLC)** A higher-intensity dietary approach for reducing risk of cardiovascular disease with defined targets for type and amount of fat and dietary fiber, physical activity, and weight reduction. This is considered the first line of treatment.

**thermic effect of food (TEF)** Energy required for the digestion, absorption, and metabolism of food; approximately 10 percent of energy needs.

**thromboxanes** Biologically active substances produced in platelets that increase platelet aggregation (and therefore promote blood clotting), constrict blood vessels, and increase blood pressure.

**thromboxane** The parent of a group of thromboxanes derived from the n-6 fatty acid arachidonic acid. Thromboxane increases platelet aggregation and constricts blood vessels, causing blood pressure to increase.

**thrombus** Blood clot.

**toddlers** Children between the ages of 1 and 3 years.

**Tolerable Upper Intake Levels** Highest level of daily nutrient intake that is likely to pose no risk of adverse health effects to almost all individuals in the general population; gives levels of intake that may result in adverse effects if exceeded on a regular basis.

**total diet approach** Guidance based on overall eating patterns that meet needs with a variety of foods over time.

**total fiber** Sum of dietary fiber and functional fiber.

**tracheoesophageal atresia** Incomplete connection between the esophagus and the stomach *in utero*, resulting in a shortened esophagus.

***trans* fat** A type of unsaturated fat present in hydrogenated oils, margarine, shortenings, pastries, and some cooking oils that increase the risk of heart disease. Fats containing fatty acids in the *trans* versus the more common *cis* form are generally referred to as *trans* fat.

***trans* fatty acids** Fatty acids that have unusual shapes resulting from the hydrogenation of polyunsaturated fatty acids. *Trans* fatty acids also occur naturally in small amounts in foods such as dairy products and beef.

**transient ischemic attacks (TIAs)** Temporary and insufficient blood supply to the brain.

**type 1 diabetes** A disease characterized by high blood glucose levels resulting from destruction of the insulin-producing cells of the pancreas. This type of diabetes was called juvenile-onset diabetes and insulin-dependent diabetes in the past, and its official name is type 1 diabetes mellitus.

**type 1 diabetes** A disease characterized by high blood glucose levels resulting from destruction of the insulin-producing cells of the pancreas. This type of diabetes was called juvenile-onset diabetes and insulin-dependent diabetes in the past.

**type 2 diabetes** A disease characterized by high blood glucose levels due to the body's inability to use insulin normally, or to produce enough insulin. This type of diabetes was called adult-onset diabetes and non-insulindependent diabetes in the past.

**type 2 diabetes** A disease characterized by high blood glucose levels due to the body's inability to use insulin normally, or to produce enough insulin. This type of diabetes was called adult-onset diabetes and non-insulin-dependent diabetes in the past. Its official name is type 2 diabetes mellitus.

**type 2 diabetes** A disease characterized by high blood glucose levels due to the body's inability to use insulin normally, to produce enough insulin, or both.

**unsaturated fats** Fats in which adjacent carbons in one or more fatty acids are linked by one or more double bonds (e.g., –C–C=C–C=C–).

**USP (United States Pharmacopeia)** A nongovernmental, nonprofit organization (since 1820); establishes and maintains standards of identity, strength, quality, purity, processing, and labeling for health care products.

**vegan diet** The most restrictive of vegetarian diets, allowing only plant foods.

**very low-birthweight infant (VLBW)** An infant weighing $<1500$ g at birth.

**viscous fiber** Types of fiber characterized by their ability to form a gel solution when combined with liquid. Formerly called soluble fiber.

**weaning** Discontinuation of breastfeeding or bottle feeding and substitution of food for breast milk or infant formula.

**work of breathing (WOB)** A common term used to express extra respiratory effort in a variety of pulmonary conditions.

**xerostomia** Dry mouth can be a side effect of medications (especially antidepressants), of head and neck cancer treatments, of diabetes, and also a symptom of Sjogren's syndrome, which is an autoimmune disorder for which no cure is known.

# Index

## A

## F

## I



## J

## N



## O

# P

## Q



## R



## S

## T



## U

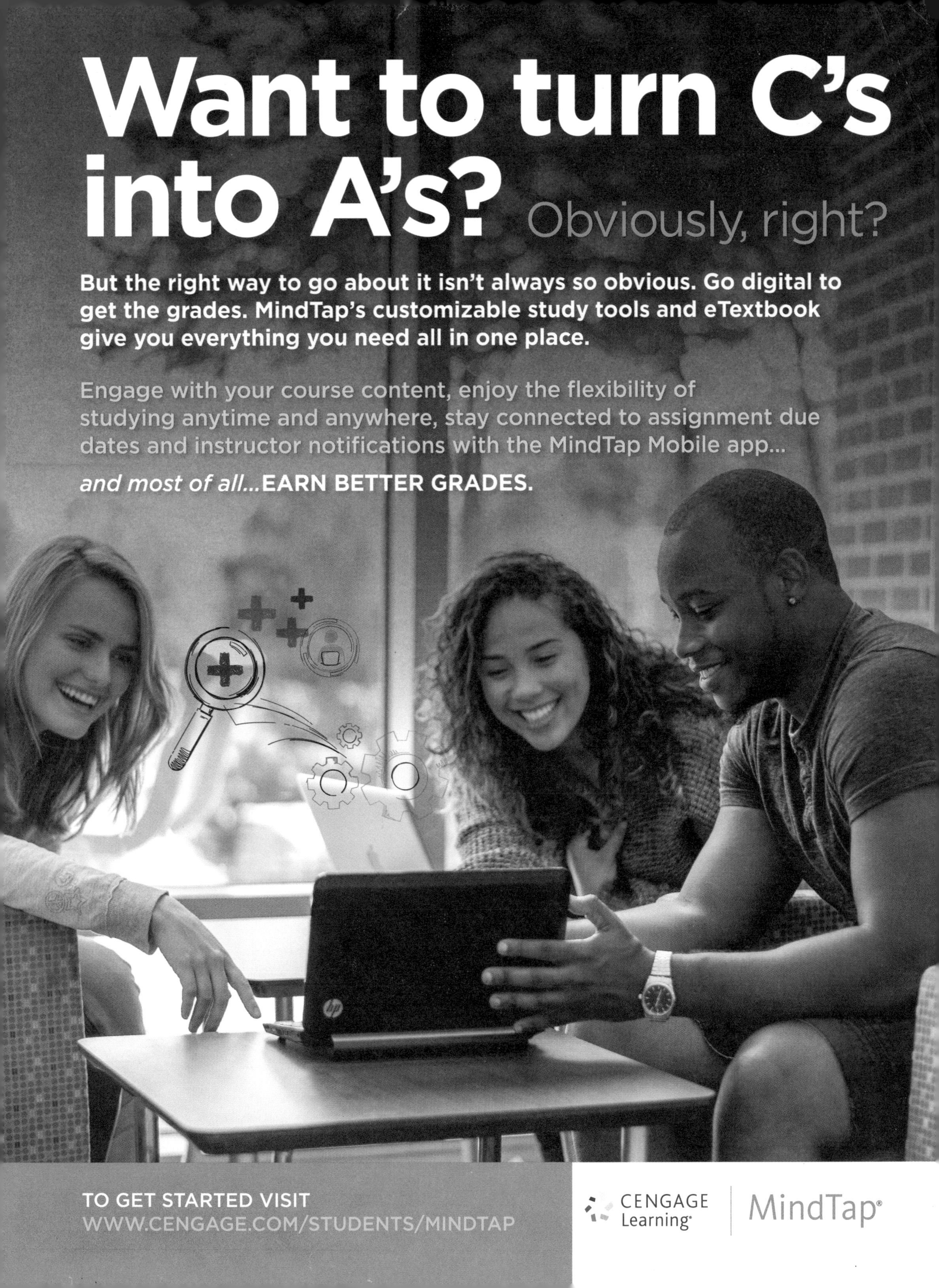

## Tolerable Upper Intake Levels (UL) for Vitamins

| Age (yr) | Niacin (mg/day)[a] | Vitamin B6 (mg/day) | Folate (μg/day)[a] | Choline (mg/day) | Vitamin C (mg/day) | Vitamin A (IU/day)[b] | Vitamin D (IU/day) | Vitamin E (mg/day)[c] |
|---|---|---|---|---|---|---|---|---|
| *Infants* | | | | | | | | |
| 0–0.5 | — | — | — | — | — | 600 | 1000 (25 μg) | — |
| 0.5–1 | — | — | — | — | — | 600 | 1500 (38 μg) | — |
| *Children* | | | | | | | | |
| 1–3 | 10 | 30 | 300 | 1000 | 400 | 600 | 2500 (63 μg) | 200 |
| 4–8 | 15 | 40 | 400 | 1000 | 650 | 900 | 3000 (75 μg) | 300 |
| 9–13 | 20 | 60 | 600 | 2000 | 1200 | 1700 | 4000 (100 μg) | 600 |
| *Adolescents* | | | | | | | | |
| 14–18 | 30 | 80 | 800 | 3000 | 1800 | 2800 | 4000 (100 μg) | 800 |
| *Adults* | | | | | | | | |
| 19–70 | 35 | 100 | 1000 | 3500 | 2000 | 3000 | 4000 (100 μg) | 1000 |
| >70 | 35 | 100 | 1000 | 3500 | 2000 | 3000 | 4000 (100 μg) | 1000 |
| *Pregnancy* | | | | | | | | |
| ≤18 | 30 | 80 | 800 | 3000 | 1800 | 2800 | 4000 (100 μg) | 800 |
| 19–50 | 35 | 100 | 1000 | 3500 | 2000 | 3000 | 4000 (100 μg) | 1000 |
| *Lactation* | | | | | | | | |
| ≤18 | 30 | 80 | 800 | 3000 | 1800 | 2800 | 4000 (100 μg) | 800 |
| 19–50 | 35 | 100 | 1000 | 3500 | 2000 | 3000 | 4000 (100 μg) | 1000 |

[a]The UL for niacin and folate apply to synthetic forms obtained from supplements, fortified foods, or a combination of the two.
[b]The UL for vitamin A applies to the preformed vitamin only.
[c]The UL for vitamin E applies to any form of supplemental α-tocopherol, fortified foods, or a combination of the two.